MW00996151

Handbook of Autopsy Practice

Handbook of Autopsy Practice

Fourth Edition

Brenda L. Waters, MD

*Department of Pathology and Laboratory Medicine,
University of Vermont and Fletcher Allen Health Care,
Burlington, VT, USA*

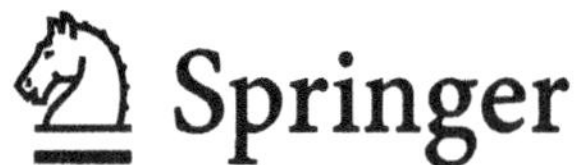

Editor
Brenda L. Waters, MD
Associate Professor
Department of Pathology and Laboratory Medicine
University of Vermont
and
Fletcher Allen Health Care
Burlington, VT, USA

ISBN 978-1-58829-841-6 e-ISBN 978-1-59745-127-7
DOI: 10.1007/978-1-59745-127-7

Printed on acid-free paper

springer.com

Dedication

I dedicate this book to Nicholas J. Hardin, teacher, mentor, colleague, and friend, who instilled in me and many others, an unwavering quest for excellence in autopsy pathology.

Preface

In the twenty-five years of my practice I have seen significant changes, many of which testify to the continued evolution of autopsy pathology. Technologic advancements such as computerized lab information systems, molecular diagnostics, immunohistochemical methods, digital imaging and the Internet have had important applications to autopsy pathology. A less welcomed change is the decline in the autopsy rate in teaching hospitals – a decline that threatens to continue. One reason for this may be the more sophisticated imaging techniques which some believe supplant the need for postmortem exam. Another may be the discomfort that house staff and attendings still experience when asking for permission. Nevertheless, the autopsy remains the diagnostic gold standard. Recent medical literature is rich with articles extolling the diagnostic power of the postmortem exam. Beyond the autopsy's critical role in transmitting information to clinicians, the postmortem examination procedure provides unrivaled opportunities for pathology residents to hone the essential skills of their trade. These skills include efficient and safe dissection techniques, appropriate handling of unexpected findings, meticulous written and photographic documentation, accurate interpretation of findings, and finally, timely, compassionate, and professional communication with families, physicians and legal counsel. This writer's view is that the future of autopsy pathology is founded on the perpetuation of these skills. It is with this vision in mind that the 4th edition of the *Handbook* is offered.

Part I of the 4th edition has six completely new chapters in which the reader will find an assortment of tools that will increase the value of the autopsy. There is a sample next-of-kin letter which is sent to the family member who authorized the autopsy, following distribution of the final report. This letter notifies the person that the report is complete and invites him/her to discuss the autopsy findings with the involved physician. The reader will find a quality assurance worksheet that can be used to check for omissions, discrepancies or insufficiently supported conclusions in the final report. A new discourse on the dissection procedure is accompanied by a worksheet and template for the gross description. There is also a new, detailed discussion of the safe handling of sharps, complete with photographs. The same superb photographs, characteristic of William Edwards, highlight the chapter devoted to the cardiovascular system. The reader will find the updated requirements of the Eye Bank of America and the U.S. Food and Drug Administration for ocular tissue transplantation. Significant advancements in cytogenetic techniques have occurred since the 3rd edition, especially with respect to the application of molecular methods using fluorescent labeled DNA probes. The updated cytogenetics chapter will help autopsy pathologists to decipher when conventional chromosome studies are useful and when molecular cytogenetic methods are more applicable.

Added to the discussion of legal aspects of autopsy practice is material on common law and statute law pertaining to dead bodies and autopsies in general. Many questions that often arise, such as who can view an autopsy, who can receive the autopsy report and how organs or tissues are donated for transplantation, are addressed.

Although a virtual gross specimen museum can be created using digital images, teaching with actual pathologic specimens may still have a role in educating medical students and in inspiring elementary and secondary school students. Therefore, the applied science of long-term organ preservation is discussed with many of the venerable fixatives from the previous editions retained. New items are a step-by-step procedure for paraffin-embedding hearts (courtesy of the Cardiac Registry at Boston Children's Hospital) and a concise description of the fascinating technique of plastination.

Part II has been updated with new diseases and recent references added. Practicing autopsy pathologists, residents and students are invited to review this alphabetical listing of disorders before each autopsy in order to re-acquaint themselves with what they might encounter.

Part III concludes the book with a series of tables providing organ weights and body measurements for fetuses, children and adults. Many of these are more recent than those of the 3rd edition. The growth charts for children are presented in a larger format to facilitate their use.

I wish to thank all the contributors to this book, past and present, who helped to maintain autopsy pathology as an important and evolving field. I am indebted to Candace LaFreniere for her secretarial help and to Raj Chawla for his expert photographic skills. I wish also to thank my longtime colleague, fellow autopsy pathologist and friend, Dr. Nicholas J. Hardin, who reviewed many of the new chapters and offered much helpful advice. His editorial skills are exceeded only by his skills as a pathologist. His thorough investigative approach to every postmortem exam thankfully rubbed off on me. To him, I dedicate this book.

Brenda L. Waters, MD

Contents

Contributors

VERNARD I. ADAMS, MD • *Medical Examiner Department, Hillsborough County, Department of Pathology and Laboratory Medicine, University of South Florida, Tampa, FL, USA*

HAGEN BLASZYK, MD • *Department of Pathology, Maine Medical Center, Portland, ME, USA*

R. JEAN CAMPBELL, MD • *Emeritus Member, Department of Laboratory Medicine and Pathology, and of Ophthalmology, Mayo Clinic, and Emeritus Professor of Pathology, College of Medicine, Mayo Clinic, Rochester, MN, USA*

KELLY L. CLASSIC, MS • *Section of Safety, Mayo Clinic, Rochester, MN, USA*

GORDON W. DEWALD, PHD • *Emeritus Member, Department of Laboratory Medicine and Pathology, Mayo Clinic, Emeritus Professor of Laboratory Medicine and Pathology, and Medical Genetics, College of Medicine, Mayo Clinic, Rochester, MN, USA*

WILLIAM D. EDWARDS, MD • *Division of Anatomic Pathology, Mayo Clinic, Professor of Laboratory Medicine and Pathology, College of Medicine, Mayo Clinic, Rochester, MN, USA*

CATERINA GIANNINI. MD • *Division of Anatomic Pathology, Mayo Clinic, Associate Professor of Laboratory Medicine and Pathology, College of Medicine, Mayo Clinic, Rochester, MN, USA*

CHERYL R. HANN, MS • *Ophthalmic Pathology Assistant, Ophthalmology Research Laboratories, Mayo Clinic, and Instructor in Laboratory Medicine and Pathology, College of Medicine, Mayo Clinic, Rochester, Minnesota, USA*

JURGEN LUDWIG, MD • *Emeritus Member, Department of Laboratory Medicine and Pathology, Mayo Clinic, Rochester, MN, USA*

DYLAN V. MILLER, MD • *Division of Anatomic Pathology, Mayo Clinic, Assistant Professor of Laboratory Medicine and Pathology, College of Medicine, Mayo Clinic, Rochester, MN, USA*

HARUO OKAZAKI, MD • *Emeritus Member, Department of Laboratory Medicine and Pathology, Mayo Clinic, Rochester, Minnesota; Emeritus Professor of Laboratory Medicine, College of Medicine, Mayo Clinic, USA*

BRENDA L. WATERS, MD • *Associate Professor of Pathology and Laboratory Medicine, University of Vermont and Fletcher Allen Health Care, Burlington, VT, USA*

Autopsy Techniques and Procedures

I

1 Ensuring Quality in the Hospital Autopsy

Brenda L. Waters

Despite an unceasing stream of publications extolling the value of postmortem examination *(1–12),* the hospital autopsy rate continues to decline. Estimates, published in the 1990s, of the overall autopsy rate in the United States are as low as 5%, with the rate in academic institutions estimated at 11% *(13,14).* Several factors contribute to this. One is the notion that the autopsy will not reveal information above and beyond that gained from current sophisticated imaging studies. Another is the clinicians' concern about resultant litigation. A more fundamental reason, however, is the lack of vigor on the part of the clinician to seek permission from the family *(15).* The physician attending the death may be too quickly distracted by other competing concerns and responsibilities, or more likely, (s)he is unfamiliar with the family of the deceased. This latter situation is frequent in teaching hospitals, where a house officer with no prior contact with the patient attends the death and feels uncomfortable in requesting permission for autopsy. These obstacles notwithstanding, it this author's opinion that any academic teaching hospital must make a genuine and persistent effort to achieve a hospital autopsy rate of at least 25%.

PATHOLOGIST'S ROLE IN PROMOTING THE AUTOPSY

Although the chairs of clinical departments must be motivated to help with this goal, autopsy personnel can take a number of steps to encourage hospital autopsy permissions. These steps involve effective and timely communication with the clinician.

Before commencing the evisceration, the prosector should call the clinical resident and/or the attending to discuss the patient's history. When the prosector is relatively inexperienced, it is preferable to have the pathology attending contact the clinical attending. Either way, this conversation allows the clinician to express any specific questions (s)he may hope to have answered by the autopsy, as well as simply to describe the events that led to the patient's death. When the initial dissection is completed, the clinicians again should be called and informed of the gross pathological findings. During that conversation, the prosector should invite the clinicians to the morgue to view the findings themselves. The examination of the organs soon after the patient's death offers a significant learning experience for clinical attendings, as well as house staff and medical students. Any digital photographs of significant abnormalities should be emailed to the clinicians within the same day of the postmortem examination. Generally, the timely receipt of these photographs is much appreciated, because the clinicians will be quickly distracted by their responsibilities to their living patients. Photographs of the gross findings are very effective teaching tools, especially in morbidity and mortality and other clinical conferences. In fact, gross photographs are probably most effective, since both autolysis and the clinicians' relative inexperience with histology lessen the value of microscopical images. Further discussion on photography may be found at the end of this chapter.

Most hospital autopsy services generate a preliminary report. This report of the major gross findings, preferably organized pathogenetically, should be distributed within 24 hours of the initial prosection. Residents should be inculcated in the importance of sending copies of this and the final report to the patient's referring physician(s) including those from outside hospitals. Lastly, a short turn-around time between initial dissection and distribution of the final autopsy report will also be much appreciated by clinicians. Many clinicians consider autopsy reports received after one month to be useless and irrelevant, as they have already had their conference with the family. Further discussion of the hospital autopsy report may be found in Chapter 12.

These efforts toward timely communication, eagerness to demonstrate the pathologic findings to the clinicians, provision of gross photographs, and prompt distribution of the final report will help treating physicians understand the value of the service and make them more receptive to seeking autopsy permissions in the future *(15).*

The permission form for autopsy should be as brief as possible, so that the family can understand it, but be as inclusive as possible to allow the pathologist to gain maximum yield from the procedure. A sample permission form is found as Fig. 1-1. It is the nearest relative who must sign the permission form. Most states have statutes that list the next of kin in descending order of priority. Generally, that list is spouse, reciprocal beneficiary, an adult child, either parent, an adult sibling, a grandparent, the individual possessing a durable power of attorney, the guardian

From: *Handbook of Autopsy Practice,* 4th Ed. Edited by: B.L. Waters

I (Print Full Name) ______ hereby grant permission for a complete postmortem examination, including the removal and retention or use for diagnostic, scientific, educational, or therapeutic purposes of such organs, tissues and parts as the physicians in attendance at (Name of Institution) _____ may deem desirable, on the remains of (Print Full Name of Deceased) _________

This authority is granted subject to the following restrictions (if none, write "none"):

____

The following special examinations are requested: _____________

I am the nearest relative of the deceased and entitled by law to control the disposition of the remains.

Signature: ______________ Date & Time: ________ Relationship: ___________

Mailing Address: ____________________

Telephone Number: _________________

Permission obtained by: (Print Full Name):________ Title: _______________

Second witness (required if telephone permission): (Print Full Name): ____________

Title: ________________ Signature: _______________ Date & Time: ___________

Fig. 1-1. Proposed text for an Autopsy Permission Form.

of the decedent, or any other individual authorized or under obligation to dispose of the body. The reader is advised to consult local and/or state statutes. In most institutions, obtaining permission over the telephone requires a witness.

Restrictions on the autopsy as set by the next-of-kin may range from "none" to one or several needle biopsies. If there is any uncertainty as to the wishes of the next-of-kin with regard to restrictions, further discussion with the family or the physician who personally obtained the permission must occur, so as to clarify the family's intent. If any doubt remains, the most restricted interpretation of the permission must be followed.

We find that it is advantageous to notify the next-of-kin by mail when the autopsy report is completed and sent to the appropriate physicians. In that letter, sympathy for the loss of the family member is expressed as well as statements made regarding the value of the autopsy to the advancement of medical knowledge. Equally important, the letter invites the family member to discuss the findings with the clinician. An example of such a letter is included as Fig. 1-2. It is advisable not to send the letter to the next-of-kin immediately after distribution of the report, but rather one to two weeks later. This will allow sufficient time for the clinician to receive and review the report. Situations will arise in which the family of the deceased person wishes to discuss the pathologic findings with the pathologist. This certainly should not be discouraged, but courtesy and collegiality compel the pathologist to notify the clinician that such a meeting has been requested. This will minimize animosity and may even help the pathologist in interacting with the family. Further discussion on meeting with the next-of-kin may be found at the end of this chapter.

IN CASES WITH THERAPEUTIC COMPLICATIONS When an autopsy is to be performed on a patient who has possibly died as a result of a medical or operative complication, communication with the clinician is even more important. Given the potential medicolegal implications, the pathology attending must discuss the case with the physician and should invite her (him) to be present during the procedure. Adequate photography is essential in these cases, and the resulting images will then be available for later reexamination and possible presentation in morbidity and mortality conferences. If the complication is of a hemorrhagic nature, photographs should be taken prior to evacuation of the blood, so as to document the extent of the hemorrhage. When a site of bleeding is found, this site must also be adequately photographed. Abnormalities encountered during the prosection should be documented with great attention to accuracy and detail. An excellent array of photographs will promote and enhance such accuracy. Therapeutic complications may be dramatically demonstrated at autopsy, and all personnel must maintain a calm and objective demeanor throughout the prosection, whether clinicians are present or not. Although clinicians may wish to help with the dissection, they should be tactfully dissuaded whenever the pathologist is concerned that tissue relationships may be altered before full understanding of the process is achieved. On the other hand, having a surgeon present during prosection of a complex operative site can be of great help.

When the final report is nearly completed, it is absolutely essential that the clinical attending be invited to review the report before its signing and distribution. This extra step will rectify any differences of opinion that exist between the clinician and

Dear (Next-of-Kin) ____________:

Let me extend my sympathy to you and your family over the death of your (Relationship to deceased)________.

The report of findings of the postmortem examination has been completed and will be forwarded to _____, the attending physician, and _______, the referring physician.

We invite you to discuss the report with these physicians. If you wish, you can obtain a copy of the report by contacting Medical Records at ______ (Institution conducting the autopsy).

Knowledge gained from such examinations helps in our efforts to treat other patients with similar problems, and may prolong a life or, someday, lead to a cure or prevention of disease. Your contribution to these efforts is deeply appreciated.

Very Sincerely,

Fig. 1-2. Letter sent to the next-of-kin (i.e., the person who signed the Autopsy Permission Form) on completion and distribution of the Autopsy Report.

pathologist. Not infrequently, these disparities of opinion indicate incomplete understanding of the nature of the complication, either by the clinician or the pathologist or both. With continued dialogue, fuller comprehension of the event is attained. Moreover, it is important for members of the family of the deceased to be spared, if possible, any differences in opinion as to what happened to their family member. To perceive contention between doctors as to the nature of their loved one's death will seriously impede the family's grieving process, as well as increase their motivation to seek litigation. Finally, when the clinician is given the opportunity to review the report before it is issued, (s)he will be left with the distinct conclusion that the pathologist is not an adversary, but rather a valued resource.

THE VALUE OF AUTOPSY CONFERENCES The postmortem examination involves, by its nature, dissection and description of a large number of organs and tissues. It is lengthy procedure, taking up to six hours and is often performed under a time constraint, since funeral home and family may be waiting for the body and a death certificate. Frequently, ancillary activities, such as photography and blood or tissue procurement for chemistry, serologic tests, or culture, are indicated. During these activities, the pathologist may be interrupted by pages, consultations with clinicians, or questions posed by other autopsy personnel. It is not inconceivable then, in this milieu of activities, certain anatomic findings may be overlooked or misinterpreted. This possibility is compounded by the copious amount of blood that one encounters during the dissection. For this reason, review of the major organs during a gross conference is important to any autopsy practice, especially if pathologists-in-training are involved. In our institution, we retain the lungs, heart, urinary system, neck block, esophagus, stomach, proximal duodenum with the extrahepatic biliary tree, the internal genitalia, and rectum for review at Gross Conference. For the liver, spleen, and the rest of the bowel, only representative portions are retained. Following at least a day's worth of fixation in formalin, the organs are washed and presented at Gross Conference.

In this setting, the prosector and attending on the case, along with other attendings and residents on the autopsy service, review the organs, discuss the findings, and not infrequently, notice lesions that were missed or misinterpreted on the day of prosection. This process has several beneficial outcomes. Residents on the service see the gross pathology of all cases that come through the service and thereby hone their observation skills. Moreover, they are able to see how fixation affects the appearance of different abnormalities, such as acute myocardial infarction, acute bronchopneumonia, and early cirrhosis. The conference provides a forum where any differences of opinion regarding interpretation of the gross findings can be addressed and discussed, to the illumination of all. These interactions cannot help but to increase the value of the final autopsy report.

It is also helpful to conduct a weekly Microscopic Conference, during which selected slides from the previous week's cases are reviewed. This meeting offers a chance to teach the residents and to discuss differences of opinion regarding interpretation of pathologic findings, with the goal of achieving consistency of diagnoses among pathologists. This type of conference is frequently found in surgical pathology services.

INTRADEPARTMENTAL REVIEW OF REPORTS Unlike the surgical pathology report, the autopsy report involves literally hundreds of datapoints. These datapoints include organ weights, descriptions, and measurements; descriptions and measurements of lesions; histological descriptions; and, finally, dozens of interpretations. Therefore, it is not unusual for even the most diligent attending pathologist to overlook small-to-significant inaccuracies in a multipage report, despite several reviews. These inaccuracies can be typographical or grammatical errors, inadequate documentation of abnormalities, omission of diagnoses, or forming conclusions that are inadequately supported by the pathologic findings. In academic institutions, where residents are the authors of much of the report, inaccuracies may be numerous. Residents are prone to make conclusions that are not adequately supported by the pathologic material to which clinicians, in certain situations, may take umbrage. Such statements must be removed from the report. To catch "errors" such as these, our institution has found it very helpful to have another autopsy pathologist review each final report before signing. With fresh eyes, this pathologist is likely to identify the errors and can bring them to the attention of the original pathologist. In our institution, this step has significantly reduced inaccuracies in the final autopsy report.

Some autopsy pathologists may find it helpful to use a quality assurance worksheet to review the autopsy reports prior to signing. Such a worksheet may be found as Appendix 1-1. This worksheet was patterned after the CAP Checklist for Autopsy Pathology *(16)*. Note that questions 8 and 9 on this form generate data that will be useful for quality assurance programs in other departments, such as surgery, medicine, and radiology.

PHOTOGRAPHY

A well-composed photograph of an autopsy specimen conveys significant and clear information to experienced clinicians and medical students alike. Digital photographs have an advantage in that they can be disseminated to clinicians within hours of the autopsy and can be readily stored and, later, incorporated into presentations for teaching. Although photographs of fresh specimens are ideal, very good images of fixed specimens are equally informative. Either way, excellent photographs that are shared with clinicians in a timely manner will further convince the clinicians of the value of their autopsy service. It is, therefore, imperative that every photograph intended for review at clinical conferences be of the highest technical quality. The sole intent of the photograph is to convey pathologic information. With a good photograph, the viewer's eye will not be distracted by puddles of blood or body fluids in the background, lack of focus, a soiled label, or an unclear presentation of the pathologic process. A good photograph is dramatic, but not lurid. The viewer quickly becomes oriented as to what he/she is viewing. A good photograph will rouse a weary intern into a moment of curiosity and attention.

A sturdy, durable and easily accessible photography stand is essential (Fig. 1-3) . The camera, ideally a digital camera with a zoom lens, should be firmly attached to a sturdy vertical pole upon which the camera may be raised and lowered. To reduce the amount of blood or tissue fluid on the support stage, we find it very useful to set a clear plastic panel, with small risers under each corner, on the support stage. This allows the specimen to be properly positioned beneath the camera without actually moving the specimen on the plastic. This avoids the formation of pools of blood or tissue fluid around the specimen.

Following the guidelines below will result in a good photograph:

1. The specimen should be thoroughly washed of blood. This critical step enhances the impact of the photograph by allowing the various colors of the tissues to be fully visible.
2. The camera should be close enough to clearly demonstrate the abnormality, but be far enough away so that the viewer can recognize the identity of the surrounding tissues. Certainly, landmarks may be pointed out by the presenter,

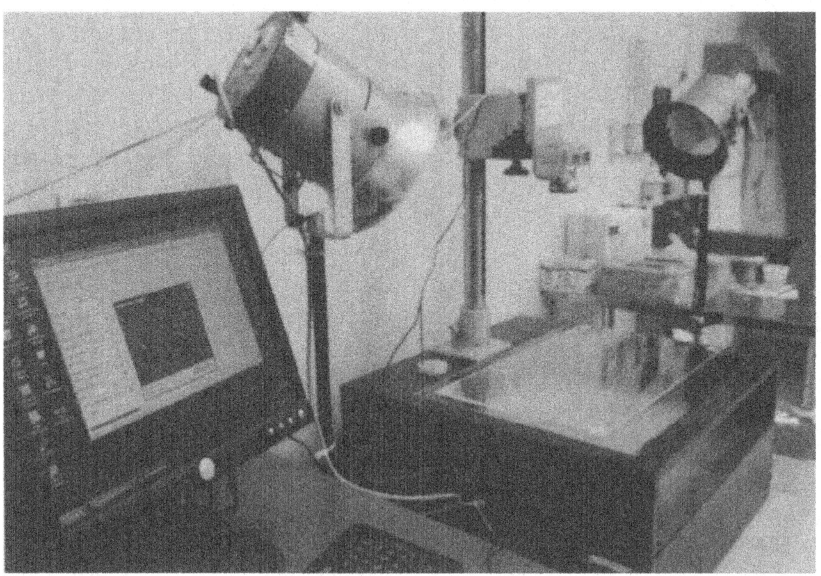

Fig. 1-3. A functional photography stand has an easily cleaned table, a camera with zoom lens, and a reliable computer program for storage of images.

but following such an introduction, the viewer should be fully oriented as to what was being photographed and at what vantage point. Fig. 1-4 demonstrates a close up image of a portal vein thrombosis. The opened gallbladder serves to orient the viewer.

3. The glass or plastic on which the specimen sits must be completely free of blood or body fluid. Puddles of fluid are distracting and thus pull the viewer's eyes away from the reason for which the photograph was taken.
4. A label should be placed in the photograph, so that no important detail of the pathologic process is obscured. The "up-and-down" orientation of the label should coincide with the generally perceived "up and down" of the organ being photographed. For instance, if one is photographing a tumor in a lung, the superior region of the lung should be positioned in the upper part of the image and the label should be placed at the bottom of the image, with the upper edge of the label being closest to the upper region of the image. Ideally, the labels should be typed, not handwritten, and should include a ruler.

A camera should also be available to take *in situ* pictures. In situ photographs may be necessary when a lesion would be significantly disrupted by the evisceration. Examples include pleural or peritoneal abscess, lung collapse, hemopericardium, and epidural hemorrhage. These photographs are much more challenging because they may, by their nature, require various machinations on the part of the photographer to get the photograph appropriately framed. Labels must be included in the framing and retracting fingers should be excluded. Finally, it is important that the unavoidably lurid nature of the autopsy be minimized by excluding skin flaps, structures not directly involved by the pathologic process and blood and body fluid accumulations from the photograph. Fig. 1-5 is an example of a good in situ picture: The rib cage serves to orient the viewer; no skin flap or retracting hands are included and the empyema is readily seen.

In some instances, it may be appropriate to include photographs in the autopsy report. Regardless, a note should be entered into the autopsy report, stating that photographs were taken and that they are on file.

MEETING WITH THE NEXT-OF-KIN In most institutions, the clinical attending physician reviews the autopsy findings with the family. Since the autopsy report is never automatically sent to the family, this conversation is of great importance. Inevitably however, there will be an occasion when the next-of-kin wishes to discuss the autopsy findings with the pathologist. The pathologist should see this request as an opportunity to provide detailed information about the autopsy findings to help clear up any miscommunications that may have occurred between the family and the clinicians, as well as to facilitate the family members in their grieving process. As mentioned earlier in this chapter, the pathologist must notify the clinical attending physician that such a meeting is planned. The clinician may be able to provide further information about the family and/or about events leading up to the death.

Before meeting with the family, carefully review both the clinical history of the deceased as well as the autopsy report. A thorough knowledge of the patient will better prepare the pathologist for any questions that may arise and, thus, allow him/her to be more relaxed during the exchange. Provide a quiet room for the meeting so that privacy will be assured. This may be the pathologist's office or a conference room. Do not meet in or near the autopsy laboratory. It is strongly recommended that, during the meeting, the pathologist make him/herself unreachable by phone or pager, so as to avoid momentary or prolonged distractions from the meeting at hand. Such a concerted effort

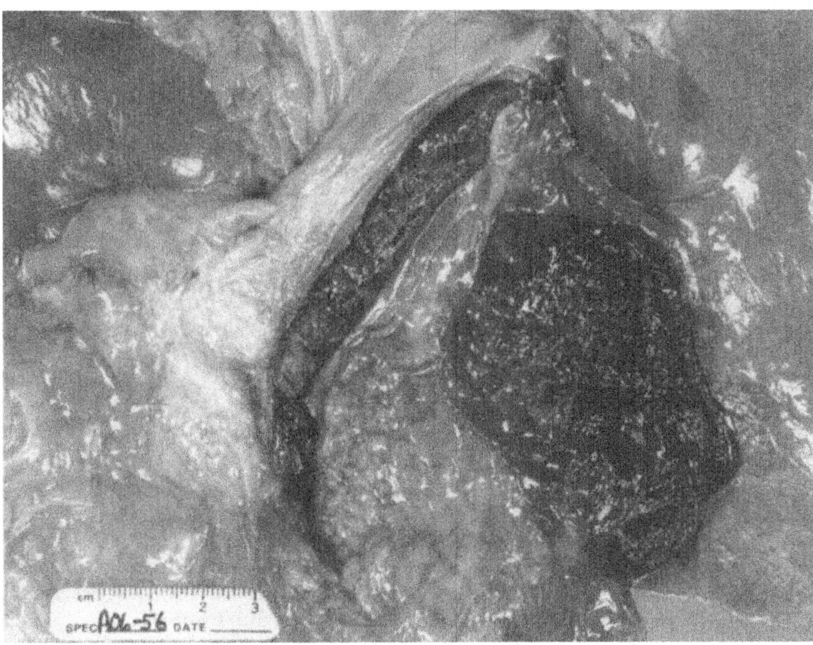

Fig. 1-4. This close-up image of a portal vein thrombosis dramatically demonstrates the pathology, while including enough of the surrounding tissue so that the viewer can readily discern the anatomic site.

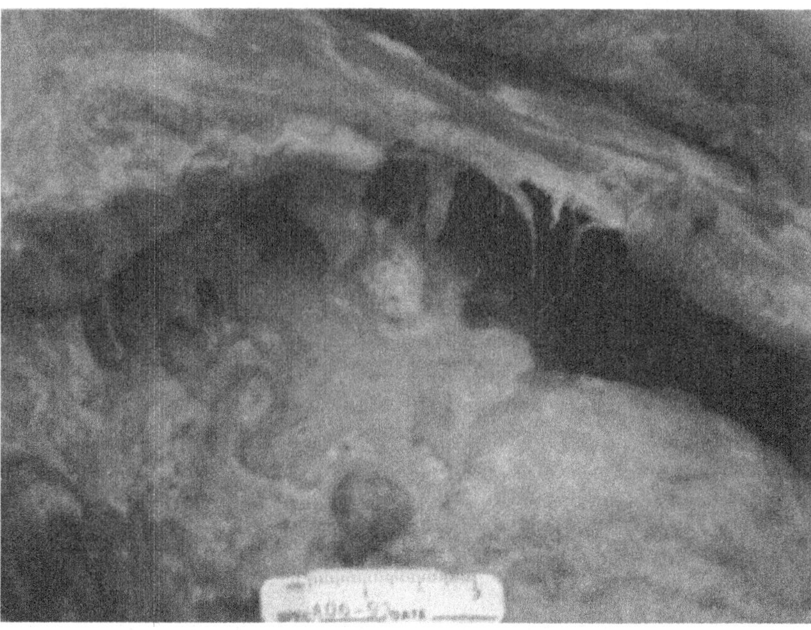

Fig. 1-5. This in situ image clearly showcases the left-sided empyema without including extraneous structures.

to give the family undivided and empathic attention cannot help but promote better communication between the pathologist and the family. It is essential that the pathologist relay information to the family in layperson's terms and to make sure that the family understands what is being said. Simple explanations of human physiology may be required. The pathologist should not hurry this conversation, as it may take the family minutes to digest what is being said and then more time to formulate questions. When adequate time has elapsed for these exchanges to occur and the family members appear satisfied with the information, the meeting may come to a close. At this point, it is very helpful to give the family a phone number by which they may reach the pathologist with further questions. This will have a comforting effect, as they will understand that the pathologist remains available to them should new questions or concerns arise.

Finally, the reader is directed to the recommendations for quality assurance and improvement in autopsy pathology from the Association of Directors of Anatomic and Surgical Pathology. These recommendations have been published in three major pathology journals *(17–19)*.

REFERENCES

1. Cardoso MP, Bourguignon DC, Gomes MM, Saldiva PH, Pereira CR, Troster EJ. Comparison between clinical diagnoses and autopsy findings in a pediatric intensive care unit in Sao Paulo, Brazil. Pediatr Crit Care Med 2006;7(5):423–427.
2. Lardenoye JH, Kastelijn KW, van Esch L, Vrancken Peeters MP, Breslau PJ. [Evaluation of the rate of autopsy and rate of disparity between autopsy results and clinical cause of death in a surgical ward, with the emphasis on necrological review]. Ned Tijdschr Geneeskd 2005;149:1579–1583.
3. Ferguson RP, Burkhardt L, Hennawi G, Puthumana L. Consecutive autopsies on an internal medicine service. South Med J 2004;97:335–337.
4. Combes A, Mokhtari M, Couvelard A, Trouillet JL, Baudot J, Henin D, Gibert C, Chastre J. Clinical and autopsy diagnoses in the intensive care unit: a prospective study. Arch Intern Med 2004;164:389–392.
5. Gibson TN, Shirley SE, Escoffery CT, Reid M. Discrepancies between clinical and postmortem diagnoses in Jamaica: a study from the University Hospital of the West Indies. J Clin Pathol 2004;57:980–985.
6. Killeen OG, Burke C, Devaney D, Clarke TA. The value of the perinatal and neonatal autopsy. Ir Med J 2004;97:241–244.
7. Dimopoulos G, Piagnerelli M, Berre J, Salmon I, Vincent JL. Post mortem examination in the intensive care unit: still useful? Intensive Care Med 2004;30:2080–2085.
8. Newton D, Coffin CM, Clark EB, Lowichik A. How the pediatric autopsy yields valuable information in a vertically integrated health care system. Arch Pathol Lab Med 2004;128:1239–1246.
9. Shojania KG, Burton EC, McDonald KM, Goldman L. Changes in rates of autopsy-detected diagnostic errors over time: a systematic review. JAMA 2003;289:2849–2856.
10. Perkins GD, McAuley DF, Davies S, Gao F. Discrepancies between clinical and postmortem diagnoses in critically ill patients: an observational study. Crit Care 2003;7:R129–132.
11. Ornelas-Aguirre JM, Vazquez-Camacho G, Gonzalez-Lopez L, Garcia-Gonzalez A, Gamez-Nava JI. Concordance between premortem and postmortem diagnosis in the autopsy: results of a 10-year study in a tertiary care center. Ann Diagn Pathol 2003;7:223–230.
12. Burton JL, Underwood J. Clinical, educational, and epidemiological value of the autopsy. Lancet 2007;369:1471–1480.
13. Hasson J, Schneidermann H. Autopsy training programs. To right a wrong. Arch Pathol Lab Med 1995;119:289–291.
14. Welsh T, Kaplann J. The role of postmortem examination in medical education. Mayo Clinic Proc 1998;73:802–805.
15. Burton EC, Phillips RS, Covinsky KE, Sands LPL, Goldman L, Dawson NV, Connors AF Jr., Landefeld CS. The relation of autopsy rate to physicians' beliefs and recommendations regarding autopsy. Am J Med 2004;117;255–261.
16. College of American Pathologists. Autopsy Pathology Checklist © 2006 College of American Pathologists.
17. Nakhleh R, Coffin C, Cooper, K. Recommendations for quality assurance and improvement in surgical and autopsy pathology. Am J Clin Path 2006;126:337–340.
18. Nakhleh R, Coffin C, Cooper, K. Recommendations for quality assurance and improvement in surgical and autopsy pathology. Am J Surg Path 2006;30:1469–1471.
19. Nakhleh R, Coffin C, Cooper, K. Recommendations for quality assurance and improvement in surgical and autopsy pathology. Hum Path 2006;37:985–988.

APPENDIX 1-1 QUALITY ASSURANCE DOCUMENT, AUTOPSY SERVICE AUTOPSY NO. _____

1.	Are all appropriate components of autopsy report included? (major diagnoses; case discussion; clinical summary, gross, micro, cultures, smears, photos, x-rays, results of special procedures, neuropathology)	YES	NO	
2.	FRONT SHEET:			
	a) Major diagnoses in logical (pathogenetic) sequence?	YES	NO	
	b) Results of special studies (micro, chem, etc.) reported and interpreted in front sheet or final note?	YES	NO	NA
	c) Major neuropath diagnoses in appropriate places in front sheet?	YES	NO	NA
	d) All major diagnoses or disease processes included on front sheet (examples: hypertension, diabetes, all previous cancers)?	YES	NO	
3.	GROSS DESCRIPTION:			
	a) Consistent with and supports each diagnosis on front sheet?	YES	NO	
4.	MICROSCOPIC DESCRIPTION:			
	a) Consistent with and supports each diagnosis on front sheet?	YES	NO	
	b) Previous surgicals and cytologies reviewed and recorded?	YES	NO	NA
	c) Consultant opinions documented in report?	YES	NO	NA
5.	NEURO GROSS AND MICRO:			
	a) Consistent with and supports diagnoses on front sheet?	YES	NO	NA
	b) Major neuropathologic diagnoses addressed in final note?	YES	NO	NA
6.	CASE DISCUSSION:			
	a) Does case discussion, in combination with front sheet, adequately address clinical questions and autopsy findings?	YES	NO	
7.	CAUSE OF DEATH:			
	a) Cause of death clearly stated on front sheet or final note?	YES	NO	NA
	b) Death certification appropriate and accurate (or amended)?	YES	NO	NA
8.	Did autopsy identify discrepancies between autopsy and clinical diagnoses?	YES	NO	
	CLINICAL DIAGNOSIS: ________________________________			
	AUTOPSY DIAGNOSIS: ________________________________			
	COMMENT: ________________________________			
9.	Did autopsy reveal (or confirm) complications of therapy or surgery?	YES	NO	
	If yes, was the complication suspected or diagnosed clinically?	YES	NO	
	SURGERY OR THERAPY: ________________________________			
	COMPLICATION: ________________________________			
	COMMENT: ________________________________			

______ ________________ ________________

Date Prosector's Signature Attending Signature

2 Principles of Dissection

Brenda L. Waters

TECHNIQUES TO ENSURE SAFETY

The principle of "Universal Precautions" is predicated on the assumption that all autopsies carry a significant risk of transmitting disease, either by aerosols or through the use of sharp instruments. To prevent exposure, the prosector is now mandated to wear surgical scrubs over which (s)he dons mask, head protection, apron, sleeve covers, and cut-resistant as well as latex (or rubber) gloves.

The elimination of cutting injuries is not guaranteed by the use of cut-resistant gloves; it requires conscious and continuous attention to the safe handling of knives and scalpels. Multiple approaches may be employed. First, the morgue should have a policy in place stipulating that all long knives be routinely sharpened. When a prosector is forced to apply excessive pressure to cut tissue, the likelihood of the knife slipping with injury resulting is increased. A serviceably sharp long knife can readily incise all the large organs, such as the lungs, kidneys, and liver, with only a modicum of pressure. The prosector will find that incising with long strokes, using as much of the length of the knife as possible, and pushing the knife through with as little pressure as possible will result in smooth slices. This type of knife is preferable to the disposable blades that are nearly as sharp as a scalpel. In addition, disposable blades are very flexible and require a handle. Both of these characteristics increase the chances of injury. Microtome blades are also undesirable because of their extreme sharpness. These blades contribute to a disproportionate percentage of cutting injuries when used at an academic pathology department *(1)*. The prosector will find that the great proportion of the dissection procedure can be done safely with simply a pair of sharp, blunt-tipped scissors. These scissors will also require careful, intermittent sharpening.

With regard to the handling of scalpels, pathology trainees should be instructed in the inherent potential of sharps to transmit a chronic and life-threatening disease, such as hepatitis or acquired immune deficiency syndrome. The trainee should develop the habit of using a scalpel only when absolutely necessary, such as while taking sections for histological examination or incising small organs, such as adrenals. The scalpel should always be set down in clear view, away from pools of blood, organs, and other instruments, preferably at the far corner of the cutting board. The scalpel blade should be used for cutting only. It should never be used to point out an item of interest or to gesticulate in any way. As a corollary, one should be vigilant in not placing one's hand in the vicinity of another hand that is wielding a blade. "Mid-air collisions" have occurred in these situations.

Insufficient data is available to determine whether using scalpel blades without handles poses a greater risk than using them with handles. Certainly, attaching a scalpel blade to and removing a blade from a handle require additional manipulation of the blade. On the other hand, using a blade without a handle may increase the risk of injury, because the blade is in close proximity to the cutting hand.

When arming a handle with a scalpel blade, the prosector should point the sharp edge away from the hands and use a minimum of force to accomplish the task. Disarming a blade handle is more dangerous, because the blade may be contaminated with blood. The handle should be held firmly in the nondominant hand, with the blade facing up. With the dominant hand, the prosector grasps the blade at its base with a sturdy pair of forceps or clamp and applies a force perpendicular to the long axis of the handle (Fig. 2-1A). This will lift the base of the blade away from the bevel. Then, with the base of the blade lifted away from the bevel, a controlled force is applied toward the end of the handle, thereby slipping the blade off the end of the handle (Fig. 2-1B). Figure 2-1 demonstrates the procedure as performed by a right-handed person. Notice that the thumb of the hand holding the handle can be used to gently push the blade off the handle by pushing on the forceps. A left-handed person would accomplish the same task with the blade facing down toward the cutting board and using the dominant hand to pull the blade off to the left. Rarely, the blade has been witnessed to inadvertently be "ejected" with a good deal of velocity, while it is removed from the handle. Thus, one must always face the tip of the blade away from people when removing it from a handle.

EVISCERATION TECHNIQUES

There are several techniques by which the organs are removed at autopsy. These have been amply discussed in previous editions of this book, as well as in other books devoted to the subject *(2,3,4)*. Briefly, many forensic pathologists use the Virchow

From: *Handbook of Autopsy Practice,* 4th Ed. Edited by: B.L. Waters

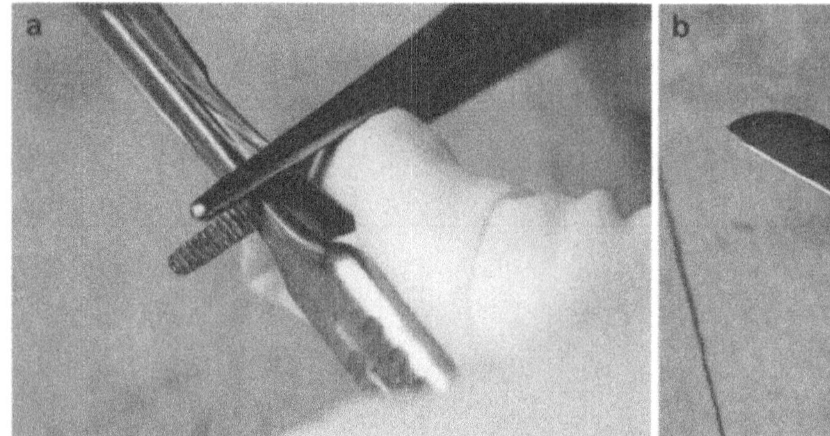
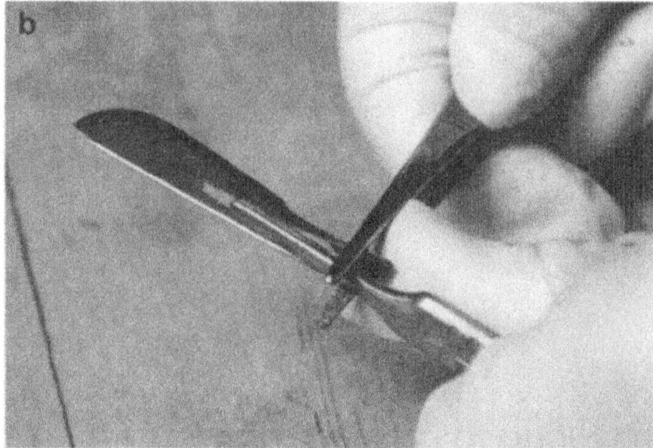

Fig. 2-1. (**a**) With the scalpel blade directed upward, the base of the blade is grasped firmly with a sturdy pair of forceps and then it is carefully pulled away from the bevel. (**b**) Both the right hand and the thumb of the left hand firmly slip the blade off the bevel.

method, by which organs are removed one at a time. In the Letulle method, the entire organ block is removed in its entirety and the dissection proceeds on the prosector's table *(5)*. This technique has a disadvantage in that the removed organ block is very heavy and may not fit on standard cutting boards. In academic settings, where pathology residents perform the autopsies with the help of a diener, the modified Letulle technique may be employed. In this approach, following removal of the anterior chest plate, the heart is removed and given to the resident to begin dissecting, while the diener removes the bowel from the region just distal to the ligament of Treitz to the distal sigmoid-proximal rectum. Then, the diener removes the cervical, thoracic, abdominal, and pelvic organs in one block. This method allows the body to be prepared for the funeral director in a timely manner, independent of the extra time needed by an inexperienced pathology resident to complete the dissection. The Rokitansky method is poorly described in the literature, but involves *in situ* dissection in combination with organ block removal. The technique of Ghon involves removal of the thoracic and cervical organs, the abdominal organs, and the urogenital system as three separate blocks.

Discussion of the various organ systems below will be predicated on the modified Letulle evisceration technique, as described above.

CARDIOVASCULAR SYSTEM

For a discussion of the cardiovascular system, *see* Chapter 3.

RESPIRATORY SYSTEM

In only the rarest of adult cases need the prosector remove the tongue, soft palate, and tonsils. In those instances, the prosector must use caution to avoid cuts through the skin of the face. To gain access to the nasal cavities and adjacent sinuses, remove the brain first so that the nasal and perinasal bony structures may be separated from the rest of the base of the skull with an oscillating saw. This must be done with meticulous attention to preservation of the contours of the face.

Generally, the larynx, trachea, and proximal esophagus are removed as one block, using a transverse cut through the esophagus and trachea 2–3 cm below the inferior margin of the thyroid gland. After the parathyroid and thyroid glands are examined, as described below in Endocrine System, the cervical esophagus is opened posteriorly. Following that, the trachea is also opened posteriorly, along the midline. The lateral portions of the larynx are pulled apart to better expose the mucosa. In adults, this maneuver may require breakage of the ossified hyoid and laryngeal cartilages. In forensic cases, where fractures of the hyoid bone are a possibility, this maneuver should not be performed.

The lungs and bronchi are then approached posteriorly, with removal of the aorta, followed by removal of the esophagus and stomach, the last two as one block. In some institutions, the heart will already have been removed, as described above. If not, the heart is removed by cutting the inferior vena cava close to the diaphragm, the pulmonary veins close to the lungs, the superior vena cava well above the right atrium, and the great vessels above the semilunar valves. The heart may then be set aside for dissection later. For dissection of the heart, *see* Chapter 3. The lungs are dissected from the diaphragm. Any pleural adhesions must be carefully transected as close to the parietal pleura as possible. If adhesions are extensive, then the prosector may find it advantageous to remove the lungs with portions of adherent parietal pleura attached. Remnants of the pericardial sac and mediastinal soft tissue are also removed. The lungs are then separated from each other by transverse cuts across the mainstem bronchi and weighed. If the lungs are to be perfused, it is advisable that the transverse cuts in the mainstem bronchi be as close to the tracheal bifurcation as possible. This will allow enough length of bronchus in which to wedge the perfusion tubing. Before perfusing the lungs, be sure that the lungs have indeed been weighed and that all cultures have been taken.

Pathologists have debated the pros and cons of lung perfusion for decades. One faction claims that a perfused lung is easier to slice and that parenchymal abnormalities, such as pneumonia, emphysema, and fibrosis are better demonstrated with perfusion. The other side states that perfusion obscures pulmonary edema. The accumulation of experience will help the prosector to resolve this dilemma. A compromise can be that only one lung is perfused or that sections of lung are taken before perfusion. It should be noted here that even in perfused lungs, pulmonary edema can still be seen histologically. Edema fluid appears as pale eosinophilic proteinaceous material that is pushed (by the formalin perfusate) against the alveolar walls. It is distinguished from the hyaline membranes of diffuse alveolar damage (adult respiratory distress syndrome), in that the edema fluid is not as condensed or as deeply eosinophilic. Pulmonary edema is very likely to be present if foamy fluid is noted to exit the bronchi prior to perfusion.

When perfusing lungs after weighing (Fig. 2-2), it is helpful to employ one clamp to hold the bronchus as the perfusate tube is inserted. Another clamp may be used to cross-clamp the bronchus when the perfusion appears to be complete. The lungs should expand fairly briskly. If there appears to be a delay, slight repositioning of the tube may help. If there is copious exudate, mucin, blood, or tumor in the bronchial tree, perfusion may be sluggish, in which case one can perfuse the arterial system instead. Although it may be convenient to set the lungs aside at this juncture, for dissection later, they may be sectioned immediately, if desired. Although rents in the pleural surfaces due to excision of pleural adhesions or procurement of lung tissue for culture will hamper lung perfusion, they do not negate the advantages of perfusion. These rents may be closed with clamps. Remember to weigh the lungs prior to perfusing. It may be a good idea to post such a reminder on the carboy that holds the formalin perfusate.

The commonly used planes of sectioning for lungs are transverse and parasagittal. The transverse plane may be preferable if the pathologist is trying to correlate the autopsy findings with the CT or MRI images. In most cases the parasagittal plane works well. The prosector begins with the hilar region facing up and the lateral pleural surface on the cutting board (Fig. 2-3A). A long, serviceably sharp knife is best. The lung sections should be no thicker than 2 cm (Fig 2-3B). When the slices are this thick, reconstruction of the lungs will not be difficult. The prosector should use long strokes of the knife, keeping the knife parallel to the cutting board. This will ensure that the slices are of uniform thickness. A succession of long back-and-forth strokes with the knife, using as little force as needed, will minimize uneven cutting. As the slices approach the hilar region, the prosector may encounter difficulty cutting through the larger branches of the

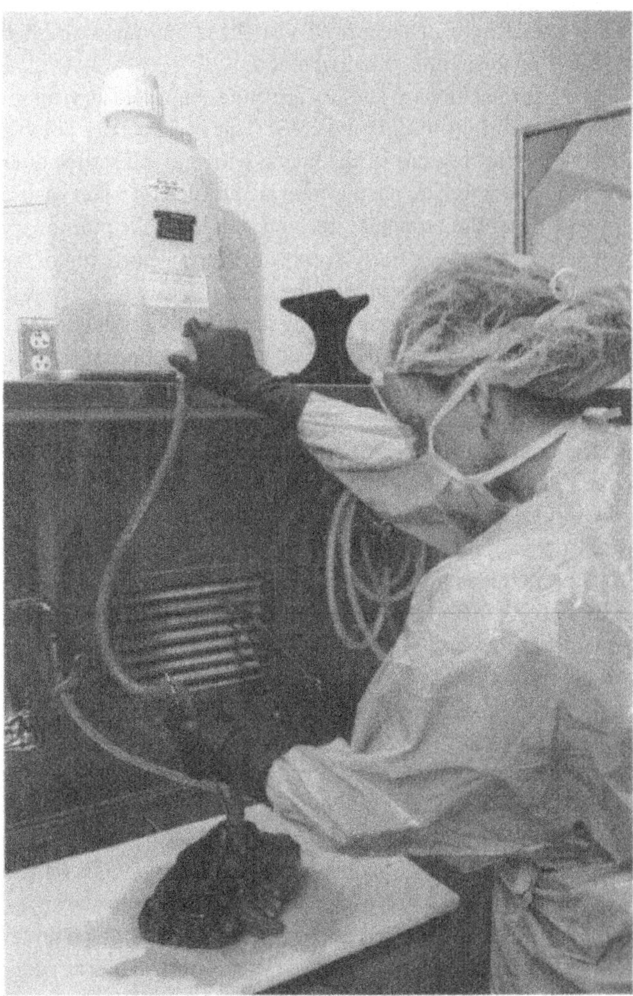

Fig. 2-2. Perfusion of a lung. The resident is holding the lung by way of a clamp attached to the mainstem bronchus and is keeping the perfusion tubing wedged into the bronchus.

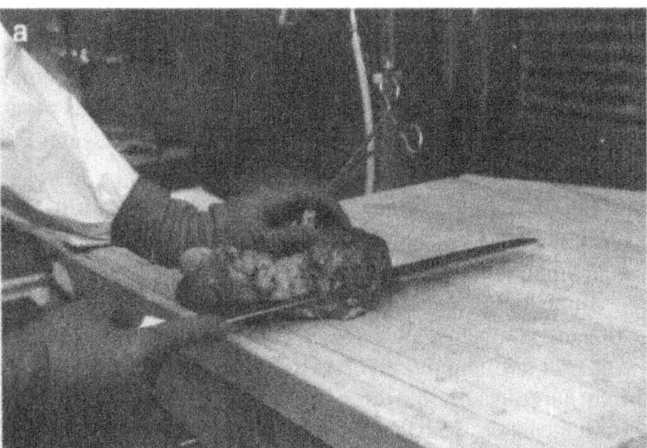

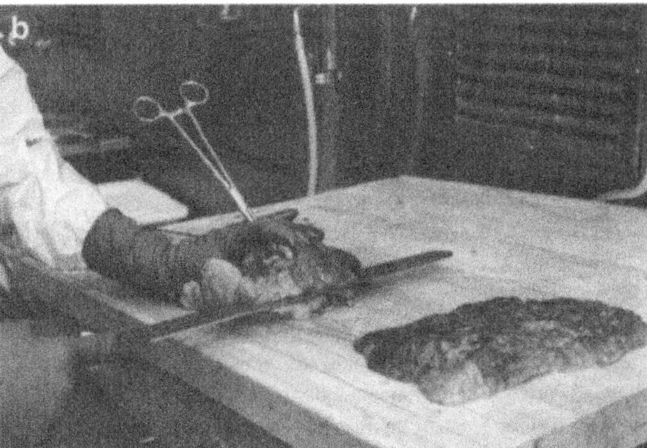

Fig. 2-3. Slicing the lung. (**a**) The lung is placed hilum up and close to the edge of the cutting board, so that the prosector can use the entire length of the knife without her hand bumping into the cutting board. (**b**) If attention is directed to keeping the knife parallel to the cutting board, uniform slices will be the result.

bronchi. Instead of adding more force to the knife, (s)he may cut the bronchi with a heavy pair of scissors and then continue with the knife. Finally, all the large vascular and bronchial branches should be opened with scissors. A good autopsy pathologist is reluctant to leave a tubular structure unopened. Pulmonary tumors and emboli can be well visualized and photographed using this parasagittal slicing method.

Most normal lungs at autopsy are quite congested and, therefore, have a bright-to-dark red color. This is especially notable in the posterior regions of the lungs, where blood settles after death. A characteristic postmortem artifact occurs when gastric contents enter the bronchial tree and settle into the pulmonary parenchyma. This generally occurs during transportation of the body to the morgue. Because of the strong acidity of the gastric fluid, the involved portions of lung are literally digested. They will appear dark gray to black but will not feel consolidated. The mucosal surfaces of the bronchi supplying these areas will often be darkened and brown-black. When actual aspiration of gastric contents occurs, the tracheobronchial mucosa will be hyperemic and thus red in the fresh state.

Useful axioms in gross lung pathology include the following: Acute pneumonia is characteristic in that its gross appearance is more pronounced after fixation. This can be of help diagnostically. Also, in lungs involved by centriacinar emphysema, acute pneumonia may not be as evident grossly. Fixation may bring out the gross features of acute inflammation, but the reduction in parenchyma as a result of emphysema may still obscure its presence or extent. Finally, pulmonary hemorrhage may often be differentiated from severe pulmonary congestion by its associated consolidation and by the continuous outpouring of blood from the lung slices, even after fixation.

Common, clinically inconsequential abnormalities of the lungs include mild artherosclerosis of the pulmonary arteries, subpleural fibrosis of the posterior aspect of the lower lobes and focal fibrosis of the apices. These generally occur in older individuals. However, in patients with pulmonary hypertension, the atherosclerosis may be accentuated.

The diaphragm need not be retained in its entirety, but it is a good idea to carefully examine it and retain a small portion of it in a "stock jar." Such containers are used to store small sections of all the major organs and are kept for a year or longer if necessary. Further comments on these jars are found in Chapter 6. Common gross abnormalities of the diaphragm include hyaline plaques on the thoracic side (due to asbestos exposure) and small foci of anthracotic pigment.

SPECIAL PROCEDURES

DEMONSTRATION OF TENSION PNEUMOTHORAX Once the skin and subcutaneous tissue is dissected laterally from the initial Y-shaped incision, water is poured into the recess lateral to the rib cage and medial to the skin flap. Then, a scalpel is placed below the surface of the water and inserted into the pleural space between two ribs. The scalpel is rotated slightly. Exiting of air bubbles establishes the diagnosis of tension pneumothorax. Another approach to observe this abnormality is to view the domes of the diaphragm from the abdominal cavity. In a tension pneumothorax, the dome may be pushed downward.

PREPARATION OF PAPER-MOUNTED SECTIONS This method was pioneered by Gough and has undergone several modifications *(6)*. The technique yields very instructive, detailed, and extremely durable views of pulmonary abnormalities. Following perfusion fixation with formalin and sodium acetate, 2-cm slices of the lungs are washed and embedded in gelatin mixture that contains a disinfectant. After the gelatin has penetrated the tissue, the block is frozen and large 400-µm sections are cut, refixed, and transferred to another gelatin mixture. They are then mounted on paper. Routine stains can be applied without difficulty. Readers will find that paper-mounting requires both skill and patience. The original method Cough required 11 days, although other authors have achieved comparable results in 2 days *(7)*. Despite this method's didactic and esthetic appeal, it has been largely replaced by photography of perfusion-fixed specimens.

PULMONARY ANGIOGRAPHY These injection procedures require inflated lungs. Therefore, careful removal of the lungs and sealing of accidental lacerations of the pleura are essential.

For arteriography, tubing is tied with glass or plastic cones into the pulmonary artery and the bronchus, respectively. The lung is inflated through the bronchus with air at a pressure of approximately 20 mm of Hg. The barium-gelatin mixture is warmed to about 60°C and injected into the pulmonary artery at a pressure of about 70 mm Hg to 80 mm Hg. Some experimentation may be necessary since required injection pressures vary depending on the viscosity and the temperature of the mixture. This method should result in filling peripheral artery branches down to vessels with an internal diameter of about 60 µm. The study of smaller vessels requires very low-viscosity gelatin or nonconsolidating contrast media. For the average-sized lung, about 150 mL of medium are needed. The injection takes 5–10 minutes. When the vascular tree is filled, the pressure increases sharply, indicating that injection is completed. The lung should be kept warm during the injection so that the gelatin does not set too quickly. A lung processed this way is depicted in Fig. 2-4. This method may be adapted to infant lungs *(8)*. Another approach is to perfusion-fix the lungs with formalin, using the pulmonary arteries and then perfuse the arteries with white contrast medium (see Fig. 2-5).

The injection technique for venography is similar, although the filling of the pulmonary veins must be accomplished from the left atrium. Thus, if this technique is planned, the heart should not be separated from the lungs, or the pulmonary veins should be kept as long as possible on the lungs. Injection pressures may vary between 20 and 70 mm Hg.

Lymphangiography requires the use of sodium tritrizoate and a no. 30 lymphangiography needle, while the lung is kept at an inflation pressure of about 18 cm H_2O *(9)*.

Bronchial arteriography may be accomplished by tying a 30-gauge polyethylene catheter to the isolated bronchial vessels. The left lung usually has two bronchial arteries, and the right lung usually has one. The left bronchial arteries arise from the anteromedial surface of the aortic arch. The superior artery ostium is just lateral to the carina and posterior to the left main bronchus. The inferior left bronchial artery ostium is just inferior to the left main bronchus. The right bronchial artery arises from the right third posterior intercostal artery or rarely

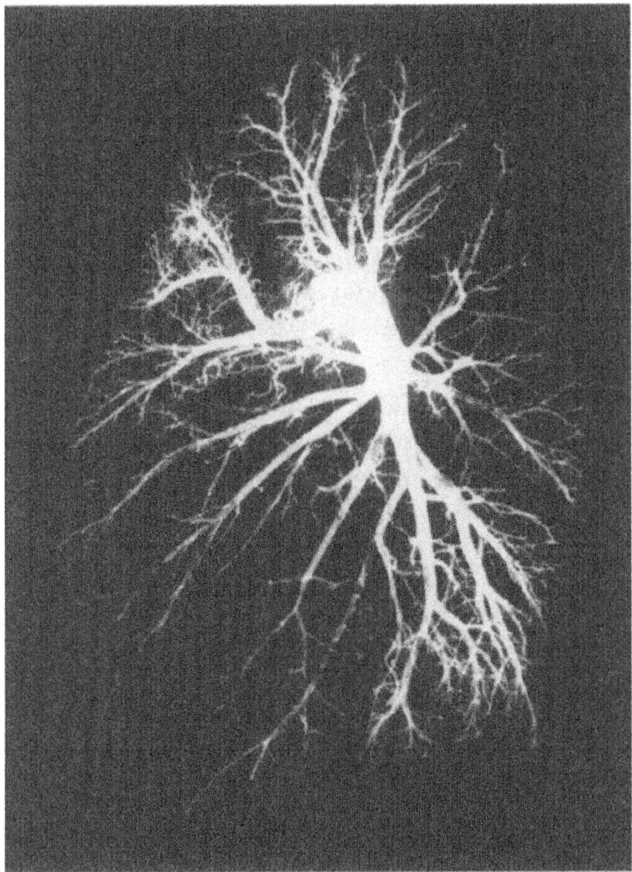

Fig. 2-4. Arteriogram of left lung. The lung was inflated with carbon dioxide and the pulmonary artery was injected with barium sulfate-gelatin mixture. Note the blunting of the arterial tree in this emphysematous lung.

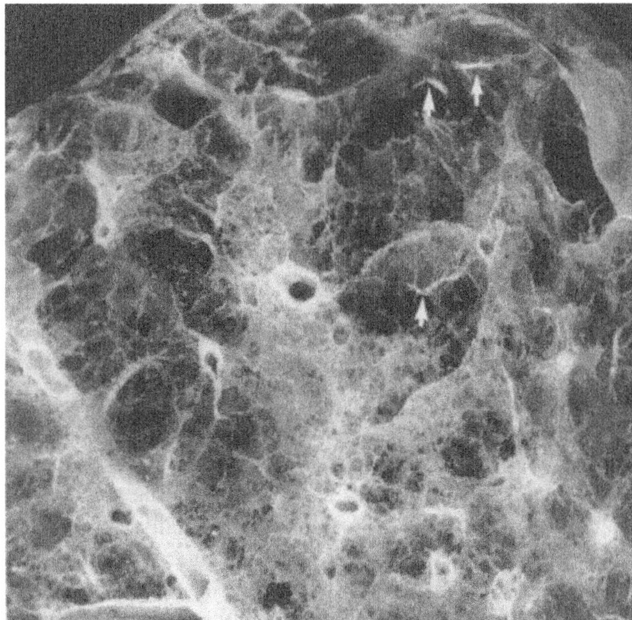

Fig. 2-5. Perfusion-fixed lung with advanced destructive centrilobular emphysema, photographed underwater. Note the pulmonary artery branches containing white contrast medium *(arrows)*.

from the thoracic aorta via the superior left bronchial artery. The path of these arteries continues to the upper esophagus, and runs along the posterior wall of the main bronchi to penetrate the lung parenchyma. The lung is first inflated with air. Then, the contrast medium, usually barium sulfate, is injected through the catheter. The injection pressure is 150 mm Hg. An example of a bronchial arteriogram is shown in Fig. 2-6.

PARTICLE IDENTIFICATION Many particles can be readily identified if they are within the resolution limits of the light microscope. The *Particle Atlas* is most helpful in such a situation *(10)*. Inorganic particles can be isolated and concentrated for morphologic study by holding an unstained, uncovered paraffin section over a flame, such as a Bunsen burner, until the organic material has been incinerated.

In most cases, light microscopic observation with polarizing lenses provides sufficient semiquantitative information. However, for research purposes, mineral particles in lung tissue can be quantitatively analyzed with macroanalytic techniques, such as X-ray diffraction, X-ray fluorescence, neutron activation analysis, atomic absorption spectroscopy, or proton-induced X-ray emission spectroscopy. Microanalytic techniques include energy dispersive X-ray spectroscopy and wave-length dispersive X-ray spectroscopy. Excellent descriptions of these methods are found in the references *(11,12,13)*.

For the quantification of asbestos, ferruginous bodies are harvested from the fixed or unfixed lungs by digesting the tissue in 5.25% sodium hypochlorite. The solid residues are collected on membrane filters. The characteristic features of asbestos bodies allow reasonably accurate counts. For a detailed description of

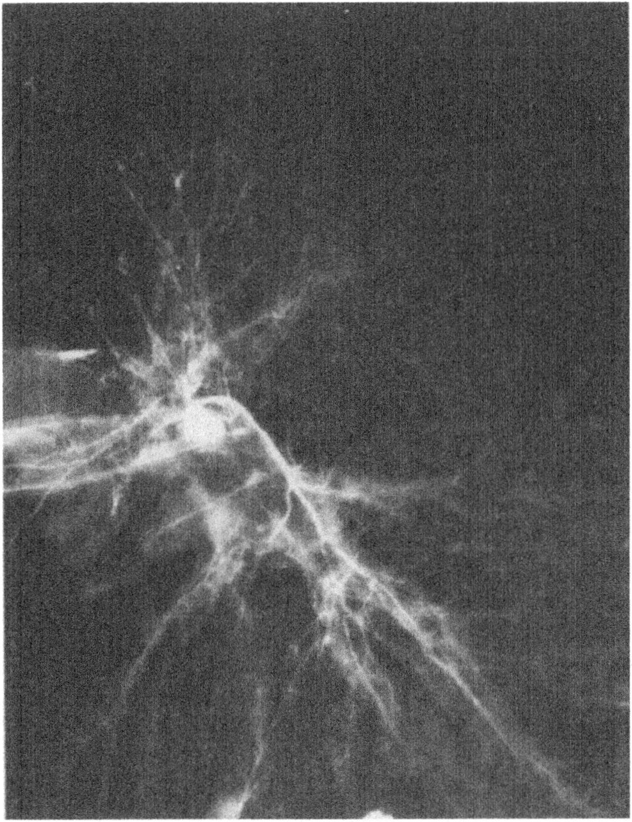

Fig. 2-6. Bronchial arteriogram.

current digestion and counting strategies, see reference *(14)*. For the semiquantitative demonstration of asbestos bodies, dried scrapings from lung sections are often studied. Ferruginous bodies also can be viewed using electron microscopy *(15,16)*.

HEMATOPOIETIC SYSTEM, SPLEEN, AND THYMUS

In patients with hematopoietic disease, the prosector should procure multiple sections of bone marrow. Sites of procurement include ribs, sternum, vertebrae, and iliac crest. Bone marrow smears may also be very useful, although they inevitably show autolysis when obtained postmortem. It is best if a hematology technician can come to the morgue to obtain the smears, as he or she is most experienced in this procedure.

The ribs are ideal sources of marrow. First, they are readily available in cases in which the autopsy permission allows examination of the thorax and, second, marrow taken from them requires little to no decalcification. With a scalpel in hand, the prosector instructs the deiner to compress the rib just below the cut end. This can be accomplished with the use of a pair of pliers, or similar tool. What generally follows is an extrusion of bone marrow from the end of the rib. The prosector uses the scalpel like a spatula and carefully gathers the marrow up and places it onto previously moistened tissue paper that lines a cassette. This method of bone marrow collection results in a beautiful display of the cytology of the hematopoietic cells, since decalcification is not required. Patients with aplastic anemia often have very watery marrow that resembles hemorrhagic serous fluid. Patients with multiple myeloma or other myeloproliferative disorders frequently have copious amounts of thick, dark brown marrow retrieved by this method.

In addition, small samples of bone from the vertebral bodies should be taken. There is a tendency to take too large of a section of bone marrow for histologic section. In actuality, multiple small sections, the size of a small pea, taken from several different sites, require less decalcification and allow for greater preservation of cells. Overdecalcified bone marrow sections appear smudgy, with the basophilia of the nuclei blending with the eosinophilia of the cytoplasm. This problem may be mitigated by rehydrating the section, immersing it in a lithium carbonate solution and then restaining with Harris hematoxylin. See the decalcification procedure under Skeletal System, at the end of this chapter.

The size of the spleen varies greatly in hematologic diseases, so it is important to record the spleen weight. The spleen may be sectioned in the coronal, parasagittal, or transverse planes. The choice of plane should be made with the intent of demonstrating the largest diameter of the organ. Because of the high content of blood in the spleen, the organ should be sliced thinly, so as to maximize fixation. The spleen may be perfused with formalin, using the splenic artery, however it is beneficial to first perfuse with normal saline so as to wash out much of the blood. In fact, the splenic reticulum can be well demonstrated by that perfusion method. If the injection pressure is about 100 mm Hg, the splenic pulp will turn white after about 1 hour. The perfusion is then continued with 10% formalin. Splenic arteriography may also be accomplished using the splenic artery.

In the fetal life and in childhood, the thymus is a prominent multilobed organ, situated partly in the neck and partly in the thorax. It rests on fascia over the great vessels and on the anterosuperior region of the pericardium. It may extend into the neck to the level of the lower border of the thyroid gland. It reaches its maximum size at puberty, weighing up to 35 grams. It then gradually decreases in size and may weigh only 6 grams at the age of 70. If it is important to examine thymic tissue at autopsy, such as in a patient with a history of thymoma.

Although formalin fixation is adequate for hematopoietic tissue, we find that B-Plus Fixative™ (BBC Biochemical) minimizes cytoplasmic retraction, and provides excellent cytologic preservation.

ENDOCRINE SYSTEM

NECK BLOCK The thyroid and parathyroid glands are part of the "neckblock," a traditional term that refers to the larynx, the proximal esophagus, and the proximal trachea extending "two fingers" (about 2-3 cm) below the inferior margin of the thyroid gland. This inclusion of the trachea below the thyroid insures that the inferior parathyroid glands will remain with the block. The dissection begins with steps to view the thyroid and parathyroid glands before opening the esophagus or trachea/larynx. The most anterior fascicles of the strap muscles may be removed. Overtrimming of muscle and connective tissue from the neck block should be avoided, since this may result in inadvertent removal of one or more of the parathyroid glands. Multiple incisions are made no more than 0.5 cm apart in the soft tissue between the esophagus and the posterior margin of the thyroid gland. In that region, using an astute and patient eye, the parathyroid glands will be found. The glands will be slightly flattened, like a lentil bean, and have a homogenous tan to golden color. With age, they become a brighter yellow. The lower glands are generally larger than the upper. Lymph nodes of comparable size will have a grayer or pink hue and small nodules of the thyroid will have a glassy, brownish-red hue. Fixing the neck block will stiffen the tissue and make the task of identification of the parathyroid glands easier.

In the great majority of patients coming to autopsy, there is no clinical suspicion of parathyroid disease. This may lull the inexperienced pathologist to erroneously conclude that it is unnecessary to search for these glands on a routine basis. In our practice, we encourage first-year pathology residents to submit all the parathyroid glands for histologic confirmation. This provides them with feedback for their developing eye. When the clinical history of the patient raises the question of parathyroid disease, then the glands should be assiduously sought out. All possible contenders for parathyroid tissue should have their location documented before they are removed from the neck block. A simple drawing or "map" is sufficient, designating each nodule with a different letter. Each possible parathyroid gland should be trimmed of fat, and individually weighed in a balance that records a weight in grams to three decimal points. Such a scale may be found in the histology or chemistry laboratory. The normal weight for four parathyroid glands is 120 mg in adult males and 142 mg in adult females. Finally, each of the specimens is separately submitted for histologic examination.

When the search for parathyroid glands is completed, the thyroid gland is either removed, weighed, and incised or just incised while still attached to the neck block. The slices should be spaced no more than 0.5 cm apart. The normal thyroid has a rich brown-gold color and a glassy sheen. The latter characteristic is the result of the colloid. Nodules of hyperplastic follicles are frequently present, as are foci of dystrophic calcification. Neoplasms are less frequent, and generally have a more tan and less glassy appearance. They may seem to be well circumscribed and may readily bulge up from the cut surface. In any of these neoplastic nodules, it is prudent to include in the histologic section both the tumor and the surrounding thyroid tissue, since issues of capsular invasion should still be dealt with in autopsy material. Regional lymph nodes need to be sampled in cases of thyroid neoplasia.

ADRENAL GLANDS The adrenal glands in most individuals may be found within the retroperitoneal fat above and/or medial to the superior poles of the kidneys. It is generally a good idea to remove them as soon as possible, as they autolyze and soften quickly, resulting in fragmentation. Also, they can be very difficult to locate later, when surrounding organs, such as the kidneys, have been removed. First, the posterior leaves of the diaphragm are cut along each side of the aorta and reflected upward and out of the way. Then, by using blunt dissection and careful palpation, the prosector should be able to locate the adrenal gland. When the borders are discerned by palpation, the prosector can begin to remove the gland by taking a cuff of fat around it. At this point, the adrenal gland may not be visualized directly, but rather palpated. If the prosector cuts into the adrenal, he or she will recognize it by its golden-to-dark brown red color. The adrenal artery may be conspicuous. Once the adrenal is removed, as much of the periadrenal fat is removed as possible. This is accomplished by holding the scissors flat and parallel to the cortical surface. Once trimmed, the organ is weighed. The average weight of a well-trimmed adrenal gland is 4-6 grams. The right adrenal is more triangular and is also flatter, as it resides between two solid organs, the right lobe of the liver and the right kidney. The left adrenal is more elongated and usually features a superior, midline upfolding of its cortex, forming a longitudinal ridge. The adrenal cortex ranges in color from yellow gold, to brown red, depending on the content of lipid and the degree of congestion in the deeper areas. The medulla, characterized by gray more solid tissue beneath the cortex, can be mistaken for metastatic cancer. Normally, the medulla is present only in the body and head of the gland.

PITUITARY Removal of the pituitary is discussed in Chapter 4.

THE GASTROINTESTINAL TRACT

ESOPHAGUS Dissection of the gastrointestinal tract begins at the esophagus, the proximal portion of which is part of the neck block. This segment of esophagus on the neck block is opened posteriorly. In most adult autopsies, the esophagus may be removed prior to opening, because there is no suspicion of any fistulous connection between it and the bronchial tree. If there is any history of pathology in the esophagus, it should be opened, examined, and fixed immediately. In cases of infiltrating carcinomas arising from or involving the esophagus, the esophagus should be opened prior to removal from the thoracic organs so as to identify and preserve any fistulae. With minimal autolysis, the mucosa will be white to gray and may show islands of acanthosis, characterized by mucosal thickening and gray-white opacification. Moderate to severe autolysis will cause areas of the mucosa to slough, leaving a darkened reddish surface. This change can be mistaken for ulceration or Barrett's esophagus if it is near the gastroesophageal junction. Early fixation, followed by procurement of a longitudinal section of esophagus containing both grossly normal and abnormal areas will allow the correct interpretation in most instances.

Esophageal varices that have eroded through the mucosa and have bled are readily seen as hyperemic ulcerations often with thickening of the wall. On the other hand, unruptured varices may be difficult to see. Even in normal patients, the submucosal veins may appear quite dilated when incised in transverse section. One strategy for improving the demonstration of varices entails turning the esophagus inside out with the aid of a long clamp prior to opening. This may be quite successful in some cases. Formalin fixation may further accentuate the varices. Injection with barium sulfate-gelatin mixture may also highlight the varices (see Fig. 2-7).

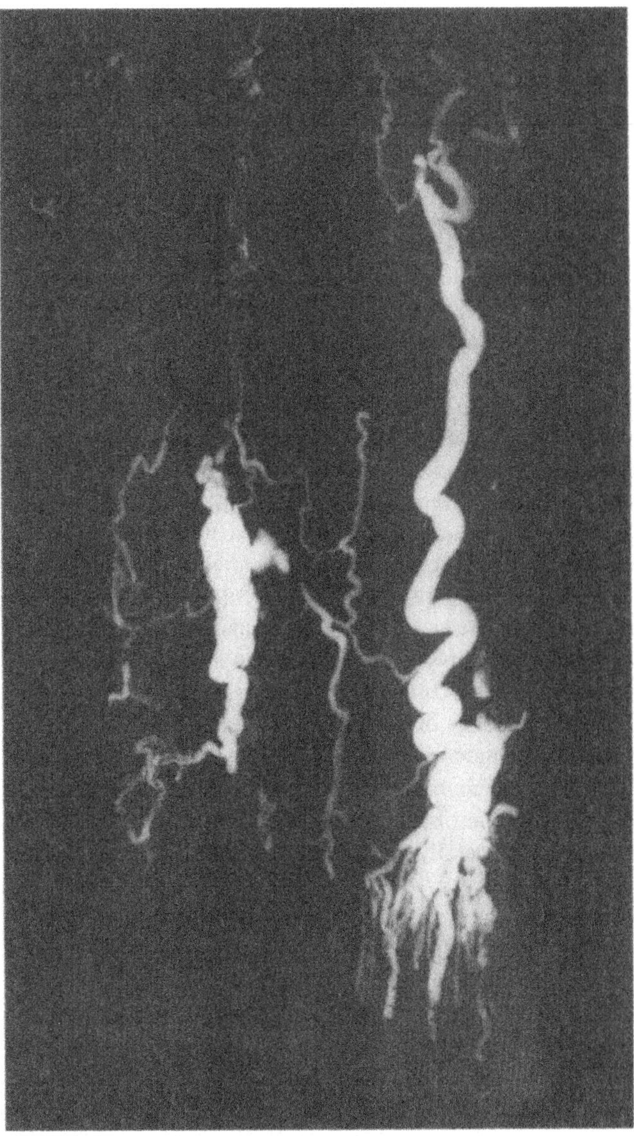

Fig. 2-7. Roentgenogram of esophageal varices injected with barium sulfate-gelatin mixture.

Although the lower end of the esophageal wall is normally thicker, some patients with a history of dysphagia may have an accentuation of this wall thickness and may appear to have stenosis of the lumen. Comparing the internal circumference of the area of suspected stenosis with that of other regions of the esophagus may help to quantify the degree of stenosis. To confirm the presence of lower esophageal rings (Schatzki rings), remove the lower half of the esophagus with the upper half of the stomach and an attached ring of diaphragm. Clamp the stomach across the corpus. The viscus is then slightly distended with a mixture of barium sulfate and 10% formalin with clamping of the esophagus. Roentgenograms should be prepared as soon as possible. Subsequently, the specimen should be fixed in the distended state in formalin until it is to be cut. This method can be used for other types of stricture of the esophagus.

STOMACH In most cases, the stomach may be separated from the pancreas and opened along the greater curvature. When penetrating ulcers or infiltrating tumors are anticipated, the stomach should remain attached to the adjacent organ involved and a plane of sectioning chosen to best demonstrate the pathologic process.

The gastric rugae stretch out and flatten soon after death. For this reason, early examination and fixation of this organ should be a priority, especially in patients with any kind of gastric disease. The pyloric region of the stomach has a characteristically flattened mucosa, as compared to the regions proximal. The muscular wall is also thicker in this region, which may resemble the gastric wall thickening in linitis plastica. The proximal duodenum should be severed about 4 cm (two prosector's finger-widths) distal to the pylorus such that any peptic ulcer adjacent to the pyloric sphincter is not transected.

Advanced autolysis results in the classic changes of mural thinning and blackening of the gastric cardia and fundus. The vessels take on a characteristic appearance, that of an increase in their diameter and exaggeration of their branching. Rarely, this autolytic process culminates into a postmortem gastric perforation, with accumulation of gastric fluid in the peritoneal cavity. The inexperienced pathologist might think this is a ruptured viscus with peritonitis. However, closer examination will reveal a complete lack of fibrinous exudate on adjacent serosal surfaces. This autolytic change can also discolor the overlying dome of the diaphragm and adjacent tissues.

In the majority of autopsies, the stomach will show multiple, minute mucosal hemorrhages, usually in the fundus and body. These hemorrhages are considered to be perimortem in onset and are attributed to the hemodynamics of the agonal state. They generally do not reflect a clinically recognizable premortem process.

The stomach wall must be carefully examined for serosal nodules, such as a metastatic implants, gastrointestinal stromal tumors and leiomyomas.

Celiac Arteriography For gastric arteriography, the organs supplied by the celiac artery should be removed en masse. The splenic and hepatic arteries are tied as far distally as possible. A barium preparation is injected through the celiac artery. After injection, the stomach is isolated, opened along the middle of the anterior surface parallel with the longitudinal axis of the organ, spread out on an X-ray cassette and radiographed.

SMALL AND LARGE BOWEL The greater omentum should be examined prior to discard. In clinical situations where there is a history of abdominal malignancy it should be fixed and retained for possible future reexamination, such as at Gross Conference.

The C-shaped proximal segment of the duodenum will be covered in the section pertaining to the hepatobiliary tree and pancreas.

The intestines autolyze quickly and thus should be examined and fixed promptly, especially in patients with intestinal disease. Opening of the bowel is greatly facilitated when the mesentery has been cut close to the wall of the intestine. Having minimal attached mesentery also allows for pinning of the bowel segments to a corkboard so as to have a flat surface for excellent, close up photography.

The color of normal bowel varies widely at autopsy. It may be tan-pink as seen in surgical specimens, or it may be dark pink, red, green, yellow, or black, the latter if the bowel was adjacent to a postmortem rupture of the gastric fundus. Despite its length, the small bowel infrequently manifests pathology at autopsy. Submucosal lipomas may be found as well as dilated lacteals. The latter are whitish and may be slightly raised as they appear through the overlying normal mucosa. When incised, they sometimes quickly collapse and spill out a milky fluid. The most common malignancy to involve the small bowel at autopsy is intraperitoneal metastatic carcinoma. This may appear as multiple rounded to flattened deposits of white, firm tissue in the bowel serosa, submucosa and/or mesentery.

Ischemic bowel, especially in its early stages, may be a difficult entity to distinguish from autolysis. The colors of ischemic bowel may resemble those of normal postmortem change. Subtle characteristics of early bowel ischemia include hemorrhage or hyperemia in the submucosa and muscularis, fine roughening of the mucosa and finally, an odor. The odor of ischemic or necrotic bowel is most characteristic and once perceived, is well remembered by alert prosectors. Any section of bowel that is suspected to be ischemic or infarcted should be fixed immediately and processed for histologic examination.

More advanced bowel necrosis is typified by a dusky blue serosal surface often with fibrinous exudate, bowel dilation, and/or darkening of the mucosa by hemorrhage or severe hyperemia. The wall may be thickened and the odor of dead bowel may permeate the room.

Small polyps frequently reside in the large bowel. They autolyze so quickly that the prosector may not consider them worthy of histologic examination. However, if the bowel is examined soon after removal, these polyps will be surprisingly well preserved such that histologic examination will allow them to be properly categorized. The diagnosis of colonic polyps is of importance to family members of the deceased.

Carcinomas of the large bowel should be photographed prior to obtaining sections for histologic examination. Careful attention should be paid to looking for mesenteric lymph nodes in the region of the carcinoma.

A modification of the placental "membrane roll" method may be employed to obtain long sections of intestinal wall for histologic examination (Fig. 2-8A-F). Following fixation, a long rectangular strip of bowel wall is cut from the organ. With the

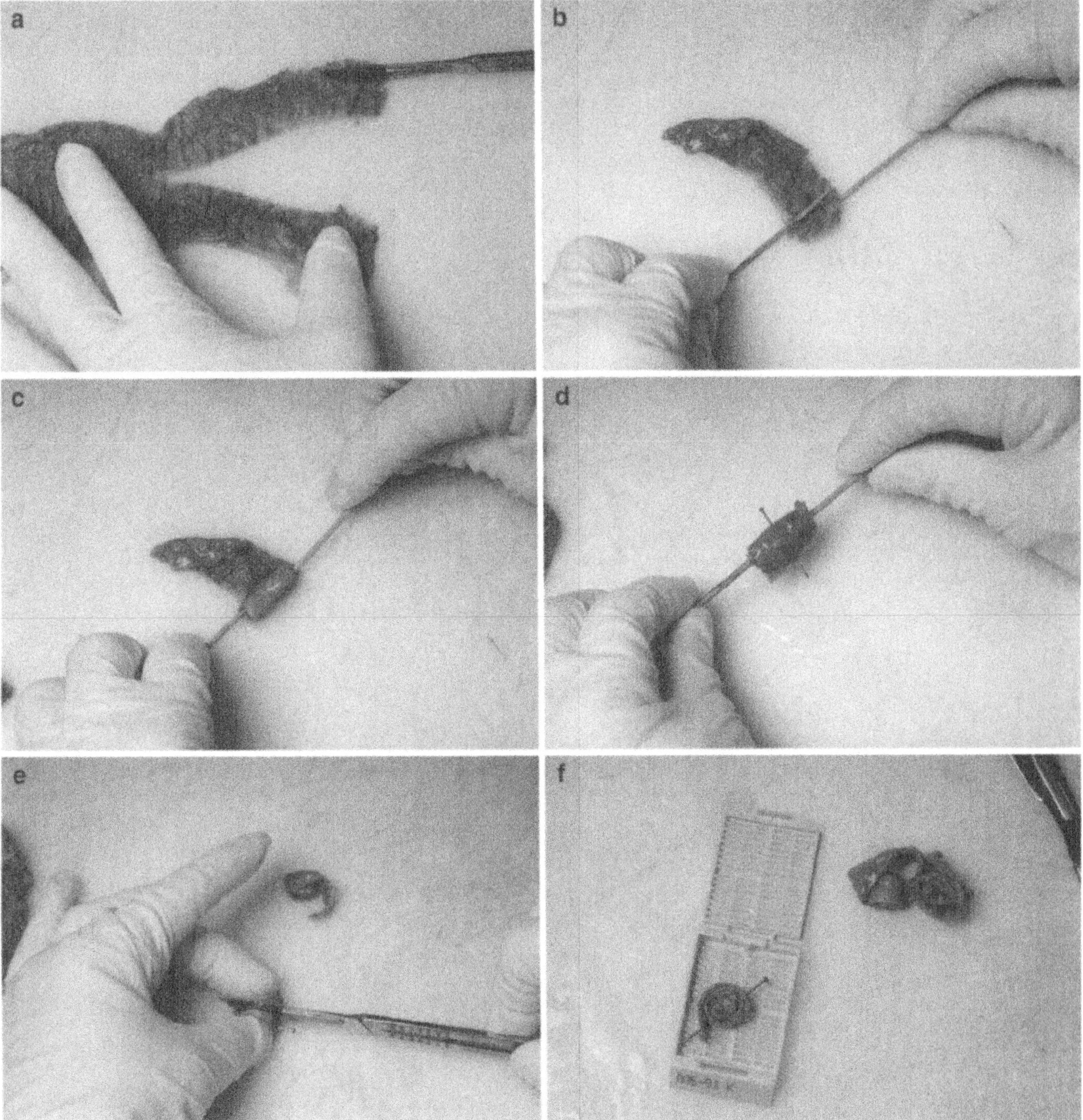

Fig. 2-8. (**a**) A rectangular strip of bowel is cut away. (**b**) With two wooden sticks, the strip is wound into a roll. (**c**) A pin is placed through the roll. (**d**) The sticks are pulled out, leaving the pin in place. (**e**) The roll is sliced on both sides of the pin to obtain a section thin enough to fit into a cassette. (**f**) The pin remains in the roll. The requisition accompanying the cassette, should have a notation warning the histology technician that there is a pin present.

use of two wooden sticks, the strip is rolled up and pierced by a straight pin between the sticks so as to hold the roll in place. Following removal of the sticks, the roll is cut on both sides of the pin to a thickness appropriate for placement in a cassette. The section is submitted to the histology laboratory, accompanied by a written warning that a pin is present in the block. What results is sampling of a large area of mucosa and muscularis.

Preparation for Study under Dissecting Microscope Inevitably, autolysis will cause flattening of the mucosal plicae. To obtain the best results, immediate processing of the tissue is essential. Opened segments of the bowel should be rinsed in saline, pinned to corkboard, mucosa side up and then fixed in 10% formalin for at least 24 hours. The tissue is then immersed in 70% alcohol for two hours and then immersed in two changes of 95% alcohol for 2 hours each. The tissue may then be stained with 5% alcoholic eosin for 4 minutes and subsequently immersed in two changes of absolute alcohol for 2 hours each. The fixed and dehydrated intestinal wall is then placed in xylol. The preparation is now ready for examination *(17)*.

Mesenteric Angiography The celiac, superior mesenteric or inferior mesenteric artery can be injected with a barium sulfate-gelatin mixture, either in situ or after en block removal of the abdominal viscera. If all three vessels are injected (Fig. 2-9), the abdominal organ block must be partitioned so that the three vascular compartments can be displayed properly (18).

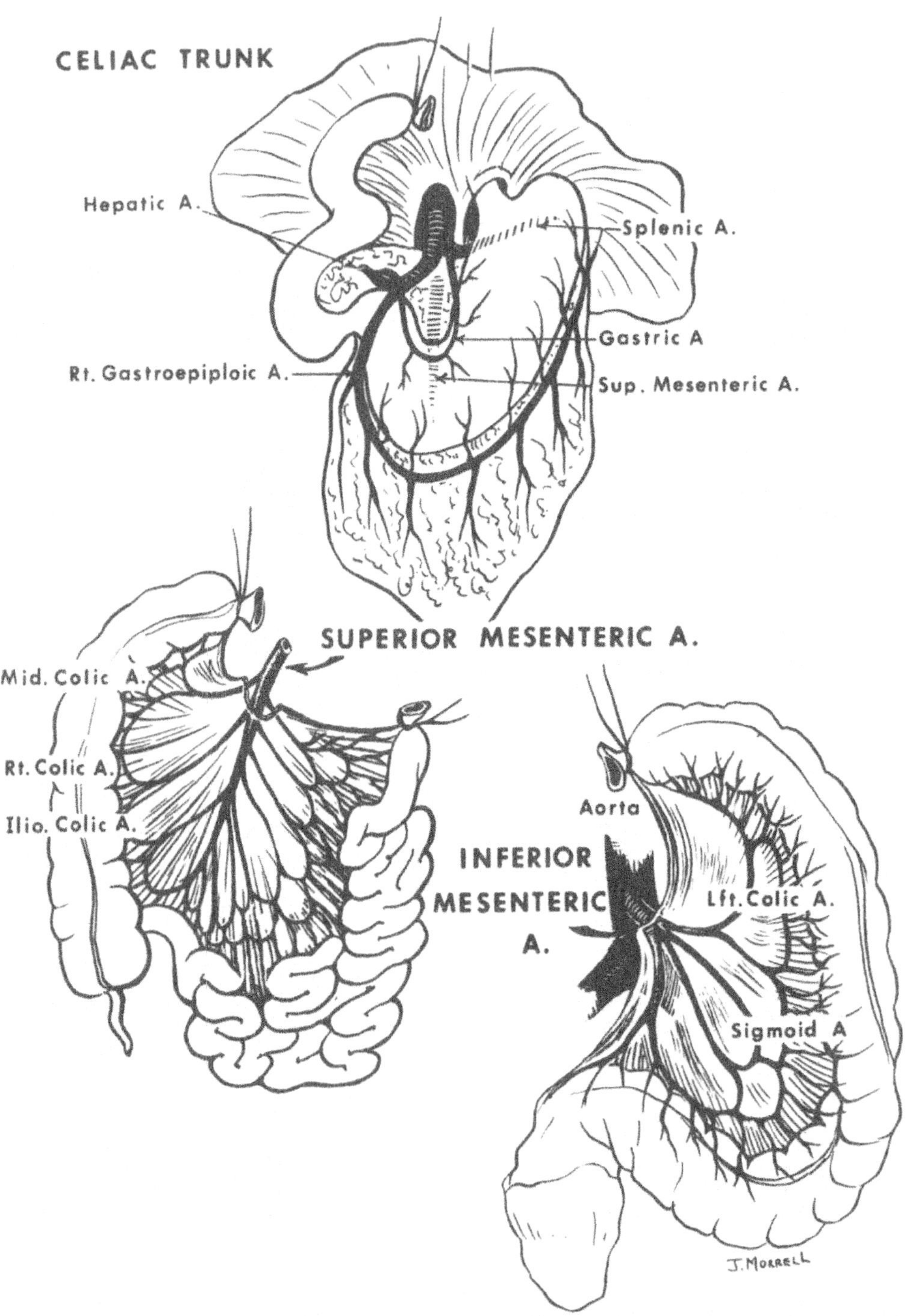

Fig. 2-9. Partitioned abdominal viscera for celiac and mesenteric arteriography. *Celiac trunk specimen*: Note the rotation and upward sweep of the duodenum. The root of the superior mesenteric artery remains with the celiac artery but is hidden behind the pancreas. *Superior mesenteric artery specimen:* This includes the intestine from the middle of the first jejunal loop to the middle of the transverse colon. *Inferior mesenteric artery specimen:* This extends from the middle tranverse colon to the anus. Adapted from ref. *(18)*.

HEPATOBILIARY TREE AND PANCREAS

The hepatobiliary block comprises the liver, gallbladder, pancreas, and the retroperitoneal "C" loop of duodenum. This block is approached from its posterior surface. Extraneous fat is removed as well as the mesentery of the small intestine. Although the mesentery may be discarded during most autopsies, multiple cuts should be made into it to reveal the luminal patency – or lack thereof – of the mesenteric arteries and portal veins. The duodenum should then be opened along its anti-mesenteric border. At this point, firm, sustained pressure on the gallbladder should express bile through the bile duct and ampulla. This maneuver does take a bit of patience. The inferior vena cava is examined and removed. Next, a superficial transverse incision across the hepatoduodenal ligament is made with the intent of entering the portal vein. Using scissors, open the portal vein toward and away from the liver to establish its patency. If it is free of pathology, then it may be transected. Then, a deeper transverse incision into the hepatoduodenal ligament uncovers the hepatic artery, on the left side. This vessel should also be opened to determine its patency. Finally, the common bile duct will be encountered to the right of the hepatic artery, with a third and deeper transverse incision. It is opened along its entire length, from porta hepatis to its entry into the duodenum. If stones are present, the prosector should document the degree of duct dilation, if any, proximal to the stone. A simple method to roughly quantify the caliber of any tube is to measure its internal circumference. Simple arithmetic calculation ($D=C/\pi$, where D = diameter, C = circumference), will approximate the luminal diameter.

Opening the cystic duct is fraught with difficulty because of its semicircular valves. However, the task can be completed with patience and a small pair of blunt-ended scissors. The gallbladder is then extricated from its bed against the liver, but left still attached to the pancreas and duodenum. It is advisable to open the gallbladder near the edge of the cutting board, toward the sink or into a container, such that the bile is does not stain the rest of the organs. However, the prosector should closely inspect the gallbladder's contents, so that any stones may be recognized, quantified, and characterized.

To maximize the exposure of the parenchyma, the pancreas may be incised along the frontal (i.e., coronal, plane). When there is suspicion that the pancreatic duct is dilated, then sagittal sections are preferred. Commonly, autolysis causes the pancreas to demonstrate a blotchy, dark red pattern. This may be confused with hemorrhagic pancreatitis by inexperienced pathologists. However, the abnormality frequently accompanying hemorrhagic pancreatitis, that is fat necrosis, is conspicuously absent. Routine sections from the pancreas should come from the tail, since a higher concentration of islets is found in that region.

The liver may be sliced in the coronal or the transverse planes. The latter approach yields the most recognizable shape of the liver, with both lobes well seen and with the porta hepatis clearly shown in at least one slice. However, the best demonstration of a pathologic process must remain the primary goal when choosing the plane of sectioning. It is best to section liver in slices that are no more than 2 cm thick. This will ensure adequate examination and proper fixation of the slices that are reserved for demonstration at a later time. To avoid leaving telltale marks of the knife, the prosector should use a long, sharp knife, with as minimal downward force as possible. The knife should be drawn in long sweeps, using the entire length of the blade, as if playing a cello. One is reminded of the adage, "Let the knife do the work." In this way, not only will the surfaces of the slices be smoother, but the prosector will reduce the risk of a cutting injury.

This author finds it useful to push the tip of her index finger through a slice of unfixed liver in every autopsy to roughly assess the degree of fibrosis. Normally with this maneuver, the liver will tear easily. In situations of chronic congestive heart failure, where there is centrilobular fibrosis, the liver will resist tearing. In cases of cirrhosis, the task is nigh impossible. This so called "finger test" can be applied to fresh slices of liver only, no more than 2–2.5 cm thick. With consistent use of this test, the pathologist may be able to recognize early hepatic fibrosis grossly.

In situations of a tumor involving the porta hepatis or of cirrhosis with a portosystemic shunt, the prosector must use ingenuity to choose the dissection approach that will best demonstrate the relationships between the pathologic process and the adjacent organs. This may require that the biliary connections be preserved and that the organ block be sliced in the coronal, transverse or even sagittal plane. Patience and possible conference with other pathologists may help to decide on which plane to use. The result will be a specimen that is dramatically instructive to both clinicians and other pathologists.

Up to 10% of patients undergoing upper GI endoscopy or radiography have a duodenal diverticulum. These diverticula are seen at autopsy at generally the same frequency. They characteristically have a large opening, are thin walled, and project into the mesentery of the proximal portion of the retroperitoneal duodenum. They are considered developmental in pathogenesis, rather than secondary to obstruction.

Gross Demonstration of Liver Staining for Iron This method *(19)* is particularly useful in cases of hemochromatosis. It can be applied to other organs, such as pancreas and myocardium. The actual staining procedure is described in Chapter 16.

Quantitative Assessment of Hepatic Iron or Copper Iron load may be quantified from fresh or paraffin-embedded tissue, using atomic absorption spectroscopy *(20)*. This method may also be applied to measure copper in tissue, such as in Wilson's disease.

Pancreatic Angiography and Duct Roentgenography Arteriograms require injection of the celiac and superior mesenteric artery system, as described earlier. The retrograde injection of radiopaque medium from the papilla of Vater provides excellent roentgenograms of the pancreatic duct system. The pancreatograms show stones and other duct abnormalities quite clearly *(21)*.

Hepatic Angiography Remove the liver together with the diaphragm, the hepatoduodenal ligament, and a long segment of the inferior vena cava. Vessels can be injected with contrast medium either before or after perfusion fixation. Fig. 2-10A shows the equipment that is needed for the infusion of the contrast medium. Fig. 2-10B shows such a nozzle in place.

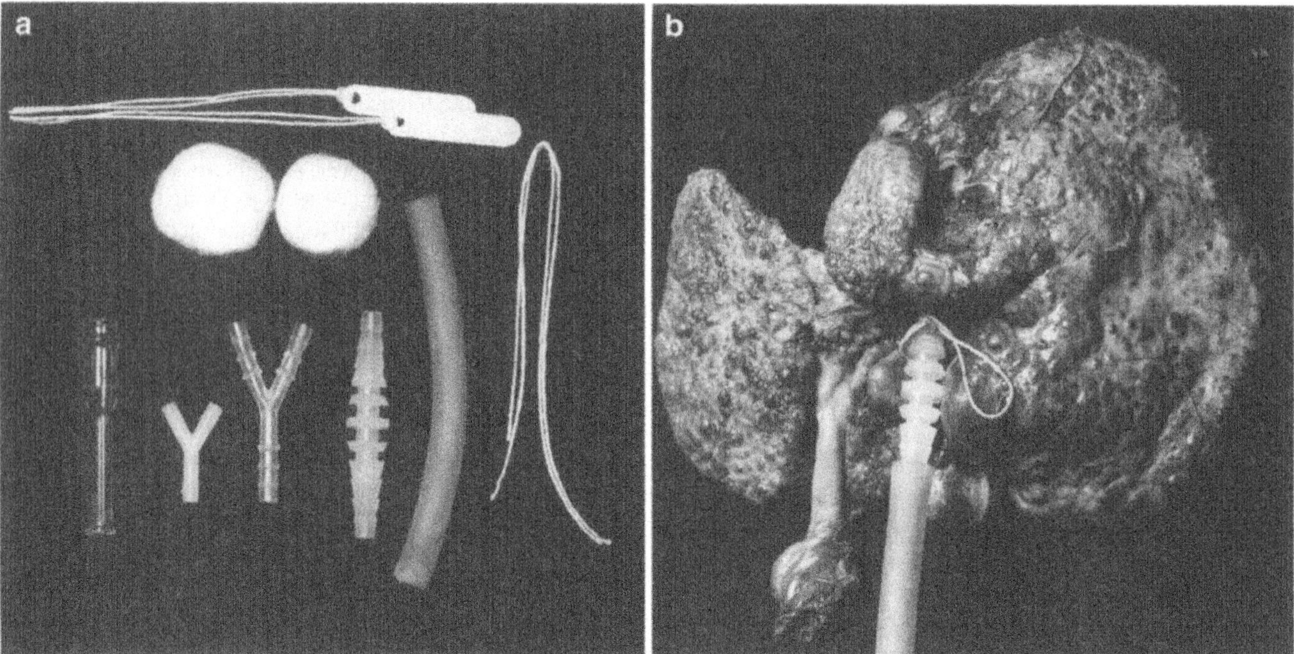

Fig. 2-10. Preparation for angiography and cholangiography. (**a**) Straight and bifurcated nozzles for hilar vessels and bile ducts; rubber hose for attaching specimens to perfusion apparatus; cotton was for plugging hepatic veins; ligature with needle to secure nozzles. Two identification tags are also shown. (**b**) Cirrhotic liver with nozzle tied into portan vein. Adapted from ref. *(22)*.

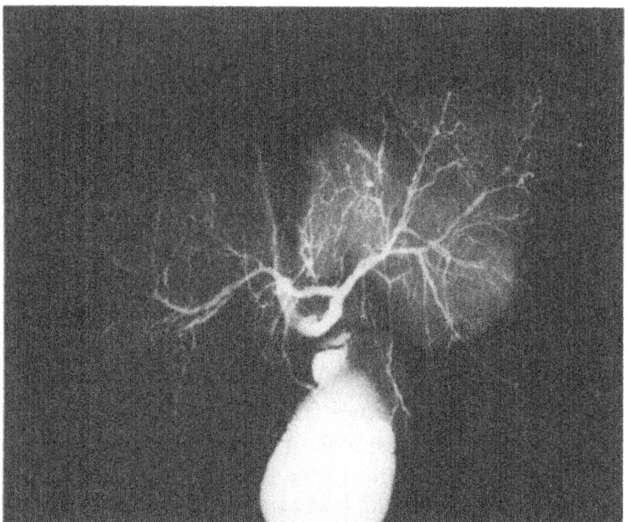

Fig. 2-11. Postmortem specimen cholangiogram. Note that in this case, the gallbladder has been left in place and is filled with contrast medium.

After the vessels have been cannulated, blood and blood clots are flushed out with saline. Perfusion can be performed with the contrast media. Barium sulfate gelatin mixtures give excellent results. Lowering the viscosity of the barium will enhance the filling of smaller vessels.

Cholangiography Cholangiography is easier if a sufficiently long sleeve of the common hepatic duct remains attached to the liver, so that a cannula can easily be tied into the lumen. Removal of the gallbladder prior to cholangiography may lead to leakage of contrast medium. Therefore, it may be substantially easier and more elegant to fill the gallbladder, still attached to the liver, along with the bile ducts (Fig. 2-11). Lowering the viscosity of the barium will enhance the filling of smaller ducts.

URINARY TRACT

RENAL ARTERIES Dissection and examination of the urinary tract are preceded by opening of the aorta and renal arteries and by removal of the adrenal glands. The inferior vena cava will be encountered on the right side and assessment of its patency can be performed at this time. Any renal artery stenosis, whether at the aortic ostium or along its length, should be searched for and documented. Then, the renal arteries may be transected either close to the renal hilum or midway along their length, with the proximal portions left attached to the aorta. The aorta may then be removed, starting at the iliac bifurcation and extending through to the aortic arch.

KIDNEYS AND BLADDER It is wise at this juncture to locate the ureters so that they are not inadvertently cut. Once they are located, removal of excess fat around the kidneys may be done. The kidneys are then dissected down towards the pelvis, with care taken not to transect the ureters. The prosector will note that the retroperitoneal ureters course anterior to the rectum, to enter the posterior wall of the bladder. Any retroperitoneal tissue that is still attached medial to the kidneys and ureters may be removed. With the organ block facing down, the rectum can then be removed. There is no easy fascial plane to guide the prosector along the anterior margin of the rectum, but if he removes the rectum by keeping the plane of dissection close to the rectum, no ureter will be cut. Once removed, the rectum is opened, rinsed, and examined.

The perirenal fat and the renal capsules are then removed and the kidneys are bivalved, leaving the anterior and posterior

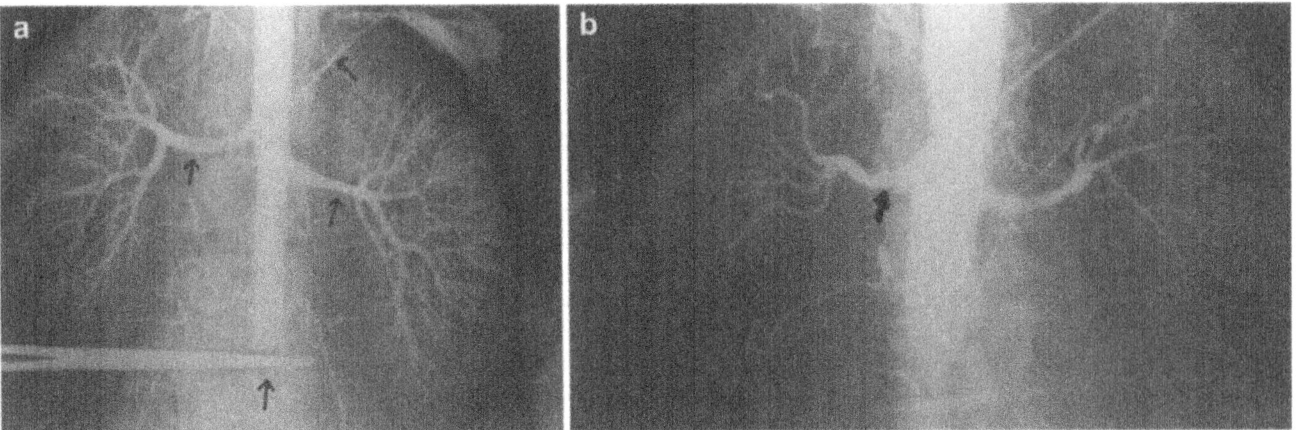

Fig. 2-12. In situ renal arteriograms. (**a**) Note the polyetheylene catheter in the superior mesenteric artery *(upper arrow)*. The main renal arteries had minimal atherosclerosis *(arrows)*. Cross-clamping of the aorta is evident at the base of the film *(arrow)*. (**b**) Evidence of narrowing in both renal arteries but more pronounced in right renal artery *(arrow)*. Histologically, the stenosis was severe. Adapted from ref. *(23)*.

halves connected at the hilum. In patients with renal tumors, hilar nodes should be sampled. If each half of the bivalved kidney is thick, then each may be incised again. The next task is to open the ureters. The easiest approach for many is to orient the urinary block such that the posterior aspect is resting on the cutting board, kidneys nearest to the prosector, and bladder farthest away. The smooth, peritoneum-covered posterior wall of the bladder should be lying against the cutting board. With a pair of blunt-tipped scissors, enter the renal pelvis and cut down each ureter to enter the anterior wall of the bladder. When this has been accomplished, the two openings are connected by a transverse cut in the anterior bladder wall. Finally, an anterior cut is made out the urethra and up the midline to the dome of the bladder.

Removal of the renal capsules will reveal the most common gross abnormality of the kidneys, that of arterial sclerosis. This is manifested by a diffuse, fine granularity of the renal cortical surface. When severe, this disorder will also feature small cortical cysts. The cut surface will often show thinning of the renal cortex. The normal thickness of the cortex is about 1.5 cm. Large areas of ischemic atrophy or old pyelonephritis will appear as broad areas of cortical thinning, surrounded by raised, more normal parenchyma. It is common to find one to several small tubular adenomas in scarred kidneys. Small, well-circumscribed tan nodules in the cortex characterize these neoplasms. Fibromas, angiomyolipomas and myelolipomas are not uncommon. Heterotopic adrenal cortex will appear as flattened foci of yellow-tan tissue on the cortical surface. Many diabetic patients at autopsy will have characteristic deep orange noncalcified atheromas in their renal artery branches. Acute tubular necrosis may be suggested when pallor and swelling of the renal cortex or obscuration of the corticomedullary junction is seen.

The bladder frequently contains slightly thick, milky fluid. This material may be mistaken for an inflammatory reaction, such as severe pyuria, but is actually just sloughed urothelium suspended in urine. A Gram, Papaniculau, or hematoxylin-eosin stained smear of this material will reveal innumerable urothelial cells. This finding is a postmortem artifact. The bladder mucosa normally has a pale tan color at autopsy. Mucosal hyperemia or hemorrhage may be found, and may be the result of bladder catheterization, severe cystitis, or profound hypotension.

Renal Perfusion Fixation In this method, a length of renal artery is left attached to the kidneys. A cannula is then tied into this vessel and the kidney is perfused first with normal saline and then with 10% formalin.

Renal Angiography Arteriograms (Fig. 2-12A and B) and venograms (Fig 2-13) may be performed either in situ or after en bloc removal of the abdominal aorta and kidneys or on isolated organs. Clinical contrast media or barium sulfate gelatin mixtures give excellent results. A catheter is tied into the celiac artery in situ or after removal of the organ block and all nonrenal arteries are ligated and both ends of the aorta are clamped. Venography is conducted by injection of contrast medium into a segment of the inferior vena cava that was sealed off by ligatures. By moving the ligatures higher, excellent hepatic venograms can be prepared.

Urography Retrograde urograms are easy to prepare with any of the conventional contrast media. The ureter is cannulated either from the urinary bladder or through the wall of the distal ureter.

Urethral valves may be demonstrated by injection of radiopaque material into the urinary bladder. The valves will prevent contrast from entering the urethra. The urethra should then be opened along the anterior midline opposite to the direction of flow of urine (Fig. 2-14). This will prevent laceration of the delicate valves.

FEMALE AND MALE REPRODUCTIVE SYSTEMS

Following removal of the rectum, the vagina, uterus, fallopian tubes, and ovaries may be examined. Separation of the uterus/vagina from the back of the bladder is not routinely required. The vagina may be opened, using scissors, with a midline posterior cut, extending to the cervix. Since the uterus and cervix are

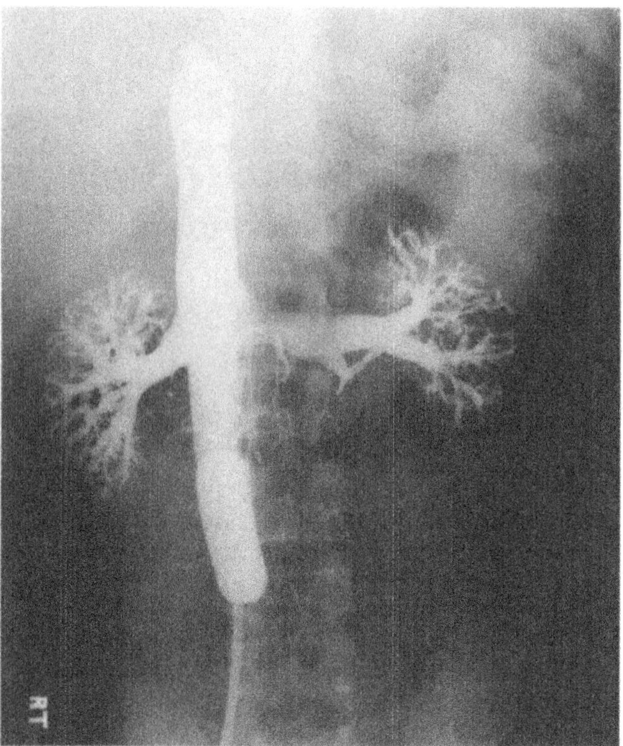

Fig. 2-13. Normal renal venogram. A rubber tube with two inflatable cuffs was introduced to seal off the inferior vena cava above and below the renal veins. Barium sulfate-gelatin mixture was injected through the midportion of the tube. There is also filling of lumbar, prevertebra, adrenal, and left testicular veins.

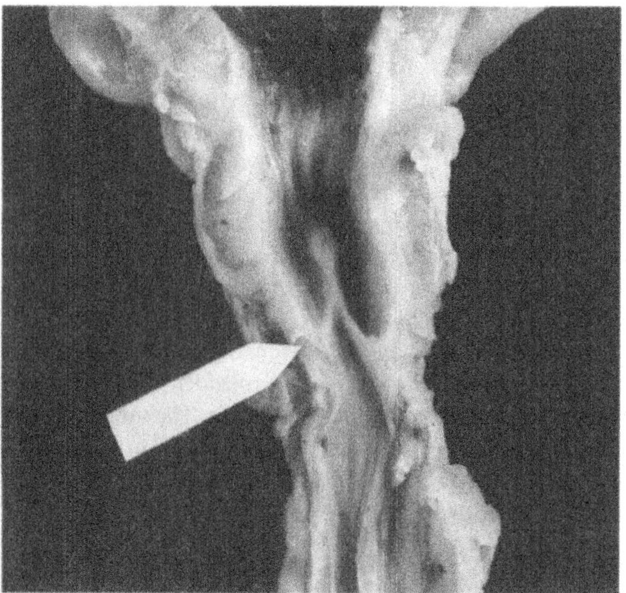

Fig. 2-14. Urethra with congenital valves. The penis and urinary bladder have been removed in continuity and have been opened in the anterior midline. The *arrow* shows the delicate urethral valves.

more muscular, opening them may require the use of a knife. Should there be suspicion of myometrial pathology, multiple transverse or coronal cuts through the uterus may be indicated. The endocervical canal often contains mucosal (Nabothian) cysts and abundant mucin. The endometrium should be assessed for polyps, atrophy, cysts and for hemorrhage. The latter finding infrequently develops in situations of profound hypotension. The ovaries in menstruating women will appear complex, with an assortment of red corpora hemorrhagica, yellow corpora lutea, and smaller, white corpora albicantia, as well as follicular cysts. Postmenopausal ovaries are smaller, have a folded, undulating, and fibrotic surface, and may contain corpora albicantia of variable sizes.

The testes are accessed through the inguinal canal. The tunica vaginalis of each of them should be opened. Any fluid exiting from this space should be documented. The tunica albuguinea normally has a smooth surface, with a slightly grayish hue. Small, polypoid structures may be seen at the cranial end of the epididymis (the appendix epididymis) and at the cranial end of the testis (the appendix testis). The former represents the most cranial end of the mesonephric (Wolffian) duct, and the latter represents the most cranial end of the paramesonephric (Müllerian) duct. The testes can then be bivalved. The cut surface of the normal testis is light brown. Fibrosis of the testis will lend a translucent gray color to the cut surface and will also prohibit the traditional "string test." This maneuver is accomplished by attempting to pull a few seminiferous tubules away from the cut surface with a pair of forceps. In normal testes, the seminiferous tubules may be pulled away for a distance of 3–4 cm. The distance is far shorter in testes with fibrosis.

Rarely in pediatric and perinatal autopsies does the prosector need to remove the penis. Congenital urethral valves, strictures and tumors are the main indications. The penis, usually without surrounding skin, should be removed with the bladder attached. Removal is achieved by either sawing out a portion of the pubic bone or by pulling the penis through the pubic arch. The urethra may then be opened lengthwise in the anterior midline. When suspecting urethral valves, be sure to open the urethra anteriorly, and in the direction opposite to that of urine flow. This will minimize disruption of the valves.

PLACENTA The placenta should be examined in autopsies on all stillbirths (*see* Part II, "Stillbirth") and neonates. The following gross features of the placenta should be documented: umbilical cord insertion site, length, diameter, surface appearance, and number of vessels; appearance and insertion pattern of the membranes (i.e.. marginal, circummarginate, and circumvallate); dimensions and trimmed weight of the placental disc; appearance of the fetal (chorionic plate) surface and appearance of the maternal surface. When examining the fetal surface, the pathologist may encounter a small, round white to slightly yellow structure that is situated on the membranes or between the amnion and chorion of the placental disc. This is the yolk sac. For expected placental weights, see Part III. The placental disc should be cut into thin slices with a long-bladed knife. Blood is wiped off and the cut surfaces are inspected.

Histologic examination of grossly normal placentas should include two rolls of membranes, two sections of umbilical cord, and two sections of placental disc. One should avoid submitting sections of the periphery of the disc, since there normally is more fibrin and calcification in these regions, which may be incorrectly interpreted as abnormal. The most common lesions found in the placental disc are infarcts and intervillous thrombi. When sectioning these lesions, the pathologist should include not only the lesion in the section, but a generous portion of the surrounding parenchyma.

When examining placentas of multiple fetuses, stillborns, or newborns, it is important to establish chorionicity. If a twin gestation with two, unfused placentas, the chance of monochorionicity is extremely unlikely. In fused twin or multiple placentas, it is important to identify the dividing membranes so that they can be examined histologically. This should be done before too much manipulation, since the dividing membranes can be pulled apart and away from the chorionic plate surface, making their identification more difficult. With any fused twin/multiple placenta, a search for vascular anastomoses on the chorionic plate should be conducted. Vascular injection may be employed by injecting milk into selected vessels. Although vascular anastomoses may not be seen on the chorionic plates of monochorionic twins, vascular injection studies will invariably demonstrate shunts within the placental parenchyma. Shunts are absent in all dichorionic twins. During the injection, blood must be allowed to escape through the severed end of the umbilical cords. Any successful vascular injection should be photographed. Following the injection study and description and removal of the umbilical cords and membranes, the placenta disc(s) can be weighed and measured.

SKELETAL SYSTEM

Portions of bone should be retained in all autopsies. Sites for sampling include ribs, sternum, vertebrae, iliac crest, and sternoclavicular joint. The vertebral column will have the greatest yield in routine cases, since common diseases such as osteoporosis, osteoarthritis, and metastatic carcinoma can be very evident and easily photographed in vertebral bodies. The anterior half of the vertebral column can be removed using an oscillating saw, such as the Stryker saw (Stryker Corporation, Kalamazoo, MI). It is a good idea to remove the bone dust left by the stryker saw, so as to better visualize the bony trabeculae and to reveal any pathologic process, such as those listed above. Gently brushing the cut surface of the bone with a small brush, such as a toothbrush, and rinsing under gently running water will remove the bone dust. This maneuver may generate aerosols, therefore the velocity of the water flow must be minimized. The brushing should not be overdone, since this could result in excessive loss of bone marrow, which may need to be sampled later.

Removal of the femur requires a long lateral skin incision. The knee joint is exposed by flexing the knee and cutting the quadriceps tendon, the joint capsule, and the cruciate ligaments. The muscular attachments are dissected from the shaft of the femur, starting at the distal end and continuing toward the hip. The capsule of the hip can be palpated and then incised by flexing and rotating the femur. Should bone marrow need to be obtained from the femur, a 5-cm portion of the anterior half of the femoral shaft can be removed with an oscillating saw. This will maintain the continuity of the long bone.

The best joint sections are prepared by shelling out the whole joint and sawing across the proximal and distal bones, staying far from the joint space so as to prevent cutting into the joint capsule. The whole specimen is then sawed, usually in the frontal plane. Good saw sections should include articular cartilage, synovium, meniscus, capsule, epiphysis, metaphysis and a small portion of diaphysis. If complete joint removal is impractical, then the joint may be opened and representative sections of articular cartilage, capsule, synovium, and other components of the joint may be obtained.

The laryngeal joins, particularly the crico-arytenoid joint, are very useful in the study of rheumatoid arthritis. Good sections of these small joints can be prepared from sagittal sections through the entire posterior wall of the larynx, in a paramedian plane. The cricoarytenoid joints are found at or just beneath the level of the vocal cords.

Skeletal contours and continuity of long bones and spinal column must be restored after the autopsy. An assortment of wooden prostheses should be available for insertion in place of the removed bone. A simple substitute is a wooden rod with two nails protruding from both ends. After the nails have been inserted into the wooden rod, the heads of the nails are sawed off. The tips of the nails are then driven into the proximal and distal portions of the bone. Complete segments of the spinal column can be replaced by such prostheses. For replacing the hip, angular metal rods are useful. Plaster of Paris provides a good prosthesis for calvarium. Simple wood dowels and plastic tubing is recommended as replacement for bones and joints of fingers and toes. However, procedures involving the extremities require special permission.

DECALCIFYING PROCEDURES

Decalcification is required when preparing histologic sections of bone, teeth, calcified vessels, and calcified lesions such as granulomas. As always, the tissues must be completely fixed before exposure to decalcifying agents. The most common methods of decalcification use a relatively weak acid solution and a chelating agent. The weak acid serves to dissolve the calcium and phosphate salts. The chelating compounds facilitate decalcification by sequestering the liberated calcium ions so as to drive the reaction to completion. The ratio of decalcifying reagent to tissue should be at least 100:1 to avoid depletion of the reagent before all the calcium is removed. Formic acid alone may be used, although it tends to take longer to decalcify tissues than reagents that include a chelating agent. Decalcification solutions are commercially available, as described below. Tissues which have been formalin-fixed overnight need to be washed with tap water for at least one hour before being placed into an HCL-containing decalcification solution. The reason for this is that if formalin comes into contact with hydrochloric acid, a carcinogen, chloromethyl ether is generated.

FORMIC ACID This reagent is easy to prepare, inexpensive, and causes little tissue distortion. It does require a longer time for decalcification than the reagent listed below.

Composition: 80 mL neutral buffered formalin, 20 mL formic acid

Formic acid decalcification should not last longer than 2 days. The formic acid must be removed by washing the specimen for 30 min in running tap water.

DECAL SOLUTION (Decal Chemical Corporation, Tallman, NY) This reagent contains both hydrochloric acid and EDTA (the chelating agent) and works well for essentially all tissues requiring decalcification. It is a corrosive and its vapors are harmful.

PROCESSING OF SPECIMENS The tissue sections should be no thicker than 3 mm. For each section, 100 mL of decalcification fluid should be used. Change and agitate the solution daily or more often. Decalcification time depends on numerous factors, such as the size and texture of the specimen, the type and temperature of the solution, and the use of agitation.

Exact end-point determination is essential because staining properties will be lost if the reagent is not washed out immediately after decalcification is completed. Bending the specimen usually permits one to judge roughly when decalcification is complete. Another indicator is the decrease or disappearance of CO_2 bubbles emanating from the specimen. If the stained histologic section appears to be over-decalcified, then the section can be rehydrated and immersed in a 0.05% lithium carbonate solution for about 30 minutes. This will raise the pH, so as to restore the basophilia of the tissue. The section can then be restained, ideally with Harris hematoxylin. The lithium carbonate solution may be made by adding 0.5 gram of lithium carbonate to 1000 ml of deionized water.

REFERENCES

1. Pritt BS, Waters BL. Cutting injuries in an academic pathology department. Arch Pathol Lab Med 2005;129:1022–1026.
2. Ludwig J. Handbook of Autopsy Practice, 3rd ed. Humana Press, Totowa, New Jersey, 2002.
3. Sheeffwill, Hopster DJ. Postmortem Technique Handbook, 2nd ed. Springer-Verlag, London Limited, 2005.
4. Finkbeiner WE, Ursell PC, Davis RL. Autopsy Pathology: A Manual and Atlas. Churchill Livingston, Philadelphia, 2004.
5. Culora GA, Roche WR. Simple method for necropsy dissection of the abdominal organs after abdominal surgery. J Clin Pathol 1996;49:776–779.
6. Cough J. Twenty years' experience of the technique of paper-mounted sections. In: Lie bow AA, Smith DE, Eds. The Lung. Williams and Wilkins, Baltimore, 1968, pp.311–316.
7. Paper mount by Marlyce George, Webb Waring Lung Institute In: Thurlbeck's Pathology of the Lung, 3rd ed. Thieme Medical Publishers. New York, 1995.
8. Davies G, Reid L. Growth of the alveoli and pulmonary arteries in childhood. Thorax 1970;25:669–681.
9. Hendin AS, Greenspan RH. Ventilatory pumping of human pulmonary lymphatic vessels. Radiology 1973;108:553–557.
10. McCrone WC, Draftz RB, Delly JC. The Particle Atlas: A Photomicrographic Reference for the Microscopical Identification of Particulate Substances. Ann Arbor Science Publishers, Ann Arbor, MI, 1967.
11. Churg A, Green, FHY. Analytic methods for identifying and quantifying mineral particles in lung tissues. In: Churg A, Green FHY, Eds. Pathology of Occupational Lung Disease, 2nd ed. Williams and Wilkins, Baltimore, 1998.
12. Roggli VL, Sharma A. Analysis of tissue mineral fiber content. In: Roggli VL, Oury TD, Sporn TA, eds. Pathology of Asbestos-Associated Diseases, 2nd ed. New York: Springer, 2004, pp.309–354.
13. Myers JK, Churg AM, Tazelaar, Wright J. Special Techniques. In: Thurlbeck's Pathology of the Lung, 3rd ed. Thieme Med Publishers, New York, 1995.
14. Roggli Vl, Greenberg SD, Pratt PC. Pathology of Asbestos-Associated Diseases. Little, Brown and Company, Boston, 1992.
15. Churg H, Sakoda N, Warnock ML. A simple method for preparing ferruginous bodies for electron microscopy. Am J Clin Pathol 1977;68:513–517.
16. Roggli VL. The role of analytical SEM in the determination of causation in malignant mesothelioma. Ultrastruct Pathol. 2006;30(1):31–35.
17. Loehry CA, Creamer B. Post-mortem study of small-intestinal mucosa. BMJ 1966;1:827–829.
18. Reiner L. Mesenteric vascular occlusion studied by postmortem injection of the mesenteric arterial circulation. Pathol Ann 1966;1:193–220.
19. Pulvertaft RJV. Museum techniques: a review. J Clin Pathol 1950;3:1–23.
20. Beilby JP, Prins AW, Swanson NR. Determination of hepatic iron concentration in fresh and paraffin-embedded tissue. Clin Chem 1999;45:573.
21. Schmitz-Moormann P, Himmelmann GW, Brandes J-W, Fölsch UR, Lorenz-Meyer H, Malchow H, et al. Comparative radiological and morphological study of human pancreas. Pancreatitis like changes in postmortem ductograms and their morphologic pattern. Possible implications for ERCP. Gut 1985;26:406–414.
22. Ludwig J, Ottman DM, Eichmann TJ. The preparation of native livers for morphological studies. Mod Pathol 1994;7:790–793.
23. Holley KE, Hunt JC, Brown Al Jr, Kincaid OW, Sheps SG. Renal artery stenosis: a clinico-pathologic study in normotensive and hypertensive patients. Am J Med 1964;37:14–22.

3 Cardiovascular System

WILLIAM D. EDWARDS AND DYLAN V. MILLER

REMOVAL OF THE HEART FROM THE CHEST

INITIAL STEPS Before the autopsy is begun, a radiogram of the chest may be performed (*see* Chapter 10). The removal of the chest plate is then performed. In patients who have had previous open-heart surgery via a median sternotomy, diffuse pericardial adhesions are common, which require careful dissection of the heart away from the sternum so as not to disrupt any surgical sites. Pericardial exudates should be cultured (*see* Chapter 7). Pericardial blood clots should be weighed. If it is necessary to distinguish between blood and serosanguinous fluid, a hematocrit can be obtained.

In cases of "sudden unexplained death" in patients from childhood through age 35 yr, consideration should be given to freezing blood in EDTA tubes and/or freezing tissue samples (heart, liver, spleen) for possible molecular studies for gene mutations. If a storage disease is suspected, tissue samples should also be processed for transmission electron microscopy. For further directions in cases of sudden unexplained death, see the section later in this chapter.

CHOOSING THE METHOD OF REMOVAL Normal hearts and most hearts with acquired disease can be excised separately. In the presence of extracardiac disorders such as pulmonary or esophageal carcinoma or ascending aortic dissection, the heart should be removed with the *thoracic organs en bloc* (*see* Chapter 2). For congenital heart disease, the thoracic contents should be removed en bloc, regardless of the age of the patient.

DESCRIPTION OF THE HEART Cardiac *size* may be normal or enlarged (cardiomegaly) due to hypertrophy or dilatation (or both) and can involve one or more chambers. Overall cardiac *shape* may be conical (normal), globoid, or irregular (as with a ventricular aneurysm), and one or more chambers may be abnormal in shape. The *color* of the subendocardial myocardium may be gray with an old infarct, pale with chronic ischemia, and mottled or hemorrhagic with an acute infarct or rupture. Left ventricular *consistency* can be firm (due to hypertrophy, fibrosis, amyloidosis, calcification, or rigor mortis) or soft (due to acute myocardial infarction, myocarditis, dilated cardiomyopathy, or decomposition).

From: *Handbook of Autopsy Practice,* 4th Ed. Edited by: B.L. Waters

PERFUSION FIXATION OF THE HEART Formalin fixation of the heart using a perfusion apparatus allows for complete fixation of specimens and simulates, in the fixed specimen, the appearance of the blood-filled heart as imaged using various modalities (CT, MRI, echocardiography) in living patients. This is recommended for dissections that are to be used for teaching purposes, including museum specimens and illustrative photographs *(10,11)*. This method is also indicated for the tomographic and window types of dissection, and several methods have been described *(27–29)*.

The intact specimen is prepared for perfusion by inserting bell-shaped rimmed glass cannulas of an appropriate diameter into the aorta, at least 2 cm above the aortic valve, and in a pulmonary vein and either the inferior or superior vena cava. These are secured in place with string cinched around the part of the vessel that overlies the rim of the cannula. Cork stoppers with glass tubing through the center may be used in place of flared glass cannulas. Cork stoppers are inserted into all other great vessels and are held in place with either straight pins or string. An identifying tag with patient number/name should be affixed to the cardiac specimen.

The heart is placed in a container with formalin. Rubber tubing is used to connect the glass cannulas to a formalin reservoir (such as a carboy or covered 10-gallon tub fitted with a spigot) at least 12 inches above the specimen. The specimen is perfused using gravity flow for at least 24 hours. Formalin flows through the coronary tree and all cardiac chambers.

Excess formalin accumulating in the specimen container can be recycled to the reservoir using a hydraulic pump (0.25 horsepower) as in Fig. 3-1A. High capacity perfusion fixation systems can be devised by connecting several tubes in parallel to a primary reservoir and/or additional subreservoir containers in series (*see* Fig. 3.1B).

Hearts may also be fixed in an apparent distended state by filling the chambers and vessels with cotton *(30)*.

EVALUATION OF THE CORONARY ARTERIES

Before any of the many forms of cardiac dissection is applied *(1–14)*, coronary arteries should be inspected for calcification and tortuosity. If postmortem angiography is indicated, the procedure must be performed before dissection of the coronary vessels and preferably before fixation of the heart.

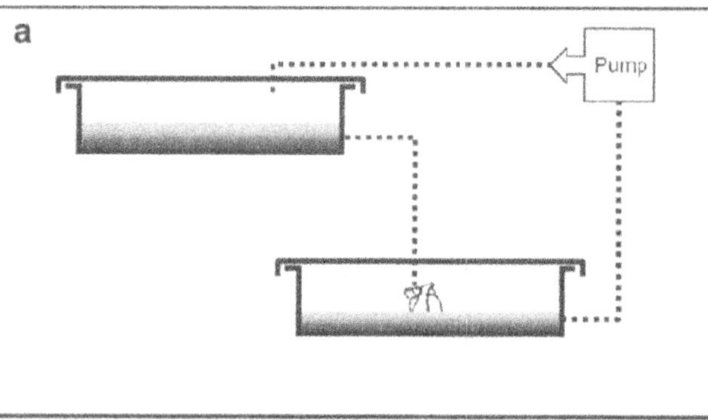

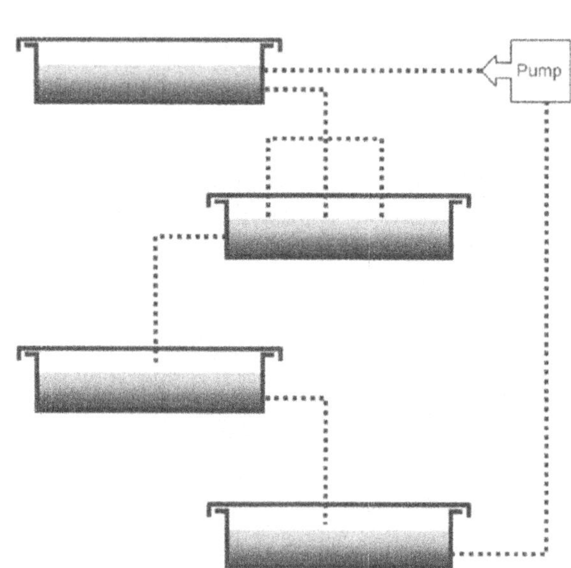

Fig. 3-1. Perfusion fixation apparatus. Gravity driven perfusion fixation through tubing connected to an elevated formalin reservoir is demonstrated in the top panel. A hydraulic pump can be used to recycle the fixative from the perfusing tub back to the reservoir. The bottom panel illustrates how several specimens can be perfused at once using additional connections to the reservoir "in parallel" and/or additional tubs (sub-reservoirs) "in series".

POSTMORTEM CORONARY ANGIOGRAPHY This important method is described in Chapter 10.

DISSECTION OF CORONARY ARTERIES In subjects younger than 30 years of age, in whom the cause of death is noncardiac, the coronary arteries may be opened longitudinally. Otherwise, the vessels should be cut in cross-section at 3-5 mm intervals. Calcified vessels that cannot be readily cut with a scalpel should be stripped off the heart and decalcified for at least 24 h before cutting.

GRADING OF CORONARY OBSTRUCTION A four-point system is applied, by 25% increments of narrowing in cross-sectional area *(15)*. A grade-4 lesion indicates stenosis of at least 75% and is considered severe, whereas a grade-4 lesion 90% represents critical stenosis. As a rule, grade-4 lesions should be documented microscopically. Depending on the number of major epicardial vessels with grade-4 lesions, a heart may have severe 1-vessel, 2-vessel, or 3-vessel disease. Severe left main disease is equivalent to 2-vessel disease, and its coexistence with grade-4 disease in the other three coronary arteries represents severe 4-vessel disease.

DISSECTION METHODS OF THE HEART

Many older methods *(7)* are impractical for routine diagnostic pathology. Only the inflow-outflow and short axis (bread slice) methods have withstood the test of time; the latter technique is applicable to virtually any form of heart disease. In addition, some recently described methods are useful for teaching purposes and correlations with current cardiac imaging *(8–14)*.

INFLOW-OUTFLOW METHOD OF CARDIAC DISSECTION This technique is suitable primarily for normal hearts. For each side of the heart, the atrium is opened first, and then the ventricle is opened along its inflow and outflow tracts, following the direction of blood flow (Fig. 3-2). Valves are cut between, not through, their commissures.

Using scissors, the initial cut is made from the inferior vena cava to the right atrial appendage, sparing the superior vena cava with the region of the sinus node. The right ventricular inflow tract is opened with a knife or scissors from the right atrium, through the posterior tricuspid leaflet, running parallel to and about 1 cm from the posterior ventricular septum. The outflow tract is opened in a similar fashion, approximately 1 cm from the anterior ventricular septum, extending through the anterior pulmonary cusp and into the main pulmonary artery.

The left atrium is opened with scissors from the tip of the appendage, across the body of the atrium, cutting between the orifices of the upper and lower pulmonary veins, to the level of the atrium septum. The left ventricular inflow tract is opened with a long knife along the lateral aspect through the left atrial wall near its appendage, through the midportion of the posterior mitral leaflet, between the two mitral papillary muscles, and through the apex. The outflow cut travels parallel to the anterior ventricular septum and about 1 cm from it. This curved cut is best accomplished with a scalpel; care should be taken not to cut into either the anterior mitral leaflet or the ventricular septum. Scissors can be used to extend the cut across the left aortic cusp and into the ascending aorta, to one side or the other of the left coronary ostium. Further slicing into the myocardium is not recommended other than for microscopic slides.

SHORT-AXIS METHOD OF CARDIAC DISSECTION This is the method of choice not only for the evaluation of ischemic heart disease *(2,15)* but for virtually any other cardiac condition, because the slices expose the largest surface area of myocardium. They correspond to the short-axis plane produced clinically by two-dimensional echocardiography *(8–14)*.

For this method, the flat diaphragmatic aspect of the heart is placed on a paper towel to prevent slippage, and cuts 1.0-1.5 cm thick are made with a sharp knife, parallel to the atrioventricular groove. One firm slice should be used, or two slices in the same direction, avoiding sawing motions that leave hesitation marks. Each slice is viewed from the apex toward the base (Fig. 3-3), analogous to two-dimensional imaging. The basal third of the ventricles is left attached to the atria. The basal portion is then opened according to the inflow-outflow method, as described earlier.

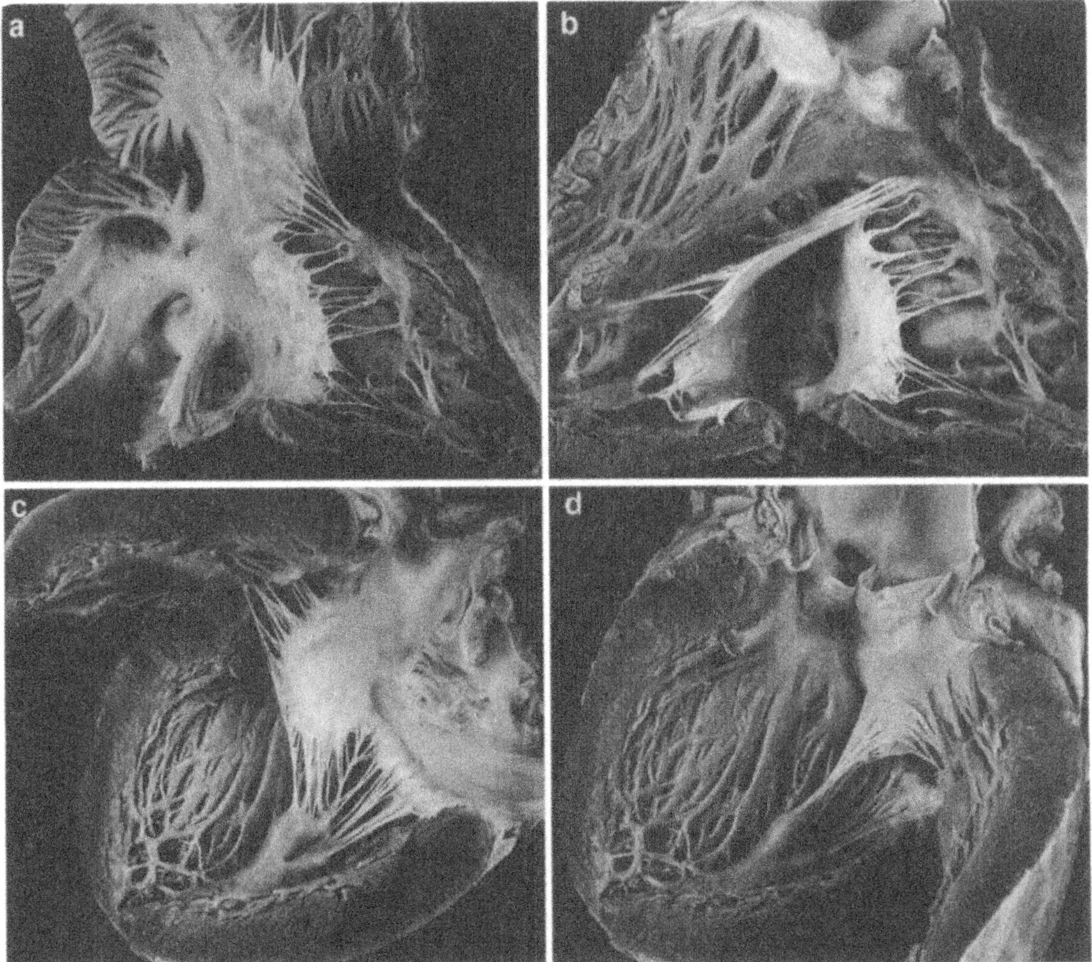

Fig. 3-2. Inflow-outflow method of cardiac dissection. The method is shown in a normal heart. (**a**) Opened right atrium and right ventricular inflow tract. (**b**) Opened right ventricular outflow tract and pulmonary artery. (**c**) Opened left atrium and left ventricular inflow tract. (**d**) Opened left ventricular outflow tract and aorta.

OTHER TOMOGRAPHIC METHODS OF DISSECTION AND REPAIRING MISTAKES For teaching purposes, the short-axis, long-axis, and four-chamber planes are ideally suited for demonstrating cardiac pathology *(10,11)*. Additional planes that have proven useful clinically and at autopsy include right ventricular long-axis, left-sided two-chamber, right-sided two-chamber, transverse (horizontal, or foreshortened four-chamber), frontal (or coronal), lateral (or parasagittal), and others. Hearts should first be fixed in a distended state, either by perfusion fixation or by chamber distention with cotton or paper towels.

Repairing Mistakes If mistakes are made in attempting tomographic dissection, pieces can be glued back together and then recut in a more desirable plane of sectioning. For most purposes, any of the commercially available cyanoacrylate glues (such as Superglue® or Krazy Glue®) will suffice *(12,13)*.

Four-Chamber Method Using a long knife and beginning at the cardiac apex, a cut is extended through the acute margin of the right ventricle, the obtuse margin of the left ventricle, and the ventricular septum (Fig. 3-4). Cutting is then extended through the mitral and tricuspid valves and through the atria. This will bisect the heart into two pieces, both of which show all four chambers. The upper half can then be opened along both ventricular outflow tracts, according to the inflow-outflow method previously described.

Long-Axis Method For this cut, the plane is best demarcated with three straight pins before making the cut. The first pin is placed in the cardiac apex, the second in the right aortic sinus (adjacent to the right coronary ostium), and the third near the mitral valve annulus, between the right and left pulmonary veins. The heart can then be cut along this plane, from the apex toward the base (or in the opposite direction), passing through both the mitral and aortic valves (Fig. 3-5).

Base of Heart Method This method displays all four valves intact at the cardiac base and thus is ideal for demonstrating anatomic relationships between the valves themselves and between the valves and the adjacent coronary arteries and the atrioventricular conduction system. The technique is best applied to hearts with prominent valvular disease, including prosthetic valves (Fig. 3-6) *(10,11)*.

The left anterior descending coronary artery can be evaluated before dissecting the base of the heart, but the right and circumflex

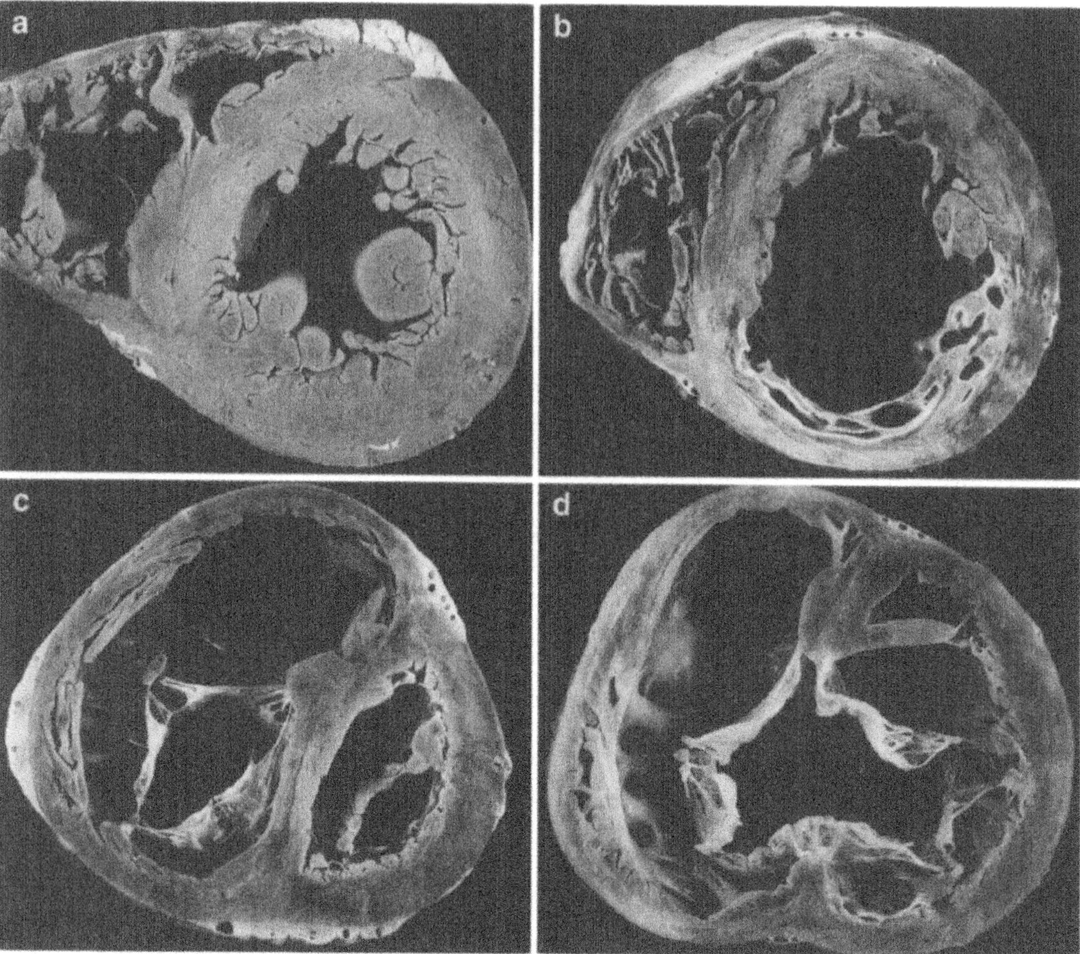

Fig. 3-3. Short-axis method of cardiac dissection. (**a**) Normal heart, with ventricular cross-section oriented for evaluation. (**b**) Old transmural myocardial infarct, involving inferior wall of left ventricle, with secondary left ventricular dilatation. (**c**) Right ventricular hypertrophy and dilatation due to chronic pulmonary hypertension. (**d**) Complete atrioventricular septal defect, showing the common atrioventricular valve.

arteries are best left uncut until afterward. The ventricles are sliced in the short-axis plane before the cardiac base is dissected, and slices can extend above the level of the tips of the mitral papillary muscles. With the cut surface of the ventricles placed on a paper towel, the atria are removed. Begin at the inferior vena cava with scissors and cut into the right atrium, staying about 0.5-1.0 cm above the tricuspid valve annulus. Cut only through the atrial free wall, taking care not to injure the adjacent right coronary artery. End the cut at the upper aspect of the atrial septum, adjacent to the ascending aorta.

For the left atrium, first locate the ostium of the coronary sinus, near the inferior vena cava, and cut in a retrograde fashion along the outer wall of the coronary sinus in the left atrioventricular groove. Then, use scissors or a scalpel to cut through both the inner wall of the coronary sinus and the adjacent left atrial free wall. This cut should extend from the lower aspect of the atrial septum to the level of the left atrial appendage. Continue the cut between the mitral valve annulus below and the appendage above, dissecting the left atrial wall away from the ascending aorta. At the upper border of the atrial septum, the left atrial cut should meet that from the right atrium. Cut through the atria septum, from its upper to lower aspects, and remove the two atria from the cardiac base.

Transect the two great arteries along their sinotubular junctions, at the level of the valve commissures. After removing the ascending aorta and pulmonary artery, the arterial sinuses can be trimmed away with scissors to better demonstrate the two semilunar valves. The aortic valve is located centrally and abuts against the other three valves. After photographs have been taken, the right and circumflex coronary arteries can be evaluated for obstructions.

Window Method This method is useful for the preparation of dry cardiac museum specimens, using paraffin and other materials *(5,16,17)* or plastination *(18)*. Hearts should be perfusion-fixed (*see* above.) Windows of various sizes can be removed from the chambers or great vessels with a scalpel (Fig. 3-7). The blocks of tissue that are removed in this manner can be used for histologic study. Windows should initially be

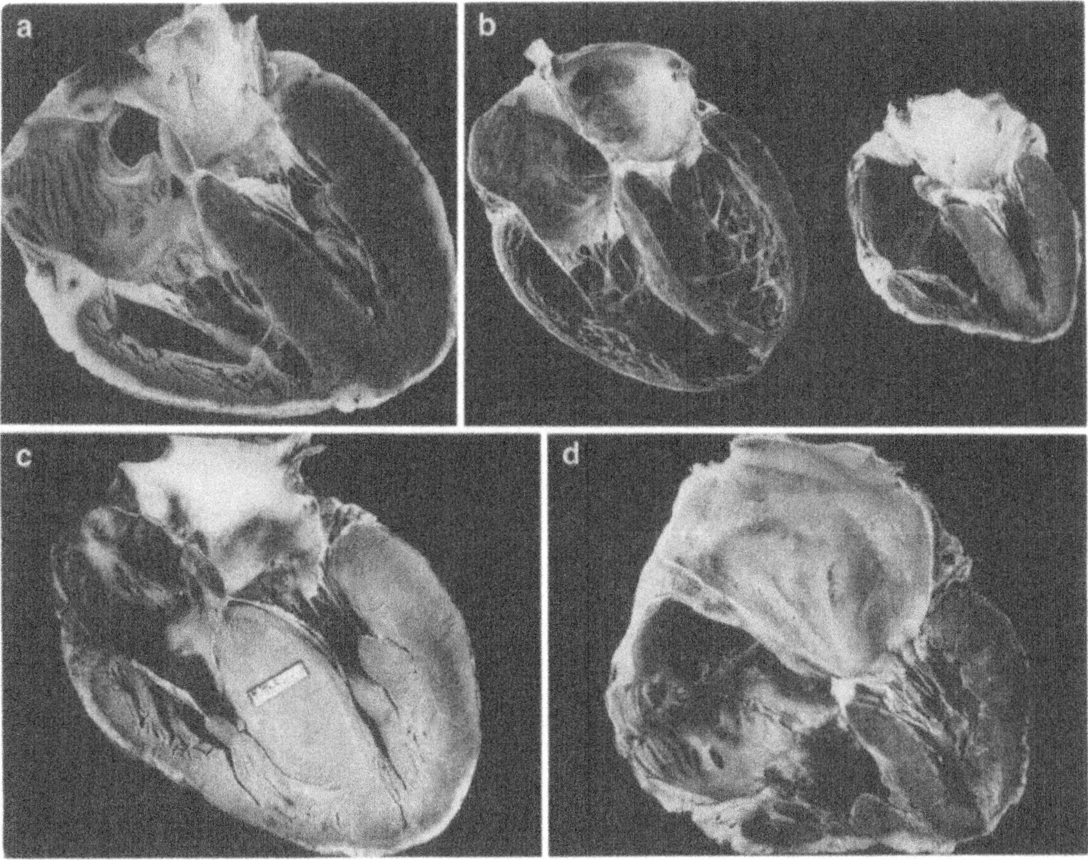

Fig. 3-4. Four-chamber method of cardiac dissection. (**a**) Normal heart, showing both atrioventricular valves and all four cardiac chambers. (**b**) Idiopathic dilated cardiomyopathy, with dilatation of all four chambers, compared with a normal heart (to the right). (**c**) Hypertrophic cardiomyopathy, with disproportionate ventricular septal hypertrophy. (**d**) Restrictive cardiomyopathy, with biatrial dilatation.

made small. Then, by looking inside the heart, one can determine how much to enlarge the opening to best demonstrate the lesion of interest.

Injection-Corrosion Method Plastic or latex is injected into the coronary vasculature or into the cardiac chambers and great vessels *(5,7,21–24)*. Casts made from silicon rubber are resilient and nonadhesive and can therefore be extracted from the coronary arteries or cardiac chambers without resorting to corrosion of the specimen *(23)*. For further details on injection-corrosion methods, *see* Chapter 16.

Dissection of the Cardiac Conduction System *In situ* demonstration of the glycogen-rich left bundle branch with Lugol's iodine solution is possible but only within 90 min after death *(5)*. The atrioventricular (AV) bundle and proximal portion of the right bundle lie too deep to be shown by this technique. However, the AV node, AV (His) bundle, and right bundle branch can be observed by gross dissection *(5,25,26)* although the procedure is of no practical diagnostic value. The sinus node cannot be identified in this manner.

Many descriptions exist of the microscopic evaluation of the conduction system in normal and abnormal hearts *(2,5,6,25,26)*. In practice, such an examination is rarely necessary, except for cases of nontraumatic death in which toxicologic studies are negative and no anatomic cause of death can be found. Another example is complete heart block. In such cases, the sinus node and the atrioventricular conduction tissues should be evaluated microscopically.

To remove a block of tissue that consistently contains the sinus node, the first cut should be made with scissors just anterior to the crista terminals, cutting through the numerous pectinate muscles (Fig. 3-8). This cut should extend to the upper border of the right atrial appendage. The second cut, perpendicular to the first, courses along this upper border and into the superior vena cava. The third cut, roughly perpendicular to the second and parallel to the first, travels along the right atrial wall, where it joins the atrial septum, and is directed from the superior vena cava toward the inferior vena cava. This cut should be about 2 cm long. The fourth cut completes the rectangular shape of the tissue block.

From this block, 6-8 sections are made with a scalpel, parallel to the second and fourth cuts. This cuts the sinus node artery, which usually can be seen grossly, in cross section. All sections can usually be submitted in 2 or 3 (consecutively labeled) cassettes. Because the node contains substantially more collagen than the adjacent myocardium, a trichrome or Verhoeff-van Gieson stain will aid in its identification. Between the ages of

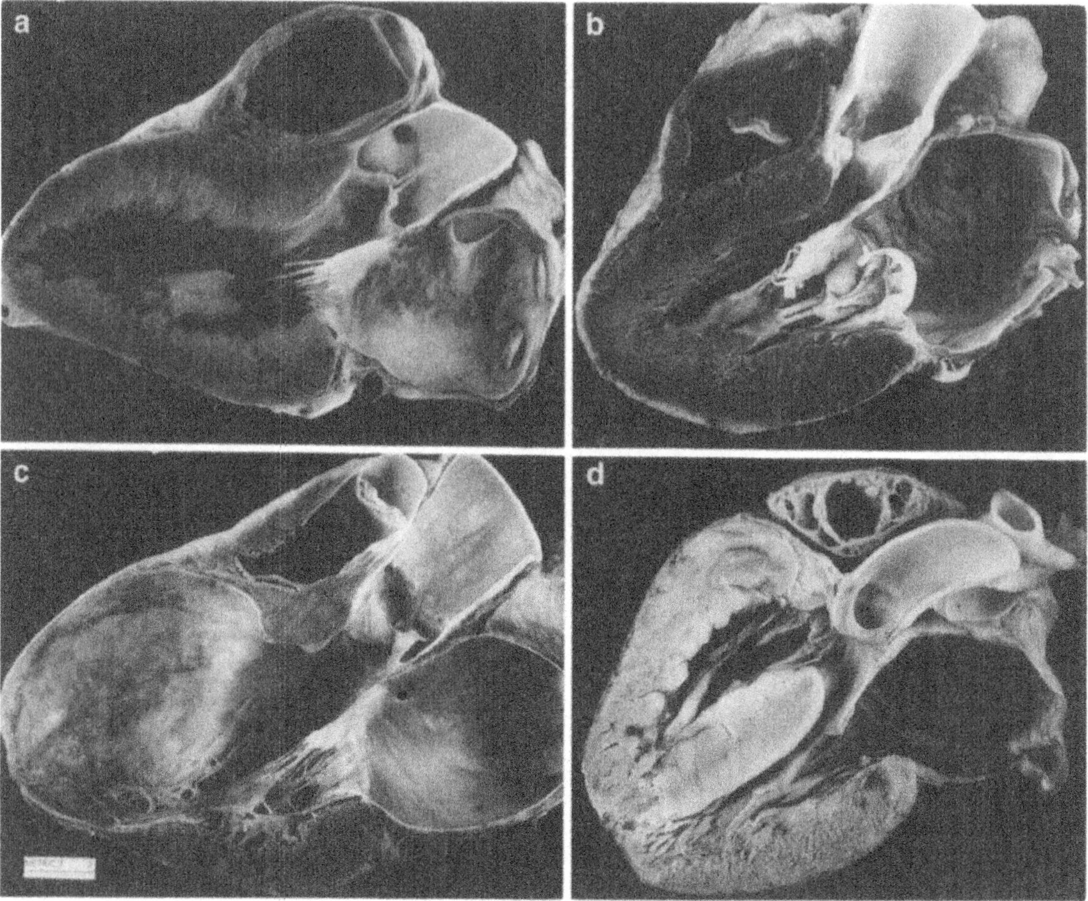

Fig. 3-5. Left ventricular long-axis method of cardiac dissection. (**a**) Normal heart, showing left ventricular inflow and outflow tracts, left atrium, ascending aorta, and right ventricular outflow tract. (**b**) Myxomatous mitral regurgitation, with prolapse of the posterior leaflet. (**c**) Old transmural myocardial infarct, with a large apical anteroseptal aneurysm. (**d**) Membranous ventricular septal defect.

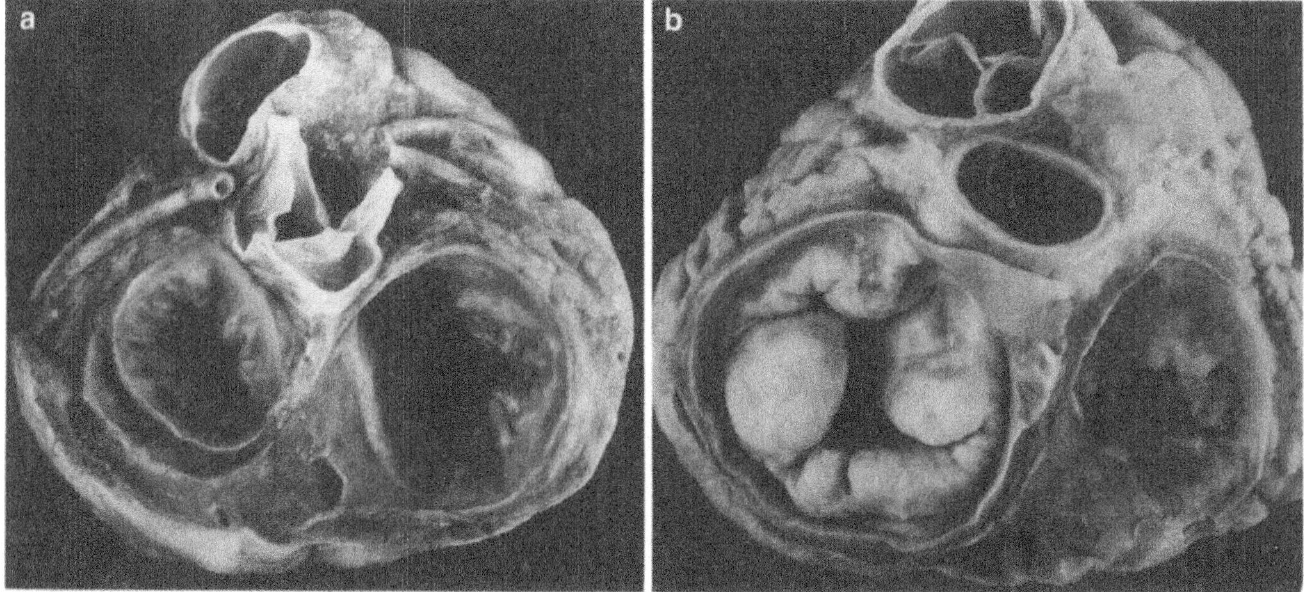

Fig. 3-6. Base-of-heart method of cardiac dissection. (**a**) Normal heart. (**b**) Myxomatous mitral valve disease.

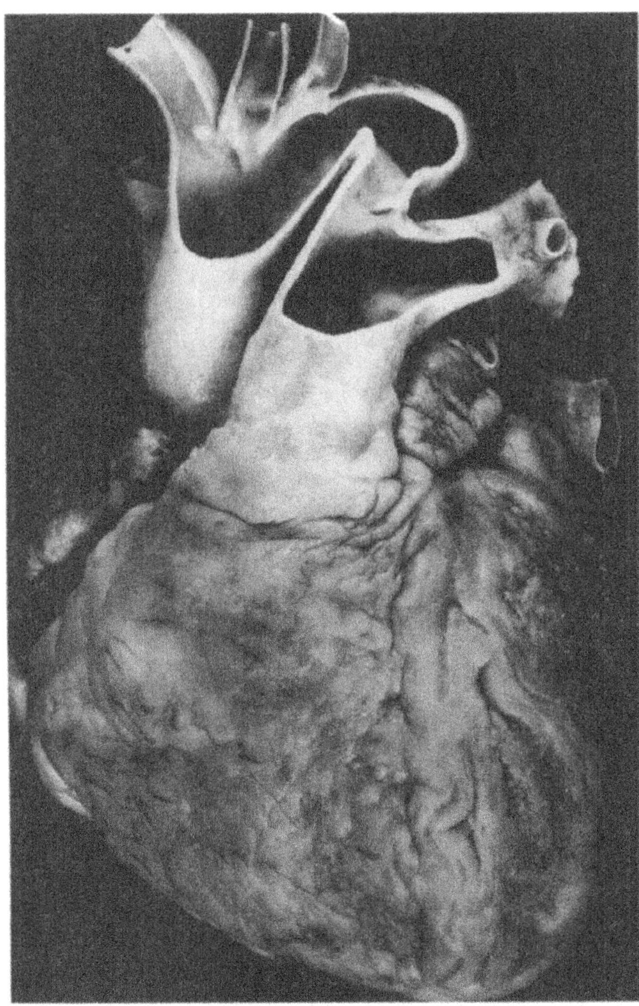

Fig. 3-7. Window method of cardiac dissection. Window in the great arteries, showing a widely patent ductal artery.

10 and 90 yr, the percentage of collagen normally expected in the sinus node is approximately the same as one's age *(25)*.

To remove a tissue block that consistently contains the AV conduction system, the dissection should commence from the right side of the heart. The AV node is located just above the tricuspid valve annulus, between the coronary sinus ostium and the membranous septum, within the triangle of Koch. First, orient the heart with the right-sided chambers opened such that the right atrium is positioned above and the right ventricle below (Fig. 3-9). Using a scalpel, remove a rectangular block of tissue, approximately 2.0 cm in height that extends laterally from the coronary sinus ostium to the far right side of the membranous septum. Within the tissue block, the tricuspid annulus should be skewed upward, such that about 1.5 cm of *atrial* septum is included at the side near the coronary ostium and 1.5 cm of *ventricular* septum is present at the side of the membranous septum.

The excised tissue block will contain much of the septal tricuspid leaflet and portions of the mitral and aortic valves; only the pulmonary valve should remain uncut. Valves can be trimmed back to within 0.5 cm of their annuli. For right-handed cutting, rotate the specimen 180°, with the right atrium closer to the prosector than the right ventricle and the left-sided chambers against the cutting board. Using a scalpel, cut 6 to 10 sections about 3 mm thick, beginning at the side nearest to the coronary sinus ostium and progressing toward the side with the membranous septum. Place tissues, in that order, into cassettes labeled AV-1, AV-2, and so on. Depending on the thickness of the ventricular septum, each cassette may hold 1-3 specimens.

Generally, each paraffin block from the conduction system needs to be cut only at one level. Trichrome or Verhoeff-van Gieson stains are most suitable to identify the conduction system because it is insulated with collagen. In rare instances, such as iatrogenic injury to the conduction system, one or two blocks may be cut at several levels to better delineate the damage, but exhausting the block to make slides from every 10th to 40th section is indicated only for detailed research investigations.

QUANTITATIVE MEASUREMENTS OF THE HEART

HEART WEIGHT *Total heart weight is the most reliable single measurement at autopsy for correlation with cardiac disease states (7).* The assessment must take into account the size of the patient. Other described measurements such as linear external dimensions, surface areas, and volume of the entire heart or myocardium *(7)* are less useful than the total heart weight.

Hearts are weighed after the parietal pericardium has been removed, the great vessels have been trimmed to about 2 cm in length, and postmortem clots have been removed from the cardiac chambers. Weights are recorded to the nearest gram *(3,6)* (or at least to the nearest 5 g in adults). For subjects younger than 1 yr, scales should be used that weigh accurately to the nearest 0.1 g. Fixation may alter heart weight by 5 to 10% *(31,32)*. Among the numerous available tables of normal values *(5–7,32–34)* the variation has generally been less than 10%.

Normal expected heart weights are related to age, gender, and body size *(32–34)* (*see* also Part III of this book). Normal heart weight usually correlates better with body weight than with age or height *(33,34)*. In some settings, for instance if patients received massive fluid therapy for shock or had a recent amputation, expected heart weight should be based on height or on the body weight before fluid therapy or amputation.

CARDIAC WALL THICKNESS Left ventricular thickness has usually been measured 1-2 cm below the mitral annulus *(5)*, but because wall thickness is greatest at the base and least at the apex, the most reliable average measurement is found at the level of the papillary muscles. The ventricular septum and the right ventricle should be measured at the same level. All three values can readily be attained from hearts dissected by the short-axis method. Trabeculations and papillary muscles should not be included in the measurements. Fixation may increase left ventricular wall thickness by 10% *(31)*. Right ventricular thickness is usually greater inferiorly than anteriorly. Normal values only apply to nondilated hearts (*see* Part III of this book) *(31,33,34)*.

There has been considerable debate whether the heart stops in systole, diastole, or asytole at death. Initially, the heart is flaccid *(7)* but within an hour, it begins to develop rigor mortis. Therefore, the left ventricular wall thickness and chamber

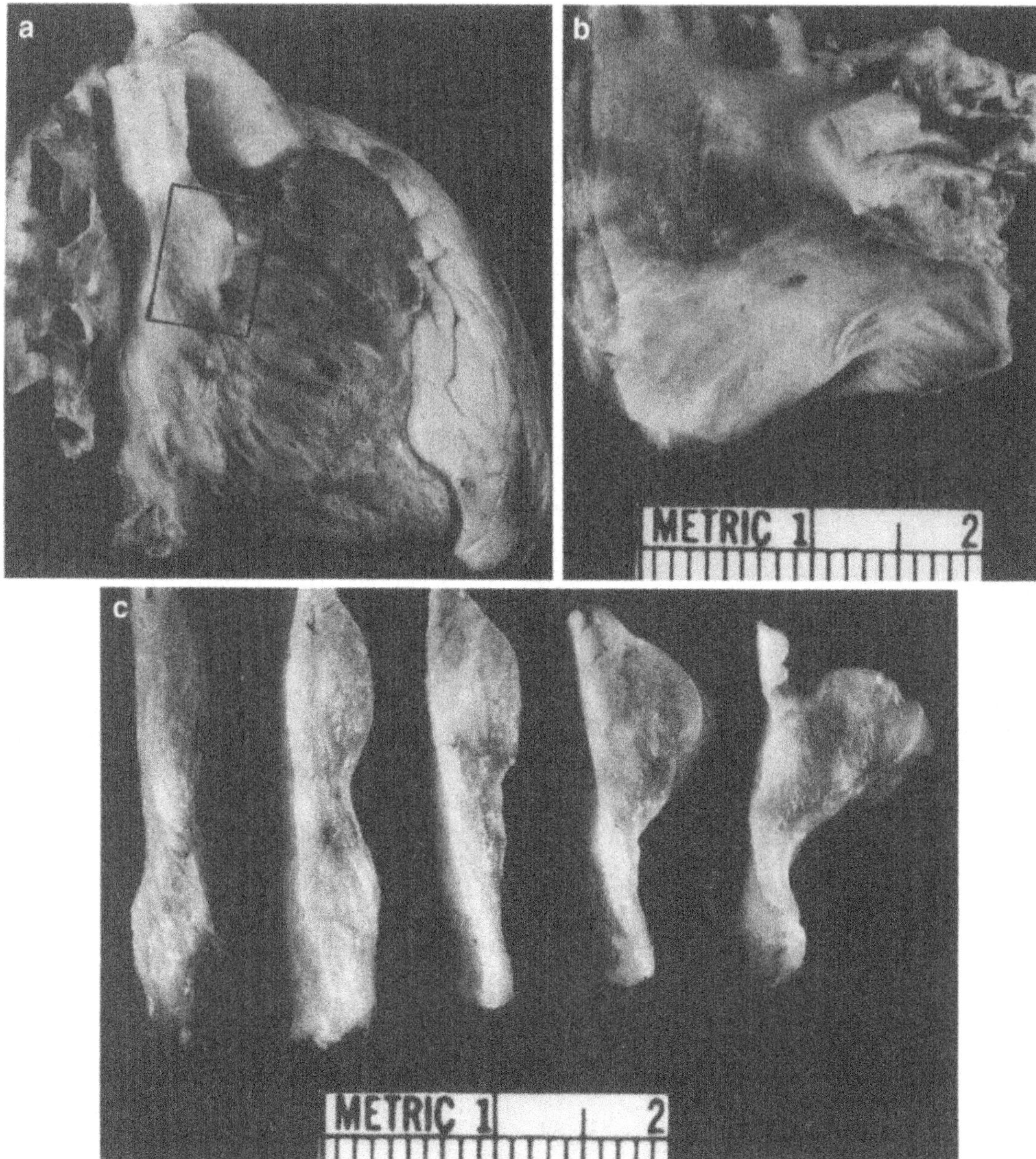

Fig. 3-8. Dissection of the sinus node for microscopy. (**a**) Right lateral view of the right atrium, showing the rectangular region (black lines) to be removed. (**b**) Excised tissue block, showing the endocardial aspect. (**c**) Sections cut for microscopy.

dimensions generally resemble those in end-systole *(35)*. About 24 h after death, rigor mortis remits, left ventricular wall thickness decreases again, and the chambers dilate, a condition not to be confused with dilated cardiomyopathy.

CARDIAC CHAMBER SIZES After death, chamber sizes may change considerably because of rigor mortis (*see* above) or fixation (which *decreases* ventricular volumes by about 50%) or because of perfusion fixation (which may *increase* them appreciably) *(36)*. This makes the interpretation of chamber volumes difficult. From the internal long-axis length (L) and short-axis diameter (D), a formula ($\pi LD^2/6$) may be used to calculate left ventricular volume.

CARDIAC HYPERTROPHY AND DILATATION For nondilated hearts from adults who show rigor mortis, hypertrophy is generally present if left ventricular wall thickness exceeds 1.5 cm or if right ventricular wall thickness exceeds 0.5 cm *(7)*. For dilated hearts, however, these measurements are not reliable. Thus, total heart weight is the best gross indicator of cardiac hypertrophy, when compared to expected normal weight (*see* Part III of this book) *(37)*. For research studies, the partition method is recommended, with comparison to tables of normal values for each chamber *(6,7,20)*.

There is no gross or microscopic difference between physiologic hypertrophy of athletes and pathologic hypertrophy that results from disease states *(6)*. However, in athletes, the heart weight is rarely increased more than 25% above the expected value. Ischemic heart disease alone, without coexistent hypertension, generally produces only mild hypertrophy, affecting all four chambers, and a heart weight of <550 g *(38)*.

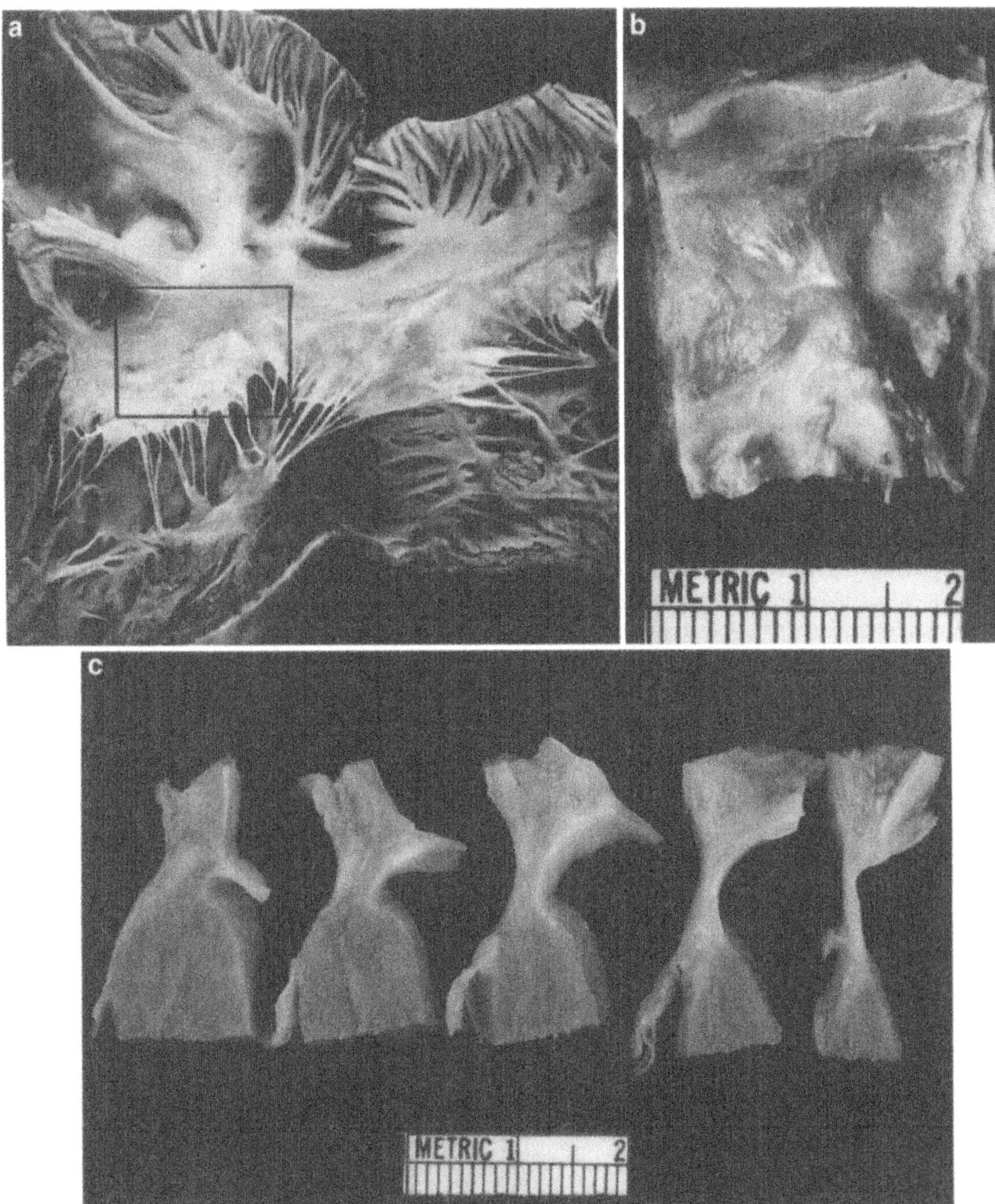

Fig. 3-9. Dissection of the atrioventricular (AV) conduction tissues for microscopy. (**a**) Opened right atrium (above) and right ventricle (below), showing the rectangular specimen (black lines) to be removed. (**b**) Excised tissue block, showing its right-sided aspect. (**c**) Sections cut for microscopy.

In chronic disorders such as systemic hypertension, aortic stenosis, dilated or hypertrophic cardiomyopathy, and congenital heart disease, the heart often weighs 2.0-2.5 times the expected value, or about 600-900 g in adults. Weights exceeding 1000 g may be found in hypertrophic cardiomyopathy, chronic aortic regurgitation, and acromegaly with hypertension. Isolated right ventricular hypertrophy due to pulmonary hypertension rarely produces a heart weight above 500 g.

Volume hypertrophy (avoid the potentially misleading term, eccentric hypertrophy *[37]*) of the left ventricle is always accompanied by chamber dilatation and secondary wall thinning. In hearts from adults of average size with rigor mortis, the short-axis internal dimension of the left ventricle is normally ≤2.5 cm. This measurement can be used to estimate the severity of left ventricular dilatation (*see* Part III of this book). The wall thickness of a *dilated* left ventricle cannot be used as an accurate indicator of hypertrophy *(37,39)*; instead, the overall heart weight is used for this purpose. The other three cardiac chambers are normally thin-walled; thus, hypertrophy and dilatation are not as readily quantitated as for the left ventricle, and pressure hypertrophy is often attended by substantial dilatation. All dilated chambers should be evaluated for mural thrombi, particularly within atrial appendages, ventricular apices, and ventricular aneurysms.

CARDIAC VALVE SIZE Valve function is difficult to evaluate at autopsy *(6)*. Regurgitation can be assessed to some extent by filling the chambers with water to check for retrograde flow through the intact valve. Stenosis is best evaluated by measuring the effective orifice size.

For intact hearts, valve *diameters* can be measured with a ruler or a calibrated cone (Fig. 3-10A) *(32)*. A cone will distort the elliptical orifices of the mitral and tricuspid valves, producing minor inaccuracies. In stenotic valves, cones measure orifice size rather than annular size.

Most pathologists measure valve *circumferences* (rather than diameters) along the annulus of the atrioventricular valves and at the arterial sinotubular junction of the semilunar valves. Measurements should be to the nearest 0.1 cm. Standard fixation may decrease valvular circumferences by 10-25% *(31)*, whereas perfusion fixation generally increases the measurements, particularly for the right-sided valves. For a given body size, women have slightly larger valves than men *(34)*. Valve circumferences, particularly those of the semilunar valves, progressively dilate during adult life *(34,40)*. The thickness and area of leaflets and cusps also increase with age. For normal values and their interpretation, and for further references, *see* Part III of this book *(32–34,40)*.

PATENCY OF THE FORAMEN OVALE Postnatally, the foramen ovale closes either anatomically or only functionally, as a flap valve. A patent foramen ovale may later serve as an avenue of paradoxical embolization and, therefore, its presence should be recorded. If an interatrial passageway is present, a probe can be passed from the right atrium between the valve and limb of the fossa ovalis, or from the left atrium from the ostium secundum. The maximum potential diameter of the foramen ovale is best established using graduated probes (Fig. 3-10B). For normal values *(41)*, *see* Part III of this book.

STANDARD GROSS AND MICROSCOPIC EXAMINATION

Many suggestions have been made for sections to be taken for microscopic examination *(3,42)*; most current policies are determined by the clinical history, the gross findings, special interests of the prosector *(7)*, and cost restraints.

GENERAL RECOMMENDATIONS For operated hearts and cases with a cardiac cause of death, a photograph of the heart should be taken before its dissection is begun. Preferably, the heart should be fixed in formalin for at least 5 min (to dull the surface) and then oriented as it is normally positioned in the chest. If it is dissected by the short-axis method, at least one photograph of the largest slice should be obtained, with the specimen viewed from the apex toward the base and with a short ruler (*see* Fig. 3-3).

For autopsy cases with a noncardiac cause of death and a grossly normal heart, no histologic slides may be needed or only a single section from the left ventricle, preferably including one of the papillary muscles. All microscopic samples should be transmural, about 1.5 cm wide and 0.3 cm thick. Rectangular sections, rather than pie-shaped, are preferred because they contain more subendocardial tissue, where ischemic injury most commonly occurs. Specimens should be labeled in detail according to their location (Fig. 3-11).

Coronary arteries and valves should be stained with Verhoeff-van Gieson. For conduction tissues, a trichrome stain is optional.

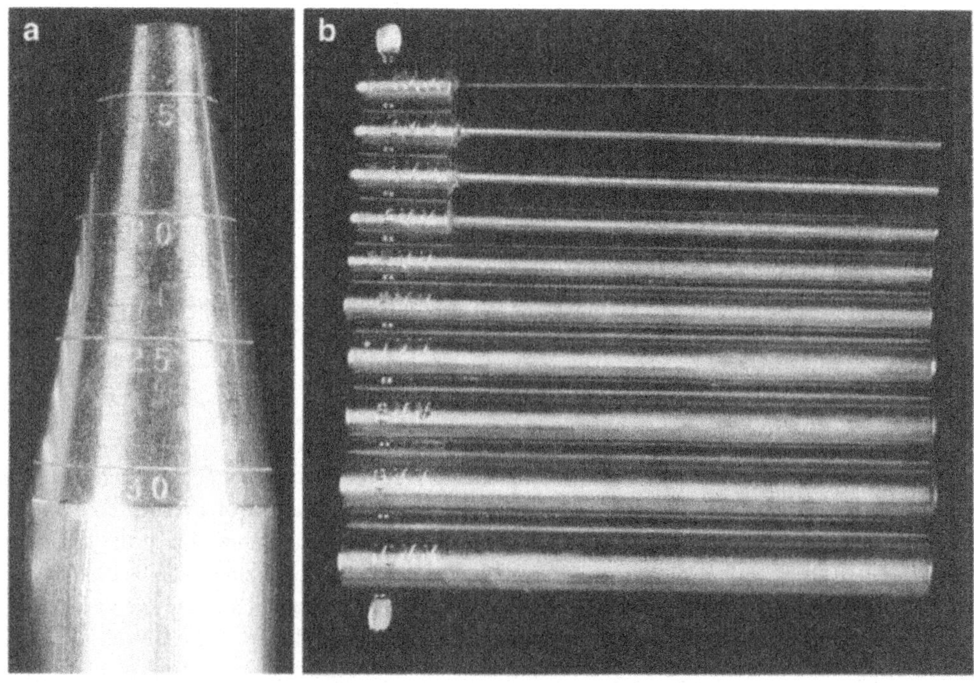

Fig. 3-10. Calibrated measuring devices. (**a**) Metal cone, with markings for diameters ranging from 1.0–3.0 cm. (**b**) Metal probes, ranging from 1–10 mm in diameter.

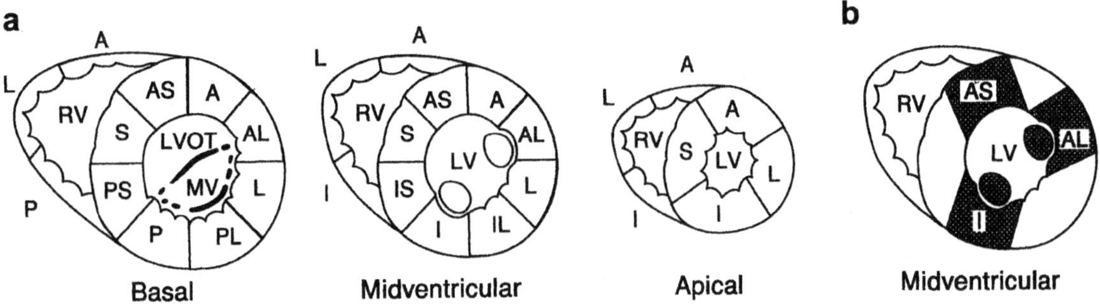

Fig. 3-11. Schematic diagram of the left (LV) and right (RV) ventricular regions. (**a**) Abbreviations for ventricular regions. (**b**) Three standard sections for microscopic evaluation. (A, anterior; AL, anterolateral; AS, anteroseptal; I, inferior; IL, inferolateral; IS, inferoseptal; L, lateral; P, posterior; PL, posterolateral; PS, posteroseptal; S, septal.)

Routine stains suffice for most other cardiac sections. In the first week after open heart surgery, low-output failure without an obvious morphologic cause, either grossly or microscopically, is common *(43)*.

ISCHEMIC HEART DISEASE Coronary artery disease, ischemic myocardial changes, and, in some cases, the effects of surgical and nonsurgical interventions must be evaluated *(2,15,44,45)*. Postmortem coronary angiography is optional; perfusion fixation is only necessary in research studies. The arteries are cut in cross sections at 3 mm to 5 mm intervals. Heavily calcified vessels should be removed and decalcified prior to sectioning. Microscopy may be performed to document chronic grade-4 obstructions and acute lesions such as plaque rupture and thrombosis (Table 3-1).

Segments with nonsurgical interventions such as percutaneous transluminal coronary angioplasty (PTCA), stent placement, or atherectomy may also be evaluated microscopically. For bypass grafts, sections should include the most obstructed areas of the graft body, coronary anastomosis, and distal coronary artery (Fig. 3-12). In most cases, all sections from one graft can be placed into one cassette (*see* Appendix 3-1). At the anastomosis, the coronary artery should be cut in cross-section, regardless of the angle of the graft.

Hearts should be dissected by the short-axis method (*see* Fig. 3-3) *(7,11,42,46,47)*. Only for teaching purposes are other methods recommended. Grossly, both old and acute infarcts should be described in terms of extent (transmural or subendocardial), location (anteroseptal, inferior, or lateral), and level (apical, midventricular, or basal).

For the macroscopic demonstration of acute myocardial ischemia, various dyes have been used, the most popular of which have been nitro-blue tetrazolium (NBT) and triphenyl tetrazolium chloride (TTC) *(46–49)*. Nevertheless, the best and least expensive method, within 4 h after injury, is a slide well-stained with hematoxylin-eosin. The microscopic features of acute and chronic myocardial ischemia *(50–53)* and of acute myocardial infarction of various ages (Table 3-2) *(54–56)*, have been described, although reperfusion alters the pattern *(15,57,58)*. All current methods of detecting early myocardial infarctions have been reviewed *(52)*.

If ischemic heart disease is suspected as the cause of death, at least three histologic sections should be taken at the midventricular level and include the anteroseptal, anterolateral, and inferior walls, with both mitral papillary muscles. If mottled or obviously infarcted areas are identified grossly, these should also be evaluated. Sections from inferoseptal infarcts should also include the inferior wall of the *right* ventricle.

VALVULAR HEART DISEASE For cases of suspected endocarditis, vegetations can be cultured as described in Chapter 7. Other disorders of native or prosthetic valves are best demonstrated using a combination of the short-axis and base-of-heart methods of dissection (*see* Fig. 3-6). For aortic and mitral valve disease, the left ventricular long-axis approach can also be used (*see* Fig. 3-5). For the distinguishing features of various prosthetic valves, see Table 3-3 *(59–62)*.

For microscopic examination of infected valves, large or multiple sections should be taken to increase the likelihood of detecting organisms. After treatment with antibiotics, a Grocott methenamine silver stain may better demonstrate dead bacteria in the vegetations than a Gram stain.

Left-sided valve disease may be associated with myocardial ischemia, due to inadequate coronary perfusion, coronary obstruction from embolic valvular vegetations, or injury to a coronary artery during valve surgery. Accordingly, the myocardial sections recommended for cases of valvular heart disease are the same as those for ischemic heart disease, particularly if there is a valvular vegetation, valvular prosthesis, or history of sudden death.

Additional recommendations for specific valvular lesions are listed in Part II of this book.

CARDIOMYOPATHIES For most cases of dilated cardiomyopathy, arrhythmogenic right ventricular cardiomyopathy, and hypertrophic cardiomyopathy, the heart should be dissected by the short-axis method. In contrast, the four chamber method is ideal for demonstrating biatrial dilatation in the eosinophilic and noneosinophilic forms of restrictive cardiomyopathy. Occasionally, it can also be used for dilated or hypertrophic cardiomyopathy (*see* Fig. 3-4). The long-axis method of dissection is useful for demonstrating the anatomic substrate for left ventricular outflow tract obstruction in some patients with hypertrophic cardiomyopathy.

The heart from any adult with suspected cardiomyopathy should be evaluated for coexistent coronary atherosclerosis. For dilated cardiomyopathy in adults, an iron stain is recommended

Table 3-1
Correlation Between Clinical Manifestation of Coronary Artery Disease and Pathologic Features of Atherosclerotic Plaques[a]

Clinical State	*Microscopic features of coronary atherosclerosis*
Asymptomatic	Stable plaques, grades 1–3; occasionally, grade 4 stable plaques (generally one-vessel disease).
Angina pectoris	
Chronic stable (exertional)	Stable grade 4 plaques (usually two-vessel or three-vessel disease).
Variant (Prinzmetal's)	Stable plaques, of any grade; evidence of plaque progression; occasionally an unstable atheroma.
Microvascular	No significant disease of epicardial coronary arteries; medial and intimal thickening of intramural arteries; swollen capillary endothelial cells.
Unstable (preinfarction)	Unstable plaque, of any grade, with rupture and acute nonocclusive platelet-rich thrombus; also stable grade 4 plaques (usually three-vessel disease).
Myocardial infarction (MI)	
Acute myocardial ischemia[b]	Unstable plaque, of any grade, with rupture and acute thrombus, either nonocclusive or occlusive; often associated with other stable grade 4 plaques.
Acute subendocardial MI	Same as for unstable angina.
Acute transmural MI	Unstable plaque, of any grade, with rupture and acute occlusive fibrin-rich thrombus; also stable grade 4 plaques (usually two-vessel or three-vessel disease).
Chronic myocardial ischemia[c]	Stable grade 4 plaques (usually two-vessel or three-vessel disease).
Old healed MI (scars >1 cm)	Stable grade 4 plaques (usually two-vessel or three-vessel disease); old organized thrombus; especially with transmural infarcts.
Chronic heart failure	Stable grade 4 plaques (usually two-vessel or three-vessel disease); old organized thrombus; evidence of plaque progression.
Sudden death	Unstable plaques, of any grade, with rupture and acute thrombus, either nonocclusive or occlusive; associated with other stable grade 4 plaques (two-vessel or three-vessel disease in 80%, one-vessel disease in 15%, and four-vessel disease in 5%).

[a] Represents autopsied cases only (a source of bias). *See* the section on "Evaluation of Coronary Arteries" for a description of the grades of obstruction. Unstable plaques are characterized by a thin fibrous cap, a large lipid-rich core, subendothelial clusters of macrophages or foam cells, atherophagocytosis, or adventitial or intimal lymphocytes.

[b] Characterized microscopically by contraction band necrosis or by nuclear pyknosis and intense sarcoplasmic staining with eosin, occurring in the absence of an infiltrate of neutrophils or, with reperfusion, macrophages. These features generally represent preinfarction changes in which the patient died before leukocytic infiltration occurred.

[c] Characterized microscopically by patchy subendocardial collections of vacuolated myocytes or by small (<1 cm) subendocardial patches of fibrosis or granulation tissue.

Adapted from Edwards *(15)*.

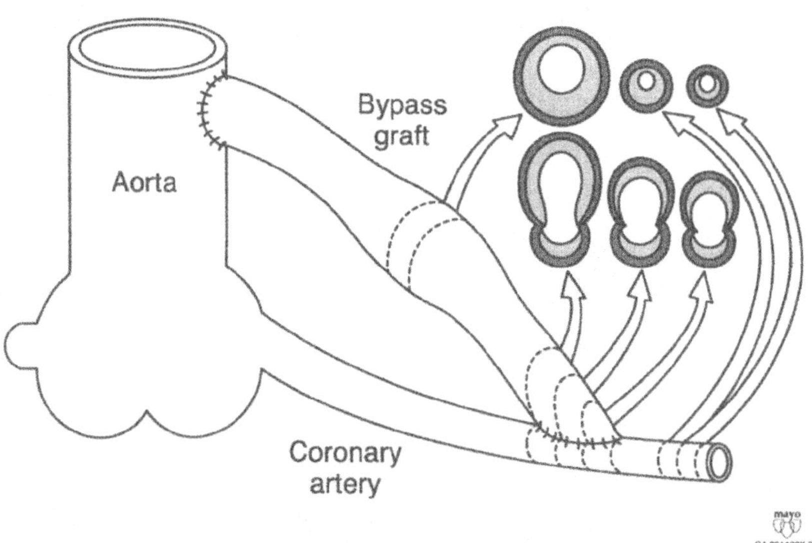

Fig. 3-12. Schematic diagram of a coronary artery bypass graft and the recommended sites for microscopic evaluation.

Table 3-2
Age-Related Features of Myocardial Infarction

Age	*Gross features*	*Light microscopy*
<4 h	No change.	No change.
4–12 h	Slight mottling, with areas of dark discoloration.	Intense sacroplasmic eosinophilia and nuclear pyknosis; contraction bands (with reperfusion).
12–24 h	Mottled and mildly edematous, with bulging cut surface.	As above, with early interstitial edema and neutrophilic infiltrates.
2–4 d	Soft yellow-tan core with mottled border.	Maximum neutrophilic infiltrate; nuclear loss and sarcoplasmic coagulation.
5–7 d	Yellow-tan core and irregular hyperemic red-brown border.	Basophilic interstitial debris; early macrophage infiltration; dilated capillaries at border.
8–10 d	Yellow-gray core and red-brown border; depressed cut surface.	Numerous macrophages, with active phagocytosis; pigmented macrophages filled with lipofuscin.
11–14 d	Yellow-gray core and red-gray border; depressed cut surface.	Granulation tissue along border; ongoing phagocytosis at core.
2–4 wk	Core becoming smaller; border becoming larger, grayer, firmer, and less gelatinous; less depressed cut surface.	Ongoing scar formation, dense at outer border; chronic inflammation; dilated peripheral small vessels; central core of necrotic tissue.
>1 mo	Firm gray-white or red-gray scar, with scar retraction and variable wall thinning.	Mature scar (dense collagen, focal elastin, and hypercellularity); focal lymphocytes.

Adapted from Edwards *(15)*.

Table 3-3
Types of Prosthetic Heart Valves Likely to Be Encountered at Autopsy

Mechanical	*Bioprosthetic*
Bileaflet	Porcine Aortic Valve
CarboMedics	Carpentier-Edwards
St. Jude	Hancock
Tilting Disk	Bovine Pericardial Valve
Bjork-Shiley	Carpentier-Edwards
Lillehei-Kaster	Ionecu-Shiley
Medtronic-Hall	Cadaveric Homograft Valve
Omniscience	CryoLife
Sorin	Red Cross
Caged Ball	Autograft
Starr-Edwards	Ross Procedure[a]

[a] Involves using the patient's own pulmonary valve in the aortic position.

for the evaluation of possible hemochromatosis, and an amyloid stain is suggested for cases with suspected hypertrophic cardiomyopathy. (For macroscopic staining methods, *see* Chapter 16.) Diffusely vacuolated myocytes may be indicative of an underlying storage disease, such as Fabry's disease; transmission electron microscopy is indicated in such cases.

Additional recommendations for specific types of cardiomyopathy are listed in Part II of this book.

CONGENITAL HEART DISEASE The evaluation should include study of the underlying malformation, its secondary effects on the heart and lungs, and review of diagnostic or therapeutic procedures and their effects or complications *(63)*. Chronic lesions such as aortic root dilatation (with conotruncal anomalies) or myxomatous valves (with single functional ventricles), in operated patients who have survived into adulthood, may also be encountered at autopsy.

Detailed descriptions of the specific forms of congenital heart disease can be found in Part II of this book. Synonyms abound for cardiovascular anomalies, and these are listed in Appendix 3-2, as well as with each individual malformation in Part II. For cardiac anatomy and for congenital cardiac anomalies, Anglicized terms rather than Latin names are currently preferred, and these are listed in Appendix 3-3. Common eponyms for various surgical procedures applied to malformed hearts, and their explanations are supplied in Appendix 3-4. In Appendix 3-5, a two-page form is provided that can be used during the autopsy evaluation of complex cases of congenital heart disease *(63–65)*.

In general, the thoracic organs should be removed en bloc but if the vascular connections are normal, the tracheobronchial tree, lungs, and esophagus can be removed from the heart. Section from the upper and lower lobes of both lungs should be evaluated for pneumonia and hypertensive pulmonary vascular disease. Note that the modified Heath-Edwards classification of plexogenic pulmonary hypertension is applicable only for subjects with congenital left-to-right shunts (*see* Table 3-4). In operated patients, the lesions of pulmonary venous hypertension are more common than plexogenic disease.

The major epicardial coronary arteries should be examined for anomalies in origin and distribution and for obstruction, especially if operative procedures have been performed nearby. Cardiomegaly is a common feature; even years after surgical repair of congenital heart disease, residual ventricular hypertrophy

Table 3-4
Modified Heath-Edwards Classification of Plexogenic Pulmonary Hypertension in Congenital Cardiac Left-to-Right Shunts

Grade	*Lesion*	*Reversible*
1A	Muscularization of arterioles	Yes
1B	Medial hypertrophy of arteries	Yes
1C	Loss of intra-acinar arteries	Yes
2	Concentric intimal proliferation	Borderline
3	Concentric laminal intimal fibrosis	Borderline
4[a]	Plexiform lesions	No
5	Dilatation (angiomatoid) lesions	No
6	Fibrinoid degeneration of arteries	No
6	Necrotizing arteritis	No

[a] Grade 4 plexiform lesions are now thought to represent the aftermath of necrotizing arteritis and microaneurysm formation and, hence, follow rather than precede grade 5 and 6 lesions.

Adapted with permission from Edwards *(63)*.

and dilatation may be striking. Asymmetric septal hypertrophy in conotruncal anomalies should not be misinterpreted as coexistent hypertrophic cardiomyopathy.

Congenitally malformed hearts may be opened by the inflow-outflow method, but in postoperative cases the short-axis method is best (*see* Fig. 3-3D). In selected circumstances (*see* Figures 3-5D and 3-7), the four-chamber, long-axis, base-of-heart, and window methods are also useful *(10)*. In general, microscopic sections should be taken from both ventricles for the evaluation of fibrosis and recent ischemic injury, particularly in the subendocardial region of hypertrophied hearts.

UNEXPLAINED SUDDEN DEATH The coronary arteries should be examined carefully throughout their length, to document any anomalies or obstructions, including ostial flaps. Hearts with appreciable ischemic, valvular, cardiomyopathic, or congenital lesions should be dissected as described earlier.

If the heart appears grossly normal, at least four slides should be taken for microscopy from the left ventricle, and two from the right ventricle. If no myocarditis or acute myocardial ischemia is detected microscopically, the cardiac conduction system should be evaluated as described earlier in this chapter. Though rare, mesothelioma of the AV node or sarcoidosis of the AV node or AV (His) bundle may cause sudden death.

The heart may be structurally normal in some fatal arrhythmic disorders such as long QT syndrome (*66*), catecholaminergic polymorphic ventricular tachycardia, and Brugada syndrome. In such cases, molecular studies for mutations in ion channel proteins or the ryanodine receptor may be informative. Because DNA fragmentation introduced by formalin fixation and paraffin processing yields suboptimal testing material for these studies, frozen tissue is ideal. Some of these syndromes have been implicated in drowning and near-drowning circumstances. If abnormalities such as cardiomyopathy (dilated or hypertrophic) or even aortic dissection are apparent, genetic studies on frozen tissue may be essential for effective screening of surviving family members (*67*) Frozen tissue can also be submitted for viral molecular studies in cases of myocarditis or dilated cardiomyopathy, especially in infants, adolescents, and young adults.

EVALUATION OF THE VASCULATURE

Examination of coronary arteries was described earlier in this chapter. For the study of vessels in other organs, see the appropriate chapter. Microscopic evaluation of vascular diseases should include a Verhoeff-van Gieson stain.

AORTA AND OTHER MAJOR ARTERIES In general, the thoracic and abdominal portions of the aorta are opened posteriorly, between the origins of the right and left intercostal and lumbar arteries. In cases of congenital heart disease, the thoracic aorta is left attached to the heart. If an acute aortic dissection is suspected, the heart and the entire aorta should be removed intact; transsection of the ascending aorta may distort or destroy the intimal tear. For the evaluation of renovascular disease, the kidneys and renal arteries are best kept together with the abdominal aorta.

Measure all aneurysms in length and diameter. They may be dissected either longitudinally or by cross-section, noting the amount of mural thrombus and the size of the residual lumen. Rupture sites should be studied microscopically for any underlying disease processes. Most forms of obstructive arterial disease are best evaluated by cross-section, but in fibromuscular dysplasia, longitudinal sections are recommended both grossly and microscopically.

Although the mesenteric arterial system can be more rapidly examined by opening the vessels longitudinally, cross-sections are better for the documentation of obstructions. If vasculitis is suspected, multiple cross-sections from the distal portion of the mesentery will reveal many small arteries for microscopic evaluation. The celiac arterial system is best demonstrated by arteriography (*see* Chapter 2), followed by dissection of the major branches.

Atherosclerosis of the longitudinally opened aorta is graded according to the percentage of intimal surface area that contains plaques. Four grades of disease exist, based on 25% increments of involvement. Grade 4 implies that more than 75% of the surface area is involved by plaques. Grade 0 indicates an absence of lesions. Mural thrombus, ulceration, calcification, and aneurysm do not affect the grade but are described individually. Usually, the grade is stated separately for the thoracic and abdominal regions (or for the suprarenal and infrarenal regions), because infrarenal disease is often more severe.

Atherosclerosis of aortic branches (such as coronary, renal, and mesenteric arteries) is graded according to the percentage of obstruction in *cross-sectional area*. Thus, a four-point grading system is applied to cross sections of these vessels, based on 25% increments of involvement. Grade-4 disease indicates a region of stenosis in which more than 75% of the expected cross-sectional area has been obstructed; this often leads to ischemic injury. Total occlusion (100% obstruction) should be specified; it is generally the result of old or acute plaque rupture and thrombosis.

Older methods of evaluating atherosclerosis require longitudinally opened vessels. The intima is stained with Sudan IV solution *(68)* to facilitate grading, or the vessels are compared with a panel of photographs prepared by the American Heart Association *(69)*. These methods still may be used for research studies.

The patency of grafts and anastomoses should be recorded. Arterial and venous anastomoses in transplanted organs should be inspected for obstruction, including internal thrombosis and external compression or stricture. Synthetic vascular grafts may also compress or erode into adjacent structures. Infected grafts or aneurysm can be cultured.

OBTAINING VESSELS AFTER EMBALMING In general, the vessels of the neck, face, arms, and legs are inaccessible to the prosector until after embalming. For removal of the neck vessels, see Chapter 4. Temporal arteries may be resected from the subcutaneous aspect of the skin flap made during removal of the brain. The femoral and popliteal vessels can be removed without having to make skin incisions along the legs *(70)*. For this method, an aluminum tube is used, which measures approx 1.5 cm in internal diameter and 75 cm in length and which has been sharpened distally to form a cutting edge (Fig. 3-13). A string is tied around the femoral artery and vein, just proximal to the inguinal ligament, and passed through the metal tube. By pulling on the string, a constant pressure is placed on the vessel, while the tubing is pushed down the thigh, with a twisting motion, toward the popliteal fossa. Then the tension on the string is released, and the vessels are cut distally by twisting the sharpened edge of the tube. Femoral and popliteal vessels are removed intact with the tube. Veins can be opened longitudinally and inspected for thrombus, particularly in the pockets of the venous valves, but arteries should be cut in cross section.

EVALUATION OF AIR AND FAT EMBOLISM Diagnostic autopsy methods are described in Part II of this book (*see* "Embolism, air" and "Embolism, fat").

EVALUATION OF LYMPHATIC VESSELS Under normal circumstances, only the thoracic duct and its main tributaries can be evaluated. Distended small lymphatic vessels can be identified in conditions such as lymphatic carcinomatosis, congestive heart failure, and cirrhosis of the liver.

The thoracic duct lies in the adipose tissue behind the descending aorta and is best dissected from the left side. It usually travels medial to the azygos vein and crosses over to the left side of the vertebral column at the level of the aortic arch. For exposure, the left lung is either lifted up (and held there by an assistant) or removed from the chest cavity. The intercostal arteries are transected close to the aorta, and the descending thoracic aorta is pulled rightward so that the thoracic duct can be dissected from the surrounding fat tissue (Fig. 3-14). Care must be taken not to lacerate it, particularly near the aortic arch, to which it is closely related. Dissection is facilitated by injecting saline or gelatin solution, with or without dye. Contrast medium may be injected for lymphangiography.

Some pathologists prefer to dissect the thoracic duct after the chest organs have been removed from the body. To avoid laceration of the duct, the mediastinal tissues must be separated from the spine immediately above the vertebral periosteum. If injection of the duct and its tributaries is planned, this must be done before the thoracic organs are removed.

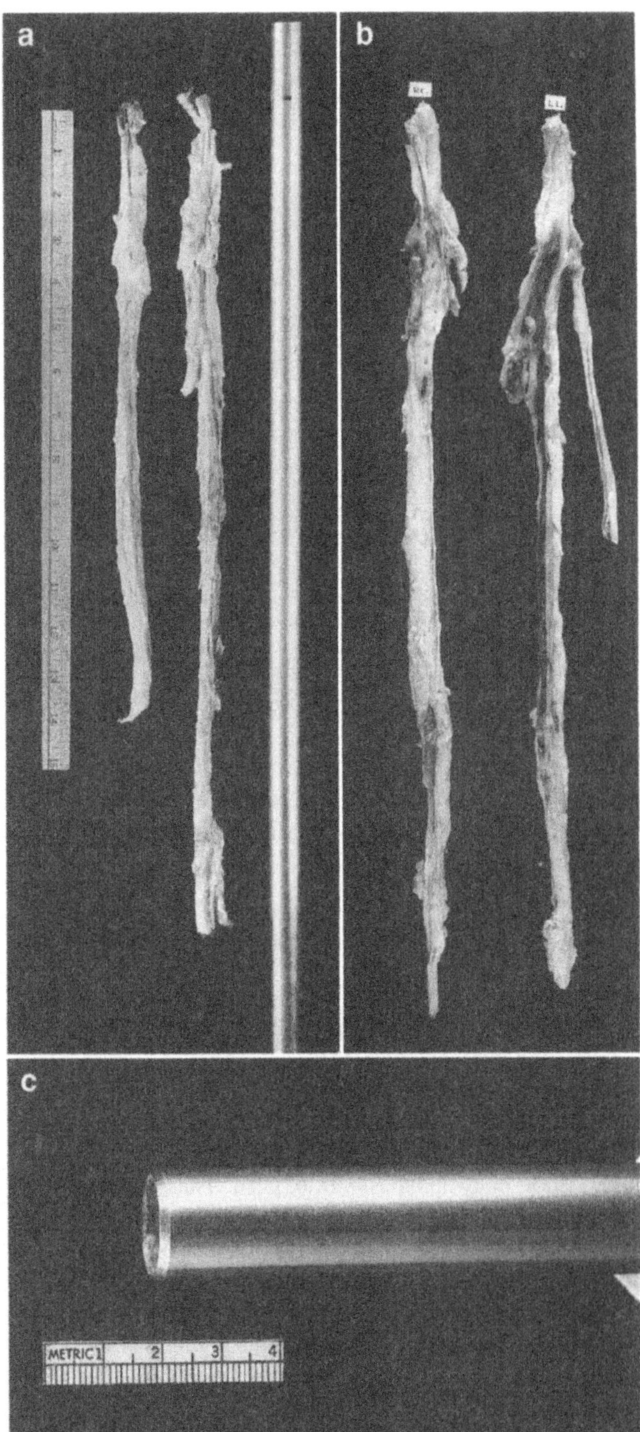

Fig. 3-13. Aluminum tube for the removal of the femoral and popliteal vessels. (**a**) Extracted femoral-popliteal vessels, with metal tube (to the right). (**b**) Bilateral venous thrombosis, in opened femoral and popliteal veins. (**c**) Cutting edge of the metal tube.

Peripheral lymphatics can be demonstrated at autopsy by lymphangiography. Because retrograde injection is rarely successful, a peripheral lymphatic channel must be identified. It is then cannulated with a 27-gauge needle. For contrast medium, one can use Ethiodol, stained with a few drops of oil paint, or a

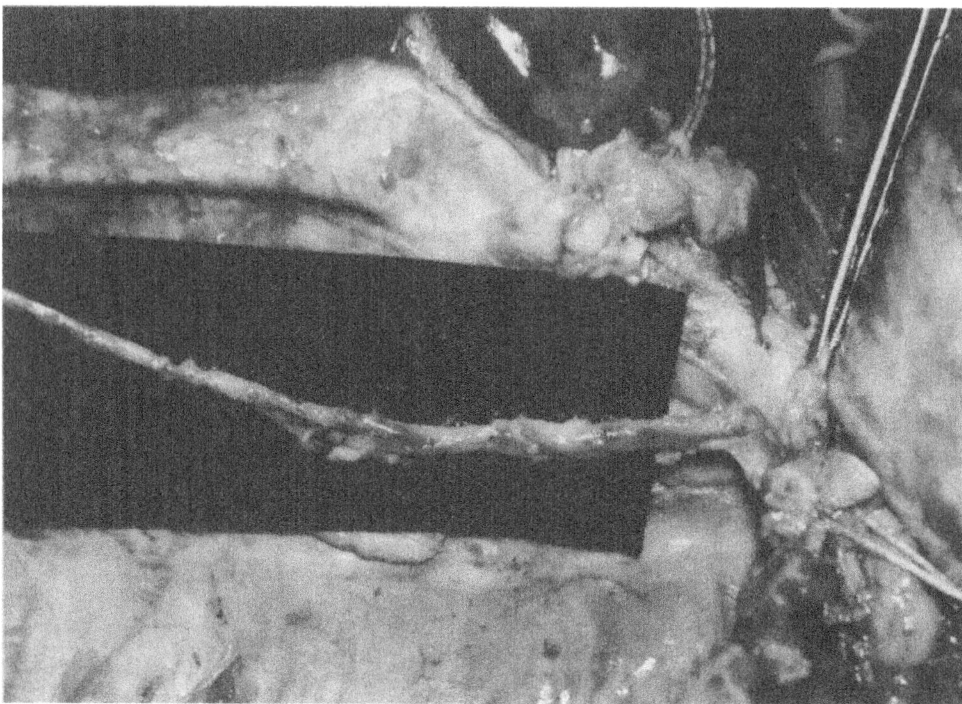

Fig. 3-14. Removal of the thoracic duct. The approach is from the left side. The left lung has been lifted out of the thoracic cavity, and the descending thoracic aorta has been dissected free and retracted rightward. The thoracic duct, displayed on black cardboard, has been dissected away from the retroaortic adipose tissue.

dilute barium sulfate mixture *(71)*. Owing to the thick medium and small needle caliber, the required injection pressure may be quite high (500–600 mm Hg).

Lymphatic channels can also be demonstrated by applying a 3% solution of hydrogen peroxide onto the surface of an organ or tissue, which will cause, after a short time, the spontaneous inflation of lymphatics with oxygen. The results may be unimpressive but can be improved if the tissues are first aged for 12–24 h and then soaked for 4–8 h in a 1:10 dilution of a stock solution of 10 gallons of water, 20 lb of crystalline phenol, 5 lb of potassium nitrate, 1.5 lb of sodium arsenite, 1.5 gallons of glycerin, 1.5 gallons of ethanol, and 0.5 gallon of formalin. After this, the samples are immersed for several minutes in 1% hydrogen peroxide *(72)*.

REFERENCES

1. Edwards WD. Cardiac anatomy and examination of cardiac specimens. In: Allen HD, Gutgesell HP, Clark EB, Driscoll DJ, eds. Moss and Adams' Heart Disease in Infants, Children, and Adolescents, 7th ed. Lippincott Williams & Wilkins, Philadelphia, 2007, pp. 1–39.
2. Virmani R, Ursell PC, Fenoglio JJ. Examination of the heart. Major Probl Pathol (Cardiovasc Pathol) 1991;23:1–20.
3. Silver MM, Silver MD. Examination of the heart and of cardiovascular specimens in surgical pathology. In: Silver MD, Gotlieb AI, Schoen FJ, eds. Cardiovascular Pathology, 3rd ed. Churchill Livingstone, New York, 2001, pp. 1–29.
4. Hutchinson GM, ed. Autopsy: Performance and Technique. College of American Pathologists, Northfield, IL, 1990.
5. Ludwig J, Lie JT. Heart and vascular system. In: Ludwig J, ed. Current Methods of Autopsy Practice, 2nd ed. W.B. Saunders, Philadelphia, 1979, pp. 21–50.
6. Davies MJ, Pomerance A, Lamb D. Techniques in examination and anatomy of the heart. In: Pomerance A, Davies MJ, eds. The Pathology of the Heart. Blackwell Scientific Publications, Oxford, 1975, pp. 1–48.
7. Reiner L. Gross examination of the heart. In: Gould SE, ed. Pathology of the Heart and Great Vessels, 3rd ed. Charles C. Thomas, Springfield, IL, 1968, pp. 1111–1149.
8. Seward JB, Khandheria BK, Freeman WK, Oh JK, Enriquez-Sarano M, Miller FA, et al. Multiplane transesophageal echocardiography: image orientation, examination technique, anatomic correlations, and clinical applications. Mayo Clin Proc 1993;68:523–551.
9. Seward JB, Khandheria BK, Edwards WD, Oh JK, Freeman WK, Tajik AJ. Biplanar transesophageal echocardiography: anatomic correlations, image orientation, and clinical applications. Mayo Clin Proc 1990;65:1193–1213.
10. Ackermann DM, Edwards WD. Anatomic basis for tomographic analysis of the pediatriac heart at autopsy. Perspect Pediatr Pathol 1988;12:44–68.
11. Edwards WD. Anatomic basis for tomographic analysis of the heart at autopsy. Cardiol Clin 1984;2:485–506.
12. Silverman NH, Hunter S, Anderson RH, Ho SY, Sutherland GR, Davies MJ. Anatomical basis of cross sectional echocardiography. Br Heart J 1983;50:421–431.
13. Edwards WD, Tajik AJ, Seward JB. Standardized nomenclature and anatomic basis for regional tomographic analysis of the heart. Mayo Clin Proc 1981;56:479–497.
14. Tajik AJ, Seward JB, Hagler DG, Mair DD, Lie JT. Two-dimensional real-time ultrasonic imaging of the heart and great vessels: technique, image orientation, structure identification, and validation. Mayo Clin Proc 1978;53:271–303.
15. Edwards WD. Pathology of myocardial infarction and reperfusion. In: Gersh BJ, Rahimtoola SH, eds. Acute Myocardial Infarction, 2nd ed. Chapman & Hall, New York, 1997, pp. 16–50.
16. Kramer FM. Dry preservation of museum specimens: a review, with introduction of simplified technique. J Tech Methods 1938;18:42–51.

17. Gross L, Leslie E. Paraffin infiltration of hearts: a permanent method for preservation. Am Heart J 1931;6:665–671.
18. Tiedemann K, von Hagens G. The technique of heart plastination. Anat Rec 1982;204:295–299.
19. Rodriguez FL, Reiner L. A new method of dissection of the heart. Arch Pathol 1957;63:160–163.
20. Bove KE, Rowlands DT, Scott RC. Observations on the assessment of cardiac hypertrophy utilizing a chamber partition technique. Circulation 1966;33:558–568.
21. Baroldi G, Scomazzoni G. Coronary Circulation in the Normal and the Pathologic Heart. U.S. Government Printing Office, Washington, DC, 1967, pp. 1–96.
22. James TN. Anatomy of the Coronary Arteries. Paul B. Hoeber, Inc./Harper & Brothers, New York, 1961, pp. 3–161.
23. Kilner PJ, Ho SY, Anderson RH. Cardiovascular cavities cast in silicone rubber as an adjunct to post-mortem examination of the heart. Int J Cardiol 1988;22:99–107.
24. Dübel H-P, Romaniuk PA. A simple technique for producing cast specimens of the cardiac ventricles. Cardiovasc Intervent Radiol 1980;3:131–133.
25. Davies MJ, Anderson RH, Becker AE. The Conduction System of the Heart. Butterworths, London, 1983, pp. 9–94.
26. Anderson RH, Becker AE. Anatomy of the conduction tissues revisited. Br Heart J 1978;40(Suppl):2–16.
27. Thomas AC, Davies MJ. The demonstration of cardiac pathology using perfusion-fixation. Histopathology 1985;9:5–19.
28. McAlpine WA. Heart and Coronary Arteries: An Anatomical Atlas for Clinical Diagnosis, Radiological Investigation, and Surgical Treatment. Springer-Verlag, Berlin, 1975, pp. 1–8, 133–209.
29. Glagov S, Eckner FAO, Lev M. Controlled pressure fixation apparatus for hearts. Arch Pathol 1963;76:640–646.
30. Rosenberg HS, Marcontell J. Whole-mount paraffin embedding as a method for preservation of congenitally malformed hearts. Am Heart J 1964;67:379–382.
31. Eckner FAO, Brown BW, Overll E, Glagov S. Alteration of the gross dimensions of the heart and its structures by formalin fixation: a quantitative study. Virchows Arch [Pathol Anat] 1969;346:318–329.
32. Hutchins GM, Anaya OA. Measurements of cardiac size, chamber volumes and valve orifices at autopsy. Johns Hopkins Med J 1973;133:96–106.
33. Scholz DG, Kitzman DW, Hagen PT, Ilstrup DM, Edwards WD. Age-related changes in normal human hearts during the first 10 decades of life. Part I (growth): a quantitative anatomic study of 200 specimens from subjects from birth to 19 years old. Mayo Clin Proc 1988;63:126–136.
34. Kitzman DW, Scholz DG, Hagen PT, Ilstrup DM, Edwards WD. Age-related changes in normal human hearts during the first 10 decades of life. Part II (maturity): a quantitative anatomic study of 765 specimens from subjects 20 to 99 years old. Mayo Clin Proc 1988;63:137–146.
35. Maron BJ, Henry WL, Roberts WC, Epstein SE. Comparison of echocardiographic and necropsy measurements of ventricular wall thicknesses in patients with and without disproportionate septal thickening. Circulation 1977;55:341–346.
36. Sairanen H. Post mortem measurement of ventricular volumes of the heart: an analysis of errors and presentation of a new method. Acta Pathol Microbiol Immunol Scand [Sect A] 1985;93:109–113.
37. Edwards WD. Applied anatomy of the heart. In: Giuliani ER, et al. eds. Mayo Clinic Practice of Cardiology, 3rd ed. Mosby, St. Louis, MO, 1996, pp. 422–489.
38. Dean JH, Gallagher PJ. Cardiac ischemia and cardiac hypertrophy: an autopsy study. Arch Pathol Lab Med 1980;104:175–178.
39. Murphy ML, White HJ, Meade J, Straub KD. The relationship between hypertrophy and dilatation in the postmortem heart. Clin Cardiol 1988;11:287–302.
40. Schenk KE, Heinze G. Age-dependent changes of heart valves and heart size. Recent Adv Studies Cardiac Structure Metabol 1975;10:617–624.
41. Hagen PT, Scholz DG, Edwards WD. Incidence and size of patent foramen ovale during the first 10 decades of life: an autopsy study of 965 normal hearts. Mayo Clin Proc 1984;59:17–20.
42. Lie JT, Titus JL. Pathology of the myocardium and the conduction system in sudden coronary death. Circulation 1975;52(Suppl III):41–52.
43. Lee AHS, Gallagher PJ. Post-mortem examination after cardiac surgery. Histopathology 1998;33:399–405.
44. Waller B. Morphology of percutaneous transluminal coronary angioplasty used in the treatment of coronary heart disease. Major Probl Pathol (Cardiovasc Pathol) 1991;23:100–133.
45. Virmani R, Atkinson JB, Forman MB. Aortocoronary bypass grafts and extracardiac conduits. In: Silver MD, ed. Cardiovascular Pathology, 2nd ed. Churchill-Livingstone, New York, 1991, pp. 1607–1648.
46. Lichtig C, Glagov S, Feldman S, Wissler RW. Myocardial ischemia and coronary artery atherosclerosis: a comprehensive approach to postmortem studies. Med Clin North Am 1973;57:79–91.
47. Baroldi G, Hatt PY, Málek P, Milam J, Paulin SJ, Pearse AGE, et al. The pathological diagnosis of acute ischaemic heart disease: report of a WHO scientific group. WHO Techn Rep Ser 1970;441:1–27.
48. Klein HH, Puschmann S, Schaper J, Schaper W. The mechanism of the tetrazolium reaction in identifying experimental myocardial infarction. Virchows Arch [Pathol Anat] 1981;393:287–297.
49. Feldman S, Glagov S, Wissler RW, Hughes RH. Postmortem delineation of infarcted myocardium: coronary perfusion with nitro blue tetrazolium. Arch Pathol Lab Med 1976;100:55–58.
50. Teraoka K, Kaneko N, Takeishi M. Clinical and pathologic studies on contraction band lesion: relation to acute myocardial infarction and unexplained sudden death. Mod Pathol 1991;4:6–12.
51. Bouchardy B, Majno G. Histopathology of early myocardial infarcts. Am J Pathol 1974;74:301–330.
52. Vargas SO, Samson BA, Schoen FJ. Pathologic detection of early myocardial infarction: a critical review of the evolution and usefulness of modern techniques. Mod Pathol 1999;12:635–645.
53. Geer JC, Crago CA, Little WC, Gardner LL, Bishop SP. Subendocardial ischemic myocardial lesions associated with severe coronary atherosclerosis. Am J Pathol 1980;98:663–680.
54. Fishbein MC, Maclean D, Maroko PR. The histopathologic evolution of myocardial infarction. Chest 1978;73:843–849.
55. Lodge-Patch I. The ageing of cardiac infarcts, and its influence on cardiac rupture. Br Heart J 1951;13:37–42.
56. Mallory GK, White PD, Salcedo-Salgar J. The speed of healing of myocardial infarction: a study of the pathologic anatomy in seventy-two cases. Am Heart J 1939;18:647–671.
57. Cowan MJ, Reichenbach D, Turner P, Thostenson C. Cellular response of the evolving myocardial infarction after therapeutic coronary artery reperfusion. Hum Pathol 1991;22:154–163.
58. Roberts CS, Schoen FJ, Kloner RA. Effect of coronary reperfusion on myocardial hemorrhage and infarct healing. Am J Cardiol 1983;52:610–614.
59. Mehlman DJ. A pictorial and radiographic guide for identification of prosthetic heart valve devices. Prog Cardiovasc Dis 1988;30:441–464.
60. Morse D, Steiner RM. Cardiac valve identification atlas and guide. In: Morse D, Fernadnez J, eds. Guide to Prosthetic Cardiac Valves. Springer-Verlag, New York, 1985, pp. 257–346.
61. Silver MD, Datta BN, Bowles VF. A key to identify heart valve prostheses. Arch Pathol 1975;99:132–138.
62. Schoen FJ. Pathologic considerations in replacement heart valves and other cardiovascular prosthetic devices. In: Schoen FJ, Gimbrone MA, eds. Cardiovascular Pathology: Clinicopathologic Correlations and Pathogenetic Mechanisms. USCAP Monograph in Pathology, No. 37. Williams & Wilkins, Baltimore, 1995, pp. 194–222.
63. Edwards WD. Congenital heart disease. In: Damjanov I, Linder J, eds. Anderson's Pathology, 10th ed. Mosby Year Book, St. Louis, 1996, pp. 1339–1396.
64. Edwards WD. Classification and terminology of cardiovascular anomalies. In: Allen HD, Gutgesell HP, Clark EB, Driscoll DW, eds. Moss & Adams' Heart Disease in Infants, Children, and Adolescents, Including the Fetus and Young Adult, 7th ed. Williams & Wilkins, Philadelphia, 2007, pp. 34–36.
65. Anderson RH, Becker AE, Freedom RM, et al. Sequential segmental analysis of congenital heart disease. Pediatr Cardiol 1984;5:281–288.
66. Ackerman MJ, Porter CJ. Identification of a family with inherited long QT syndrome after a pediatric near-drowning. Pediatrics 1998;101:306–308.
67. Tester DJ, Ackerman, MJ. The role of molecular autopsy in unexplained sudden cardiac death. Curr Opin Cardiol 2006;21:166–172.

68. Guzman GA, McMahan CA, McHill HC Jr, Strong JP, Tejada C, Restrepo C, et al. Selected methodologic aspects of the International therosclerosis Project. Lab Invest 1968;18:479–497.
69. McGill HC, Brown BW, Gore I, McMillan GC, Paterson JC, Pollak OJ, et al. Grading human atherosclerotic lesions using a panel of photographs. Circulation 1968;37:455–459.
70. Becking RE Jr, Titus JL. Laboratory suggestion: a method for the autopsy study of the femoral-popliteal vessels. Am J Clin Pathol 1967;47:652–653.
71. Ludwig J, Linhart P, Baggenstoss AH. Hepatic lymph drainage in cirrhosis and congestive heart failure: a postmortem lymphangiographic study. Arch Pathol 1968;86:551–562.
72. Parke WW, Michels NA. A method for demonstrating subserous lymphatics with hydrogen peroxide. Anat Rec 1963;146:165–171.

Appendix 3-1
Examples for Abbreviations Used for Labeling Microscopic Slides[a]

Abbreviation	Meaning
Aorta and Selected Arteries (Excluding Coronaries)	
Br-Ceph Art	Brachiocephalic (innominate) artery (or BCA or Innom Art)
Ductal Art	Patent ductal artery (patent ductus arteriosus) (or PDA)
Ductal A Lig	Ductal artery ligament (ligamentum arteriosum)
Asc Aorta	Ascending aorta
Desc Thor Ao	Descending thoracic aorta
Abd Aorta	Abdominal aorta
Truncal Art	Persistent truncal artery (truncus arteriosus)
Cardiac valves	
Ao Valve-L	Left cusp of aortic valve (or AV-L)
Ao Valve-P	Posterior cusp of aortic valve (or AV-P)
Ao Valve-R	Right cusp of aortic valve (or AV-R)
Aortic Valve	Aortic valve
Com AV Valve	Common atrioventricular valve (or CAVV)
Mitral Valve	Mitral valve
Pulm Valve	Pulmonary valve
Pulm Valve-A	Anterior cusp of pulmonary valve (or PV-A)
Pulm Valve-L	Left cusp of pulmonnary valve (or PV-L)
Pulm Valve-R	Right cusp of pulmonary valve (or PV-R)
Tric Valve	Tricuspid valve (or TV)
Tric Valve-A	Anterior leaflet of tricuspid valve (or TV-A)
Tric Valve-P	Posterior leaflet of tricuspid valve (or TV-P)
Tric Valve-S	Septal leaflet of tricuspid valve (or TV-S)
Trunc Valve	Truncal valve (or Truncal Valv)
Coronary arteries	
AVNA	AV nodal artery
LAD	Left anterior descending
LAD-D	Unspecified diagonal branch of LAD
LAD-D1	First diagonal branch of LAD
LAD-FSP	First septal perforating branch of LAD
LCX	Left circumflex
LCX-OM	Unspecified obtuse marginal branch of LCX
LCX-OM1	First obtuse marginal branch of LCX
LCX-OM2	Second obtuse marginal branch of LCX
LCX-PD	Posterior descending branch of LCX (with left dominance)
LMA	Left main coronary artery
IA	Intermediate artery (with trifurcating LMA)
RCA	Right coronary artery
RCA-PD	Posterior descending branch of RCA
Coronary arteries *(continued)*	
RCA-PL	Posterolateral branch of RCA
SNA	Sinus nodal artery
Coronary artery bypass grafts	
LAD-GEA	Gastroepiploic artery to LAD
LAD-LIMA	Left internal mammary (thoracic) artery to LAD
LAD-LIMA-RA	LIMA to radial artery segment to LAD
LAD-SVG	Saphenous vein graft to LAD
LAD-D1-SVG	Saphenous vein graft to LAD-D1
LCX-SVG	Saphenous vein graft to LCX
LCX-OM1-SVG	Saphenous vein graft to LCX-OM1
RCA-RIMA	Right internal mammary (thoracic) artery to RCA
RCA-SVG	Saphenous vein graft to RCA
RCA-PD-SVG	Saphenous vein graft to RCA-PD
RCA-PL-SVG	Saphenous vein graft to RCA-PL
Myocardium	
Atrial Sept	Atrial septum
AV-1	Atrioventricular conduction tissue (first cassette); AV-2 (second cassette), etc.
LA	Left atrial free wall
LAA	Left atrial appendage
LA-MV-LV	Left atrium, mitral valve, and left ventricle (one specimen)
LV-AV-Ao	Left ventricle, aortic valve, and ascending aorta (one specimen)
LV-I apex	Inferior wall of left ventricle at apical level
LV-PS base	Posteroseptal wall of left ventricle at basal level
LV-S mid	Ventricular septum at midventricular level
RA	Right atrial free wall
RAA	Right atrial appendage
RA-TV-RV	Right atrium, tricuspid valve, right ventricle (one specimen)
RV-A base	Anterior wall of RV at basal level (or RVOT, for RV outflow tract)
RV-A,L mid	Anterior and lateral walls of RV at midventricular level
RV-I mid	Inferior wall of right ventricle at midventricular level
RV-PV-PA	Right ventricle, pulmonary valve, pulmonary artery (one specimen)
SN-1	Sinus node (first cassette); SN-2 (second cassette), etc.

[a]All abbreviations listed above have 12 or fewer characters, in accordance with automated slide labeling systems that generally allow only 12 characters per line.

For abbreviations for veins, find their arterial counterpart and replace "Artery, Art, or A" with "Vein or V."

Appendix 3-2
Synonyms for Commonly Used Diagnostic Terms in Congenital Heart Disease

Preferred term	*Synonyms*
Anomalous pulmonary venous connection	Anomalous pulmonary venous drainage or return (not always anatomically accurate).
Aortopulmonary septal defect	Aortopulmonary window or fenestration; aorticopulmonary window or septal defect.
Asplenia syndrome	Right isomerism; visceral heterotaxy; Ivemark's syndrome (eponyms should be avoided).
Atrioventricular discordance	Ventricular inversion; L-loop ventricles.
Atrioventricular septal defect	AV canal defect; endocardial cushion defect; AV commune; common AV orifice.
Common inlet right ventricle	Cor biloculare (no longer an acceptable term).
Complete transposition of the great arteries	D-transposition; d-loop transposition; simple regular transposition; transposition of the great vessels.
Congenitally corrected transposition of the great arteries	L-transposition; corrected transposition of the great arteries; physiologically corrected transposition.
Double outlet right ventricle with subpulmonary VSD	Taussig-Bing heart (eponyms should be avoided).
Double chamber left atrium	Subdivided left atrium; triatrial heart; cor triatriatum (a term to avoid).
Double inlet left ventricle	Single left ventricle; univentricular heart; common ventricle (exceedingly rare); cor triloculare biatriatum (no longer an acceptable term).
Double inlet left ventricle with normally related great arteries	Holmes heart (eponyms should be avoided).
Extrathoracic heart	Ectopic heart; ectopia cordis.
Inlet VSD	Subtricuspid, AV canal, or AV commune VSD.
Membranous VSD	Paramembranous, perimembranous, or infracristal VSD.
Muscular VSD	Persistent bulboventricular foramen.
Outlet or infundibular VSD	Subarterial, subaortic, subpulmonary, supracristal, conal, or doubly-committed juxta-arterial VSD.
Patent ductal artery	Patent arterial duct; patent ductus arteriosus; persistent ductus arteriosus.
Persistent truncal artery	Persistent arterial trunk; truncus arteriosus; truncus arteriosus communis.
Polysplenia syndrome	Left isomerism; visceral heterotaxy.
Primum ASD	Ostium primum ASD; partial AV septal defect.
Pulmonary atresia with VSD	Tetralogy with pulmonary atresia (pseudotruncus and type IV truncus are no longer acceptable terms).
RPA or LPA from ascending aorta	Hemitruncus (no longer an acceptable term).
Secundum ASD	Ostium secundum ASD, or fossa ovalis ASD.
Sinus venosus defect	Sinus venosus ASD, Juxtacaval ASD; sinoseptal defect.
Superoinferior ventricles	Over-and-under heart; upstairs-downstairs heart.
Tricuspid atresia	Single inlet left ventricle; absent right atrioventricular connection.
Twisted atrioventricular connection	Criss-cross heart.

ASD, atrial septal defect; AV, atrioventricular; d, dextro; l, levo; LPA, left pulmonary artery; RPA, right pulmonary artery; VSD, ventricular septal defect.

Adapted from Edwards *(63)*.

Appendix 3-3
Latin Terms and Their Anglicized Equivalents for Cardiovascular Structures

Latin term (Plural)	*Anglicized equivalent (Plural)*
Annulus (annuli); anulus (anuli)	Annulus (annuluses), or anulus, or ring
Aorta (aortae)	Aorta (aortas)
Atrium (atria)	Atrium (atriums)
Chorda tendinea (chordae tendineae)	Tendinous cord (cords)
Conus arteriosus	Right ventricular outflow tract, or infundibulum
Cor triatriatum	Triatrial heart, or double chamber left atrium
Cor triatriatum dexter	Double chamber right atrium
Crista supraventricularis	Supraventricular crest or ridge
Crista terminalis	Terminal crest or ridge
Ductus arteriosus (ductus arteriosi)	Ductal artery, or arterial duct
Ductus venosus	Ductal vein, or venous duct
Ectopia cordis	Ectopic heart, or extrathoracic heart
Foramen ovale	Oval foramen
Fossa ovalis	Oval fossa
Inferior vena cava	Inferior caval vein
Infundibulum (infundibula)	Infundibulum (infundibulums)
Ligamentum arteriosum	Arterial ligament, or ductal artery ligament
Ligamentum venosum	Venous ligament, or ductal vein ligament
Limbus fossae ovalis, or annulus ovalis	Limb or rim of the oval fossa
Ostium (ostia)	Ostium (ostiums), or orifice
Ostium primum	First ostium or orifice
Ostium secundum	Second ostium or orifice
Patent ductus arteriosus	Patent ductal artery
Patent foramen ovale	Patent oval foramen
Septum (septa, not septae or septi)	Septum (septums)
Septum primum	First septum
Septum secundum	Second septum
Sinus venosus	Venous sinus, or sinus vein
Situs ambiguous	Isomerism, or indeterminate sidedness
Situs inversus	Mirror-image sidedness
Situs solitus	Normal sidedness
Superior vena cava	Superior caval vein
Trabecula septomarginalis	Septal band, or moderator band
Trabecula carnea (trabeculae carneae)	Trabeculation(s)
Truncus arteriosus	Truncal artery, or arterial trunk

Adapted from Edwards *(63)*.

Appendix 3-4
Eponyms for Surgical Procedures for Congenitally Malformed Hearts

Eponym	*Description of procedure*	*Cardiovascular anomalies*
Blalock-Hanlon shunt	Partial atrial septectomy (posterosuperior region).	Complete TGA with intact ventricular septum.
Blalock-Taussig shunt	Subclavian-to-pulmonary artery (classic: end-to-side anastomosis; modified: interposed synthetic graft).	Conditions with decreased pulmonary blood flow (tetralogy, PA-VSD, and DORV or DILV with PS).
Damus-Kaye-Stansel procedure	Proximal PT to ascending aorta (end-to-side anastomosis); conduit from RV to distal PT; VSD closure.	Complete TGA without PS and with or without VSD.
Glenn anastomosis	SVC to RPA (end-to-side); ligation of SVC at RA; ligation of proximal RPA (bidirectional Glenn: no ligation of RPA).	Tricuspid atresia, or DILV with PS.
Fontan procedure (modified)	Anastomosis of SVC, RA, or RV to RPA or LPA; may include intra-atrial conduit from IVC to SVC.	Hearts with single functional ventricle (e.g., tricuspid atresia or DILV).
Jatene procedure	Transection and switching of great arteries and coronary arteries.	Complete TGA, and DORV with subpulmonary VSD.
Konno procedure	Outlet (infundibular) septostomy, with patch enlargement of LV and RV outflow tracts, and aortic valve replacement.	Tunnel subaortic stenosis, and severe hypertrophic cardiomyopathy.
Mustard procedure	Resection of atrial septum; intra-atrial baffle directing caval blood flow to LV, and pulmonary venous blood to RV.	Complete TGA.
Norwood procedure	*Stage 1* (atrial septectomy; PDA ligation; PT transection; aortic incision; reconstruction of aorta with allograft; aorta-PT shunt). *Stage 2* (modified Fontan operation).	Aortic atresia (hypoplastic left heart syndrome).
Potts shunt	Descending thoracic aorta to LPA (side-to-side anastomosis).	Same as for Blalock-Taussig shunt.
Rastelli procedure	VSD closure directing LV blood to aorta; conduit from RV to distal PT; ligation of proximal PT.	PA-VSD, PTA, complete TGA with VSD and PS, and DORV with PS.
Senning procedure	Use of atrial septum to fashion intra-atrial baffle, similar to Mustard procedure.	Complete TGA.
Waterston shunt	Ascending aorta to RPA (side-to-side anastomosis).	Same as for Blalock-Taussig shunt.

DILV, double inlet left ventricle; DORV, double outlet right ventricle; IVC, inferior vena cava; LPA, left pulmonary artery; LV, left ventricle, PA-VSD, pulmonary atresia with a ventricular septal defect; PDA, patent ductal artery; PS, pulmonary stenosis; PT, pulmonary trunk; PTA, persistent truncal artery; RA, right atrium; RPA, right pulmonary artery; RV, right venricle; SVC, superior vena cava; TGA, transposition of the great arteries; VSD, ventricular septal defect.

Adapted with permission from Edwards *(63)*.

Appendix 3-5 Standardized Form for the Autopsy Evaluation of Congenital Heart Disease

GENERAL INFORMATION CASE NO.: ____________

Patient Name: ______________________________ Age, Gender: ____________

Patient I.D. No.: ______________________________ Date of Death: ____________

CARDIAC ARRANGEMENT

Thoracic Position ☐ Left-Sided ☐ Right-Sided ☐ Midline ☐ Unknown ☐ Ectopic ________

Apical Direction: ☐ Left-Sided ☐ Right-Sided ☐ Midline ☐ Other: ____________

Displacement: ☐ None ☐ Leftward ☐ Rightward ☐ Midline ☐ Unknown

Morphologic RA: ☐ Right-Sided ☐ Left-Sided ☐ Bilateral ☐ Absent ☐ Indeterminate

PULMONARY ARRANGEMENT

Morphology of Right-Sided Lung: ☐ Right ☐ Left ☐ Indeterminate No. of Lobes: ________

Morphology of Left-Sided Lung: ☐ Left ☐ Right ☐ Indeterminate No. of Lobes: ________

ABDOMINAL ARRANGEMENT

Spleen: ☐ Single ☐ Accessory ☐ Polysplenia ☐ Asplenia ☐ Unknown

Liver: ☐ Right-Sided ☐ Left-Sided ☐ Midline ☐ Unknown ☐ Other: ____________

Bowel: ☐ Normal ☐ Malrotation: ______________________________

VISCERAL SIDEDNESS

Cardiac: ☐ Normal ☐ Mirror-Image ☐ R. Isomerism ☐ L. Isomerism ☐ Indeterminate ________

Pulmonary: ☐ Normal ☐ Mirror-Image ☐ R. Isomerism ☐ L. Isomerism ☐ Indeterminate ________

Abdominal: ☐ Normal ☐ Mirror-Image ☐ R. Isomerism ☐ L. Isomerism ☐ Indeterminate ________

ATRIUMS

Right-Sided: ☐ RA ☐ LA ______________________________

Left-Sided: ☐ LA ☐ RA ______________________________

Septum: ☐ Intact ☐ POF ☐ ASD: ______________________________

Cor. Sinus: ☐ Present ☐ Absent ☐ Other: ______________________________

ATRIOVENTRICULAR VALVES

Right-Sided: ________ % to RV ________ % to LV Morphology: ____________________

Left-Sided: ________ % to RV ________ % to LV Morphology: ____________________

Common: ________ % to RV ________ % to LV Morphology: ____________________

VENTRICLES

Morphologic RV: Orientation: ☐ Normal ☐ Mirror-Image Position: ____________

Morphologic LV: Orientation: ☐ Normal ☐ Mirror-Image Position: ____________

Hypoplastic: ☐ RV ☐ LV ______________________________

Septal Position: ☐ Vertical ☐ Angled ☐ Horizontal ☐ Twisted ☐Other: ____________

Septum: ☐ Intact ☐ VSD: ______________________________

SEMILUNAR VALVES

Pulmonary: ________ % to RV ________ % to LV Morphology: ____________________

Aortic: ________ % to RV ________ % to LV Morphology: ____________________

Truncal: ________ % to RV ________ % to LV Morphology: ____________________

AORTIC VALVE POSITION RELATIVE TO PULMONARY VALVE

☐ R. Post. ☐ Dextroposed ☐ R. Lat. ☐ R. Ant. ☐ Ant. ☐ L. Ant. ☐ L. Lat. ☐ L. Post. ☐Post.

GREAT ARTERIES

Pulm. Artery: ☐ Present ☐ Atretic ☐ Hypoplastic ☐ Absent ☐ Other: ____________

Systemic Collaterals: ☐ Absent ☐ Present: ______________________________

Thoracic Aorta: ☐ L. Arch ☐ R. Arch ☐ Coarctation ☐ Other: ____________

Ductal Artery: ☐ Patent ☐ Absent ☐ Ligament ☐ Other: ____________

CORONARY ARTERIES

Ostiums: ☐ Normal ☐ Other: ______________________________

Distribution: ☐ Normal ☐ Mirror-Image ☐ Other: ______________________________

CONNECTIONS

Venoatrial	(Systemic Veins):	☐ Normal Veins	☐ Other: ______		
	(Pulmonary Veins):	☐ Normal Veins	☐ Other: ______		
Atrioventricular	(Biventricular):	☐ Concordance	☐ Discordance	☐Ambiguous:	______
	(Univentricular):	☐ Double Inlet	☐ Single Inlet	☐ Common Inlet	______
Ventriculoarterial	(Two Arteries):	☐ Concordance	☐ Discordance	☐ Double Outlet	______
	(One Artery):	☐ Single Outlet (Atretic PT)		☐ Common Outlet (Truncal Artery)	

CARDIAC MEASUREMENTS

Body Size:	Height (cm) ______	Weight (kg) ______	BSA (m2) ______
Weights (g):	Heart & Lungs ______	R. Lung ______	L. Lung ______
	Heart ______	(Normal Mean ______	and Range ______)
Wall Thickness (cm):	LV ______	RV ______	VS ______
Valves (cm):	Aortic ______	Pulmonary ______	Truncal ______
	Mitral ______	Tricuspid ______	Common ______

Shunts (cm): POF ______ ASD ______ AVSD ______ VSD ______ PDA ______

SECONDARY CARDIAC EFFECTS

	Hypertrophy	Dilation	Atrophy	Fibrosis	Mural Thrombus
LV:	______	______	______	______	______
RV:	______	______	______	______	______
LA:	______	______	______	______	______
RA:	______	______	______	______	______

SECONDARY PULMONARY EFFECTS

Plexogenic Pulmonary Hypertension: ______

Pulmonary Venous Hypertension: ______

Other Pulmonary Hypertension: ______

Pulmonary Infection: ______

Other Microscopic Features: ______

INTERVENTIONAL PROCEDURES

Procedure (Date): ______

Appearance at Autopsy: ______

Procedure (Date): ______

Appearance at Autopsy: ______

Procedure (Date): ______

Appearance at Autopsy: ______

4 Nervous System

CATERINA GIANNINI AND HARUO OKAZAKI

REMOVAL OF BRAIN IN ADULTS

INCISION OF SCALP The head is elevated slightly with a wooden block or a metal headrest attached to the autopsy table. The hair is parted with a comb along a coronal plane connecting one mastoid with the other over the convexity (Fig. 4-1). A sharp scalpel blade can then be used to cut through the whole thickness of the scalp from the outside. The incision should start on the right side of the head (the "viewing-side" in most American funeral parlors) just behind the earlobe, as low as possible without extending below the earlobe, and extend to the comparable level on the other side. This will make reflection of the scalp considerably easier. Sufficient tissue should be left behind the ear to permit easy sewing of the incision by the mortician.

The anterior and posterior halves of the scalp are then reflected forward and backward, respectively, after short undercutting of the scalp with a sharp knife, which permits grasping of the edges with the hands. The use of a dry towel draped over the scalp edges facilitates further reflection, usually without the aid of cutting instruments. If the reflection is difficult, a scalpel blade can be used to cut the loose connective tissue that lags behind the reflecting edge as the other hand continues to peel the scalp. The knife edge should be directed toward the skull and not toward the scalp. The anterior flap is reflected to a level 1 cm or 2 cm above the supraorbital ridge. The posterior flap is reflected down to a level just above the occipital protuberance.

SAWING OF CRANIUM The cranium is best opened with an oscillating saw. Because aerosolization of bone dust poses a risk of infection, the procedure should be done using protective devices, such as inside a plastic bag *(1,2)*. (Fig. 4-2). If Creutzfeldt-Jakob disease or other prion-related disease is suspected, we follow standard prion disease procedures including removal of the brain under a tent apparatus, placement of a wet paper towel on the calvarium (the dissector sawing through the towel) and use of appropriate respiratory protection with a powered-air purifying respirator (PAPR). Alternatively, a handsaw can be used in these cases *(3,4)*. Helpful information and detailed discussion of procedures in autopsies of patients with suspected prion disease can also be found in the Centers for Disease Control Web site (http://www.cdc.gov/ncidod/dvrd/cjd) and related links from the Biosafety in Biomedical and Microbiological Laboratories (http://bmbl.od.nih.gov/contents.htm) and National Prion Disease Pathology Surveillance Center (http://www.cjdsurveillance.com).

Various saw cuts are in use but we recommend the method illustrated in Fig. 4-3. The configuration of the saw cut minimizes slippage of the skull cap during restoration of the head by the embalmer. Naturally, the saw cut may have to be modified after some neurosurgical procedure(s) or in the presence of skull fracture(s). The temporalis muscle should be cut with a sharp knife and cleared from the intended path of the saw blade. Ideally, sawing should be stopped just short of cutting through the inner table of the cranium, which will easily give way with the use of a chisel and a light blow with a mallet. Leaving the dura and underlying leptomeninges intact allows viewing of the brain with the overlying cerebrospinal fluid (CSF) still in the subarachnoid space. To obtain this view, after removal of the skull cap, the dura must be cut with a pair of scissors along the line of sawing and reflected.

To protect the brain, the extended index finger of the hand that holds the neck of the oscillating saw should gauge the distance of the blade penetration. The oscillating blade should be moved from side to side during cutting to avoid deep penetration in a given area. Our saw (Lipshaw Co.) is equipped with a guard and can be used with little training, without fear of deep penetration.

The frontal point of sawing should start about two fingerbreadths above the supraorbital ridge. While the lateral aspects of the skull are being cut, turning the head to the opposite side permits the brain to sink away from the cranial vault and thereby diminishes the chance of injury to the brain.

When the dura is left intact, as in the method described earlier, the skull cap can be peeled away easily. A twist of a chisel placed in the frontal saw line will admit the fingers inside the skull cap. A blunt hook may be used to pull the skull cap away from the underlying dura. A hand inserted between the skull and the dura (periosteum) helps the blunt separation of these while the other hand is pulling the skull cap. If the dura adheres too firmly to the skull, it can be incised along the line of sawing and the anterior attachment of the falx to the skull can be cut

From: *Handbook of Autopsy Practice,* 4th Ed. Edited by: B.L. Waters

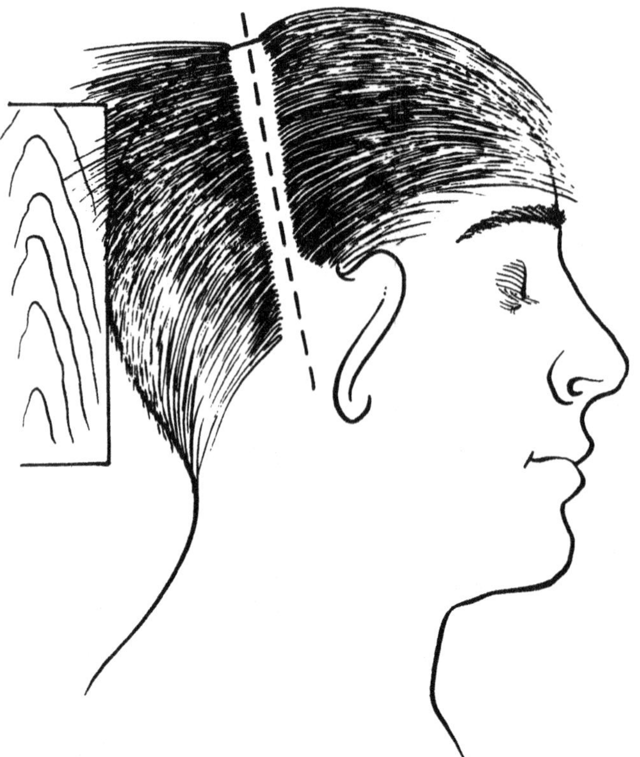

Fig. 4-1. Scalp incision. Dotted line indicates coronal plane of the primary incision. It starts on right side over the mastoid just behind earlobe and passes over palpable posterolateral ridges of parietal bones to reach opposite mastoid. This line is slightly tilted backward from plane parallel with face.

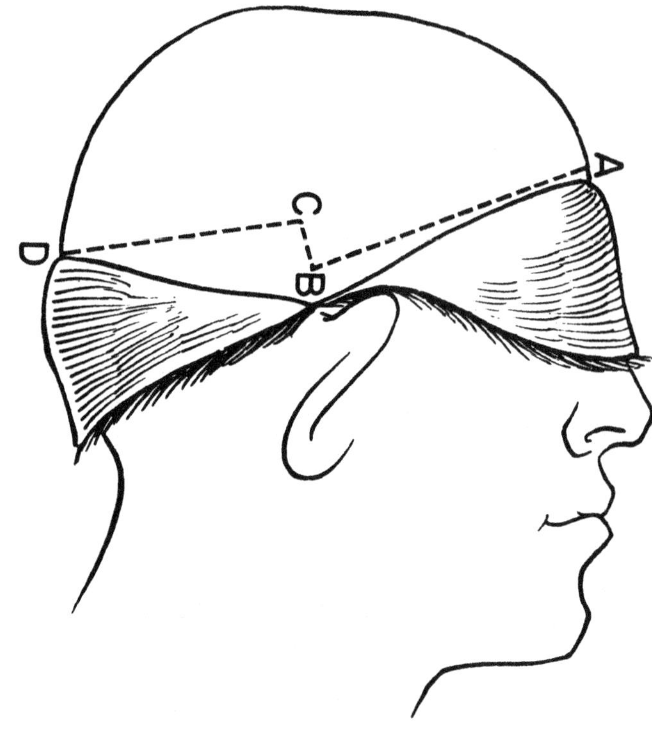

Fig. 4-3. Lines of saw cuts for skull cap removal. Frontal point (A) is approx two fingerbreadths above supraorbital ridges. Temporal point (B) is at the top of ear in its natural position before scalp reflection. Point (C) is approx 2 cm above (B). Occipital point (D) is approx two fingerbreadths above external occipital protuberance (inion). If (A) is too low, there is danger of cutting into the roof of the orbit; if (B) is too low, saw will enter petrous portion of temporal bone. Either of these will make removal of skull vault difficult. When (D) is too low, saw line will be below attachment of the tentorium.

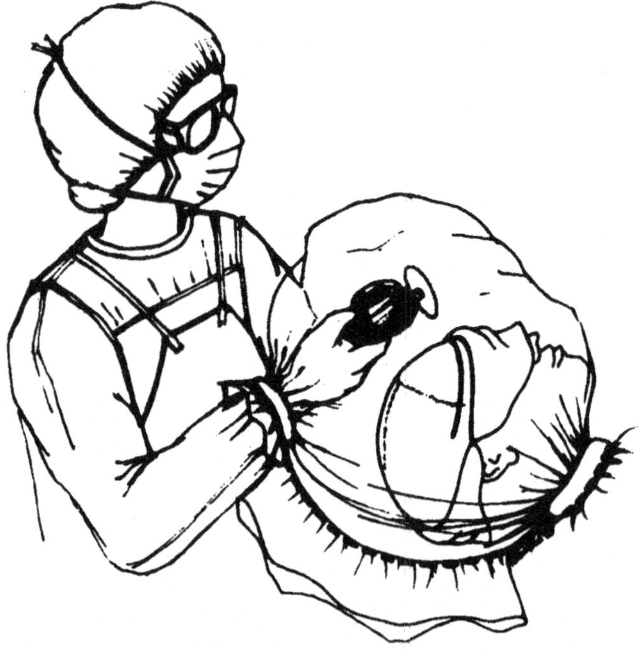

Fig. 4-2. Protective device. Prosector's hand holds saw inside bag. Dashed line indicates tape-seal of bag to, from left, prosector's gown, opposite side of the bag and neck of deceased. Adapted from ref. (1).

between the frontal lobes. The posterior portion of the falx can be cut from inside after the skull cap is fully reflected. The dura is then peeled off the skull cap. The superior sagittal sinus may be opened with a pair of scissors at this time. Routinely, the dorsal dural flaps on both sides can be removed easily from the brain by severing the bridging veins. In the presence of epi- or subdural hemorrhage and neoplasia, it is best to leave the dural flaps attached to the dorsal brain and section them together.

DETACHMENT OF BRAIN The frontal lobes are gently raised and the olfactory bulbs and tracts are peeled away from the cribriform plates. The optic nerves are cut as they enter the optic foramina. Under its own weight, the brain is allowed to fall away from the floor of the anterior fossa, while it is being supported with the palm of one hand. The pituitary stalk is cut, followed by the internal carotid arteries as they enter the cranial cavity. Cranial nerves III, IV, V, and VI are severed as close to the base of the skull as possible. Subdural communicating veins are also severed. Next, the attachment of the tentorium along the petrous ridge is cut on either side with curved scissors. At this time, the brain must not drop backward excessively because this will cause stretch tears in the cerebral peduncles. This can be prevented by raising the head very high from the beginning, with pronounced flexion of the neck, using a wooden pillow or a metal support attached to the table.

Cranial nerves VII, VIII, IX, X, XI, and XII are then cut identifying each one in sequence. The vertebral arteries are severed with scissors as they emerge into the cranial cavity. Then, the cervical part of the spinal cord is cut across as caudally as possible, but too oblique a plane of sectioning should be avoided. Curved scissors will be best for this purpose. If a critical lesion exists in the region, a cross-section perpendicular to the neuroaxis at the pontomedullary junction or higher may be elected in order to preserve the integrity of the abnormality.

The brain can then be reflected further back by using the support hand to deliver the brain stem and cerebellum from the posterior fossa without causing excessive stretching at the rostral brain stem level. The brain is pulled away from the base of the skull after cutting the lateral attachment of the tentorium to the petrous bones. The pineal body must not be left behind during this maneuver.

REMOVAL OF BRAIN IN FETUSES AND INFANTS

When the sutures are not closed and the cranial bones are still soft, Beneke's technique is used to open the cranium. The scalp is reflected as in adults. Starting at the lateral edge of the frontal fontanelle, the cranium and dura on both sides are cut with a pair of blunt scissors along the line indicated in Fig. 4-4A. (In this age group, the skull is often difficult to separate from the underlying dura in the manner described for adults.) This cut leaves a midline strip approx 1 cm wide, containing the superior sagittal sinus and the falx, and an intact area in the temporal squama on either side, which serves as a hinge when the bone flap is reflected. The older the infant, the narrower the sagittal strip will be because ossification advances toward the midline.

An alternate method of cutting, which follows the cranial suture lines, is illustrated in Fig. 4-4b and b'. With this method, fracture lines will be created along these bone flaps on their reflection; an optional cut along the posterior base of the frontal bone on either side will facilitate the procedure. The falx is then sectioned in a manner similar to that described for adults.

To minimize brain distortion during removal, several methods have been proposed *(5–9)*. In an early stage of the autopsy, fixatives such as 10% formalin in 70% alcohol can be infused through the neck arteries; this increases the consistency of the brain and facilitates its removal *(7)*. The fixative also can be injected percutaneously into the lateral ventricles, through the lateral margin of the anterior fontanelle, while the CSF fluid is allowed to exit via an intrathecal spinal needle *(5,7)*. Zamboni's fixative, which is yellow, shows whether the injection is sufficient. All these methods interfere with microbiologic examination.

In a modification of Beneke's method the skull is incised lightly along the cranial sutures and at the fontanelles *(7)*. By reversing the scalpel and passing it under the bones, the bones are separated from the underlying dura. The bone flaps are reflected after a small nick is made at the base in each of the bones. This procedure is similar to the method illustrated in Fig. 4-4 and B'. The dura is then cut as close to the base of the skull as possible. This method has the advantage of protecting the usually friable surface of the infant brain from damage during its removal. Damage to the brain can be minimized further if the

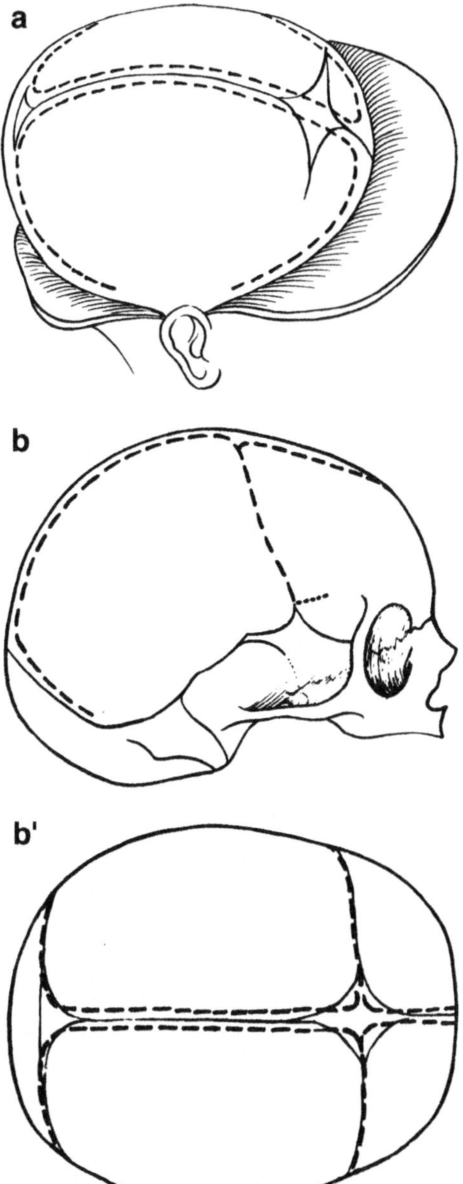

Fig. 4-4. Two methods of opening the calvarium in fetus and neonate. (a) illustrates Beneke's technique as described in text. In method shown in (b) and (b'), reflection of frontal bone flaps will result in fracture lines along their base. Optional cut may be made into posterior portion of these flaps as indicated by dots in (b).

scalp and calvarium are opened and the falx sectioned with the body in a sitting position and the infant's head being supported by an assistant. The tentorium and vein of Galen are transected in this position by gently separating the parieto-occipital lobes. After the tentorium is sectioned, the body is suspended upside down by the assistant, the brain being supported during the movement by the hand of the prosector.

The brain is cut away from the base of the skull in this upside-down position, which minimizes movement of the brain and damage to the brain substance and its surfaces. The bone flaps can be repositioned in their normal position on one side;

supporting the head with the hand on this side, the brain can be freed on the other side. This is repeated on the opposite side. The brain is not touched directly during these procedures and, when all attachments are severed, it is allowed to fall free, preferably into a body of water and not on to a hard surface.

Beneke's method of leaving the tentorium and removing the cerebral hemispheres from the brain stem and cerebellum is controversial *(9)*. We keep the brain as intact as possible at this stage but inspect the tentorium and neighboring structures during the removal procedure.

REMOVAL OF SPINAL CORD IN ADULTS

Removal of the spinal cord has been traditionally neglected by general pathologists but can be accomplished very easily within 10–15 min by the use of an oscillating saw, as described below. This should be part of every autopsy.

POSTERIOR APPROACH The body should be placed in the prone position with blocks under the shoulders. The head is rotated forward in a flexed position. Towels are placed under the face to avoid damage. A midline incision is placed over the spinous processes, muscles are resected, and bilateral laminectomies are made with the use of a saw (Fig. 4-5).

This methods allows easy exposure of the uppermost cervical spine and allows direct visualization of the craniocervical junction; it is therefore recommended in cases in which neck injuries are suspected (flexion and extension neck injuries), in cases of craniocervical instability and in special situations, for example, when an occipital encephalocele needs to be excised or *in situ* exposure of an Arnold-Chiari malformation is required. A myelomeningocele also can be removed more easily by the posterior approach. Since many morticians object to the routine use of this method, because embalming fluids tend to leak from the incision on the back, we reserve this method largely to the above mentioned special occasions. Therefore, if embalming is planned, this approach should be chosen only when strictly indicated. Posterior dissection reveals the posterior muscles of the neck, ligaments, vertebrae (spinous and transverse processes as well as the vertebral bodies), and vertebral arteries. Deep contusions with blood extravasation, injuries to ligaments, and fractures of posterior parts of vertebral bodies also are demonstrated by this method *(10)*. After the spinal cord has been removed, the spinal canal can be readily examined. With this approach, continuity between lower brainstem and upper cervical cord can be maintained, if indicated. To study sites of compression and related histologic abnormalities in the area, the cervical spinal cord and medulla may be removed inside the bony column, in continuity with the foramen magnum *(11)*. At our institution, we use a home developed device made of a simple hollow cylinder machined from steel and nickel plated for corrosion, with an arbor (for a drill) on one end and a cutting edge impregnated with natural and industrial diamond grit on the other end (Dr. EA Pfeifer, personal communication). The device, attached to an air drill, is centered around the foramen magnum and used to cut through the base of the skull and around the cervical spine. When using the adult size device, which is 3 and 3/8 inches in diameter, the transverse processes of the cervical vertebrae along with the spinal cord will slip into the cylinder undamaged.

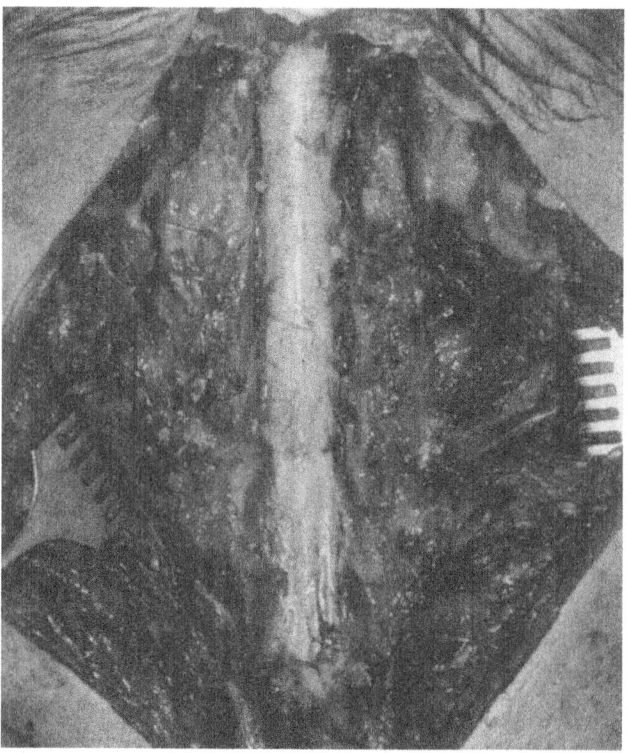

Fig. 4-5. Posterior approach to spinal cord. The spinal cord inside the dura after the removal of vertebral arches C1–C7 is shown.

Posterior dissection of the spinal cord may be limited to the upper thoracic and cervical cord or extended down to the sacral segments. However, compared with the anterior approach, this dissection method is much less suited for pursuing the course of peripheral nerves for any length in contiguity with the spinal cord.

ANTERIOR APPROACH The anterior approach is simple and quick and does not require turning the body over. It also permits removal of the spinal cord and peripheral nerves in continuity when indicated. Immediate examination of the vertebral bodies is an added advantage. We prefer not to use Kernohan's hemivertebral section method, devised as a quick anterior approach with the advantage of providing rigidity to the spinal column, since it fails to expose one side of the spinal cord *(7)* and consequently restricts removal of the spinal cord, nerve roots, and dural covering.

For complete removal of these structures, we proceed as follows. After evisceration is completed, the first cut is made across the uppermost part of the thoracic region (T-1 or T-2). The head is dropped back by removing the head support or placing a wooden block behind the back under the midthoracic region, which straightens the spinal column and facilitates the procedure. The next cut is placed on either side of the upper thoracic spine, caudal to the first, for approximately 10–15 cm along the line indicated in Fig. 4-6A. The sawing should be stopped as soon as one feels a "give," to prevent cutting into the spinal cord. Sectioning over the proximal ends of the ribs *(7)* has the advantage of creating a wider opening for the spinal

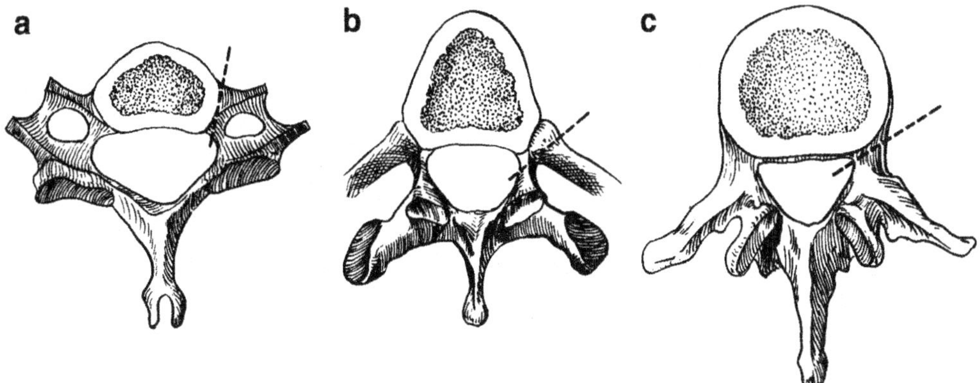

Fig. 4-6. Anterior approach to spinal cord. Dotted lines between vertebral body and arch indicate planes of saw cut adjusted to shapes of different levels of vertebral column. (a) Cervical. (b) Thoracic. (c) Lumbar.

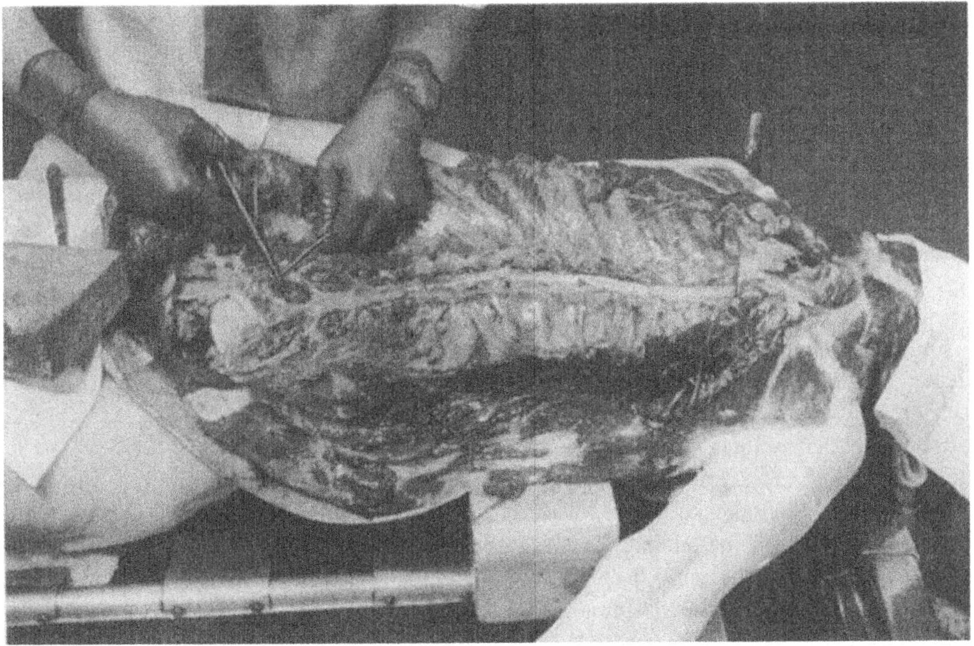

Fig. 4-7. Freeing of lumbar roots and plexus. It is convenient at this time to place a string and label around L4 or L5 root for future identification of spinal cord segments.

cord and of giving easier access to the spinal ganglia and the peripheral nerves. The freed portion of the thoracic spine readily snaps up toward the prosector, especially when the spine has been straightened as described earlier.

It is better to saw both sides of the spine for short distances, instead of one side all the way down to the lumbar area, followed by the other side. With the latter technique, one cannot be certain whether the line of cut is being placed properly. If the upper thoracic spine fails to snap up because of faulty sectioning, a remedial cut can be placed at this early stage. Grasping the freed spine with the left hand and pulling it toward the prosector makes the caudal extension of the cuts easier.

As one proceeds toward the lumbar area, the angle of the blade should be changed by adjusting to the shape of the vertebrae as illustrated in Fig. 4-6B and C. The muscles in this area should be cut away from the spine, down to the level of emerging nerves but without dividing them before sawing. Since removal of the L-5 body with the rest of the spine is often difficult because of the angulation of the spine at this level, L5 can be removed separately from the sacral bone with relative ease but first, the lumbar spine at the L4-5 interspace must be transected with a slightly curved short knife. Twisting a broad chisel in the saw tracts helps to separate the vertebral bodies away from the rest of the spine. In most instances, the cauda equina roots can be transected at either L-4 or L-5.

Freeing the rest of the cauda equina from the sacral bone is time-consuming, because it is difficult to manipulate the saw within the pelvic cavity. In rare instances, one has to cut a wedge of bone near the midline with an oscillating saw blade and remove the remaining lateral portion of the sacral bone with a rongeur to avoid damage to the nerve roots in the foramina.

The exposed portion of the spinal cord and the cauda equina encased by the dura mater are lifted away from the spinal canal with as many spinal ganglia as possible. When indicated, the spinal cord can be removed with all spinal ganglia and the nerves of the lumbar plexuses and beyond by extending the process of freeing these structures from the bony and soft-tissue encasement more peripherally (Fig. 4-7). A string with a label tied to one of the lumbar roots allows future identification.

The cervical spinal cord can be removed by Kernohan's extraction technique, without removing the cervical spine. To extract the spinal cord by *Kernohan's method*, first the dura is cut circumferentially at the exposed edge and opened longitudinally along the anterior midline below this level, second the spinal cord and dura are wrapped in a moist towel. The right hand grasps the lower portion of the spinal cord and provides a gentle, steady, caudal pull while the fingers of the left hand are placed close to the top of the exposed spinal cord to minimize angulation at this point. Although some plucking of the nerve roots (especially the posterior ones) from the cord occurs, the often expressed fear that the cord itself may be seriously damaged by this method is unfounded, based on our experience. The most frequent damage is caused by an inexperienced prosector who places the right thumb over the upper thoracic cord and proceeds to bend the cord at this level instead of pulling it caudally along the long axis. This extraction method is a compromise to encourage the routine removal of the entire length of the cord.

However, cervical spinal roots or posterior spinal ganglia cannot be obtained by this technique and therefore, when these structures must be examined, the dissection of the spine must be extended upward. The carotid arteries are pushed to the side and the cervical plexuses are exposed in the same manner as used in lumbar area. The spine is then cut along the plane shown in Fig. 4-8 on either side up to the level of C2-3 interspace, where it is transected with a scalpel blade (Fig. 4-8 upper). Alternatively, the cervical spine is simply reflected cephalad and fractured (Fig. 4-8 lower). This method should only be applied in the absence of important antemortem bony lesions in this area.

A slight lateral tilting of the blade facilitates the removal of the spinal ganglia in this region. With excessive tilting, accidental cutting of the spinal cord may occur. Another common mistake is to deviate the line of cutting toward the midline cephalad, ending up with the pointed tip. This easily results in damage to the underlying cervical cord. To facilitate the insertion of the oscillating saw blade underneath the skin flap, we have cut off the top portion of the circular blade. Adequate exposure of the neck region requires a primary chest incision from shoulder to shoulder and freeing the skin flap from the underlying muscles and connective tissue.

In order to remove the upper cervical cord and its roots from the intact bony canal one needs to approach it from the cranial cavity to free the dural attachment from the foramen magnum as high as possible. First, one makes a circular cut here. The dura is then peeled away from the bones caudad. Holding the freed dura taut with a hemostat or forceps facilitates this procedure. Usually, no special tools are required other than a pair of long scissors. On occasion, we have made use of semicircular chisels.

If the remaining portion of the spine needs to be removed, one can use a wire-saw passed through the spinal canal or a jigsaw with a long blade to complete the section. The latter instrument may injure the spinal cord, whereas the wire-saw can be used safely while the cervical cord is still in place. This will permit removal of the cervical spine in one piece. Although the upper cervical cord can be safely removed by the anterior approach, we would advocate the safer posterior approach if examination of higher cervical segments is critical.

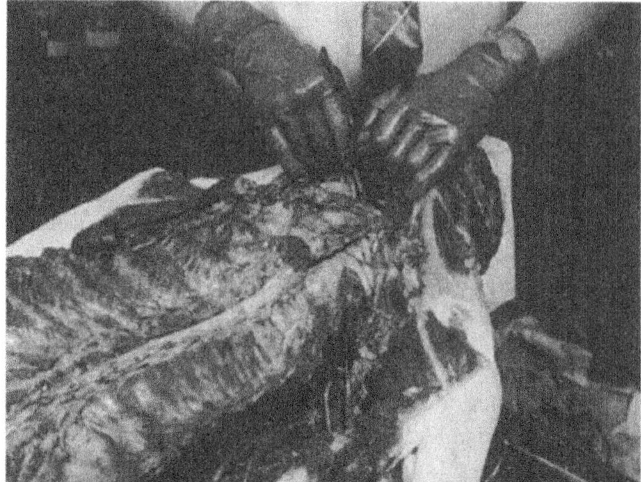

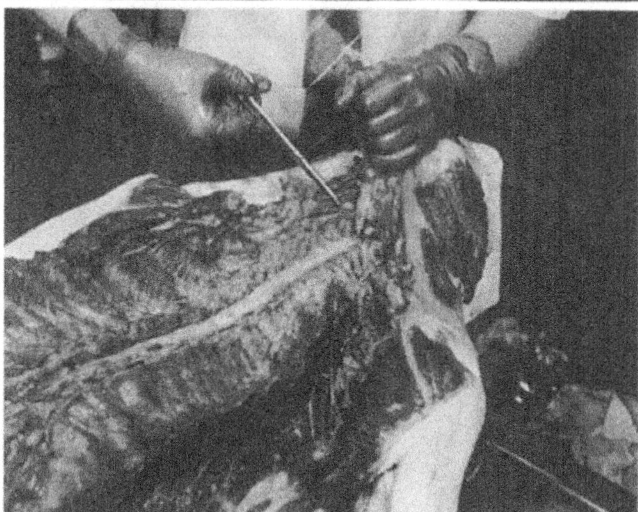

Fig. 4-8. Removal of cervical spine. Upper, scalpel blade is used to separate bone block at an intervertebral disk. Lower, bone block to be removed is reflected upward forcefully to break off at high cervical level. This method is faster, but not suitable when examination of the cervical spine (e.g., for fractures or disk protrusion) is necessary. Notice continuity of cervical roots with spinal cord.

After the cervical spine has been removed and the cervical cord exposed, the spinal cord and brain can be removed in continuity. This may be desirable in rare situations, as in the case of a tumor of the medulla and spinal cord. Of course, the usual transection at the lower medulla should not be made earlier. In this situation, it is better to expose and loosen the spinal cord completely before working on the removal of the brain *(7)*.

Finally, the posterior base of the skull also can be removed together with the cervical spine and spinal cord *(11)*. For removal of the central nervous system in toto, undisturbed within the bony cage, *see* ref. *(12)*.

REMOVAL OF SPINAL CORD IN INFANTS

ANTERIOR APPROACH The basic principle is the same as in adults. The incomplete calcification of the spinal column permits the use of a scalpel blade instead of an oscillating saw blade.

COMBINED APPROACH For complete removal of a meningocele, meningomyelocele, or other lesion related to a midline fusion defect, it is best to combine the anterior and posterior approaches. After evisceration, the body is turned over and an incision is made around the meningomyelocele or other defect to allow en bloc removal of the lesion with the entire spinal column and cord. That task can be approached either posteriorly by extending a midline incision over the spinous processes, or anteriorly. In either case, the ribs are separated from the spine and the sacral bone is cut away from the rest of the pelvic bones. A transection is made across the upper thoracic spine and the entire block is freed from soft-tissue attachments. For retaining the continuity of the cervical spine, the posterior approach obviously is the method of choice. The method can be used regardless of the position of the midline defect. A similar approach is suitable for the removal of an occipital meningocele or encephalocele. An Arnold-Chiari malformation should be exposed with its posterior aspect within the bony cavity and for this, the posterior portion of the occipital bone is cut off, followed by laminectomy of the upper cervical spine. The skull is opened in a routine fashion.

EXAMINATION AND REMOVAL OF STRUCTURES AT BASE OF THE SKULL

VENOUS SINUSES, GANGLIA, AND DURA The venous sinuses including the cavernous sinuses are opened with curved scissors after removal of the brain. The Gasserian ganglia can be removed at this time. The dura at the base of the skull should be thoroughly stripped. This procedure is essential for exposing fracture lines. Before the dura is stripped, chisel and hammer should be used with caution because they may create artifactual fractures. Removal of the cavernous sinuses with their contents may be indicated, as in a case of aneurysm of the internal carotid artery, and in such a case, the method described next for the *in situ* removal of the pituitary gland can be used.

PITUITARY GLAND The margins of the diaphragma sellae should be incised before the posterior clinoid is knocked off with a small chisel. The tip of the chisel is placed at the crest of the dorsum sellae. The chisel can be directed either posteriorly (downward) over and nearly parallel to the midline anterior fossa or nearly perpendicular to it. If the chisel is placed perpendicularly, the pituitary remains visible during the procedure but a tap is needed over the broad side of the chisel near the tip, instead of a tap on the end of it. The diaphragma must be freed first or the tension on it may result in squeezing of the tissue in the pituitary fossa. A pair of forceps is applied to the edge of the diaphragma and the pituitary is dissected out, with a sharp blade, away from the base of the fossa. The pituitary gland may be removed with its bony encasement, for example, in a case of pituitary adenoma. For this, saw cuts are made along the lines indicated in Fig. 4-9 and the entire block is lifted off the base of the skull. With normal pituitary glands, removal from the fossa becomes more difficult after fixation, because the gland enlarges and the dura adheres firmer to the sella. For histologic examination, it is best to cut the pituitary gland after fixation.

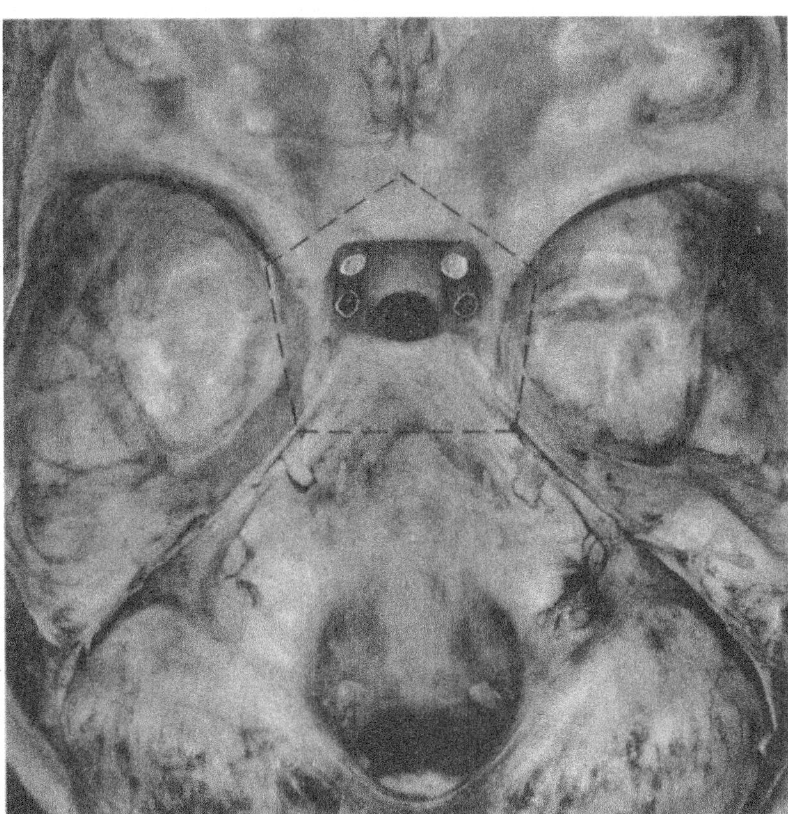

Fig. 4-9. Removal of pituitary gland with its bony encasement. Pentagonal block is cut out along the lines indicated, with saw blade directed roughly perpendicular to bone surfaces.

A method to remove the hypothalamus and the pituitary gland and its bony encasement in continuity is available also *(13)*. Should this be indicated, most of the brain is resected and only the hypothalamus and pituitary gland are left *in situ*. The block is lifted with the cavernous sinuses and posterior lining of the sella attached. For better preservation of the cerebral tissue, one can remove the frontal lobes, along the coronal plane at the level of the lamina terminalis, and free the pituitary from the pituitary fossa by sharp dissection and, if necessary, with use of a small rongeur to chip some of the bones. The remainder of the brain is removed as usual.

PARANASAL SINUSES AND NASOPHARYNX

Various paranasal sinuses can be entered intracranially for inspection or removal of specimens for histologic observation. The ethmoid sinuses can be approached by breaking the cribriform plate with a chisel and mallet. Continued chiseling leads into the maxillary sinuses. The frontal sinuses are entered by chiseling away their posterior walls close to the midline. The sphenoidal sinuses can be inspected after the anterior wall and the floor of the pituitary fossa have been exposed. If the block of bone containing the pituitary fossa is removed (Fig. 4-9) with an oscillating saw, the sphenoidal sinuses are exposed even better. The nasopharynx and the throat can be entered by extending this dissection. For an excellent review of nasopharyngeal dissection methods, *see* ref. *(14)*. More recently, en bloc resection of all ENT-relevant organs without disfiguring the body has been described *(15)*.

EAR

Even when there is no indication for removing the auditory and vestibular apparatus in one piece, it is still a good practice to look into the middle and inner ear, particularly in the presence of an inflammatory process within the cranial cavity. This can be done simply by the use of a large rongeur over the posterolateral portion of the petrous ridge. A primary focus of infection may be found within the ear structures. When total removal of the ears is indicated, we apply the method described in the pamphlet from the Temporal Bone Bank *(16)*. The use of an oscillating saw facilitates the procedure.

The cut is made along the lines indicated in Fig. 4-10. The block of bone thus sectioned is lifted with a bone-holding forceps, and the connective tissue bands anchoring the block are cut with curved scissors. When the temporal bone is freed, chisel and hammer should be used with caution. The internal carotid artery stump should be ligated or, simpler still, plugged with clay to help the embalmer. Alternatively, a bone-plug cutter attached to the vibrating saw (Fig. 4-10) can be used. The Temporal Bone Bank recommends the use of 20% formalin

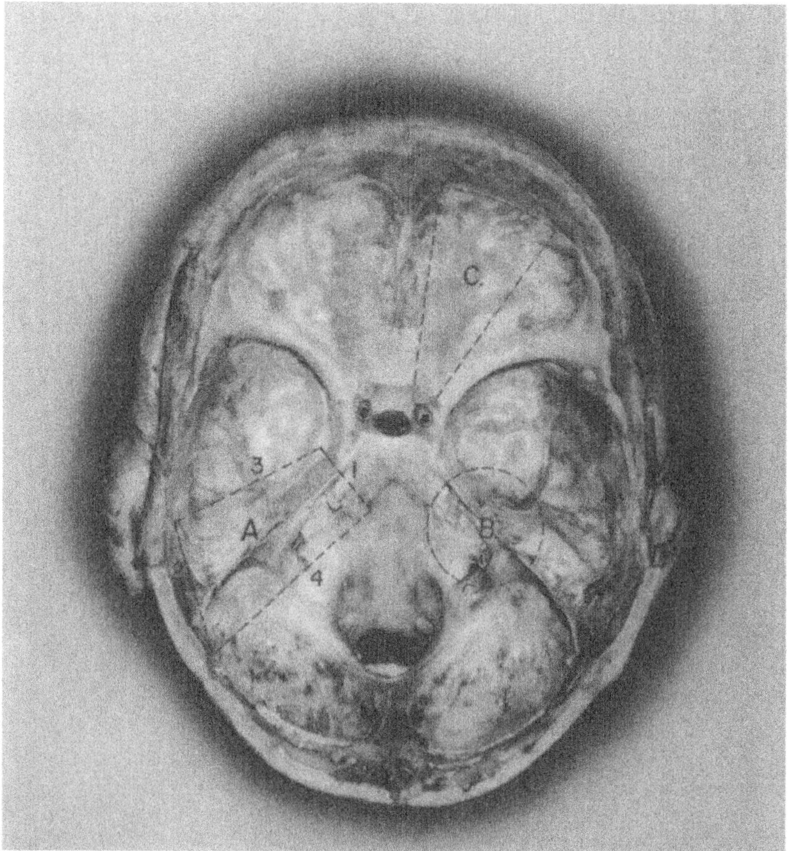

Fig. 4-10. Removal of inner and middle ear and eye. (A) line 1 is placed near the apex of petrous bone as possible, roughly at right angle to superior edge of petrous bone. Line 2 is over mastoid region, as close to lateral wall as possible. Line 3 is placed, with blade held vertical to floor. (B) Circle indicates block to be removed with bone-plug cutter. (C) Dotted line indicates area of bone removal to approach orbital content intracranially.

solution, approximately 400 mL, for fixation in a refrigerator for 1 d and fresh 10% formalin solution daily for two additional days. Refrigerated specimens can be saved indefinitely. Following a short decalcification, the specimen can be sliced and processed for light microscopy *(17)*.

FIXATION

The best routine fixative that allows the widest choice of stains for the nervous tissue is formalin, usually as a 10% solution (*see* Chapter 14). In fetuses and infants, the addition of acetic acid to the fixative solution appears to be helpful. Acetic acid increases the specific gravity of the fixative and allows the brain to float in the solution; it also makes the tissue firmer without altering its histologic characteristics *(18)*.

IMMERSION METHODS For detailed anatomic studies of the nervous system it is best to fix the specimen, with a minimum of prior handling, in a large amount of freshly prepared 10% formalin solution. We use plastic buckets that hold 8 L. These are readily available at local stores at a considerably lower price than traditional glass or earthenware jars, which also are heavier and break more easily. We suspend the brain to prevent distortion during fixation by passing a thread underneath the basilar artery in front of the pons. Inevitably, the vessel is slightly pulled away from the brain substance. If this is undesirable, as in the case of pontine infarcts or other lesions in this region, a thread can be passed under the internal carotid or middle cerebral arteries on both sides, provided that no pathologic lesions are suspected in these regions.

Alternatively, the dorsal dura can be used as an anchoring point. A thread is passed through the short dural flaps on either side of the falx, and the brain is suspended right-side-up. However, a minor pull may deform the parasagittal brain tissue and cause an abnormally pointed dorsal midline surface of the brain. Generally, suspension from blood vessels deforms the parenchyma less than dural suspension. In rare instances, we suspend the brain upside down with a pair of threads tied to the edge of the entire dorsal dural flap on either side. With all these methods, the ends of the thread(s) are tied to the attachments of the bucket handle, care being taken not to allow the specimen to touch the bottom or sides of the bucket. Another safe method makes use of the plastic brain support described below for perfusion. Placing several holes in the dome-shaped receptacle will ensure proper fixation of the contact surface of the brain.

We do not recommend any method based on tying a thread around any portion of the brain substance, such as the stump of the medulla or the midbrain, nor do we recommend sectioning of the corpus callosum for alleged improved entry of fixative into the ventricles.

Formalin solution should be replaced within the first 24 h, but this not mandatory if a large amount of fixative is used. If the fixative becomes very bloody, prompt replacement with fresh solution is indicated; this also prevents undue discoloration of the specimen.

Approximately 10 to 14 days are required for satisfactory fixation. If the brain is dissected earlier, the central portion may still be pink, even though the consistency may be satisfactory.

PERFUSION METHODS The brain can be perfused with fixative through the arterial stumps before further fixation by immersion, as described earlier. This shortens the fixation time and ensures adequate fixation of deeper portions of the brain. When it is necessary to dissect the brain at the time of autopsy, this preliminary fixation method makes the tissue firmer and thus facilitates the dissection and decreases the surface wrinkling and tissue warping that are inevitable under these circumstances.

Large volumes of formalin (for example, 1,000 mL) improve fixation but with too much fixative, large lakes of fluid may accumulate, particularly in the areas weakened by a pathologic process (e.g., infarct, hemorrhage, metastasis), and the specimen may become asymmetric because of uneven perfusion. Even without these gross distortions, excessive volumes of fixative may produce annoying perivascular zones of tissue rarefaction microscopically, in addition to artifactual dilatation of small blood vessels. Obstructing emboli or thrombi also might be obscured. The weight changes induced by perfusion fixation are described in Part III of this book. Injection of 150 mL of isotonic saline followed by 150 mL of 10% formalin solution causes the least problems *(19)*. This can be done manually with a syringe connected to a simple tubing system *(7)*. For easy handling and better preservation of the contour of the specimen, we use a plastic holder during the procedure. Satisfactory fixation for dissection can be obtained in 7 d to 10 d. However, earlier dissection may be possible if one can tolerate some degree of incomplete fixation, which is manifested mainly by central areas of softness and pink coloration. For perfusion of a large amount of fixative, an embalmer's pump may be used. For a simple gravity-feed method, one may use an infusion bottle raised 150 cm to 180 cm above the specimen.

DISSECTION OF BRAIN AND SPINAL CORD

Brain weight in the fresh and fixed state should be recorded. It is not necessary to use a very large knife to dissect the brain. We prefer a single-blade autopsy knife about 25 cm long and 2 cm wide.

DISSECTION OF FRESH BRAIN IN ADULTS The most accurate examination of brain in terms of recognition of lesions and correlation of their topography with clinical symptoms and images generated by computerized trans-axial tomography (CT) or magnetic resonance imaging (MRI) techniques can be achieved only when the brain is sectioned after adequate fixation *(20–22)*. At times, however, the fresh brain must be dissected, particularly when microbiologic and chemical investigations are of prime importance or when an immediate diagnosis is needed (this speed unfailingly leads to distortion of the cut surface during subsequent fixation). As a compromise, we limit fresh dissection to three or four coronal cuts through the cerebral hemispheres, leaving more complicated anatomic structures such as the basal ganglia and upper brain stem (thalamus and midbrain) as undisturbed as the circumstances permit. This preliminary dissection usually reveals the presence of large lesions, directly or indirectly, by showing distortion of the ventricular system or other anatomic landmarks.

Further judiciously selected sections may be made into the primary slices of the brain tissue to expose the suspected hidden lesions. The central portion of the cerebral hemispheres is left connected with the brain stem, and this block is suspended by a string, as described earlier. It may be necessary to sever the brain stem and cut into the infratentorial structures; one horizontal cut through these structures usually suffices for preliminary examination. Even with several cuts, one should not be satisfied solely with fresh dissection of the brain because many small lesions are easily missed and subtle lesions such as an early infarct, small or large, can be overlooked. Every brain should be reexamined with new dissection after adequate fixation.

Preliminary perfusion or cooling of the brain in a refrigerator for about 30 min, preferably in a contoured support as described earlier, makes the brain firmer and dissection easier. If diffuse, roughly symmetric lesions are expected, as in lipidoses, "degenerative diseases," "demyelinating" disorders, other inborn or acquired toxic-metabolic diseases, or widespread infectious conditions, the brain may be bisected along the sagittal plane, one half being further sectioned and submitted for chemical or microbiologic investigations while the other half is retained for later sectioning and histologic examination. This latter half must be fixed either by suspension or by letting it lie on its midsagittal plane to avoid undesirable distortions.

Dissection of fresh brain (according to the aforementioned procedure) may be required by brain-banking protocols or specific research protocols (e.g., Alzheimer's disease), in order to provide adequate material for histological, immunocytochemical, biochemical, and molecular biology studies. References *(23)* and *(24)* provide a general overview regarding procedures involved in "brain banking."

We find no use for the classical *Virchow method* of fresh dissection. Any brain subjected to this method would look, after adequate fixation, like a book immersed in water and subsequently dried.

DISSECTION OF FRESH BRAIN IN FETUSES AND INFANTS Without an overriding need to secure unfixed samples for chemical or microbiologic examination, fetal and infantile brains are best kept intact until after proper fixation, because of their pronounced softness and ease of bruising. Our method is essentially similar to that described for adult brains. To increase consistency to fetal or infantile brains, we use as fixative 20% formalin solution containing 1% glacial acetic acid. No additional measures such as one or two changes of alcohol are needed.

DISSECTION OF FIXED BRAIN After a careful inspection of the external surface of the brain, the arteries at the base of the brain may be exposed through tears made into the arachnoid membrane and followed for a short distance distally to check for pathologic conditions such as thrombosis, embolism, or aneurysm. This procedure should be omitted when pathologic processes in this region may be disturbed. Routine removal of the arterial tree from the brain substance has no merit in a thorough pathologic examination because this separates vascular lesions from the resulting areas of parenchymal damage.

After adequate external examination, the brain stem and the cerebellum are separated from the cerebral hemispheres. In rare instances, it is better to retain this continuity, for example, for display of the distorting effect of a supratentorial lesion on the brain stem. It is essential to section through the midbrain along a flat surface perpendicular to the neuroaxis. For this purpose, with the brain placed upside down, the cerebellum should be held between the index finger of the one hand with the tip in proximity of the pineal gland and the thumb on the inferior surface of cerebellum (Fig. 4-11). With the scalpel in a pen-holding position, the cutting hand rests on the ventral aspect of the frontal lobes to provide the proper angle. The blade is held toward the prosector with its tip in front of the distant cerebral peduncle a few millimeters above the tip of the mammillary body. The blade enters the midbrain in the midline, aiming toward the pineal gland until the scalpel barely passes through the thickness of the brainstem; the blade is then brought toward the prosector (resulting in sectioning through half of the midbrain). The scalpel is now flipped over and moved forward along the same

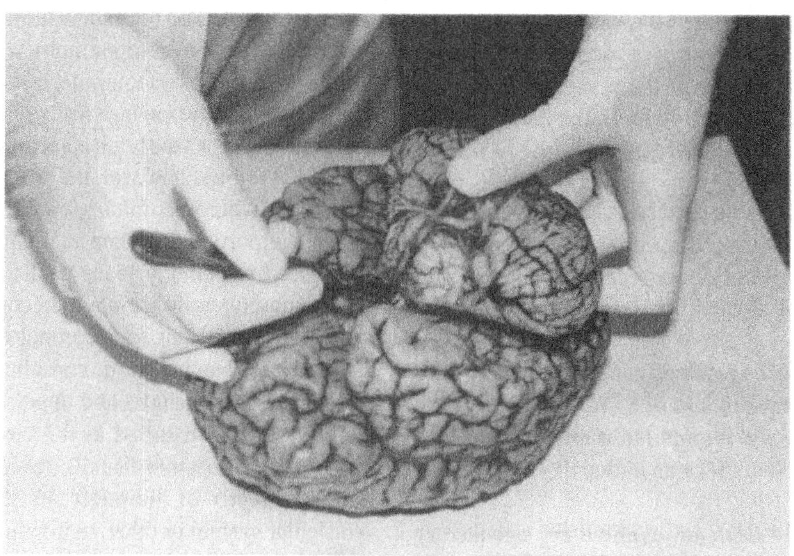

Fig. 4-11. Sectioning brain stem at midbrain level.

plane cutting the other half of the midbrain. A gentle pull with the holding hand on the brain stem and cerebellum during the procedure helps to complete the sectioning. Placing a knife over the temporal lobe and cutting the midbrain from the side should be avoided since this will result in a roof-shaped midbrain, making impossible its complete cross-sectional representation on histologic slides.

Attempts to sever the midbrain too rostrally often result in an uneven or incomplete cut because the cerebral peduncles widen rapidly in the rostral portion. In order to avoid this, one may place a preliminary section close to the pontomesencephalic junction; then, under direct visualization, a parallel slice of the midbrain can be removed more rostrally.

Coronal sectioning of the cerebral hemispheres is the most common and safest method for any contingencies. We prefer free cuts, without use of a cutting apparatus. Before sectioning, the central sulci should be marked by carefully cutting, with the tip of a scalpel blade, into the leptomeninges bridging over them, without injuring the underlying brain substance. This gives a valuable point of reference on multiple coronal sections.

As an initial step we hold the brain on its convexity with the orbital lobes and occipital poles in an horizontal plane. The first section is made through the mammillary bodies and cut surfaces are examined for symmetry (Fig. 4-12a). Attempts to slice with a single motion of the knife often exerts undue pressure toward the cutting board, which may squash or tear various structures, while the vessels are dragged into the softer brain tissue. Multiple slicing excursions without undue downward pressure produce a clean-cut surface more effectively. The knife handle should be held lightly, as this will facilitate smooth gliding movements of the blade. A firm grip tends to cause knife marks on the surfaces of brain slices.

Alternatively, the first cut can be made just in front of the temporal poles, exposing the anterior ventricular horns. This may be important in cases of hydrocephalus, in which this view may disclose an obstruction of the foramen of Monro (e.g., by a colloid cyst or a third ventricular tumor) and still allow a change in sectioning technique to better demonstrate the obtruction *(25)*.

Brain slices should be approximately 1 cm thick. We like to section the halved brain pieces by holding them down on the cut surface and by moving the knife side to side from the inferior surface of the brain toward the convexity (Fig. 4-12 b,c). A slicing guide (below) can be used for particularly delicate specimens. It is also important to examine each new cut surface before the next slice is made so that any necessary adjustment can be made in the next plane of section. The slices are displayed on a board, with the right side of the specimen on the left side of the prosector. Although the classical pathologists' approach to the brain corresponded to viewing one's own brain from behind (and therefore, right side of the specimen on the right side of the prosector), we prefer the frontal view because of current neuroimaging practice, which is similar to that of the physician who sees the living patient face to face. A large cutting board is needed because slices should not overlap. Sufficient space for display is mandatory for adequate examination of the brain.

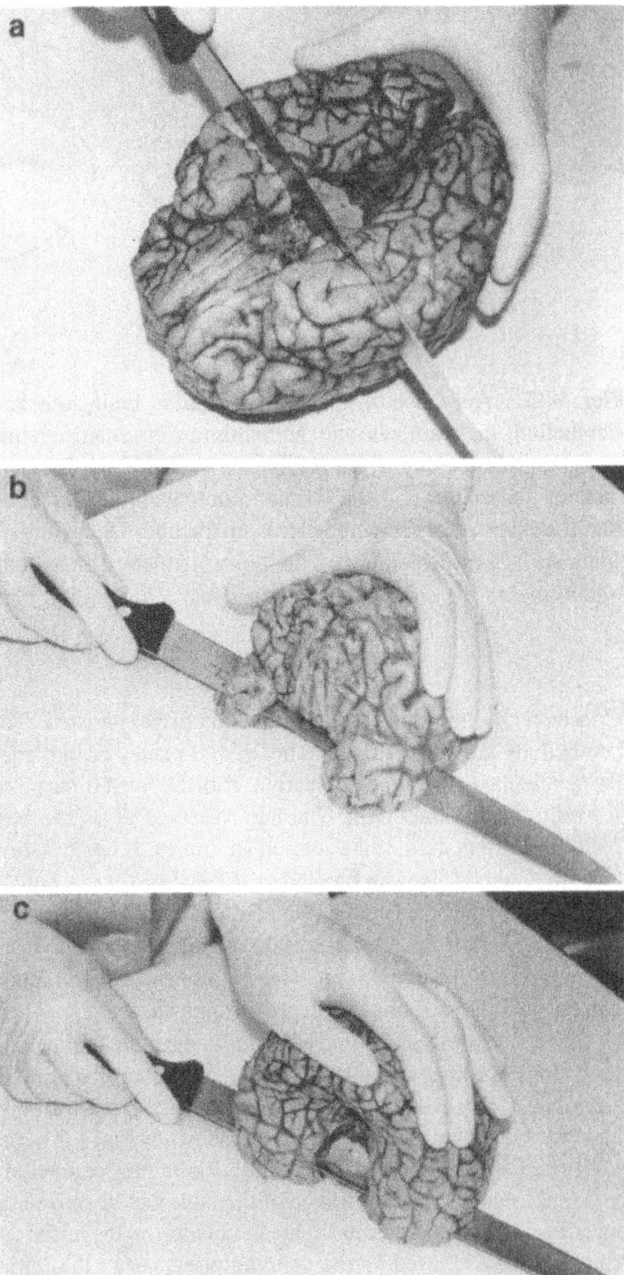

Fig. 4-12. Sectioning of cerebral hemispheres. (a) initial cut is placed through mammillary bodies. (b,c) the halved brain pieces are held down on the cutting board and sliced from the inferior surface toward the convexity. Cloth or paper towels under the brain will prevent the board surface becoming slippery from fluid dripping from the brain. When slicing cerebral hemispheres in this fashion, the "limp" optic nerves need to be propped up to avoid cutting them longitudinally.

Several different approaches can be used in routine dissection of the brain stem and cerebellum (Fig. 4-13). The brain stem is best sectioned perpendicular to its axis, which is slightly curved.

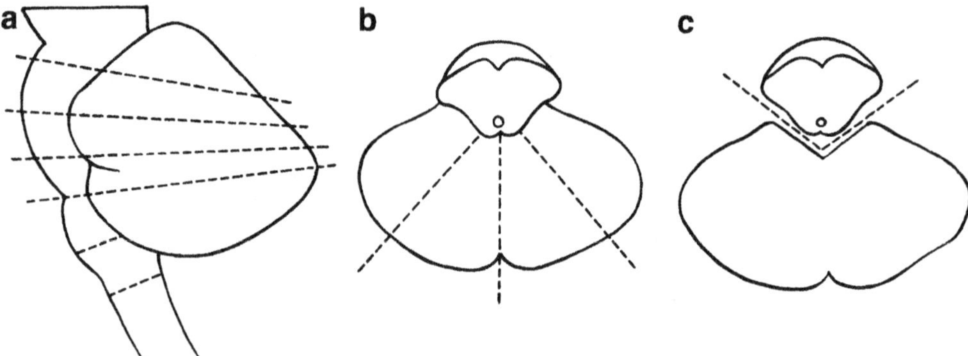

Fig. 4-13. Approach to routine dissection of brain stem and cerebellum. (a) Brain stem and cerebellum are dissected together by series of cuts roughly perpendicular to neuroaxis. For consistency, base line is made through pontomedullary junction and posterior ridges of cerebellar hemispheres. This will give a flat surface on which to rest the brain stem and cerebellum, which makes the subsequent sections easy. (b) Midline incision is made in vermis, and wedge of tissue is removed from each cerebellar hemisphere. Hemispheres are further sectioned through vertical planes perpendicular to external lines of cerebellar cortex. Brain stem and rest of cerebellum are sectioned as in (a). (c) Cerebellum is separated from brain stem. Latter is sectioned as in (a). Cerebellum is sectioned either horizontally or vertically as in (b).

Consequently, the planes of section should be adjusted. The cerebellum can be sectioned in horizontal planes or in planes perpendicular to the folial orientation, with the converging point in front of the cerebellum. The latter method gives the best histologic orientation of the cortical structures. A combination of both methods also can be used.

Display of the brain stem and cerebellum should be consistent with the principle used for the cerebral hemispheres. There are two options to achieve this end (*see* below) and either method can be suitably used under different circumstances.

Since the advent of CT and MRI, sections of the brain along the planes of tomography have become important for clinicopathologic correlation *(26)*. For this purpose, we use a simply constructed device made of plexiglass, shown in Fig. 4-14. The table (Fig. 4-14A) has a small opening to admit the cerebellum and brain stem. The guide on top of the table can be moved up and down so that the most desirable inclination on the initial cut can be selected, based on the imaging prints. After the initial cut (Fig. 4-14B), the halved brain pieces are sectioned serially on the board (Fig. 4-14C), which has 10-mm guides on its edge. Guides half as tall as these can be attached on the other side of the board. The display slices should correspond to the printed CT images.

We consider the coronal sectioning of the cerebral hemispheres and the horizontal sectioning of the brain stem and cerebellum the best routine method for the brain in that the slices obtained will display most advantageously the pattern of vascular supplies and the relationship of the internal structures. This holds true even in the absence of corresponding neuroimages.

DISSECTION OF SPINAL CORD For routine examination, after the dura has been opened along the anterior midline and the cord surface has been examined, series of cross-sections are prepared. Marking the right side of the cord with India ink may help later when segmental and long pathway pathology need to be reconstructed. The dura should be left attached to the cord to keep the sectioned spinal cord and roots together. This allows to orient roots for cross sections during embedding. When specific radicular level involvement has been reported premortem, the involved roots should be identified and processed separately (*see* "Peripheral Nerves"). With a sharp scalpel blade, the spinal cord is sectioned approx at 1-cm intervals. Occasionally, longitudinal sections can be made to emphasize the rostral-caudal extent of the lesion, such as in traumatic contusion. However, it is often difficult to get a straight plane of section. In most instances, the cross-sectional extent of the lesion at any given segmental level is more important for understanding clinical symptoms. A combination of the two methods may be used by taking a cross-sectional slice at the point of maximal damage and slicing the rest longitudinally along the frontal plane. Of course, unorthodox and creative sectioning may, in rare instances, display some lesions at their best.

SELECTION OF TISSUE BLOCKS FOR HISTOLOGIC EXAMINATION

BRAIN AND SPINAL CORD When the lesions in the brain are obvious, selection of the appropriate blocks is simple. For orientation and for possible evidence of pathologic involvement, some recognizable structures from the surrounding and presumably normal areas should be included. When gross lesions cannot be found despite the presence of clinical neurologic signs or symptoms, one must be familiar with the topographic distribution of the lesions expected in a given disease or syndrome to be able to select appropriate sections. Familiarity with the patient's clinical history must be accompanied by some basic knowledge of where the lesions are to be expected.

It is difficult to define what constitutes adequate selection of sections in "routine normal cases." No universally accepted standards exist, but whatever choices are made, selections should be consistent topographically. The areas shown in Fig. 4-15 are our minimal requirements; the reasons for this selection are given in the legend. Standardized specific research protocols

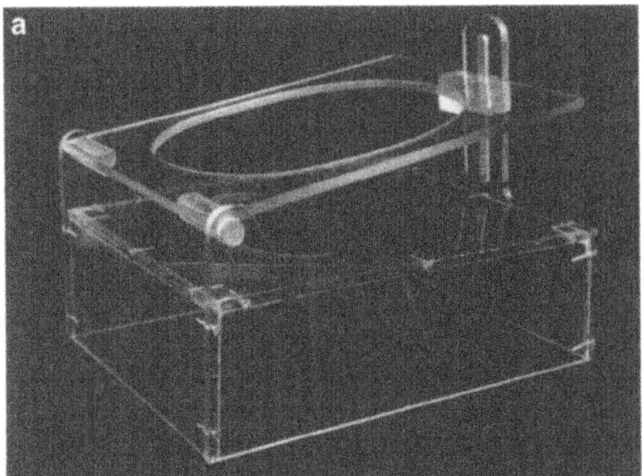

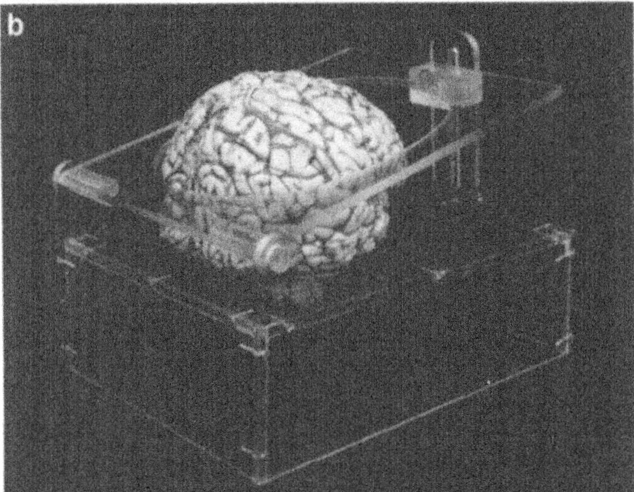

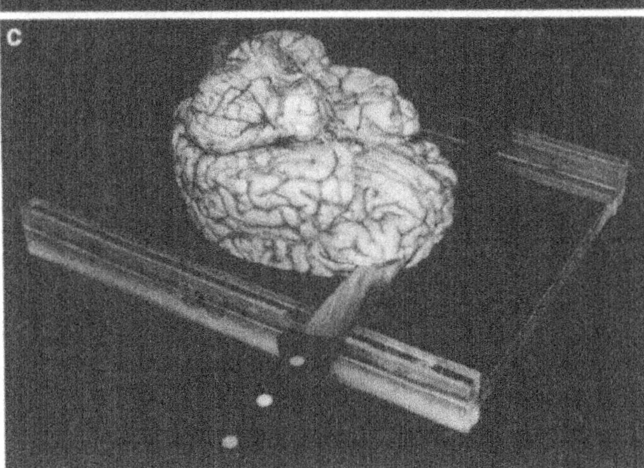

Fig. 4-14. Device for sectioning brain along planes of tomography. (a) Plexiglass table with opening for cerebellum and brain stem and movable guide. (b) Brain in position for initial cut. (c) Halved brain positioned on board for serial sectioning.

in order to provide adequate histological sampling for neurodegenerative diseases (e.g., Alzheimer's disease) are available *(27, 28)*. Reference *(29)* provides useful general guidelines to the postmortem sampling of the brain and other tissues in a variety of neurodegenerative disorders. It is best to store the whole brain until the microscopic examination is completed and the clinicopathologic correlation is satisfied.

In most cases, the size of the sections can be limited so as to fit in the standard plastic cassettes and applied to the 1- by 3-inch glass slides. For larger sections, such as a full cross section of pons, larger metal cassettes and glass slides are used. We try not to "mutilate" the original brain slices and therefore, if photographs are taken of cross-sectional surfaces, we select tissue blocks from the same surface of the adjoining slice so that photography can be repeated. Alternatively, the brain slab can be sliced thinly up to the area of block removal while the knife blade protects the lower half of the slab and vertical cuts are made into the upper slab. Experienced prosectors can prepare complete thin slices and lay them on the cutting board before blocks are removed. It is not a good practice to hold a thick slab in the hand and to try to undercut a centrally located block through one of the vertical cuts, as this will invariably result in an uneven "dig" into the remaining tissue.

In the absence of known *spinal cord* abnormalities, one section each from the cervical, thoracic, and lumbosacral levels is appropriate. When spinal cord lesions are expected, pathologists should attempt to localize the "radicular-segmental" or "vertebral body" level of the lesion. Keeping in mind that the conus medullaris generally ends at the level of the upper part of the L2 vertebral body, the L1 and L2 dural root exits can be localized. Cephalad from this point, spinal cord roots and vertebral body levels can be counted. For correct localization of the levels, the dural sac and the exit zones must be intact (*see* "Removal of spinal cord" and "Dissection of the spinal cord").

PERIPHERAL NERVES The cervical and lumbar plexuses can be removed totally and in continuity with the spinal roots and ganglia, as outlined for removal of the spinal cord. As a routine procedure, this is too time-consuming.

A quicker method is to cut the nerves as they emerge from the intervertebral foramina and to sample selected nerves as the clinical signs dictate. Routinely, lengths of the sciatic and femoral nerves or any other portions of the lumbosacral plexuses proximal to their exits from the pelvic and abdominal cavities can easily be removed without creating new incisions. Similarly, sampling of the brachial plexuses and their distal extensions can be achieved from the supraclavicular axillary regions. Care should be exercised to preserve the brachial arteries for embalming.

In cases in which detailed clinical studies were performed on the peripheral nervous system, the affected nerves should be sampled at autopsy. When incisions are made in the extremities for sampling of muscles, as described in the next section, the nerves innervating them can be removed conveniently. In a diffuse neuropathic condition, one may select the sciatic nerve and its distal ramifications for detailed studies. To this end, the body is turned over and an incision is made in the back of the thigh to free the sciatic nerve, which has been severed previously at its pelvic exit. The incision may be extended caudally to allow the removal of the peroneal and tibial nerves in the leg. More conservatively, a 15-cm longitudinal incision in the popliteal region exposes these nerves at their bifurcation. The arteries in the vicinity must not be lacerated, as this would interfere with the embalming procedure. To assist the embalmer, we have also

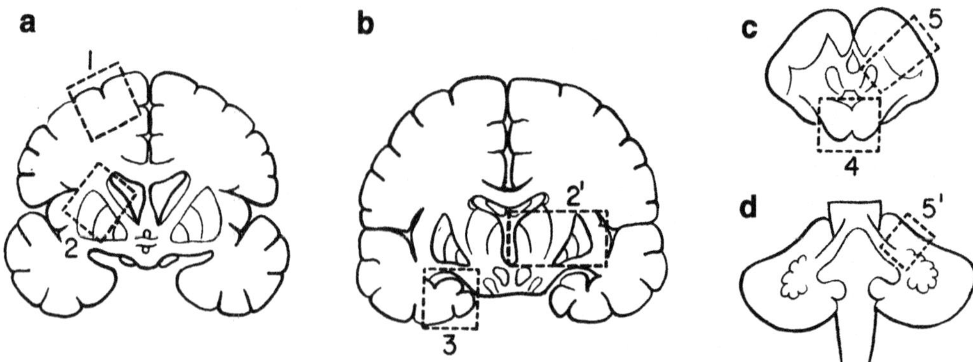

Fig. 4-15. Selection of tissue blocks. (a) 1 = superior and middle frontal gyri. This is an arterial border ("water-shed") zone most likely to harbor small ischemic lesions. This also may reveal atrophic or "senile" changes such as senile plaques or neurofibrillary tangles. 2 = basal ganglia. Vascular changes and their effects on parenchyma are likely to be found here, as are other "degenerative changes." (b) 2' = basal ganglia together with thalamus. 3 = hippocampus and adjacent neocortex. This is often a sensitive indicator of anoxic-ischemic changes. Neurofibrillary tangles, neuritic plaques, and the "aging" changes make their first appearance here. (c,d) 4 = pons. Vascular (particularly small arterial) changes are found more frequently here than in other portions of brain stem. 5 and 5' = cerebellum. Ischemic and toxic metabolic conditions are often reflected in cerebellar cortex.

removed the sciatic nerve by incising the anterior surface of the thigh and leg. Sawing away a portion of the pelvic bone (mainly the ischium) helps to free the nerve without pulling it up or down behind the bone. This approach is cumbersome, but a bonus is the easy removal of the femoral nerve and its branches.

One of the most accessible peripheral nerves is the sural nerve, which has been biopsied in many clinical studies. Therefore, its removal at autopsy through a small incision behind the lateral malleolus gives an excellent base for comparison. For removal and fixation techniques, *see* ref. *(30)*. A useful adjunct to diagnostic studies of the peripheral nervous system is a fiber-teasing method that has become a standard procedure in many research laboratories. After fixation, a portion of nerve is stained with 1% osmium tetroxide and macerated in 60% glycerol, and individual fibers are teased out under a dissecting microscope. This method allows to examine fibers three dimensionally and to evaluate axonal degeneration and demyelination *(30)*. For best preservation of these nerves, autopsies should done within 6 h after death.

SKELETAL MUSCLE In the absence of specific diseases affecting the neuromuscular system, skeletal muscle is rarely sampled. One or two specimens should be stored in the "routine" autopsy. The ileopsoas muscle is easily accessible and shows the effects of general systemic disease on the skeletal muscles.

In cases of known or suspected neuromuscular diseases, more extensive sampling is required. For primary myopathies, the selection has to be based on clinical findings and the status of the muscles at the time of autopsy. Sections should be taken from muscles that are severely affected, that show early but active involvement, and that are grossly uninvolved. A list of muscles to be sampled in cases of neurogenic muscle atrophy is shown in ref. *(31)*. Table 4-1 lists muscles that are accessible without major procedures and will give an adequate diagnostic sampling.

The specimens should be cleanly excised or neatly trimmed to about 3.0 × 1.0 × 0.5 cm. Placing the samples on a piece of cardboard does not completely prevent shrinkage of the tissue during fixation. A corkboard with two narrow strips of cork fastened to it provides ridges to which multiple muscle samples can be pinned. This eliminates the problem of poor fixation of the underside of the specimens. Parts of wooden applicator stick may be used to support smaller pieces of muscle, which are tied to it with suture material at both ends. We consider 10% neutral formalin solution

Table 4-1
Suggested Muscles for Sampling at Autopsy

Muscle	*Comment*
Extraocular muscles	Obtained through orbital plate intracranially or anteriorly with or without the globe.
Tongue	Removed with pharynx and larynx; small pieces can be removed through mouth.
Sternocleidomastoid; pectoralis diaphragm; major	No new incision required; pectoralis major is preferred over deltoid because previous intramuscular injection into deltoid may have caused abnormalities.
Biceps; triceps	Removed through incision in axillary aspect of upper arm or by subcutaneous extension of primary incision into arm.
Forearm muscles	Morticians generally consider skin incision on the forearm undesirable, particularly in females. Incision in ulnar side of palmar aspect of forearm is least objectionable.
Intercostal; psoas major	No new incision required.
Quadriceps	Removed through incision in ventral aspect of thigh.
Anterior tibialis; gastrocnemius	Removed through incision in lateral aspect of lower leg

the most satisfactory all-purpose fixative, particularly if staining of the nervous tissue elements in the specimen is important. Additional pieces can be fixed in Bouin's solution to improve trichrome stains; fresh-frozen cryostat sections can be prepared for Gomori's trichrome stain and for staining with hematoxylin and eosin, after 2 min fixation in 10% formalin solution on a cover slip (Engel AG, personal communication).

Teasing the removed specimens lengthwise after fixation, rather than cutting with a knife blade, sometimes produces a better longitudinal arrangement of the muscle on histologic slides. As with peripheral nerves, both cross and longitudinal aspects of the muscle should be represented.

SPECIAL TECHNIQUES

ARTERIOGRAPHY Adequate examination of the extracranial portions of the cerebral arteries is important. The simplest method consists of injecting water through the proximal stumps to test patency. This test is conclusive only when vessels are completely occluded; luminal narrowing cannot be appreciated by this method.

Many postmortem angiographic studies of cerebral arteries have been described *(31-34)*. We remove the neck vessels in most instances and thus, angiographic studies are not performed routinely. When indications for them do arise, to opacify the intracranial cerebral arteries, we prefer to inject them after removal of the brain, so that the lesions can be inspected first. We routinely use a barium sulfate-gelatin mixture (Chapter 2), with or without addition of red or blue dye. When a cerebral aneurysm or vascular malformation is suspected but not immediately visualized by external inspection and careful flushing of the blood from the basal subarachnoid space, we prefer to inject the opacifying material before attempting to "dig out" the lesion. Successful roentgenographic demonstration (Fig. 4-16) obviates excessive "picking" of the brain substance. After roentgenographic demonstration of these lesions, the brain is best left intact until fixation is completed. Postmortem angiography is also useful in cases of surgically treated vascular lesions, for example, clipping of an aneurysm. Angiography shows whether the vascular system is patent, that is, whether contrast medium appears beyond the site of clipping.

Postmortem angiogram can be performed before removal of the brain. We carefully clamp the external carotid arteries and inject 5–10 mL of warm barium sulfate-gelatin mixture into the common carotid arteries and roentgenograms are made in the autopsy room. In a similar fashion, the vertebral arteries can be injected at their origins. Injection from the intracranial stumps of the internal carotid arteries also has been described *(32)*. We have injected a 40% solution of potassium iodide in Karo corn syrup, approximately at systolic pressure. The contrast medium temporarily distends the injected vessels and then dissipates rapidly, which does not interfere with satisfactory embalming of the face and with proper evaluation of the arteries and brains by the pathologist.

VENOGRAPHY Injection of the venous system *in situ* or after removal of the brain appears to have little diagnostic use, although it provides background information for neuroradiologists who study the deep cerebral venous system in order to localize lesions. Radiopaque material is injected into the straight sinus or vein of Galen, preferably through a burr hole, before the brain is removed from the cranial cavity. The external venous system of various cranial sinuses and the superficial cerebral veins can be examined directly.

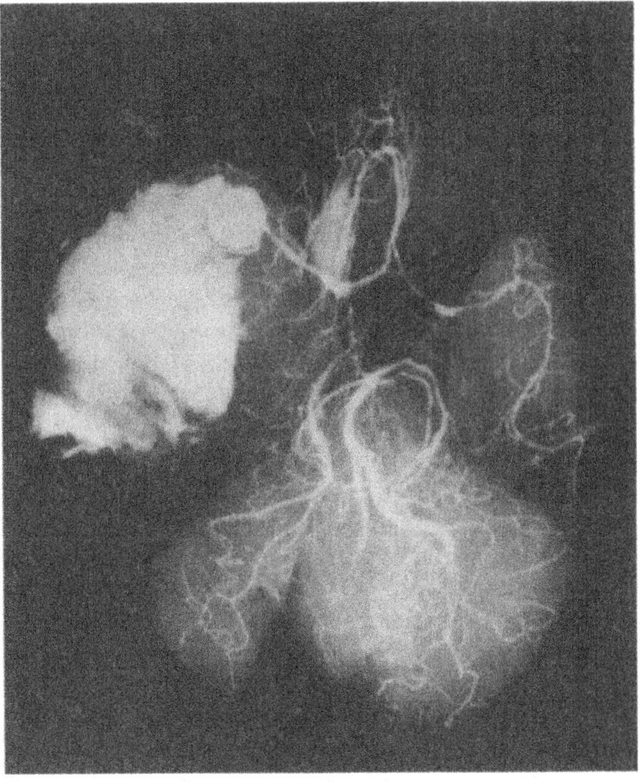

Fig. 4-16. Postmortem angiography. Usefulness of the method is demonstrated by this case in which large temporal lobe hematoma is associated with ruptured saccular aneurysm of right middle cerebral artery at "trifurcation".

VENTRICULOGRAPHY Outlining the ventricular system of the brain by injection of various materials has been attempted in the past mostly for preparation of anatomic specimens. Because pneumoencephalography and ventriculography are of historical interest only, these casting methods have ceased to be of interest for diagnostic neuropathology. For the technique of making casts, *see* ref. *(35)*.

REMOVAL OF NECK VESSELS For fear of interfering with subsequent embalming, neck vessels are rarely removed completely in the United States. We remove the neck organs and arteries after the embalming procedure, which is performed by private morticians in rooms adjoining the autopsy room. In some institutions, the common and internal carotid arteries are removed from the neck and a small rubber or plastic catheter is placed in the proximal external carotid artery for subsequent embalming at funeral homes *(33)*.

After the primary incision, the skin flap is reflected over the face while subcutaneous tissue is severed by blunt dissection with scissors. Keeping the neck straight or slightly overextended facilitates the approach to the arteries. The common carotid arteries are followed upward by blunt dissection, with occasional snips of scissors, up to the bifurcation. Then, the external and internal carotid arteries are isolated and the dissection is continued along the latter up to as close to the base of the skull as possible. If indicated, the cavernous and petrous portions of the arteries are freed from the bony enclosure intracranially by chiseling or rongeuring the bone away. First, portions of the occipital and temporal bones above the lateral and posterior parts of the atlas are removed intracranially by chiseling along the line shown in Fig. 4-17. The carotid canal may be enlarged and the artery freed from the soft tissue in this region. This can be accomplished by removing a vertical strip of bone medial to the canal and just above the entrance of the vertebral artery. Use of an oscillating saw in part will facilitate the procedure. Then, the neck arteries can be pulled down from below.

Dissection of the vertebral arteries is a little more time consuming *(36)*. The posterior process of the superior articular surface of the atlas, which hides the artery, is chiseled away. The artery is then dissected free from the dura to the transverse process of the atlas. Second, in the neck (Fig. 4-18), the transverse foramina of the cervical spine up to the C-3 level are opened with a chisel; the transverse processes are broken, exposing the vertebral artery. The chisel should now be directed upward and laterally to follow the course of the artery in C-2. Because of the fibrous fixation of the artery to the transverse process of the atlas, the process is chiseled off medial to the artery and removed with the latter. Fig. 4-19 illustrates a lateral view of a vertebral artery dissection

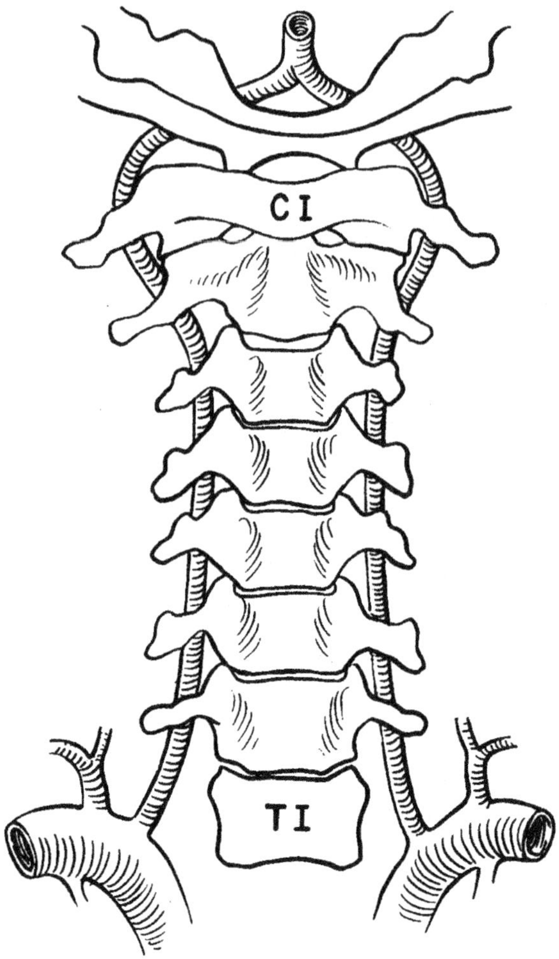

Fig. 4-18. Course of vertebral artery in neck.

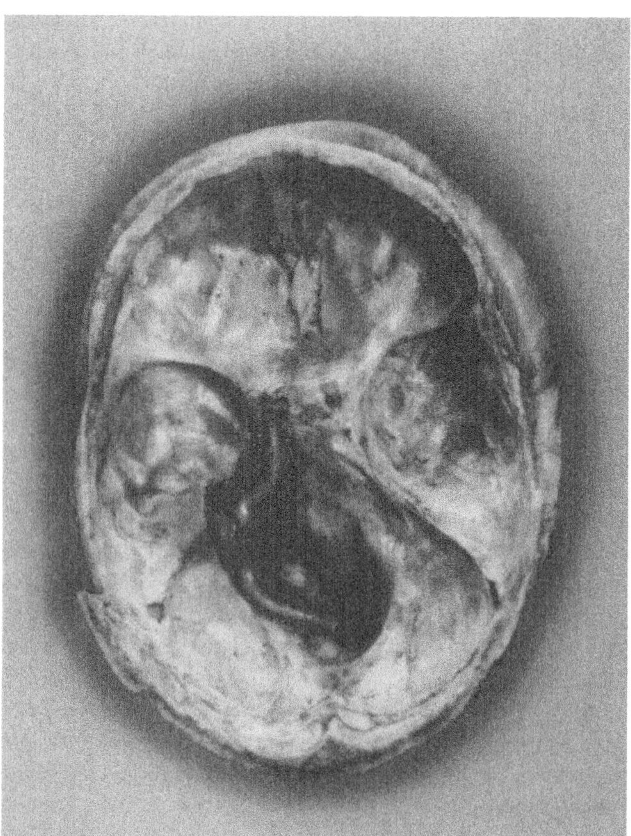

Fig. 4-17. Intracranial freeing of internal carotid and vertebral arteries. Portion of basal cranial bones to be removed is shown. Horizontal portion of carotid artery is exposed first down to carotid canal. Later it is exposed along with entrance of vertebral artery.

following removal of cervical spinal cord and medulla inside the bony column, in continuity with the foramen magnum, described above and used to document the focal thrombosis of the vertebral artery in a case of Wegener's granulomatosis *(37)*.

Alternatively, the cervical portion of the carotid and vertebral arteries can be removed together with the cervical spine (from the atlas to the seventh cervical vertebra), preceded by the injection of a barium sulfate-gelatine mixture into these arteries *(7)*. Because this interferes with the embalming procedure, the method proved impractical in our institution.

The removed arteries are examined either before or after adequate fixation. A method of perfusing the neck arteries under constant pressure (120–150 mm Hg) *(38)* supposedly preserves the vessels in the shape and degree of distention present in the systolic phase. Longitudinal sections of these vessels reveal the nature and extent of an atheromatous process, but the degree of narrowing of affected arterial segments cannot be assessed by this method. Also, this method of opening will create artifactual fractures on the surface of extensive plaques, and the condition of the luminal surface will be difficult to evaluate. Some particularly fragile atheromatous material will be lost. Of course, when occlusion is complete, this method of opening cannot be continued

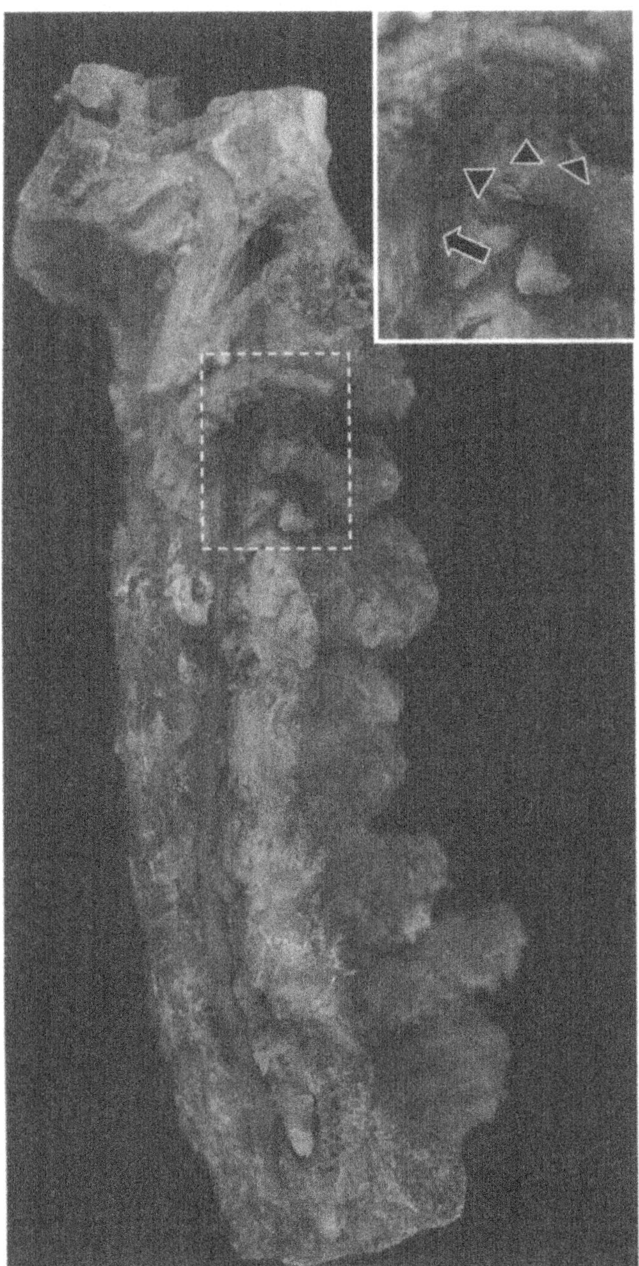

Fig. 4.19. The figure shows a lateral view of the all cervical column and base of skull with the fully exposed vertebral artery. The inset shows in high power the site of thrombosis. Reprinted with modifications from Maramattom BV, Giannini C, Manno EM, Wijdicks EF. Wegener's granulomatosis and vertebrobasilar thrombosis Cerebrovasc Dis 2005;20:65–68.

without destroying the pathologic process. To avoid these difficulties and to demonstrate the degree of luminal narrowing or the presence of thrombotic occlusion, submission of a transverse section of the artery is preferred and generally causes less regret.

Calcified neck vessels can be fixed in a formalin solution containing ethyl enediamine tetraacetic acid (EDTA). This decalcification step greatly reduces crush artifacts at the time of sectioning.

ACKNOWLEDGMENT

The authors would like to thank Drs. Vincenzo Caronia and Fabio Ricagna for their help with some of the illustrations.

REFERENCES

1. Mac Arthur S, Jacobson R, Marrero H, Rahman Z, Schneiderman H. Autopsy removal of the brain in AIDS. A new technique (Correspondence). Hum Pathol 1986;17:1296–1297.
2. Towfighi J, Roberts AF, Foster NE, Abt AB. A protective device for performing cranial autopsies. Hum Pathol 1989;20:288–289.
3. Brown P. Guidelines for high risk autopsy cases: special precautions for Creutzfeldt-Jakob disease. In: Autopsy Performance and Reporting. College of American Pathologists, Northfield, IL, 1990, pp. 68–74.
4. Budka H, Aguzzi A, Brown P, Brucher JM, Bugiani O, Gullota F, Haltia M. Tissue handling in suspected Creutzfeldt-Jakob disease and other human spongiform encephalopathies. Brain Pathol 1995;5:319–322.
5. Isaacson G. Postmortem examination of infant brains (techniques for removal, fixation and sectioning). Arch Pathol Lab Med 1984;108:80–81.
6. Bass T, Bergevin MA, Werner AL, Liuzzi FJ, Scott DE. In situ fixation of the neonatal brain and spinal cord. Ped Pathol 1993;13:699–705.
7. Okasaki H. Nervous system. In: Ludwig J, ed. Current Methods of Autopsy Practice. W.B. Saunders, Philadelphia, PA, 1979, pp. 96–129.
8. Wigglesworth JS. Performance of perinatal autopsy. In: Bennington JL, ed. Perinatal Pathology, vol. 15. Major Problems in Pathology. W.B. Saunders, Philadelphia, 1984, pp. 37–39.
9. Towbin A. Neonatal neuropathologic examination. In: Tedeschi CG, ed. Neuropathology: Methods and Diagnosis. Little, Brown, Boston, 1970, pp. 215–224.
10. Adams VI. Autopsy technique for neck examination II. Vertebral column and posterior compartment. Pathol Annu 1991;26:211–226.
11. Geddes JF, Gonzales AG. Examination of spinal cord in diseases of the craniocervical junction and high cervical spine. J Clin Pathol 1991;44:170–172.
12. Laurence KM, Martin D. A technique for obtaining undistorted specimens of the central nervous system. J Clin Pathol 1959;12:188–190.
13. Sheehan HL. Neurohypophysis and hypothalamus. In: Bloodworth JMB Jr, ed. Endocrine Pathology. Williams & Wilkins, Baltimore, MD, 1968, pp. 12–74.
14. Szanto PB. A modified technique for the removal of the nasopharynx and accompanying organs of the throat. Arch Pathol 1944;38:313–320.
15. Lamprecht J, Hegemann S, Hauptmann S. Advantages of ENT-specialty-specific autopsy technique [German] HNO 1994;42:233–235.
16. Temporal Bone Banks Program for Ear Research. Technique for acquiring and preparing the human temporal bone for the study of middle and ear pathology. Tran Am Acad Ophthalmol Otolaryngol 1966;70:871–878.
17. Michaels L, Wells M, Frohlich A. A new technique for the study of temporal bone pathology. Clin Otolaryng 1983;8:77–85.
18. Thompson SW. Selected Histochemical and Histopathological Methods. Charles C. Thomas, Springfield, IL, 1966, pp. 13–14.
19. Tedeschi CG. Neuropathology: Methods and Diagnosis. Little, Brown and Co., Boston, MA, 1970.
20. Simpson RHW, Berson SD. The postmortem diagnosis of diffuse cerebral injuries, with special reference to the importance of brain fixation. S Afr Med J 1987;71:10–14.
21. Katelaris A, Kencian J, Duflou J, Hilton JMN. Brain at necropsy: to fix or not to fix? J Clin Pathol 1994;47:718–720.
22. Powers JM. Practice guidelines for autopsy pathology. Autopsy procedures for brain, spinal cord and neuromuscular system. Autopsy Committe of the College of American Pathologists. Arch Pathol Lab Med 1995;119:777–783.
23. Alafuzoff I, Winblad B. How to run a brain bank: potentials and pitfalls in the use of human post-mortem brain material in research. J Neural Transm 1993;39:235–243.
24. Jean Paul G. Vonsattel Æ Maria Pilar del Amaya Æ Christian E. Keller Twenty-first century brain banking. Processing brains for research: the Columbia University methods. Acta Neuropathol 2007 Nov 6 (Epub ahead of print)

25. Lindenberg R. Forensic neuropathology. In: Minckler J, ed. Pathology of the Nervous System. McGraw-Hill, New York, 1972, pp. 2726–2740.
26. Nguyen JP, Gaston A, Louarn F, Marsault C, Bargiotas E, Wallman J, Poirier J. CT of brain: technique for comparative postmortem slicing. Am J Neuroradiol 1983;4:191–193
27. Braak H, Braak E Neuropathological stageing of Alzheimer-related changes. Acta neuropathologica. 1991; 82: 239–259
28. Newell KL, Hyman BT, Growdon JH, Hedley-Whyte Application of the National Institute of Aging (NIA)-Reagan Institute criteria for the neuropathological diagnosis of Alzheimer disease J Neuropathol Exp Neurol 1999;58:1147–1155.
29. Love S Postmortem sampling of the brain and other tissues in neurodegenerative disease Histopathol 2004;44:309–17.
30. Dyck PJ, Dyck PJB, Engelstad J. Pathologic Alterations of Nerves. In: Dyck PJ, Thomas PK. Peripheral Neuropathy, 4th ed. Elsevier, Philadelphia, 2005, pp. 733–830.
31. Beckwith JB. Sampling of muscle at autopsy in cases of lower motor neuron disease. Am J Clin Pathol 1964;42:92–93.
32. Choi SS, Crampton A. Atherosclerosis of arteries of neck: postmortem angiographic and pathologic study. Arch Pathol 1961;72:379–385.
33. Stein BM, Svare GT. A technique of postmortem angiography for evaluating arteriosclerosis of the aortic arch and carotid and vertebral arteries. Radiology 1963;81:252–256.
34. Karhunen PJ, Mannikko A, Penttila A, Liesto K. Diagnostic angiography in postoperative autopsies. Am J Forens Pathol 1989;10:303–309.
35. Thompsett DH, Tedeschi CG. Museum preparations of brain and spinal cord. In: Tedeschi CG, ed. Neuropathology: Methods and Diagnosis. Little, Brown, Boston, 1970, pp. 215–224.
36. Bromilow A, Burns J. Technique for removal of the vertebral arteries. J Clin Pathol 1985;38:1400–1402.
37. Maramattom BV, Giannini C, Manno EM, Wijdicks EF Wegener's granulomatosis and vertebro-basilar thrombosis Cerebrovasc Dis. 2005;20:65–8
38. McCormick WF, Stein BM. Technique for study of extracranial arteries. Arch Pathol 1962;74:52–56.

5 Eye and Adnexa

R. Jean Campbell and Cheryl R. Hann

INTRODUCTION

The eye and the adnexal structures may be affected by systemic disease, as well as by direct extension of pathologic processes from adjacent structures. Thus, it is important to consider their removal and study during autopsy *(1,2)*. Such primary pathologic conditions embrace not only neoplasms but also congenital abnormalities, primary open-angle glaucoma, and a host of retinal diseases for which the pathogenesis may not have been described. In addition to the value of correlative information, the eyes provide valuable teaching material. The use of fresh tissue allows research studies of the corneal endothelium, cells of the trabecular meshwork, and the retina.

Forensic investigation may require sampling the vitreous for toxicologic and biochemical studies *(3,4)*. Sampling the vitreous for toxicologic and other forensic investigations *(3,4)* or for microbiologic studies *(5)* is best performed on an intact eye that is without structural intraocular pathology, such as a retinal detachment. A 15-gauge needle is inserted at an oblique angle through the sclera at a point 5 mm lateral to the limbus (corneoscleral junction) (Fig. 5-1). The needle traverses the pars plana and enters the vitreous body. Gentle aspiration of 2 to 3 mL of vitreous is drawn into a 10-mL sterile syringe; this aspirate may be stored at 4°C for up to 48 hours. The correct concentration of potassium within the vitreous can be used for a rough estimation of the postmortem interval. A traumatic aspiration will result in damage to the retinal cells and result in a falsely high potassium value.

The eye may also be injured directly or show the effects of a nonaccidental death such as that caused by child abuse *(1,2,6)*. In cases of suspected child abuse, vitreous should never be aspirated because there is a risk of artifactual damage to the retina. Prior to removal of the eye (see below), the fundus should be photographed. The retina bears the brunt of injury in child abuse, and the assessment and identification of the position of retinal hemorrhages are of prime importance *(2)*.

REMOVAL OF THE EYE

ANTERIOR APPROACH In most instances, the entire eye is removed by the anterior approach. The eyelids are held apart with the aid of retractors (Fig. 5-2). Tenon's capsule is left intact to avoid leakage into the empty socket. The four rectus muscles are cut, leaving approximately 5.0 mm of each muscle attached to the globe. This allows for subsequent orientation of the globe. The inferior oblique muscle is then severed. Rotation of the eye temporally by traction on the stump of the inferior oblique muscle allows access to the optic nerve and ensures that a long piece of the intraorbital portion of the optic nerve is obtained. It is not necessary to ligate the optic stalk, because only a portion of the leakage after enucleation arises from the severed end of the optic nerve. The socket is dried with a towel and a silastic mold is placed in position (Fig. 5-3) *(7)*. Alternatively, the empty socket is packed with gauze. The disadvantage of the anterior approach is that it excludes adequate examination of the orbital contents and the lacrimal gland.

INTRACRANIAL APPROACH (EXENTERATION PROCEDURE) This method is advisable when there is pathology that involves the orbit and the eye. Such pathology includes neoplasia, vascular disease, and disease of the orbital portion of the optic nerve. This method consists of first cutting the conjunctival attachments at the limbus by the anterior approach (as outlined earlier), then using the intracranial approach to expose the orbital contents.

After removal of the brain, two saw cuts are made, first vertically downward opposite the cribriform plate of the ethmoid bone and the second downward and medially, immediately anterior to the lateral end of the lesser wing of the sphenoid bone. The orbital plate is broken with a chisel and hammer, and the bone is removed piecemeal with the aid of bone forceps. Care must be taken not to damage the optic nerve and other contents of the optic foramen when this area is exposed. Curved scissors are used to free the globe and its attached muscles. Freeing of the conjunctival attachment at the limbus must proceed with caution to avoid damage to the eyelids and the anterior chamber of the eye. The superior oblique muscle is cut from the body of the sphenoid bone and the inferior oblique muscle is cut from the floor of the medial orbit.

The eye with the optic nerve and its surrounding nerves, muscles, and fat are freed from the walls of the orbit. Tenon's capsule is left intact to avoid leakage into the empty socket. The orbit and lacrimal fossa should be palpated after exenteration to determine the presence or absence of any abnormality, such as a neoplasm.

From: *Handbook of Autopsy Practice,* 4th Ed. Edited by: B.L. Waters

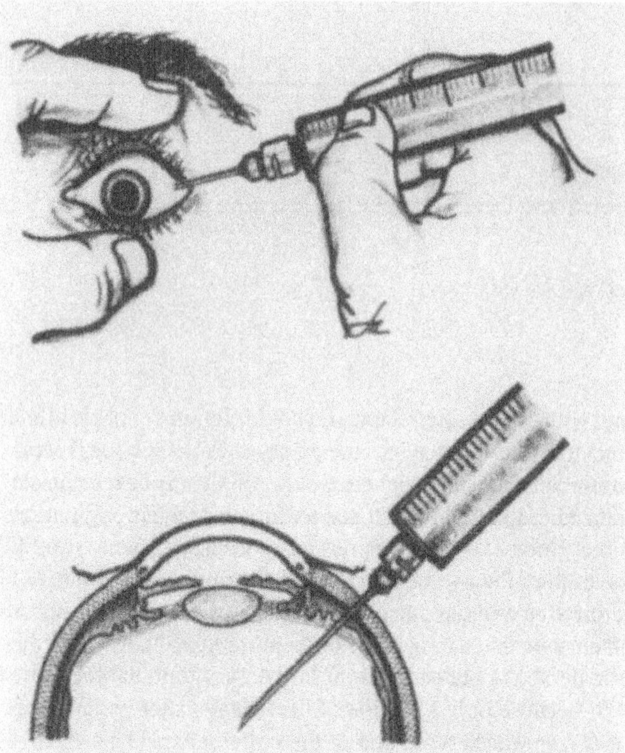

Fig. 5-1. Aspiration of vitreous. *Top,* Needle is inserted 5 mm lateral to limbus (corneoscleral junction). *Bottom,* Needle enters vitreous through pars plana of ciliary body.

REMOVAL OF THE LACRIMAL GLAND The lobulated, bean-shaped lacrimal gland lies in the lateral part of the upper orbit in the hollow of the medial side of the zygomatic process of the frontal bone, adjacent to the roof (Fig. 5-4). The gland may be obtained either before or after removal of the globe. The lacrimal nerve and artery, which lie in the fat at the junction of the roof and the lateral wall of the orbit, may be traced to the lacrimal gland. The concave medial surface of the gland lies on the superior levator and lateral rectus muscles; these may also be traced to the gland. Curved scissors are used to free the gland from the adjacent muscles and the short fibrous bands that bind it to the orbital margin.

If only a limited autopsy is permitted, a specimen of lacrimal gland may be obtained by inserting a biopsy needle beneath the upper eyelid and aiming it upward and laterally toward the gland.

PROCESSING OF OCULAR SPECIMENS

FIXATION, ORIENTATION, SECTIONING, AND DOCUMENTATION OF LESIONS The enucleated eye is placed in 20–25 times its volume of 10% buffered formalin for 48 hours of fixation. The neck of the container should be approximately twice the diameter of the globe. Injection of fixative is not necessary because it introduces artifact into the globe.

If the eye and the orbital contents have been removed in toto, the eye should be dissected from the orbital contents and placed in a separate container; otherwise, fixation will be delayed. The orbital contents should be fixed separately.

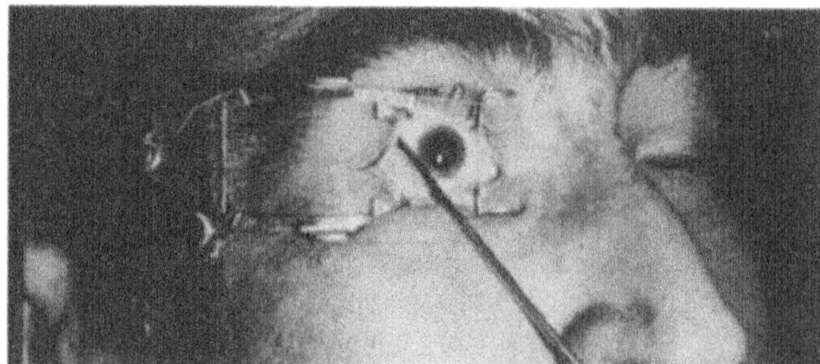

Fig. 5-2. Eyelids held apart by a Weeks speculum to allow enucleation or biopsy of lacrimal gland.

After 48 hours of fixation, the eye is rinsed in running water to allow easier handling by personnel sensitive to formalin. Orientation with regard to side is determined by observation of the following (Fig. 5-5):

1. The horizontal plane is characterized by the posterior ciliary vessels; the more prominent vessels lie on the nasal side.
2. The temporal side is characterized by the insertion of the inferior oblique muscle, which is usually fleshy and extends inferiorly from the optic nerve.
3. The superior aspect is characterized by the tendinous insertion of the superior oblique muscle, which underlies the superior rectus muscle.

The superior pole is marked with a grease pencil to allow continued quick orientation during subsequent handling (Fig. 5-6). The anteroposterior, horizontal, and vertical planes are measured with a caliper (Fig. 5-7). If the presence of calcium, bone, or a foreign body is suspected, a radiograph of the globe can be helpful (Fig. 5-8).

A phthisical eye contains bone and thus requires decalcification. The rapid method using RDO (Rapid Decalcifier, Apex Engineering Products Corp, Aurora, IL) *(8)* is effective. The endpoint is determined by the ease of cutting. Orbital bone requires a stronger decalcification solution. The rapid method with Decalcifier II (Surgipath Medical Industries, Inc, Richmond, IL) is effective, but after the bone is placed in this solution, it must be examined every 2 hours and cannot be left in the solution overnight. Adequate decalcification is determined by a repeat radiograph. The external appearance of the eye should be documented. Surgical and accidental penetrating or perforating wounds should be noted. Transillumination of the globe is then performed. If a defect in transillumination is present, such as may be caused by an intraocular tumor, the area is outlined with a grease pencil, the size of the opacity determined, and the plane of section is made accordingly to provide the best information. A transverse section of the optic nerve is made only if the length of the optic nerve is such that the back of the globe will not be opened by the cut (Fig. 5-9).

Sectioning is performed on a piece of dental wax, to which the escaping vitreous does not adhere; thus, the attachment of the retina to the choroid is maintained. The eye is positioned so that the cornea is against the wax and the optic nerve projects upward. The inferior "cap," or calotte, is removed by placing a blade immediately

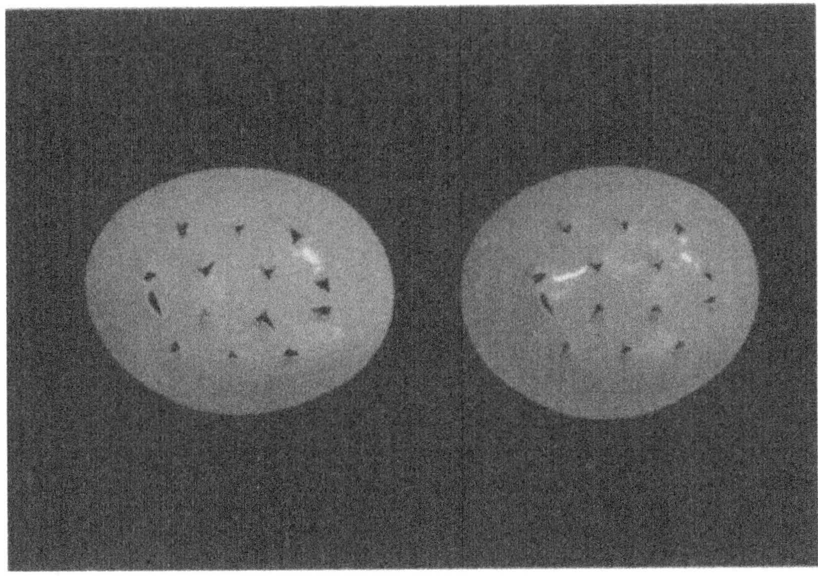

Fig. 5-3. Prosthetic molds used for empty sockets.

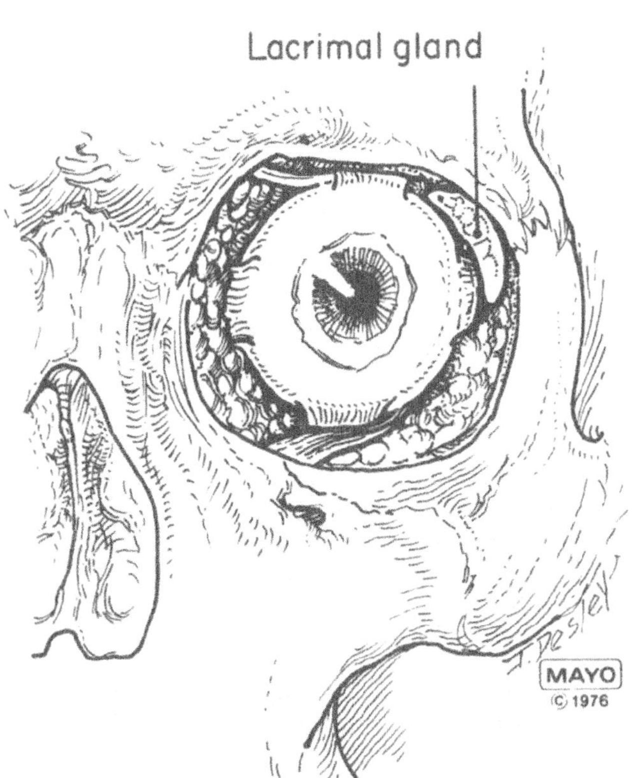

Fig. 5-4. Diagram of left orbit viewed from front shows lacrimal gland in lacrimal fossa. (Used with permission of Mayo Foundation for Medical Education and Research.)

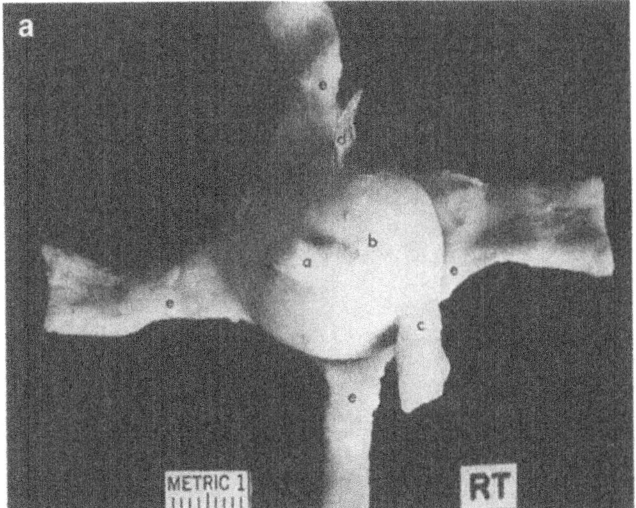

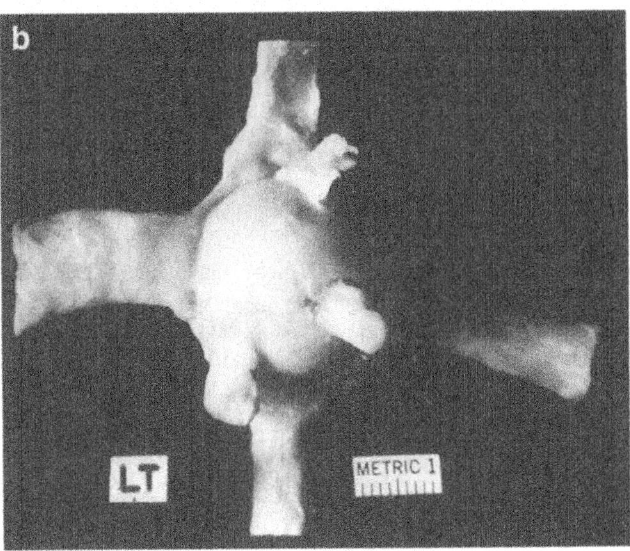

Fig. 5-5. *A*, Right eye and, *B*, left eye enucleated at autopsy. In, *A*, note (a) optic nerve, (b) posterior ciliary vessels running horizontally, (c) inferior oblique muscle, (d) superior oblique muscle, and (e) rectus muscles.

abutting the inferior aspect of the optic nerve (Fig. 5-10). With a smooth motion, the blade is directed toward the limbal edge of the cornea. The inferior calotte, together with the remaining globe, is examined under a dissecting microscope (Fig. 5-11). Pathologic conditions are noted at this time and photographs are taken. Most

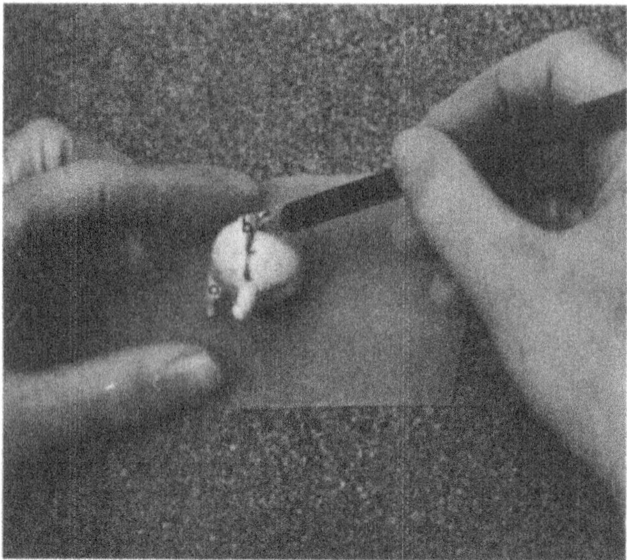

Fig. 5-6. Left eye in position on dental wax shows inferior oblique muscle (A) and superior oblique muscle (B) marked with grease pencil.

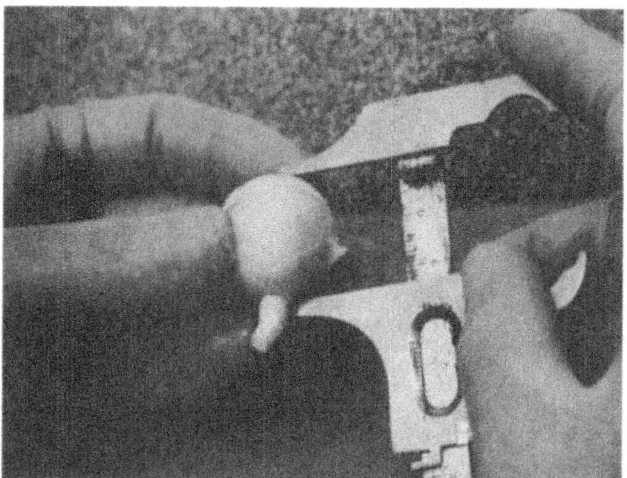

Fig. 5-7. Globe is measured in anteroposterior, horizontal, and vertical planes.

eyes are sectioned in the horizontal plane (Fig. 5-12). For eyes that have been traumatized or contain a neoplasm, such a horizontal cut may not show the pathologic findings to best advantage; thus, an oblique or vertical cut may be required.

The larger portion of the globe with the superior pole is then placed on the dental wax with its flat surface down. The blade is placed immediately adjacent to the optic nerve, and the second cut is made parallel to the first; this mid section of the globe, approximately 3 mm thick, is submitted for processing. The section obtained is known as the PO (pupil-optic disk) section and it will show the macula as well as the pupil and the optic disk. A diagram for sectioning the globes is shown in Fig. 5-13. The instruments used in sectioning are shown in Fig. 5-14.

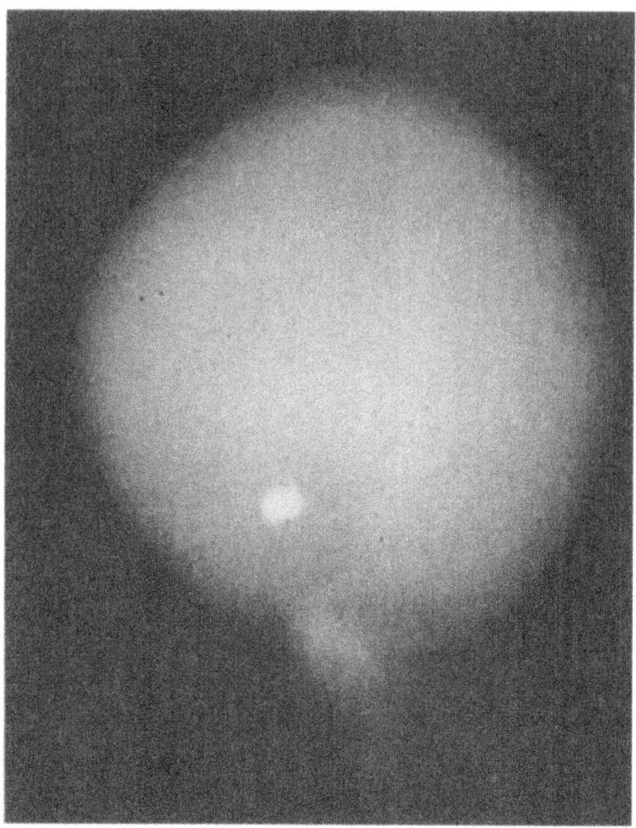

Fig. 5-8. Radiograph of globe shows foreign body (bullet fragment).

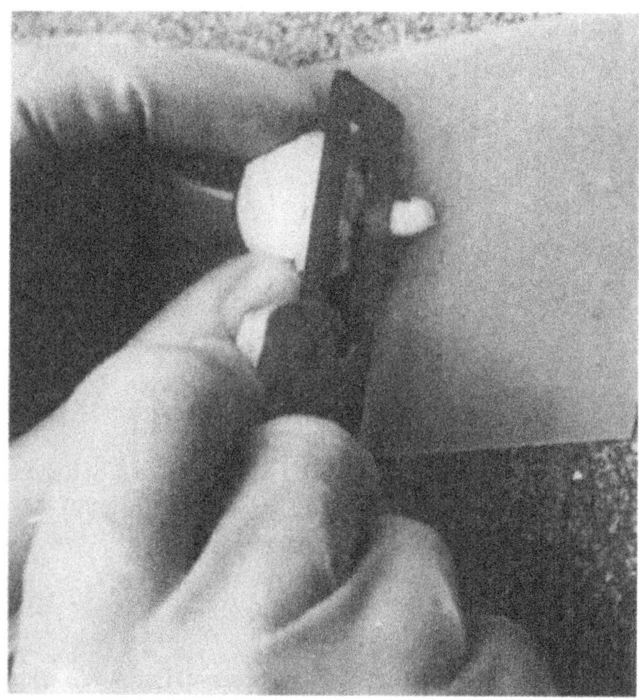

Fig. 5-9. Eye is placed on dental wax for transverse section of optic nerve.

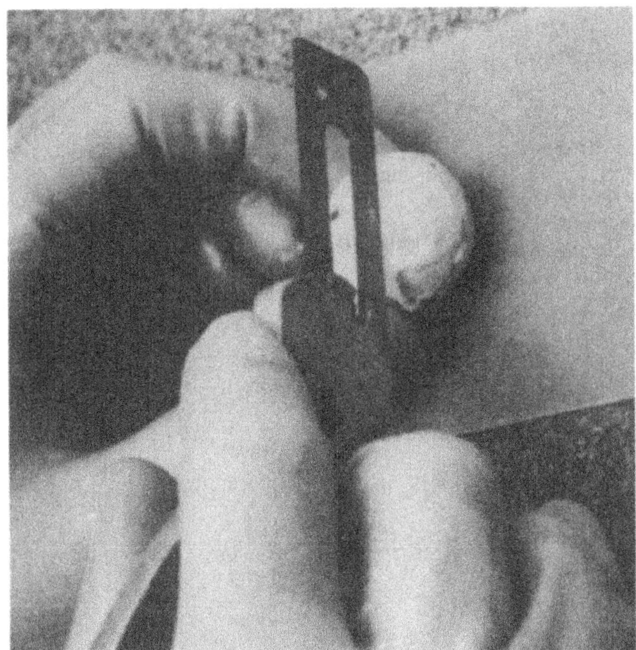

Fig. 5-10. For sectioning, globe is positioned with cornea facing down on dental wax and superior pole with grease pencil mark to left. For removal of inferior calotte, blade is placed parallel to horizontally running posterior ciliary vessels and immediately abutting optic nerve.

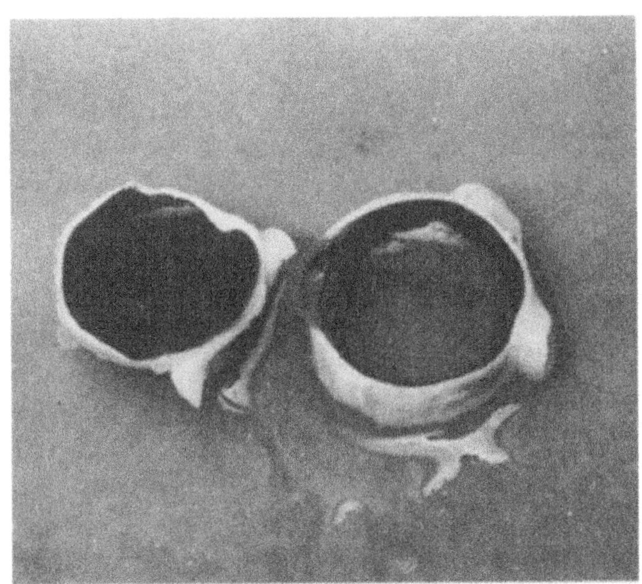

Fig. 5-12. Sectioned globe with 3-mm thick horizontal section on right and superior calotte on left.

EYES CONTAINING AN INTRAOCULAR PROSTHESIS Specimens with an intraocular prostheses should be opened in the coronal plane. The anterior segment is processed as a whole. Chloroform is used as the clearing agent and will dissolve plastic prostheses and other plastic substances, such as a scleral buckle or a Molteno shunt.

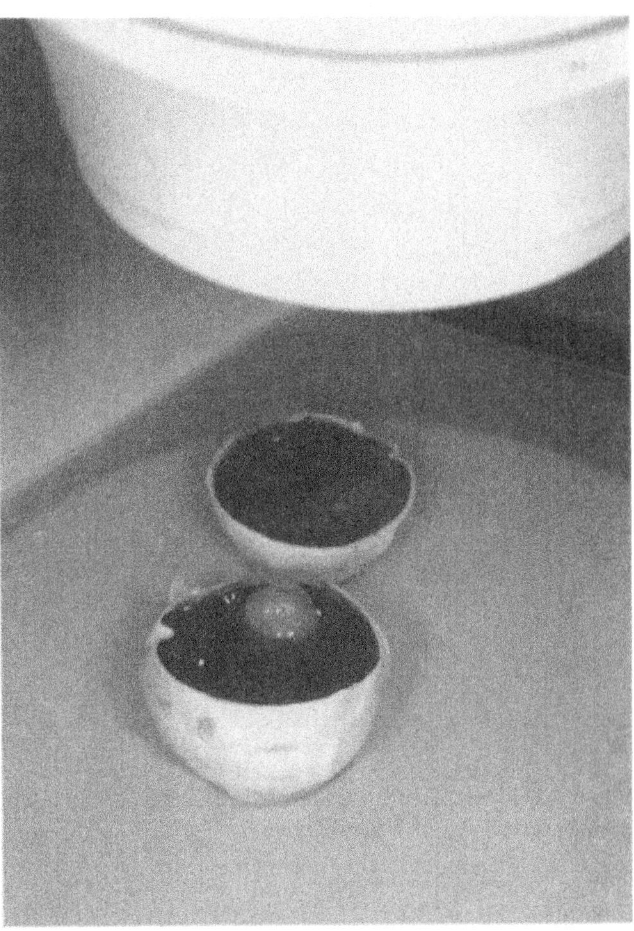

Fig. 5-11. After globe is sectioned, inferior calotte and remaining globe are examined under a dissecting microscope.

The paraffin-infiltrated specimen is then trisected to display the position of the haptics that have anchored the prosthesis within the eye. All sectioned pieces are embedded. The posterior portion of the globe is sectioned in the horizontal plane.

STAINING PROCEDURES

Routine stains include hematoxylin and eosin and the periodic acid-Schiff reaction. The latter gives adequate examination of Descemet's membrane, the lens capsule, Bruch's membrane, and other materials with carbohydrate groupings (CHO) such as glycogen.

PREPARATION FOR ELECTRON MICROSCOPY

The eye is opened immediately after removal from the body, and the specimen is placed promptly in Trumps solution. This fixative is a combination of 4% formaldehyde and 1% glutaraldehyde. With the aid of the dissecting microscope, 1-mm square sections are cut from the area selected for examination *(9)*.

REMOVAL OF CORNEA FOR TRANSPLANTATION

CONTRAINDICATIONS The Eye Bank Association of America *(10)* and the U.S. Food and Drug Administration *(11)* have established stringent standards and regulations for

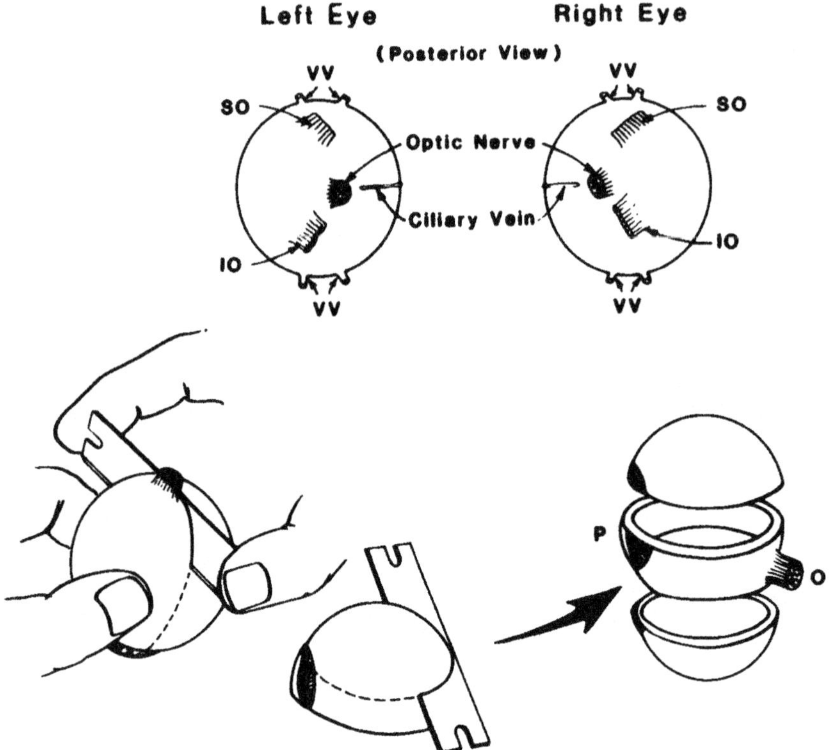

Fig. 5-13. Diagram shows steps in sectioning of globe. IO, inferior oblique insertion; PO, pupil-optic section; SO, superior oblique insertion; and VV, vortex veins.

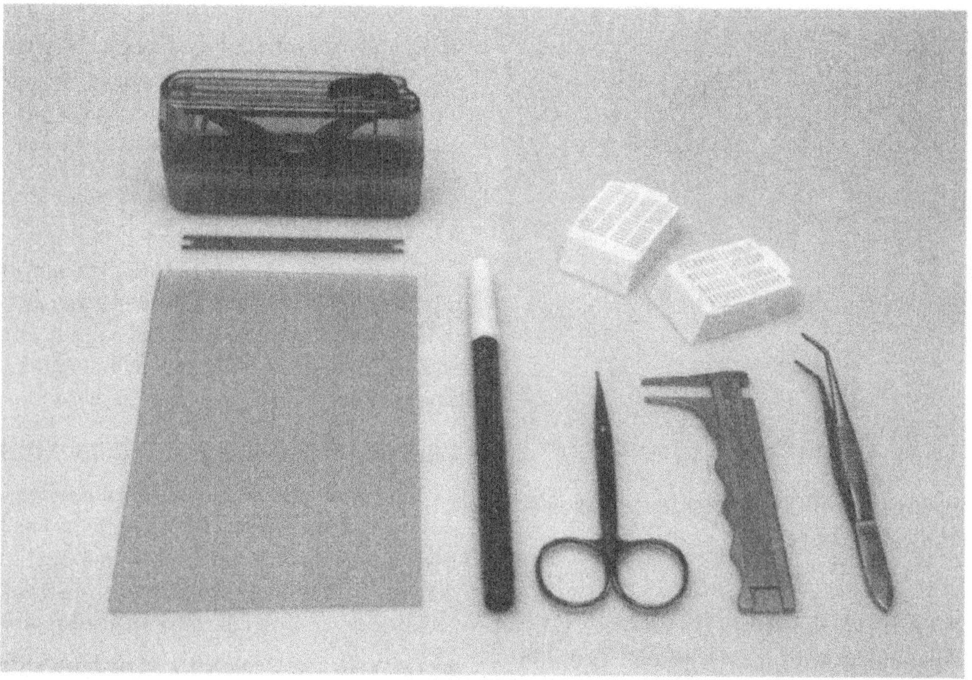

Fig. 5-14. Instruments for sectioning globe include *(from lower left)* plastic dental wax and blades *(upper left)* for sectioning, marking pen, scissors, calipers, forceps, and macrocassettes.

tissue that is to be used for transplantation. These standards have made it necessary for trained personnel who are aware of the ever-changing requirements to be responsible for the retrieval and processing of such tissue. As of this writing, the list of absolute contraindications from the Eye Bank Association of America included the human immunodeficiency virus, hepatitis B, and hepatitis C (or social conditions that put the donor at risk for these entities) *(10)*. Also considered to be contraindications are Creutzfeldt-Jakob disease, ocular and intraocular inflammation, rabies, malignant tumors of the anterior segment, leukemia, lymphoma, and retinoblastoma. Previous corneal surgery, refractive surgery, and intravenous drug abuse are other contraindications. The medical standards of the Eye Bank Association of America define the minimum standards of practice for the procurement, preservation, storage, and distribution of eye tissue for transplantation as determined by the ophthalmic medical community.

TECHNICAL ASPECTS Preferably, the enucleation is performed before the general autopsy procedure commences. The eye is removed by the anterior approach under aseptic conditions within 24 hours of death and preferably as soon as possible after death. The eye is placed with the cornea directed upward in a sterile plastic container filled with sterile saline (Fig. 5-15). The specimen is refrigerated at 2° to 6°C. If the eye is to be transported out of town, the moist chamber jar is placed in an insulated container with plastic bags that contain chipped ice. Blood is collected from the donor (7–10 mL) for the necessary serologic testing.

Some corneas are now obtained by *in situ* excision, during which trained personnel excise the corneoscleral rim but leave the rest of the globe within the orbit. Rapid transportation of the donor tissue is handled by the local eye bank staff, volunteers, and transportation companies (airlines and taxicabs).

REMOVAL OF SCLERA FOR TRANSPLANTATION

Banked sclera may be used to wrap porous orbital implants or to serve as spacer material for eyelid surgery, particularly for correction of eyelid retraction caused by Graves disease. In addition, sclera may be used in patients with severe scleral thinning, either as a consequence of rheumatoid arthritis or as a consequence of mitomycin therapy. It is a fairly routine procedure during glaucoma surgery to use sclera to cover the drainage tube at the limbus; on occasion, donor pericardium is used.

The requirements for removal of sclera are the same as those used for retrieval of other tissues for transplantation. For example, when an autopsy is to be performed, the eye is removed before commencement of the general autopsy procedure. Enucleation is performed by either method outlined above. After removal of the corneoscleral rim for transplantation under a laminar flow hood, the global contents are removed and any excess tissue is removed with sterile gauze and sterile saline. The remaining sclera is left whole or cut into suitable portions (halves or quarters) for surgical use. Each portion is preserved in 95% ethyl alcohol in a sterile jar.

The Eye Bank Association of America allows scleral preservation in a 70% or greater concentration of ethyl alcohol, or in sterile glycerin, or by cryopreservation or gamma radiation. After completion of sterilization, a batch of sclera is cultured to determine whether sterilization is adequate.

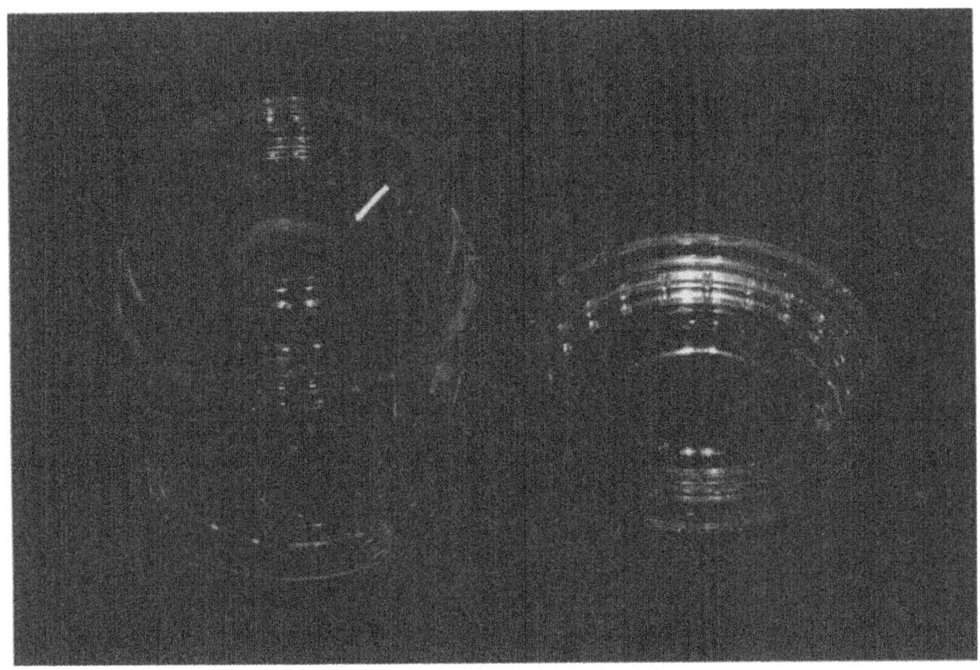

Fig. 5-15. For maintenance of moisture, cornea (*arrow*) is placed in a sterile plastic receptacle of sterile saline.

REFERENCES

1. Lee WR. Examination of the globe: technical aspects. In: Lee WR, ed. Ophthalmic Histopathology. Springer-Verlag, London, 1993, pp. 1–23.
2. Parsons MA, Start RD. ACP Best Practice No. 164: necropsy techniques in ophthalmic pathology. J Clin Pathol 2001;54:417–427.
3. Forrest AR. ACP Broadsheet no. 137: April 1993. Obtaining samples at post mortem examination for toxicological and biochemical analyses. J Clin Pathol 1993;46:292–296.
4. McKinney PE, Phillips S, Gomez HF, Brent J, MacIntyre M, Watson WA. Vitreous humor cocaine and metabolite concentrations: do postmortem specimens reflect blood levels at the time of death? J Forensic Sci 1995;40:102–107.
5. Mietz H, Heimann K, Kuhn J, Wieland U, Eggers HJ. Detection of HIV in human vitreous. Int Ophthalmol 1993;17:101–104.
6. Green MA, Lieberman G, Milroy CM, Parsons MA. Ocular and cerebral trauma in non-accidental injury in infancy: underlying mechanisms and implications for pediatric practice. Br J Ophthalmol 1996;80:282–287.
7. Kelco Supply Company [homepage on the Internet]. Minneapolis (MN): Kelco Supply Company c2004 [cited 2006 May 3]. Available from http://www.kelcosupply.com
8. Apex Engineering Products Corporation [homepage on the Internet]. Aurora (IL): Apex Engineering Products Corp. Rapid decalcifier for preparation of histological materials [updated 2004 Mar 25; cited 2006 Apr 4]. Available from http://www.rdo-apex.com/
9. Trump BF, Jones RT. Diagnostic Electron Microscopy, vol. 2. John Wiley & Sons, New York, 1978, p. 118.
10. Eye Bank Association of America [homepage on the Internet]. Washington (DC): Eye Bank Association of America. Medical standards and procedures manual [cited 2006 Apr 4]. Available from http://www.restoresight.org/
11. Food and Drug Administration, HHS. Current good tissue practice for human cell, tissue, and cellular and tissue-based product establishments; inspection and enforcement. Final rule. Fed Regist 2004;69:68611–68688.

6 Autopsy Laboratory

Brenda L. Waters

THE FACILITIES

The environs devoted to autopsy activities should be large enough to comfortably house evisceration tables, dissection tables, a cooler for storage of bodies and supplies, cabinets for equipment, shelving for fixed specimens and unused containers, a photography stand (*see* Chapter 1), an X-ray machine and view box, sinks for rinsing organs, sinks for washing hands, and sufficient office space for all related paper work. The laboratory must be well lit, amply ventilated *(1)* and minimally cluttered. Step stools and wastebaskets should be situated away from the main routes of traffic. If possible, shelving for containers with fixed specimens should not be placed above eye level. A sturdy cart should be available for transferring large, heavy containers from one place in the laboratory to another. Frequently used equipment, such as scissors, knives, scalpels, specimen containers, pencils, tissue cassettes, and labels, should be readily accessible, free of gross contamination, and neatly arranged. Balances must be available that can accurately weigh specimens as large as livers and as small as parathyroid glands. They must be calibrated on a routine basis, such as every six months. Telephones should be abundantly installed throughout the area to allow for ready access when answering pages.

Some designs of evisceration tables allow for height adjustment (Fig. 6-1), while other tables are designed to transport the body to and from the cooler (Fig. 6-2). This latter style eliminates the need to transfer the body from one table to another. Either way, it is preferable to have the evisceration tables sufficiently distanced from the dissection tables, so as to provide adequate room for both diener and prosector to perform their separate duties. The dissection tables may use wood or plastic cutting boards. This author prefers wood cutting boards, since they are less slippery than plastic and their light brown color produces less glare. They can be adequately sanitized with soap and water, 10% bleach and air-drying.

The autopsy area should be restricted to authorized personnel only. This may be accomplished by using either card keys or combination locks at the entry door. A telephone may be installed outside the door and set up such that clinicians seeking entry may simply pick up the phone, causing the phone to ring inside the lab.

From: *Handbook of Autopsy Practice,* 4th Ed. Edited by: B.L. Waters

Some laboratories may find it advantageous to have a viewing room, in which the family of the deceased view the body in a quiet and private space (Fig. 6-3) If such a viewing room is installed, it is important to provide a route by which the family may enter and leave without seeing the rest of the laboratory.

CLEANING PROCEDURES Although the hospital's housekeeping department may be responsible for routinely cleaning the floors, it is essential that mops be available in the lab to clean up puddles of water or body fluids, since these can make the floor very slippery.

The walls should be washed regularly with soft brushes and disinfected with a 10% solution of sodium hypochlorite (household bleach—1 part bleach to 9 parts water). For the floors, a germicidal solution is required. Evisceration and dissection tables must be decontaminated after each autopsy with soapy water and then with bleach. Instruments should be washed in hot, soapy water, then immersed in a 10% solution of bleach and finally, thoroughly dried. It is particularly important that these steps are undertaken for any equipment that is intended to leave the autopsy laboratory area. If reliable decontamination cannot be achieved with any instrument, then a warning label "CONTAMINATED" should be affixed to the item (Fig. 6-4).

While cleaning up grossly contaminated equipment, personnel should don full protective gear (i.e., use universal precautions) (*see* Prevention of Injury below). If a small formalin spill occurs, the fluid can be absorbed into paper or cloth towels. This absorbent material must then be tightly enclosed in a biohazard bag, so as to prevent evaporation of the formalin into the room. The floor should then be wet-mopped and the mop thoroughly rinsed. If a large formalin spill occurs, personnel should leave the area and institute the hospital's appropriate procedures.

Broken glassware should never be picked up with the hands, but rather with mechanical devices such as a dustpan and cardboard pusher. The broken glass must be placed in a sharps container. If contamination with radioactive material occurs, follow the recommendations in Chapter 11.

WASTE DISPOSAL Of course, all sharps (i.e., scalpels and needles) must be disposed of in rigid plastic "sharps" containers that are specifically designed for this purpose. When these containers are filled to about three fourths of their capacity, they must be discarded in red biohazard bags. This is to avoid the tendency of someone to push the blade into the container rather than drop it.

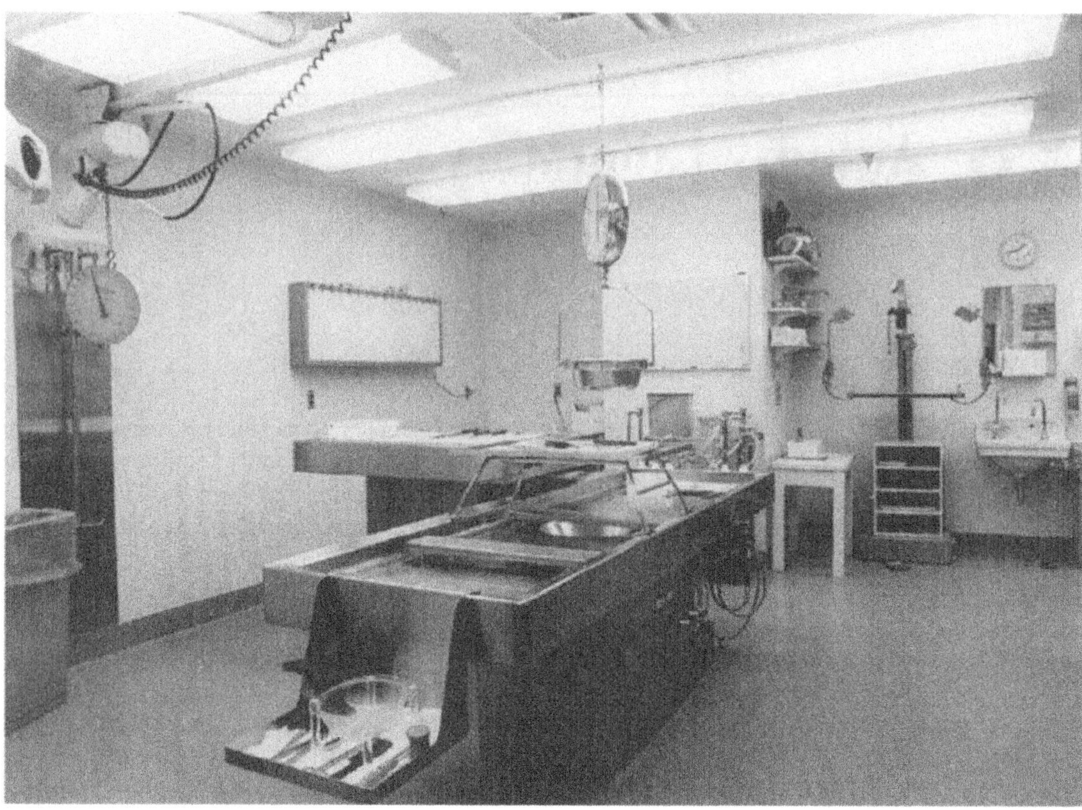

Fig. 6-1. Note the spacious and well-lit layout of the room. This type of evisceration table allows for height adjustment, but does require that the body be transferred to and from it.

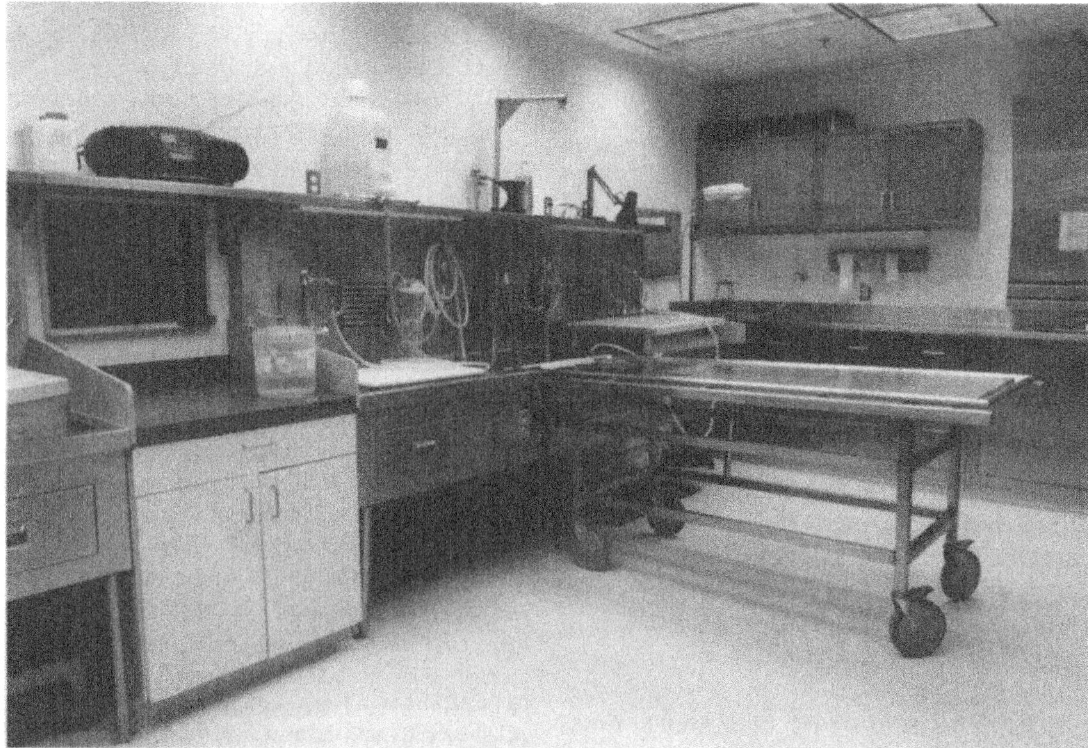

Fig. 6-2. The evisceration table pictured here is fixed in height, but has the capacity to carry the body to and from the cooler. The wheels have locking devices to immobilize the table during the procedure.

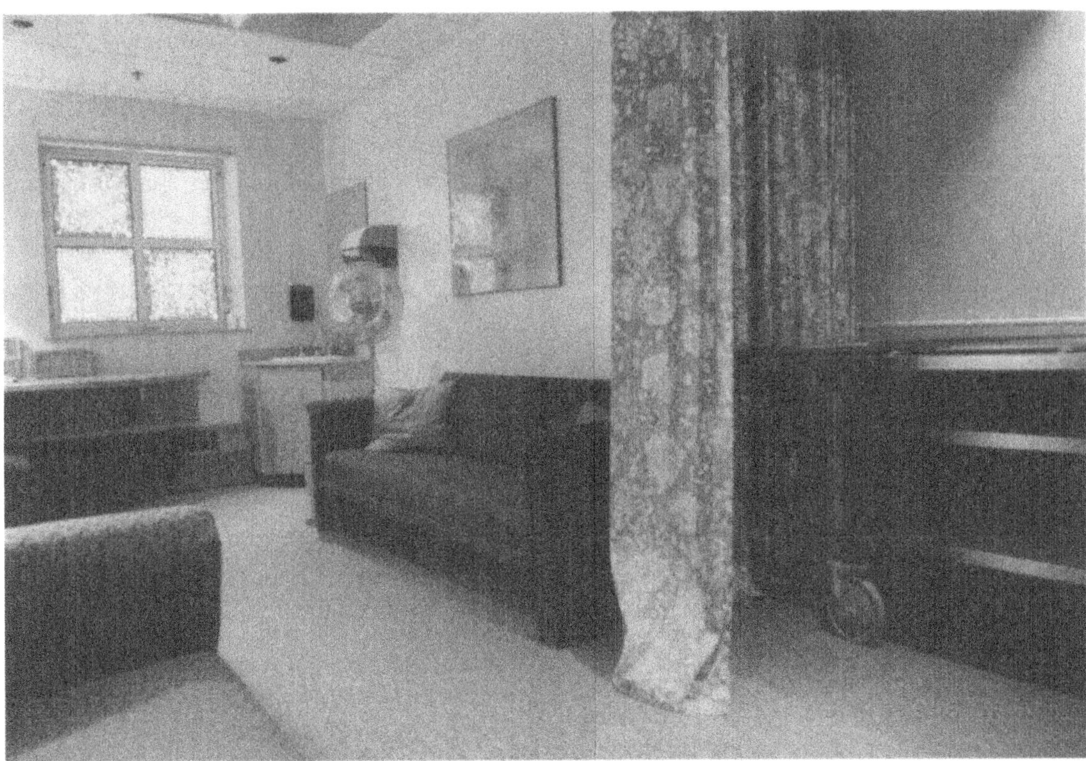

Fig. 6-3. A room for families to view the body of their loved-one. Note how the table bearing the body is rolled into the room, and a curtain pulled around the table. The room is equipped with comfortable furniture, a sink, telephone and plenty of tissues.

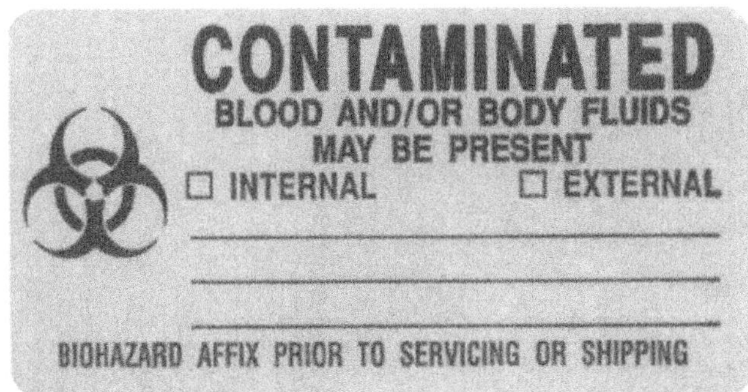

Fig. 6-4. This, or similar sticker should be affixed to any piece of equipment leaving the autopsy suite that cannot be adequately decontaminated.

All disposable devices that are contaminated with blood or other body fluids must be placed in biohazard bags. Such material includes venous and arterial lines, foley catheters, endotracheal tubes, dressings, gauze pads, stoma bags and grossly contaminated protective gear worn by autopsy personnel. Pacemakers and defibrillators must never be discarded, since incineration may cause them to explode. These devices should be removed, ideally with their leads uncut, cleaned, and set aside for pickup by the manufacturer.

The biohazard bags may be placed in biohazard cardboard boxes so as to facilitate transport to the incinerator (Fig. 6-5). The surgical cotton scrubs, which should not be contaminated

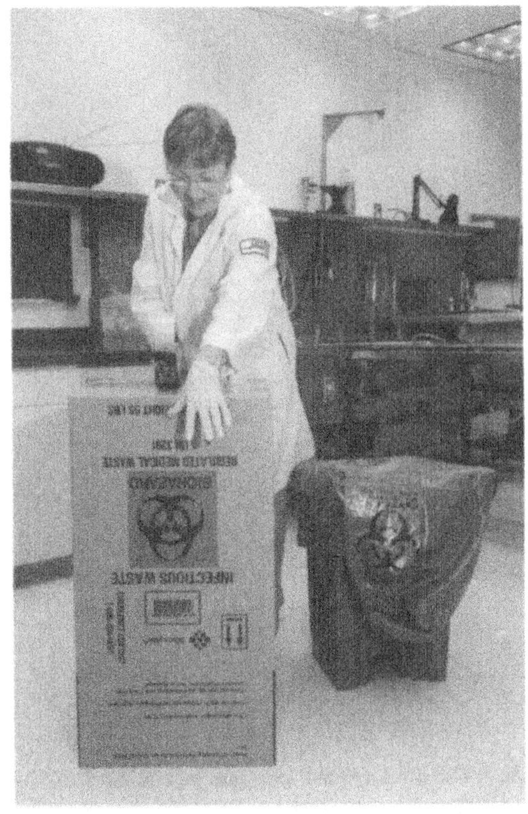

Fig. 6-5. Here, the diener is preparing a biohazard box into which a biohazard bag will be placed.

because of the required protective wear, may be placed in the hospital laundry bin

STORAGE AND DISPOSAL OF ORGANS For initial fixation and storage of retained organs, we find it useful to place the organs in large enamel pots (nicknamed "lobster pots" in our laboratory) (*see* Fig. 6-6), which are filled to about one third capacity with 10% formalin. When scheduled for review at Gross Conference, the organs are washed in this receptacle for several hours and then, after the conference, they are placed in a smaller container (*see* Fig. 6-6). The smaller container provides less volume of fixative, but this is acceptable, since most of the fixation already occurred in the larger pot. The organs are retained in these containers until they are discarded. In our laboratory, we retain these fixed organs until 3 months after the case has been signed out. Representative portions (2–3 cm in diameter) of all major organs (including nerve, skin, diaphragm, and rib) are placed in a smaller container (sometimes called a "stock jar"), and these are generally retained for a year. These jars are depicted in Fig. 6-7. Fresh tissues that are not retained, such as slices of liver, segments of bowel or fat, must be discarded in red biohazard bags.

The College of American Pathologists stipulates that wet tissue from nonforensic autopsies must be retained until three months after completion of the final report. At that time, they may be discarded, but they must be placed in Biohazard bags and sent for incineration. Paraffin blocks, slides, and reports are retained for 10 years. Accession log books should be retained for 2 years *(2)*.

PERSONNEL

THE VALUE OF THE DIENER No single individual is more important to the smooth, safe, and pleasant running of an autopsy service than the diener. The term diener comes from the German word, "leichendiener" which means, literally "servant of the dead." This position lies at the core of all autopsy activities and therefore, assumes responsibilities that are many and varied. A diener not only must eviscerate and prepare the bodies for release, but must also interact directly with funeral directors, clinicians, pathologists, residents from all specialties, medical students, and families of the deceased. He or she is the first line of defense against the malfunctioning of telephones, computers, cameras, dictating machines, scales, and light fixtures. A diener is responsible for maintaining sufficient supplies in the autopsy laboratory, keeping the areas safe and the instruments in good functioning order. This person must be resourceful and persistent in locating misplaced items of all kinds. He or she must be welcoming to newcomers, soothing to stressed residents, and entertaining when the situation demands. The diener may be the first staff person in the autopsy service to orient new residents to the autopsy service, to calm visiting medical students, or to field questions from seasoned clinicians and pathologists. When recruiting for this position, one should look for a person with maturity, motivation to learn, attention to detail, and a sense of humor.

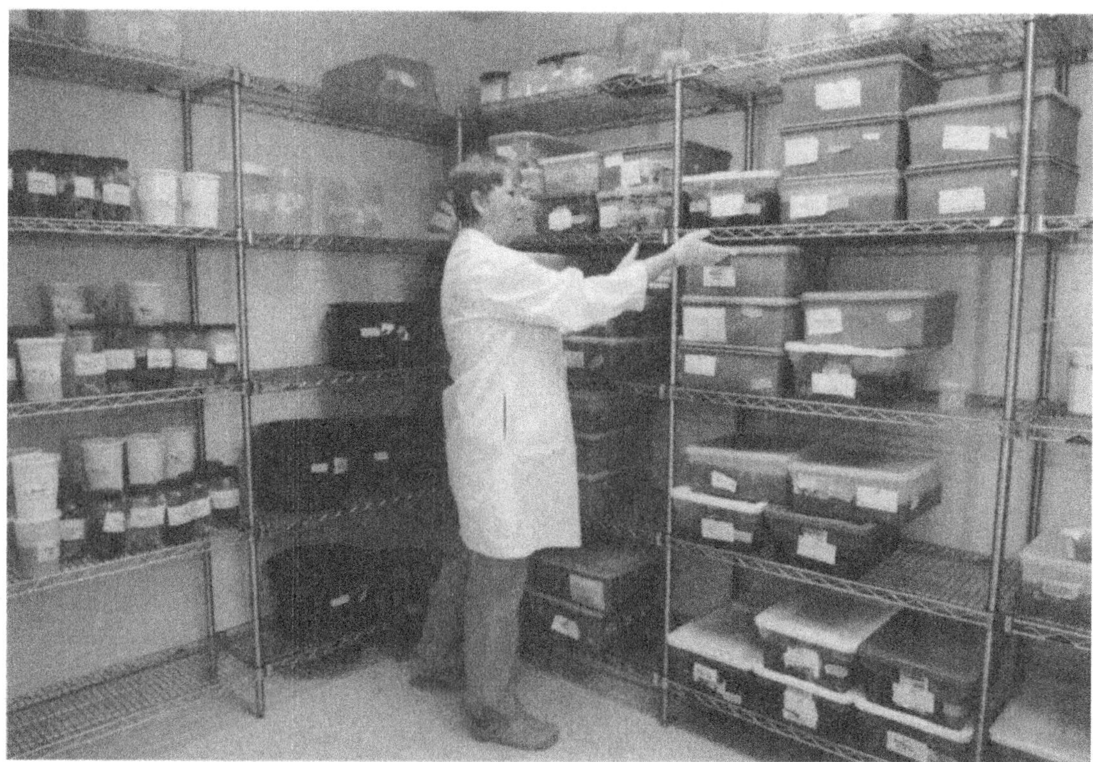

Fig. 6-6. The large enamel pots are seen just behind the diener. These are used for initial fixation of organs. The smaller plastic boxes, in front of her, are used to store the organs after review at Gross Conference. These boxes should have tightly fitted lids, to minimize formalin evaporation.

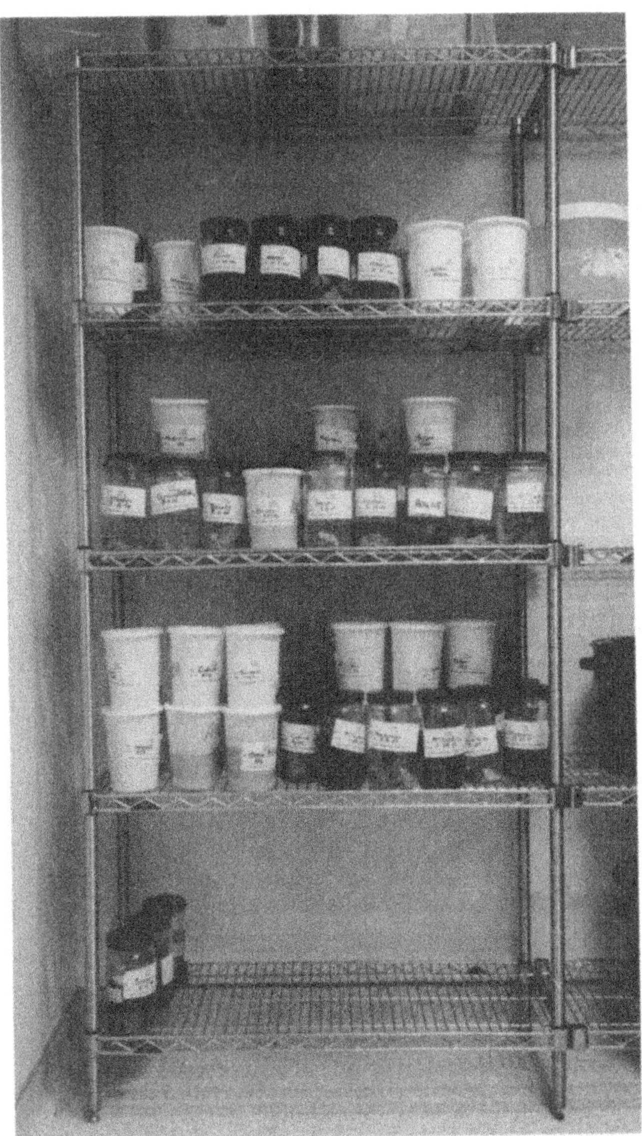

Fig. 6-7. These smaller containers are used to retain small sections of all the major organs. They are retained for one year.

MEASURES TO AVOID INJURY As mentioned in the first chapter, the concept of "universal precautions" assumes that all autopsies are potentially infectious. Thus, persons engaged in postmortem examinations must be protected from splatter, direct skin exposure, and cuts. To comply with this standard, all people engaged in evisceration and dissection activities must wear surgical scrubs, face protection (safety goggles and mask or plastic face shield), head cover, double latex or nonlatex gloves in between which is a cut-resistant glove on both hands, sleeve covers, an apron (or equivalent), and shoe covers (Fig. 6-8).

Steel-mesh gloves are available and do provide the most effective protection against cuts. However, they greatly reduce the "feel" that is needed to evaluate the texture of organs and lesions. This author believes that strict and consistent attention to safe handling of sharps is the best method for preventing cutting injuries. The reader is directed to the discussion of safe handling of sharps in Chapter 2. If both the diener and prosector are working inside the body cavity of the deceased, such as blunt dissection of abdominal adhesions, no scalpels are to be used. If use of a scalpel is required, then the person not wielding the blade must remove his(her) hands from the area and wait until the specific task is completed. Proper maintenance of other cutting instruments can also reduce the chance of injuries. Knives, if serviceably sharp, are far safer than dull knives, since the latter require greater force during cutting and thus are more prone to slip. Scissors, most of which should be blunt tipped, must be routinely sharpened. A good set of sharp scissors will encourage prosectors to use them rather than scalpels. To maintain the sharpness of the scissors as long as possible, all users should desist from using them to cut bone. The dieners should set aside either a dull pair of scissors or a bone-cutting instrument to be used for that purpose.

If a Faxitron® (225 Larkin Drive, Wheeling, IL) is utilized in the laboratory, it will require yearly safety checks by the radiation safety group in the hospital. Handling of radioactive isotopes is discussed in detail in Chapter 11.

The concentration of formalin fumes in the air must be monitored intermittently, as directed by Occupational Safety and Health Administration (OSHA) formaldehyde standard (29CFR1910.1048) and required by the College of American Pathologists (CAP) *(2)*. Good ventilation, tight fitting covers on specimen containers and a safety-oriented approach will reduce the exposure to acceptable levels.

Review of the patient's medical record may suggest that (s)he had an infection that if transmitted to autopsy personnel, would pose a significant threat of chronic disease or death. Such a postmortem exam has been termed "high risk autopsy" *(3)*. Infectious diseases included in this group are tuberculosis, acquired immunodeficiency syndrome, Creutzfeldt-Jakob disease, Hantavirus pulmonary syndrome, Neisseria meningitis and hepatitis (See these entries in Part II.) Cutting injuries *(4)* and other forms of exposure are documented to transmit these diseases *(5–9,17)* and even cause fatalities. It is estimated that the risk of developing tuberculosis in autopsy personnel is 100–200 times greater than the risk in the general population *(15)*. Risks and safety precautions have been discussed in numerous publications, particularly for HIV *(4,6–9,11)*, tuberculosis *(10,12–15)*, Creutzfeldt-Jakob disease *(9,16)*, and Hantavirus *(2)*.

In high-risk autopsies such as these, we recommend limiting the number of persons in the autopsy room to the prosector, the deiner and a "clean" assistant who completes paper work and performs all duties that do not require contact with body fluids, tissues, and contaminated surfaces or instruments. Proper face protection, gloves, and garments, cleaning procedures, and waste disposal are discussed above. The cut end of the ribs should be covered with cloth so as to prevent punctures. Scalpels should be used only when absolutely necessary and as with all autopsies.

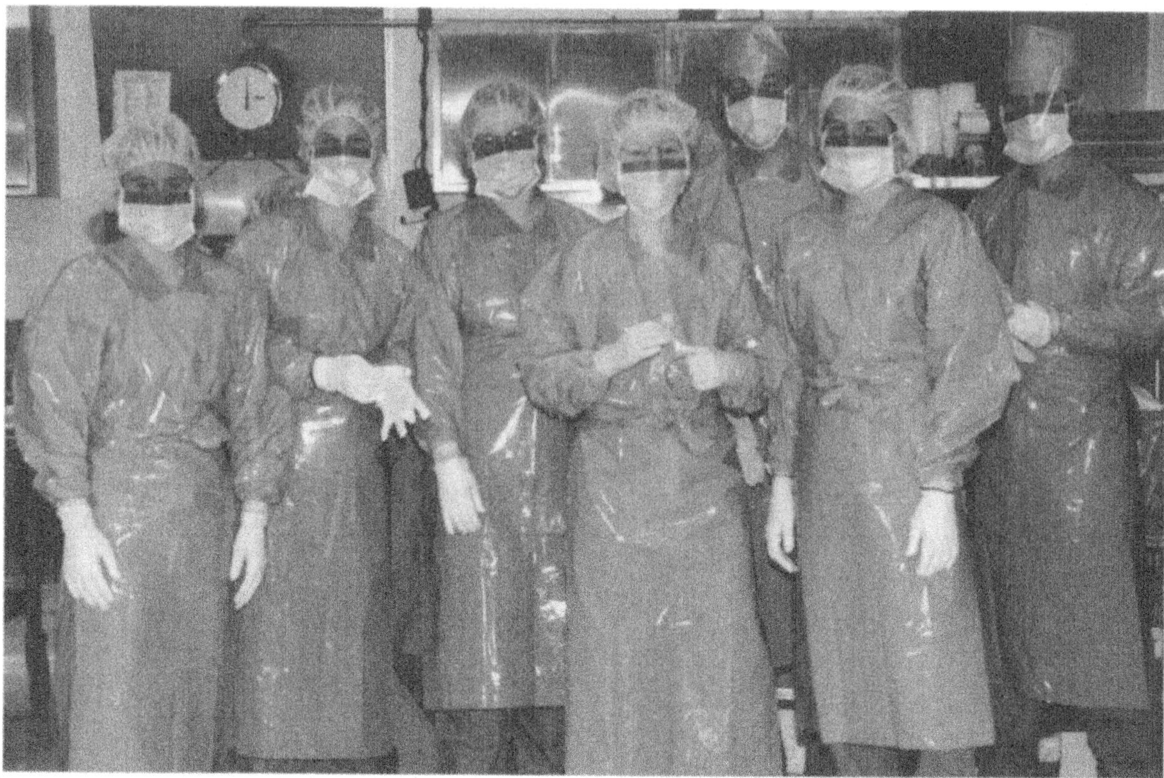

Fig. 6-8. Personal Protective Equipment. Not pictured are the required shoe covers.

During autopsies on patients with tuberculosis or other airborne infectious agents, morgue personnel must use powered, high-efficiency particulate air (HePa) filters (Fig. 6-9). The latter must be individually fitted and training for using this equipment must be provided. Face protection is particularly important when aerosol hazards are great, such as during the opening of the cranial vault. For additional protection, this latter procedure should be performed with the saw inside a plastic bag as discussed in Chapter 4 (Nervous System).

Before leaving this topic, it is important to emphasize that the most effective strategy for preventing transmission of infection during any autopsy is assiduous attention to safe scalpel handling. As Geller states in his article *(6)*, "the greatest danger in most settings is not the patient or the autopsy facility, but the pathologist's lack of regard for the potential risk inherent in every autopsy"

Finally, all autopsy personnel must receive appropriate immunizations and tests for organisms to which they may be exposed (e.g., hepatitis B vaccine and skin testing for tuberculosis).

RESPONDING TO INJURIES One should never ignore the presence of blood beneath a glove. The glove must be removed, as well as the cut–resistant glove, so as to make sure that the glove immediately next to the hand is not cut

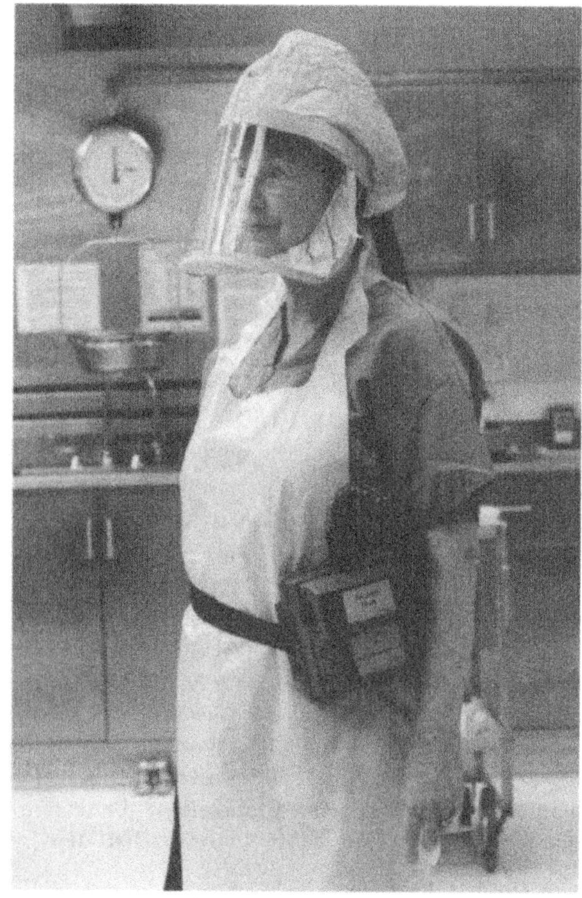

Fig. 6-9. Here the diener sports the Hepa filter apparatus. Of course, during an autopsy, she would be wearing all components of personal protective equipment.

as well. If the integrity of this glove indeed is breached, then one must immediately investigate the possibility of a cutting injury. Should a cut injury be discovered, then the wound must be thoroughly washed and the incident reported to the institution's Employee Health Department as soon as possible.

If potentially contaminated material makes contact with the eyes, the eyes should be flushed immediately, under a properly installed eye flush device. Flushing should be continued for 15 min. Incidents such as these must also be reported to the Employee Health Department for further advice, observation (e.g., repeated testing for HIV), and/or treatment. A detailed Employee Incident—Injury/Illness Investigation Report must be filed. Workmen's compensation and other proceedings may rely on such records.

REFERENCES

1. al-Wali W, Kibbler CC, McLaughlin JE. Bacteriological evaluation of a down-draught necropsy table ventilating system. J Clin Pathol 1993;46:746–749.
2. College of American Pathologists. Anatomic Pathology Checklist #ANP.33500, 2006. Northfield, IL
3. Claydon SM. The high risk autopsy. Am J Forensic Med Pathol 1993;14(3):253–256.
4. Johnson MD, Schaffner W, Atkinson J, Pierce MA. Autopsy risk and acquisition of human immunodeficiency virus infection: a case report and reappraisal. Arch Pathol Lab Med 1997;121:64–66.
5. Nolte KB, Taylor DG, Richmond JY. Biosafety considerations for autopsy. Am J Forensic Med Pathol 2002;23(2):107–122.
6. Geller AS, The autopsy in acquired immunodeficiency syndrome. How and why. Arch Pathol Lab Med 1990;114:324–329.
7. Karhunen PJ, Brummer-Korvenkontio H, Leinikki P, Nyberg M. Stability of human immunodeficiency virus (HIV) antibodies in postmortem samples. J Forensic Sci 1994;39:129–135.
8. Douceron H, Deforges L, Gherardi R, Sobel A, Chariot P. Long-lasting postmortem viability of human immunodeficiency virus: a potential risk in forensic medicine practice. Forensic Sci Int 1993;60:61–66.
9. Ironside JW, Bell JE. The 'high-risk' neuropathological autopsy in AIDS and Creutzfeldt-Jakob disease: principles and practice. [Review] Neuropathol Appl Neurobiol 1996;22:388–393.
10. Ussery XT, Bierman JA, Valway SE, Seitz TA, DiFerdinando GT Jr, Ostroff SM. Transmission of multidrug-resistant Mycobacterium tuberculosis among persons exposed in a medical examiner's office, New York. Inf Contr & Hosp Epidemiol 1995;16:160–165.
11. McCaskie AW, Roberts M, Gregg PJ. Human tissue retrieval at post-mortem for musculoskeletal research. Br J Biomed Sci 1995;52:222–224.
12. Kappel TJ, Reinartz JJ, Schmid JL, Holter JJ, Azar MM. The viability of mycobacterium tuberculosis in formalin-fixed pulmonary autopsy tissue: review of the literature and brief report. [Review]. Hum Pathol 1996;27:1361–1364.
13. Wilkins D, Woolcock AJ, Cossart YE. Tuberculosis: medical students at risk. Med J Austral 1994;160:395–397.
14. Lundgren R, Norrman E, Asberg I. Tuberculosis infection transmitted at autopsy. Tubercle 1987;68:147–150.
15. Collins CH, Grange JM. Tuberculosis acquired in laboratories and necropsy rooms. Commun Dis Public Health 1999;2(3):161–167.
16. Budka H, Aguzzi A, Brown P, Brucher JM, Bugiani O, Collinge J, Diringer H, et al. Consensus report: tissue handling in suspected Creutzfeldt-Jakob disease (CJD) and other spongiform encephalopathies (prion diseases) in the human. Brain Pathol 1995:5:319–322.
17. Healing TD, Hoffman PN, Young SE. The infection hazards of human cadavers. Commun Dis Rep. CRD Review. 1995;5:R61–R68.
18. Nolte KB, Foucar K, Richmond JY. Hantaviral biosafety issues in the autopsy room and laboratory: concerns and recommendations. Hum Pathol 1996;27:1253–1254.

7 Autopsy Microbiology

Brenda L. Waters

GENERAL COMMENTS

The pathologist may be tempted to obtain multiple cultures while performing an autopsy, considering the variety of tissues and fluids that are available to him or her. However, the medical literature is replete with examples of discrepancies between clinical evidence of infection and postmortem culture results *(1–6)*. These discrepancies are attributed to contamination during specimen collection *(5, 6)*, transmigration of bacteria from the gut into surrounding tissues and blood *(2, 4)*, and even the presence of indigenous bacteria in normal, healthy tissue *(7)*. Of these explanations, contamination is most frequently implicated and remains a major obstacle in meaningful postmortem microbiology. The theory of transmigration has never been substantiated. Articles published as early as 1921 offered evidence to disprove it *(8)*. As for the presence of indigenous bacteria in normal tissue, this theory has never gained much support. An exhaustive review of postmortem bacteriology can be found in references *9* and *10*.

Given the lack of specificity inherent in postmortem microbiology, it is necessary for the prosector to be very careful in her selection of specimens for culture. This approach will optimize the information obtained as well as limit the cost of microbiologic assessment. Moreover, judicious use of cultures in the autopsy service fosters a good working relationship with the microbiology laboratory.

A thorough knowledge of gross pathology is the best tool for determining what specimens to submit for culture. In most patients whose immunologic status is intact, a grossly visualized host response, such as pneumonia, abscess, caseating granuloma, or cloudy, foul-smelling fluid is the best indication for culture. As a rule, one should not culture if there is no grossly evident host response or no clinical information to raise suspicion of infection. Positive cultures from tissues that show no inflammation histologically generally are the result of contamination and, thus are meaningless.

CONSIDERATIONS IN IMMUNOCOMPROMISED PATIENTS Immunocompromised patients require a different approach at autopsy. Since their inflammatory response is blunted or absent, their infections may not be grossly evident. Thus, the selection of specimens for microbiological assay must be directed by a thorough understanding of the clinical history, close communication with the physicians who cared for the patient, and a carefully thought out differential diagnosis of possible etiologic agents. At the autopsy table, the pathologist should carry a higher index of suspicion and be prompted to submit cultures from organs that show no gross features of infection. Furthermore, the variety of organisms to which these patients are susceptible is greater, requiring a larger scope of microbiological methods to isolate and characterize them. As a result, specimens might be collected for bacterial, mycobacterial, and fungal culture, and tissue submitted in transport media for viral culture. Immediate placement of tissue in fixative for electron microscopy, freezing of tissue at –70°C, and obtaining air-dried smears or touch preparations also may be indicated.

THE VALUE OF THE GRAM STAIN A powerful tool in the autopsy pathologist's armamentarium is the Gram stain. This stain is inexpensive, easy to perform, and can be done by the pathologist with little inconvenience to the clinical laboratory staff.

With just a brief examination of the smear, an experienced pathologist can characterize the inflammatory response or identify neoplasia. Such findings may direct the focus of further investigation. Gram stains of smears and touch preps are superior to those of paraffin-embedded tissue in demonstrating bacterial morphology.

If the presence of an infection is in doubt, tissue or fluid samples may be submitted to the clinical microbiology laboratory with the instruction to "culture for bacteria if Gram stain shows inflammation." Although this instruction may sound vague, it encourages dialog between the microbiology staff and the autopsy physicians and demonstrates the commitment of the autopsy service to minimize unnecessary cultures.

Touch preparations of tissue for Gram staining are best obtained from a 1-cm^3 tissue block from which excess blood and tissue fluid are removed by dabbing the specimen once or twice on a paper towel. Then, the tissue fragment is blotted 2 or 3 times onto different areas of a slide. Following air-drying and heat fixation, the touch preparations are ready to Gram stain and examine. The "pull-prep" method is useful in preparing smears of fluid or pus for Gram staining. In this procedure, a single drop of fluid is placed onto the center of a slide. A second slide

From: *Handbook of Autopsy Practice*, 4th Ed. Edited by: B.L. Waters

is pressed against the first, keeping the slides nearly congruent, and then the two are pulled apart, thereby spreading the fluid into a thin layer. It is best to place the drop of fluid in the center of the slide so as to maximize the area over which the fluid will be spread. In most cases, a single small drop of fluid is sufficient, despite the temptation to add more.

PRINCIPLES OF SPECIMEN COLLECTION In the setting of an autopsy, as well as thc great majority of clinical situations, the use of swabs for collecting material is inadequate. Fluids or exudates should be collected in needleless syringes, which may be conveniently sealed with the cap that accompanied them. Two to three milliliters of fluid are sufficient. This volume allows storage of leftover fluid for future use, should new questions arise. Tissue specimens should measure at least 1–2 cm^3. If the sample is too small, it may dry out during transportation to the microbiology laboratory. Some laboratories freeze and store unused tissue for several weeks in case histologic examination reveals an unexpected finding, such as viral inclusions or granulomatous inflammation.

The tools needed to obtain specimens for culture at autopsy (Fig. 7-1) include a Bunsen burner, matches, spatula, forceps that can be sterilized in the flame, scalpels, sterile syringes and needles, sterile specimen containers, blood culture bottles, povidone iodine and alcohol swabs, an appropriate container for disposal of sharps, and the necessary writing utensils to label the containers and requisition slips. Protective eyewear and gloves are also required. Glass slides should be available for smears and touch preparations. Any grinding or surface decontamination of tissues is best performed in a biosafety cabinet by the microbiology technologists.

Finally, both safety and courtesy demand that all specimen containers departing the autopsy suite be clean and dry on the outside. Given the nature of the autopsy procedure, this standard may take more effort to achieve but it must be no less inviolable. It may be helpful to have an assistant with clean, gloved hands who can fill the blood culture bottles and handle the containers while the prosector procures the specimens.

SPECIMEN COLLECTION

BLOOD CULTURES Postmortem blood cultures infrequently provide useful information. A study *(5)* from a general hospital showed that in 54% of patients with negative antemortem blood cultures, positive blood cultures were obtained postmortem although the patients had no infectious disease that could be implicated as a cause of death. Of patients with confirmed antemortem bacteremia/fungemia, only 34% had a postmortem blood culture from which the same organism was isolated. Moreover, of patients without cultures or with negative or contaminated antemortem blood cultures, all had positive postmortem cultures; 76% of the isolates were considered contaminants and 22% of the isolates were of indeterminate significance *(5)*. Thus, the decision to obtain a blood culture at autopsy should rely on a strong clinical suspicion of sepsis in the absence of an isolated pathogen ante-mortem. Given the poor reproducibility of postmortem blood cultures, there is little utility in trying to reisolate a known bloodstream pathogen at autopsy. Hospitalized patients commonly receive antibiotics prior to phlebotomy for blood cultures. This is frequently prompted by new fever spikes or acute deterioration in clinical status. Despite such treatment, organisms may still be isolated at autopsy from these patients *(1)*.

Although the theory of bacterial transmigration through the bowel wall is largely dismissed, traditional autopsy protocol recommends that blood be obtained prior to manipulation or

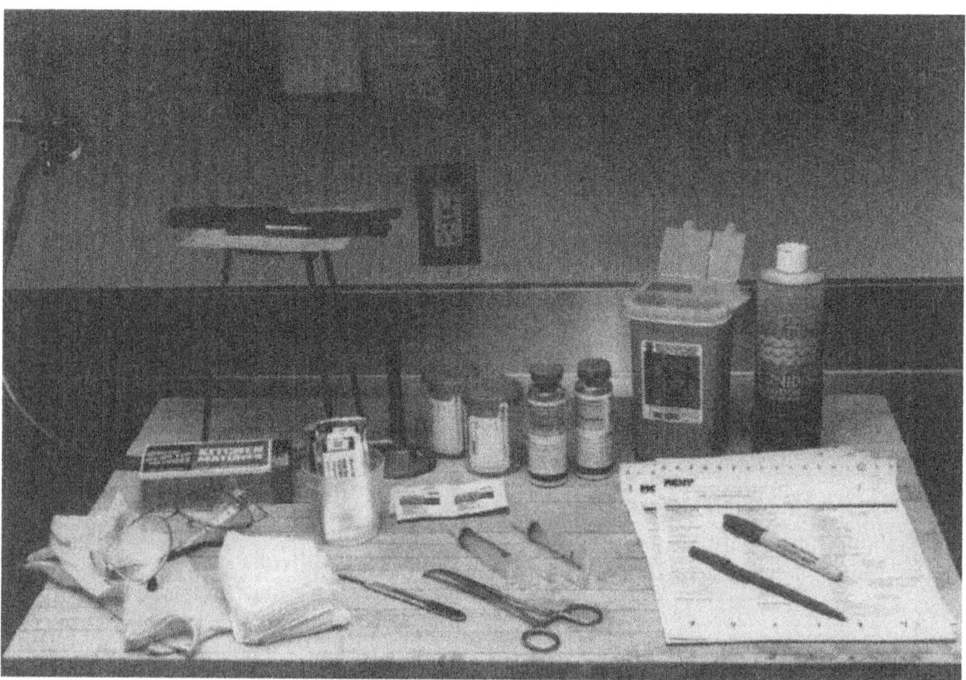

Fig. 7-1. Equipment need for collecting autopsy specimens for culture. These tools should be readily available in the autopsy laboratory. See text for details.

removal of the bowel. Blood may be obtained from the right atrium, inferior vena cava, or from the aorta. Searing the area with a hot spatula will sterilize the site of needle entry. In cases requiring a femoral stick, sterilize the skin with povidone iodine. In fetuses and neonates, a portion of liver may be submitted in place of blood, since searing of the heart or great vessels may cause significant damage.

LUNG CULTURES The lungs' gross appearance should direct the pathologist to the best site for culture. The most common evidence of infectious pneumonia is parenchymal consolidation and less often fibrinous pleuritis. Observation and palpation of the lungs while they are still *in situ* is the best method for detecting these changes. The surface of the lungs may be sterilized by searing with a heated spatula. Four stabbing motions, 90° to each other with a sterile blade, will mobilize a cube of tissue that can then be lifted up with a sterile forceps. The blade can then make the final cut to free the tissue block. The tip of the forceps should not be too hot as the tissue will stick, making it difficult to drop the specimen into the container. Providing that the lung has not been perfused with formalin, areas of consolidation may still be cultured after the lung is sliced. Again, the surface should be sterilized by searing. In patients with moderate to severe emphysema, pneumonia may be more difficult to visualize grossly. Thus, in these patients, the prosector's index of suspicion should be raised.

It is standard practice in most microbiology laboratories that with all cultures of tissue a Gram stain is performed as well. If the prosection occurs in the morning, the results of the Gram stain may be available to be included in the preliminary autopsy report.

Oral and gastric contents may enter the bronchial tree agonally or during transit of the body to the autopsy room. This contamination may darken the pulmonary cut surface as well as add more bacteria to the lung parenchyma. However, the lack of consolidation will help the pathologist to conclude that the discoloration is not pneumonia. Should the pathologist obtain a lung culture of such an area, the Gram stain will yield the correct interpretation.

ABSCESSES During evisceration or dissection of organs, abscesses may be found unexpectedly. In such cases, the prosector should immediately aspirate some of the pus into a syringe. An attempt should be made to take material from the center of the abscess. Even though an abscess may be inadvertently opened prior to culturing, an aspirate of the material is still quite acceptable since any organisms in the abscess will far outnumber those introduced during the course of the dissection. The Gram stain will aid in this interpretation.

There is no reason to culture acute perforations of bowel since both Gram stain and culture will point to fecal flora. Only when a host response is seen, such as an abscess, should a culture be deemed appropriate.

VALVULARVEGETATIONS The microbiologic investigation of endocarditis is a special challenge for the pathologist, because it competes with the other components of a complete examination, that of, photography and histology. If a vegetation is suspected clinically, the task is easier. In the case of an aortic or pulmonic valve vegetation, the ascending aorta or main pulmonary artery may be cut carefully away so as to visualize the valve leaflets (Fig. 7-2). Following photography, a portion of the vegetation may be removed with sterile forceps and scalpel or scissors and sent for culture. Enough material should be collected to allow for an adequate Gram stain to be prepared as well. Since the amount of tissue is usually scant, it should be sent to the microbiology laboratory as soon as possible to prevent drying.

In a patient with suspected infective endocarditis of the mitral or tricuspid valve, the outside of the heart need not be seared as this would cause unnecessary disfigurement of the heart. Rather, begin the cut at the corresponding atrium and extend it into the ventricle along the acute or obtuse margin (right or left ventricles, respectively) with a sterile scalpel until the ventricular chamber is entered and the valve is visualized (Fig. 7-3). With the help of an assistant to keep the ventricle open, the prosector may take photographs and procure a portion of the vegetation for culture and Gram stain.

If coronary atherosclerosis and myocardial infarctions are anticipated, the prosector may find it more appropriate to examine (or remove) the coronary arteries prior to addressing the valve pathology. Manipulation of the heart should be minimized. The pathologist may then begin to "breadloaf" the heart, keeping the slices at a 1-cm thickness. This approach ensures good demonstration of myocardial infarctions, should they be present. When the slices have reached the tip of the papillary muscles, the valve may be viewed from below and specimens may be procured for Gram stain and culture. When infective vegetations are encountered unexpectedly, the pathologist should submit tissue

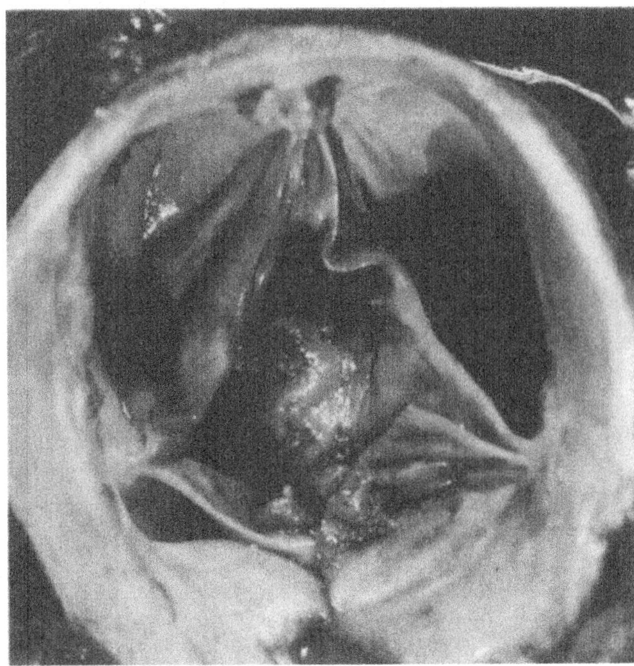

Fig. 7-2. Aseptic exposure of aortic valve vegetation. The aorta has been trimmed away to allow good visualization of the aortic valve. Photography and collection of a portion of the vegetation for culture and Gram stain was easily accomplished. (Courtesy D. W. D. Edwards)

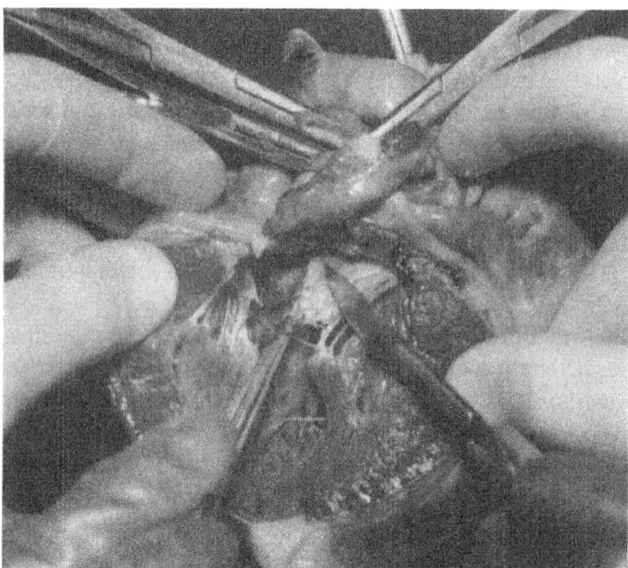

Fig. 7-3. Aseptic exposure of a mitral valve. With an incision into the left ventricle along the obtuse margin, the valve is adequately exposed for photography and sampling of a vegetation for culture and Gram stain.

for culture and Gram stain, despite the expected contamination. Important information can still be obtained because the repertory of expected pathogens is limited and the Gram stain will aid in the interpretation of the culture results.

DRAINING SINUSES Since draining sinuses are usually continuous with the skin surface, they may be heavily contaminated with skin flora. Thus, the material closest to the skin surface should be wiped away with sterile gauze. The purulent material that is present in the deeper sections of the sinus will be much more informative. This material may be aspirated with a large bore needle and syringe, a scalpel or, as a last resort, a swab. The Gram stain is critically important in the interpretation of the organisms isolated. The presence of acute inflammation will differentiate true infection from colonization. When the clinical history suggests *Actinomyces*, the prosector should examine a portion of the pus for "sulfur granules." If they are found, they may be pressed between two slides and then the two slides may be pulled apart, as with the "pull-prep." Since sulfur granules are more solid and require more force to spread out, it is safer to press the two slides together on a counter top, so as to avoid breaking the slides.

CEREBROSPINAL FLUID (CSF) When infectious meningitis is suspected but not confirmed prior to death, the prosector may find it necessary to procure CSF. This is most easily accomplished by performing a cisternal tap. The procedure entails placing the body in a prone position making sure that there is adequate padding under the face so as to avoid disfigurement. After vigorous cleansing of the skin with iodine and then alcohol, insert a 12-gauge needle at the midline below the base of the occipital bone and directed slightly superiorly, toward the eyes. Advance the needle slowly and carefully, with frequent attempts to aspirate fluid. Unnecessary movement of the syringe should be avoided so as to prevent bleeding. If no or only blood-tinged CSF is aspirated, it is still possible to collect a satisfactory specimen after removal of the calvarium. A needle may be inserted in the subarachnoid space. Should this fail, a tissue specimen of meninges and a small amount of underlying brain may be taken. Pus tends to collect in the inferior aspect of the brain, thus making collection of material possible.

If a brain abscess is suspected, the prosector can try to localize the lesion by palpation. Should the site be determined, the brain surface can be sterilized by searing and aspiration can be attempted with a long, large-bore needle. In certain situations, hemisection of the brain (*see* Chapter 4) and fresh cutting of one half may be indicated.

REFERENCES

1. Koneman EW, Minckler TM, Shires DB, de Jongh DS. Postmortem bacteriology: II. Selection of cases for culture. J Clin Pathol 1971;55:17–23.
2. Nehring JR, Sheridan MF, Funk W. Postmortem bacteriology: II. The use of tracer organisms to evaluate the possibility of postmortem bacterial transmigration. Am J Clin Pathol 1971;56:133–134.
3. Koneman EW, Davis MA. Postmortem bacteriology: III. Clinical significance of microorganisms recovered at autopsy. Am J Clin Pathol 1974;61:28–40.
4. Kellerman GD, Waterman NG, Scharfenberger LF. Demonstration *in vitro* of postmortem bacterial transmigration. Am J Clin Pathol 1976;66:911–915.
5. Wilson SJ, Wilson ML, Reller, LB. Diagnostic utility of postmortem blood cultures. Arch Pathol Lab Med 1993;117:986–988.
6. Wilson ML. Clinically relevant, cost-effective clinical microbiology. Strategies to decrease unnecessary testing. Am J Clin Pathol 1997;107:154–167.
7. Minckler TM, Newell GR, O'Toole WF, Niwayama G, Levine PH. Microbiology experience in collection of human tissue. Am J Clin Pathol 1966;45:85–92.
8. Giordano AS, Barnes AR. Studies in postmortem bacteriology. Value and importance of cultures made postmortem. J Lab Clin Med 1921;7:538–546.
9. Morris JA, Harrison LM, Partridge SM. Postmortem bacteriology: a re-evaluation. J Clin Pathol 2006; 59:1–9.
10. Morris JA, Harrison LM, Partridge SM. Practical and theoretical aspects of postmortem bacteriology. Curr Diagn Pathol 2007;13:65–74.

8 Autopsy Chemistry

Vernard I. Adams

DEFINITION, INDICATIONS AND LIMITATIONS OF THE METHOD

Autopsy chemistry, or postmortem chemistry, is the term applied to the measurement of endogenous constituents in dead bodies. Toxicological tests, which measure concentrations of exogenous drugs and toxins, are discussed in Chapter 13. Postmortem chemical studies provide *direct* information concerning derangements of physiology. In contrast, customary gross and histological autopsy examinations are primarily tests of structural derangements, from which physiologic derangements may sometimes be inferred. Chemical testing may not only establish the cause of death but may contribute to the evaluation of the physiologic effects of recognizable anatomic lesions. For example, the extent of uremia can be determined in a case of polycystic kidney disease.

Although any clinical laboratory test may be applied to postmortem material, only a limited number of tests yield interpretable results. Useful tests fall into two groups; those which measure analytes which are stable after death, and those which measure a diagnostically useful postmortem rise or fall in the concentration of the analyte. For many biochemical substances, interpretation of postmortem tests is precluded by the total absence of published data.

Our understanding of postmortem chemistry was considerably enhanced by the pioneering work of J. L. Coe *(1)*, a forensic pathologist who showed that the vitreous, a specimen unavailable for clinical testing, is the substrate of choice for what have become the most frequently used postmortem chemical tests. Because the eye is mechanically isolated and protected by the orbit, vitreous humor is usually preserved even if serious trauma to the head has occurred. Vitreous humor is less subject to putrefaction than is blood, and is not subject to diffusion of drugs and alcohols from the stomach. Like cerebrospinal fluid, it is nearly free of erythrocytes, but is more accessible, and the artifacts produced by its procurement are easier to recognize as such.

In this chapter, we give only an overview of autopsy chemistry. For methodological details, the reader should consult standard textbooks and manuals of laboratory medicine and the references in the review articles by Coe *(1)* and Kleiner et al. *(2)*. Many of the data presented here are derived from Coe's work.

From: *Handbook of Autopsy Practice,* 4th Ed. Edited by: B.L. Waters

SELECTION AND COLLECTION OF SPECIMENS FOR ANALYSIS

Specimens for postmortem biochemical analysis must be retrieved, labeled, stored, and analyzed under established, standardized conditions *(3)*. In most cases, the time of sample procurement is the documented time of autopsy. For this reason, the recorded time of the autopsy should be the time that the internal examination is commenced. If a postmortem sample is drawn either before or after the internal autopsy examination, the time of procurement should be separately noted. Interpretation of postmortem chemistry reports is aided by the routine recording of early putrefactive changes.

BLOOD This is the substrate of choice for testing for hemoglobin S, hormones, cholinesterase, and abnormal metabolites in infants with suspected inborn errors of metabolism. Blood can be used to measure the concentrations of creatinine, urea nitrogen and bilirubin if vitreous, the specimen of choice, has not been procured. For glucose quantification, vitreous is superior. All postmortem serum or plasma samples have some degree of hemolysis, and laboratories differ in their tolerance for specimens of this type. The sampling and labeling policies required for toxicologic analysis are more than adequate for postmortem chemical analysis. The choice of container is dictated by the test to be undertaken, as in clinical testing. A common screening panel for inborn errors of metabolism requires drops of blood and bile on filter paper *(4)*.

VITREOUS This is the most frequently used specimen for postmortem chemical analysis. Typically a panel of six tests is run, comprising sodium, potassium, chloride, urea nitrogen, creatinine, and glucose. Bilirubin may be added to the panel if the gross autopsy is equivocal for the diagnosis of jaundice. If no postmortem chemical testing is contemplated, routinely drawn vitreous specimens can be sent to the toxicologist, who will use them for volatiles analysis and drug screening. Drug screening is described in Chapter 13. Depending on the analytical technique, centrifugation of the vitreous may be required to obtain a supernatant sample and thus avoid clogging the analytical instrument.

Table 8-1
Common Changes of Postmortem Chemical Values[a]

Substances	*Body fluids or tissues analyzed*	*Interpretation*
Bilirubin	Serum	Slight increase after death.
Chloride	Serum and vitreous	Serum chloride values decrease after death; vitreous sodium is stable. (*See* Table under "Dehydration" and "Uremia.")
Cholesterol	Serum	Stable after death (but *not* cholesterol esters).
Cholinesterase (true and pseu-do-cholinesterase)	Serum	Stable after death (important for diagnosis of organic phosphorus or carbofuran poisoning).
Creatinine	Serum and vitreous	Values stable after death.
Glucose	Serum and vitreous	High values in vena cava and right heart chambers; vitreous values rapidly drop to near zero except when blood glucose is pathologically elevated or when body is rapidly chilled. (*See* Table under "Diabetes mellitus" and "Hypoglycemia.")
Hypoxanthine	Vitreous	Values increase steadily after death; has been proposed to determine postmortem interval *(9)*. (*See* also "Potassium.")
Lactic acid	Serum and vitreous	Values increase after death.
Lipoproteins		(*See* "Triglycerides and lipoproteins.")
Potassium	Vitreous	Values increase steadily after death; has been proposed to determine postmortem interval. (*See* also "Hypoxanthine.")
Proteins	Serum	Electrophoretic patterns remain stable.
Sodium	Serum and vitreous	Serum sodium values decrease after death; vitreous sodium is stable until the onset of putrefaction.
Triglycerides and lipoproteins	Serum	Erratic changes after death.
Urea nitrogen	Serum and vitreous	Values stable after death.

[a] Data from refs (1) and (2) except as separately cited. Numerous other substances (e.g. ammonia, amino acids, creatine, magnesium, phosphates, sulfates, trace elements, uric acid, xanthine) have been studied in various body fluids but are not listed here because tests in the postmortem setting are unreliable or are rarely of practical importance.

Table 8-2
Postmortem Chemical Changes in Pathological Conditions[a]

Diseases or conditions	*Body fluids analyzed*	*Interpretation*
Acidosis and alkalosis	Serum	Postmortem pH diminishes. Not reliable for antemortem diagnosis. For ketoacidosis, see "Diabetes mellitus."
Dehydration	Vitreous	High sodium (>155 mEq/L) and chloride (>135 meq/L) values with increase (above 40 mg/dL) of urea nitrogen concentration.
Diabetes mellitus	Vitreous	High glucose (>200 mg/dL or >11.1 mmol/L) and ketone concentrations in diabetic ketoacidosis. Ketones can be detected by tablet screening, and by gas chromatography in the course of routine alcohol testing.
Endocrine disorders	Serum and other body fluids	The concentrations of many pituitary, adrenal cortical, and some other hormones *(10)* reflect the antemortem values. Epinephrine and insulin are unstable.
Hepatic coma	Cerebrospinal fluid	Glutamine concentrations increased.
Hyperglycemia		See "Diabetes mellitus."
Hypoglycemia		No reliable way to diagnose hypoglycemia from postmortem specimens.
Inborn errors of metabolism[b]	Blood and bile	Abnormal metabolites are found.
Liver diseases (*See* also "Hepatic coma")	Serum	Aminotransferases and other enzyme activities increase erratically after death and cannot be used for diagnosis. The albumin-globulin ratio can be estimated reliably.

(continued)

Table 8.2
(continued)

Diseases or conditions	*Body fluids analyzed*	*Interpretation*
Low-salt pattern	Vitreous	Low sodium, chloride, and potassium concentrations common in fatty change or cirrhosis of the liver.
Postmortem change unrelated to clinical disease (decomposition pattern)	Vitreous	Low sodium and chloride concentrations but *high* potassium values (>20 mEq/L).
Uremia	Vitreous	Marked increase of urea nitrogen and creatinine concentrations with sodium and chloride values near the normal range. (*See* also "Dehydration.")

[a] Based on data from ref (1) except as separately cited.

[b] Examples are maple syrup urine disease, methylmalonic acidemia, medium chain acyl-Co-A dehydrogenase deficiency.

INTERPRETATION OF POSTMORTEM CHEMICAL DATA

The most important changes of body fluid components after death are compiled in Table 8-1. A synopsis of postmortem chemical findings in diseases such as diabetes mellitus is shown in Table 8-2. The tables show that glucose is best determined in vitreous because blood glucose values may increase dramatically in the agonal period, particularly after resuscitation attempts *(1)*. Hyperglycemia and diabetic ketoacidosis can be diagnosed readily. Hypoglycemia cannot be confirmed by postmortem testing, but the ratio of insulin to C-peptide has been suggested for the postmortem diagnosis of insulin overdose *(5)*. The dehydration pattern (Table 8-2) provides a compelling basis for the diagnosis of dehydration in cases of homicidal deprivation of food and water *(6)*.

ADVANCED ANALYTICAL METHODS

Postmortem adrenaline and noradrenaline concentrations have been determined by high performance liquid chromatography *(7)*. Atomic absorption spectroscopy, together with inductively coupled plasma emission spectroscopy and inductively coupled plasma mass spectroscopy can quantify iron, copper, and other essential elements in fresh and formalin-fixed autopsy tissues *(8)*.

REFERENCES

1. Coe JL. Postmortem chemistry update. Emphasis on forensic application. Am J Forensic Med Pathol 1993;14:91–117.
2. Kleiner DE, Emmert-Buck MR, Liotta LA. Necropsy as a research method in the age of molecular pathology. Lancet 1995;346:945–946.
3. Forrest AR. Obtaining samples at post mortem examination for toxicological testing and biochemical analyses. ACP Broadsheet no 137: April 1993. J Clin Pathol 1993;46:292–296.
4. Chace DH, DiPerna JC, Mitchell, BL, Sgroi B, Hofman LF, Naylor EW. Electrospray tandem mass spectrometry for analysis of acylcarnitines in dried postmortem blood specimens collected at autopsy from infants with unexplained cause of death. Clin Chem 2001;47:1166–1182.
5. Iwase H, Kobayashi M, Nakajima M, Takatori T. The ratio of insulin to C-peptide can be used to make a forensic diagnosis of exogenous insulin overdose. For Sci Int 2001;115:123–127.
6. Madea B, Lachenmeier DW. Postmortem diagnosis of hypertonic dehydration. For Sci Int 2005; 155:1–6.
7. Hirvonen J, Huttunen P. Postmortem changers in serum noradrenalin and adrenalin concentrations in rabbit and human cadavers. Int J Legal Med 1996;109:143–146.
8. Bush VJ, Moyer TP, Batts KP, Parisi JE. Essential and toxic element concentrations in fresh and formalin-fixed human autopsy tissues. Clin Chem 1995;41:284–294.
9. Munoz JI, Suarez-Penaranda JM, Otero XL, Rodriguez-Calvo MS, Costas E, Miguens X, Concheiro L. A new perspective in the estimation of postmortem interval (PMI) based on vitreous. J Forensic Sci 2001;46:209–214.
10. Edston E, Druid H, Holmgren P, Ostrom M. Postmortem measurements of thryoid hormones in blood and vitreous humor combined with histology. Am J Forensic Med Pathol 2001;22-78–83.

9 Chromosome Analysis of Autopsy Tissue

Gordon W. Dewald

INDICATIONS

IN ADULTS Various aneuploidies of the sex chromosomes are the most common chromosome abnormalities encountered in autopsies of adults. The Turner (usually 45,X but mosaicism is common) and Klinefelter (47,XXY) syndromes are two examples *(1)*. Deletions or unbalanced translocations and inversions are rarely seen in autopsies of adults because patients with these abnormalities seldom survive into adulthood. Approximately 1/500 adults carries a genetically balanced abnormality of chromosome structure. These balanced chromosome anomalies may affect the reproductive history of an individual, but rarely affect the phenotype *(2)*. Some adults have sporadic chromosome changes as part of a chromosome breakage syndrome such as Fanconi anemia *(3)*, ataxia-telangiectasia *(4)*, Bloom syndromes *(5)*, and others.

Chromosome analysis may be done at autopsy to eliminate a specific clinical diagnosis. Thus, establishing that the karyotype of the deceased is normal can be useful. Chromosome studies may be done at autopsy to establish the karyotype of specific tissues when chromosome mosaicism is suspected *(6)*. Cytogenetic studies may be useful in the same setting to help resolve issues of malignant disorders. Chromosome studies can help establish the presence of an abnormal clone, classify neoplastic disorders, assess disease progression, and detect the emergence of therapy-related neoplasms. More than 200 different chromosome abnormalities have been strongly associated with specific malignant disorders *(7–9)*. In these cases, it is important that the tissue(s) selected for chromosome studies be derived from the neoplasm in question. Sometimes autopsy chromosome studies are done as part of research protocols.

IN NEONATES, INFANTS, AND CHILDREN Chromosome analysis should be done when malformations correspond to well-established chromosome syndromes, especially when the diagnosis is doubtful. The syndromes associated with aneuploidy are the most common and easily recognized at autopsy. Three of the more frequently encountered conditions in autopsies of newborns are the Down (trisomy 21) *(10)*, Patau (trisomy 13), and Edwards (trisomy 18) syndrome *(11)*. Presence of ambiguous genitalia is also a common indication of a genetic problem and may be a clue to gonadal dysgenesis, true hermaphroditism, and other abnormalities or gene mutations involving the sex chromosomes *(1,12)*.

As a group, deletions, translocations, and inversions are the most common chromosome abnormalities in newborns; they also are the most difficult to recognize clinically. Anomalies of chromosome structure can involve more than one chromosome and they can involve any part of any chromosome. Structural anomalies in neonates are often private mutations (i.e., found only in the deceased or some of their blood relatives). For this reason, genetic imbalances resulting from structural anomalies are inconsistent among individuals and the clinical presentation is generally nonspecific. Because structural anomalies usually are associated with multiple congenital anomalies, postmortem chromosome analysis may be done in severely malformed neonates. Three rare syndromes that involve abnormalities of chromosome structure and may be encountered at autopsy of neonates are Cri du Chat *(13)*, Wolf-Hirschhorn *(14)*, and Langer-Giedion syndromes *(15)*, but many others are known.

It is particularly important to do chromosome studies of a neonate when the family has a history of frequent spontaneous abortions, as the results can be useful in genetic counseling of living relatives *(2)*. Structural abnormalities of chromosomes can be familial when one of the parents is a balanced carrier. When this occurs, the parents of the deceased and other relatives may be at considerable risk to produce abnormal offspring and this information is important in family planning and the application of prenatal genetic testing with future pregnancies *(2)*.

IN SPONTANEOUS ABORTIONS Chromosome analyses on spontaneous abortuses can be an emotional benefit to patients, both in having the cause of death explained or in ruling out an identifiable inherited abnormality. Chromosome studies of spontaneous abortions may be done to define the cause of fetal demise, collect information on familial chromosome anomalies, and identify molar pregnancies *(16,17)*.

From 1991 to 1993, we studied 1,502 spontaneous abortuses; some were associated with recognizable fetal tissue but others did not contain discernible fetal tissue. We successfully completed chromosome studies on 1,164 of these specimens: 414 (36%) had a chromosome abnormality. Chromosome anomalies in abortuses with identifiable tissue included any

From: *Handbook of Autopsy Practice*, 4th Ed. Edited by: B.L. Waters

kind of autosomal trisomy (47%), triploidy (17%), and 45,X (Turner syndrome, 16%). The remaining chromosome anomalies included unbalanced translocations, aneuploidy of multiple chromosomes, mosaicism, tetraploidy, and balanced translocations. These results are consistent with other investigations of spontaneous abortions *(16)*.

Of the 33 abnormal spontaneous abortuses without recognizable fetal tissue, we found 5 that had triploid karyotypes. This karyotype is often associated with partial hydatidiform moles. In the remaining 28 spontaneous abortuses, 6 carried anomalies which could have been familial. Familial chromosome anomalies would include any unbalanced or balanced structural abnormality. In these cases, family members and subsequent pregnancies should be studied because of the risk that a similar chromosome abnormality will recur. Chromosome abnormalities identified in the remaining cases included trisomies and monosomies, and were the probable cause of fetal demise.

It is possible to calculate the statistical probability that future pregnancies of a couple will involve a chromosome abnormality based on the karyotype of the spontaneous abortus and the parents. In general, if the spontaneous abortus has an abnormal karyotype and the parents have a normal karyotype, the risk for a future abortion due to chromosome abnormalities is about 1%. Prenatal studies are often recommended in subsequent pregnancies when the spontaneous abortus has a trisomy or monosomy that has been associated with a classic syndrome.

Complete and partial hydatidiform moles are genetically aberrant conceptuses that have the potential to develop into malignancies *(17)*. Usually, complete moles have a diploid karyotype with only paternal chromosomes. Most partial moles have 69 chromosomes (triploidy), including 23 of maternal origin and 46 of paternal origin. Differentiation between complete and partial moles is important, as the two entities have different potentials for clinical persistence, malignant transformation, recurrence, and presence of a fetus. The complete mole consists of abnormal, cystic chorionic villi with no fetal tissue present. Retained fragments after an incomplete spontaneous abortion may evolve into choriocarcinoma. The risk of recurrence is about 1%. The partial mole also has cystic chorionic villi, but a fetus is always present initially. The fetal tissue may or may not survive up to the time of diagnosis. The recurrence risk for triploid partial hydatidiform moles is unknown. Subsequent pregnancies should be studied with either finding.

Any structural chromosome abnormality found in a spontaneous abortion requires chromosome studies on the parents to determine whether the abnormality is familial or a de novo mutation *(2)*. When the spontaneous abortus has a duplication or deletion not found in the parent, the recurrence risk is <0.5%. Thus, during subsequent pregnancies, studies are not strongly indicated. When the spontaneous abortus has an unbalanced inversion, and one parent is the carrier, recurrence risk in subsequent pregnancies ranges from 0.5% with a paracentric inversion to 5–10% with a pericentric inversion. In the latter case, prenatal studies are indicated for all future pregnancies. If the spontaneous abortion has a translocation, either balanced or unbalanced, prenatal studies would be indicated only if one of the parents carries the balanced translocation.

Approximately 80% of spontaneous abortions without recognizable fetal tissue in our study were chromosomally normal females. We suspect many of these studies were done on maternal cells. This potential for maternal contamination points out the importance of attempting to collect specimens that contain fetal tissues. When unidentifiable tissue is all that can be collected, the cytogenetic laboratory should attempt to further isolate embryonic or extra-embryonic tissue using a dissecting microscope. The rationale to do chromosome analyses on unidentified tissue is not always clear. In our study, only 11 of the 33 products of conception had chromosome anomalies, which may have explained the fetal demise or may have led to useful chromosome studies on the parents.

COSTS

Since cytogenetic studies are expensive, they should be applied to autopsies in a frugal manner, but they certainly are indicated if chromosome analysis is the only means to obtain pertinent medical information. The cost of chromosome analysis varies among cytogenetic laboratories and ranges from a few hundred dollars to over $1,000, depending on the type of tissue studied.

SPECIMEN COLLECTION, TRANSPORT, AND PROCESSING

Most cytogenetic studies require living tissues to obtain successful cell culture for chromosome studies *(18)*. For this reason, it is important to use sterile procedures to collect specimens. Whole blood and other tissues have been cultured successfully from mailed-in specimens for clinical purposes. Thus, it is not necessary for the autopsy pathologist to have ready access to a cytogenetic laboratory. Since living cells are involved, it is important to transport specimens to the cytogenetic laboratory within 1 or 2 d. Moreover, exposure of the specimen to temperature extremes (freezing or >30°C) can prevent a successful chromosome study. The specimens should not be frozen or packed on ice for delivery.

The cytogenetic laboratory is often used to culture cells from autopsies with evidence of a molecular or biochemical genetic disorder. In these cases, it is important that the prosector informs the cytogenetic laboratory about the need for molecular or biochemical genetic testing. This will ensure that the cytogenetic laboratory processes the specimen correctly and forwards the cultured cells to another laboratory for appropriate genetic or biochemical testing.

The following procedures may be used to prepare and mail specimens collected at autopsy for cytogenetic studies. When other tissues are needed, the collection procedure and mode of transportation should be discussed with personnel from the cytogenetic laboratory to enhance chances of a successful result.

BLOOD Blood is generally the preferred specimen for chromosome analysis when a congenital disorder is suspected and it is possible to collect an appropriate specimen. Obtain 5–10 mL of unclotted, uncontaminated blood in a sterile fashion. Mix the blood sample with 1 mL of sodium heparin in a small sterile vial and send it to the cytogenetic laboratory.

In the cytogenetic laboratory, the cells are incubated for 66–72 h at 37°C with a T-cell mitogen such as phytohemagglutinin to induce mitosis. The cells are then harvested for chromosome analysis using ethidium bromide, colcemid, and hypotonic solution and fixed with glacial acetic acid and methanol.

A few factors may interfere with processing blood for chromosome analysis. Cells may be lysed due to forcing the blood quickly through a needle. An improper anticoagulant (sodium heparin is best) or inadequately mixing the blood with the anticoagulant can cause the blood cells to clot. Rare patients have circulating T-lymphocytes that do not respond to mitogens.

FIBROBLASTS Specimens for fibroblast cultures should be collected at autopsy when a congenital disorder is suspected and blood is either unavailable or alternative tissues are needed to answer a medical question. Fibroblast cultures are generally more expensive than other chromosome studies because they require more time and culture maintenance. The prosector should make a longitudinal incision through disinfected skin of the lateral thigh and dissect down to the fascia lata. A 5–15 mm^2 sample of the fascia lata is then removed, together with about 2–3 mm thickness of underlying muscle. The tissue is wrapped in sterile gauze moistened with Hank's balanced salt solution (HBSS) and placed in a small sterile vial for transportation to the chromosome laboratory. Some laboratories have vials of Hank's solution already made up for use.

Upon arrival in the cytogenetic laboratory, the specimen is cut into small pieces and treated with enzymes *(19)*. The tissue is then placed into a culture flask with Chang and MEM-alpha-medium containing 20% fetal bovine serum (FBS) and antibiotics. After 5–14 d, the fibroblasts are processed for chromosome analysis with ethidium bromide, colcemid, hypotonic solution, and fixed with glacial acetic acid and methanol.

The most common problems with these specimens are lack of viable cells and bacterial contamination. These problems can interfere with attempts to establish fibroblast cultures.

BONE MARROW Bone marrow specimens may be required for chromosome studies at autopsy when a question of malignant hematological disorder is involved. Approximately 1 mL of bone marrow should be obtained in a sterile fashion and mixed with 1 mL of sodium heparin in a small sterile vial, and then sent to the cytogenetic laboratory.

In the cytogenetic laboratory, bone marrow specimens may either be processed for chromosome analysis directly or by a short-term (24–72 h) culture method *(19,20)*. In either case, the bone marrow is harvested for chromosome analysis by using ethidium bromide, colcemid, and hypotonic solution and then fixed with glacial acetic acid and methanol.

PRODUCTS OF CONCEPTION OR STILLBIRTHS These specimens should be collected when a congenital disorder is suspected and blood is unavailable. A 1-cm^3 biopsy of muscle and fascia from the thigh, a 1-cm^3 biopsy of lung, or 20–30 mg of chorionic villi should be obtained. Each biopsy sample is placed in a separate 15 mL sterile centrifuge tube with 10 mL of transfer culture media. In situations where the fetus is not identifiable, the specimen is placed in a single sterile container with 10 mL of HBSS or a similar solution.

Upon arrival in the laboratory, these specimens are cut into small pieces and treated with enzymes *(19)*. The tissues are then placed into separate tissue flasks with Chang and MEM-alpha-medium containing 20% FBS and antibiotics to establish a fibroblast culture. After 5–14 d, the fibroblasts are processed with ethidium bromide, colcemid, hypotonic solution, and fixed with glacial acetic acid and methanol.

Chromosome analysis may be unsuccessful because of a lack of viable cells or bacterial contamination. In our experience, this occurs in up to 20% of cases and is usually due to a lack of viable cells. If the fetus shows any degree of autolysis, it is recommended to take the sample from the placenta, preferably from the region just beneath the chorionic plate surface.

SOLID TUMORS The submitter of the tissue must make certain that only tumor is submitted for analysis. Normal cells are often present in and around tumor tissue, and in culture, these cells may grow better than neoplastic cells and overgrow them, resulting in the study of normal somatic cells.

Neoplastic chromosomal abnormalities are rarely present in normal tissues. Necrotic areas of the tumor should also be avoided. Using sterile procedures, a 5-mm^3 or larger tumor biopsy is submitted. The specimen is placed in a transport container with 5 mL of HBSS or a similar solution.

In the cytogenetic laboratory, the tissue is dissociated using enzymes and/or mechanical means and then transferred to culture flasks *(19)*. The cultures are incubated at 37°C with 5% C02, 5% O2 and 90% N2 for 1–2 d depending on cell growth. The cells are harvested for chromosome analysis with ethidium bromide, colcemid, hypotonic solution, and fixed with glacial acetic acid and methanol.

PARAFFIN EMBEDDED TISSUES These specimens are not suitable for conventional cytogenetic studies. However, methods are now available to detect chromosome anomalies in paraffin embedded tissues using fluorescence-labeled DNA probes and in situ hybridization (FISH). The FISH studies can be performed on extracted individual nuclei or on thin section preparations *(21)*. These methods are particularly useful for studying specimens that may involve neoplastic disorders or do not have viable cells for conventional chromosome studies such as products of conception *(22)*.

METHODS OF CHROMOSOME ANALYSIS AND INTERPRETATION OF RESULTS

The methods to analyze chromosomes are numerous, sophisticated, and vary among laboratories. Today, the cytogenetic laboratory must be proficient with many forms of culture techniques, more than 20 different chromosome staining methods, and have expertise with FISH *(18,23–25)*. Typical examples are shown in Fig. 9-1. Metaphases are usually stained with G-banding, but other staining methods are frequently employed as needed. Twenty metaphases are typically examined for structure and number of chromosomes, but structural chromosome abnormalities are subtle and can be missed. In cases where mosaicism is suspected, 30 or more metaphases are often analyzed. Nevertheless, true mosaicism is sometimes missed because of metaphase sampling error. Representative metaphases are photographed and karyotypes are prepared from at least two cells.

In the case of malignant neoplasms, two or more metaphases with the same structural abnormality or extra chromosome, or three or more metaphases lacking the same chromosome, are

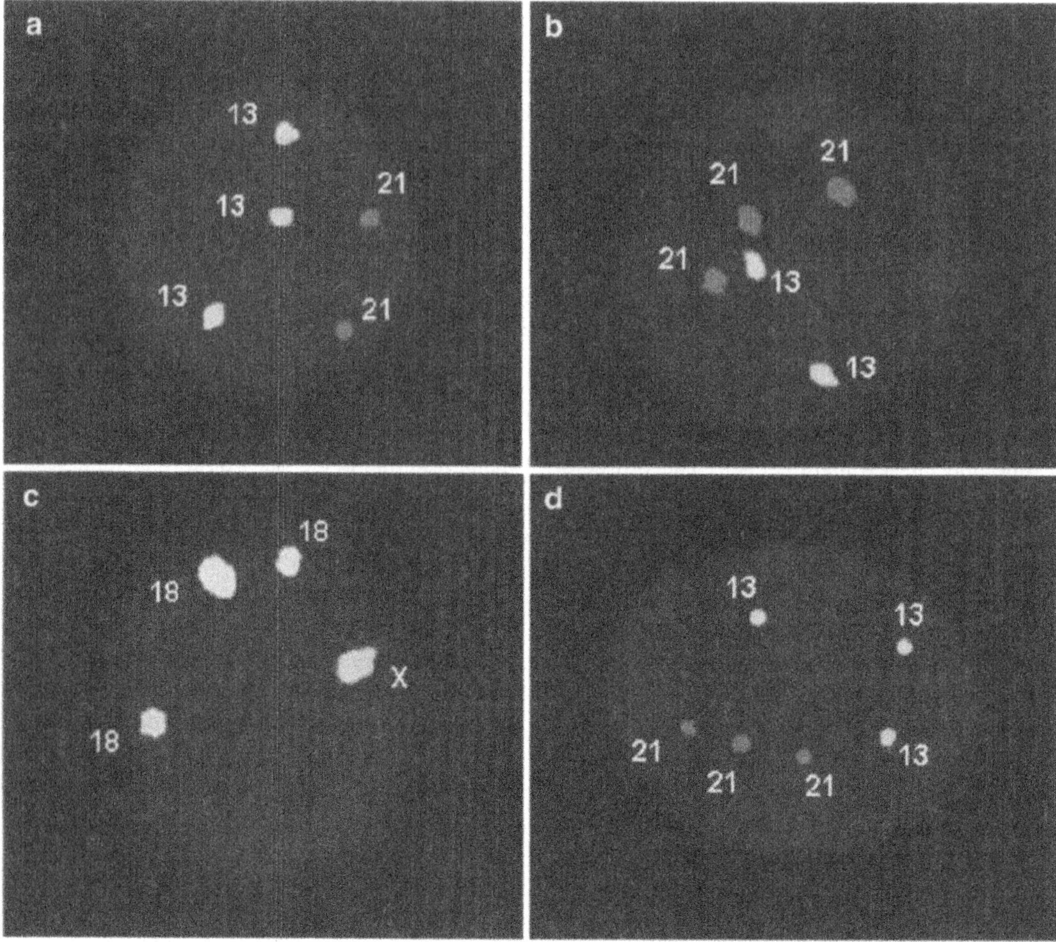

Fig. 9-1. Utility of fluorescence *in situ* hybridization (FISH). (**a**) FISH with locus-specific DNA probes for chromosome 13 band q14 and chromosome 21 band q11.2-q22.2 in an interphase cell with trisomy 13. (**b**) FISH with locus-specific DNA probes for chromosome 13 band q14 and chromosome 21 q11.2-q22.2 in an interphase cell with trisomy 21. (**c**) FISH with centromere-specific DNA probes for the X chromosome and chromosome 18 in an interphase cell with monosomy X and trisomy 18. (**d**) FISH with locus-specific DNA probes for chromosome 13 band q14 and chromosome 21 band q11.2-q22.2 in a triploid interphase cell.

regarded as minimal evidence for the presence of an abnormal clone *(26)*. In some neoplastic disorders, abnormal clones may be missed when the malignant cells are not dividing *(9)*. In solid tumors, numerous complex chromosome anomalies sometimes make it difficult to identify specific chromosome abnormalities, but it is usually possible to identify the presence of an abnormal clone *(27)*.

The results of chromosome studies are usually provided according to a complicated but well-defined nomenclature *(28)*. In addition, cytogeneticists usually provide a narrative report that may be readily appreciated by a physician who is not an expert in genetics. A cytogenetic report is usually issued after 5–7 days for peripheral blood and bone marrow, 15 days for fibroblast cultures, and about 10 days for solid tumors.

REFERENCES

1. Dewald G, Spurbeck JL. Sex chromosome anomalies associated with premature gonadal failure. Semin Reprod Endo 1983;1:79–92.
2. Dewald GW, Michels VV. Recurrent miscarriages: cytogenetic causes and genetic counseling of affected families. Clin Obstet Gynecol 1986;29:865–885.
3. Kuffel DG, Lindor NM, Litzow MR, Zinsmeister AR, Dewald GW: Mitomycin C chromosome stress test to identify hypersensitivity to bifunctional alkylating agents in patients with Fanconi anemia or aplastic anemia. Mayo Clin Proc 1997, 72:579–580.
4. Dewald GW, Noonan KJ, Spurbeck JL, Johnson DD: T-lymphocytes with 7;14 translocations: frequency of occurrence, breakpoints, and clinical and biological significance. Am J Hum Genet 1986, 38:520–532.
5. Dicken CH, Dewald G, Gordon H. Sister chromatid exchanges in Bloom's syndrome. Arch Dermatol 1978;114:755–760.
6. Lindor NM, Devries EM, Michels VV, Schad CR, Jalal SM, Donovan KM, Smithson WA, Kvols LK, Thibodeau SN, Dewald GW. Rothmund-Thomson syndrome in siblings: evidence for acquired in vivo mosaicism. Clin Genet 1996;49:124–129.
7. Dewald GW, Schad CR, Lilla VC, Jalal SM. Frequency and photographs of HGM11 chromosome anomalies in bone marrow samples from 3,996 patients with malignant hematologic neoplasms. Cancer Genet Cytogenet 1993;68:60–69.
8. Mahaffey VJ, Spurbeck JL, Carlson RO, Dewald GW. Hematologic malignancies, critical genes and representative pictures for 166 chromosome anomalies. Leuk Res 2004;28:1351–1356.
9. Dewald GW, Ketterling RP. Conventional Cytogenetics and Molecular Cytogenetics in Hematological Malignancies. In: Hoffman R, Benz E, Shattil S, Furie B, Cohen H, Silberstein L, McGlave P, eds. Hematology:

Basic principles and practice. Churchill Livingston, Philadelphia, 2005, pp. 928–939.

10. Rex AP, Preus M. A diagnostic index for Down syndrome. J Pediatr 1982;100:903–906.
11. Nagahana H, Haamoto Y, Takeuchi T. An autopsy case of the 18 trisomy syndrome. Bull Osaka Med Sch 1974;20:2633.
12. Dewald G, Haymond MW, Spurbeck JL, Moore SB. Origin of chi46,XX/46,XY chimerism in a human true hermaphrodite. Science 1980;207:321–323.
13. Niebuhr E. The Cri du Chat syndrome: epidemiology, cytogenetics, and clinical features. Hum Genet 1978;44:227–275.
14. Tachdjian G, Fondacci C, Tapia S, Huten Y, Blot P, Nessmann C. The Wolf-Hirschhorn syndrome in fetuses. Clin Genet 1992;42:281–287.
15. Fryns J, Emery L, Timmennans J, Pedersen J, Van den Bergh P. Trichorhino-phalangeal syndrome type 11: Langer-Giedion syndrome in a 2.5-year-old boy. Am J Hum Genet 1980;28:53–56.
16. Warburton D, Kline J, Stein Z, Hutzler M, Chin A, Hassold T. Does the karyotype of a spontaneous abortion predict the karyotype of a subsequent abortion? Evidence from 273 women with two karyotyped spontaneous abortions. Am J Hum Genet 1987;41:465–483.
17. Lindor NM, Ney JA, Gaffey TA, Jenkins RB, Thibodeau SN, Dewald GW. A genetic review of complete and partial hydatidiform moles and nonmolar triploidy. Mayo Clin Proc 1992;67:791–799.
18. Dewald G. Modern methods of chromosome analysis and their application in clinical practice. Clinical Laboratory Annual. Edited by Homberger H, Batsakis J. Norwalk, CT, Appleton-Century Crofts, 1983, pp 1–29.
19. Spurbeck JL, Carlson RO, Allen JE, Dewald GW. Culturing and robotic harvesting of bone marrow, lymph nodes, peripheral blood, fibroblasts, and solid tumors with in situ techniques. Cancer Genet Cytogenet 1988;32:59–66.
20. Dewald GW, Broderick DJ, Tom WW, Hagstrom JE, Pierre RV. The efficacy of direct, 24-hour culture, and mitotic synchronization methods for cytogenetic analysis of bone marrow in neoplastic hematologic disorders. Cancer Genet Cytogenet 1985;18:1–10.
21. Paternoster SF, Brockman SR, McClure RF, Remstein ED, Kurtin PJ, Dewald GW. A new method to extract nuclei from paraffin-embedded tissue to study lymphomas using interphase fluorescence in situ hybridization. Am J Pathol 2002;160:1967–1972.
22. Dewald G, Brockman SR, Paternoster SF: Molecular cytogenetic studies in hematological malignancies. Hematopathology in Oncology. Edited by Finn W, Peterson L, Kluwer Academic Publications, 2004, pp 69–112.
23. Crifasi PA, Michels VV, Driscoll DJ, Jalal SM, Dewald GW. DNA fluorescent probes for diagnosis of velocardiofacial and related syndromes. Mayo Clin Proc 1995;70:1148–1153.
24. Jalal SM, Law ME, Carlson RO, Dewald GW. Prenatal detection of aneuploidy by directly labeled multicolored probes and interphase fluorescence in situ hybridization. Mayo Clin Proc 1998;73:132–137.
25. Jalal S, Law M, Dewald G. Atlas of Whole Chromosome Paint Probes: Normal Patterns and Utility for Abnormal Cases. Rochester, MN, Mayo Foundation for Medical Education and Research, 1996, pp 145.
26. Mitelman F, ed. International system for cytogenetic nomenclature. Basel, S. Karger, 1995.
27. Kimmel DW, O'Fallon JR, Scheithauer BW, Kelly PJ, Dewald GW, Jenkins RB. Prognostic value of cytogenetic analysis in human cerebral astrocytomas. Ann Neurol 1992;31:534–542.
28. Shaffer LG, Tommerup N, eds. ISCN An International System for Human Cytogenetic Nomenclature. Farmington, CT, Karger, 2005.

10 Postmortem Imaging Techniques

Jurgen Ludwig

Roentgenology provides an important supplement to modern autopsy technology. Several applications of postmortem roentgenography, in particular, angiographic procedures, have been described in Chapter 2. In addition, numerous indications for the use of autopsy roentgenography are listed throughout Part II. Therefore, in this chapter, only a brief overview shall be provided.

COMMON APPLICATIONS

MEDICOLEGAL CASES Roentgenographs in medicolegal autopsies *(1)* are used primarily for:

- Identification purposes;
- The diagnosis of traumatic bone lesions;
- The identification of bullets and other foreign bodies; and
- Identification of gas in body cavities, vessels, and other sites.

Comparison of postmortem dental roentgenograms with in vivo films is the most common method of identification, particularly in the presence of advanced decomposition. Fractures and other bone lesions generally can be identified with greater accuracy in roentgenograms than by dissection. In fact, bone lesions of the extremities often cannot be studied in any other way. Most important, bullets and other radiodense objects may be impossible to find by any method other than roentgenography (Fig. 10-1). It should be noted, however, that a prosector still may have difficulty in finding a small metallic object such as a bullet, even if it is clearly visible in the roentgenogram. In such an instance, the tissue with the foreign object should be removed and subdivided. Roentgenograms of the smaller samples will allow location of the area where the object can be found. If the tissue with the foreign object cannot be removed, additional roentgenographs with placement of radiodense markers is helpful. Finally, roentgenograms are most helpful in identifying gas, for example, if one wants to determine whether a newborn was breathing and thus has air in the lungs and the gastrointestinal tract *(1)*. For other examples, see below.

From: *Handbook of Autopsy Practice,* 4th Ed. Edited by: B.L. Waters

CLINICAL CONDITIONS DEMONSTRABLE BY POSTMORTEM ROENTGENOGRAMS

The most important indications and methods are listed here. It should be noted that many of the indications may have medicolegal implications.

- Gas embolism, pneumothorax, pneumomediastinum, and pneumoperitoneum generally are easy to identify in appropriate roentgenograms. Without this technique, these conditions may be missed or the diagnosis must be based on a fleeting impression because only roentgenograms can provide a permanent record. However, the important distinction between air and putrefaction gases must be made. Whereas the changes in a tension pneumothorax are diagnostic (for an illustration, *see* "Pneumothorax" in Part II), air embolism may be simulated by putrefaction gases. The presence of other putrefactive changes and the analysis of the gas should provide the correct diagnosis;
- Angiographically demonstrable vascular abnormalities. Coronary artery disease (*see* below), congenital coronary abnormalities, pulmonary vascular disease *(2),* mesenteric, splenic *(3),* or hepatic artery occlusion, cerebral artery aneurysm, or arteriovenous malformations *(4),* renal artery stenosis or renal vein thrombosis, vascular tumors, and many other arterial and venous lesions that can be demonstrated *in situ* or on isolated organs;
- Cholangiography. Typical indications are primary sclerosing cholangitis and Caroli's disease *(5)*;
- Postoperative autopsies. Roentgenographic techniques, including angiography *(6),* may be most helpful to find and document operative mishaps or postoperative complications such as anastomotic arterial occlusion or iatrogenic tension pneumothorax as described earlier;
- Postinfectious, dystrophic calcification as in pulmonary tuberculosis *(1)* or parasitic diseases, or metastatic calcifications (e.g., in lungs, stomach, or kidneys) in hyperparathyroidism;
- Traumatic, neoplastic, metabolic, and other skeletal diseases.

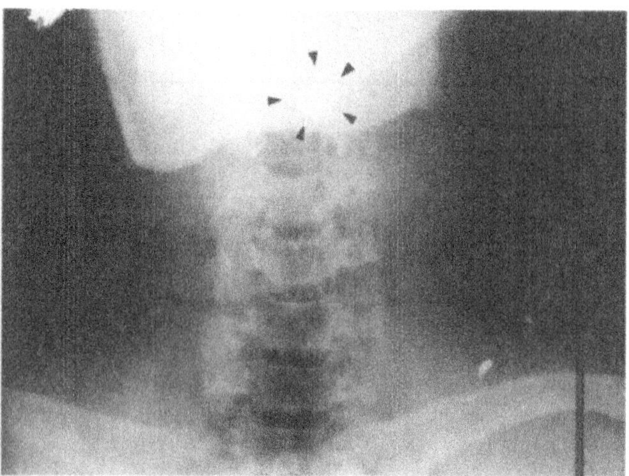

Fig. 10-1. Use of roentgenogram in medicolegal cases: deflected bullet lodged at base of skull. The entrance wound of this 38 caliber bullet was found on the back, over the left scapula, but during dissection at autopsy, the bullet could not be found. The roentgenogram shows two small bullet fragments, clearly visible in the soft tissue of the left shoulder but the remainder of the bullet had been deflected upward and was found in a deformed state at the level of the foramen magnum (arrow heads), just to the left of the midline.

EQUIPMENT IN THE AUTOPSY ROOM

We use a modified and shielded autopsy room as shown in part in Fig. 10-2. A Machlett Super Dynamax Tube (1-mm and 2-mm focal spots) has been installed. We are using a Picker X-ray table. A 300-mA Keleket machine (140-kV generator) is in an adjacent room. Films are processed in a small darkroom with a Kodak RP X-OMAT processor, which permits one to monitor injection procedures by reviewing films while the injection is still under way.

We use this facility for chest roentgenography before most autopsies, for roentgenographic surveys in medicolegal cases, and occasionally for *in situ* angiographic or other studies. In the last case, the autopsy or parts of the autopsy are done on the X-ray table. Most angiographic or cholangiographic studies are carried out on isolated organs such as heart, lungs, liver, kidneys, or brain.

The modifications of an autopsy room with shielding and new installations may be forbiddingly expensive. However, less elaborate setups are available. For years we worked with an old transportable Keleket machine and had satisfactory results. In order to bring the cassette into proper position, we used a special sturdy rack, on which bodies' autopsies could be done. It consisted of an aluminum frame with channels at the inside, for sliding cassettes back and forth, and a top layer of X-ray Bakelite (Fig. 10-3).

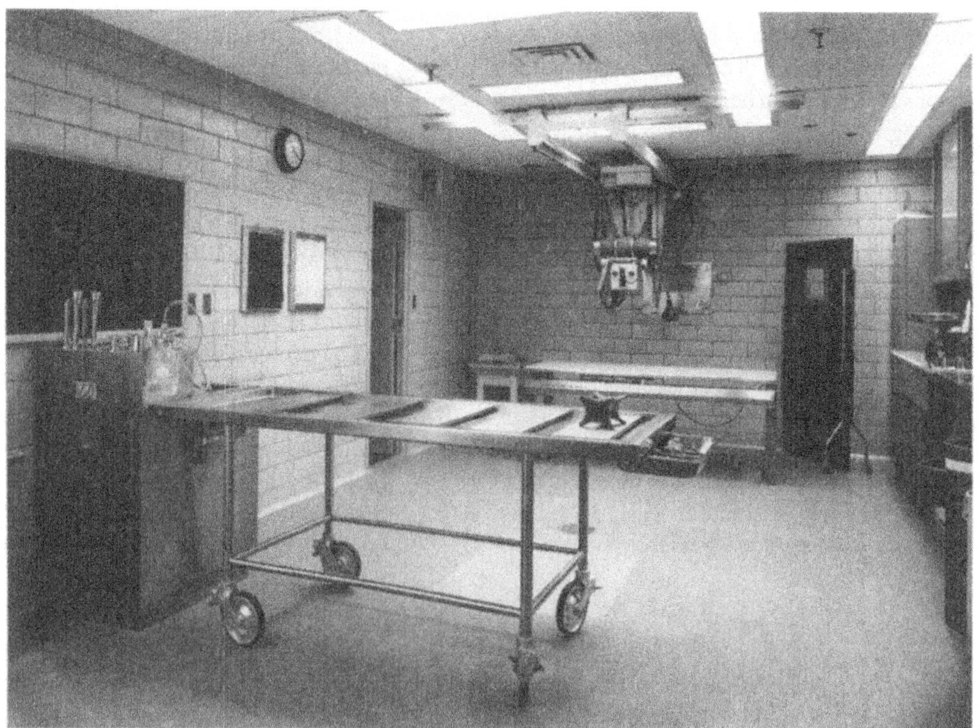

Fig. 10-2. Shielded autopsy room for roentgenologic examination. In the background is a Machlett Super Dynamax Tube and a Picker X-ray table. In adjacent room to the left, a 300-mA Keleket X-ray machine with a 125-kV generator is installed. In the foreground is a mobile autopsy table with a separate service island.

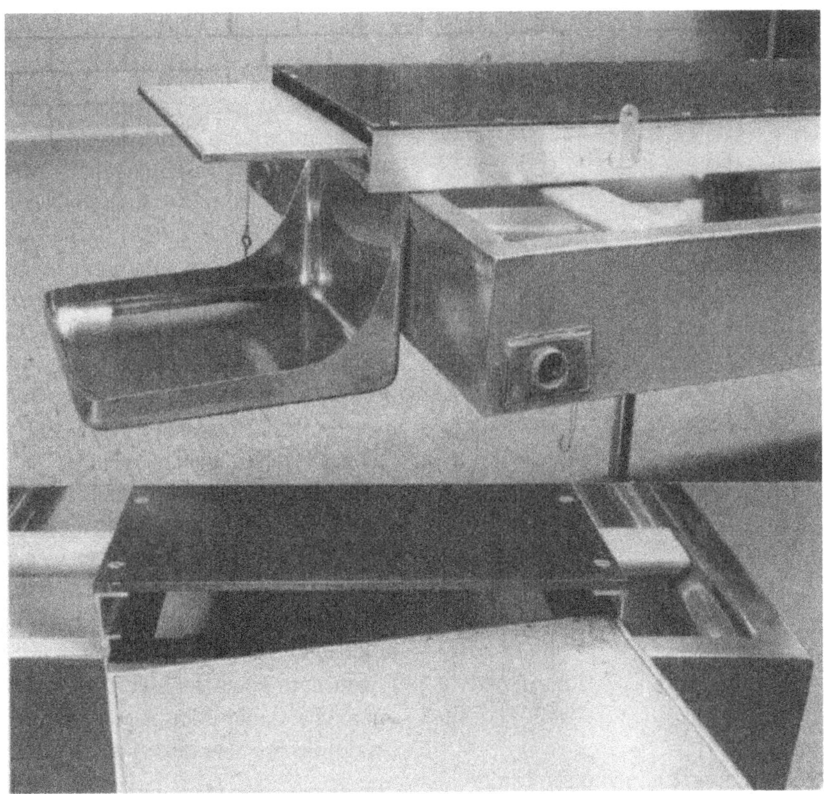

Fig. 10-3. Autopsy rack for postmortem roentgenography with transportable X-ray machines. This rack is 198 by 40 cm and consists of an aluminum frame (upper) with channels that permit the X-ray casette to slide to the desired position. The casette is inserted at the end of the rack and can be moved by hand from below (lower). The rack is covered with X-ray Bakelite, 0.64 cm thick. The Bakelite seams are watertight so that autopsies can be done on this rack and contamination of the inside can be kept to a minimum.

If X-ray equipment is used by the autopsy service, the facilities and procedures must be reviewed and approved by a radiation safety officer. For the decontamination of X-ray tables, racks, cassettes, and other tools for autopsy roentgenology, the principles apply that are described in Chapter 6.

ANGIOGRAPHIC TECHNIQUES

Postmortem angiography is one of the most important applications of roentgenologic methods in the autopsy room. For contrast media, see Chapter 16. Because of its importance, postmortem coronary angiography is described here. Similar methods, applied to other organ systems, have been presented in Chapter 2.

POSTMORTEM CORONARY ANGIOGRAPHY Many contrast media have been used in the past *(7,8)* but barium sulfate with gelatin is preferred (9,10), although iodinated dyes can also be used *(11)*. For quantitative studies, a radioisotope dilution method has been reported *(12)*. Double-contrast techniques and *in situ* angiography (Fig. 10-4) have also been described *(13–15)*. Radiopaque dyes used clinically are applicable to the coronary arteries at autopsy. A setup for controlled-pressure coronary angiography is shown in Fig. 10-5. For this procedure, the heart is removed with 2–4 cm of the major vessels attached. Postmortem clots are removed by irrigation with saline. Cannulas of suitable size are placed into the coronary ostia. Care is taken to identify an independent ostium. Ligatures are placed around the coronary arteries and are tied as near as possible to the origins.

The cannulated heart is suspended in isotonic saline or Kaiserling I solution at about 45°C. The coronary arteries are perfused at a low pressure with isotonic saline. This is continued for several minutes, with use of 100–200 mL, until the return through the coronary sinus is free of blood.

The previously prepared barium-gelatin mixture (Chapter 16) is drawn into two 30-mL syringes. These are attached, via three-way stopcocks, to the apparatus shown in Fig. 10-5, and the actual injection is begun. Care is taken to avoid introduction of air bubbles at any stage of the procedure. While the system is kept supplied with contrast medium by way of the syringes, the pressure is increased almost simultaneously to a maximum of 110 mm Hg. Lacerated vessels may require ligation at this stage, but these are rare in my experience. A control roentgenogram can be prepared at this time. The heart chambers may be irrigated to remove any contrast material that enters into the lumens. With the coronary cannulas still in place and maintaining a pressure of 100–120 mm Hg, the chambers are packed with formalin-soaked cotton to their approximate normal size and shape and the specimen is immersed in cold Kaiserling I or formalin solution (Chapter 15). The heart is cooled for 1–3 h to permit the gelatin to set and then roentgenograms are prepared.

Angiography may underestimate the severity of obstruction if the narrowed region is compared to an adjacent segment

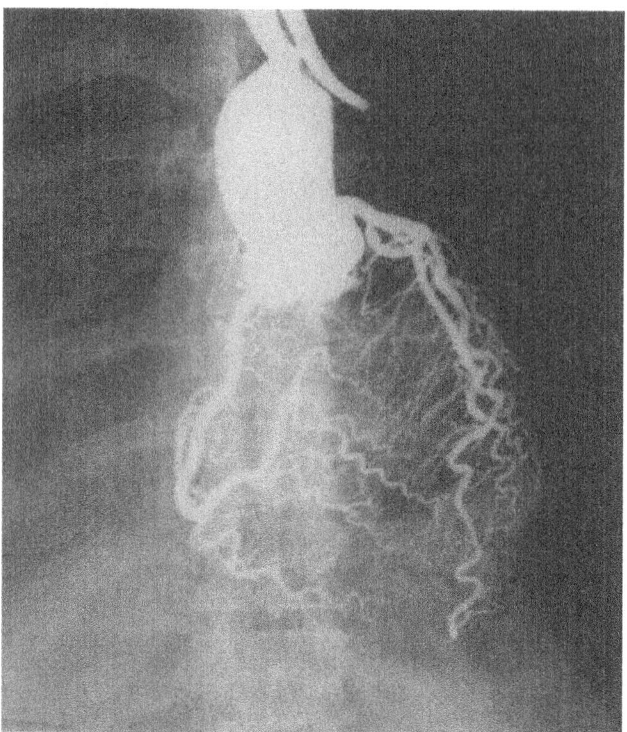

Fig. 10-4. Normal coronary angiogram in situ. The sternum was split in the midline and about 300 mL of barium sulfate-gelatin mixture was injected into the ascending aorta without pressure regulation, by hand with a large syringe. Superior portion of ascending aorta has been clamped off.

that is considered normal but is actually stenotic. Conversely, microscopy can overestimate the degree of narrowing if the effect of compensatory dilatation of atherosclerotic segments is not considered *(16)*. Thus, coronary angiography does not replace microscopy. Although arteriography localizes obstructive lesions, microscopy is still necessary to determine its nature—for example, chronic atherosclerosis vs acute plaque rupture with stenosis.

The arteries of the extremities can be studied by angiography with a pressure-controlled system *(17)*, resembling the system used with coronary arteries. As mentioned in Chapter 2, phlebography and lymphangiography (Fig. 10-6) can also be performed at autopsy *(18)*. Intra-osseous phlebography can be used for the evaluation of thrombosis of deep leg veins, but the method is a bit cumbersome *(19)*.

ANGIOGRAPHY OF OTHER ORGANS Pulmonary angiography and bronchography is described in Chapter 2; the demonstration of esophageal varices and mesenteric angiography is presented in Chapter 2; in Chapter 4, cerebral arteriography, venography, and ventriculography are discussed; and in Chapter 16, the use of angiographic methods in the study of museum specimens is shown. Roentgenologic and other imaging techniques in specific clinical or forensic diseases and conditions are also shown in Part II.

OTHER IMAGING TECHNIQUES

Except for ultrasonography which probably could be used in many autopsy settings without too much difficulty, other imaging techniques have also been widely used in recent years.

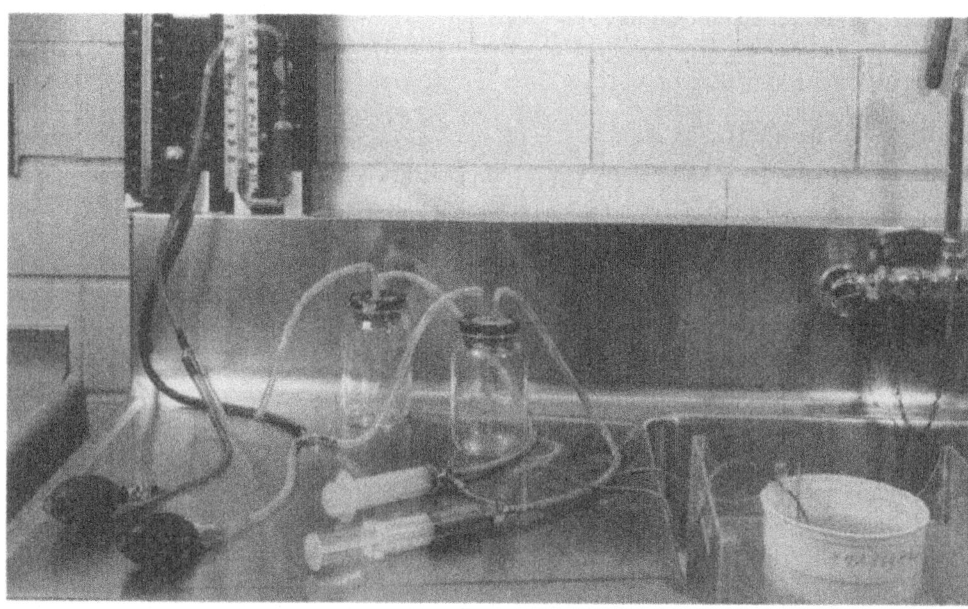

Fig. 10-5. Setup for controlled pressure injection of contrast medium into coronary arteries. In this instance, each syringe contains chromopaque of a different color and is connected to one of the coronary orifices and the pressure-regulating system. The heart is suspended in Kaiserling solution or saline in the container on the right, which is in an ice-water bath. The two independent pressure-regulating systems with manometers are on the left.

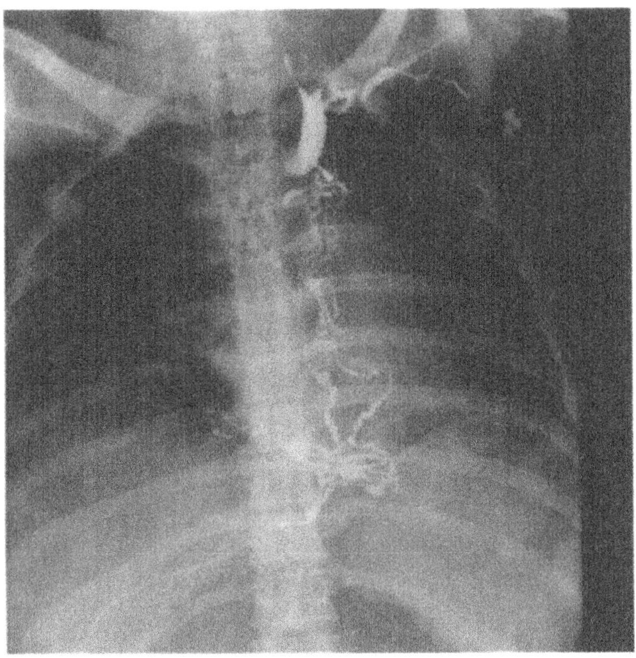

Fig. 10-6. Postmortem lymphangiography showing dilated lymphatics in the hepatoduodenal ligament and the anterior mediastinum in a patient with liver cirrhosis and congestive heart failure. The lymphatics drain in the subclavian vein as shown by the presence of contrast medium in this vessel. Adapted with permission from ref. (18).

MAGNETIC RESONANCE IMAGING (MRI) This has been used particularly as a supplement to perinatal autopsies *(20)*, autopsies in stillbirth *(21)*, and pediatric autopsies in cases of suspected child abuse *(22)*. MRI was useful in directing the autopsy and, particularly, the brain cutting to focal areas of abnormality *(22)*. In a limited number of comparisons which included two adults, MRI was equal to autopsy in detecting gross cranial, pulmonary, abdominal, and vascular pathology, and superior in detecting air and fluid in potential body spaces *(21)*.

COMPUTERIZED TOMOGRAPHY (CT) CT images produced in vivo are widely used in autopsy studies, primarily in brain cutting. The method also has been used to compare diagnostic yields of CT and MRI (*see* above) (23) and other research endeavors but we are not aware of routine use in autopsy settings.

ULTRASONOGRAPHY This is an underutilized modality. In the hands of a motivated pediatric radiologist, multiple anomalies can be discerned in a fetus with a crown-rump length of 4.1 cm, such as a small posterior fossa cyst, platyspondyly, small thoracic cavity, abnormally shaped scapulae, curved clavicles, curved femurs and absence of fibulae. (Brenda L. Waters, MD)

REFERENCES

1. Schmidt G, Kallieris D. Use of radiographs in the forensic autopsy. Forensic Sci Int 1982;19:263–270.
2. Resnik JM, Engeler CE, Derauf BJ. Postmortem angiography of catheter-induced pulmonary artery perforation. J Forensic Sci 1992;37:1346–1351.
3. Karhunen PJ, Penttila A. Diagnostic postmortem angiography of fatal splenic artery haemorrhage. Zeitschrift für Rechtsmedizin.J Legal Med 1989;103:129–136.
4. Karhunen PJ, Penttila A, Erkinjuntti T. Arteriovenous malformation of the brain: imaging by postmortem angiography. Forensic Sci Int 1990;48:9–19.
5. Terada T, Nakanuma Y. Congenital biliary dilatation in autosomal dominant adult polycystic disease of the liver and kidneys. Arch Pathol Lab Med 1988;112:1113–1116.
6. Karhunen PJ, Manniko A, Penttila A, Liesto K. Diagnostic angiography in postoperative autopsies. Am J Forensic Med Pathol 1989;10:303–309.
7. Reiner L. Gross examination of the heart. In: Gould SE, ed. Pathology of the Heart and Great Vessels, 2nd ed. Charles C. Thomas, Springfield, IL, 1968, pp.1111–1149.
8. Saphir O. Gross examination of the heart: injection of coronary arteries; weight and measurements of heart. In: Gould SE, ed. Pathology of the Heart and Great Vessels, 2nd ed. Charles C. Thomas, Springfield, IL, 1960, pp. 1043–1066.
9. Schlesinger MJ. A new radiopaque mass for vascular injection. Lab Invest 1957;6:1–11.
10. Hales MR, Carrington CB. A pigment gelatin mass for vascular injection. Yale J Biol Med 1971;43:257–270.
11. Suberman CO, Suberman RI, Dalldorf FG, Gabrielle OF. Radiographic visualization of coronary arteries in postmortem hearts: a simple technic. Am J Clin Pathol 1970;53:254–257.
12. Davies NA. A radioisotope dilution technique for the quantitative study of coronary artery disease postmortem. Lab Invest 1963;12:1198–1203.
13. Ludwig J, Lie JT. Heart and Vascular System. In: Ludwig J, ed. Current Methods of Autopsy Practice, 2nd ed. W.B. Saunders, Philadelphia, 1979, pp. 21–50.
14. Rissanen VT. Double contrast technique for postmortem coronary angiography. Lab Invest 1970;23:517–520.
15. Davies MJ, Pomerance A, Lamb D. Techniques in examination and anatomy of the heart. In: Pomerance A, Davies MJ, eds. Blackwell Scientific Publications, Oxford, 1975, pp. 1–48.
16. Edwards WD. Pathology of myocardial infarction and reperfusion. In: Gersh BJ, Rahimtoola SH, ed. Acute Myocardial Infarction, 2nd ed. Chapman & Hall, New York, 1997, pp. 16–50.
17. Ross CF, Keele KD. Post mortem arteriography "normal" lower limbs. Angiology 1951;2:374–385.
18. Ludwig J, Linhart P, Baggenstoss AH. Hepatic lymph drainage in cirrhosis and congestive heart failure. A postmortem lymphangiographic study. Arch Pathol 1968;86:551–562.
19. Lund F, Diener L, Ericsson JLE. Postmortem intraosseous phlegogaphy as an aid in studies of venous thromboembolism. Angiology 1969;20:155–176.
20. Brookes JA, Hall-Craggs MA, Sams VR, Lees WR. Non-invasive perinatal necropsy by magnetic resonance imaging. Lancet 1996;348:1139–1141.
21. Ros PR, Li KC, Baer H, Staab EV. Preautopsy magnetic resonance imaging: initial experience. Magn Reson Imaging 1990;8:303–308.
22. Hart BL, Dudley MH, Zumwalt RE. Postmortem cranial MRI and autopsy correlation in suspected child abuse. Am J Forensic Med Pathol 1996;17:217–224.
23. Westesson PL, Katzberg RW, Tallents RH, Sanchez-Woodworth RE, Svensson AS. CT and MR of the temporomandibular joint: comparison with autopsy. Am J Roentgenol 1987;148:1165–1171.

11 Autopsies of Bodies Containing Radioactive Materials

KELLY L. CLASSIC

The current practice of medicine uses a variety of radioactive sources. These sources are introduced into a human body intentionally for medical research, diagnosis and therapy, or accidentally when there is an incident involving radioactive materials. Because incidents involving uptakes of radioactive materials are rare, medical procedures are the primary source of origin when a body is radioactive. Each year there are nearly ten million medical procedures performed involving injection, ingestion, or implantation of radioactive materials by patients *(1)*. Predominant studies are those of the liver, bone, respiratory system and heart, accounting for nearly 60% of the studies performed. As more radiopharmaceuticals are developed for diagnosis and with continued progress in new radionuclide-based therapies, individuals performing autopsies, embalming or cremating bodies have significant probability to perform these activities on a radioactive cadaver.

BACKGROUND

Some patients who have been administered therapeutic radiopharmaceuticals must remain under the control of the licensed facility *(2)*. In these cases, immediate notification of the person in charge of the radiation safety program (usually designated as the radiation safety officer) would occur prior to release of the body to a morgue or funeral home. The radiation safety officer or designee would attach a label to the body indicating the body is radioactive and whether special precautions are necessary (Fig. 11-1). However, today, fewer patients remain in the hospital after radiopharmaceutical therapy due to newer regulations and regulatory guidance *(2,3)* allowing more of these patients to go home with restrictions. Patients administered liquid radiopharmaceuticals for diagnostic purposes are rarely under the control of a licensed facility. Diagnostic procedures are outpatient procedures and patients are not considered a hazard to other members of the public under normal circumstances.

Patients containing radioactive implants (radioactive material in a solid form) may or may not remain under the control of a licensed facility. Those who do remain and die while in a facility will have the implant removed prior to release of the body. The body is no longer radioactive after removal of the implant and no special precautions are required while working on or around it. Under certain circumstances *(3)*, patients containing permanent radioactive implants can be released from a medical facility. Radiation exposure from these patients is not considered hazardous to the general public, however, family members are instructed to contact the prescribing radiation oncologist if the patient dies at home or in another hospital to assure that appropriate measures are taken with regard to the implant.

HAZARD TYPES

Radioactive bodies present two types of hazard: external exposure and radioactive contamination. The level of each of these is dependent upon the type and activity of radiation in the body, whether the body will be opened, days since administration of the radioactive material, and time to be spent in the vicinity of the body. External exposure is the primary concern if the body will not be opened. Individuals will rarely encounter high exposure rates around bodies of patients that were released from a hospital; however, bodies from a medical center with the appropriate tag attached may have appreciable exposure rates. Table 11-1 shows unshielded dose rates at two distances for some radionuclides that may be encountered. The radioactivity level chosen for the first entry (^{99m}Tc) is typical administered activity in diagnostic nuclear medicine and the level chosen for the last four entries is activity below which a patient can be released from hospital confinement *(3)*. Beta-emitting radionuclides (^{32}P, ^{89}S, ^{90}Y) are not considered external exposure hazards when the body cavity will not be opened so are not addressed in the table. The listed dose rates will decrease rapidly over time for radioactive materials with short half-lives (6h and 2.7d for ^{99m}Tc and ^{198}Au, respectively) and for those that would have rapidly metabolized prior to death (^{99m}Tc and ^{131}I). Activity in implants will decrease only by half-life.

Radiation exposure limits for members of the general public have been determined by federal regulatory agencies and radiation protection consensus groups *(4,5)*. Members of the public who may be exposed to sources of radiation can receive 1 mSv (100 mrem) to their whole body annually. Family members or caregivers of patients receiving some form of radionuclide therapy can receive up to 5 mSv (500 mrem) whole body.†

† In the International System (SI) of Units, the Sievert (Sv) represents effective radiation dose. In this chapter, SI units will be used followed in parenthesis by conventional units. One Sv = 100 rem; 1 mSv = 100 mrem). Becquerel (Bq) is the SI unit of radioactivity; 3.7×10^7Bq = 1 millicurie (mCi).

From: *Handbook of Autopsy Practice,* 4th Ed. Edited by: B.L. Waters

RADIOACTIVITY

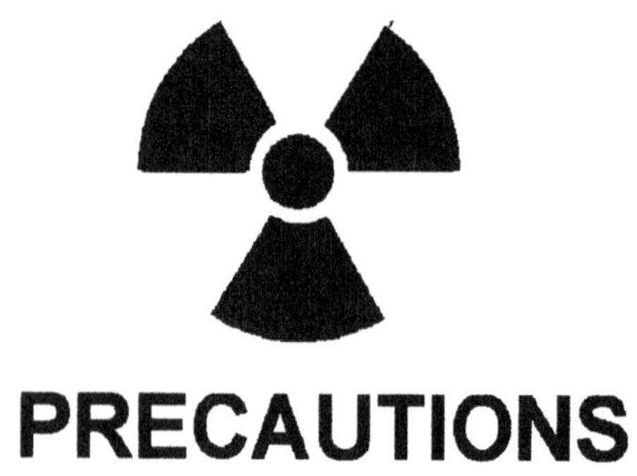

PRECAUTIONS

Radionuclide ____________________

Administered Activity ____________________ mCi

Final Measured Dose Rate ______________ mR/h

Date ____________________

Tag is not to be removed until:

1) Radioactive material is removed from patient, or

2) Authorization is received from Radiation Safety Officer.

Signature ____________________
Radiation Safety Officer

Fig. 11-1. Example of a body tag for a cadaver containing radioactive material.

Table 11-1
Unshielded Radiation Dose Rates at 30 and 100 cm for Common Radioactive Materials

		Dose Rate in mSv/h (mrem/h)	
Radionuclide	*Activity in GBq (mCi)*	*30 cm*	*100 cm*
^{99m}Tc	1.48 (40)	0.32 (32)	0.04 (4)
^{103}Pd (implant)	1.48 (40)	0.33 (33)	0.03 (3)
^{125}I (implant)	0.33 (9)	0.11 (11)	0.01 (1)
^{131}I	1.22 (33)	0.78 (78)	0.07 (7)
^{198}Au	3.44 (93)	2.33 (233)	0.21 (21)

If the body will be opened for an autopsy or other procedure, both external exposure and radioactive contamination are of concern. The dose rates in Table 11-1 still apply but in addition, precautions to minimize or prevent contamination must be practiced.

GENERAL PRECAUTIONS

Reducing time, increasing distance and using shielding are methods to decrease radiation exposure. Minimizing time will be the principal external exposure reduction method for individuals performing autopsies. Time is linear with exposure; decreasing time to perform a procedure by half will reduce exposure by half.

Extremity exposure can be reduced through the use of long-handled instruments because of the additional distance. Distance is inversely proportional to the square of the exposure; increasing distance by a factor of two will decrease exposure by a factor of four. Shielding, such as a radiology lead apron (0.5 mm lead equivalent thickness) will provide some protection for gamma radiation from ^{99m}Tc and ^{125}I but will do little for highly penetrating gammas from ^{103}Pd, ^{131}I, ^{182}Ta, and ^{198}Au.

Common barrier protection as determined by consensus standards *(6)* includes numerous items that minimize external radiation exposure from beta-emitting radionuclides (when the body cavity is opened) and assist in prevention of personal contamination. These include double-gloves, hair covers, long-sleeved jump suits that are fluid resistant, foot covers and facial protection (splash guards). Any wound sustained during procedures on a radioactive body should be attended immediately. The wound should be debrided if necessary and rinsed thoroughly to remove as much radioactivity as possible.

Plastic-backed paper for the floor around the autopsy table will facilitate decontamination of the facility and prevent further spread of contamination. Autopsy tools can be wrapped in plastic for the same reasons.

PROCEDURE SPECIFIC TECHNIQUES

If a patient contains therapeutic amounts of radionuclides, is hospitalized and subsequently dies, it is likely that a knowledgeable person (radiation safety officer or designee) will accompany the body to the funeral home or morgue. This individual will be able to provide specific direction for the prevention of contamination and reduction of exposure. Hospitalized patients containing implants will have the implant removed; no residual radioactivity remains in these patients' body fluids. Patients who have permanent implants will have sources imbedded in the body but body fluids are not radioactive.

EMBALMING For cadavers containing liquid radionuclides, simple embalming using standard aspiration and injection methods can minimize the likelihood of contamination if a significant amount of the radioactivity is in the body fluids. Fluids should be removed by means of a trocar and tubing in a manner that does not require an individual to hold either item or be close to the body while the fluid is draining. Fluids from the body can be drained directly into the sewage system unless directed otherwise by the attending radiation safety officer. Collection and handling of collected body cavity fluids should be done only under the direction of a knowledgeable person as both can result in higher radiation exposures. Depending on the radionuclide and route of administration, the fluid may contain high radioactivity levels and must be handled accordingly (e.g., shielded containers).

In cases where radioactivity is no longer in the body fluids, embalming may not significantly reduce activity levels. Early after administration, ^{131}I is circulating throughout the body, but twenty-four hours after administration, only trace amounts are circulating with much of the material either having been excreted or taken up by the thyroid. Similarly, all remaining (not excreted) ^{89}Sr is found in the skeleton after only a few days. Therefore, 2–3 days after administration, these radionuclides would be found only in minimal concentrations in embalming fluid. However, patients who have received interstitially or intraperitoneally administered radionuclides (e.g., ^{32}P, ^{198}Au) will have a large portion of the activity removed with the ascitic and pleural fluids *(7)*.

URINE The urine may contain some radioactivity depending upon time since administration, radionuclide administered, and route of administration. Within a few days of administration, the urine may contain a significant amount of radioactivity and, as with the cavity fluids removed with embalming, it should be drained directly to the sewer system unless directed otherwise.

Like embalming, activity levels may or may not be reduced by removal of residual urine. Within the first two days of the administration of ^{131}I and ^{89}Sr, more than half the activity would normally be excreted through the urine *(8)* though the patient's medical condition may sometimes alter metabolism. Draining urine from the bladder of these patients within a few days of the radionuclide administration prior to autopsy procedures can result in a concomitant reduction in radiation exposure. Radionuclides metabolized more slowly or administered interstitially will be less affected by removal of urine.

AUTOPSY - LIQUID RADIONUCLIDES Radionuclides administered intraperitoneally (^{32}P, ^{90}Y, ^{198}Au) will have some remaining activity on serous surfaces though much activity will be removed with pleural and ascitic fluids *(7)*. Drying the open cavity with sponges can reduce the radioactivity level. Gloves must be used and double gloving or rubber gloves should be considered with the final determination based on whether necessary procedures can be performed with thicker gloves without increasing hand time in the cavity. Table 11-2 shows dose to the hands from work performed in the peritoneal cavity. The use of long-handled devices is recommended if they do not impede the work. With beta emitters, distances of as little as six inches of air or an inch of tissue can appreciably reduce extremity exposure.

An article published by Parthasarathy, et al. discusses procedures for handling a cadaver with a high ^{131}I radioactivity burden *(9)*. Emphasis was placed on reducing external exposure levels and contamination potential of the cadaver while at the hospital prior to release of the body to a local funeral home because of regulatory exposure limits for the general public *(4)*. These procedures included identification and removal of organs with high radioactivity burdens. During organ removal external exposure was monitored by issuing each individual one dosimeter to be worn on the torso of the body and one to be worn on the dominant hand under gloves. The highest doses were received by the lead pathologist (who worked on the cadaver with high radioactivity organs still in place) and were 0.22 mSv (22 mrem) whole body and 5.5 mSv (550 mrem) hand. Radiation dose reduction precautions included the use of personal protective equipment, limiting personnel time (20 minute staff rotations), instructing staff to maintain increased distance from the cadaver when feasible, and general methods to reduce room contamination. Employees other than the lead pathologist received a maximum of 0.13 mSv (13 mrem) whole body and 0.59 mSv (59 mrem) hand.

A paper by Johnston, et al. dealing with a similar circumstance included preselection of surgical instruments that were either easy to clean or disposable, controlled access to the autopsy room and complete stocking of the room so personnel did not exit for supplies in addition to some precautions stated previously *(10)*. These authors also describe action specific procedures similar to those used at a decontamination facility: correct donning and removal of personal protective equipment, use of a "clean" area (not radioactively contaminated), and frequent personal surveys with a portable radiation detection monitor. The pathologist received 0.2 mSv (20 mrem) whole body and 0.7 mSv (70 mrem) hand. In this circumstance, radioactive organs were not removed nor was the body embalmed. At the direction of the funeral director, the body was placed directly into a commercial casket liner made of steel and sealed shut. Although radiation levels could still be detected through the

Table 11-2
Radiation Dose To Hands In Peritoneal Cavity*

	Radiation Dose in mSv/minute (mrem/minute)					
	^{198}Au			*^{32}P or ^{90}Y*		
Activity in GBq (mCi)	*No Gloves*	*Surgical Gloves*	*Double Gloves*	*No Gloves*	*Surgical Gloves*	*Double Gloves*
0.037 (1)	0.12 (12)	0.07 (7)	0.02 (2)	0.13 (13)	0.08 (8)	0.05 (5)
0.19 (5)	0.6 (60)	0.35 (35)	0.1 (10)	0.65 (65)	0.4 (40)	0.25 (25)
0.37 (10)	0.1 (10)	0.7 (70)	0.2 (20)	1.3 (130)	0.8 (80)	0.5 (50)
0.93 (25)	3.0 (300)	1.75 (175)	0.5 (50)	3.25 (325)	2.0 (200)	1.25 (125)
1.85 (50)	6.0 (600)	3.5 (350)	1.0 (100)	6.5 (650)	4.0 (400)	2.5 (250)

*Adapted from Reference 7.

casket, they diminished rapidly due to the short (8d) half-life. Another paper suggesting similar radiation safety precautions shows measured doses to pathology staff to be less than 0.1 mSv (10 mrem) from an autopsy procedure *(11)*.

A more recent article suggests that embalming not be performed within 48 h of the administration of ^{131}I for therapy unless there are extenuating circumstances *(12)*. These authors also report estimated pathologist radiation doses at 0.4 mSv (40 mrem) body while performing the necessary procedures on a cadaver containing approximately 407 MBq (11 mCi) ^{131}I. Questioning the need to an autopsy on cadavers with recently administered ^{131}I therapy is also discussed n a paper by Wallace and Bush *(13)*. They go on to suggest, for these cadavers, that many dose rate measurements of the body be taken to preplan who can perform what task and how long they can perform it.

Based on these experiences and consensus standard recommendations *(7)*, the following procedures should be followed when an autopsy is to be performed on bodies containing high levels of liquid radioactivity:

1. Supervision by an individual knowledgeable in radiation (radiation safety officer from a local licensed facility)
2. External exposure monitoring of personnel (whole body and hand)
3. Preselection of tools
4. Anticipated supplies in room
5. Secured area access
6. Personnel time limits (rotation of personnel)
7. Bioassay of personnel at conclusion of procedure (to assure radioactivity was not inhaled, absorbed or ingested)
8. Surveys of personnel with portable instrumentation upon exit from procedure area
9. Survey and decontamination of area and all equipment
10. Disposal of contaminated waste items as radioactive
11. Use of personal protective equipment:
    - double gloves
    - face mask
    - eye (splash) protection
    - surgical hats
    - plastic gowns
    - plastic shoe covers or rubber boots
    - lead aprons (where they might reasonably reduce exposure levels)

Removal of highly radioactive organs is dependent upon anticipated disposition of the body. If a full autopsy will be performed, removal of the organs is encouraged to limit pathologist exposure. If there will only be embalming, removal of organs could reduce exposures. However, because embalming involves only short periods of time next to the cadaver and greater distances during the procedure itself, the embalmer would receive minimal exposure with the organs in place while an individual removing the organs could receive higher exposure. Staff must consider exposure to all personnel during each procedural step to keep collective exposure as low as possible. If the embalmer will do cosmetic restoration of the face and the thyroid is the highly radioactive organ, consideration should be given to removal of the thyroid and adjacent contaminated tissue.

AUTOPSY - IMPLANTS Radioactive implants, sometimes referred to as seeds, are generally either small pieces of radioactive wire or small capsules containing the radioactivity. If the location of the implant is known and will not be disturbed during the autopsy, the decision whether to remove the sources will be based on expected external exposure to personnel. Removal of the sources may involve more radiation exposure than leaving them undisturbed and working quickly when near them. Table 11-3 shows unshielded and shielded (with body tissue) radiation exposure rates at chosen distances for two activities from radionuclides commonly permanently implanted. The numbers represent possible hand exposures. Permanent implants of beta emitters and low energy gamma emitters, e.g., ^{125}I or ^{103}Pd, do not normally present significant radiation hazards and therefore typically do not require removal for an autopsy to be performed *(14)*.

If removal of sources or tissue containing the sources is deemed most practical, a radiograph of the area should be performed to show current location since the sources may have shifted since implant. After removal of the sources or tissue, a second radiograph or a survey with a portable radiation detection instrument will confirm removal of all sources. Source removal should be done rapidly and with long-handled instruments. If an

Table 11-3
Radiation Dose Rates From Unshielded Radioactive Implants

	Dose Rates in mSv/h (rem/h) For 1.85 GBq (50 mCi)							
	^{125}I		*^{103}Pd*		*^{182}Ta*		*^{198}Au*	
<Diistance (cm)	*No Shielding*	*Tissue Shielding**	*No Shielding*	*Tissue Shielding*	*No Shielding*	*Tissue Shielding*	*No Shielding*	*Tissue Shielding*
3	39 (3.9)	12 (1.2)	1.7 (0.17)	1.2 (0.12)	378 (37.8)	288 (28.8)	155 (15.5)	111 (11.1)
8	5.5 (0.55)	0.2 (0.02)	0.2 (0.02)	0.08 (0.008)	53 (5.3)	26 (2.6)	18 (1.8)	7.4 (0.74)
13	2 (0.2)	0.01 (0.001)	0.09 (0.009)	0.02 (0.002)	21 (2.1)	6.6 (0.66)	7 (0.7)	1.7 (0.17)
20	0.8 (0.08)	negligible	0.04 (0.004)	negligible	8.3 (0.83)	1.3 (0.13)	2.8 (0.28)	0.3 (0.03)
30	0.4 (0.04)	negligible	0.02 (0.002)	negligible	3.8 (0.38)	0.2 (0.02)	1.3 (0.13)	0.05 (0.005)

*Tissue shielding assumes that the distance in column 1 is all body tissue

entire organ or section of tissue can be removed with the sources intact, individuals performing the procedure would receive much less exposure. Laughlin, et al. reports that exposures to pathologists at an institution performing sixteen procedures each year on cadavers with permanent implants remain below maximum permissible radiation limits for the general public *(15)*.

If sources are explanted, they should be placed together in a container and located in an area not frequented by personnel and not near areas where personnel may linger. Disposal of active sources should be by approved methods *(4,16)*. This can be accomplished by contacting and returning the sources to the institution where they were implanted, contacting a local institution licensed to receive and dispose of the radionuclide, or contacting the local regulatory radiation control department.

CREMATION Cremation of bodies containing radionuclides will contaminate the crematorium and, in most cases, will leave contaminated ashes. Removal and handling of the ashes must be performed with appropriate personal protective equipment. In a report of three crematorium contamination incidents, the ash collection worker wore a heat resistant jacket, leather gloves and a dust mask, and used long-handled (3–4 m) tools to rake and sweep the ashes toward the front of the oven *(17)*. Because this individual was still found to have internal contamination, most likely from inhalation, it is recommended that personnel wear respirators while collecting ash.

If procedures to reduce the radioactive burden can be performed prior to cremation, the decision to perform them should be based on level of radioactivity remaining in the cadaver. One radiation protection consensus group states that no radiation hazard would exist if a crematorium were to handle a total of up to 7.4 GBq (200 mCi) ^{131}I or 74 GBq (2,000 mCi) of all other radionuclides annually *(7)*. Another indicates no special precautions for cremation of individual cadavers containing less than 1.11 GBq (30 mCi) ^{131}I or ^{198}Au, or 370 MBq (10 mCi) ^{32}P *(18)*. Both groups state that attempts should be made to remove permanent implants prior to cremation.

An article by Que offers precautions for the handling of cremated remains *(19)*. These include the wearing of a mask by the cremationist, no further processing of the cremated remains – they should simply be put in an urn for storage or burial, no scattering of remains of a cadaver that contained radioactive implants until ten half-lives postimplant date have passed, and that knowledgeable radiation safety staff be consulted before, during, and after the cremation.

Both the Nuclear Regulatory Commission and the International Commission on Radiological Protection have indicated that cremation of cadavers that had previously received radionuclide therapy with a "bone seeker" such as ^{89}Sr can be more of a problem *(20,21)*. Within a few days of administration, the radionuclide is in the bone and decays with a longer half-life (50.5 days). Thus, the ash and bone fragments in the ash contain the radioactivity. Although neither make specific recommendations regarding the reduction of exposure for the individual handling the ash of a ^{89}Sr cadaver, measures should be taken to prevent inhalation of ash dust during ash collection.

RADIOACTIVE TISSUES - SECTIONING AND STORAGE

Tissue removed from a radioactive cadaver may contain some of the radionuclide if it was not a seed implant. If the removed tissue was the location of a radionuclide implant, it likely will contain all of the radioactive material.

Liquid radioactive materials tend to localize in one or two primary organs (i.e., the thyroid is the primary organ for administered ^{131}I). Other tissues would contain negligible amounts of the radioactive material and would be of little hazard. However, prudent precautions should still be taken that include minimal handling time, double gloving, and wearing splash protection and protective gowns to prevent personnel contamination. If the primary organ will be handled and death occurred within only a few days of the radionuclide administration, tools should be used as much as possible minimizing direct organ contact. One paper states that tissue samples for sections taken from a patient who received ^{131}I therapy, placed in formalin-containing jars read a maximum of 0.05 mSv/h (5 mrem/h) on the surface of the jars *(10)*.

In the case of a radionuclide implant, only the tissue site of the implant will contain the radioactive material. Other tissues would contain no radiation and would have no handling restriction. If the implant site needed to be sectioned, removal of the implanted seeds from the tissue prior to sectioning is recommended even if it has been more than 10 half-lives of decay of the radionuclide since the implant date. Implanted seeds would likely be in a cadaver only if the individual had a permanent implant (e.g., ^{125}I seeds for prostate cancer) and was released from the hospital. In the case of temporary implants, where the patient would be hospitalized during treatment, the implant would be removed before the body was transferred to the morgue or funeral home.

If radioactive tissues will be stored, the type of container used for storage will depend on radioactivity levels in the tissue sample or organ. Most samples will be of little hazard although primary organs or primary organ tissue may need leaded containers available from a local radiation safety professional. Radioactivity will diminish with storage time eventually eliminating need for lead containers.

INSTRUMENT AND CLOTHING DECONTAMINATION

Instruments and clothing that must be decontaminated (versus becoming radioactive waste) can generally be cleaned by repeated soaking in water with regular detergents. Some items, as determined by the radiation safety professional, may need to be held for decay of the radionuclide. Items held for decay should be placed in a plastic bag and properly marked with the radionuclide, date and level of activity, and projected date the item(s) can be removed from storage (typically ten half-lives *(4)* or a point when the radioactivity on the items can no longer be detected on a radiation contamination survey instrument). Storage of these items should be in a location remote from where routine daily work takes place.

CONTAMINATED WASTE PRODUCTS

Items to be disposed as radioactive waste must be bagged and properly marked with the radionuclide, date, and amount of radioactivity. If the half-life is short, the materials can be held for decay and disposed as nonradioactive *(4)*. If the half-life is long, a radiation safety professional should determine the most appropriate way to dispose of the materials.

REFERENCES

1. Institute of Medicine. Radiation in Medicine: The need for regulatory reform. National Academy Press, Washington, DC, 1996.
2. U.S. Nuclear Regulatory Commission. Code of Federal Regulations, Title 10, Part 35. U.S. Government Printing Office, Washington, DC, 2003.
3. U.S. Nuclear Regulatory Commission. Regulatory Guide 8.39: Release of patients administered radioactive materials. U.S. Government Printing Office, Washington, DC, 1997.
4. U.S. Nuclear Regulatory Commission. Code of Federal Regulations, Title 10, Part 20. U.S. Government Printing Office, Washington, DC, 1992.
5. National Council on Radiation Protection and Measurements. Limitation of exposure to ionizing radiation. Bethesda, NCRP, Report No. 116, 1993.
6. National Committee for Clinical Laboratory Standards. Protection of laboratory workers from infectious disease transmitted by blood, body fluids, and tissue. NCCLS Document M29-T2:62–70;1991.
7. National Council on Radiation Protection and Measurements. Precautions in the management of patients who have received therapeutic amounts of radionuclides. Bethesda, NCRP Report No. 37, 1970.
8. International Commission on Radiological Protection. 1990 Recommendations of the International Commission on Radiological Protection. Pergamon Press, Oxford; ICRP Publication 60; Ann. ICRP 21(1–3);1991.
9. Parthasarathy KL, et.al. Necropsy of a cadaver containing 50 mCi of sodium ^{131}iodide. J Nucl Med 1982;23:777–780.
10. Johnston AS, Minarci J, Rossi R, Pinsky S. Autopsy experience with a radioactive cadaver. Health Phys 1979;37:231–236.
11. Griffiths PA, Jones GP, Marshall C, Powley SK. Radiation protection consequences of the care of a terminally ill patient having received a thyroid ablation dose of ^{131}I-sodium iodide. BJR 2000;73:1209–1212.
12. Greaves CD, Tindale WB. Radioiodine therapy: Care of the helpless patient and handling of the radioactive corpse. J Radiol Protection 2001;21:381–392.
13. Wallace AB, Bush V. Management and autopsy of a radioactive cadaver. Australasian Phys Engineering Sci Med 1991;14:119–124.
14. National Council on Radiation Protection and Measurements. Protection against radiation from brachytherapy sources. Bethesda, NCRP, Report No. 40, 1972.
15. Laughlin JS, Vacirca SJ, Duplissey JF. Exposure of embalmers and physicians by radioactive cadavers. Health Phys 1968;15:451–455.
16. National Council on Radiation Protection and Measurements. Radiation protection for medical and allied health personnel. Bethesda, NCRP, Report No. 105, 1989.
17. Kaufman KA, Hamrick B. Contamination events in crematoriums. RSO Magazine 1997;January/February:23–25.
18. International Commission on Radiological Protection. The handling, storage, use and disposal of unsealed radionuclides in hospitals and medical research establishments.Pergamon Press, Oxford; ICRP Publication 25; Ann. ICRP 1(2); 1977.
19. Que W. Radiation safety issues regarding the cremation of the body of an I-125 prostate implant patient. J Appl Cl Med Phys 2001;2:174–177.
20. U.S. Nuclear Regulatory Commission. Issues associated with use of strontium-89 and other beta emitting radiopharmaceuticals. Information Notice 94–70, September 29, 1994.
21. International Commission on Radiological Protection. Release of patients after therapy with unsealed radionuclides.Pergamon Press, Oxford; ICRP Publication 94, Vol. 34(2); 2004.

12 The Hospital Autopsy Report, Death Certification

Brenda L. Waters

The prime goal of the hospital autopsy report is to provide easily accessible and concise information to the treating physician(s), and through them, the family *(1)*. It should address whatever clinical questions arose during the care of the patient, as well as correlate autopsy findings with clinical radiographic and other diagnostic studies. A well-written autopsy report adequately prepares the clinician for a discussion with the family and enables the clinician to answer most of the questions that may be posed. In academic institutions, a second goal of the autopsy report is to teach pathology residents how to write clear and accurate descriptions of abnormalities and to organize those pathologic findings into an understanding of the pathogenetic sequences that led to the morbidity and death of the patient.

The components of the autopsy report usually include the: (1) Preliminary Autopsy Report (PAR) and (2) Final Autopsy Report (FAR). The latter contains a Clinical Abstract, Gross Description, Microscopic Description, Case Discussion, and List of Final Diagnoses. In most cases, the pathologist upon completion of the autopsy will be responsible for filling out a death certificate. These shall be discussed below.

PRELIMINARY AUTOPSY REPORT

The first autopsy report to be sent to the clinician is the Preliminary Autopsy Report (PAR). It comprises the gross autopsy diagnoses arranged in two lists: the Major Diagnoses and Additional Diagnoses. It should be issued within 24 hours of the initial dissection. The following demographic information should head the report:

- Name, age, medical record number and autopsy number of patient.
- Date of admission (if admitted).
- Date and time of death.
- Date and time of autopsy.
- Name of clinician(s) to which the report will be sent.
- Restrictions (if any).

From: *Handbook of Autopsy Practice,* 4th Ed. Edited by: B.L. Waters

In the PAR, the major diagnoses may be listed by organ system (i.e., cardiovascular, respiratory, digestive, etc.) or in outline form in order of causal sequence. This latter format is preferred, especially in academic settings, since it ties pathologic findings together into an understandable pathogenetic sequence. All diagnoses in the PAR should be based on the gross findings alone and not on what one expects to see on histologic examination or on what the clinicians suspected. For example, a subarachnoid hemorrhage should be listed as such, without adding the diagnosis of "ruptured Berry aneurysm" until the latter has actually been identified. If the clinicians collected chemical evidence of an acute myocardial infarction, but no infarct is seen at the time of the initial gross examination, then the diagnosis should not appear on the PAR. Clinicians are more accepting of new diagnoses appearing in the Final Report based on the microscopy, rather than of diagnoses disappearing. Moreover, the clinician may have relayed the preliminary diagnoses to the family, so that, if one of those diagnoses proves to be false, confusion may arise. The role of the autopsy is not to perpetuate a clinical diagnosis in the absence of a pathologic correlate.

There will be instances in which the pathologist may wish to use the modifier "probable" in front of a diagnosis, to reflect a lack of certainty. This temptation should be resisted. It is best to withhold the "probable" diagnosis until histologic review can allow the pathologist to either dispense with the qualifier "probable" or with the diagnosis itself. Again, this minimizes confusion for the clinician and family.

Below the Major Diagnoses, there can be a list of Additional Diagnoses. These abnormalities are those considered worthy of mention but not contributory to death. They may be listed by organ system. Examples include such entities as Meckel's diverticulum, cholelithiasis, and nodular hyperplasia of the prostate. Any "non-Major Diagnosis," such as mild atherosclerosis, may be included under a Major Diagnosis, such as "Atherosclerotic and Hypertensive Cardiovascular Disease," because the two are pathogenetically related. At the end of the PAR, beneath the Major and Additional Diagnoses, the ancillary tests should be listed. These may include microbiologic tests, radiographic imaging, karyotype analysis or blood serology. Although the results may be pending at the time of issue of the PAR, the mention of the tests on the preliminary report will remind the pathologist to search for the results and include them in the final report. There should also be documentation of any photographs taken.

FINAL AUTOPSY REPORT

CLINICAL SUMMARY The next component of the Autopsy Report is the Clinical Abstract. This is a distillation of the clinical history, with emphasis on the patient's significant signs, symptoms, and laboratory and radiographic abnormalities leading up to death. The abstract, written in complete sentences, should document any questions that the clinicians may have had while caring for the patient. An example would be whether the X-ray findings in a lung represented aspiration pneumonia or a mass with distal obstructive pneumonitis. Writing this abstract familiarizes the pathologist with the patient and thus enables her or him to better correlate the clinical history with the pathologic findings. This part of the Final Autopsy Report serves to teach a pathologist-in-training to efficiently review a medical record, glean important information from it, and paraphrase the patient's clinical history into a few concise, well-written paragraphs.

GROSS AND MICROSCOPIC DESCRIPTION It is on the basis of both the gross and microscopic descriptions that all autopsy diagnoses are established. Therefore, these two important sections must be complete, accurate, and concise.

There are several tools available to record gross findings at the time of initial dissection. They include chalkboards, white boards, and various styles of dictating machines. Our laboratory has found that during the dissection, writing the findings on the steel cabinets above the dissection tables, using a Sharpie® permanent marker (Sanford Corporation, Oak Brook, IL) works quite well. The jottings (i.e., weights, measures, descriptions of abnormalities) are easily wiped away with an alcohol-soaked cloth. If the gross description is not then directly dictated, the pathologist may wish to use a worksheet on which to write the data. An example of such a worksheet may be found in Appendix 12.1. This data must then be transferred into the Gross Description section of the Final Autopsy Report. Laboratories may choose to use one of a variety of templates in which to record this data. Hand drawings, photographs, or computer-generated outlines of organs may enhance any autopsy report, but templates that use pictures as the main form of documentation do not encourage complete description of lesions. Purely narrative descriptions, as promulgated by Virchow *(2)*, permit detailed description of complicated findings. However, good narrative protocols can be expected only from experienced pathologists whose style is lucid and whose descriptions of abnormalities are brief, yet complete. Probably the most suitable protocol for gross descriptions is one that is based on sentence completion (See Appendix 12.2). This format can be dictated with ease and yet it allows extra descriptions to be inserted as needed. Importantly, this type of protocol ensures uniformity in the layout of the reports, and encourages inexperienced pathology residents to include all the important information.

The Microscopic Description follows the Gross Description. Again, brevity as well as complete documentation of findings is the goal. These descriptions may be in phrase form, so as to minimize unnecessary words such as "This section shows ..." or "no other abnormalities." The pathologist may find it helpful, however, to use full sentences when writing more complex descriptions, such as the cytologic appearance and infiltrative pattern of a malignancy. Significant negatives are also important, such as "no tumor" in lymph nodes that were taken from a patient with carcinoma, or "no amyloid present" in a patient who has amyloidosis in other organs. If tissues or organs were removed from the patient, premortem, and submitted to surgical pathology, it is our practice to have those slides reviewed by the autopsy pathologist. This review allows the trainee to correlate the premortem pathologic abnormalities with those found at autopsy. Mention of this review can be placed in the Microscopic Description, with brief comments stating the diagnosis rendered on this review. Should there be disagreement between the surgical pathologist's and autopsy pathologist's diagnoses, then a discussion must take place between the autopsy pathologist and the sign-out surgical pathologist. Such interchanges have a valuable role in quality assurance.

LIST OF FINAL DIAGNOSES Once the Gross and Microscopic Descriptions are completed, the list of diagnoses that were recorded in the Preliminary Autopsy Report may be amended, so as to generate the list for the Final Autopsy Report. Again, the same guidelines apply: Arrange the major diagnoses pathogenetically where appropriate; include only diagnoses that are substantiated by the Gross or Microscopic Descriptions; and with any malignancies, state whether or not there are metastases. At the bottom of the List of Final Diagnoses, the results of ancillary tests that were conducted on postmortem tissue can be reported.

CASE DISCUSSION Of all sections of the autopsy report, the Case Discussion is the most controversial. Especially with trainees, this section tends to encourage merely a repetition of much of the data in the Final List of Diagnoses and thus rightfully, may be considered to be a waste of space. However, an informative Case Discussion will include statements that correlate the pathologic findings with the patient's signs, symptoms, and radiographic and laboratory abnormalities. Specifically, if chest radiographs suggest infiltrates or masses, and they are not found at autopsy (despite careful repeated examination), or if pulmonary abnormalities are identified at autopsy, but were not recognized radiographically, these discrepancies should be mentioned in the Case Discussion.

This section should never be used as a forum to comment on clinical management. In the case of significant therapeutic complications, the pathologist must be very careful to not attribute excessive or unnecessary blame to the clinician. Any statements made about therapeutic complications must be firmly substantiated by the gross and microscopic findings. If there is any doubt regarding the occurrence or mechanism of a therapeutic complication, that doubt must be duly expressed in the Case Discussion. In these cases, as stated in Chapter 1, it is critically important that the pathologist invites the clinician to read the entire Final Autopsy Report before the report is finalized. This will ensure that both pathologist and clinician are in agreement with the conclusions made.

Finally, the Case Discussion serves as an important teaching tool for the pathology resident. It compels the trainee to organize a collection of pathologic findings into a coherent series of pathophysiologic events leading up to death. It provides practice in good writing and forces the resident to demonstrate full understanding of the case. It also offers the resident a chance to review and cite recent literature on any aspect of the patient's disease(s). However, the resident must be reminded that a Case Discussion is not a short term paper on basic pathology, but rather it is a brief series of cogent statements directed to a clinician.

The Case Discussion is probably the most difficult part of the Autopsy Report for the resident, simply because it requires a higher level of critical thinking than all the other sections. If only for that reason, it may serve a purpose in academic pathology departments.

DEATH CERTIFICATE

Death certificates are important documents for vital statistics and are required for the processing of burial permits, life insurance claims, estate settlements, and claims for survivorship benefits. They must be filed for all deceased individuals who legally lived and/or were given birth certificates (i.e., stillborns do not require a death certificate, per se, but do require a Report of Fetal Death). Death certificates generate important information for public health statistics, but physicians frequently fill them out inaccurately. In a series of 50 patients who died and did not receive an autopsy, 34% of the death certificates that were completed by nonpathologists at an academic institution contained either a wrong cause or manner of death *(3)*. Even when autopsies were performed, substantial discrepancies persisted between the diagnoses on the death certificate and those generated by the autopsy *(4)*. Thus, there remains significant room for improvement in the accuracy of death certification. All physicians who fill out Death Certificates should read the instructions provided by the College of American Pathologists *(5)*.

COMPONENTS OF THE U.S. STANDARD CERTIFICATE OF DEATH The **Decedent section** contains the necessary demographic information of the decedent, such as name, dates of birth and death, Social Security number, place of death, marital status, occupation, residence, and ethnic and racial background. The funeral director fills in this part of the certificate.

The **Cause of Death section** contains boxes in which to enter the cause of death, circumstances of injury, if any, and the manner of death. This section is the responsibility of the physician certifier. **Part I** of this section is devoted to the Immediate Cause of Death (line a.) and the Underlying Causes (lines b., c., d.), if any, that directly led to the Immediate Cause. The Immediate Cause of Death is defined as the disease, injury, or complication that directly led to death. In some cases, the Immediate Cause of Death (line a.) is also the Underlying Cause, such as death occurring right after a gunshot injury. Here, only one line is necessary. Other scenarios require use of the Underlying Cause lines (lines b., c. and d.) in order to document a series of pathogenetically related conditions that finally culminated in death. For example, an Immediate Cause would be acute myocardial infarction and the Underlying Cause, written on line b., would be coronary atherosclerosis. Three lines in Part 1 may be required to document a scenario such as upper gastrointestinal hemorrhage as the Immediate Cause (line a.), due to portal hypertension (line b), due to alcoholic cirrhosis (line c.). No matter how many lines are used in Part 1, the bottom line should contain the underlying disease that culminated in the patient's death.

All too frequently, physicians list the *mechanism* of death in Part I, rather than the *cause* of death *(6)*. Mechanisms of death include entities such as cardiopulmonary arrest, heart failure, and renal failure. If these phrases are listed in Part I, in the absence of an underlying cause, such certification is so vague and nonspecific as to be meaningless. For example, a mechanism of death, such as congestive heart failure could be caused by a large number of different diseases, such as aortic dissection, myocardial infarction, tumors, or trauma. Statements of mechanism of death are acceptable only if they are followed by an etiologically specific underlying cause. Ideally, statements of mechanism of death should be avoided.

Part II of the Cause of Death section documents the conditions that contributed to death, but were not related to the underlying cause given in Part I. For the patient with an acute myocardial infarction, a contributory condition may be metastatic cancer, or cirrhosis. A patient dying of diabetic nephropathy may have contributory factors such as pneumonia or hepatitis.

The final important component of the Cause of Death section is the **Manner of Death** and **Injury** section. The possible Manners of Death are natural, accident, suicide, homicide, pending, and undetermined. All deaths resulting from accident, suicide, or homicide must be reported to and certified by the medical examiner, coroner, or their designee. If the certifier is contemplating using any manner of death besides "natural," then he or she should discuss the case with the Medical Examiner. Clinicians sometimes erroneously certify a patient as dying of natural causes, when in fact the patient died of complications stemming from an accident or act of violence that occurred weeks or even years previously. Proper certification requires careful review of the patient's chart to determine whether the immediate cause of death can be attributed to that event. If the connection is established, then the manner of death is not natural and the case must be reported to the Medical Examiner. If the manner of death is accident, then the injury section of the certificate must be filled in. This section is also the responsibility of the medical examiner, and not of the hospital or office physician.

The physician signs and dates the Death Certificate in the **Certifier section.**

The **Disposition section** contains information on the method of disposition, places of temporary and final disposition of the body, and the signature of the funeral director or designee.

The **Registrar section** is signed by the person, often a Town Clerk, who files the death certificate.

To aid in the proper completion of Death Certificates, the U.S. Department of Health and Human Resources has published a list of instructions *(7)*. They are paraphrased below:

- Use the current form designated by the state.
- Type all entries whenever possible. If a typewriter is not available, then print legibly in *black* ink.

- Make every entry legible and fill in all applicable boxes.
- Do not make alterations, cross-outs, or erasures. If a correction is needed, start with a fresh form.
- All signatures must be written. Rubber stamp or other facsimile signatures are not acceptable.
- Do not use abbreviations except those recommended in the specific item instructions.
- Spell entries correctly. Verify all place names.
- The registrar will accept originals only. Do not submit carbon copies, reproductions, or duplicates for filing.

USE OF THE TERM "PENDING" FOR CAUSE OR MANNER OF DEATH Use of the term "Pending" in the Cause of Death section is intended only for cases in which there is expectation that additional information will establish the cause of death. This additional information may be histologic findings and toxicology or microbiology results. Deaths in which intoxication by alcohol or drugs is suspected may need to have the death certificate pended in order to await the results of laboratory testing. In the case of a natural death, such as an elderly person with fever who dies at home but the autopsy fails to show gross evidence of infection, the use of "Pending" may be warranted, while waiting for slide review or culture results. In other situations, incomplete details of the death need not delay certification. For example, if a patient died of "cancer of the stomach," reporting the cause should not be deferred while the histologic type of the cancer is determined, because the vital statistics nosologists code such a death simply as "malignant neoplasm of stomach." Similarly, if a death results from "influenza," there is no need to delay certification because a virological test is being carried out.

In many of these instances, it still may be appropriate to certify the manner of death as "Natural", as long as there is no evidence to suggest accident, homicide or suicide.

All Death Certificates with the term "Pending" in the Cause and/or Manner of Death sections must be amended as soon as possible. Local laws or customs of the registrar's offices determine the time allowed to finalize a "Pending" Death Certificate.

REFERENCES

1. Bayer-Garner IB, Fink LM, Lamps LW. Pathologists in a teaching institution assess the value of the autopsy. Arch Pathol Lab Med 2002;126:442–447.
2. Virchow R. Post-mortem examinations with especial reference to medico-legal practice. Fourth German edition. (English translation by TP Smith.) P. Blakiston, Son, Philadelphia, 1885.
3. Pritt BS, Hardin NJ, Richmond JA, Shapiro SL. Death certification errors at an academic institution. Arch Pathol Lab Med 2005;129: 1476–9.
4. Sington JD, Cottrell BJ. Analysis of sensitivity of death certificates in 440 hospital deaths: a comparison with necropsy findings. J Clin Pathol 2002;55:499–502.
5. Hanzlick, RL. Cause-of-Death statements and certification of natural and unnatural deaths. College of American Pathologists, Northfield, IL, 1997.
6. Hanzlick RL. Principles for including or excluding "mechanisms" of death when writing cause of death statements. Arch Pathol lab Med 1997;121:377–380.
7. National Center for Health Statistics, Public Health Service: Physicians' Handbook on Medical Certification of Death. Publication No. (PHS) 2003–1108.

Appendix 12.1 Autopsy Gross Description Worksheet

Restrictions:

External Examination:

Sex: ______________

General description (development, nutrition, clothing):

____

Body length: __________________ Body weight: __________________ Body temp: ______________

Lymphadenopathy: ______________________

Hair description: ____ Hair length:

Iris color: ____________________ Pupil diameter: ___________________ Sclera color: __________________

Teeth condition: ____________________________

Evidence of Therapy/Injuries:

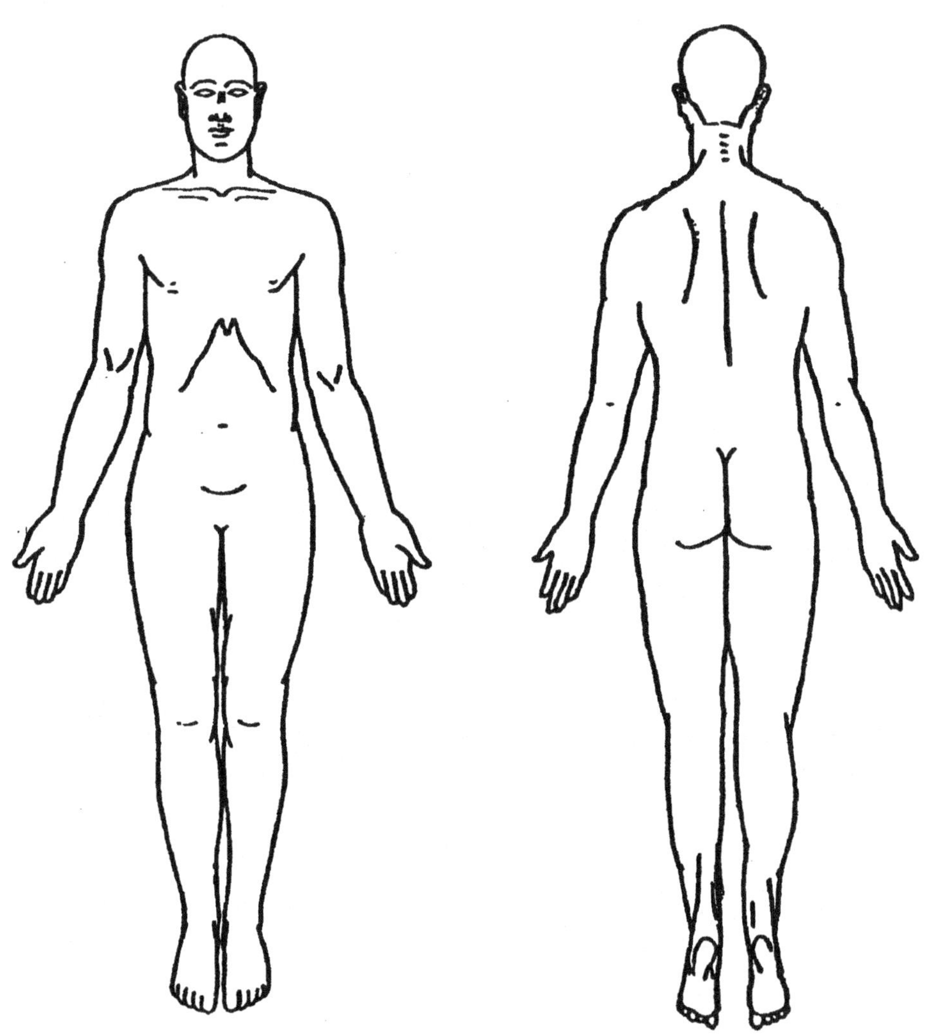

Internal Examination:

Pannus: __________________cm

Thoracic cavity:

____

- R pleural cavity fluid: ______________________ml Character: ______________________
- L pleural cavity fluid: ______________________ml ______________________
- Mediastinum: ______________________ Diaphragm: ______________________

Abdominal cavity:

____

- Abdominal cavity fluid: ______________________ml Character: ______________________

Pericardial cavity:

____

- Pericardial cavity fluid: ______________________ml Character: ______________________
- Abnormalities of pleura, pericardium, or peritoneum: ______________________

Heart:

____

- Weight: ____________g RV thickness: ________________cm LV thickness: ______________cm
- Valve circumference: T: __________cm P: _________cm M: _________cm A: __________cm
- Valve cusps: ____
- Pap muscles and chordae: ____
- Coronary artery description: ____
    - Left main: ____
    - First Diagonal: ____
    - Circumflex: ____
    - Obtuse marginal: ____
    - Right coronary artery: ____
    - PDA: ____

Foramen ovale: ______________________ Septum: IA: __________________________cm IV: ____________________cm

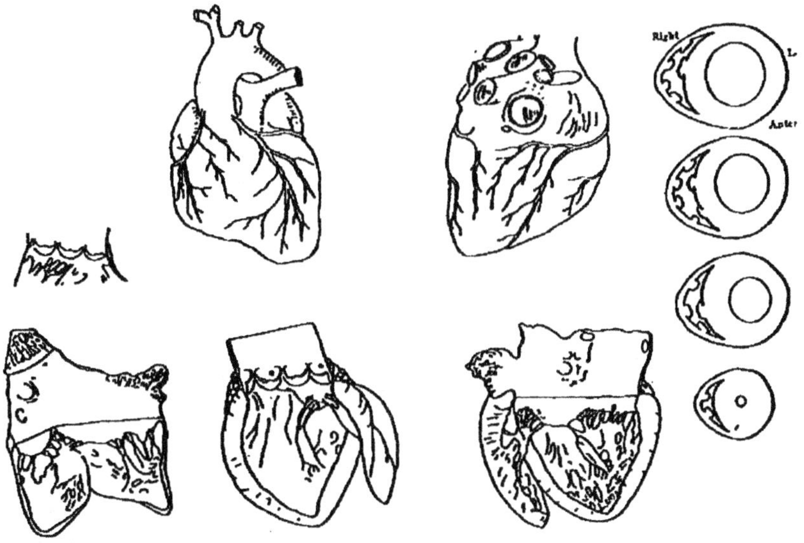

Aorta and Major Branches:

____

- Intimal description:
____
- % involvement: ____________________

SVC and IVC and Branches:
- Patency: ___________________ Thrombi: _________________

Larynx and Trachea:
- Airway patency: ______________________________
- Mucosa (intact, edema, exudates):
____
- Paratracheal LN:
____

Lungs and Pleura:

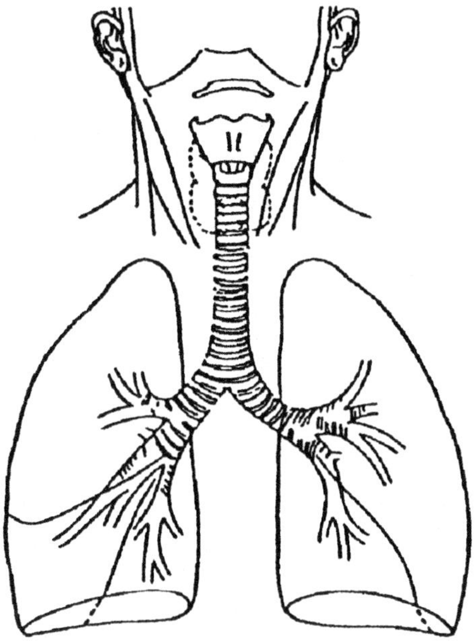

____

- R lung weight: _____g
- L lung weight: _____g
- Visceral pleura:
____
____
____

- Gross appearance: ______________________________________
  ____
- Sectioning: ______________________________________
  _____ ______________________________________
- Bronchovascular pattern: ______________________________
- Bronchi: ______________________________________
  ____
- Hilar and bronchial LN: ______________________________

Digestive System:

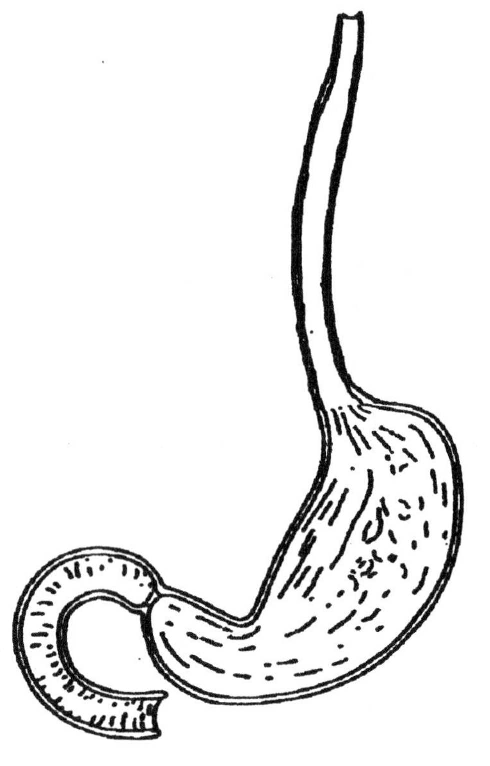

- Esophagus:

____

- Stomach: ______________________________________
  ____
  ____
  - Stomach contents: ____________cc
  - Character: ______________________________
- Small and Large Intestine: ______________________
  ____
- Appendix: ______________________________________
  ____
- Rectum: _____ ______________________________
  ____

Pancreas:

Liver:

- Weight: ______________________g
- Capsule:
  ____
- Parenchyma:
  ____
- Portal and hepatic veins:
  ____
- Intrahepatic biliary ducts:
  ____

Gallbladder and Biliary Ducts:

____

- Contents: _____________cc Character:
  ____
- Wall: _________________ Mucosa:
  ____
- Extrahepatic ducts:
  ____

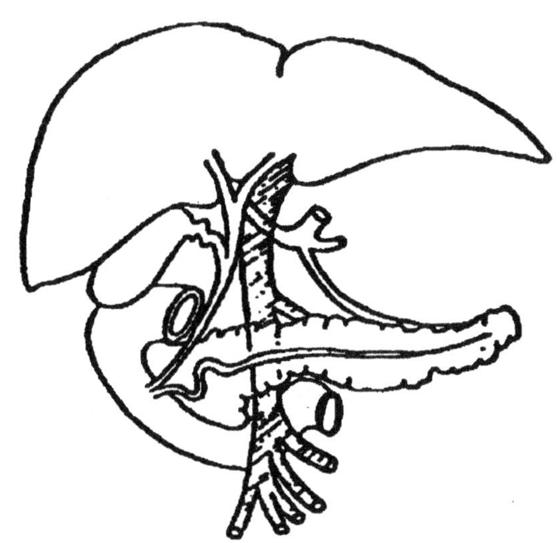

Urinary System:

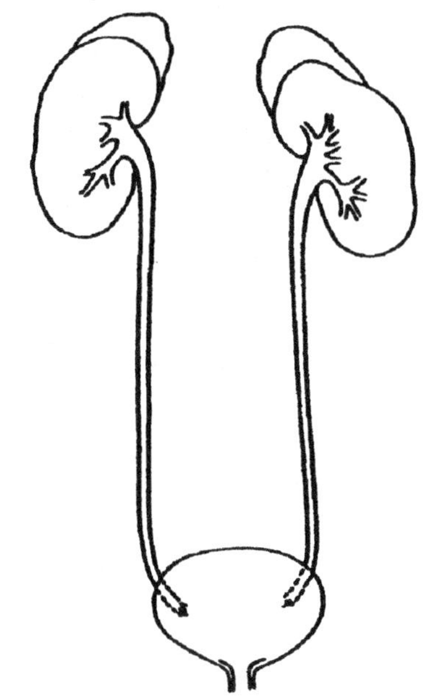

- L Kidney: _______g R Kidney: __________g
  - Cut section:
    ____
- Cortex thickness: ________________cm
- Vessels: _________________________________
- Ureters: _________________________________
- Bladder mucosa: ___________________________
- Bladder contents: ________________cc
- Urethra: _________________________________

Male Reproductive System:

____

- Testes position: ____________________ Length pole-to-pole: L: ___________cm R: ___________cm
- Prostate:

  ____

Female Reproductive System:

____

- Vaginal mucosa:

  ____

- Uterus:

  ____

  - Dimensions: __________________ × ______________________ ×______________________
- Cervix:

  ____

- Endometrium:

  ____

  - Thickness: ____________________cm
- Myometrium:

  ____

- Fallopian tubes:

  ____

- Ovaries: R: __________cm L: ________________cm

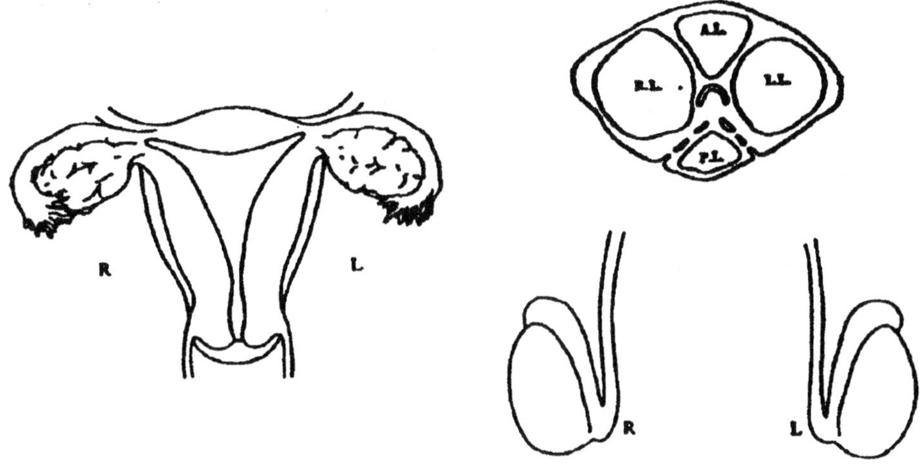

Thyroid Gland:

____

- __________ × __________ × __________

Parathyroid Glands:

____

Pituitary:

____

Adrenal Glands:

____

- L: __________g R: __________g
- Cortices:

  ____

  - Thickness: __________cm

Spleen:

____

- Weight: __________g
- Capsule:

  ____

- Cut surface/follicles/trabeculae:

____

Thymus:

____

Lymph Nodes:

____

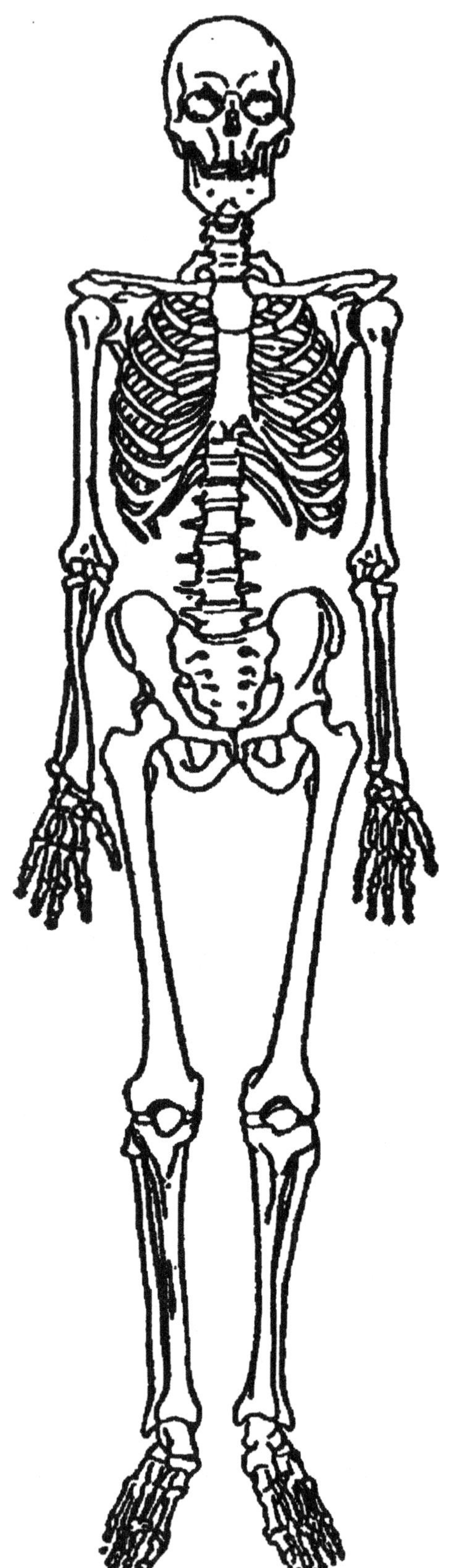

Bone Marrow: ____________________

- Location examined: ____________________

Musculoskeletal:
- Vertebrae: ____________________
- Skeletal abnormalities: ____________________

Sternum and Ribs: ____________________

Meninges: ____________________

Brain: *See neuropathologic description*
- Weight prior to fixation: ____________________

Spinal Cord: ____________________

Tongue and Salivary Glands:
Eyes and Paranasal Sinuses:

Appendix 12.2 Example of a Gross Description Template

External Examination:

This is the body of a #, # dressed in a #. The body length is # inches. The body weight is # pounds. There is no palpable lymphadenopathy. The hair is # measuring up to # in length. The irides are # and the pupils are fixed measuring # in diameter. The sclerae are white. There is no discharge from the ears, nose or mouth. Natural teeth are present in the mouth in # condition. The neck is symmetrical and without masses. The chest is symmetrical and # muscled. The breasts are symmetrical and without masses. The abdomen is flat and without scars. The external genitalia are those of an adult # without abnormality. The upper and lower extremities are symmetrical and # developed and without edema. There is a # on the # identifying the body by name and medical record number. The back is without abnormality. There is # developed rigor of the jaw, upper and lower extremities and neck. There is #, dependent # livor mortis. The body temperature is #.
Evidence of therapy: #.
External injuries: #.

Internal Examination:

Panniculus: The abdominal panniculus is # cm thick.

Thoracic Cavity: The serosal surfaces are smooth and glistening with no fluid, hemorrhage or adhesions. There is no evidence of pneumothorax.

Mediastinum: The soft tissues are unremarkable. The thoracic organs are in the usual anatomic position.
Diaphragm: Unremarkable.

Peritoneal Cavity: The serosal surfaces are smooth, and glistening, with # fluid, adhesions or hemorrhage. The viscera are positioned normally. The omentum and mesentery are not unusual.

Pericardial Cavity: The pericardial sac contains # of serous fluid. The serous surfaces are smooth and glistening, with no adhesions.

Heart: The heart weighs # grams. It has a normal external configuration. The great vessels are normally aligned and positioned. The coronary circulation is # dominant. The coronary arteries contain # plaques with luminal stenoses as follows: left main, # %; left anterior descending, # %; diagonal, #%; circumflex, # %; obtuse marginal branch, #% and right coronary artery, # %. The epicardium is glistening and contains the usual amount of fat. The atria are of usual size, each with a smooth, thin endocardium. The interatrial and interventricular septa are intact. The foramen ovale is #. The ventricles are of the usual size. The ventricular endocardium is thin, smooth and glistening. The left ventricular wall is # cm thick, and the right is # cm thick. The myocardium is homogeneously firm, reddish-brown, and there are no apparent infarcts or fibrosis. The valve circumferences are as follows: tricuspid, # cm; pulmonic, # cm; mitral, # cm; and aortic, # cm. The valve cusps are smooth, pliable, and have an appropriate architecture. The papillary muscles and chordae are unremarkable.

Aorta and Major Branches: Normal course and caliber. There is atherosclerosis characterized by # involving an estimated #% of the aortic intimal surface.

Superior and Inferior Vena Cavae and Branches: Usual caliber. Patent. No thrombi.

Larynx and Trachea: The airway is patent. The mucosa is intact, and there is no appreciable edema or exudate. The paratracheal lymph nodes are #.

Lungs and Pleura: The right lung weighs # grams, and the left lung weighs # grams. The visceral pleura is smooth and glistening. The lungs have a # appearance and are # crepitant to palpation. Sectioning of the # lungs reveals # of the left and # of the right. The bronchovascular pattern is normal. The major vessels are patent. The bronchi are # in color and are patent and free of mucus and exudate and show no grossly evident airway dilation. The hilar and bronchial lymph nodes are #.

Digestive System: The esophagus is of normal course, caliber, and thickness. The mucosa, muscular wall, and serosa are normal. The stomach contains # and is the usual size and shape. The mucosa and muscular wall are unremarkable. The small and large intestines are of usual course and caliber. The mucosa, muscular wall, and serosa are unremarkable. The appendix is present and #. The rectum is free of polyps or other lesions.

Pancreas: The pancreas is of usual size with the usual tan color and lobular architecture. The pancreatic duct is of normal caliber and not obstructed.

Liver: The liver weighs # grams. The capsule is smooth and glistening. The parenchyma has a uniform, firm consistency. The cut surface is red-brown with the normal sinusoidal pattern. The portal and hepatic veins are patent. The intrahepatic biliary ducts are not dilated.

Gallbladder and Biliary ducts: The gallbladder is of normal size and contains # of # bile. The wall is thin. The mucosa is green and velvety. There are no stones. The extra-hepatic ducts are #.
Urinary System: The left kidney weighs # grams, and the right kidney weighs # grams. The capsules strip with ease revealing smooth cortical surfaces. Cut section reveals the cortices to be # cm in thickness, with distinct corticomedullary junctions. Calyces and pelves are of the normal caliber, and the epithelium is smooth and glistening. The vessels are patent. The ureters have a normal course and caliber and are patent throughout. The bladder contains # urine and has a smooth and intact mucosa with a normal trabecular pattern. The muscular wall is of normal thickness. The urethra is patent with # mucosa.

Male Reproductive System: The testes are descended. They measure # cm pole to pole. The seminiferous tubules and epididymis appear normal. The prostate gland is symmetrical with typical gray-white parenchyma and contains # nodules. The seminal vesicles are usual in appearance on cut section.

Female Reproductive System: The vaginal mucosa is intact and #. The uterus # has an appropriate shape, and measures # x # x # cm. The cervix is # and is unremarkable. The endometrium is pale pink, velvety and glistening, and measures # cm thick. The myometrium is pink-red and firm. The fallopian tubes and ovaries are of usual size, shape, and development for this age. There are no tubal or ovarian adhesions. The ovaries measure in maximum dimension # cm on the left and # cm on the right.

Thyroid Gland: Symmetrical, # with the usual firm consistency and glossy, reddish-tan cut surface.

Parathyroid Glands: # glands are identified in their usual locations. Not enlarged.

Pituitary: Normal size, shape, and color.

Adrenal Glands: The left weighs # grams, and the right weighs # grams. Good corticomedullary differentiation. The cortices are yellow-orange and # mm in thickness.

Spleen: Weighs # grams. The capsule is smooth and grayish-blue. The parenchyma has a # consistency. The cut surface is the normal red-purple color with #distinct follicles and trabeculae.

Thymus: No thymic remnant is identified.

Lymph Nodes: No lymphadenopathy.

Bone Marrow: # bone marrow is homogeneous, red-brown and unremarkable.

Musculoskeletal: The vertebrae have normal strength and structure, without palpable fractures. No skeletal abnormalities are present.

Sternum and Ribs: Unremarkable.

Meninges: The dura and leptomeninges are normal.

Brain: Weighs # grams prior to fixation. See neuropathologic description.

Spinal Cord: Unremarkable.

Tongue and Salivary Glands: Not examined.

Eyes and Paranasal Sinuses: Not examined.

13 Medicolegal Autopsy and Postmortem Toxicology

Vernard I. Adams

MEDICOLEGAL AUTOPSIES

DEFINITION In the broadest sense, a medicolegal autopsy is any autopsy that generates an evidentiary document that forms a basis for opinions rendered in a criminal trial, deposition, wrongful death civil suit, medical malpractice civil suit, administrative hearing, or workmen's compensation hearing. Because any autopsy report can become such a document, all autopsies should be considered medicolegal. However, for the purposes of this chapter, a medicolegal autopsy is more narrowly defined as an autopsy that is performed pursuant to the provisions of a medical examiners or coroners act of a state.

FORENSIC PATHOLOGISTS, MEDICAL EXAMINERS, AND CORONERS Ideally, medicolegal autopsies should be carried out by trained forensic pathologists, that is, experts in the physical effects of mechanical, chemical, baro-, and electrical trauma. This ideal is met in several states but other states are woefully underserved. The United States has approximately 400 board-certified forensic pathologists working full-time (Hanzlick R, personal communication, 2005). Florida, the largest state with complete coverage, has nearly 70 (17%) of them *(1)*, despite having only 6% of the population. In underserved states general pathologists still perform many of the medicolegal autopsies, when they are done at all.

ACTIVITIES RELATED TO MEDICOLEGAL AUTOPSIES Particularly challenging are death investigations involving blunt impact to the head or neck, infant deaths, postoperative deaths, and drug-related deaths. Investigation of the last group has become easier with the advent of sophisticated methods of toxicologic analysis as mentioned later in this chapter. Medical examiner autopsies sometimes are requested by next-of-kin who are dissatisfied with the medical care that was rendered to a decedent. Life insurance companies also rely on medicolegal autopsies. Finally, both plaintiff and defense attorneys in the medical malpractice field and hospital risk managers prefer to have autopsies in as many deaths as possible.

ERRORS IN MEDICOLEGAL INVESTIGATION In many instances a seemingly trivial error can have unforeseen disastrous consequences. Every pathologist who works in this field should benefit enormously by reading and rereading the examples given in Moritz' classic paper *(2)*. Although nonforensic pathologists generally understand the purpose of the descriptive (objective) part of the autopsy report, they have little or no training in opinion formation. The essentials are set forth in the following paragraphs.

First, one must understand the terms "cause of death," "manner of death," and "mechanism of death." The *cause of death* is the disease or injury which sets in motion the physiologic train of events culminating in cerebral and cardiac electrical silence. "Carcinoma of the Pancreas," and "Gunshot Wound of the Head with Perforation of the Skull and Brain" are underlying causes of death. "Bronchopneumonia" and "Pulmonary Embolism" are *immediate* causes of death, being in almost all cases the consequence of underlying injuries or diseases such as femoral neck fracture or Alzheimer's Disease. If the time between the initiation of disease or injury and the death is short, the underlying cause and the immediate cause of death may be the same.

The *manner of death* is a pseudojudicial classification of deaths dating back to Norman England, when the property of suicide victims was seized by the Crown. The four manners of death are natural, accident, suicide, and homicide. *Natural* deaths are caused exclusively by disease. *Accidents* are deaths in which trauma causes or contributes to the cause of death, and the harm inflicted is not intentional. A *homicide* is death at the hands of another person, with intent to cause harm. *Suicide* is the intentional unnatural death of one's self, by one's self.

The *mechanism of death* is the physiological derangement set in motion by the causes of death that leads to cessation of cellular electrical activity. Mechanisms of death include entities such as ventricular fibrillation, neurogenic shock, cerebral concussion, cardiac concussion, adult respiratory distress syndrome, sepsis, and cerebral edema. The mechanism of death is more closely linked to the immediate cause of death (if any) than to the underlying cause of death.

The cause and the mechanism of death are interrelated and one may explain the other. For example, an autopsy reveals arteriosclerotic heart disease, and the toxicological studies reveal concentrations of benzodiazepines and opioid narcotics somewhat above the therapeutic ranges. If the history is that of

From: *Handbook of Autopsy Practice,* 4th Ed. Edited by: B.L. Waters

a man who was alert and oriented and who suddenly collapsed in view of witnesses, one may infer a ventricular arrhythmia as the mechanism and arteriosclerotic heart disease as the cause of death. If, for the same set of findings, the history is that of a man who became somnolent, gradually comatose, and then had a diminishing tidal volume followed by respiratory arrest, and then a brief period of persistent cardiac activity, then one may infer that the mechanism is respiratory depression and the that cause of death is intoxication by the effects of the drugs. When clinicians use the term "cause of death," they usually mean the immediate cause of death or the mechanism of death.

DEGREE OF CERTAINTY In a criminal proceeding, opinions must be to a *reasonable degree of certainty*. This means that there can be no other reasonable possibilities—that is, the opinion is beyond a reasonable doubt. Speculation is not admissible in court. For example, it is *conceivable* that the man who collapsed in the previous paragraph was surreptitiously injected with an exotic poison by a foreign agent, but such a possibility is obviously speculative and inadmissible in the absence of any circumstances or history pointing to such a scenario.

In a civil proceeding, the opinion by an expert is to the standard of *probable*, that is, *more likely than not*. Under this standard, one need not eliminate competing reasonable possibilities. It is necessary only that the competing possibilities be less likely than the favored one. Speculation is not allowed in civil proceedings either.

For death certificates, the standard is not well defined, but is generally understood to require a more-likely-than-not probability. In the case of homicide, it is good practice to meet the criminal-law standard of reasonable medical certainty on the death certificate, to avoid having the death certificate be used to impeach one's trial testimony.

In the formation of opinions, three principal errors are often made. First, a pathologist will seize onto one particularly interesting finding but ignore equally compelling evidence pointing to a contrary opinion. Unwarranted criminal or civil suits may result. Moritz described this approach as the substitution of intuition for a scientifically defensible interpretation (2). Second, some errors are caused by the failure to appreciate the distinction between various degrees of opinion and probability. Thus, a mere reasonable possibility is introduced as if it were a probability, or a speculative idea is presented as a reasonable possibility. Third is the failure to appreciate the unspoken underlying assumptions that can help guide a pathologist to a defensible opinion when facts are meager. For instance, a pathologist conducting a second autopsy must start with the rebuttable presumption that the findings of the first autopsy are correct, because the autopsy is a destructive test and many findings cannot be replicated at a second autopsy. Likewise, in the absence of facts, or in the presence of conflicting facts, a decedent is entitled to the rebuttable presumption of a natural death for the purpose of the formation of the final cause of death opinion. This is perfectly compatible with an initial investigative presumption of homicide because this ensures a careful investigation. A violent death creates the rebuttable presumption of an accidental manner, as opposed to suicide or homicide. For example, in the case of a death caused by intoxication by heroin, one should opine the manner as accident unless circumstances clearly point to injection by another person or suicide. The practice of certifying the manner of all recreational drug deaths as undetermined serves no useful public purpose.

PRONOUNCEMENT OF DEATH Failure to ascertain that death has in fact occurred has on occasion led to serious embarrassments and repercussion. The findings supporting a pronouncement of death are briefly recapitulated here. With few exceptions—for example, mitochondrial poisoning by cyanide, the majority of deaths occur by either a rapid cardiac mechanism or a slow central nervous system mechanism *(3)*.

Medical professionals such as nurses who attend deaths uninterrupted by resuscitation efforts will observe the following:

1. Cessation of respiration. As a slow death approaches, the person frequently breathes in gasps. The intervening apneic periods rarely last for more than 30 s; their presence can be ruled out by extending the examination over a 10-min period.
2. Cessation of circulation. In slow deaths, the lack of a peripheral pulse does not necessarily denote cardiac arrest, and the heartbeat does not necessarily cease as soon as breathing stops *(4)*. In contrast, in persons with a rapid cardiac death, ventricular fibrillation or asystole leads to immediate cessation of blood flow to the brain and immediate cessation of the pulse. Cessation of respiratory efforts, voluntary muscle activity and consciousness all follow within 13 s.

DEATHS FROM NATURAL CAUSES. Not all medicolegal autopsies concern violent or unnatural deaths. For example, in two major medical examiner districts in Florida, 40% of the autopsies conducted involved deaths ultimately deemed to be from natural causes that had occurred suddenly, unexpectedly, or in an unusual manner *(5)*. Arteriosclerotic and hypertensive vascular diseases in their cardiac and cerebral manifestations were the most common diseases causing natural deaths *(6)*. The experiences of forensic pathologists working in other cities of the world have been similar. One cannot necessarily conclude that the manner of death is natural merely because a natural disease is demonstrated, because the natural disease may be an immediate cause of death that resulted from an underlying traumatic cause of death. Table 13-1 provides a checklist of natural diseases that can be the sequelae of mechanical or chemical trauma.

EVALUATION OF THE SCENE AND CIRCUMSTANCES OF DEATH Investigation of the scene where the body was found may provide critical environmental evidence, allow the preservation of medicaments, and allow the medical examiner to take witness accounts that are crucial to interpreting the autopsy findings. A body thought by police to have bled from a homicidal wound can be determined to be a putrefied body with pulmonary purging, dead from apparent natural causes. In this situation, an opinion by a medical examiner at the scene prevents an unnecessary full-scale criminal investigation.

TABLE 13-1
Some Common Natural Diseases and Their Possible Violent Antecedents

Disease	*Possible Underlying Injury, Acute or Chronic*
Central Nervous System	
Meningitis; cerebral abscess	Fracture of skull, jaw, facial bones; injuries to middle ear, nasopharynx, air sinuses; infection introduced by surgical, anesthetic, roentgenologic, chemotherapeutic, diagnostic procedures
Intracerebral hemorrhage	Cerebral contusion enlarged by alcoholic coagulopathy, masquerading as hypertensive bleed
Subarachnoid hemorrhage	Blunt impact to head or neck; laceration of vertebral artery
Subdural hematoma	Blunt impact to head from fall
Cardiovascular System	
Coronary artery insufficiency	Emotional or strenuous physical effort related to occupation, or threat of assault
Ruptured heart valve; aortic aneurysm	Strenuous physical effort or blunt impact
Congenital anomalies	Teratogenic drugs
Seizure disorder, syncope	Shock; fright; impact to chest
Respiratory System	
Pneumothorax; subcutaneous and mediastinal emphysema; hemopneumothorax	Traumatic intubation, artificial ventilation with bag-mask, aspiration of foreign body, SCUBA diving, premature putrefaction in the setting of sepsis
Pneumonia; pulmonary embolism	Trauma, immobilization
Pulmonary fibrosis; mesothelioma; pneumoconiosis	Exposure to radiation; drugs; asbestos; industrial exposure
Alimentary System	
Ruptured viscus; perforated ulcer; peritonitis; intestinal obstruction	Impact to abdominal wall ; burns; strenuous physical effort; foreign bodies by mouth or rectum, or left at laparotomy; diagnostic or therapeutic endoscopy; paracentesis; peritoneal dialysis
Fulminant toxic hepatitis; massive hepatic necrosis	Exposure to drugs; poison, anesthetic agents; pesticides; shock
Genitourinary System	
Renal tubular necrosis; papillary necrosis	Poisons; drugs; heavy metals; burns; shock; dehydration
Cystitis; pyelonephritis; ruptured bladder; ruptured uterus; ruptured ectopic pregnancy	Impact to abdomen; abortion; injudicious instrumentation
Hematopoietic & Reticuloendothelial system	
Hemolytic anemia	Incompatible blood transfusion
Aplastic anemia; agranulocytosis; thrombocytopenia; leukemia	Drugs; poisons; pesticides; industrial and laboratory chemicals; antibiotics
Miscellaneous	
Malnutrition; failure to thrive	Negligence; parental cruelty; eccentric or unusual religious beliefs
Crib death	Accidental or homicidal suffocation

Physicians responsible for investigating scenes of violent death should encourage the police to develop policies ensuring that nothing in the vicinity of the body is disturbed before their arrival. The uninstructed patrolman will instinctively remove a firearm from the body of a suicide. On the other hand, such a policy need not be transmitted to the fire department. A well-trained firefighter will pull a freshly dead, viewable body off a pile of smoldering tires, making identification easy, whereas a well-trained detective will not disturb the scene. If the medical examiner arrives at a death scene before the police technicians and detectives, masterly inactivity is required until they are ready for the body to be disturbed. In jurisdictions with few homicides, the medical examiner will often be summoned immediately by the first uniformed police officer to arrive at the scene.

The position of the body, the distribution of blood lost by the victim or the assailant, or objects in the vicinity of the body may offer important clues for the reconstruction of the fatal events, especially in cases of blunt impact or bludgeoning, and in cases of industrial accidents. Scene investigation is much more apt to yield clues as to the approximate time of death than is the autopsy (see below) and may help in the estimation of the interval between injury and death.

Pathologists without significant forensic experience should not hesitate to secure help from statewide law enforcement agencies. Homicide detectives and crime scene technicians from large police departments are familiar with death scene investigations; patrolmen and detectives from small police jurisdictions usually have very limited experience in this area.

Pathologists who do not examine the site where the body was found must rely on the written or oral reports of the circumstances of death, and photographs or illustrating sketches, if they are available.

A forensic autopsy should not begin before the known circumstances surrounding the death are reviewed. The quantity of historical and circumstantial information available in accidental, suicidal, and natural deaths is generally greater than that available in homicides.

ESTIMATION OF THE TIME OF DEATH The postmortem interval is determined by asking the police investigator when the decedent was last known to be alive and when the decedent was found dead. An opinion can be given with assurance that the subject died in that time frame. Because the onset of signs of death varies widely, the physician can only in some cases opine that death occurred more toward one end of that time spectrum than the other. The physical signs that may help in this regard are described in the following paragraphs.

Livor Mortis (Postmortem lividity) After cessation of circulation, the blood drains to the most dependent vessels and becomes deoxygenated. The external manifestation of this process is the appearance of a faint pink erythema of the dependent skin surfaces, visible after 30–60 min in bright light in Caucasians, and later with poor lighting or when the skin is pigmented.

As the blood continues to pool under the influence of gravity, a distinct purple appearance develops on the dependent surfaces. Up until roughly 12–24 h after death, the livor can be blanched by pressing a finger or instrument against the skin surface. Livor is usually absent at pressure points, such as the skin over the scapulas and buttocks in a supine body.

Then, as autolyzing red cells stack in distended capillaries or blood pigment migrates extravascularly, the lividity becomes fixed. In a body whose position is changed before the onset of fixation of livor, the blood will shift to the newly dependent areas. If the livor has become entirely fixed, it will not shift, and the pattern of the livor will be inconsistent with the position of the body.

Livor mortis is of most use in determining that death has in fact occurred. It is occasionally helpful in determining whether the body has been moved after death. Less commonly is it of use in determining the postmortem interval. The full fixation of livor, in the experience of the author, usually coincides with the passing of rigor and the onset of the earliest signs of putrefaction. Livor mortis is red-pink in the presence of substantial concentrations of carboxyhemoglobin. Refrigeration of bodies frequently induces a similar change in parts exposed fully to air. However when this occurs the fingernail beds and the surfaces of the body in contact with the tray or slab typically remain purple.

Rigor Mortis (Postmortem Rigidity) The maintenance of a loose, supple quality in muscle fibers requires energy in the form of adenosine triphosphate and glycogen. The low-energy state of muscle fibers is manifested by stiffness. In dead bodies the stiffness is customarily termed rigor mortis. The strength of the rigor is entirely dependent on the mass of muscle. Grading rigor as weak, moderate and strong is a useless exercise. Thus, a muscular young man who is dead will have impressively strong rigor mortis that is difficult to break, whereas a frail elderly woman with little muscle mass will seem to have weak rigor mortis. More important to note is whether the rigor is present or absent, and if present, whether it is oncoming, fully developed, or passing.

Rigor mortis ordinarily makes its first appearance 2–4 h after death. Its detectable appearance is hastened by antemortem depletion of muscular energy stores. Thus, vigorous physical activity or convulsions immediately before death can result in the almost instantaneous onset of muscle stiffening. Rigor may begin at identical times in two bodies, but will be apparent earlier in the body with the greater muscle mass. It becomes fully developed in roughly 4–10 h. The onset and passing of rigor are hastened by high ambient temperatures and delayed by cold ambient temperatures. This is most often manifested by the maintenance of rigor in bodies maintained under refrigeration. Rigor begins to fade simultaneously with the onset of putrefaction. Rigor is easily and reliably ascertained by attempting to open the mouth by pressing on the mandible. In the extremities, especially the upper limbs, rigor often has been broken prior to transport because the elbows, hips, and knees had to be straightened.

Algor Mortis (Postmortem Cooling) The rate of cooling of a dead body is dependent on the temperature gradient between the body and the environment; the body mass in relation to its surface area; the rate at which air or water moves across the body surfaces; and the extent to which insulation is afforded by shelter, clothing, and adipose deposits. This multiplicity of variables results in wide variation in the rate of cooling. Published tables and formulas for estimating the postmortem interval generally take into account only the temperature gradient. Such formulae seem to enjoy popularity in cool climates where most people die indoors in structures with indoor heating and fairly uniform temperatures. In Florida, where outdoor deaths occur throughout the year, the formulas are largely ignored. The author's practice is to palpate the torso with the back of the gloved hand, and to estimate whether the body is warm, cool, cold, or at ambient temperature. In most cases, warm bodies are either recently dead; hyperthermic from sepsis, cocaine intoxication or neuroleptic medication; or have retained heat because of obesity. Cool bodies of adults usually have been dead for some time, and often have livor or rigor mortis.

Stomach Contents and State of Digestion Under normal conditions, the stomach empties a medium weight meal in approx 3 h. Emptying time is delayed by a heavy meal. Significant craniocerebral trauma can delay gastric emptying for days. Carbohydrate foods such as potatoes and bread are readily dissolved by swallowed salivary amylase. Vegetable matter and meat are recognizable for a few hours. Mushrooms seem to stand up to gastric juices the longest.

In a homicide for which the time of injury is not known, the gastric contents not needed for toxicologic analysis can be strained and rinsed to facilitate naked-eye identification of food matter. The information gained can be correlated with investigative information to help establish whether or not the decedent was alive at certain times or present at certain meals.

Autolysis Within 3 or 4 hours after death the corneas begin to cloud. This effect is most useful in determining whether death was very recent. The degree of cloudiness if no real use. Corneal clouding is extreme in burned bodies, in which the corneas have been baked. Such high temperatures tend to render all irises a cloudy blue, regardless of the initial color.

Skin slippage, or postmortem blistering, is a sign of autolysis that develops simultaneously with putrefaction. But under subtropical sun, or if the skin is near a heat source, slippage can be evident within a half hour after death.

Putrefaction Putrefaction comprises the changes consequent to the migration of bacteria from the gut into the blood, where they multiply, consume the blood, and produce a variety of gases as metabolic products. The volume of gases produced can be enough to float submerged bodies that have been tied down with iron weights. In most cases hydrogen sulfide is produced. This gas combines with the iron in hemoglobin and myoglobin to produce black-green discoloration of the blood, viscera, and cutaneous livor.

The earliest visible effect of putrefaction is often blue staining of the skin of the right lower quadrant of the abdomen, over the cecum, and black staining of the inferior aspect of the right lobe of the liver, adjacent to the hepatic flexure of the colon. Because putrefaction follows the blood, it is most pronounced in areas of dependent lividity, where it first manifests as ruddy and then green-black marbling, also termed venous suggillations. With fully developed putrefaction, the face and genitalia become grotesquely swollen with gas, the eyes bulge, the skin acquires extensive green-black discoloration, and a foul, putrid odor becomes evident. The body cavities are filled with putrid gases under tension, which escape with a rush when the cavities are opened. The soft tissues and viscera are softened, darkened, mottled, and riddled with gas bubbles.

Exsanguination removes the principal nutrient source for bacteria and greatly retards putrefaction. In temperate climates, putrefactive changes begin to be evident roughly 3 d after death. In subtropical climates, they can be evident within 24 h. Putrefaction is hastened by obesity because the viscera are insulated from cooling, and delayed in infants, whose bodies cool rapidly.

Mummification When the body cools rapidly, the warmth needed to sustain putrefactive bacterial growth is denied. The ears, nose, lips, toes and fingers, and in extreme cases, the calves and forearms shrivel and darken as the water content evaporates from the tissue. This change is of little use in determining the postmortem interval. Mummification is more common with children, small-framed adults, and in a cold or dry environment.

Adipocere This substance is a rancid semisolid product of fat decomposition. Adipocere is found most often on bodies that have decomposed without having been exposed to air. It is not useful in determining postmortem interval.

Entomologic Evidence Dead bodies attract flies, which lay eggs, particularly near the eyes, nares, mouth, genitalia, and wounds. The larvae that hatch from fly eggs are called maggots. Maggots consume soft tissue, leaving behind bone, cartilage, gristle, and some, but not all, dermis. The maggots molt one or more times, going through stages of development termed *instars*, and finally crawl off the body to pupate in nearby soil. The maggots are eaten by other insects. When the soft tissues have been largely removed and the partly skeletonized remains have dried somewhat, beetles move in to consume the cartilage, gristle and dried dermis. The order of their appearance depends on the local fauna present at that particular time of year, and can be used to infer how long a body has been dead, largely based on the fact that insects mature more rapidly in warm weather. A forensic entomologist can make these interpretations, but generally requires baseline data for the local area, including the time of appearance of local species and data on degree days. An entomologist can narrow the date-of-death window down to a few days in some cases, whereas the forensic pathologist working with the signs of decomposition can only give broad estimates of numbers of weeks or months in cases of advanced decomposition.

Chemical Evidence Mathematical formulas have been devised to estimate the postmortem interval from the concentration of nitrogenous compounds in cerebrospinal fluid, and from potassium in vitreous humor. In practice, the formulas produce wider time frames than are provided by acquiring from the police the times last known alive and found dead, and are of academic interest only.

IDENTIFICATION OF THE BODY An instant photograph of the face is useful for the purpose of identification of a viewable body by friends or relatives. Burned bodies often have one or two printable fingers and may be identifiable by dental comparison or comparison of antemortem and postmortem somatic radiographs. Dismembered bodies that are recovered piecemeal require the separate identification of the major elements. The head can be identified by dental comparison or plain radiographs that portray the unique outlines of the frontal sinuses. The upper extremities can be identified by fingerprinting. The torso can be identified by chest, abdominal, and pelvic radiographs if antemortem films exist. Virtually any part of the body can be used for a DNA match. Serologic studies performed by the crime laboratory can differentiate human from animal blood or tissue.

Fingerprinting may become difficult if the skin is shriveled, macerated from immersion, or charred. If there is no ridge elevation, but the pattern is visible, the whorl pattern can be photographed with a macro lens. If there are ridges, but the finger pads do not roll well because of maceration or desiccation, the finger pads can be built up with injectable compounds, including formalin.

Identification by DNA matching can be done by the crime laboratory in cases such as bludgeonings, where the laboratory is conducting tests to put a suspect at the scene. Because such laboratories often have case backlogs that are too long for the purposes of identifying and releasing a body, private laboratories must often be used when DNA is required for identification. DNA testing can be done on the same blood samples used for toxicological testing. In the author's office, blood stains on filter paper are prepared for all autopsied bodies, whether dead from natural or unnatural causes. The dry stains are stored at room temperature in the regular case file, and can be used for DNA identification years after the liquid and solid tissue specimens have been discarded.

Sex determination can be made from most skeletal remains from the contours of the pelvis and skull. Age determination can be based on evaluation of epiphyses, laryngeal and sterno-costal cartilages, sacral, hyoid, and cranial bone sutures, and the condition of joints and teeth. Stature is reconstructed by anthropologic measurements and formulas *(7)*.

THE FORENSIC AUTOPSY PROTOCOL The subjective and objective sections of the autopsy report should be clearly separated from each other. The subjective portion comprises the cause of death opinion, the diagnoses, and the prose summary and opinion if there is one. The objective portion comprises the macro- and microscopic descriptions. The macroscopic descriptions constitute what is commonly called the autopsy protocol.

The subjective sections should be clearly labeled as opinion. The opinions contained in these sections are based on all the available information, including medical history and circumstantial information. Unlike the data in the gross protocol, which should never change, the opinions *can* change if there are changes in circumstantial and historical information on which the opinions are based.

The gross protocol should contain objective descriptions with which no reasonable, trained pathologist would disagree. Ideally, the findings should be dictated so that no revision of the gross description is necessary after the microscopic slides are reviewed and further medical history and investigative information becomes available. Diagnostic terms may be used if the diagnosis will never be in question. For instance, if the lungs have obvious bronchopneumonia, and it is clear that the diagnosis will not be changed by subsequent microscopic studies, the end of communication is best served by including the term "bronchopneumonia" in the description of the lesion.

A pathologist who wants to ensure that all details, no matter how irrelevant, are captured, will dictate concurrently with the evisceration and dissection. However, many experienced pathologists make notes on a body diagram, and then dictate the external and internal examinations after the completion of the internal examination. This style tends to produce a concise, well-organized prose narrative.

If the protocol is dictated directly at the time of examination, and there are no handwritten notes, it should be promptly typed and proofread. If notes have been made, the need for a prompt proofing is still apparent for lengthy protocols with multiple gunshot wounds, or combinations of injurious modalities, such as impact, strangulation, and stabbing. The most common error made by experienced pathologists is the transposition of the words "left" and "right."

Because it is the testimony that is offered into evidence at trial, and not the autopsy report, mistakes in the protocol can be corrected at any time. However, the concerned attorneys must be notified immediately of any change that affects an opinion. If a change is cosmetic, it is sufficient to notify the attorney who has called the pathologist, just before going on the witness stand. The attorney can choose whether to elicit testimony concerning the change on direct examination, or to ignore it.

Identifying features must be recorded in detail for bodies which are unidentified. In contrast, a brief mention of iris color, hair color and distribution, facial hair, and significant scars is adequate for bodies for which identification is not in question. For instance, this author is satisfied to estimate the length of scars as small, medium, and large in relation to the body region in the description for identified bodies.

Descriptions of endotracheal tubes, central venous catheters, and other devices of therapy are best clustered in a single paragraph that has both the external and internal aspects of the descriptions of the locations of the devices. For example, "An endotracheal tube runs from the mouth to the trachea." The observations in this paragraph need not be repeated in the external and internal sections of the report.

Penetrating wounds, including gunshot wounds, should be described in such a way that the correlation of the external and internal aspects is readily apparent to the reader. This is elegantly accomplished by the use of a separately titled section for all the external and internal data for such wounds. The same device can be used for blunt impact wounds, with separate sections for head and neck, torso, and extremities. In this format, the wound descriptions are *not* repeated in the customary sections for external examination and internal examination.

Measurements are made metrically or in the English system, depending on the purpose to which the measurements will be put. Lesions caused by disease and anatomical measurements of interest only to physicians should be measured metrically. Wounds can be measured metrically or by the English system, at the discretion of the pathologist. The author measures wounds metrically, unless the wound is patterned, and is being matched to an impacting object that was manufactured to English system specifications. It can no longer be presumed that a vehicle which strikes a pedestrian and leaves the scene of an accident in the United States is of American manufacture. The old axiom that wounds must be measured in inches no longer holds; jury pools now contain citizens educated in the metric system.

In the United States, distances between wounds and anatomic landmarks such as the top of the head, the median sagittal plane, and the soles of the feet should be made in inches, because police investigators will be using feet and inches to measure the distances between bullet holes in walls and floors.

In the United States, body length and weight should be in the English system, because the parties who use this information are most often attorneys. Readers of the autopsy report who must perform physiologically oriented calculations based on body weight or length will be capable of converting the English measurements to metric measurements.

Measurements should be preceded by a qualifying adjective to indicate whether the number is actually measured, or is estimated (e.g., "The left pleural cavity has a measured 1200 ml of dark red clot," "The subdural space on the left has a measured 85 grams of clot," and "The retroperitoneal soft tissues have estimated 100 ml of liquid blood") Blood accumulations in the retroperitoneal or mediastinal soft tissues must be estimated because they cannot be readily measured.

"Normal, "Unremarkable," and "Within normal limits" may be used for descriptions of organs that are not pertinent to the cause of death, such as the prostate gland or the thymus.

The written description of external wounds should be supplemented by photographs and sketches on pre-printed diagrams. Suitable diagrams of the external surface anatomy, the skeleton, dentition, and organs are available from the Armed Forces Institute of Pathology and the College of American Pathologists. Diagrams are particularly useful in jogging the memory while reviewing old cases, because they depict the wounds not as the camera saw them, but as the pathologist perceived them. Standards and guidelines for the performance and reporting of medicolegal autopsies are available from the National Association of Medical Examiners and the Florida Association of Medical Examiners *(8,9)*.

THE CHAIN OF CUSTODY In all criminal or noncriminal cases, medicolegal or hospital-derived, the chain of custody of the body should be documented by a record which includes the names of the transport driver, the log-in technician, the log-out technician, and the driver for the funeral home to which to body is released; and the dates and times of each transfer. Care must be taken that no one tampers with the body without authorization. If possible a lock should be put on the cooler in which the body is kept.

Likewise, a record of the chain of custody must be kept of physical evidence such as bullets, hair and fingernail exemplars, trace evidence, and toxicological specimens. (For the chain of custody of toxicologic evidence, *see* also below under "Autopsy Toxicology.") Such material should be saved in containers labeled with the case number, the name of the deceased if known, the date the specimen was impounded, the name of the specimen and the site from which it was removed, and the name of the medical examiner.

Bullets can be inscribed on the base or nose, but not on the sides. Any inscribed mark or symbol serves to take a bullet out of the legal category of fungible items. Pathologists in court frequently recognize their bullets not by the faded, tarnished inscriptions made months before, but by the writing on the evidence envelope or by comparing the bullet to photographs taken of the bullet before it was sealed in the evidence envelope. The author routinely photographs all removed bullets with a macro lens.

THE EXTERNAL EXAMINATION When available, clothing from victims of gunshot wounds and pedestrians struck by vehicles that fled the scene should be examined for soot and gunpowder, and transfer of paint and trace evidence, respectively. Victims of bludgeoning, brawls, and strangulation should be examined for transferred hairs and fibers before the body is stripped and cleaned. Clothing can be examined at the scene and placed into police custody there, or transported on the body to the autopsy facility and reexamined in good light, at the discretion of the pathologist. For apparent natural deaths, the clothing can be stripped by the autopsy room technicians, and retained for later examination by the pathologist in the unlikely event that it becomes necessary.

The inspection of the external body surfaces and orifices should be sufficient to detect old suicidal wrist scars, partial finger amputations, needle tracks, conjunctival petechiae, cutaneous contusions, and open wounds of the hair-bearing aspects of the scalp. However, when the hair is thick and tightly curled, perforations of the scalp are easily obscured. Cutaneous contusions are made less evident by skin pigmentation.

Roentgenographs The availability of roentgenographs varies with the equipment and personnel of the facilities in which autopsies are conducted (*see* Chapter 10). All bullets should be located by roentgenographs. Bullets in the head, neck, and torso are most easily located if both anteroposterior and lateral films are made. Radiographs should be taken of stab wounds to locate broken bits of blades.

Head, neck, chest, abdominal, and pelvic radiographs should be taken before the internal examination in unviewable bodies, because they may be needed for identification purposes. If an unviewable body has decomposed to the extent that trauma cannot be ruled out with confidence, then roentgenographs of the extremities should be prepared also.

Chest roentgenographs should be obtained in cases of motor vehicle accidents with head trauma, and in victims of stabbing of the neck, to detect venous air embolism, unless the victim has lived long enough to have had spontaneous circulation of blood. The common portals of air entry are dural sinuses lacerated by skull fractures, and penetrating wounds of the jugular and subclavian veins. (For the detection of pneumothoraces, *see* under that heading in Part II and below under "Internal Examination.")

Pelvic roentgenographs are helpful in traffic fatalities, because they are more sensitive than the autopsy in detecting pelvic fractures. Chest roentgenographs are not needed to detect rib fractures because the autopsy is more sensitive in this regard. Likewise, roentgenographs are less sensitive for the detection of skull fractures than is direct observation after reflection of the galea and stripping of the dura. Cervical roentgenographs will show cervical dislocations that are obvious at autopsy, but are inferior to posterior neck dissection in detecting lethal craniocervical derangements in which there is no residual static dislocation.

Photographs Photographs of external wounds should be taken with a 35-mm camera or the digital equivalent. Traditionally, pathologists used Ektachrome or Kodachrome transparency film because the slides were small and stored easily, there was no need to develop prints, and the images were suitable for projection at lectures. Police customarily used print film, and developed the prints only if a court appearance was anticipated. However, many, if not most pathologists and law enforcement agencies now use digital photography, which meets all the needs just listed.

It is useful to have an internal scale near a lesion being photographed to get a sense of scale, but the internal scale cannot be used to measure the lesion in the picture, owing to the distorting effect of photographing a curved surface. Attorneys have at times raised the question of what lesions might be obscured by the scale, so it is good practice to have a companion photograph without a scale or other objects.

THE INTERNAL EXAMINATION A postmortem examination should include examination and removal of the thoracic, abdominal, pelvic and neck organs, and the intracranial contents. So-called limited autopsies, which omit the opening of the skull, examination of the neck organs, or examination of the chest or abdominal organs, permit only limited opinions to be made, and are only specimen retrievals. An autopsy conducted pursuant to statute should never be limited. It is often preferable to have no postmortem examination at all than to be responsible for an examination that cannot answer the anticipated questions.

The standard Y-shaped incision will permit a thorough examination of the anterior neck organs, and removal of the tongue. After retracting the skin and muscles of the anterior aspect of the chest, a pleural window should be created to detect prevmothorax by scraping the intercostal muscle off the external aspect of the parietal pleura. This should be done on both sides of the anterior aspect of the chest, usually near the third ribs.

For special procedures for the diagnosis of arterial and venous air embolism or pneumothorax, see under these headings in Part II.

In cases of third and fourth degree burns it is usually necessary to make a European-style midline incision to the chin, because the tissue is contracted and indurated. For the same reason, the testes must often be removed through scrotal incisions in these bodies. This is not a problem for the undertaker because these bodies are not viewable.

Layerwise examination of the anterior neck structures is desirable in all cases, and is accompanied by sequential in-situ photography in cases of suspected strangulation *(10)*. Layerwise examination of the posterior neck structures is required for traffic fatalities in which there is insufficient trauma elsewhere to account for death, or in which there is an unexplained laceration of the brainstem, or hemorrhage in the prevertebral fascia *(11)*. Posterior neck dissection is necessary to rule out craniocervical derangement in cases of suspected suffocation in traffic accidents, and is recommended in all infant deaths that occur outside the hospital. The pathologist opening an infant spinal canal for the first time may be surprised to find that the delicate and loosely supported epidural venous plexus has become so hypostatically congested that the blood has extravasated into the loose fibrofatty tissue of the epidural compartment. The absence of sprain hemorrhages in the supporting ligaments and muscles of the vertebral column permits the exclusion of the diagnosis of true epidural hemorrhage.

The method of evisceration should be the one with which the pathologist is most comfortable. Some experienced forensic pathologists remove thoracic and abdominal organ blocks prior to dissection but others remove organs in sequence (Virchow's technique), with equally good results. Many crucial observations can be made only during the evisceration. Therefore it is important for the pathologist not to delegate the evisceration procedure. If this is neglected, an attorney might convince the judge, the jury, and the press that the autopsy was actually performed by the technician, and that the doctor merely looked at removed specimens. The helper in these cases may be called to testify, because the observations that he has passed on to the pathologist are hearsay.

The order of examination of the organs is not critically important. The pathologist who does only occasional autopsies should use the same order consistently so that no change of dissection techniques is necessary. Some pathologists prefer to dissect the heart first, arguing that the most important findings in an apparent cardiac death should be brought to light first. The author's preference in such cases is to dissect the heart last, to decrease the time interval between the observations and the recording of these observations.

EMBALMING For the autopsy pathologist, embalming is much to be desired in an exhumed body, but much to be avoided in a fresh body. Embalming involves two phases.

Arterial embalming involves the introduction of a catheter into a common carotid artery, usually the right, following which the blood vessels are flushed with embalming fluid. An embalmer who observes that the embalming fluid is not perfusing an extremity will expose the brachial and femoral arteries as necessary. Poor perfusion generally results from luminal obstruction by postmortem clots. In the United States, embalming fluid is generally a mixture of methanol, ethanol, formaldehyde, and red dye.

Obviously, embalming creates challenges for the toxicologist. After the arteries have been thoroughly flushed, the arterial and venous contents are not blood but, rather, some combination of blood-tinged embalming fluid, blood diluted by embalming fluid, and fixed clots. Ocular fluid, bile, and urine are available as liquid specimens, but will have artifactual concentrations of methanol appearing in the gas chromatograph. Technical problems abound in these situations.

Arterial embalming produces soft formalin fixation and artifactual pink coloration of the tissues. It produces artifactual effusions in the body cavities, and hardens intravascular clots. At the same time, it induces contraction of the tunica media in the walls of blood vessels, which then contract around any postmortem clots, producing an appearance similar to or indistinguishable from that of a distending thrombus.

Trocar embalming involves the introduction of a sharp-tipped hollow metal pipe through the abdominal wall. The trocar is used to aspirate any liquids and to inject concentrated embalming fluid. This fluid has no dyes and has a higher concentration of fixatives than does the arterial fluid. After trocar embalming, the liver, stomach, mesenteries, and loops of bowel have numerous perforations. The lungs and heart usually have fewer perforations, depending on the diligence of the embalmer. The tissue along the perforations is firm and gray, unlike the tissue fixed only by the arterial embalming fluid. The perforations of the diaphragm and pericardial sac produce communication paths among body cavities. The body cavities can contain substantial formalin collections mimicking effusions. More troublesome are real effusions and blood collections that are diluted by the embalming fluid. Fixed feces is often found floating in the peritoneal fluid.

The practice of permitting arterial embalming before an autopsy is mentioned only to discourage it. At the Mayo Clinic, where the autopsy suite includes an embalming room, the neck organs are removed after arterial embalming has been accomplished, which facilitates the work of the embalmer. Embalming before examination of the neck organs should not be permitted for medicolegal autopsies.

EXHUMATION AND OTHER SPECIAL PROCEDURES Recently exhumed bodies differ from the embalmed bodies described above only by the presence of colorful growths of mold on the skin surfaces. The internal findings are similar to those of yet-to-be-buried embalmed bodies. Long-buried bodies have variable degrees of decomposition, and can be virtually skeletonized.

Many special procedures, from "Abortion" to "Strangulation" are listed in Part II in alphabetical order of the condition.

AUTOPSY TOXICOLOGY

Most autopsies in which toxicological analysis is performed are autopsies conducted pursuant to statute, toward the end of determining the cause of death.

INVESTIGATION OF CIRCUMSTANCES OF POISONING Frequently, medical examiner investigators or police detectives can use directed interview questions to elicit information which is helpful to further a toxicological investigation, once poisoning is suspected. The questions are focused on meals, beverages, and exposure to herbicides and pesticides.

CONTAINERS To prevent contamination of specimens by cleaning or embalming agents, previously unused polyethylene or glass containers are preferable in most situations. With time, highly volatile compounds, such as the accelerants used by arsonists, will diffuse through polyethylene and escape the container. When arson is suspected, metal cans are often used. The pathologist should always have control over the selection, use, and labeling of syringes and specimen containers. This can be an issue for itinerant autopsy pathologists who work in funeral homes.

The label for each specimen container should state the date the material was secured, the name of the decedent, the case number, and the name of the organ or liquid sample. Samples added to containers with preservatives should be inverted several times to disperse the preservative through the sample. Samples should be kept refrigerated before and during transport to the toxicology laboratory. After analysis, deep-freeze storage is preferable to refrigeration.

ROUTINE SAMPLING OF TOXICOLOGIC MATERIAL In the author's office, it is usual practice in all autopsies to save central blood, bile, urine, gastric contents, liver, brain, available femoral vein blood, all retrievable vitreous humor, and nasal swabs. Most but not all the blood is placed in commercial blood collection tubes with sodium fluoride as a preservative. Sodium fluoride inhibits both bacterial growth and serum esterases which hydrolyze cocaine postmortem. If commercially available gray-top tubes are not used, 250 mg of NaF can be added to 30 ml containers. Urine and bile are placed in 10 mL polypropylene centrifuge tubes, and the specimens of gastric contents, liver, brain are placed in 50 mL polypropylene centrifuge tubes. Because blood specimen collection protocols must also anticipate the needs of the DNA laboratory, which can detect a few molecules of contaminant DNA, all containers and syringes must be unused.

Urine Urine is aspirated with a syringe through the dome of the bladder after the peritoneal cavity has been opened. If the bladder is nearly empty, it can be secured by hemostats before incising the dome to facilitate aspiration of the bladder lumen under direct vision. Toxicologists often prefer urine as a specimen for immunoassay drug screening, because it can be analyzed without extraction. NaF as a preservative is optional; as an inhibitor of cocaine hydrolysis NaF is unnecessary because the immunoassays detect cocaine metabolites rather than parent cocaine.

Blood Central luminal blood is preferred to cavity (pleural, pericardial, peritoneal) blood. Central ("heart blood") specimens are aspirated from any chamber of the heart, or from the ascending aorta, pulmonary artery, or vena cava. For a growing number of analytes, most notably tricyclic antidepressants, peripheral blood is preferred over central blood. Peripheral blood is aspirated by percutaneous puncture before autopsy, from the femoral vein or the subclavian vein. The author prefers the femoral approach in order to avoid any question of artifact in the diagnosis of venous air embolism. Peripheral blood can be obtained by a technician as soon as the body is received. If cocaine intoxication is likely, it is highly desirable to obtain this specimen in a tube with NaF as soon as possible, in order to inhibit post-mortem hydrolysis of cocaine. The term, "cavity blood" is used for blood ladled or aspirated from a hemothorax, hemopericardium, hemoperitoneum, or from the pooled blood left in the common cavity after removal of the heart and lungs. Cavity blood analyses should be supplemented by peripheral blood, vitreous, or solid tissue analyses, because of the real possibility of contamination by diffusion from the stomach.

Vitreous Vitreous is an excellent specimen for alcohol and drug analysis. The protected location in the orbit renders the fluid less susceptible to putrefaction than blood, and the problem of site-dependent variation in concentrations in blood specimens is avoided. Two to three ml of vitreous humor from one or both eyes is gently aspirated from the lateral angle of the eye with a 5 mL clean syringe (See Fig. 5-1). The tip of the needle should lie near the center of the eyeball. Forceful aspiration must be avoided because it may detach retinal cells, which cloud the specimen and give spuriously high potassium values. In infants, vitreous collection is often delayed until the pathologist has opened the head and knows whether the eyes will be needed for histopathological examination for retinal hemorrhage. Before analysis, the laboratory analyst must invert the specimen 10 or 12 times to ensure thorough mixing.

Gastrointestinal Tract After removal of the stomach, duodenum, pancreas, and esophagus, the gastric contents are squeezed out the esophagus, or through an incision in the stomach, into a 1-L container. A representative 50 ml specimen is satisfactory for the toxicologist, unless the stomach contents have a non-uniform slurry of solid and liquid elements, in which case a higher volume is desirable. If the solid elements seem to be fragments of medicaments, then nearly all the contents should be saved for the toxicologist, except for what is needed to strain and inspect the material to identify food matter. In suspected suicides, in which death may have followed ingestion by several hours, it can be useful to ligate a length of jejunum before removing it and draining it into a specimen container. The jejunum in such circumstances may have a higher concentration of analyte than the stomach.

The establishment of the diagnosis of intoxication in adults cannot be done from analysis of gastric contents; investigative information and analysis of tissue or body fluids are needed. Analysis of gastric contents may help to establish suicidal intent and to investigate poisoning in infants. In infants, testing of gastric contents also can be used as a screening tool to save the limited quantities of blood for quantitative analysis.

Cerebrospinal Fluid (CSF) The practice of removing CSF by suboccipital or lumbar puncture is mentioned only to discourage it. Although pathologists certainly vary in their skill levels, and some can make a clean puncture more often than not, even in the best hands blind punctures often produce blood-lined tracks that render the interpretation of posterior neck and vertebral dissections problematic. Vitreous, like CSF, is a low-protein erythrocyte-free substitute for blood, and is preferred to CSF in most situations. If CSF must be drawn, it is best taken from the cerebral cisterns after the skull has been opened in such a fashion that the leptomeninges are relatively intact and the CSF has not run out. The situation most often calling for a CSF specimen is the meningitis autopsy with no urine available for a latex agglutination test for bacterial antigens.

Bile Bile is aspirated by needle after the abdomen is opened and before the organs are removed. Because the mucosa of the gallbladder is lush and easily becomes ensnared in the needle tip, it is helpful to aspirate with gentle vacuum and to move the needle tip slightly within the gallbladder. Bile is a useful substitute for blood when the analyte of interest is an opiate or an alcohol. In rapidly fatal opiate intoxications, the offending opiate may be detectable only in bile.

Other Liquid Specimens In hospitalized decedents, the highest concentrations of toxic substances may be found in dialysis and lavage fluids, if they have not been discarded after death.

Solid Organs Liver is the solid organ of choice when no liquid specimens are available. Reference values are available for the lethal concentrations of numerous types of drugs in liver tissue. Specimens from the right lobe of the liver are preferred to specimens from the left lobe, to help avoid spuriously high concentrations caused by diffusion from the stomach *(12)*. Brain tissue can be used for alcohol determination in the absence of a useful liquid specimen. Many reference values for drug concentrations are also available for brain tissue.

In fully putrefied bodies blood and bile are usually absent, and the only specimens available may be solid organs such liver, brain and skeletal muscle. Skeletal muscle from the least decomposed extremity is preferred.

In fire deaths, arson investigators occasionally request specimens for accelerant analysis. For this purpose, a lung is sealed in an unused lidded metal can of the style used by paint manufacturers.

Hair Hair is a useful specimen in suspected chronic arsenic poisoning, and may be useful in the determination of chronic drug abuse. Hair should be pulled from the scalp so as to include the roots. A large sample, about 10 grams, should be tied in a lock to identify the root end of the specimen.

Skin If one suspects that a poisonous substance has been injected, the skin around the needle puncture site can be excised at a radius of 2–4 cm from the injection site. If a poisonous substance might have been taken up by absorption, the skin is excised in the area where the absorption is thought to have occurred, and from a distant, preferably contralateral area as a control. Skin samples are saved with the expectation that the toxicologist will prefer to obtain the information necessary to opine the cause of death by first analyzing the customary liquid specimens.

CHAIN OF CUSTODY The continuity of the custody of the specimens should be documented. A blank space on the specimen transmittal form (see next paragraph) can be used for tracking custody from the pathologist to an in-house toxicology laboratory.

Transmittal Sheet If a courier is used to transport a sealed container with multiple specimens from multiple cases to an outside laboratory, an additional, separate, single transmittal form can be devised which lists all the case numbers, omits specimen details, and which has signature/date lines for the in-house technician, the courier, and the receiving clerk at the laboratory (*see* Table 13.2).

METHODOLOGY

Volatiles by Gas Chromatography The analyte most frequently tested is ethyl alcohol. Toxicologists in medical examiner offices generally detect and quantify ethyl alcohol by gas chromatography, as part of a general panel designed to capture numerous volatile compounds, including ethyl, methyl and isopropyl alcohols, and ketones. A few toxicologists now link the gas chromatograph to a mass spectrometer for analyte confirmation. Tertiary butyl alcohol is often used as an internal standard, because it does not occur naturally. Hospital and clinical laboratories most often use the alcohol dehydrogenase method, which measures any substance capable of being dehydrogenated by the enzyme. It does not distinguish methyl, ethyl, and isopropyl alcohols and it has a larger experimental error than does gas chromatography. The dichromate method, which measures oxidizing activity, is nonspecific and mainly of historical interest.

Specific Drug Screening by Immunoassay Drugs of abuse are commonly detected but not quantified by enzyme-linked immunosorbent assay (ELISA), which has largely supplanted EMIT (Enzyme Multiplied ImmunoTechnique). Immunoassays measure the activities of selected families of drugs by antibody interaction. The panels are selected depending on local drug abuse patterns. Panels are available for cocaine metabolites, tricyclic antidepressants, barbiturates, cannabinoids, amphetamines, opiates and propoxyphene and many others, including fentanyl.

Drug Screening by Thin-Layer Chromatography (TLC) Although immunoassay panels detect the most commonly occurring abused drugs, they are not general drug screens. The technically simplest general drug screen utilizes the TLC so familiar to high school chemistry students. Specimens

TABLE 13-2

TOXICOLOGY SPECIMEN TRANSMITTAL SHEET

Toxicology Specimen Transmittal Sheet

(Name of Medical Examiner Agency)

(Address and Telephone Number of Medical Examiner Agency)

Medical Examiner Case Number: 06-*012345*

Name of Decedent: *John Doe*

Date Specimens Obtained: *5/3/2006*

Duration of Hospitalization: *36 hours* Embalmed? *No* Transfused? *No*

Decomposition (circle): None 1+ 2+ 3+ 4+

[*X*] Check here to retain specimens and issue a report that states "Toxicology Testing Not Indicated"

X	Blood, heart*
X	Blood, peripheral
	Blood, cavity
	Liquid from heart or vessels (embalmed)
X	Bile
X	Urine
X	Gastric content
	Bowel content
X	Vitreous Humor
X	Liver
	Lung
X	Brain
	Kidney
	Skeletal muscle
	Nasal swabs
	Other:_____

Other information or instructions:

Pathologist name and date:

Laboratory receipt of specimen; name and date:

*An "X" indicates specimen collected.

are prepared for TLC by extracting into solvents under acidic, neutral, or basic conditions, in order to bring different classes of drugs into the extraction solvents.

Specific Drug Identification and Quantitation by Chromatography Linked to Mass Spectrometry Gas chromatography uses a very long, very thin, coiled column. The output of the column is fed into a mass spectrometer that breaks compounds into ionic subunits, whose weights form a bar-graph spectrum which can be specific for each compound. Formerly, the gold standard for identifying drugs was gas chromatography linked to mass spectroscopy (GC/MS). GC utilizes a gas solvent to separate the analyte drugs. GC/MS is being supplanted for many tests by high performance liquid chromatography in tandem with mass spectroscopy (HPLC/MS). HPLC uses a liquid carrier solvent in a short narrow linear tube. Because the carrier is liquid, the instrument has a cool injection port that causes much less analyte degradation than the hot injection port of a gas chromatograph.

Carbon Monoxide Tests Carboxyhemoglobin is detected in most medical examiner toxicology laboratories by visible spectrophotometry. In hospitals, carboxyhemoglobin is frequently detected and reported in the course of routine arterial blood gas analysis. Some medical examiner laboratories use GC for the determination of carboxyhemoglobin.

Metals Heavy metals can be detected by qualitative tests. For example, the Reinsch test primarily detects arsenic, and is an insensitive test for mercury, antimony and bismuth. Quantification and specific metal identification is done by atomic absorption spectroscopy, usually by a reference laboratory.

Cyanide A good screen for cyanide is the nose of a person who capable of smelling hydrogen cyanide. Because only a minority of persons can smell cyanide, it is helpful to know in advance if any person in an office or laboratory can smell hydrogen cyanide. Textbooks state that hydrogen cyanide gas smells like bitter almonds; forensic pathologists who can smell the compound state that it has its own specific odor that is not comparable to any other (Davis JH, personal communication, 1984).

Sampling for Specific Toxicologic Substances Pertinent procedures have been listed in Part II, under the name of the substances involved, from "Alcohol Intoxication and Alcoholism: to "Poisoning, Thallium."

ACKNOWLEDGMENT

Wayne Duer, PhD, and Jacqueline Lee, MD, reviewed the manuscript, suggested improvements, and corrected errors in the toxicology and autopsy sections, respectively. Any remaining errors are those of the author.

REFERENCES

1. From data on the web site of the Florida Medical Examiners Commission (http://www.fdle.state.fl.us/cjst/MEC/AMEList.pdf).
2. Moritz AR: Classical mistakes in forensic pathology. Am J Clin Pathol 1956;26:1383–1397. Reprinted in the Am J Forensic Med and Pathol 1981;2:299–308.
3. Davis JH, Wright RK. The very sudden cardiac death syndrome - a conceptual model for pathologists. Human Pathol 1980;11:117–121.
4. Atlee WL, the Medical Faculty of Lancaster. Report of a series of experiments made by the medical faculty of Lancaster, upon the body of Henry Cobler Moselmann, executed in the jail yard of Lancaster County, Pa., on the 20th of December, 1839. Am J Med Sci 1840;51:13–34.
5. 2004 Annual Report. Medical Examiners Commission, Florida Department of Law Enforcement, p 8.
6. Medical Examiner Department database for 2005, Public Records of Hillsborough County, Florida.
7. White TD. Human Osteology. San Diego, Academic Press, 2000.
8. Forensic Autopsy Performance Standards. National Association of Medical Examiners, 2005, at http://www.thename.org/ (*select* Download).
9. Practice Guidelines for Florida Medical Examiners. Florida Association of Medical Examiners, 2006, at http://fameonline.org/ (*select* Download).
10. Adams VI. Autopsy Technique for Neck Examination: I. Anterior and Lateral Compartments and Tongue. Pathol Ann 1990;25(2): 331–349.

11. Adams VI. Autopsy Technique for Neck Examination: II. Vertebral Column and Posterior Compartment. Pathol Ann 1991;26(1): 211–226.
12. Pounder DJ, Fuke C, Cox DE, Smith D, Kuroda N. Postmortem Diffusion of Drugs from Gastric Residue. Am J Forensic Med Pathol 1996;17:1–7.

AN ANNOTATED REFERENCE LIST FOR THE OCCASIONAL FORENSIC PATHOLOGIST

Baselt RC. Disposition of Toxic Drugs and Chemicals in Man, 7th ed. Biomedical Publications, Foster City, CA, 2004.

Has well-organized descriptions of metabolism, procedures, therapeutic concentrations, and concentrations found in fatalities.

Bass WM. Human Osteology: A Laboratory and Field Manual, 5th ed. Missouri Archaeological Society, Columbia, MO, 2005.

Useful manual for identifying isolated bones.

Dolinak D, Matches E, Lew E. Forensic Pathology: Principles and Practice. Elsevier, Burlington, MA, 2005. *Lavishly illustrated and practically oriented.*

Froede RC, ed. Handbook of Forensic Pathology. College of American Pathologists, Northfield, IL, 2003. *A brief reference on applied forensic pathology.*

Spitz WU, ed. Spitz and Fisher's Medicolegal Investigation of Death: Guidelines for the Application of Pathology to Crime Investigation, 4th ed. CC Thomas, Springfield, IL, 2006.

A standard textbook of forensic pathology.

14 Legal Aspects of Autopsy Practice

Vernard I. Adams

This chapter focuses on general legal principles pertaining to autopsies in the United States.

In the United States, the legal basis for the transportation, refrigeration, chemical preservation, and dissection of human bodies, as well as the retention and postmortem use of body parts, organs, tissues, and fluids, rests largely on common law as it has evolved from its 1776 basis in English common law. Statute law has superseded much of the common law in Great Britain and Australia, but in the 50 states of the United States coverage by statute law is incomplete and common law continues to be made by judicial opinions. Pathologists should familiarize themselves with the laws and judicial decisions that govern the performance of autopsies in the states in which they practice. Laws governing autopsies in other nations are beyond the scope of this chapter.

Under 17th century common law no property right inhered in a dead human body and it could not be willed. This concept has softened. Some courts have held that although a dead body is not considered property in the commercial sense, the next-of-kin have a right to possess the body for the purpose of burying it and a right to maintain a claim for disturbance of the body *(1)*. This quasi-property right has been applied to a stillborn fetus *(2)* and has been additionally interpreted to mean that the next-of-kin have a right to claim the body in the same condition as when death occurred *(3)*. Other courts, recognizing that any right to possess a body for disposition is limited by state laws and ordinances, have recognized the right of the *decedent* to have a decent burial. This right is known as the right of sepulcher (or sepulture) *(4)* and has been articulated as a presumption against disturbing the repose of the dead *(5)*.

These common law precepts were articulated during an era when a dead body had no commercial value. Now, a brain-dead body with a beating heart may contain organs that can be transplanted into another human being. Similarly, tissue banks find value in skin, corneas, bones, dura, and cardiac valves from dead bodies with no cardiovascular circulation. As a result, the no-property concept has been eroded. All states now permit the donation of organs from dead bodies under provisions of their various enactments of the Uniform Anatomical Gift Act *(6)*.

From: *Handbook of Autopsy Practice*, 4th Ed. Edited by: B.L. Waters

AUTOPSIES BY STATUTE

AUTHORIZATION In most states, autopsies in cases of suspicious deaths are authorized by medical examiners or coroners. Many states also invest this authority in prosecuting attorneys. In a few instances, autopsies may be ordered by the sheriff or county manager. A statutory autopsy may be performed without the consent or even against the expressed will of the surviving spouse or next-of-kin. A medical examiner or coroner usually has the discretion to perform an autopsy in any case that falls under the jurisdiction of the enabling statute, but is required to perform autopsies in only some specified categories such as deaths caused by criminal agency.

Outside the military services, no federal law supersedes state authority to order autopsies or move bodies. Within the United States, military law, not state law, applies on those military bases with exclusive federal jurisdiction over the land on which the bases sit. Some installations have concurrent jurisdiction or partial legislative jurisdiction. Medical examiners and coroners who have federal military bases within their areas of jurisdiction can contact the Directorate of Engineering and Housing and the legal office at the military base to ascertain the style of jurisdiction *(7)*.

The Federal Bureau of Investigation (FBI) is charged by federal law with the investigation of the death of a President or other specified dignitaries *(8,9,10)* and, as such, displaces the sheriff or police department that would ordinarily conduct the criminal death investigation. Although these laws have no provision that overrides the authority of the local medical examiner or coroner to move or autopsy the body, they have been so interpreted.

OBJECTIONS TO STATUTORY AUTOPSIES Objections based on religious views must be handled with sensitivity. In Dade County, Florida, the Orthodox Rabbinical Council has rabbis who are specifically delegated to attend autopsies; they discuss the procedures to keep them down to the minimum needed to serve the public interest *(11)*. This usually entails the use of *in-situ* dissection as much as possible. Rather than relying on medical examiners and coroners to voluntarily respect religious sensibilities, California *(12)*, New Jersey *(13)*, New York *(14)*, Ohio *(15)*, and Rhode Island *(16)* have enacted statutes to achieve the same end. *In these states, if the next-of-kin express a religious objection to autopsy, the coroner or* *medical examiner must petition for a hearing before a judge to overturn a statutory prohibition of autopsy unless the death is caused by criminal agency or an immediate threat to the public health.* Maryland has a simple statute that states that an autopsy may not be performed in the face of a religious objection by the next-of-kin unless the autopsy is authorized by the chief medical examiner or his designee *(17)*.

Sensitivity in these situations can mean delaying the autopsy until the family members have had time to discuss the matter and consult with an attorney, or it can mean omitting the autopsy when the public interest is outweighed by the private interest, as in the case of a fractured femoral neck caused by a fall at home.

WHO MAY PERFORM AN AUTOPSY In most states, autopsies conducted pursuant to statute may be performed by medical examiners and their deputies, coroners and their deputies, and physicians working under the authority of a coroner. Autopsies performed outside the purview of medical examiner or coroner statutes are conducted by permission of the person who claims the remains for burial (*see* below).

CIRCUMSTANCES UNDER WHICH AN AUTOPSY MAY BE PERFORMED In most states, the law authorizes autopsies when the medical examiner or coroner deems them necessary as part of the statutory duty to determine the cause of death. This duty generally arises when a death occurs unexpectedly while in apparent good health, or under violent, suspicious, or unusual circumstances. Some state laws require the medical examiner to determine cause of death when death occurs in a penal institution, is caused by criminal abortion, or involves a possible threat to the public health; or when cremation is intended. In some states, statute or administrative code requires autopsies in certain types of deaths, such as sudden infant death syndrome.

AUTOPSIES BY CONSENT

WHEN IS AN AUTOPSY INDICATED? Ideally, autopsy permission should be sought in all hospital deaths for two main reasons: (1) For reliable data analysis, the number of cases should be large and the selection as random as possible; and (2) the most interesting and important findings may be totally unexpected and thus are often missed if authorization is requested only for defined groups of deceased patients. Despite these compelling reasons, financial, legal, and other constraints often cause institutions to seek autopsy permission only under specific circumstances. Thus, the College of American Pathologists *(18)* recommends including in such a list: (1) unknown or unanticipated complications; (2) unknown causes of death; (3) special concerns of the next-of-kin or the public; (4) deaths following diagnostic procedures and therapeutic interventions; (5) deaths of patients who have participated in clinical trials; (6) unexpected or unexplained deaths which are apparently natural; (7) deaths from environmental or occupational hazards; (8) deaths resulting from high-risk infectious and contagious diseases; (9) all obstetric deaths; (10) all perinatal and pediatric deaths; and (11) deaths in which it is believed that autopsy would disclose a known or suspected illness that may have a bearing on survivors or recipients of transplant organs. For several of these categories the medical examiner or coroner may have jurisdiction, depending on the locality.

AUTHORIZATION In some institutions a specially trained representative of the autopsy service or the transplant service asks the next-of-kin to authorize an autopsy. In institutions without such persons, a physician should seek permission for autopsy. Although autopsy permission usually must be requested at what appears to be the most inappropriate time for the next-of-kin, a tactful explanation of the benefits for the family of the deceased, and for other patients will usually be successful in securing permission.

Referring a death to the medical examiner or coroner to obtain an autopsy after the next-of-kin have denied permission engenders ill will and only rarely results in an autopsy. Unless the autopsy is required by law the medical examiner will usually respect the wishes of the next-of-kin and certify the death based on the medical record.

PERSONS WHO MAY AUTHORIZE AUTOPSY The right to grant, restrict, or withhold authorization for an autopsy rests with the surviving spouse, or, if there is no surviving spouse, the next-of-kin. In the absence of known kin, autopsy permission may often be granted by the person who has custody of the body. Authorization of an autopsy should be documented on a form designed for the purpose so that there will be no dispute over what was authorized. Some states require the authorization to be written *(19)*.

Surviving Spouse The wishes of the surviving spouse clearly override those of the next-of-kin *(20)*. However, divorce terminates the spouse's authority. Separated couples are considered legally married; a separated surviving spouse has the same right to claim the remains as does a cohabiting spouse. In other words, "separated" is a living arrangement, not a civil status.

Next-of-Kin After the surviving spouse, the order of priority in any given state depends on whether the applicable statute is an autopsy law, a funeral directing act, or the probate act. State law should be consulted before an autopsy service develops an institutional policy regarding the priority of the classes of next-of-kin. If several persons have an equal degree of kinship it would be wise to obtain a statement that the contact person is acting on behalf of all members of the group. If two parties claim equal priority, the best approach is usually to wait until the family sorts out the issue.

The following order often applies:

1. Children of the deceased, if they are of age
2. Parents
3. Relatives of lesser degree
4. Friends or any person of legal age who assumes responsibility for the burial. The institution or person obtaining permission may ask for an affidavit stating the facts of the friendship or other relation, and stating that the person in question will assume the costs of the burial.

Persons Entitled by Statute Autopsy authorization by medical examiners and coroners is discussed in the beginning of this chapter. In addition, statutes in some states provide that hospitals or physicians may give permission for an autopsy on a body when no one is known who would be legally entitled to take custody of the body for burial *(21)*. Depending on the state in which the death occurs, autopsies may be done on such bodies or they may be required to be surrendered to a medical school for scientific studies. In all these instances, reasonable efforts must be made to communicate with relatives or friends who might want to assume custody of the body and the costs of burial. Most hospital administrators are reluctant to exercise the option to authorize an autopsy and will attempt to refer such cases to the medical examiner.

In some states, workmen's compensation laws authorize an industrial commission to order autopsies *(22)*. In some of these states, if the next-of-kin do not consent to the autopsy, compensation is denied. Similarly, a state law might give life insurers the right to have autopsies *(23)*, or policies may require autopsies. In either case the right seems not to be absolute, and refusal by the next-of-kin may trigger denial of a claim.

Permission from Decedent In many states, a person may authorize an autopsy on himself or herself. However, relying on such a permission in the face of objections from the next-of-kin who are claiming the remains is not recommended.

PERMISSION FOR SPECIAL PROCEDURES Authorization for an unrestricted autopsy assumes the understanding that the autopsy will be carried out in the usual manner - that is, the chest and abdominal cavities will be examined and the brain and neck organs will be removed. For any procedures that require additional incisions, particularly of the face, neck, or hands, or that may interfere with embalming, it is prudent to secure a special permission specifying the nature of the intended maneuver. This also holds true for removal of the eyes. A medical examiner or coroner who intends to perform these extended procedures must be sure that they serve the public interest and are not conducted solely for research or educational purposes.

RESTRICTED AUTHORIZATION FOR AUTOPSY The place, manner, and extent of the autopsy may be stipulated for any reason by the person who has the right to refuse an autopsy *(24)*. Restrictions regarding the place of autopsy generally are intended to secure privacy, which is discussed below. The extent of the autopsy may be restricted to the abdominal or chest cavity, to exploration through an operative incision, or to inspection of the organs without permission to remove samples for histologic study, to name only a few examples. Whether an autopsy should be done at all under such circumstances must be carefully considered by the pathologist because restricted examinations may lead to highly misleading results—for example, if potentially fatal coronary artery disease is found but a ruptured berry aneurysm is not detected because no permission had been obtained to inspect the cranial cavity. The hospital may also be restricted from retaining entire organs at the option of the family.

AUTOPSY CONSENT FORM A two-page model consent form recently developed by the medical examiner and the public health officer of Oregon is available on the Internet *(25)*. It can be modified to conform to the laws of other states (*see* Figure 14-1). The Oregon form explains the purpose of a hospital autopsy, and gives the choice of an unlimited autopsy, a limited autopsy, or no autopsy at all. If a limited autopsy is chosen, the form has check-off lists for restricting the extent of autopsy, the disposition of organs, the exclusion of research procedures unrelated to determination of cause of death, and who may attend the autopsy. Commonly, hospitals obtain permission by fax or telephone when the next-of-kin are physically unavailable, using the same form as would be otherwise used.

UNAUTHORIZED AUTOPSIES The performance of an unauthorized autopsy or the violation of an autopsy restriction may be construed as mutilation of the dead body. The next-of-kin typically claim that a violation of sepulcher has caused them mental anguish *(26)*. The person to recover for the mutilation of the dead body generally will be the one who had the right to custody of the body and who therefore has the right to restrict or withhold authorization for an autopsy.

Many insurance policies providing indemnity of accidental death contain clauses that give the insurer the right to demand an autopsy. However, the question of whether the economic interest of the insurance carrier overrides the right of the next-of-kin to control the disposition of the body is not a settled matter. To avoid becoming embroiled in a lawsuit, the pathologist should insist on authorization from the next-of-kin.

PREVENTION OF WRONGFUL AUTOPSY If a body is released from a hospital to the medical examiner or coroner, the hospital should notify the next-of-kin that the medical examiner has custody of the body. The hospital should verbally notify the medical examiner if an objection to autopsy is known to prevent the hospital being held liable for the performance of a medicolegal autopsy.

The following three steps should be taken by the hospital pathologist and not delegated to other personnel:

1. Contact the medical examiner or coroner if the jurisdiction of the death or the identify of the deceased is in doubt.
2. Review all name tags and identification bracelets to ascertain that the body is in fact the one for which an autopsy permission has been granted. The apparent age, sex, wounds, and therapeutic apparatuses should be consistent with the information available in the medical history.
3. Ascertain that the autopsy authorization form is properly completed and signed. Possible restrictions must be noted and conveyed to technicians, residents, or other persons who may help with the autopsy. If a signed authorization form is not used, a form containing all pertinent information should, nevertheless, be used to avoid errors and misunderstandings.

ANATOMICAL GIFTS AND SPECIMEN RETENTION

DONATION OF BODY, ORGANS, AND TISSUES

Under the provisions of the Uniform Anatomical Gift Act, a driver's license or wallet-size card carried by the decedent serves as a substitute for a will for the limited purpose of donation. However, organ procurement organizations and tissue banks usually will not proceed without consent from the next-of-kin.

Anatomical gifts fall into three categories. The explantation of organs such as the heart, liver, and kidneys from a brain-dead body with a beating heart is called *vascular organ* donation. Organ procurement organizations refer to long bones, skin, and

[LETTERHEAD OF AUTOPSY SERVICE OR INSTITUTION]

CONSENT FOR AUTOPSY

An autopsy is an examination of a dead human body in order to determine the cause, seat, or nature of disease or injury and customarily includes the retention of small samples of tissues for diagnostic purposes.

Authority to Consent to Autopsy. With respect to the deceased, I am:

[ ] The health care surrogate; *or if no surrogate is legally designated;*
[ ] The surviving husband or wife; *or if no spouse survives,*
[ ] A son or daughter 18 years or older; *or if no children of age,*
[ ] Either parent or guardian; *or if no parents are alive or no guardian,*
[ ] A brother or sister aged 18 years or older; *or if no siblings survive,*
[ ] The nearest living relative; *and if no relatives are known,*
[ ] The person assuming custody of the body for purposes of burial.

I, ______________________________ (print name), have been informed about the purpose of an autopsy. I consent to and authorize a physician from [name of autopsy service or institution] to complete the type of autopsy checked below on the body of ________________________ (name of deceased). I understand that any information gained form the autopsy will be put in the deceased's medical record and that I will be able to view the autopsy report.

I hereby give permission for the following type of autopsy OR deny permission for an autopsy (check only one box).
Please ask staff to clarify any terms you do not understand. If no boxes are checked, an autopsy will not be performed.

[ ] **UNLIMITED AUTOPSY**. This autopsy will be used to determine the cause of death and to obtain information that may be used to improve medical knowledge. All organs, tissues, and fluids may be removed, examined, and retained for education or research.

[ ] **LIMITED AUTOPSY**. A partial autopsy will be done to determine the cause of death. This means that organs, tissues and fluids may be removed and examined or tested but limits what the physician can do based on my wishes. <u>If this box is checked an autopsy is allowed with the following limitations</u>:

PART 1. I have limited the autopsy to a portion of the body.

( ) Restricted to brain and spinal cord only.	( ) Restricted to the chest and abdomen only.
( ) Restricted to the chest cavity.	( ) Restricted to the abdominal cavity.

( ) Other: *(specify)*

PART 2. I direct the physician to return, dispose of, or retain tissues as follows:

( ) Organs, tissue, and fluids may be retained for education and research purposes and discarded when their purpose has been served.

( ) All organs must be returned to the body, except the samples needed to make a diagnosis. Tissues and fluids may not be used for research and will be discarded when the report is completed.

( ) Other: *(specify)*

PART 3. Additional instructions for limited autopsy:

( ) No procedures or tests unrelated to determining the cause of death or seat of disease or injury may be performed.

( ) Attendees at the autopsy are restricted to those involved with the procedure.

( ) Other: *(specify)*

I would like receive a copy of the autopsy report: **[ ] No. [ ] Yes:** *Send the report to the address below:*

[ ] **PERMISSION DENIED.** *Checking this box means that an autopsy will not be performed.*

______________________ *Signature of person authorizing autopsy*	__________ *Date*	
______________________ Signature of w*itness Date*	__________ *Date*	*Facility where autopsy will be performed.*

Fig. 14-1. Autopsy Consent form. (After Oregon).

corneas recovered from a dead body with a non-beating heart as *tissue*. The third category, popularly known as donation of a body to science, usually means donation to the anatomy laboratory of a medical school for dissection.

If a death comes under the jurisdiction of the medical examiner or coroner, the organ procurement organization interested in vascular organ or tissue donation must obtain permission from this official in addition to the permission from the next-of-kin. Denial of permission for vascular organ donation may result in the death of an identified, matched, potential recipient in the case of a heart or a liver. For this reason, many medical examiners adopt a zero-denial policy for vascular explantation. Flexibility of both parties makes this possible. Thus, the organ procurement organization will do studies such as coronary angiography if they are requested by the medical examiner. The medical examiner will sometimes perform an external inspection at the hospital or attend the subsequent surgical explantation. The author knows of no murder prosecution failing because organ harvesting was permitted. Death by criminal agency is no bar to organ donation.

In the case of postmortem tissue donation of long bones, corneas, and skin, no life is lost if the medical examiner denies permission; the denial merely reduces the shelf inventory of the tissue bank.

Some states such as Florida and Ohio permit the medical examiner or coroner to give permission for harvesting of corneas if the next-of-kin cannot be located with reasonable effort. However, the medical examiner or coroner should not knowingly refuse to read available copies of hospital records in order to avoid discovering an objection to such a donation. Such behavior may incur liability *(27)*. To avoid legal entanglements, some tissue banks do not take advantage of such laws. Instead, they focus on potential donors with known kin and medical histories, and use the donor cards only as evidence of the antemortem intentions of the decedent during discussion with the next-of-kin.

RETENTION OF ORGANS AND TISSUES FOR STUDY Removal of organs and tissues for histologic study is accepted as a normal part of the autopsy. It appears reasonable to include here non-destructive procedures such as organ angiography. Permanent retention of entire organs may not be contemplated by the next-of-kin and thus, the authorization that has been obtained should be broad enough to permit the procedure. Most permission forms used by hospitals have a specific clause that grants permission to retain organs and tissues for the purposes of education and research. In the absence of such a clause the organs should be returned to the body.

After autopsies performed pursuant to statute, only those organs are retained that serve a public purpose—for example, for cause-of-death determination, identification, or testing by other experts. However, case law on retention of organs by medical examiners and coroners is spotty. In a 2005 ruling limited to southern Ohio, a federal judge held that the next-of-kin have a constitutionally protected property right in the dead body, and further ruled that the coroner could not retain a fixed brain after releasing the body without first notifying the next-of-kin. Three years later, the federal court for Southern Ohio clarified the issue by holding that the next of kin do not have a protected right under Ohio law to organs or other body parts retained by the coroner at autopsy *(28)*.

DISSEMINATION OF AUTOPSY FINDINGS AND OPINIONS

WHO MAY WATCH AN AUTOPSY? Privacy issues must be considered if persons other than physicians are allowed to view an autopsy. Polices in this regard vary widely. In some institutions, only physicians and medical students are allowed to view autopsies because of unwelcome experiences with curiosity seekers and the resulting gossip. Others consider the educational value worthwhile and will admit nurses, law enforcement officers, or other persons who have a plausible professional relationship. Such sessions should be scheduled, and the professional standing of the attendees should be ascertained in each instance. A compromise between the opposing views in this matter is to admit nurses and other qualified persons in the medical field to organ reviews rather than to the autopsy itself.

ADMISSIBILITY AS EVIDENCE Depending on the jurisdiction, the death certificate may or may not be a public record. In almost all states a certified copy is admissible in court as evidence that death in fact occurred. In some but not all states, the cause-of-death opinion on the certificate is similarly admitted.

Autopsy protocols and diagnoses may or may not be admitted into evidence, depending on the state concerned. In most states, the protocols and diagnoses are not admissible by themselves as evidence. Rather, an expert who may or may not be the autopsy pathologist who signed the report, must give opinions under oath. This allows for cross examination, which is a right of criminal defendants in the United States.

Hospital records, including autopsy records, may be treated as business records, that is, an expert may rely on this material as foundation for opinions and the hearsay rule does not apply.

In medical malpractice suits, the testimony of the autopsy pathologist may be taken in deposition, but if there is a trial, the courtroom testimony will be provided by experts hired by the plaintiff and the defendant. If no deposition is given, the hospital pathologist may never be aware that the autopsy played a role in a lawsuit. Autopsy pathologists, like other expert witnesses, are allowed to refer to their file notes and reports when testifying.

CONFIDENTIALITY OF AUTOPSY RECORDS In most jurisdictions, information gained at autopsy is not privileged because a dead body is not considered a patient. Under common law, no rights of confidentiality inhere in a dead body. However, statute law may supersede this rule. For example, under New York law, medical examiner autopsy reports are available only to the district attorney, the family, or a person with a court order *(29)*. Hospital records are usually considered confidential, and hospital autopsy reports are part of the hospital record. In the absence of a statute that explicitly states that hospital records are public records, the pathologist wishing to avoid uncharted legal waters will probably opt to treat the hospital autopsy report as confidential. Like ordinary hospital records, hospital autopsy reports are discoverable by subpoena.

Diagnoses or opinions concerning autopsy findings are often sought by private insurance carriers. Generally, such information should be released to outside parties only after a signed authorization has been obtained from the person who had custody of the body and gave permission for the autopsy, or in response to a subpoena. However, if the autopsy was performed pursuant to statute in a state with a "sunshine" public records law, the autopsy report is considered a public record unless it concerns an active criminal investigation or if related exceptions apply *(30)*.

THE FAMILY The foremost reason for families to authorize autopsies is their desire to have the findings explained to them, either in an interview or in writing. Recommendations for such interviews have been described in detail in Chapter 1. As stated, care must be taken that the findings are disclosed primarily to the person who had custody of the body and therefore, interviews should be conducted in person rather than by phone. With consent from the custodian of the body, an interview may be held with a friend of the family or their clergyman. Letters with autopsy findings must be addressed to the person who consented to the autopsy.

Medical examiners and coroners sometimes receive requests from the spouse or next-of-kin to do an autopsy because of some suspicion of malpractice and the fear that the hospital pathologist might not render an independent opinion. An example would be a request to do an autopsy to determine if a decedent received an overdose of a particular drug two weeks prior to death. Although the autopsy may not answer the posed question, its performance may let the requestors feel that they received information concerning medical care.

Statutory autopsies also may be explained to relatives of the deceased. If such autopsies involve criminal cases, the prosecuting attorney or lead detective should be consulted first. Interviews concerning autopsies in criminal cases should usually be limited to the cause-of-death opinion as it appears on the death certificate. In suicide or accident cases it seems humane not to elaborate on suffering that the deceased may have endured. In homicide cases, that opinion is best reserved for trial, because testimony about pain and suffering may affect the penalty.

THE FUNERAL DIRECTOR

STORAGE OF BODIES Decomposition resulting from failure of a refrigeration unit has been asserted as the basis of violation of sepulcher *(31)*. However, the most common reasons for a body to decompose while lying in a refrigerated storage room are obesity and sepsis, each of which promotes decomposition. Subcutaneous fat insulates the viscera and blood from the ambient temperature. In sepsis, bacteria are already resident in the blood and need not propagate from the bowel. To mitigate liability the autopsy report should document decomposition and sepsis if present.

RELEASE OF BODIES TO FUNERAL DIRECTORS In order to reduce liability for releasing the body to the wrong claimant, a hospital, medical examiner, or coroner should require the funeral director to present a signed release from the person authorized to claim the remains that also names the funeral director as the representative who will take the body. In general, it seems prudent to delay a nonstatutory autopsy whenever more than one party seeks to claim the body and a risk of litigation exists. In the author's experience, such custody issues usually sort themselves out with time. Commonly, the claimant with the best legal claim lacks funds to bury the body and yields to a claimant with lower priority but greater financial resources.

EMBALMING In the United States, embalming is widely practiced. An important exception involves the burial practices of Orthodox Judaism, which forbids embalming. Embalming may be required by some states in certain circumstances. For example, in Minnesota, embalming is required unless the person dead of a noncommunicable disease is buried within 72 hours after death.

Embalming consists of arterial infusion of embalming fluid and trocar perforation of viscera. In bodies without extensive postmortem clotting, the arterial infusion is typically through a right subclavian skin incision, with access to the right common carotid artery after division of the sternocleidomastoid muscle. If a body does not perfuse well, the brachial arteries may be accessed through axillary incisions, or the femoral arteries may be accessed through incisions below the inguinal ligaments. After autopsy, the aortic arch vessels and external iliac arteries are accessed directly.

In the second stage of embalming, a trocar is used to perforate the left side of the abdomen, and then to aspirate any liquids from the chest, abdomen and pelvis, followed by infusion of concentrated embalming fluid. Arterial embalming fluid has a large concentration of methanol, formalin, and orange dye. Trocar work is not necessary after autopsy.

AUTOPSY TECHNIQUES AND THE WORK OF THE FUNERAL DIRECTOR In order to maintain good professional relationships, extended autopsy procedures should be discussed with the funeral director first, and every effort should be made to avoid interfering with the embalming. Funeral directors who understand and support the objectives of the autopsy may be expected to make their skills available when defects from extended autopsies must be reconstructed or when an occasional technical mishap must be repaired. Such goodwill requires that prosectors help the funeral director by identifying the vessels needed for arterial embalming. This can be accomplished by placing clearly visible ligatures around the carotid, axillary, and femoral arteries. If it is necessary to remove these arteries for examination or if there is a risk that they might be damaged during dissection on an extremity, the dissection procedure should be done in the funeral home after embalming. Proper procedures for removal of the brain, dissection at the base of the skull, and removal of the eyes are described in Chapters 4 and 5. It is obvious that technical mishaps in the head area are particularly distressing.

In areas with vigorous organ and tissue procurement agencies, complaints by funeral directors related to autopsies generally are limited to genuine grievances. Preparing a body for viewing after harvesting of long bones is considered more challenging than preparing a body that has been autopsied.

TRANSPORTATION OF BODIES Autopsy pathologists should be familiar with the laws concerning the transportation of bodies in or from their state by motor vehicle, aircraft, or other means. In some states remains must be embalmed if they are shipped by public transport *(32),* but others have no such requirement. Depending on the state, the business of transporting dead bodies may be regulated by the health department, transporters may be required to have funeral director's licenses, and a death certificate or a burial-transit permit may be required for transportation to the site of disposition.

If a body is to be shipped out of the country, the pathologist is often asked by the funeral director to supply a letter stating that the autopsy showed no evidence of any infectious or communicable diseases. The letter should have enough identifying information such as name and date of death to match it to a death certificate or transit permit, but need not offer any cause-of-death opinion. The following letter represents a useful sample.

"To Whom It May Concern:

[Name of deceased] died on [month, day year]. The autopsy revealed no evidence of any communicable or infectious disease. The remains may be transported out of the country.

[Name of physician], MD"

State regulations concerning embalming, caskets, containers, transportation, and disinterment vary. These regulations are usually the province of the funeral director.

Final disposition of the body is by burial, cremation, and uncommonly, burial at sea or donation for anatomic dissection. Removal of a body from the state is considered a form of disposition for the purposes of the death certificate. The bone fragments left after cremation are ground into small pieces to help perpetuate the illusion of ashes; this material, known as cremains, is not subject to state rules pertaining to disposition of human bodies. However, some municipalities have enacted ordinances to regulate and reduce the numbers of bone fragments strewn from airplanes, bridges and watercraft.

EXHUMATION Exhumation requests most often come from surviving relatives who want to move the remains to a more favored burial site, or who want to cremate long-buried remains. If other relatives do not object, disinterment is easily accomplished. In the case of a dispute over whether to exhume and re-inter, legal tradition has established a presumption against disturbing the repose of the dead *(5).* In criminal investigations exhumation is unusual, and in the absence of permission from the surviving spouse or next-of-kin it usually requires a court order. Such an order must be based on the reasonable expectation that the examination will yield important evidence for the prosecution or defense of a criminal charge. In areas with competent medicolegal systems, the majority of such exhumations will be for suspected poisoning. A policy of retaining toxicology specimens on all deaths that come under medical examiner jurisdiction can help reduce the number of exhumations.

In areas with low rates of medicolegal autopsies, exhumation may be for the purpose of performing a primary autopsy to detect a homicide that may have been masquerading as an accident or a suicide. Or, exhumation may be to complete an autopsy, identify the deceased, develop evidence in a medical malpractice case, or search for lost objects. Autopsies on exhumed bodies may be done both in criminal and in civil court cases.

State laws define who may authorize disinterment and under what circumstances this may be done. If the exhumation is pursuant to court order, the prosecuting attorney or civil attorney with the interest in the exhumation will draw up the order and make application to a court. If the judge approves, he merely signs the order prepared by the attorney. The interested parties, including the pathologist, will normally be informed about the date, time, and other particulars before the order is signed. After the autopsy, the remains are re-interred, the pathologist prepares a report, and makes copies as he would for a routine autopsy.

The principal participants in the exhumation are the petitioner, the cemetery director, the funeral director, and the pathologist. For the pathologist, the procedures differ little from any other autopsy. The pathologist's assistant usually removes the body from the casket, undresses it, and may redress it after the autopsy. The funeral director arranges with the cemetery director for the timely arrival of the equipment operators.

REFERENCES

1. Crocker v. Pleasant. 778 So. 2nd 978 (Fla 2001)
2. Emeagwali v. Brooklyn Hosp. Center, 11 Misc. 3d 1055(A), 2006 WL 435813, at *7 (N.Y. Sup. 2006).
3. Whack v. St. Mary's Hospital of Brooklyn, N.Y. City Civ. Ct. 2003, not reported in N.Y.S. 2d, 2003 WL, 230702.
4. Klaiman MH. Whose brain is it anyway? The comparative law of post-mortem organ retention. J Legal Med 2005;26:475–490.
5. Maffei v. Woodlawn Memorial Park (2005) June 10 CA1/1 A105260
6. Uniform Anatomical Gift Act of 1987, drafted by the National Conference of Commissioners on Uniform State Laws. http://www.law.upenn.edu/bll/ulc/fnact99/uaga87.htm.
7. Shemonsky NK, Reiber KB, Williams LD and Froede RC. Jurisdiction on military installations. Am J Forensic Med Pathol 1993;14:39–42.
8. 18 USC 1751.
9. 18 USC 351.
10. 18 USC 1116.
11. Mittleman RE, Davis JH, Kasztl W, Graves WM Jr. Practical approach to investigative ethics and religious objections to the autopsy. J Forensic Sci 1992;37:824–829.
12. Section 27491.43, California Government Code.
13. Section 42:17B-88.2, New Jersey Statutes Annotated.
14. Section 4210-C, New York Public Health Law.
15. Section 313.131, Ohio Revised Code.
16. Section 23-4-4-4.1, Rhode Island General Laws.
17. Section 5-310(b)(2), Maryland Health Codes.
18. CAP documents pertaining to the autopsy. In: Collins KA, Hutchins GM, eds. Autopsy Performance & Reporting, 2nd ed. College of American Pathologists, Northfield, IL, 2003, p. 39.
19. Section 872.04, Florida Statutes.
20. 22A Am Jur 2d, §86
21. Section 872.04, Florida Statutes.
22. Section 820 ILCS 310l, Illinois Compiled Statutes.
23. Section 627.615, Florida Statutes.
24. 22A Am Jur 2d, §64.
25. http://www.oregon.gov/MortCem/Compliance_Issues_Related/Autopsy.pdf
26. 22A Am Jur 2d, §152.
27. Brotherton v. Cleveland, 923 F. 2d 477 (6th Cir. 1991) (Ohio)
28. Albrecht v. Treon, 118 Ohio St.3d 348, 2008-Ohio-2617.
29. Section 677.3(b), New York County Law.
30. Chapter 119, Florida Statutes
31. Whack v. St. Mary's Hospital of Brooklyn, N.Y. City Civ. Ct. 2003, not reported in N.Y.S. 2d, 2003 WL, 230702.
32. Section 149A.93, Subd 9, Minnesota Statutes 2005.

15 Fixation and Transport of Autopsy Material

Brenda L. Waters

GENERAL CONSIDERATIONS

Several factors inherent in autopsy pathology conspire to prevent or diminish good tissue preservation. There is the delay in starting the dissection, which may be hours to several days in duration. In many instances, the body will remain unrefrigerated on the clinical floor during part of that delay. Autolysis is further hastened in obese patients because of decreased dissipation of body heat. Second, the autopsy procedure takes several hours and is often conducted under bright lights, providing a setting for continued autolysis. Third, the large amount of blood accompanying the organs can significantly reduce the efficacy of fixatives and finally, adequate fixation, using a fixative-to-tissue ratio as low as 5–10 to 1 still requires large containers and prohibitively large quantities of fixative.

Some of the factors mentioned above are beyond the control of the pathology department. Nevertheless, there are steps that can be taken to maximize preservation of autopsy material. When the organ block is removed from the body cavity, it should be thoroughly washed of blood, using cool or cold water. Hot water should never be used. This rinsing step will maximize the efficacy of the fixative and minimize the blood staining of organs, thereby providing more accurate representation of the specimens for description and photography. If a lesion is encountered in the initial stages of the dissection, such as hepatic cirrhosis or tumor, a section of the abnormality should be obtained early and placed in fixative before the organ is fully incised.

In our laboratory, we routinely retain the lungs, heart, neck block, esophagus, stomach, duodenum, pancreas, adrenals, urinary tract, and genital tract in their entirety, along with representative sections of liver and intestine. These are placed in a large enameled pot containing about 2 gallons (7.57 liters) of 10% formalin. If the organs are adequately rinsed of blood prior to immersion, quite good fixation will result.

FIXATIVES

For routine purposes, excellent fixation can be achieved with all the mixtures listed below. The choice depends on availability, cost, technical help, and environmental concerns. The ideal ratio of fixative-to-volume of tissue is about 15–20 to 1. This ratio is not achievable for primary fixation of the organs, but it can be attained when submitting sections for histological analysis. Regardless of the type of fixative used, the tissues should not be pressed against each other or the bottom or walls of the container. Some laboratories may find it advantageous to use refrigerated fixative, to slow down autolysis while the fixative is penetrating the tissue.

FORMALIN Formalin remains the mainstay for preservation of routine autopsy material. It is inexpensive, easy to make, penetrates readily and may be used for preservation of tissues without loss of cytologic detail. However, gross specimens after long periods of storage in formalin tend to fade in color and become homogeneously grey-tan. It is thought that formalin, like other aldehydes, forms methyl cross-links between the side chains of amino acids, thereby retaining the cellular constituents in their in vivo configuration. It has a rate of penetration of 10 mm/hour. Although formalin is not the ideal fixative for the preservation of carbohydrates, its preservative effects on proteins tend to trap the glycogen and thus prevent it from leaching from the tissue. It is also quite suitable for *in situ* hybridization and immunohistochemical methods. It is a good fixative for complex lipids, but has no effect on neutral fats *(1)*. Some laboratories use a 15% concentration for the fixation of whole brains. It should be noted that formalin-fixed tissue should not be frozen, since, during thawing, the tissue cannot absorb water and thus, extracellular ice crystals persist and severely interfere with subsequent microscopic study *(2)*. With very prolonged storage, formalin acidifies as it oxidizes to formic acid. This reduces its preservative properties. When the solution becomes acidic, formalin will precipitate out as formalin-hematin pigment. This pigment will appear as shard-like, variably sized black to brown, refractile particles within cells, especially macrophages. It needs to be distinguished from bacteria and from anthracotic and dust pigment in macrophages. Especially congested organs, such as spleen and liver, tend to promote precipitation of formalin-hematin. For this reason, unbuffered solutions of formalin should be avoided and washing of the organs prior to immersion is emphasized.

Formalin is irritating to the eyes, the upper respiratory tract as well as the skin. It should be used in well-ventilated areas and formalin-fixed tissues should be handled with gloves.

From: *Handbook of Autopsy Practice,* 4th Ed. Edited by: B.L. Waters

A 10% buffered formalin solution, the formulation most frequently used, is equivalent to 4% formaldehyde. It may be prepared by adding 100 ml of 40% formaldehyde to 900 ml of water with 4 g sodium phosphate, monobasic and 6.5 g sodium phosphate, dibasic (anhydrous). Formalin is also supplied as a concentrated neutral buffered solution (Richard-Allan Scientific, Kalamazoo, MI), from which a 10% solution is made up by simply adding 4 gallons of tap water to 1 gallon of the concentrated solution. Frozen sections with formalin-fixed tissue may be done, although the tissue may not stick reliably to the glass slide. Formalin may be stored at room temperature.

GLUTARALDEHYDE Like formaldehyde, glutaraldehyde (glutaric dialdehyde) fixes tissue by forming methyl cross-links between proteins. It actually has a greater potential for forming the crosslinks, since the molecule has more sites that can participate in the crosslinking reaction than does formaldehyde. It produces less irritating fumes than formalin and yields excellent cytological detail with increased dye uptake. Connective tissue stains are well differentiated and sectioning artifacts are less frequent. Glutaraldehyde does inhibit the activity of catalase, thus making it a good fixative for the demonstration of the peroxidase activity in peroxisomes *(3)*. It remains an excellent fixative for electron microscopy and is quite suitable for most histochemical methods. The disadvantages are its slow penetration into tissue (2–3 mm/hr), higher cost and its requirement for refrigerated storage.

1. Composition. This preparation results in a 2% glutaraldehyde solution: 50 mL purified 25% glutaraldehyde, 575 mL Sorenson's phosphate buffer 0.1 M, pH 7.4 (Electron Microscopy Sciences, Hatfield, PA).
2. To make Sorenson's phosphate buffer 0.1 M, pH 7.4: Mix 40.5 ml of 0.2 M dibasic sodium phosphate and 9.5 ml of 0.2 M monobasic sodium phosphate.
3. Procedure. Fix slices no thicker than 2 mm in 20 volumes of glutaraldehyde solution. The fixation time at room temperature will be 6–24 h. Cold fixation with glutaraldehyde yields complete fixation after 6 h but only in the outer 1 mm of tissue.
4. Storage. Store at 4°C.

ABSOLUTE ETHANOL This solution accomplishes fixation by disrupting the hydrophobic bonds that maintain the tertiary structure of proteins. Ethanol fixation causes less denaturation than other fixatives and so it has good applicability to immunofluorescent technologies. This fixative penetrates tissue relatively quickly and is indicated when preservation of water-soluble compounds, such as urates, glycogen, sulfhydryl groups of protein, and water-soluble pigments, is required. One must remember that if alcohol is used to fix water-soluble substances, no aqueous staining procedures can be employed. Prolonged storage of tissue in absolute alcohol will result in removal of histones from the nuclei as well as RNA and DNA. An advantage of ethanol is that its fumes are far less noxious than those of formalin. However, it is more expensive. Absolute ethanol's major role lies in fixation of small portions of tissue for specific histochemical or immunofluorescent assays.

1. Fix slices, no thicker than 5 mm, in 20 volumes of absolute alcohol. The fixation time will be about 4 h.
2. Transfer to 70% ethyl alcohol for another 72 h. For enzyme studies and for demonstration of urates, 70% alcohol should not be used, but instead use two additional treatments (12 h each) with absolute ethyl alcohol.
3. Fixed tissue should be stored in 70% alcohol.

CARNOY'S FIXATIVE Carnoy's is an alcohol-containing fixative with a very rapid rate of action. Thin sections may be fixed in minutes, rather than hours. It preserves organelles rich in nucleic acids especially well, along with protein sulfhydryl groups and glycogen. When beginning the staining procedure, it is important to transfer the tissue directly to absolute alcohol since dehydration has already been initiated. Moreover, delicate tissues taken from an aqueous solution may be damaged when transferred to this fixative, since the strong hydrophobicity of the chloroform will cause rapid tissue dehydration.

1. Composition: 60 mL absolute ethanol, 30 mL chloroform, 10 mL glacial acetic acid. Prepare fixative just befor use and use only glassware since this solution can dissolve some plastics. An older formulation, known as Clark's solution, contains only a 3:1 ratio of absolute alcohol and glacial acetic acid. It is claimed to work just as well, if not better than Carnoy's.
2. Slices up to 1.5 cm in thickness can be fixed. After one hour of fixation, the tissue may be transferred to absolute alcohol.

BOUIN'S FIXATIVE Picric acid-containing fixatives penetrate well and, in combination with other ingredients, leave tissue relatively soft. Bouin's solution is useful for the demonstration of glycogen, but does cause significant tissue shrinkage. It is an excellent fixative for trichrome staining and for the demonstration of edema fluid. It lyses erythrocytes and lends a yellow color to the tissues. The yellow discoloration may be removed by rinsing with aqueous solutions (50% or 70%) of alcohol. Tissue should not be stored in Bouin's since there will be continual loss of cellular basophilia. Bouin's is quite amenable to immunohistochemical studies (*see* below).

1. Composition: 75 mL saturated aqueous picric acid, 25 mL 40% formaldehyde solution, 5 ml glacial acetic acid.
2. To prepare saturated aqueous picric acid solution, combine 2 g picric acid (trinitrophenol, USP) and 100 mL distilled water. Heat until picric acid dissolves. Cool and decant the supernate.
3. Fix slices no thicker than 3–5 mm. If the tissue is very soft, thin slices can be cut from larger pieces after about 2 hours of fixation. Complete fixation will take up to 18 hours. Transfer tissue to 50% ethyl alcohol for another 6–24 h. The alcohol should be changed when it becomes yellow.
4. Fixed tissue should be stored in 70% alcohol.
5. Picric acid, if not well saturated with water, will explode. Thus, it should be stored with an overlay of water.

HOLLANDE'S The addition of copper acetate distinguishes Hollande's from Bouin's fixative. Hollande's serves as a primary fixative for GI and prostate biopsies. It provides bright staining with hematoxylin and eosin and it leaves the tissue more resistant to cracking. The copper acetate tends to stabilize red cell membranes as well as granules within eosinophils and endocrine cells. Because Hollande's will form a blue phosphate precipitate when exposed to phosphate buffered formalin, tissues primarily fixed in Hollande's must be washed prior to exposure to formalin. The glacial acetic acid provides a mild decalcifying effect.

1. Composition: 25 g copper acetate, 1000 ml distilled water, 40 gm picric acid, 100 ml formalin, 15 ml glacial acetic acid.
2. To prepare: Dissolve copper acetate in water without heat. Add picric acid slowly, stirring until dissolved. Add formalin and acetic acid.
3. When fixation is complete, the tissue should be retained in 70% alcohol.

ZAMBONI'S SOLUTION Zamboni's is a general purpose fixative. It allows secondary fixation with osmium, making it suitable as a primary fixative for electron microscopy.

1. Composition. Stock solution: 20.0 g paraformaldehyde, 150 mL saturated aqueous (double filtered) picric acid.
2. Heat solution to 60°C. After the paraformaldehyde is dissolved, add drops of 2.5% aqueous sodium hydroxide to render the solution alkaline. Filter solution and allow to cool.
3. Add phosphate buffer to solution to make 1,000 mL. Composition of phosphate buffer: 3.32 g monobasic sodium phosphate ($NaH_2PO_4 \cdot H_2O$), 17.88 g dibasic anhydrous sodium phosphate (Na_2HPO_4), 1,000 mL distilled water. If the final pH is not 7.3, the value must be adjusted.
4. Store at room temperature.

FIXATIVES FOR HEMATOPOIETIC TISSUES The mercuric chloride-containing fixatives, namely B-5, Helley's, and Zenker's solution will not be addressed in this edition, given their unacceptable levels of toxicity to the environment. An excellent fixative for hematopoietic tissue and lymph nodes is B-Plus™ manufactured by BBC Biochemical (Stanwood, WA). This fixative contains no mercury and has a long shelf life. It is also quite suitable for tissues intended for study using immunochemical methods. Small biopsies should be fixed for at least 2 hours. Larger blocks of tissue will require 3 to 12 hours. The sections may be processed using the same staining schedule that is routinely used for formalin-fixed tissues.

FIXATIVES THAT HIGHLIGHT SPECIFIC ORGANELLES

Orth's Solution This fixative is most suitable for the demonstration of chromaffin granules in adrenal medulla and pheochromocytoma.

1. Composition: 2.5 g potassium dichromate ($K_2Cr_2O_7$), 1.0 g sodium sulfate (Na_2SO_4), 100 mL distilled water. Just before use, add 10 mL concentrated formalin.
2. Procedure. Immerse slices no thicker than 4 mm in 20 volumes of fixative. The fixation time will be about 24–48 h. Wash in running water for 24 h. Transfer to 70% ethyl alcohol.
3. Store fixed tissue in 70% alcohol.

Regaud's Fixative This fixative is useful for the demonstration of rickettsiae and mitochondria.

1. Composition: 80 mL potassium dichromate ($K_2Cr_2O_7$), 20 mL of 3% aqueous solution formalin.
2. Procedure. Fix slices no thicker than 4 mm in 20 volumes of fixative. The fixation time will be 24–48 h. Wash in running water for 24 h. Transfer to 70% ethanol.
3. Store fixed tissue in 70% ethanol.

FIXATION BY MMICROWAVE IRRADIATION In conventional, domestic microwave ovens, microwaves are generated by a magnetron, which uses electricity and magnetism to produce an alternating electric field. When exposed to this radiation, dipolar molecules, such as water and polar side chains of proteins, oscillate through 180° at a rate of 2.5 billion cycles per second. This results in very rapid heating and fixation of the tissue. Optimal fixation with minimal artifact occurs when the temperature of the tissue in normal saline reaches 70° and 85° C. This technique has been used successfully for both light and electron microscopy *(4,5,6,7)*. For electron microscopy, samples should be placed in 2.5% glutaraldehyde and irradiated for 90 s to achieve a temperature of 58°C.

FIXATION FOR ELECTRON MICROSCOPY Karnovsky's glutaraldehyde/formaldehyde fixative combines the rapid fixation properties of formaldehyde with the slower, but permanent fixative properties of glutaraldehyde. It is very good for preservation of cellular ultrastructure when harsh treatments are anticipated, such as those encountered with transmission electron microscopy. Fresh tissue specimens should be less than 0.3 cm in diameter and be fixed within 15 minutes of removal from the patient. The volume of the solution should be at least 10 times that of the volume of the specimen. At least 3 hours of refridgerated fixation is best, but overnight fixation will not adversely affect the specimen.

1. Combine 11.6 gm sodium phosphate monobasic and 2.7 gm sodium hydroxide in 100 ml of 40% formaldehyde in a 250 ml Erlenmeyer flask. Add 20 ml 50% glutaraldehyde to the mixture and swirl to dissolve solids as much as possible.
2. Pour 880 ml of distilled water into a 1000 ml Erlenmeyer flask into which has been placed a magnetic stir bar. Reserve the rest of the water.
3. Pour the glutaraldehyde/formaldehyde mixture into the 1000 ml flask using the reserved water to rinse out the 250 ml flask repeatedly until all solids and liquid have been transferred completely to the large flask. Place flask on magnetic stirrer and stir until all solids have been dissolved.

4. Pour solution into a clean, plastic bottle. Store at 4 degrees C.
5. Karnovskys' fixative is stable for six months only when refrigerated. At room temperature, shelf life is one to two weeks.

For comprehensive discussions of fixatives in electron microscopy, see refs. *(9)* and *(10)*.

If no tissue was initially fixed for electron microscopy, tissue from the exposed surfaces of formalin-fixed tissue can be obtained and postfixed prior to processing. The same can be done with tissue from paraffin blocks after deparaffinization. Obviously, the quality of the electron micrographs suffers considerably under these circumstances, but, depending on the questions at hand, answers still can be obtained in some instances.

HISTOCHEMISTRY Most histochemical stains are readily applicable to autopsy tissues that were obtained after the usual postmortem intervals and were fixed in formalin solution. If new histochemical applications are used on postmortem material, pilot experiments will need to be carried out to determine their efficacy.

IMMUNOHISTOCHEMISTRY Tissue samples should be obtained as soon as possible after death and placed in formalin or Bouin's solution. The sections should be thin enough to permit rapid penetration of the fixative. If formalin is used, the sections should be processed after 12–18 h and if Bouin's solution is used, after 4–6 h. If the tissue sample is thick, a thin slice should be obtained from the exposed tissue surface after the recommended fixation time. If antigens need to be identified that are sensitive to the chemical action of fixatives or if immunofluorescent staining is intended, snap-freezing is the method of choice *(11)*. Other related analytical methods are presented in Chapter 8.

***IN SITU* HYBRIDIZATION** Buffered formalin, pH 7.0, serves as an excellent fixative for this technology. Fixatives with picric acid (Bouin's) may interfere with subsequent *in situ* hybridization. Paraffin-embedded tissue is quite suitable for many commercially available DNA probes.

X-RAY MICROANALYSIS (ENERGY-DISPERSIVE X-RAY MICROANALYSIS) Conventional transmission or scanning electron microscopes are also able to identify elements such as copper, iron, sulfur, or thorium *(11)* (elements 5–99 can be identified in this fashion). It is best to use glutaraldehyde-fixed tissue but formalin-fixed tissue can also be used, including, as a last resort, tissue from paraffin blocks, or tissues lifted from hematoxylin-eosin stained slides. For further applications, see ref. *(12)*.

AUTORADIOGRAPHY Postmortem material can be used for the identification and localization of radioactive material. Autolytic changes and choice of fixative have little effect on the quality of the autoradiograms. The demonstration of thorium dioxide contrast medium (Thorotrast) used to be the main application of this method. Presently, electron micrography with energy-dispersive X-ray microanalysis (*see* above) is a faster and more specific method. For the preparation of autoradiograms, the reader is referred to appropriate textbooks.

DECALCIFICATION PROCEDURES These procedures are described in Chapter 2, under Skeletal System.

SHIPPING OF AUTOPSY MATERIAL

Several agencies regulate the shipment of biological material. The agencies having the most stringent regulations are the International Air Transportation Association (IATA) and the International Civil Aviation Organization (ICAO). IATA regulations are followed by most of the major airlines and air carriers, including FedEx. The IATA is not an enforcement agency, however. Enforcement is under the jurisdiction of the Federal Aviation Administration (FAA) through the Department of Transportation (DOT). The shipper is responsible for all shipments until they arrive at their destinations. Anyone who prepares biological specimens for shipment must be trained every 24 months in the latest changes of the IATA Dangerous Goods Regulations. These rules are under continuous revision and the updated versions are published every January. Violation of these regulations could result in a civil penalty of up to $27,500 per offense and criminal prosecution.

The IATA groups specimens into five categories, A through E. Any biological material obtained during an autopsy would come under the rules pertaining to Category A or B. Category A infectious substances are defined as those which, when exposure to them occurs, are capable of causing permanent disability or life-threatening or fatal disease in humans or animals. These substances are assigned the number UN 2814. Category B infectious substances do not meet the criteria for inclusion in Category A. Category B material would include blood, tissue and body fluids that are being transported for purposes of research, diagnosis or disease treatment or prevention. These substances are assigned the number UN 3373. Specimens that have been treated such that the suspected pathogens have been neutralized or deactivated so that they no longer pose a health risk are not included under Category B.

Assiduous attention must be paid to proper labeling of all specimens destined for shipment. Each type of specimen requires a specific numerical designation. The details of proper labeling of the containers will not be discussed here, since the regulations are in continuous flux. The reader is advised to consult the IATA directly and to assign specific personnel in the pathology laboratory to be trained in the current regulations.

Both Category A and B specimens are shipped using the triple package system. The inner package (i.e. the primary receptacle) must be made of leak-proof glass or plastic vial, preferably with the lid taped in place. Absorbent material must be placed around the primary receptacle. The absorbent material should be of sufficient volume to take up all liquid in case the primary receptacle breaks or leaks. The absorbent material is also useful for cushioning the inner container. The primary receptacle and absorbent wrap are then placed in a second leak-proof container. Solid specimens do not require the placement of absorbent material between the primary and secondary containers. The outer packaging must be made of fiberboard, wood, metal, or rigid plastic. An itemized list of contents must be enclosed between the secondary and outer containers. The minimum package size is 4 in. If the container is smaller than this, an overwrap (plastic clinical wrap) must be used. Tissue samples that have been fixed must also be shipped using the triple packaging system. A minimum amount of fixative should be used so as to reduce the extent of any leakage.

Both Category A and B specimens must be accompanied by three forms during shipment. They are (1) a Reference Laboratory Requisition form (every reference lab has its own form), (2) a Shipper's Declaration for Dangerous Goods form, and (3) a Fed Ex USA Air Bill form.

Generally, tissue for toxicologic, biochemical or molecular testing must be shipped frozen. Dry ice will be effective for about 24 h. The dry ice should completely surround the specimen. The mailing container should be well insulated, such as with styrofoam. Durable shipping cartons, wooden boxes, or metal containers may be used as mailing containers. Affixed to the outside of the container should be a Dry Ice Sticker, which will indicate the amount of dry ice that is in the package.

Readers are again implored to consult their Environmental Safety Office for the latest regulations.

SHIPPING BLOCKS AND SLIDES Paraffin blocks previously subjected to microtomy may be sealed with paraffin to prevent the tissue from drying out. The blocks can then be wrapped in paper or plastic, but cotton or gauze should not be used because cotton fibers may stick to the paraffin and cause knife lines and abrasions. Glass slides should be shipped in unbreakable slide containers cushioned with cotton, gauze or other material. Padded envelopes are suitable for shipping both blocks and slides. The envelopes should be sealed with tape rather than staples, since the latter may injure personnel in the receiving laboratory.

PROVIDING SUFFICIENT CLINICAL INFORMATION Each shipment of autopsy material must be accompanied by enough clinical information so that the recipient of the material can proceed with the requested testing with minimal delay. This information should be placed in a water-resistant envelope, if necessary, and include: (1) name and address of the submitter, (2) name and address of receiver of the shipment, (3) name, medical record number, and autopsy number of the patient from whom the material came, (4) type of specimen sent, (5) name of examination requested, and (6) any pertinent clinical data. Telephoning the receiving laboratory at the time of shipment may facilitate proper and timely handling of the specimen upon arrival.

SHIPPING AND LABELING FOR MEDICOLEGAL MATERIAL (BY DR. VERNARD I. ADAMS) Medicolegal material is sent by messenger, registered mail, or air express. The receipt provided by such couriers is sufficient to document that the chain of custody remained uninterrupted (*see* Chapter 13). Medicolegal material will often be passed through local police authorities to the state bureau of criminal identification or investigation laboratory.

Specimen labels should contain: (1) name and address of the submitter, (2) name and address of the receiver of the shipment, (3) description of the container and the source and nature of its contents, (4) a tag describing the shipment as "evidence," and (5) if applicable, a request for specific examination.

Containers with medicolegal material should be sealed with evidence tape before shipping, so that any attempts made to open the package will be evident. The most convenient source of evidence tape for those who use it infrequently is a local law enforcement agency.

SHIPPING BLOOD AND TISSUE FOR CARBON MONOXIDE DETERMINATION For blood, a standard gray-top vacuum-collection tube (those containing fluoride-oxalate preservative) is optimal. Tissues can be packed in plastic and shipped in dry ice in an insulated mailing container.

REFERENCES

1. Prophet EB, Mills B, Arrington JB, Sobin LH, eds. Laboratory Methods in Histotechnology. Armed Forces Institute of Pathology. American Registry of Pathology, Washington, DC, 1992.
2. Rosen Y, Ahuja SC. Ice crystal distortion of formalin-fixed tissues following freezing. Am J Surg Pathol 1977;1:179–181.
3. Herzog V, Fahimi HD. The effect of glutaraldehyde on catalase. J Cell Biol 1974;60:303–311.
4. Leong AS, Daymon ME, Milios J. Microwave irradiation as a form of fixation for light and electron microscopy. J Pathol 1985;146: 313–321.
5. Leong AS-Y, Milios J, Duncis CG. Antigen preservation in microwave-irradiated tissues: a comparison with formaldehyde fixation. J Pathol 1988;156:275–282.
6. Leong AS-Y, Duncis CG. A method of rapid fixation of large biopsy specimens using microwave irradiation. Pathology 1986;18:222–225.
7. Leong AS-Y. Microwave fixation and rapid processing in a large throughput histopathology laboratory. Pathology 1991;23:271–273.
8. Baker PB. Electron microscopy. In: Hutchins GM, ed. Autopsy, Performance and Reporting. College of American Pathologists, Northfield, IL, 1990, pp. 138–140.
9. McDowell EM, Trump BF. Histologic fixatives suitable for diagnostic light and electron microscopy. Arch Pathol Lab Med 1976;100:405–414.
10. Robards AW, Wilson AJ (principal eds.). Procedures in Electron Microscopy. Centre for Cell & Tissue Research, The University, York, UK, John Wiley & Sons, New York, 1993.
11. Baker PB. Special autopsy studies. In: Hutchins GM, ed. Autopsy, Performance and Reporting. College of American Pathologists, Northfield, IL, 1990, pp. 142–146.
12. Landas S, Turner JW, Moore KC, Mitros FA. Demonstration of iron and thorium in autopsy tissues by X-ray microanalysis. Arch Pathol Lab Med 1984;108:231–233.
13. Sigee DC, Morgan AJ, Sumner AT, Warley A, eds. X-ray Microanalysis in Biology: Experimental Techniques and Applications. Cambridge University Press, Cambridge, UK, 1993.

16 Museum Techniques

Brenda L. Waters

THE PATHOLOGY MUSEUM

With increasing reliance on digital imaging in medical education, the pathology museum has suffered a decline in importance. Nonetheless, organ demonstrations still hold value for teaching. Autopsy laboratories inevitably receive requests to demonstrate gross anatomy or pathology to students in the allied health sciences and even in the primary and secondary schools. When the autopsy permit allows, these uses of autopsy material should be welcomed. The pathology museum also serves as an important repository for hearts with developmental anomalies. The heart specimens can be used to teach clinicians and pathologists who are interested in congenital heart disease and, therefore, they are a priceless component of any pathology department.

The ultimate use of the teaching specimens will determine the best way to preserve the specimen. For instance, specimens intended for demonstration to primary and secondary school children should be completely enclosed in portable, nonbreakable containers, such as plastic bags, or they may be embedded in plastic or paraffin. On the other hand, fixed and washed specimens are suitable for examination by pathologists-in-training, clinicians and medical students. In this chapter, a few basic techniques for the preservation of autopsy material are discussed. For comprehensive reviews of classic museum techniques, see refs. *(1–3)*.

COLOR-PRESERVING FIXATION MIXTURES

Most formalin-based fixatives turn the natural color of organs into a uniform gray-tan. Fortunately, there are several mixtures that better preserve the original color of the organs. Kaiserling's and Jores' solutions still are used in some institutions. Modifications of the Kaiserling solution have been published by Lundquist *(4)*, Meiller *(5)*, and others. Modifications of Jores' solution exist also *(6)*.

KAISERLING'S SOLUTIONS

1. Composition:
   a. Kaiserling I: 85 g potassium acetate, 45 g potassium nitrate (KNO_3), 4,800 mL formalin solution (3–4%).
   b. Kaiserling II: ethyl alcohol, 80–95%.
   c. Kaiserling III: 200 g potassium acetate, 300 mL glycerin, 900 mL tap water.
2. Procedure. Fix specimen for 1–5 d in Kaiserling I. Fixation time will vary with the thickness of the organ. Excessive fixation with Kaiserling I solution causes loss of natural color. Transfer to Kaiserling II for a few hours. Acid hematin will turn into alkaline hematin, which approximates the color of hemoglobin.
3. Mounting: Use Kaiserling III solution.

MODIFIED KAISERLING'S SOLUTION AFTER LUNDQUIST

This method was developed to avoid the use of alcohol, which tends to stiffen and cause contraction of the specimens *(4)*.

1. Composition:
   a. Kaiserling I: 200 g potassium acetate, 45 g potassium nitrate (KNO_3), 80 g chloral hydrate, 444 mL formalin, 4,000 mL tap water.
   b. Kaiserling III: 10 g potassium acetate, 5 g chloral hydrate, 10 mL glycerin, 90 mL tap water.
2. Procedure: Suspend the specimen in 10–20 times its volume of fluid. Just after the fixation is completed (avoid overfixation), wash thoroughly in running water and retrim so that all cut surfaces are resurfaced. Transfer to mounting solution for 12 h. Replace the mounting solution for permanent mounting.
3. Mounting: Use Kaiserling III solution.

JORES' SOLUTION

1. Composition: 10 g sodium chloride (NaCl), 20 g magnesium sulfate ($MgSO_4$), 20 g sodium sulfate (Na_2SO_4), 1,100 mL formalin solution (2–4%).
2. Procedure: Fix specimen for 1- 2 days. Rinse in 95% ethyl alcohol. Leave in 95% ethyl alcohol for 24 h or until red color has returned.
3. Mounting: Mount specimen in a solution of equal parts glycerin and water.

PRAGUE SOLUTION

1. Composition: 128 g Prague powder*, 25 g erythorbic acid (*L*-ascorbic acid), 10,000 mL distilled water, 1,000 mL con-

*Great American Spice Company, 628 Leesburg

From: *Handbook of Autopsy Practice,* 4th Ed. Edited by: B.L. Waters

centrated formalin, 4,000 mL solution A (*see* below), 4,000 mL solution B (*see* below).

a. Solution A: 47 g sodium phosphate (Na_2HPO_4), 10% formalin solution, to make 5,000 mL.
b. Solution B: 45 g potassium phosphate (K_2HPO_4), 10% formalin solution, to make 5,000 mL. Solutions A and B must be stored in separate containers.

REJUVENATION SOLUTION

1. Composition: 100 g sodium chloride (NaCl), 5 g sodium sulfate (Na_2SO_4), 50 mL glycerin, 1,000 mL tap water.
2. Procedure: Sodium chloride and sodium sulfate are dissolved in the water and the solution is filtered. Then the glycerin is added. Just before the jar containing this solution is resealed, a few drops of alcoholic camphor are added. There will be a temporary cloudiness of the solution. For another rejuvenation fluid, see ref. *(6)*.

REHYDRATION OF MUMMIFIED TISSUES

Rehydrate with modified Ruffer's solution (see ref. *7*): 3 parts ethyl alcohol, 5 parts 2% formalin, and 2 parts aqueous sodium carbonate, 5%.

SPECIMEN CONTAINERS

JARS In the past, thick-walled glass jars epitomized the traditional organ museum. Glass is attractive because it is inert to fixatives and aggressive mounting fluids, such as oil of wintergreen. However, glass jars are heavy and cumbersome to transport. Most importantly, they break easily and thus can cause serious injury. Glass jars may still have a use for those specimens that are intended to remain in the museum.

Containers made of acrylic resins are preferable, since they have excellent optical properties, low weight, minimal breakability, and chemical stability to most mounting fluids. Using acrylic sheets, museum jars can be prepared in many sizes and shapes. The material is easy to cut, machine, and assemble. Fusion of the plates is accomplished with WELD•ON 4™ (IPS Corporation, Compton, CA). Plastics of this type are easily scratched and thus may need to be repolished on occasion. As stated above, oil of wintergreen as well as benzyl benzoate cannot be used as mounting fluid because both solutions dissolve plastics. Alcohol is also not suitable since it crazes the surface of the plastic. Prague solution works well with acrylic containers. Its composition is provided above.

PLASTIC BAGS Although mounting museum specimens in plastic bags is convenient and inexpensive (Figs. 16-1 and 16-2), the method does have its drawbacks. The specimens cannot be palpated and they may not display the abnormalities as clearly as with other methods. Nevertheless, organ slices mounted in this way are quite portable and do generate great interest amongst students in primary and secondary schools.

PARAFFIN EMBEDDING

This method works beautifully for whole heart specimens and results in an attractive and fairly sturdy specimen that may be handled without gloves (Fig. 16-3). This procedure is generously provided by Amy Juraszek M.D. of the Cardiac Registry at Boston Children's Hospital.

1. At autopsy, be sure that the prosector does the following:
   a. Tie off all four brachiocephalic vessels, leaving them as long as possible.
   b. Cut the superior vena cava (SVC) and inferior vena cava (IVC) as far away from the heart as possible. Remove a cuff of diaphragm with the IVC.
   c. Avoid any needle punctures into the heart or great vessels. If a blood culture is required, obtain from the high SVC or IVC, below the diaphragm.

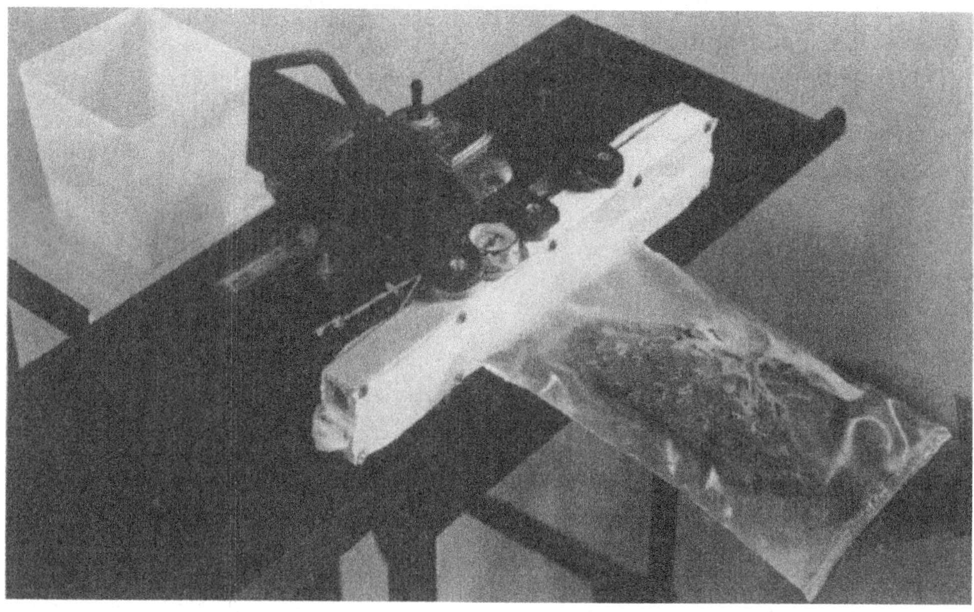

Fig. 16-1. Slices of completely fixed organs may be heat-sealed in plastic bags with a small amount of formalin included.

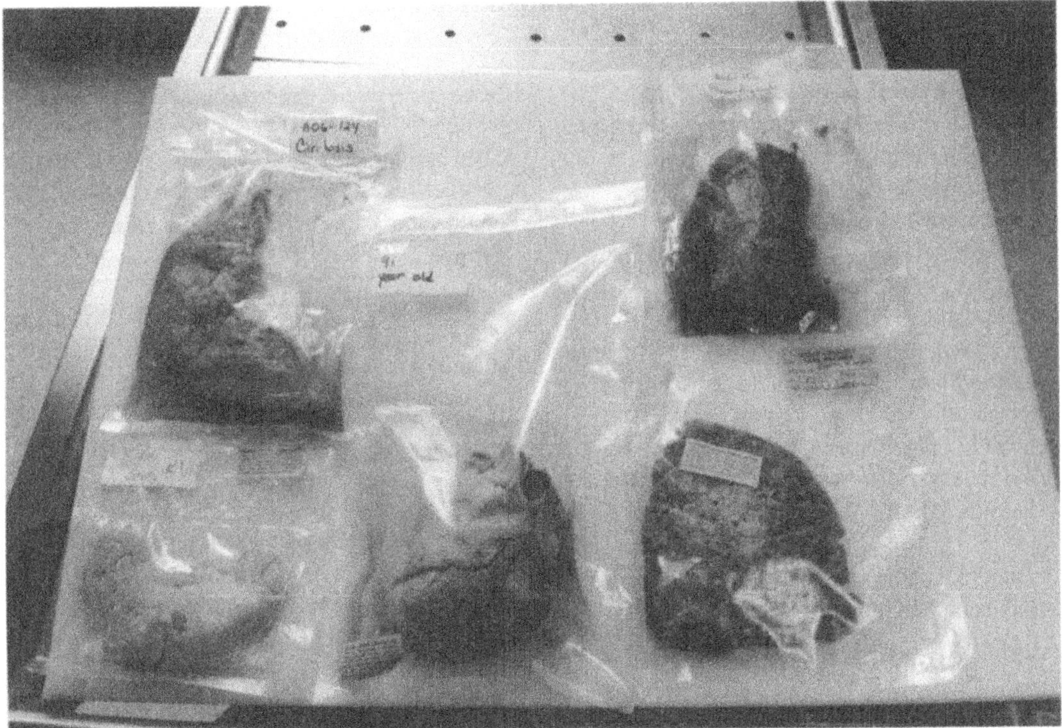

Fig. 16-2. These specimens in plastic bags are easily stored and very portable, making them ideal for teaching purposes outside of the hospital.

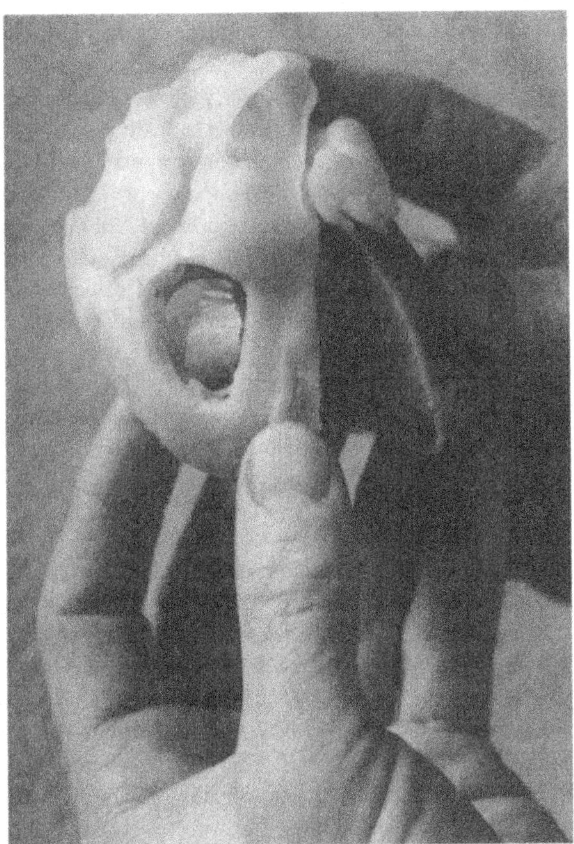

Fig. 16-3. This paraffin-embedded neonatal heart has a window cut in the right ventricle and the free wall of the left ventricle slightly lifted away from the septum. Not pictured are windows cut into the right and left atria.

   d. Cut but do not tie off the descending aorta at level of diaphragm.
   e. Remove heart and lungs en bloc.
2. Tie off and cut each pulmonary artery and pulmonary vein branch as distally as possible and remove the lungs.
3. Place the largest possible cannula in the SVC and tie it in place as high and tightly as possible.
4. Place the largest possible cork in the IVC and tie in place tightly.
5. Before tying off the descending aorta, in hearts with an opening between the atria (eg. foramen ovale or atrial septal defect) perfuse the specimen through the SVC cannula with saline several times until most blood has been washed out. During the saline rinse, small leaks can be located and the vessels tied. For hearts with no inter-atrial continuity, saline perfusion of the left heart must be done via a pulmonary vein.
6. After washing thoroughly, empty the heart of saline and tie off the descending aorta.
7. Perfuse the heart, via a pulmonary vein and/or the SVC with a mixture of formalin and alcohol (1 part 40% formalin and 4 parts 95% alcohol). Be sure that the specimen is completely submerged in a formalin-alcohol solution and that gravity pressure perfusion is maintained for at least two hours. Keep ahead of any leaks for that period of time.
8. Allow the heart to remain in the formalin-alcohol solution for at least 12 hours. Then cut off all ties, remove the cannulas and the cork.
9. Transfer to 80% alcohol – 1 day.
   Transfer to a new bath of 80% alcohol – 1 day.

Transfer to 95% alcohol – 1 day.
Transfer to a new bath of 95% alcohol – 1 day.

10. At this point, limited dissection may be carried out, such as cutting windows into the chambers.
11. After limited dissection:
    Transfer to 100% alcohol – 1 day.
    Transfer to a new bath of 100% alcohol – 1 day.
    Transfer to xylene – 1 day.
    Transfer to a new bath of xylene – 1 day.
12. Remove specimen from xylene and place in a beaker and cover with melted paraffin. Place in a 60°C oven. Change paraffin after 12–24 hours.
13. When the heart no longer smells of xylene, heat the paraffin bath over a bunsen burner. Remove specimen and drain the paraffin from the chambers.
14. Cool.
15. Trim the specimen as needed to best display the anatomy and pathology.

PLASTINATION This method of organ preservation was invented in 1978 by Gunther von Hagens, who published a clear description of the procedure in 1987 *(8)*. The method is widely popularized in Dr. von Hagens' Bodyworld® exhibitions. Four steps are involved. The first is fixation, which generally is done with formalin. The second step is dehydration using freeze substitution, by which the specimen is immersed in cold (–25° C) acetone for days to weeks. The third is called forced impregnation, by which the specimen is placed in a vacuum chamber in a special polymer solution. The vacuum causes the acetone to vaporize and draw the polymer into the cells. Curing, or hardening of the polymer is the last step and is done by exposure to a gas. All the reagents are commercially available at BIODUR™ Products, (Dr. Andrea Whalley, Heidelberg, Germany). The materials used for the plastination procedure vary, depending on the intended end product. Company directions must be followed closely for a good result. The end product is a plastic-embedded specimen that is durable, washable and suitable for handling without gloves, making it most suitable for teaching *(9)*.

INJECTION, CORROSION, AND CLEARING TECHNIQUES

Blood vessels, airways, hollow viscera, and cavities can be injected with a great variety of materials. If injection is combined with corrosion, excellent casts may be prepared. The major disadvantage of these methods is that they leave no tissue available for histologic study.

BARIUM SULFATE MIXTURES These are probably the most widely used reagents to produce radiopaque media for vascular injection. Some dry powder preparations are commercially available (Sigma B-3758, Sigma, St.. Louis, MO). The viscosity of the solution can be reduced by decreasing the amount of gelatin or by adding more water. This solution should fill vessels as small as 30–60 μm in luminal diameter. The actual viscosity of the medium within the vessels depends on the speed of injection and the temperature of the tissues to be injected. Therefore, each laboratory will have to standardize its own techniques. The injection often is done using quite elaborate methods, but injection by hand with a large syringe gives excellent results.

Barium sulfate	*Iothalamate-meglumine*
500 mL distilled water	500 mL distilled water
650 g barium sulfate[a]	OR 100 mL iothalamate meglumine (Conray®30)[b]
15 g gelatin[c]	15 g gelatin[c]
3 g thymol[d]	3 g thymol[d]

[a]Barosperse® Mallinckrodt Inc., Hazelwood, MO

[b]Conray®30 (iothalamate meglumine injection U.S.P. 60[c]) Mallinckrodt Inc.m Hazelwood, MO

[c]Gelatin (laboratory grade, 275 bloom), Thermo Fisher Scientific, Waltham, MA.

[d]Thymol Thermo Fisher Scientific, Waltham, MA.

To prepare, heat the distilled water to about 45°C in a beaker on a magnetic stir plate. Add the gelatin and stir until completely dissolved. Then add the contrast agent (barium sulfate or Conray®30), with thymol as a preservative to retard bacterial or fungal growth. Stir for approx 30 min until the solution is smooth. Divide the mixture into aliquots of 50–60 mL. These may be stored unrefrigerated in capped bottles for up to 1 yr.

In rare instances, staining of the injection fluid may be indicated, for example, for differential display of the right and left coronary artery systems. Barium sulfate can be stained with carmine, Berlin blue, naphthol green, or acridine yellow.

CLINICAL CONTRAST MEDIA These media (e.g., Ethiodol®, Savage Laboratories, Melville, NY) or Sodium Diatrizoate (Sigma-Aldrich, St. Louis, MO) are expensive and cannot be recognized histologically. However, they are readily available in most hospitals and are recommended for pathologists who do injection work only on occasion. Coloring agents can be added to these media for macroscopic and microscopic identification.

INDIA INK This material is used primarily for microscopic study of the microvasculature. The black pigment stands out readily before and after histologic processing. India ink can be mixed with gelatin and water. Thick sections usually are studied.

PLASTICS Excellent casts of vessels and cavities can be prepared with vinyl-acetate plastic mixtures (Sigma-Aldrich, St. Louis, MO), as shown in Fig. 16-4. Some of these have also been made radiopaque.

CORROSION METHODS

Vascular or other casts of plastic or metal can be viewed in roentgenograms or after corrosion of the organ (Fig. 16.4). Concentrated hydrochloric acid or 40% potassium hydroxide is used for this purpose. The duration of the process depends on the size of the specimen and may last several days. An alternative to the use of aggressive chemicals is prolonged cooking, followed by repeated rinsing in a strong jet stream of water. Placing the untreated specimen in an anthill probably gives good results but the logistics and esthetics of such an undertaking are a major obstacle.

CLEARING TECHNIQUES

Clearing techniques demonstrate bones or injected blood vessels without destroying the outline of the surrounding tissue. The clearing medium is benzene or oil of Wintergreen, both of which are skin irritants, have an unpleasant smell, and

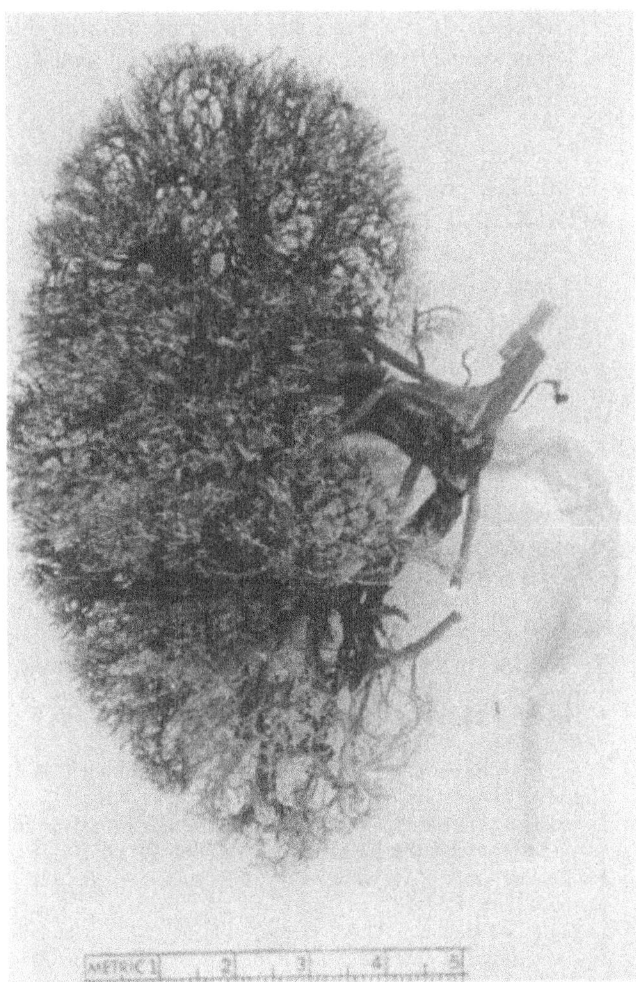

Fig. 16-4. Vinyl plastic cast of a normal kidney. Red, blue, and yellow plastic was used so that, following corrosion, the arteries, veins and collecting system were highlighted in different colors.

dissolve plastic and most sealants. These disadvantages and the availability of computed tomography and related methods have made the techniques *(2,3)* largely obsolete. Only one method shall be described here.

CLEARING METHOD AFTER SPALTEHOLZ

- Fix specimen in 10% formalin or Kaiserling I solution.
- Wash in tap water.
- Dehydrate in changes of 80 and 95% ethyl alcohol for 24 h at each change and in absolute alcohol for 48 h.
- Soak in benzene for 24 h.
- Mount in a glass jar with oil of Wintergreen.
- Seal with the following mixture: Cabinetmakers' glue sticks 80 g; powdered arabic gum 20 g; glycerin 10 g; tap water 150 mL; acetic acid 5 mL; and thymol crystals 0.05 g.

STAINING OF GROSS SPECIMENS AND SELECTED TUMORS

Historically, gross staining of tissues was used to enhance the quality of museum specimens. In current autopsy practice, stained specimens are photographed, shown at a conference, and then stored or discarded.

HEMATOXYLIN OR EOSIN STAINS Tissues such as the intestinal mucosa can be stained with alcoholic eosin or hematoxylin *(9,10,11)*.

FAT AND LIPID STAINS Fat stains are used either as differential tissue stains—for example, to outline malignant lesions infiltrating fat tissue—or to identify fat and lipids in organs or pathologic lesions.

When differential fat staining is desired, the freshly trimmed, fresh or formalin-fixed specimen is immersed in a saturated solution of Sudan III or Scharlach R in 70% alcohol *(12)*. The fat will stain bright red. Non-fatty structures are decolorized by placing the specimen in 95% alcohol. After the differentiation is complete, the tissue is washed and mounted in formalin solution. A variant of this method uses formalin-fixed specimens, which are soaked for 1 d in 50% alcohol, followed by staining for 1 or 2 d in a saturated solution of Sudan III in 70% alcohol. After the fat has become deep orange red, the specimen is returned to 50% alcohol solution until all nonfatty tissues return to their normal color.

STAIN FOR IRON (Hemosiderin) The reaction of Fe^{3+} with ferrocyanide has been used most widely for the demonstration of tissue iron in hemochromatosis and other iron overload states. Slices of liver, pancreas, heart, or other tissues are placed for several minutes in a 1–5% aqueous solution of potassium ferrocyanide and then are transferred to 2% hydrochloric acid. One can also use a solution of equal parts of 10% HCl and 5% aqueous ferrocyanide *(2)*. The specimens are then washed for 12 h in running water. In the presence of abundant hemosiderin, the tissue will turn dark blue rapidly. Mount in 5% formalin-saline. It should be noted that in hemochromatosis specimens the color tends to fade out.

STAINS FOR AMYLOID

1. Iodine stain. Immerse the specimen in a solution made up of 1 g of iodine, 2 g of potassium iodide, 1 mL of sulfuric acid, and 100 mL of water. Amyloid will turn blue. The specimen is then washed in tap water. Museum specimens are mounted in liquid paraffin. This technique is said to prevent fading of the stained amyloid; without sulfuric acid, amyloid will turn brown. Edwards and Edwards *(13)* suggest that the specimen should not be washed but should be put in 70% alcohol until the differentiation is complete. The specimen is then removed from the jar and the alcohol is allowed to evaporate. Subsequently, the nearly dried tissue is placed in liquid paraffin until it is completely soaked, which may take 8 wk or more. Liquid petrolatum appears to be the best preservative for iodine-stained amyloid containing tissues.
2. Congo red stain *(2)*. The specimen is fixed in Kaiserling I solution (*see* above) and then immersed for 1 h in 1% Congo red. It is transferred to a saturated solution of lithium carbonate for 2 min and differentiated in 80% alcohol. Normal arteries and veins tend to retain their color. The specimen is mounted in a variation of Kaiserling III solution (glycerin 300 mL, sodium acetate 100 g, 0.5% formalin solution to a final volume of 1,000 mL; adjust to pH 8.0; if necessary, filter to clear the solution).

STAINS FOR CALCIUM

1. Silver nitrate method *(12)*. Wash the formalin-fixed specimen under running water for 24 h and then in several changes of distilled water for 24 h. In a darkroom, immerse the specimen in a 1% solution of silver nitrate in distilled water and stain for 6–15 h. Rinse in distilled water and then place the specimen in 5% sodium hydrosulfite solution for 24 h. The specimen can now be exposed to light, washed, and mounted in 50% alcohol or Kaiserling solution.
2. Alizarin method. Immerse the specimen for 12 h in a 1:10,000 solution of alizarin red S with just enough potassium hydroxide to render the solution basic. For differentiation, transfer the specimen to a solution of equal parts of alcohol and glycerin and expose the jar to sunlight. Alizarin dyes stain calcium pink. After several days, mount the specimen in Kaiserling solution that is made alkaline by adding a small amount (1:1,000) of potassium hydroxide.

STAINS FOR URATES For the demonstration of gouty deposits, the murexide test is used. Murexide is the purple dye formed when uric acid is exposed to nitric acid and then to ammonia. A sample of finely dispersed tissue fragments is heated with an equal volume of 25% nitric acid until the acid has evaporated. To the dry residue add 2–3 drops of 25% ammonium hydroxide solution and then the same amount of 20% sodium hydroxide solution. In the presence of urates, the dry residue will be bright red or orange, purple after addition of ammonium hydroxide, and blue-violet after addition of sodium hydroxide. For the preparation of museum specimens, the sample is dehydrated over 2 wk in several changes of absolute alcohol. Transfer into mounting fluid (*see* below). Deposits also can be displayed in their native state.

1. Fix specimen, preferably in an anhydrous fixative such as alcohol. Although urate crystals are freely soluble in water, crystalline deposits may be identifiable in the center of the specimens even after aqueous formalin fixation. The crystals may resist the dehydration and staining procedure.
2. Mount in plastic jar with undiluted glycerin. Seal, leaving no air under the lid.

TUMORS

CHLOROMA (13)

1. The specimen should be fixed without previous washing and then placed for 24 h in methyl alcohol. Place the specimen for 24 h in the following solution: 0.5 g sodium hydrosulfite ($Na_2S_2O_4$), 1 g sodium hydroxide (NaHO), 100 mL tap water. The container with this fluid should be filled to the brim, and the lid should be sealed with petroleum jelly.
2. Mounting fluid is composed of: 0.1 g sodium hydrosulfite ($Na_2S_2O_4$), 30 mL glycerin, 10 g sodium acetate, 0.5 mL formalin, 70 mL tap water.

MELANOMA AND MELANIN-CONTAINING TISSUE

1. Thin slices (about 6 mm) of fixed tissue are kept in methyl alcohol for 12 h. Transfer into acetone for another 12–18 h and then into xylol for about 2 h. Remove when shrinkage begins and put into mounting fluid.
2. Mount in liquid paraffin.

LABELING OF MUSEUM SPECIMENS Since any label affixed to the outer surface of a container is exposed to the vicissitudes of handling, one must always attach a label directly to the specimen. These labels must be made of material capable of resisting the chemical action of the mounting fluid and must not unnecessarily obscure the specimen.

REFERENCES

1. Tompsett DH. Anatomical Techniques. E & S Livingstone, Edinburgh, 1956.
2. Pulvertaft RJV. Museum techniques: a review. J Clin Pathol 1950;3:1–23.
3. Edwards JJ, Edwards MJ. Medical Museum Technology. Oxford Uni-versity Press, London, 1959.
4. Lundquist R. A proposed modification of the Kaiserling method for preserving gross specimens. Int Assoc Med Mus Bull 1925;11:16–18.
5. Meiller FH. A method for preserving gross specimens in color. J Tech Methods 1938;18:57–58.
6. Legault JM, Huang S. Color preservation of gross specimens for teaching and medical illustration. Arch Pathol Lab Med 1979;103:300–301.
7. Allison MJ, Gerszten. Paleopathology in Peruvian Mummies: Application of Modern Techniques. Virginia Commonwealth University, Medical College of Virginia, Richmond, 1975, p. 17. 65–73.
8. von Hagens G, Tiedemann K, Kritz W. The current potential of plastination. Anat Embryol 1987;175:411–421.
9. Enhancing the value of organ silicone casts in human gross anatomy education. Aultman A, Blythe J, Souder H, Trotter R, Raoof A. J Intl Soc Plastination 2003;189.:9–13.
10. Loehry CA, Creamer B. Post-mortem study of small-intestinal mucosa. BMJ 1966;1:827–829.
11. Dymock IW, Gray B. Staining method for the examination of the small intestinal villous pattern in necropsy material. J Clin Pathol 1968;21:748–749.
12. Kramer FM. Macroscopic staining of anatomic and pathologic specimens. J Tech Methods 1939;19:72–78.Kramer FM. Dry preservation of museum specimens: a review with introduction of simplified technique. J Tech Methods 1938;18:42–50.
13. Edwards JJ, Edwards MJ. Medical Museum Technology. Oxford Uni-versity Press, London, 1959.

II Alphabetic Listing of Diseases and Conditions

Organization of Part II

Part II begins with a list of special histologic stains, their indications for use and their corresponding references. At the end of this list is a procedure for removal of formalin precipitate from tissue sections.

The bulk of Part II is devoted to a listing of major diseases for which pathologic findings have been described. The main entries are in bold print and are arranged in alphabetical order of the noun. "Viral hepatitis" will be found under "Hepatitis, viral"; "Legionnaire's disease" will be found under "Disease, Legionnaire's"; "Zellweger syndrome" will be found under "Syndrome, Zellweger" and so on. Findings related to operative procedures are listed under the alphabetized entry of the "Surgery…" or "Transplantation. …" Immediately following the disease entry, there may be a listing of synonyms and related diseases. There may also be a list of *Possible Associated Conditions*. These entities are generally linked pathogenetically to the main disease entry. Any asterisk after a related disease indicates that that disorder is also listed as a disease entry.

Many disease entries will be followed by a three-column table that provides the reader with a listing of the pathologic findings to be expected with the disease as well as the prosection and dissection procedures necessary to demonstrate those findings. It is expected that routine hematoxylin-eosin stains will be done on all sections submitted for histologic examination. Special stains will be recommended in the *Procedures* column of the tables, when indicated. Any table immediately following the two columns of disease entries always refers to the disease in the right column.

From: *Handbook of Autopsy Practice,* 4th Ed. Edited by: B.L. Waters

Special Histological Stains[a]

Name of Stain (as used in text)	*Complete Designation and/or Purpose of Stain*	*Source and Comments*
Alcian blue stain	For demonstration of sulfated mucosubstances (at pH 1.0) or acid mucopoly-saccharides (at pH 2.5).	Ref. *(1)* Also used with periodic acid Schiff stain (Alcian blue/PAS).
Alcian blue and phloxine-tartrazine stain of Lendrum	For demonstration of mucus and squamous epithelial cells in one section.	Ref. *(2)* See also below under Lendrum's stain.
Alcian blue/H&E Stain/ Metanil yellow	For the demonstration of mucinous crypts in Barrett's esophagus.	Ref. *(3,10)*
Aldehyde-Fuchsin stain	For staining of beta cells of pancreatic islets, of elastic fibers, and of cells of adenohypophysis.	Ref. *(3)* Aldehyde fuchsin also stains sulfated mucosubstances and hepatitis B surface antigen.
Aldehyde-thionin stain	For staining of cells of adenohypophysis.	Ref. *(3)* Can be combined with periodic acid Schiff stain (PAS) and with Luxol fast blue (LFB).
Auramine-rhodamine	Truant's fluorescent method for tubercle and Leprae bacilli.	Ref. *(2)*
Azure-eosin stain	Routine stain (can be substituted for the hematoxylin and eosin methods).	Ref. *(3)* The Giemsa stain and the Wright stain for blood cells also are azure-eosin stains.
Best's carmine stain	Best's carmine method for glycogen.	Ref. *(2)*
Bielschowsky stain	Bielschowsky's method for axis cylinders and dendrites.	Ref. *(2)*
Bodian stain	Bodian's method for nerve fibers and nerve endings.	Ref. *(2)*
Colloidal iron stain	Acidic mucins adsorb colloidal ferric irons in acidified, colloidal solution of ferric hydroxide. The bound ferric ion is then demonstrated through the Prussian Blue reaction.	Ref. *(3, 11)*
Congo red stain	Bennhold's method for amyloid.	Ref. *(2)*
Cresyl echt violet stain		See Luxol fast blue stain.
Crystal violet stain	Lieb's method for amyloid (crystal violet).	Ref. *(2)*
Cyanuric chloride stain	Cyanuric chloride method of Yoshiki for osteoid.	Ref. *(4)*
Ferric ferricyanide reduction test	Schmorl's ferric ferricyanide reduction test for the demonstration of melanin and other reducing substances.	Ref. *(3)* See also Fontana-Masson silver stain.
Fluorochrome stain for acid fast bacteria	Truant's fluorescent method for acid fast organisms	Ref. *(2)*
Fontana-Masson silver stain	Fontana-Masson silver method for demonstration of argentaffin granules and melanin.	Ref. *(2)* See also Ferric ferricyanide reduction test and Grimelius silver stain.
Giemsa stain	May-Grünwald Giemsa method for hematologic and nuclear elements.	Ref. *(2)* Several modifications of this methods are in use.
Gomori's chromium hematoxylin phloxine stain	Gomori's method for pancreatic islet cells.	Ref. *(2)*
Gomori's iron stain	Gomori's method for iron.	Ref. *(2)*
Gram stain	Brown and Benn, Brown-Hopps, Maccallum-Goodpasture, or Taylor's method for demonstration of Gram positive and Gram negative bacteria.	Ref. *(2)* As shown in the middle column, several modifications of this method are in use. The Gram-Weigert stain (ref. *[3]*) also stains fungi and *Pneumocystis carinii.*
Grimelius silver stain (Grimelius' argyrophil stain)	For demonstration of argyrophil neurosecretory granules (e.g., in pancreatic islets).	Ref. *(1)* The Fontana-Masson stain for melanin and argentaffin granules can also be used.
Grocott's methenamine silver stain (GMS stain)	Grocott's method for fungi.	Ref. *(2)* Also stains *Pneumocystis carinii.*
Hale's colloidal iron stain	The Hale colloidal ferric oxide procedure for acid mucopolysaccharides.	Ref. *(5)* The alcian blue stain at pH. 2.5 (see above) also can be used.
Holzer stain	A crystal violet stain for glia.	Ref *(12)*
Jones' silver stain	Jones' method for reticulum and basement membranes.	Ref. *(3)* See also methenamine silver stain.

Name of Stain (as used in text)	*Complete Designation and/or Purpose of Stain*	*Source and Comments*
Kinyoun's stain	Kinyoun's method for acid-fast bacteria.	Ref. *(2)*
Leder stain	This stain identifies naphthol AS-D chloroacetate esterase, found in granulocytes.	Ref (12)
Lendrum's stain	Lendrum's method for inclusion bodies.	Ref. *(2)* For use with alcian blue, see above.
Levaditi's stain	Levaditi-Manovelian method for spirochetes.	Ref. *(2)*
Luxol fast blue stain (LFB stain)	Klüver-Barrera method for myelin and nerve cells.	Ref. *(2)* Also used with periodic acid Schiff stain (LFB/PAS) or with cresyl echt violet stain (ref. *[1]*).
Masson's trichrome stain	Masson's trichrome method.	Ref. *(2)* Used to distinguish between collagen (blue) and smooth muscle fibers (red).
Methenamine silver stain	Chromotrope silver methenamine stain of glomerular lesions.	Ref. *(6)* See also Jones' silver stain.
Methyl violet stain	Highman's method for amyloid (methyl violet).	Ref. *(2)*
Mucicarmine stain	Mayer's mucicarmine method for mucin and *Cryptococcus*.	Ref. *(1)*
Oil red O stain	This stain highlights simple lipids in frozen sections.	Ref (3) Paraffin sections are unsuitable, since the lipids are already extracted.
Periodic acid-Schiff stain (PAS stain)	The periodic acid, Schiff Reagent (PAS) for demonstration of polysaccharides, neutral mucosubstances, and basement membranes.	Ref. *(1)* Also used with diastase digestion (diastase digests glycogen, e.g., in liver tissue). For use with alcian blue, see under that heading.
PAS-alcian blue stain (PAS/alcian blue)	PAS-alcian blue method for mucosubstances.	See above under "Alcian blue stain."
Perl's stain for iron	Perl's method for iron.	Ref. *(2)*
Peroxidase reaction	Immunoenzymic staining methods for the detection of antigens or antibodies.	Ref. *(3)* Direct and indirect staining methods can be applied, usually with horseradish peroxidase (HPR).
Phosphotungstic acid hematoxylin stain (PTAH stain)	Mallory's phosphotungstic acid hematoxylin method.	Ref. *(2)* Stains skeletal muscle with cross striations (blue), collagen (red), nuclei, and fibrin (both blue).
Reticulum stain	Gomori's method for reticulum.	Ref. *(2)*
Rhodanine stain	Rhodanine method for copper.	Ref. *(3)* Rhodanine should not be confused with rhod*am*ine, which is a fluorochrome, e.g., for the detection of mycobacteria.
Shikata's orcein stain	Orcein method for demonstration of hepatitis B surface antigen in paraffin sections of liver biopsy specimens.	Ref. *(3)* Orcein also is an excellent stain for elastic fibers.
Sirius red stain	Sweat-Puchtler method for amyloid (Sirius red).	Ref. *(2)*
Steiner stain	Will stain spirochetes, Legionella, Helicobacter and fungi dark brown, grey to black.	Ref *(13)*
Sudan stain	Sudan black B method for fat (in frozen sections). For other Sudan stains, see right-hand column.	Ref. *(2)* Oil red O solution also can be used; it gives better results than either Sudan III or Sudan IV (ref. *[5]*).
Sulfated alcian blue	Sodium sulfate alcian blue (SAB) method for amyloid.	Ref. *(8)*
Thioflavine S	Fluorochrome technics for acid fast bacteria and protozoa.	Ref. *(7)*
Thioflavine T stain	Vassar-Culling method for amyloid (thioflavine T).	Ref. *(2)*
Toluidine blue O stain	Toluidine blue O nuclear stain.	Ref. *(3)* Toloidin blue can be used for mast cells, mucin, nerve cells and glia.
Trichrome stain		See Masson's trichrome stain.

Name of Stain (as used in text)	*Complete Designation and/or Purpose of Stain*	*Source and Comments*
Van Gieson's stain	Van Gieson's method for collagen fibers.	Ref. *(2)* See also Verhoeff-van Gieson stain.
Verhoeff-van Gieson stain	Verhoeff-van Gieson technic.	Ref. *(3)* Stains elastic fibers black, collagen red, nuclei blue to black, and other tissue elements yellow. See also Shikata's orcein stain.
Von Braunmühl's stain	Von Braunmühl's stain for senile plaques.	Ref. *(9)*
Von Kossa's stain	Von Kossa's silver test for calcium.	Ref. *(3)*
Warthin-Starry stain	Warthin-Starry method for spirochetes and Donovan bodies.	Ref. *(2)* Also stains *H. pylori.*
Wright stain	Wright stain for blood smears.	Ref. *(3)* Also used with Giemsa stain.
Ziehl-Neelsen stain	Ziehl-Neelsen method for acid-fast bacteria.	Ref. *(2)*

[a]Most of these stains are recommended with appropriate entries in Part II. Some of them can be used for more purposes than stated in the middle column. For alternative stains and recommended fixatives, see current staining manuals.

Removal of Formalin Pigment from Histological Sections *(2)*

1. Deparaffinize sections through two changes each of xylene, absolute alcohol, and 95% alcohol.
2. Rinse well in distilled water.
3. Place slides for 5–10 min in *freshly made up* bleaching solution, consisting of 25 mL hydrogen peroxide 3%, 25 mL acetone, and 1 drop ammonium hydroxide.
4. Wash well in running tap water and distilled water.
5. Stain as desired.

References

1. Carson FL. Histotechnology. A Self-Instructional Text. ASCP Press, American Society of Clinical Pathology, Chicago, IL, 1990.
2. Luna LG. Histopathologic Methods and Color Atlas of Special Stains and Tissue Artifacts. Johnson Printers, Downer's Grove, IL, 1992.
3. Sheehan DC, Hrapchak BB. Theory and Practice of Histotechnology, 2nd ed. CV Mosby Company, St. Louis, MO, 1980.
4. Clark WE. Osteomalacia, histopathologic diagnosis made simple (letter to the editor). Am J Clin Pathol 1976;66:1025–1026.
5. Lillie RD. Histopathologic Technic and Practical Histochemistry, 3rd ed. McGraw-Hill, New York, 1965.
6. Ehrenreich T, Espinosa T. Chromotrope silver methenamine stain of glomerular lesions. Am J Clin Pathol 1971;56:448–451.
7. Bancroft JD, Stevens A. Theory and practice of histological techniques. Churchill Livingstone, New York, 1982.
8. Thompson SW, Hunt RD. Selected Histochemical and Histopathological Methods. Charles C. Thomas, Springfield, IL, 1966.
9. Putt FA. Manual of Histopathological Staining Methods. John Wiley & Sons, New York, 1972.
10. ASCP National Meeting (1993). Seminar on Endoscopic biopsies of the esophagus and stomach. Roger C. Haggitt, MD.
11. Carson, F. Histotechnology: a self instructional text. ASCP Press 1990.
12. Prophet EB, Mills B, Arrington JB, Sobin LH. Laboratory Methods in Histotechnology. AFIP Press, Washington D.C. 1992.
13. Elias JM, Green C. Modified Steiner method for the demonstration of spirochetes in tissue. Am J Clin Path 1979;71:109–11.

A

Abetalipoproteinemia

Synonyms and Related Terms: Acanthocytosis; Bassen-Kornzweig syndrome.

NOTE: Autopsies on patients with this rare genetic disease should be considered research procedures.

Possible Associated Conditions: Hemolytic anemia;* malabsorption syndrome.*

Organs and Tissues	*Procedures*	*Possible or Expected Findings*
External examination	Record body weight and length. Prepare chest roentgenogram (frontal and lateral view).	Below-normal weight in infants. Kyphoscoliosis.
Blood	Submit for serum lipid analysis.	Very low concentrations of cholesterol and decreased triglycerides; serum β-lipoprotein or absent; α-lipoproteins present.
	Prepare smears of undiluted blood.	Acanthocytosis (spiny red cells).
	Obtain blood for molecular studies	Gene mutations *(4)*.
Small bowel	For preservation of small intestinal mucosa and for preparation for study under dissecting microscope, see Part I, Chapter 2. Submit sample for histologic study.	Abnormal shape of villi; vacuolation of epithelial cells.
Large bowel	Submit stool for chemical analysis.	Fatty stools
Liver	Record weight and submit sample for histologic study.	Fatty changes.
	Freeze liver for molecular studies	Gene mutations *(4)*
Other organs		Systemic manifestations of malabsorption syndrome* and of vitamin A deficiency.*
Spine	Record appearance of spine (see also chest roentgenogram).	Kyphoscoliosis.
Brain, spinal cord, peripheral nerves	For removal and specimen preparation, see Chapter 4. Request Luxol fast blue stain.	Axonal degeneration of the spinocerebellar tracts; demyelination of the fasciculus cuneatus and gracilis *(2)*. Possible involvement of posterior columns, pyramidal tracts, and peripheral nerves.
Eyes	For removal and specimen preparation, see Chapter 5.	Atypical retinitis pigmentosa *(2)* with involvement of macula. Angioid streaks *(3)*.

References

1. Case records of the Massachussetts General Hospital. Case 35-1992. N Engl J Med 1992;327:628–635.
2. Rader DJ, Brewer HB Jr. Abetalipoproteinemia. New insights into lipoprotein assembly and vitamin E metabolism from a rare genetic disease [clinical conference]. JAMA 1993;270:865–869.
3. Gorin MB, Paul TO, Rader DJ. Angioid streaks associated with abetalipoproteinemia. Ophthalmic Genet 1994;15:151–159.
4. Schonfeld G, et al. Familial hypobetalipoproteinemia: genetics and metabolism. Cell Mol Life Sci 2005;62:1372–1378.

From: *Handbook of Autopsy Practice,* 4th Ed. Edited by: B.L. Waters

Abortion

NOTE: If a fetus is present, follow procedures described under "Stillbirth." If no recognizable fetal tissue is found, an indication might exist to submit material for chromosome study as decribed in Chapter 9. If attempts to induce abortion appear to have caused the death of the mother, see "Death, abortion-associated."

Abscess, Brain

Synonym: Cerebral abscess.

NOTE: For microbiologic study of tissues and abscesses, see Part I, Chapter 7. Include samples for anaerobic culture. It is best to study the brain after fixation but if specimen is examined fresh, aspirate and prepare smears of abscess content. Photograph surface and coronal slices of brain. Request Giemsa stain, Gram stain, PAS stain, and Grocott's methenamine silver stain for fungi.

Organs and Tissues	*Procedures*	*Possible or Expected Findings*
External examination	Record presence or absence of features listed in right-hand column.	Skin infections in upper half of face. Edema of forehead, eyelids, and base of nose, proptosis, and chemosis indicate cerebral venous sinus thrombosis.* Trauma; craniotomy wounds.
	If there is evidence of trauma, see also under "Injury, head." Prepare roentgenograms of chest and skull.	Skull fracture and other traumatic lesions. For possible intrathoracic lesions, see below under "Other organs."
Cerebrospinal fluid	Submit for microbiologic study.	
Brain and spinal cord	For removal and specimen preparation, see Chapter 4. For microbiologic study, photography, and special stains, see under "Note."	Traumatic lesions of brain. Foreign body.
Base of skull with sinuses and middle ears	For exposure of venous sinuses, see Chapter 4. Sample walls of sinuses for histologic study.	Cerebral venous sinus thrombosis* or thrombophlebitis.
	For exposure of paranasal sinuses, mastoid cells, and middle ears, see Chapter 4.	Paranasal sinusitis and mastoiditis. Subacute and chronic otitis media.* Osteomyelitis* and fractures of base of skull may be present.
Eyes	For removal and specimen preparation, see Chapter 5.	Thrombosis of angular and superior ophthalmic veins, associated with cavernous sinus thrombosis.*
Other organs	Procedures depend on suspected lesions as listed in right-hand column.	Congenital heart disease with right-to-left shunt; infective endocarditis.* Bronchiectasis;* lung abscess;* pleural empyema.* *Entamoeba histolytica* abscesses in liver and lung.

Abscess, Epidural

Synonym: Epidural Empyema.

NOTE: Procedures are the same as those suggested under "Empyema, epidural."

Abscess, Lung

Synonym: Pulmonary abscess.

NOTE: For microbiologic procedures and related suggestions, see also under "Pneumonia."

Organs and Tissues	*Procedures*	*Possible or Expected Findings*
External examination	Prepare chest roentgenogram.	Pulmonary cavities and infiltrates; foreign body.
	Record appearance of oral cavity.	Periodontal infection.
	If peripheral veins contain potentially infected catheters, see below under "Central veins."	Infected intravenous catheter.
Chest cavity	Before chest is opened, puncture pleural cavity and submit exudate for microbiologic study.	Empyema;* pleural effusion or exudate.*
	Prepare smears of exudate and request Gram, Kinyoun, and Grocott methenamine silver stains.	Bacteria or fungi in exudate.

Organs and Tissues	Procedures	Possible or Expected Findings
Central veins	If a metastatic abscess from an infected intravenous catheter is suspected, ligate appropriate vein proximal and distal to catheter tip and submit for microbiologic study.	Infected intravenous catheter.
Heart	See "Endocarditis, infective."	Infective endocarditis* of tricuspid or pulmonary valve.
Lungs	For bronchography and pulmonary arteriography, see Part I, Chapter 2. If abscess contents are aspirated or microbiologic studies are not crucial, perfuse intact lung with formalin.	Tumor of lung,* foreign body, or other obstructive bronchial lesion.
Other organs	Procedures depend on expected sources of infection.	Manifestations of possible underlying conditions such as acquired immunodeficiency syndrome.*

Abscess, Subdural (See "Empyema, epidural.")

Abscess, Subphrenic (See "Empyema, subphrenic.")

Abuse, Child (See "Infanticide.")

Abuse, Drugs or Other Chemicals (See "Abuse, hallucinogen(s)," "Abuse, marihuana," "Dependence,..." "Poisoning,..." See also "Alcoholism and alcohol intoxication.")

Abuse, Hallucinogen(s)

Related Terms: Diethyltryptamine (DET); dimethyltryptamine (DMT); lysergic acid diethylamide (see "Poisoning, LSD"); marihuana;* mescaline; psilocin; psilocybin ("magic mushrooms"); psychedelics; psychotomimetics; and others *(1)*.

NOTE: See also under "Dependence, drug(s), all types or type unspecified." For routine toxicologic sampling, see p. 16. There are no specific morphologic findings related to hallucinogen intake.

Reference

1. Baselt RC, Cravey RH. Disposition of Toxic Drugs and Chemicals in Man, 4th ed. Chemical Toxicology Institute, Foster City, CA, 1995.

Abuse, Marihuana

Synonyms: Cannabis; hashish; ganglia; weed.

NOTE: The tissues at autopsy show no specific changes. Tetrahydrocannabinol is routinely detected by the EMIT screen-ing procedure (*see* Part I, Chapter 2) in urine, and is confirmed and quantitated by specific assays on a variety of body fluids, including blood. However, these latter procedures are rarely needed. If abuse of other drugs is suspected, see under "Dependence, drug(s), all types or type unspecified."

Accident, Aircraft

The National Transportation Safety Board (NTSB)* has authority over aircraft wreckage and the legal authority to investigate and to determine the cause of air crashes. *(1)* The dead are the responsibility of the medical examiner or coroner. Local police will seal off the area of the crash. Other than for the purpose of determining that death has occurred, no one should be allowed to approach the bodies or any objects until the identification teams and the medical examiner or coroner have taken charge.

The sudden influx of bodies after a commercial air carrier accident and the request for speedy identification of the victims would overburden almost any institution. Managing such a disaster is eased by writing a contingency plan beforehand. Temporary morgue facilities may have to be established near the scene of the crash. Refrigerated trucks may serve as storage space. A practical approach is to deal first with those bodies that seem to be the easiest to identify, in order to narrow the field for the more difficult cases.

If bodies are scattered, their locations can be referenced to stakes in the ground or spray paint on pavement; only then should these bodies (or parts) and personal effects be collected. For large-scale crashes a locations can be referenced to a string-line grid benchmarked to GPS coordinates. Records and diagrams of the relative positions of victims are prepared during this phase. If bodies are still within the airplane, their positions are recorded, and photographed.

The personnel of the medical examiner or coroner can augmented by D-MORT team staffed by forensic pathologists, anthropologists, dentists, morgue technicians, and investigators supplied by the National Disaster Medical System.** The airline will provide a list of the passengers and the Federal Bureau of Investigation (FBI) disaster team will make itself available to take and identify fingerprints and aid in the acquisition of other identifying data such as age, race, weight, height, and hair color and style. If dental records can be obtained, this provides one of the most certain methods of identification. A medical history indicating amputations, internal prostheses, or other characteristic surgical interventions or the presence of nephrolithiasis, gallstones, and the like will be helpful. Fingerprints (and footprints of babies) should be taken in all instances. Wallets with identification cards, jewelry, name tags in clothing, or other personal belongings may provide the fastest tentative identification.

The medical examiner may elect to autopsy only the flight crew but not the passengers of an aircraft crash. However, the grossly identifiable fatal injuries should be described, photographed, and x-rayed. This may reveal identifying body changes. If comparison of somatic radiographs, dental records, fingerprints, or photographs do not identify the victim, DNA comparison must be considered. Burned or fragmented bodies of passengers and the bodies of crew members, and particularly the pilots, must have a complete autopsy, including roentgenographic and toxicologic examinations, which must always include alcohol and carbon monoxide determinations. Internal examination might reveal a coronary occlusion, or roentgenograms may disclose a bullet as evidence that violence preceded the crash. In some airplane crashes, particularly in light airplane accidents, suicide must be considered. In such cases police investigation is required to determine if the pilot exhibited suicidal ideation in the recent past.. When resources permit, autopsies should be performed on all deceased occupants of aircraft crashes, including passengers, in order to distinguish among blunt impact trauma, smoke inhalation, and flash fires as causes of death, and to answer future questions concerning pain and suffering, intoxication, and sequence of survivorship.

After a crash victim has been identified, the coroner or medical examiner will issue a death certificate. If remains of a decedent cannot be found, a judge can, upon petition, declare a passenger dead and sign a death certificate prepared by a medical examiner.

*Phone # of NTSB Command Center: 202-314-6000
**Phone # of DMORT: 800-872-6367.

References

1. Cimrmancic MA, Gormley WT, Cina SJ, Aviation pathology, in Handbook of Forensic Pathology, RC Froede, ed (College of American Pathologists, Northfield, Ill., 2003), p. 301.

Accident, Automobile (See "Accident, vehicular.")

Accident, Diving (Skin or Scuba) and Decompression Sickness (Caisson Disease)

NOTE: *Skin* diving fatalities are usually caused by drowning,* and autopsy procedures described under that entry should be followed. Usually, the circumstances that led to drowning are not apparent from the autopsy findings but can be reconstructed from reports of witnesses and the police. Because the reflex drive to seek air is triggered by hypercarbia, not hypoxia, loss of consciousness and drowning can ensue after hyperventilation and breath-holding by experienced swimmers who then drown without a struggle. There are no specific autopsy findings. A search for trauma, including a posterior neck dissection, should be made in all instances. Head and cervical injuries may be responsible for loss of consciousness and drowning, usually in individuals diving into shallow water. Toxicologic examination as described below for scuba diving accidents is always indicated.

With *scuba* diving fatalities, investigation of the equipment and circumstances is usually more important than the autopsy. Scuba fatalities should be studied by or with the aid of diving experts—for instance, members of a diving club or shop (not the one providing the gear used by the decedent) or the U.S. Navy. *(1)* Careful investigation of the scene and study of reports of witnesses and the police are essential. The investigation should ascertain the site of diving (currents and other underwater hazards), the estimated depth, the water temperature (exposure to cold), and a description of water clarity. Electrocution should be considered if the site has electric underwater cables (see "Injury, electric"). Cerebral concussion should be considered if explosives were used in the vicinity. Knowledge of the method of recovery of the body and the type of resuscitation efforts can aid in the interpretation of apparent wounds. The medical history of the diving victim should be sought, as it may lead to a diagnosis for which the autopsy is typically silent, such as seizure disorder, or may reveal asthma, emphysema, or chronic bronchitis, all of which increase the risk of air trapping and arterial air embolism.

Although drowning may be the terminal event in some scuba deaths, the investigation should be focused on the adverse environmental and equipment factors that place a capable swimmer at risk of drowning (see "Embolism, air" and "Sickness, decompression"). Because scuba divers risk arterial air embolism if they ascend with a closed glottis, on can attempt to document gas bubbles at autopsy, but their interpretation is problematic: Bodies recovered immediately are subjected to resuscitation efforts, which can by themselves produce extra-alveolar air artifacts, and bodies not recovered immediately tend to be found in a putrefied condition, full of postmortem gas. In the remaining cases, the pathologist must consider the potential of introducing artifactual gas bubbles by the forcible retraction of the chest plate and by sawing the calvarium. The following procedures apply primarily to scuba diving accidents. Interrogation of witnesses is important; the behavior and complaints of the decedent, if any, might help distinguish between a natural death by heart disease and an unnatural death by air embolism.

Organs and Tissues	Procedures	Possible or Expected Findings
External examination	Photograph victim as recovered and after removal of wet suit and other diving gear. Record condition of clothing and gear. Impound all diving equipment for study by experts, particularly scuba tank, breathing hoses, and regulators. Residual air in tank should be analyzed.	Mask, fins, weight belt, life vest, scuba tank and regulator, watch, depth gauge, or other gear may be missing. Clothing may be torn. Quick-release mechanisms of scuba tank or of weight belt may have been improperly adjusted and may not work. Mask, mouthpiece, regulator, or exhalation hose may contain vomitus. Air supply may be contaminated
	Record color of skin (including face, back, soles, palms, and scalp).	Cyanosis after hypoxia,* cherry-red color after CO poisoning,* or marbling after air embolism.*
	Palpate skin and record presence or absence of crepitation. Record extent and character of wounds. Prepare histologic specimens.	Crepitation from subcutaneous emphysema. Antemortem and postmortem abrasions, lacerations, contusions, bites, or puncture wounds (marine life—for instance, coelenterate stings). Electrocution marks, blast injuries.
	Record appearance of face (including oral and nasal cavities) and of ears.	Froth on mouth and nares. Facial edema and edema of pinnae. ("Facial squeeze" and "external ear squeeze" occur during descent.) Vomitus in mouth and nose.
	Prepare roentgenograms. If air embolism must be expected, as in the presence of pneumomediastinum, follow procedures described under "Embolism, air." For evaluation of findings, see also above under "Note." If decompression sickness (Caisson Disease) is suspected, also prepare roentgenograms of the elbows, hips, and knees.	Fractures—for example, of cervical spine in skin diving accidents (see above); bone necroses (see below); foreign bodies. Pneumothorax,* pneumoperitoneum, pneumopericardium, and mediastinal and subcutaneous emphysema (all indicating rapid ascent).
Eyes and ears	Otoscopic examination.	Otitis externa. Rupture of tympanic membrane.
	Funduscopic examination. Save vitreous for possible toxicologic and other studies.	Gas in retinal vessels after air embolism.
Head (skull and brain)	For removal of brain, see Chapter 4. Record contents of arteries of the circle of Willis and its major branches and basilar artery.	Gas bubbles in cerebral arteries after air embolism* (after rapid ascent). Nitrogen bubbles in cerebral vessels are found in victims who had "staggers." Subdural and subarachnoid hemorrhages. Cerebral edema, with ischemic necroses and focal hemorrhages, after air embolism.
	Strip dura from base of skull and from calvarium.	Skull fracture.
Middle ears	For removal and specimen preparation, see Chapter 4.	Edema and hemorrhage. ("Middle ear squeeze" occurs during descent; hemorrhage occurs in drowning.) Ruptured tympanic membranes.
Chest	For demonstration of pneumothorax, see under "Pneumothorax".	Pneumothorax; pneumomediastinum. Petechial hemorrhages of serosal surfaces.
Blood (from heart and peripheral vessels)	If gas is visible in coronary arteries, photograph. Photograph and aspirate gas in heart chambers. Submit samples of heart blood and peripheral blood for toxicologic study and drug screen.	Air embolism.* Alcohol intoxication (see "Alcoholism and alcohol intoxication"); carbon monoxide poisoning.*
Heart		Ischemic heart disease;* patent oval foramen.
Tracheobronchial tree and lungs	Examine lungs *in situ*. Save bronchial washings for analysis of debris. Fresh dissection is recommended. If decompression sickness is suspected, prepare Sudan stains from fresh-frozen lung sections.	Foam, aspirated vomitus, or other aspirated material in tracheobronchial tree. Pulmonary lacerations, bullae, and atelectases. Pulmonary edema and hemorrhage. "Pulmonary squeeze" develops during descent; nitrogen bubbles in precapillary pulmonary arteries develop during rapid ascent ("chokes"). Pulmonary fat embolism in decompression sickness.

Organs and Tissues	*Procedures*	*Possible or Expected Findings*
Other organs	Complete toxicologic sampling should be carried out (see Chapter 13). Record nature of gastric contents.	In decompression sickness, fatty change of liver, and ischemic infarctions of many organs.
Neck organs and tongue	Remove neck organs toward end of autopsy. For posterior neck dissection, see Chapter 4. Incise tongue.	Interstitial emphysema. Aspiration (see above). Trauma to cervical spine. Mottled pallor of tongue after air embolism. Contusion of tongue after convulsive chewing.
Spinal cord	For removal, see Chapter 4.	Nitrogen bubbles in spinal cord arteries may occur after rapid ascent.
Brain	For removal, see Chapter 4.	Air embolism;* cerebral edema in decompression sickness.
Bones and joints	For removal, prosthetic repair, and specimen preparation, see Chapter 2. Consult roentgenograms.	Aseptic necroses (infarcts, "dysbaric osteonecrosis"), most often in head of femur, distal femur, and proximal tibia. Infarcts indicate repeated hyperbaric exposures. Nitrogen bubbles in and about joints and in periosteal vessels ("bends") occur during rapid ascent.

References

1. Gallagher TJ. Scuba diving accidents: decompression sickness, air embolism. J Florida Med Assoc 1997;84:446–451.
2. Blanksby BA, Wearne FK, Elliott BC, Blitvich JD. Aetiology and occurrence of diving injuries. A review of diving safety. Sports Med 1997;23:228–246.
3. Arness MK. Scuba decompression illness and diving fatalities in an overseas military community. Aviation Space Environm Med 1997; 68:325–333.
4. Hardy KR. Diving-related emergencies. Emerg Med Clin North Am 1997;15:223–240.
5. Caruso JL, Bodies found in water, in Handbook of Forensic Pathology, Froede RC, ed. (College of American Pathologists, Northfield, Ill, 2003), p. 207

Accident, Vehicular

Related Terms: Automobile accident; motorcycle accident.

NOTE: A visit to the *scene* can make the interpretation of the autopsy findings easier. The vehicle can also be inspected in a more leisurely fashion at the impound lot. This is particularly useful for correlating patterned injuries with objects in the vehicle. Most vehicular crashes occur as intersection crashes or because a vehicle with excessive speed left a curved road.

The *medical examiner or coroner* should gain a basic understanding of the crash mechanism so that informed descriptions can be rendered, e.g., "Impact to the B pillar of the decedent's automobile by the front of a pickup truck which failed to stop for a stop sign at an intersection, resulting in a 2-feet intrusion into the cabin; restraint belts not employed; air bag deployed; extrication required which took 15 minutes."

Police are responsible for determining mechanical and environmental risk factors for the crash and for determining some human risk factors such as suicidal or homicidal intent. The *pathologist* determines other risk factors for crashes such as heart disease, a history of epilepsy, and intoxication by carbon monoxide, drugs, and alcohol.

Suicide as a manner of death should be considered when a single-occupant vehicle strikes a bridge abutment or a large tree head-on, with no evidence of evasive action or braking. In such a situation, the standard police traffic investigation should be supplemented of interviews of the victim's family and friends.

The *ambulance run sheet* is an invaluable source of observations that often are not available from the police. This document should be acquired in all instances, even if the paramedics determined that death occurred and did not transport.

The basic *autopsy* procedures are listed below. Most traffic victims who die at the scene or who are dead on arrival at the hospital died from neurogenic shock caused by wounds of the head or vertebral column, or from exsanguination from a torn vessel or heart. As such, they have little lividity, and little blood is found in the vehicles. Presence of intense lividity may indicate suffocation or heart disease as a cause of death.

If postural *asphyxia* is suspected, the first responders to the scene should be interviewed to determine the position of the decedent in the vehicle, and the vital signs, if any, of the decedent from the time of the crash to the time of extrication. Posterior neck dissection is indicated in these instances.

If manifestations of heart disease, intense lividity, and absence of lethal wounds suggest that a *crash occurred because the driver was dead*, other drivers on the road may have observed that the victim was slumped at the wheel before the crash. The determination of heart attack at the wheel is usually simple, because most such victims realize that something is wrong, and bring the vehicle to a stop at the side of the road, or coast gently into a fixed object. In such instances, damage to the vehicle is minor, and wounds to the decedent are usually trivial.

While *patterned wounds* can often be matched to objects (see below), patternless wounds usually cannot be visually matched to specific objects, although an opinion can sometimes be given as to what object was struck, based on the direction of motion and position of the body with respect to the vehicle. Impacts with the A-pillar produce narrow vertical zones of facial laceration and fractures extending from forehead to jaw. Tempered glass shatters into small cubes on impact, and leaves so-called "dicing" wounds, which are abraded cuts arranged in a somewhat rectilinear pattern. Windshield glass leaves shallow, abraded, vertically oriented cuts on the face or scalp.

With *pedestrians*, the lower extremities are of particular forensic interest, to determine the height and direction of impact from vehicles that left the scene. Scalp hair and blood should be collected from such "hit and run" victims and from occupants of a suspect car if police have a question as to which occupant was the driver; these exemplars can be compared to fibers and tissue recovered from the vehicle in question. Likewise, foreign material in wounds can sometimes be matched to suspect vehicles, and should be sought and retained as evidence. For pedestrians, the distance between the impact point on the lower extremities and the soles of the feet should be recorded. The legs should be opened to inspect tibial fractures; cortical fractures initiate propagation opposite to the side of impact, where they usually have a pulled-apart appearance, and then splinter the cortex at the side of impact. Abrasions are better impact markers than contusions, because subcutaneous blood extravasation can be caused not only by impact to the skin, but also from blood extravasating from underlying fractures. If no cutaneous abrasions or fractures of the leg bones are found, the skin of the legs should be incised to expose contusions.

Fracture descriptions should include location in the bone (e.g., proximal metaphysis or shaft), whether the fracture is complete or incomplete, and whether the fracture is displaced or distracted. Lacerations of intervertebral disks, facet joint capsules, and ligamenta flava should not be loosely termed "fractures." The presence or absence of blood extravasation in soft tissue adjacent to the fractures should be recorded, and its volume estimated if it appears severe enough.

Venous air embolism from torn dural sinuses cannot be diagnosed without a pre-autopsy chest radiograph or an *in situ* bubble test. If an X-ray machine is readily available, an anterior-posterior chest radiograph should be obtained in every traffic victim who dies at the scene or after a failed resuscitation attempt.

If a *hemothorax* is suspected, the rib cuts should be placed further lateral and the chest plate reflected so that the internal mammary vessels can be inspected before the chest plate is removed. After measuring and removing the bloody effusion, the underlying serosal surfaces should be inspected for defects. Lacerations of the heart and aorta will be obvious. Tamponaded lacerations of the aorta, around which the adventitia still holds, must be noted as such. If no lacerations are found at the usual sites, lacerations of the azygous veins must be considered, especially in association with fracture dislocations of the thoracic vertebral column; other sites are the internal mammary arteries, especially with fractures of ribs 1 and 2 or of the sternum, and intercostal arteries with displaced rib fractures. Only after the serosal defect is identified should the organs be removed, because that procedure creates many more holes in the serosa. For that reason, as much information as possible should be gained by *in situ* observation.

The only evidence of *concussion of the heart* may be a cardiac contusion or a sternal fracture. The usual clinical history suggests cardiovascular instability that is not associated with craniocerebral trauma and which does not respond to the infusion of intravenous volume agents.

The autopsy assistant may saw but should not retract the skull cap and remove the brain. The pathologist should observe *in situ* whether shallow lacerations of the pontomedullary junction with stretching of the midbrain are present. These lesions cannot be distinguished from artifact by examining the brain later. Thus, only after appropriate *in situ* inspection should the pathologist remove the brain.

A *posterior neck dissection* is required if no lethal craniocerebral or cardiovascular trauma is found, or if suffocation is suspected; neck trauma must be ruled out to diagnose suffocation in a traffic fatality. Sudden death in a patient with seemingly trivial wounds may be caused by undiagnosed trauma of the craniocervical articulation. A posterior neck dissection is required in these instances.

The diagnosis of diffuse axonal injury of the brain in victims with no appreciable survival interval requires that suffocation be ruled out and that no resuscitation from a cardiac arrest has been attempted. Clinicians are quick to apply the label "*closed head injury*" when a victim of a traffic crash has cerebral edema on a computerized axial tomogram of the head, even if no cerebral contusions, scalp contusions, or skull fractures are evident. This may be a misinterpretation, because cerebral edema can be caused by hypoxic encephalopathy made evident after resuscitation from a cardiac arrest, or from hypoxia caused by suffocation.

Organs and Tissues	*Procedures*	*Possible or Expected Findings*
External examination	Record presence of lividity.	Intense lividity and absence of lethal wounds may indicate that the crash occurred because the driver was dead from heart disease or suffocation.
	Photograph all external wounds; measure all lacerations and any abrasions or contusions with a pattern.	Wound documentation. Patterned injuries often sometimes be matched to objects in or about the vehicle (the most common patterned wound is that from tempered glass; see above under "Note"). Impact patterns in pedestrians may help to reconstruct the accident.
	Collect scalp hair and blood (see below) from victims of hit and run accidents. Collect foreign material in wounds.	Hair and blood of the victim may be matched to transfer evidence on a vehicle suspected of having left the scene.

Organs and Tissues	Procedures	Possible or Expected Findings
	Prepare roentgenograms of chest is cases with head impact and skull fractures.	Venous air embolism.*
Internal examination of body cavities	Collect samples for toxicologic study from all victims, including passengers.	Evidence of alcohol or drug intoxication.
	Create pleural window to detect pneumothorax. If blood is seen, examine internal mammary vessels (see under "Note").	Pneumothorax, hemothorax, e.g., after laceration of internal mammary vessels.
	Measure volume of blood in cavity bleeds, and note whether chambers of heart and great vessels are collapsed or filled.	Evidence of significant hemorrhage.
Heart and great vessels	Record evidence of cardiac contusion, sprain of intracardiac inferior vena cava, laceration of pericardial sac, and fracture of sternum.	Indirect evidence of cardiac concussion.
	Laceration of heart or great vessels (measure volume of blood). Follow routine procedures for dissection of heart and great vessels (see Chapter 3).	Evidence of exsanguinating wounds. Evidence of cardiovascular disease that may have felled the driver before the crash.
	In situ bubble test to confirm venous air embolism.	Air embolism.*
Abdomen	Record evidence of trauma and volume of blood in peritoneal cavity; estimated volume of blood in retroperitoneal soft tissues.	Laceration of solid organs; rupture of hollow viscera or vessels, other evidence of trauma and hemorrhage into the abdominal cavity or soft tissues.
Skull and brain; neck	Autopsy assistant may saw the skull but pathologist should inspect brain *in situ* and remove it personally. For removal and specimen preparation of brain, see Chapter 4. Record brain weight. Posterior neck dissection is indicated if there is no craniocerebral or cardio-vascular trauma, or if suffocation is suspected.	Cerebral lacerations at the pontomedullary junction. Cerebral edema. Trauma to the craniocervical articulation.
Soft tissue compartments at any location	Record evidence of trauma and estimate volume of blood.	

Achalasia, Esophageal

Synonyms and Related Terms: Cardiospasm; diffuse esophageal spasm; primary symptomatic achalasia; secondary achalasia.

Possible Associated Conditions: Chagas disease;* gastric malignancies; irradiation; lymphoma.*

Organs and Tissues	Procedures	Possible or Expected Findings
Larynx, trachea, bronchi, and lungs		Airway obstruction;* aspiration bronchopneumonia.
Esophagus	Remove esophagus together with stomach. Photograph esophagus and record diameter of lumen at various levels.	Segmental dilatation and hypertrophy of esophagus. Accumulation of ingested food and esophagitis. Squamous cell carcinoma is a possible complication *(1)*.
	Prepare histologic sections (cut on edge) of narrow and dilated segments.	Barrett's esophagus* with or without adenocarcinoma may be found *(2)*.
	Request Bodian stains and Verhoeff–van Gieson.	Loss of myenteric ganglion cells; partial replacement of myenteric nerves.

References

1. Streitz JM Jr, Ellis FH Jr, Gibb SP, Heatley GM. Achalasia and squamous cell carcinoma of the esophagus: analysis of 241 patients. Ann Thorac Surg 1995;59:1604–1609.
2. Ellis FH Jr, Gibb SP, Balogh K, Schwaber JR. Esophageal achalasia and adenocarcinoma in Barrett's esophagus: a report of two cases and a review of the literature. Dis Esophagus 1997;10:55–60.

Achondroplasia

Synonyms: Chondrodystrophia fetalis; Parrot syndrome.

NOTE: The appropriate resource is the International Skeletal Dysplasia Registry

(Cedars-Sinai Medical Center, 444 S. San Vincente Blvd, Ste. 1001, Los Angeles, CA 90048. Phone #310-423-9915).

Organs and Tissues	*Procedures*	*Possible or Expected Findings*
External examination	Record body length, head circumference, length of extremities, and abnormal features. Prepare skeletal roentgenograms. Photograph head, thorax, hands, and all abnormalities. Radiographs should be reviewed by a pediatric radiologist.	Dwarfism;* micromelia with pudgy fingers; frontal bossing; depressed nasal bridge. Bowing of legs; kyphosis; short pelvis; broad iliac wings; horizontal acetabular roofs; narrowed vertebral interpedicular distance; shortened tubular bones of hands and feet; precocious ossification centers of epiphyses.
Base of skull and spinal canal; brain and spinal cord; pituitary gland	For removal and specimen preparation of brain and spinal cord, see Chapter 4, respectively. For removal of pituitary gland, see Chapter 4. Record appearance and photograph base of skull; record diameter of foramen magnum *(1)*. Submit sections of spinal cord at sites of compression.	Growth retardation of base of skull with compression of foramen magnum. Internal hydrocephalus.* Narrow spinal canal with compression of spinal cord (and clinical symptoms of paraplegia). Atrophy of pituitary gland.
Bones	Submit samples (especially of epiphyses) for histologic study. Snap-freeze tissue for molecular analysis.	Dorsolumbar kyphosis and lumbosacral lordosis; short iliac wings; short and thick tubular bones; excessive size of epiphysis in long bones; elongated costal cartilage. Decreased cartilage cell proliferation at costochondral junction and at epiphyses of long bones.

Reference

1. Knisely AS, Singer DB. A technique for necropsy evaluation of stenosis of the foramen magnum and rostral spinal canal in osteochondrodysplasia. Hum Pathol 1988;19:1372–1375.

Acidosis

NOTE: Acidosis cannot be diagnosed from postmortem blood pH values. Ketone values remain fairly constant in blood and vitreous and may thus support the diagnosis—for instance, of diabetic acidosis. See also under "Disorder, electrolyte(s)".

Acromegaly

Synonyms and Related Terms: Familial acromegaly; hyperpituitary gigantism.

Possible Associated Condition: Multiple endocrine neoplasia 1 (MEN 1)* *(1)*. See also below under "Other organs."

Organs and Tissues	*Procedures*	*Possible or Expected Findings*
External examination, skin and subcutaneous tissue	Record body length and weight, length of extremities, and abnormal features.	Gigantism in younger persons; coarse facial features with prominent eyebrows and prognathism; maloccluded, wide-spaced teeth. Large, furrowed tongue with tooth marks. Parotid enlargement. Narrow ear canal.
	Prepare sections of skin and subcutaneous tissue.	Increased subcutaneous tissue; thickened skin; hypertrichosis; acanthosis nigricans.
	Prepare skeletal roentgenograms, including skull.	Osteoporosis;* kyphosis. See also below under "Bones and joints."

Organs and Tissues	Procedures	Possible or Expected Findings
Breast	Incise and prepare sections.	Lactating breast tissue.
Blood	Submit sample for calcium analysis and radioimmunoassay of plasma growth hormone.	Hypercalcemia in MEN 1 syndrome. Growth hormone excess.
Other organs	Record organ sizes and weights.	Splanchnomegaly, involving heart ("acromegalic heart disease"), liver, spleen, intestine, kidneys, and prostate.
	Sample all endocrine glands for histologic study. See also below under "Pituitary gland."	Endocrine organs may be enlarged (diffuse or nodular goiter; adrenal cortical hyperplasia; enlarged gonads; and parathyroid hyperplasia or adenoma).
	Other procedures depend on expected findings or grossly identified abnormalities as listed in right-hand column.	Pulmonary infections. Nephrolithiasis.* Manifestations of congestive heart failure,* diabetes mellitus,* hyperparathyroidism,* hypertension,* and pituitary insufficiency.* Tumors of breast, colon, thyroid gland, and other organs *(1–4)*.
Pituitary gland	For *in situ* cerebral arteriography and removal of pituitary gland, see Chapter 4. Weigh and photograph gland (include scale). Snap-freeze tumor tissue for histochemical study and hormone assay. Submit tissue for electron microscopic study.	Usually, pituitary adenoma with predominantly eosinophilic or with mixed eosinophilic-chromophobe cells. Enlargement or destruction of pituitary fossa. Tumor growth (see also "Tumor, pituitary") or hemorrhage may be the cause of death. Tumors may be ectopic (sphenoid sinus or parapharyngeal).
Skeletal muscles	For sampling and specimen preparation, see Chapter 4.	Proximal myopathy.
Bones and joints		Overgrowth of facial bones and enlarged sinuses (best seen in roentgenogram); thickening of long bones and of clavicles. Periosteal growth of metacarpal and metatarsal bones. Osteoporosis* (primarily of spine). Hypertrophy of costal cartilages. Acromegalic arthritis.

References

1. The BT, Kytola S, Farnebo F, Bergman L, Wong FK, Weber G, et al. Mutation analysis of the MEN 1 gene in multiple endocrine neoplasia type 1, familial acromegaly and familial isolated hyperparathyroidism. J Clin Endocrinol Metabol 1998;83:2621–2626.
2. Melmed S. Acromegaly. N Engl J Med 1990;322:966–971.
3. Cheung NW, Boyages SC. Increased incidence of neoplasia in females with acromegaly. Clin Endocrinol 1997;47:323–327.
4. Barzilay J, Heatley GJ, Cushing GW. Benign and malignant tumors in patients with acromegaly. Arch Intern Med 1991;151:1629–1632.
5. Horvarth E, Kovacs K. Pathology of acromegaly. Neuroendocrinology 2006;83:161–165.

Actinomycosis

Synonym: *Actinomyces* infection.

NOTE: (1) Collect all tissues that appear to be infected. (2) Request anaerobic cultures for *Actinomyces*. (3) Request Gram stain. (4) No special precautions are indicated. (5) Serologic studies are not reliable at present. (6) This is not a reportable disease.

Organs and Tissues	Procedures	Possible or Expected Findings
External examination	Prepare roentgenograms and photographs of fistulas.	Fistulas to skin of face, neck, and other sites. Periostitis or osteomyelitis of mandible. Extension of fistulas into orbits or paranasal sinuses. Mixed infections (microaerophilic streptococci, *Bacteroides* spp.).
	Submit samples of infected tissue for histologic study. For culturing fistules, see Chapter 7.	Suppurative fibrosing reaction with "sulfur granules" or gram-positive filaments of bacteria.

Organs and Tissues	*Procedures*	*Possible or Expected Findings*
Chest organs	Submit samples of infected tissue for histologic study.	Chronic cavitary pneumonia; empyema; fistulas through chest wall, pericardium, or diaphragm or into thoracic vertebrae.
Gastrointestinal tract	Submit samples of infected tissue for histologic study. For proper tracing of fistulas, *in situ* dissection is recommended.	Inflammatory masses. Fistulas through abdominal wall, to kidneys or pelvic organs (rare), or ileocecal and anorectal fistulas.
Other organs	Procedures depend on expected findings or grossly identified abnormalities as listed in	Rare manifestations include cerebral, renal, or hepatic abscess, abscesses in other or-
gans	right-hand column.	or tissues, endocarditis,* or periostitis and osteomyelitis* with fistulas to skin.

Addiction (See "Abuse, hallucinogen(s)," "Abuse, marihuana," "Dependence,..." and "Poisoning,..." See also "Alcoholism and alcohol intoxication.")

Adenoma (See "Neoplasia, multiple endocrine" and "Tumor...")

Adenomatosis, Multiple Endocrine (See "Neoplasia, multiple endocrine.")

Afibrinogenemia (See "Dysfibrinogenemia.")

Agammaglobulinemia (See "Syndrome, primary immunodeficiency.")

Agenesis, Renal

Synonym: Renal aplasia.

Organs and Tissues	*Procedures*	*Possible and Expected Findings*
External examination	Photograph infant. Record anomalies.	Evidence of oligohydramnios: flattened nose; prominent palpebral folds; flattened low set ears; flattened hands; recessed chin; joint contractures.
Lungs	Weigh lungs; calculate ratio of lung weight to body weight. (For expected weights, see Part III.)	Pulmonary hypoplasia. Normal LW/BW ratio is greater than 0.015, less than 28 wk gestation and 0.012, older than 28 wk gestation.
Abdominal cavity	Record presence or absence of renal arteries and veins, as well as of ureters, urinary bladder, and internal genital organs. Ascertain patency of the lower urinary tract.	Absence of kidneys and associated malformations (see middle column).
Placenta	Weigh and photograph fetal surface.	Amnion nodosum.

Agranulocytosis (See "Pancytopenia")

AIDS (See "Syndrome, acquired immunodeficiency.")

Alcohol, Ethyl (Ethanol) (See "Alcoholism and alcohol intoxication.")

Alcohol, Isopropyl (See "Poisoning, isopropyl alcohol.")

Alcohol, Methyl (See "Poisoning, methanol (methyl alcohol).")

Alcohol, Rubbing or Wood (See "Poisoning, isopropyl alcohol.")

Alcoholism and Alcohol Intoxication

Synonyms and Related Terms: Alcoholic cirrhosis; alcoholic liver disease;* ethanol intoxication; ethyl alcohol intoxication; fetal alcoholic syndrome;* Wernicke-Korsakoff syndrome.*

NOTE: Interpretation of alcohol concentrations can be problematic if body has been embalmed or is putrefied.

Organs and Tissues	*Procedures*	*Possible or Expected Findings*
External examination		Malnutrition; signs of cold exposure, injuries.
Specimen collection	Collect specimens of body liquids and tissues, and any subdural hematomas.	No detectable ethyl alcohol in sudden death from withdrawal. Intoxication after drinking. Alcohol dissipates more slowly from a sequestered subdural hematoma than from vascular blood. *(1)*
Vitreous	Request determination of potassium, sodium, and chloride concentrations.	Low sodium and chloride.
Stomach	Record character and volume of contents. Submit samples for histologic study.	Gastritis.
Heart	Record weight. Submit samples for histologic study.	Alcoholic cardiomyopathy.*
Lungs	Submit for microbiologic study.	Aspiration of vomitus. Lobar pneumonia. Tuberculosis.*
Liver	Record weight and submit samples for histologic study.	Alcoholic liver disease.*
Pancreas		Acute or chronic pancreatitis.*
Brain	Submit samples for histologic study.	Cerebellar cortical degeneration;* Marchiafava-Bignami disease;* Wernicke- Korsakoff syndrome.*
Peripheral nerves and skeletal muscles		Alcoholic neuropathy or alcoholic myopathy (or both).
Bones		Osteonecrosis* ("aseptic necrosis of bone").

INTERPRETATION OF LABORATORY REPORTS IN ALCOHOL INTOXICATION

How Are Alcohol (Ethanol) Concentrations in Body Fluids Expressed?

In European countries, the concentration is expressed in promille (grams per liter). In the United States, it has become customary to refer to concentration by percentage (grams per deciliter), and values in these units have been written into legislation and included in the uniform vehicle codes. Unless qualified, the use of promille or percentage does not indicate whether the result of the analysis is weight/weight, weight/volume, or volume/volume. Another common way of expressing concentration, milligrams per deciliter, has also been used to indicate alcohol concentrations. The method of expressing concentration must be clearly specified whenever the alcohol level is mentioned. The desired expression canbe derived from the toxicologic report by using the following equation:

$$1{,}000\,\mu g/mL = 100\,mg/dL = 0.10\,g/dL = 21.74\,mmol/L = 1.0\ \text{promille} = 0.10\%$$

What Are the Effects of Alcohol (Ethanol) Intoxication? Physiologic Effects:*

Blood-Alcohol Concentration g/dL	*Stage of Alcoholic Influence*	*Clinical Signs/Symptoms*
0.01–0.05	Subclinical	No apparent influence. Behavior nearly normal by ordinary observation. Slight changes detectable by special tests.
0.03–0.12	Euphoria	Decreased inhibitions. Increased self-confidence. Diminution of attention, judgment, and control. Beginning of sensory-motor impairment. Slowed information processing. Loss of efficiency in finer performance tests.
0.09–0.25	Excitement	Emotional instability; loss of critical judgment. Impairment of perception, memory, and comprehension. Decreased sensory response; increased reaction time. Reduced visual acuity, peripheral vision, and glare recovery. Sensory-motor incoordination; impaired balance. Drowsiness.
0.18–0.30	Confusion	Disorientation, mental confusion; dizziness. Exaggerated emotional states (e.g., fear, rage, sorrow). Disturbances of vision (e.g., diplopia) and of perception of color, form, motions, dimensions. Increased pain threshold. Increased muscular incoordination; staggering gait; slurred speech. Apathy; lethargy.
0.25–0.40	Stupor	General inertia; approaching loss of motor function. Markedly decreased response to stimuli. Marked muscular incoordination; inability to stand or walk. Vomiting; incontinence of urine and feces. Impaired consciousness; sleep or stupor.
0.35-0.50	Coma	Complete unconsciousness; coma; anesthesia. Depressed or abolished reflexes. Subnormal temperature. Incontinence of urine and feces. Impairment of circulation and respiration. Possible death.
0.45+	Death	Death from respiratory arrest.

*Reprinted by permission from KM Dubowsky. Copyright 1987, *(2)*.

Biochemical effects:

Hyponatremia and hypochloremia are common in the chronic alcoholic *(3)*. Hyperlipidemia also may be found.

What Is the Legal Interpretation of Alcohol (Ethanol) Intoxication?

Objective impairment of driving ability is observed at threshold blood alcohol concentrations of .035–.040 g/dL. As of August 2005 all states and the District of Columbia have adopted laws that make it criminal offense for a driver to operate a motor vehicle with a blood alcohol concentration of 0.08 g/dL or greater. Many states have an enhanced penalty for high concentrations such as 0.15 g/dL or above. Several states have zero tolerance laws, under which drivers who are minors are legally operating only if their blood alcohol concentration is 0.02 g/dL or less, and in some states, not detectable at all.

Can Postmortem Changes and Specimen Storage Affect Blood Alcohol (Ethanol) Concentrations?

Blood alcohol concentrations obtained at autopsy are valid until putrefaction begins. Specimen tubes with sodium fluoride should be used, and the specimen should be stored in the refrigerator. If the air space above the blood samples in the container is large, alcohol can evaporate and a falsely low blood alcohol level can result. Putrefactive changes before autopsy or during storage may cause a falsely high blood alcohol concentration. Ethanol can be produced in the specimen container; this is more likely in the absence of a preservative. Because fluoride inhibits bacteria far more than fungi, higher fluoride concentrations are required for the inhibition of fungal growth *(4)*.

Can the Sites Where Blood Was Withdrawn Affect Alcohol (Ethanol) Concentrations?

Although there is no major difference in the alcohol concentrations of blood samples from the intact heart chambers and the femoral vessels *(5)*, autopsy samples from pooled blood in the pericardial sac or pleural cavity are unsatisfactory. We therefore recommend that blood be withdrawn from peripheral vessels.

Is There Normal "Endogenous" Blood Alcohol (Ethanol) in a Living Person?

Blood alcohol concentrations are generally believed to be negligible in the absence of ingested alcohol. "Endogenous" ethanol in human blood exists at a concentration of about 0.0002 g/dL, which is below the limit of detection for most methods *(6)*.

Which Conditions or Factors May Lower the Tolerance to Alcohol (Ethanol) So That Death May Occur at Levels That Are Not Usually Fatal?

First in such a list would be postural asphyxia, for example, in drunks who fall asleep face down. Also, depressant drugs in the tricyclic, analgesic, barbiturate, and benzodiazepine classes all potentiate the effect of alcohol *(7)*. Also included in such a list would be infancy and childhood; ischemic heart disease;* chronic bronchitis and emphysema;* other chronic debilitating diseases; poisoning with carbon tetrachloride* or carbon monoxide;* and other causes of hypoxia.*

How Can One Estimate Blood Alcohol (Ethanol) Concentrations From Vitreous, Urine, or Tissue Alcohol Levels and From Alcohol in Stomach Contents?

The ratio of serum, plasma, urine, vitreous, and various tissues has been compiled by Garriot *(8)*. The values may vary considerably. For vitreous, the ratios varied from 0.46–1.40. These variations may depend on whether blood alcohol concentrations were increasing or decreasing at the time of death. Most other body fluids and tissues showed ranges closer to 1. Most urine values were above the blood alcohol concentrations. In another study *(9)*, the blood/vitreous (B/V) ratio in the early absorption phase was 1.29 (range, 0.71–3.71; SD 0.57) and in the late absorption and elimination phase, the B/V ratio was 0.89 (range, 0.32–1.28; SD 0.19). Blood ethanol concentrations probably can be estimated using B = 1.29V for early absorption and B = 0.89V for later phases. A urine/blood ethanol ratio of 1.20 or less indicates that the deceased was in the early absorption phase.

How Can One Use Alcohol (Ethanol) Concentrations in Postmortem Specimens to Estimate the Blood Alcohol Concentration at Various Times Before Death?

With certain limitations, one can base calculations of this kind on the assumption that the blood alcohol level decreases from its peak at a fairly constant rate of 0.015–0.018 g/dL/h until death *(10)*. If blood is not available, conversion factors (see above) must be used. Alcoholics have been reported to metabolize at a rate of up to 0.043 g/dL/h *(6)*.

Example: The driver of an automobile drinks at a party until midnight. He leaves his host at about 1:30 a.m. and is involved in a head-on collision at 2:15 a.m. He dies in the emergency room at 6:35 a.m. There are multiple injuries and the patient exsanguinates. The autopsy is done at 1:30 p.m. Although this appears quite unlikely, let us assume that no satisfactory blood sample was obtained before death and that no blood or plasma expanders were given. If under such circumstances the alcohol concentration in the vitreous was found to be 0.157 g/dL, what was the alcohol concentration in the blood at the time of the accident?

Vitreous and blood alcohol concentrations may be assumed to have remained unchanged after death. Therefore, the blood alcohol level at the time of death must have been approx 0.157 (vitreous humor alcohol) × 0.89 (conversion factor, see above) = 0.14 g/dl. The time interval between the accident (2:15 a.m.) and death (6:35 a.m.) is 4 h and 20 min or 4 1/3 h. If we assume that the decedent was not an alcoholic and that the blood alcohol concentration was decreasing from its peak at a constant rate of 0.015 g/dL/h, then the concentration at the time of the accident is estimated to have been 0.14 (concentration at time of death)

+ (4 1/3 × 0.015) = 0.140 + 0.065 = 0.205 g/dL or 0.2%.

The blood alcohol concentration at the time of the accident could have been lower if the victim stopped drinking later than 1 h or 1 1/2 h before the accident. In the latter case, the peak alcohol level would have occurred after the accident, reflecting the time to absorb the latest drink.

The blood alcohol concentration at the time of the accident could have been lower or higher if the time when the patient stopped drinking, the time of the accident, or the time of the death is uncertain.

The blood alcohol concentration at the time of the accident could have been higher if the victim was a chronic alcoholic. The elimination rate in such persons may be as high as 0.040 mg/dL, which would change the figures in our example above to 0.140 + (4 1/3 × .040) = 0.140 + 0.173 = 0.313 g/dl or 0.3%.

How Can One Use Alcohol (Ethanol) Concentrations in Postmortem Specimens To Estimate How Much the Victim Had Been Drinking?

Only rough estimates are possible. First, the peak blood alcohol level must be determined or calculated, as described in the previous paragraphs. Tables (see below) are available that relate blood alcohol level to the minimal amounts of whiskey, wine, or beer that must have been consumed *(10)*. However, tables of this type are often based on the minimum amount of alcohol circulating in the body after specific numbers of drinks; such tables do not yield reliable results if used conversely. Furthermore, inasmuch as drinking and elimination of alcohol may take place concomitantly, over a longer period the total amount of alcohol consumed may have been much greater than the tables would indicate. It cannot be lower. According to these tables, 6 pints of ordinary beer or 8 fl oz of whiskey would be the minimal amounts needed to produce a blood alcohol level of about 200 mg/dL in a person weighing 140–180 pounds. The total body alcohol can be calculated from the blood alcohol level by using Widmark's formula:

Average concentration of alcohol in entire body = .68
Concentration of alcohol in the blood

In a person weighing 70 kg, the blood alcohol concentration would be increased 50 mg/dL (0.05%) by the absorption of 1 oz of ethanol (2 oz of 100-proof whiskey).

What Is the Alcohol (Ethanol) Content of Various Beverages?

Strength of alcohol is measured in "proof"; absolute alcohol is 200 proof. Therefore, in the United States, alcohol content as volume percent is half the proof (for example, 100-proof whiskey contains 50% alcohol by volume). The alcohol content of various beverages is shown in the following table.

Approximate Alcohol Content in Various Beverages[†]

Beverage	*Ethanol Content in %*
Whiskey and gin	40
Brandy	45.5–48.5
Sherry and port wines	16–20
Liqueurs	34–59
Rum	50–69.5
Beers (Lager)	2–6
Light wines	10–15

[†]Data from Glaister, Rentoul E. Medical Jurisprudence and Toxicology, 12th ed. E & S Livingstone, Edinburgh, 1966 with permission.

What Blood Alcohol (Ethanol) Concentrations Can Be Predicted From a Known Amount and Type of Alcoholic Beverage?

Number of Drinks and Predicted Blood Alcohol Concentrations[†]

Drinks (no.)[‡]	*Predicted Blood Alcohol Level (mg/dL)*
1	10–30
2	30–50
3	50–80
4	80–100
5	100–130
6	130–160
8	160–200
10	190–230
12	250–320

[†]Within 1 h after consumption of diluted alcohol (approx 15%) on an empty stomach, assuming body weight of 140–180 pounds (63.6–81.7 kg) reproduced from (11) with permission.

[‡]One ounce (about 30 mL) of whiskey or 12 oz (about 355 mL) of beer.

What Is the Toxicity of Alcohol Other Than Ethanol?

In general, the toxicity increases as the number of carbon atoms in the alcohol increases. Thus, butyl alcohol is two times as toxic as ethyl alcohol,* but isopropyl alcohol is only two-thirds as toxic as isobutyl alcohol and one-half as toxic as amyl alcohol. Primary alcohols are more toxic than the corresponding secondary isomers *(10)*.

References

1. Hirsch CS, Adelson L. Ethanol in sequestered hematomas. Am J Clin Pathol 1973;59:429–433.
2. Dubowsky KM. Stages of acute alcoholic influence/intoxication. In: Medicolegal Aspects of Alcohol. Garriott JC, ed. Lawyers & Judges Publishing Co., Phoenix AZ, 1997, p. 40.
3. Sturner WQ, Coe JI. Electrolyte imbalance in alcoholic liver disease. J Forensic Sci 1973;18:344–350.
4. Harper DR, Corry JEL. Collection and storage of specimens for alcohol analysis. In: Medicolegal Aspects of Alcohol. Garriott JC, ed. Lawyers & Judges Publishing Co., Phoenix, AZ, 1997, pp. 145– 169.
5. Garriott JC. Analysis for alcohol in postmortem specimens. In: Medicolegal Aspects of Alcohol. Garriott JC, ed. Lawyers & Judges Publishing Co., Phoenix, AZ, 1997, pp. 87–100.
6. Baselt RC, Danhof IE. Disposition of alcohol in man. In: Medicolegal Aspects of Alcohol. Garriott JC, ed. Lawyers & Judges Publishing Co., Tuscon, AZ, 1993, pp. 55–74.
7. Garriott JC. Pharmacology of ethyl alcohol. In: Medicolegal Aspects of Alcohol. Garriott JC, ed. Lawyers & Judges Publishing Co., Phoenix, AZ, 1997, pp. 36–54.
8. Caplan YH. Blood, urine and other tissue specimens for alcohol analysis. In: Medicolegal Aspects of Alcohol. Garriott JC, ed. Lawyers & Judges Publishing Co., Phoenix, AZ, 1997, pp. 74–86.
9. Chao TC, Lo DS. Relationship between postmortem blood and vitreous humor ethanol levels. Am J Forens Med Pathol 1993;14:303– 308.
10. Larson CP. Alcohol: fact and fallacy. In: Legal Medicine Annual 1969. Wecht CH, ed. Appleton-Century-Crofts, New York, 1969, pp. 241–268.
11. Camps FE. Gradwohl's Legal Medicine, 2nd ed. Williams & Wilkins Company, Baltimore, MD, 1968, p. 554.

Aldosteronism

Synonyms and Related Terms: Bartter's syndrome; Conn's syndrome; hyperaldosteronism; idiopathic aldosteronism; primary aldosteronism; secondary aldosteronism.

Organs and Tissues	*Procedures*	*Possible or Expected Findings*
External examination	Record presence or absence of edema.	Edema of lower extremities (absent in most uncomplicated cases).
Vitreous	Submit for sodium and potassium determination.	Changes reflecting high sodium and low potassium concentrations in the blood.
Heart	Weigh heart and measure thickness of ventricles.	Prominent left ventricular hypertrophy *(1)*.
Adrenals	Dissect, weigh, and photograph both adrenal glands. Place portion (including tumor, if present) of gland in deep freeze for hormone assay. Submit samples for light and electron microscopic study.	Aldosterone-secreting adrenal cortical adenoma (Conn's syndrome), adrenal cortical nodular hyperplasia, or, rarely, adrenal carcinoma. Primary aldosteronism may be present in all these instances. Idiopathic aldosteronism is characterized by normal adrenal glands.
Kidneys	Weigh, measure, photograph. Submit samples for histologic and electron microscopic study. If there is a renal tumor, place portion in a deep freeze for hormone assay.	Vacuolar (osmotic) nephropathy due to hypokalemia. Various renal diseases may be associated with secondary hyperaldosteronism; features of juxtaglomerular cell hyperplasia may be present.
Other organs	Procedures in secondary aldosteronism depend on expected cause.	Manifestations of hypertension.* Cirrhosis,* nephrotic syndrome,* toxemia of pregnancy,* and many other conditions that may be associated with secondary aldosteronism, adrenal nodular hyperplasia *(3)*.
Brain	For removal and specimen preparation, see Chapter 4. For cerebral angiography, see Chapter 4.	Ruptured intracranial aneurysm* and hemorrhagic stroke *(2)*.

References

1. Tanabe A, Naruse M, Naruse K, Hase M, Yoshimoto T, Tanaka M, et al. Left ventricular hypertrophy is more prominent in patients with primary aldosteronism than in patients with other types of secondary hypertension. Hypertension Res 1997;20:85–90.
2. Litchfield WR, Anderson BF, Weiss RJ, Lifton RP, Dluhy RG. Intracranial aneurysm and hemorrhagic stroke in glucocorticoid-remediable aldosteronism. Hypertension 1998;31:445–450.
3. Valdes G, Roessler E, Salazaar I, et al. Association of adrenal medullae and cortical nodular hyperplasia: a report of two cases with clinical and morpho-functional consideration. Encodrine 2006; 30: 389–396

Alkalosis

NOTE: There are no diagnostic findings. Postmortem chemical analysis is of limited value in these instances. See also under "Disorder, electrolyte(s)".

Alkaptonuria

Synonyms and Related Terms: Alkaptonuric ochronosis *(1)*; familial (hereditary) ochronosis *(2)*.

Organs and Tissues	*Procedures*	*Possible or Expected Findings*
External examination and skin	Record extent of discoloration of skin and eyes. Photograph these features. Prepare histologic sections of pigmented areas. Record appearance of joint deformities. Prepare skeletal roentgenograms.	Brown-black pigment in skin, eyes (conjunctivas, corneas, scleras), and external ears. Pigment in dermal sweat glands. Deformities of knees and other joints. Ochronotic arthropathy, particularly of knee joints; spondylosis and disk calcification with fusion of vertebrae.
Urine	Submit sample for biochemical study.	Hemogentisic aciduria.
Heart and large arteries	Prepare histologic sections of pigmented areas. If electron microscopic study is intended, see Chapter 15.	Pigmentation of heart valves (e.g., with stenosis *[2]*), endocardium, and intima of large arteries.

Organs and Tissues	Procedures	Possible or Expected Findings
Larynx and trachea	Prepare histologic sections of pigmented cartilage.	Pigmentation of laryngotracheal cartilage.
Kidneys and prostate	Submit samples for histologic study.	Nephrolithiasis;* prostatitis; ochronotic pigmentation.
Other organs and tissues	Submit samples for histologic study.	Pigmentation in islets of Langerhans, pituitary gland, and other endocrine organs; pigment in reticuloendothelial system.
Middle ears	For removal and specimen preparation, see Chapter 4.	Pigmentation of tympanic membranes and ossicles of middle ears.
Eyes	For removal and specimen preparation, see Chapter 5.	See under "External examination and skin."
Bones and joints	Submit samples of cartilage of diarthrodial joints and from adjacent tendons for histologic study. Prepare frontal section through spine.	Ochronotic arthropathy (see above under "External examination and skin"). Fragments of pigmented cartilage may be found in the synovia.

References

1. Gaines JJ Jr. The pathology of alkaptonuric ochronosis. Hum Pathol 1989;220:40–46.
2. Cortina R, Moris C, Astudillo A, Gosalbez F, Cortina A. Familial ochronosis. Eur Heart J 1995;16:285–286.

Aluminosis (See "Pneumoconiosis.")

Alveolities, Extrinsic Allergic (See "Pneumoconiosis" and "Pneumonia, interstitial.")

Amaurosis Fugax

Organs and Tissues	Procedures	Possible or Expected Findings
Eyes		Papilledema.
Brain	Other procedures depend on expected findings or grossly identified abnormalities as listed in right-hand column.	Tumor of the brain or other cause of intracranial hypertension, including benign intracranial hypertension (pseudotumor cerebri*).

Amblyopia, Nutritional

Related Terms: Alcohol amblyopia; retrobulbar neuropathy; tobacco amblyopia.

NOTE: If chronic malnutrition is associated with corneal degeneration, glossitis, stomatitis, and genital dermatitis, the condition is referred to as Strachan's syndrome.

Organs and Tissues	Procedures	Possible or Expected Findings
Brain	Leave optic nerve attached when removing brain.	See below under "Eyes with optic nerves."
Eyes with optic nerves	For removal and specimen preparation, see Chapter 5. Request Luxol fast blue stain of optic nerves.	Bilateral symmetric loss of myelinated fibers in central parts of optic nerves. Ganglion cells in macula may be lost.
Other organs	Procedures depend on expected findings or grossly identified abnormalities as listed in right-hand column.	Manifestations of alcoholism,* diabetes mellitus,* malnutrition,* megaloblastic anemia,* tobacco dependence, and tuberculosis* (isoniazid treatment may cause the optic nerve damage).

Amebiasis

Synonym: *Entamoeba histolytica* infection.

NOTE: (1) Collect all tissues that appear to be infected. (2) Request parasitologic examination as well as aerobic and anaerobic cultures. Bacterial infections may be associated with amebiasis. (3) Request Gram and Giemsa stains. (4) No special precautions are indicated. (5) Serologic studies are available in many local and state health department laboratories. (6) This is a **reportable** disease.

Possible Associated Conditions: Acquired immunodeficiency syndrome (AIDS)* *(1)*.

Organs and Tissues	*Procedures*	*Possible or Expected Findings*
External examination and skin	Photograph and prepare sections of cutaneous or mucosal lesions.	Perianal and perineal ulcers after extension of amebic colitis; rarely, destruction of external genitalia. Cutaneous amebiasis from fistulas after hepatic abscess, laparotomy, or, rarely, distant spread.
Chest organs, abdominal cavity, retroperitoneal space, and pelvic organs	Record presence and course of fistulas before removal of organs. Material for parasitologic study and bacterial cultures is best removed at this time.	Amebic pneumonia, often associated with hepatic abscess (see below). Pleuropulmonary amebiasis, with or without empyema. Amebic pericarditis or amebic peritonitis is rare. Intestinal perforation into peritoneal cavity, retroperitoneal space, or other hollow viscera.
Intestine	Examine as soon as possible so as to reduce the effects of autolysis.	
	Photograph ulcers and collect samples for smears and histologic study. Specimens should include cecum; ascending, sigmoid, transverse, and descending colon; appendix; and ileum.	Buttonhole or flask-shaped mucosal ulcers are always present, in an order of involvement as listed in the middle column.
Liver	If there is a hepatic abscess with fistulas, record their course before removal of liver. Use Letulle technique (see Chapter 2) for organ removal, and open inferior vena cava along posterior midline.	Hepatic abscess(es) with or without perforation and fistula(s). Hepatic fibrosis and necroses. Portal vein thrombosis can occur. Abscess may communicate with inferior vena cava, gallbladder, bile ducts, and other structures.
	Aspirate abscess contents and submit for microbiologic study. Prepare smears and sections from periphery of abscess.	Amebae are difficult to demonstrate in amebic hepatic abscesses.
Urinary tract	If urinary tract system appears involved, incise kidneys *in situ*, in frontal plane from periphery toward pelvis (leave vessels attached); open renal pelves, ureters, and urinary bladder *in situ*.	Rarely, ascending amebic infection associated with amebic colitis and perianal spread.
Other organs	Procedures depend on expected findings or grossly identified abnormalities as listed in right-hand column.	Rarely, spread to spleen, aorta, or larynx. Other sites may be affected by systemic hematogenous dissemination.
Brain		Cerebral abscess* almost always associated with hepatic abscess and pulmonary amebiasis.

Reference

1. Fatkenheuer G, Arnold G, Steffen HM, Franzen C, Schrappe M, Diehl V, Salzberger B. Invasive amebiasis in two patients with AIDS and cytomegalovirus colitis. J Clin Microbiol 1997;35:2168–2169.
2. Ventura-Juarez J, et al. Immunohistochemical characterization of human fulminant amoebic colitis. Parasite Immunol 2007;29:201–209.

Aminoaciduria

Related Terms: Proprionic acidemia; methyl malonic acidemia; isovaleric acidemia; cystinuria; homocystinuria;* maple syrup urine disease;* urea cycle disorders; tyrosinemia; phenylketonuria.*

NOTE: Aminoaciduria is a collective name for all the conditions mentioned under "Related Terms." Because few autopsy studies of aminoaciduria have been done, each case should be considered a potential source of new, unpublished information. Multiple abnormalities of virtually all organ systems are possible.

Organs and Tissues	Procedures	Possible or Expected Findings
Blood, cerebrospinal fluid, and urine	Freeze samples for biochemical study.	Many abnormalities may be present. For specific enzyme defects, see ref. *(1)*.
Fascia lata, liver, spleen, or blood	These specimens should be collected using aseptic technique for tissue culture for chromosome analysis and biochemical studies (see Chapter 9).	Rare translocations are described *(2)*.

References

1. Chalmers RA, Lawson AM. Organic Acids in Man: The Analytical Chemistry, Biochemistry and Diagnosis of the Organic Acidurias. Chap-man and Hall, London, 1982.
2. Hodgson SV, Heckmatt JZ, Hughes E, Crolla JA, Dubowitz V, Bobrow M. A balanced de novo X/autosome translocation in a girl with manifestations of Lowe syndrome. Am J Med Gen 1986;23:837–847.

Ammonia (See "Poisoning, gas" and "Bronchitis, acute chemical.")

Amphetamine(s) (See "Drug abuse, amphetamine(s).")

Amyloidosis

Related Terms: Familial amyloidosis (multiple forms, including familial Mediterranean fever and familial amyloid nephropathy with urticaria and deafness; hereditary cerebral angiopathies); idiopathic or primary amyloidosis (AL protein) *(1)*; localized or isolated amyloidosis (amyloid in islets of Langerhans and insulinoma; congophil cerebral angiopathy;* isolated atrial amyloid; medullary carcinoma of thyroid); reactive or secondary amyloidosis (AA protein); systemic senile amyloidosis.

Possible Associated Conditions: Alzheimer's disease;* Behçet's disease;* bronchiectasis;* chronic dialysis;* Creutzfeldt-Jakob disease;* Crohn's disease;* diabetes mellitus type II; Down's syndrome;* leprosy;* malignant lymphoma, Hodgkin's type; macroglobulinemia; multiple myeloma;* osteomyelitis;* paraplegia; Reiter's syndrome;* rheumatoid arthritis* and other immune connective tissue diseases (all types); syphilis;* tuberculosis;* Whipple's disease.*

NOTE: Stain 15-micron tissue sections with Congo red and examine under polarized light for green birefringence. In AA-type amyloid but not in AL amyloid, pretreatment of tissue with permanganate, followed by routine staining with Congo red, will abolish the green birefringence. An immunohistochemistry panel is available to differentiate the subtypes of amyloidosis. Crystal violet, methyl violet, Sirius red, sodium sulfate alcian blue, and thioflavin T also stain amyloid in many instances. Electron microscopic studies *(2)* are particularly useful if routine stains are negative or controversial. For macroscopic staining of amyloid, e.g., in the heart, see Chapter 16.

Organs and Tissues	Procedures	Possible or Expected Findings
External examination and skin	Submit grossly involved and uninvolved skin for histologic study (look for amyloid in subcutaneous fat). For special stains, see above under "Note."	Papules or plaques, particularly around eyes, ears, axillae, inguinal regions, and anus. Papules may be tumorous or pigmented. Periorbital ecchymoses may be present.
Mouth	Submit gingiva, palate, and tongue for histologic study.	Amyloid infiltrates; macroglossia.
Blood and urine	In unsuspected cases, submit samples for immunoelectrophoresis and immunofixation.	Presence of monoclonal light chain.
Heart	Submit tissue from atria and myocardium of ventricles. Photograph endocardial lesions. For gross and microscopic staining, see above under "Note."	Amyloid deposits may be identifiable under endocardium of left atrium. Nonischemic congestive heart failure *(1)*.
Liver	Record size and weight. For gross and microscopic staining, see above under "Note."	Hepatomegaly with amyloid infiltrates.
Gastrointestinal tract	Take sections of all segments of the gastro-intestinal tract.	Amyloid infiltrates with ulcerations and hemorrhages.
Other organs	Microscopic samples should include respiratory system with larynx, gallbladder, pancreas, spleen, all portions of urogenital system, including prostate, seminal vesicles, and vasa deferentia, and all endrocrine glands, blood	Almost all organs and tissues may be involved. Diffuse, nodular, or primary vascular deposits may predominate. Evidence of portal hypertension* may be found but splenomegaly also may be caused

Organs and Tissues	Procedures	Possible or Expected Findings
	vessels, lymph nodes, and other tissues, such as omentum. For gross and microscopic staining methods, see above under "Note."	by amyloid infiltrates. Nephrotic syndrome;* renal involvement also may be associated with renal vein thrombosis.* See also above under "Possible Associated Conditions."
Eyes	For removal and specimen preparation, see Chapter 5.	Ocular amyloidosis *(3)*.
Brain, spinal cord, and peripheral nerves	For removal and specimen preparation, see Chapter 4.	Amyloid associated with senile plaques or neurofibrillary tangles; congophilic angiopathy *(4)*. Spinal cord compression *(5)*. Peripheral amyloid neuropathy.
Bones and bone marrow, joints, tendons		Amyloid in bone marrow, synovium, and carpal tunnel. Bone may contain osteolytic tumor (multiple myeloma*).

References

1. Gertz MA, Lacy MQ, Dispenzieri A. Amyloidosis: recognition, confirmation, prognosis, and therapy. Mayo Clin Proc 1999;74:490–494.
2. Lin CS, Wong CK. Electron microscopy of primary and secondary cutaneous amyloidosis and systemic amyloidosis. Clin Dermatol 1990; 8:36–45.
3. Gorevic PD, Rodrigues NM. Ocular amyloidosis. Am J Ophthalmol 1994;117:529–532.
4. Duchen LW. Current status review: cerebral amyloid. Intern J Exp Pathol 1992;73:535–550.
5. Villarejo F, Perez Diaz C, Perla C, Sanz J, Escalona J, Goyenechea F. Spinal cord compression by amyloid deposits. Spine 1994;19:1178–1181.
6. Picken MM, Herrera GA. The burden of "sticky" amyloid: typing challenges. Arch Pathol Lab Med 2007;131:850–851.
7. Wilcock DM, Gordon MN, Morgan D. Quantification of cerebral amyloid angiopathy and parenchymal amyloid plaques with Congo Red histochemical stain. Nat Protoc 2006;1:1591–1595.

Amyotonia Congenita

NOTE: Amyotonia congenita encompasses several different neuromuscular disorders. See under "Disease, motor neuron."

Anaphylaxis (See "Death, anaphylactic.")

Ancylostomiasis

Synonyms: Hookworm disease; miners' anemia; uncinariasis.

NOTE: (1) Collect all tissues that appear to be infected. (2) Cultures are usually not necessary, only parasitologic examination. (3) Request azure-eosin stains. (4) No special precautions are indicated. (5) Serologic studies are available at the state health department laboratories. (6) This is not a reportable disease.

Organs and Tissues	Procedures	Possible or Expected Findings
Small intestine	Request PAS with diastase treatment, azure-eosin, Perl's (or Gomori's) stain for iron, and Verhoeff– van Gieson stains.	Erosions; hemorrhages *(1)*; mucus in lumen; thickening of wall. Sprue-like mucosal changes (atrophy of villi) with deposition of hemosiderin, necrosis of mucosa, eosinophils in wall, and fibrosis of submucosa. Worms in second and third portions of jejunum.
Mesentery	Submit lymph nodes for histologic study.	Mesenteric lymphadenitis.
Liver and spleen	Submit tissue samples for histologic study.	Myeloid metaplasia.
Other organs	Procedures depend on expected findings or grossly identified abnormalities as listed in right-hand column.	Manifestations of iron deficiency anemia,* hypoproteinemia, and congestive heart failure.*

Reference

1. Kuo YC, Chen PC, Wu CS. Massive intestinal bleeding in an adult with hookworm infection. J Clin Gastroenterol 1995;20:348–350.

Anemia (See under specific designations.)

Anemia, Aplastic (See "Anemia, Fanconi's" or "pancytopenia.")

Anemia Associated With Chronic Systemic Diseases

Related Term: Normochromic normocytic anemia.

NOTE: This type of anemia occurs with chronic inflammatory conditions such as endocarditis,* osteomyelitis,* or tubercu-losis* but may also be associated with connective tissue disorders such as lupus erythematosus* or rheumatoid arthritis.* Malignancies, uremia, chronic liver disease, endocrine disorders (e.g., Adrenal insufficiency,* hypothyroidism,* or pituitary insufficiency*), or poisoning with chemicals or drugs and radiation injury may also be involved.* The anemia in some of these con-ditions may be slightly microcytic or macrocytic.

Organs and Tissues	Procedures	Possible or Expected Findings
All organs	Request iron stain.	See above under "Note." Extramedullary hematopoiesis and hemosiderosis, particularly of liver and spleen.
Bone marrow	Procure sections and smears.	Frequently hyperplastic. Hypoplastic in bone marrow failure (pancytopenia*).

Anemia, Fanconi's

Synonyms: Congenital aplastic anemia; congenital pancytopenia; constitutional infantile panmyelopathy; familial panmyelophthisis; Fanconi's pancytopenia; Fanconi's syndrome (see also under "NOTE"); pancytopenia-dysmelia syndrome.

NOTE: Another disease group, also named "Fanconi's syndrome," is marked by proximal renal tubular transport defect; this latter syndrome is unrelated to Fanconi's anemia.

Organs and Tissues	Procedures	Possible or Expected Findings
External examination	Record and photograph abnormalities. Request radiographs of skeleton.	Short stature; microcephaly; café au lait spots; dyskeratosis congenita; absent/hypoplastic thumbs; hyperpigmentation; nail dystrophy; hypogonadism; microphthalmia.
Blood, fascia lata, or liver (liver obtained by percutaneous biopsy)	These specimens should be collected using aseptic technique for tissue culture for chromosome analysis (see Chapter 9).	Chromosomal breaks.
Other organs	Culture any sites suggestive of infection. Record and photograph sites of bleeding. Record weight of spleen. Request iron stains.	Hemosiderosis. Small spleen. Small pituitary gland. Evidence of infection or hemorrhage at various sites. Solid tumors *(1)* (liver and other organs or tissues, including eyes and bones).
Bone marrow	Procure sections and smears.	Pancytopenia;* myelodysplastic syndromes and leukemia* *(1)*.
Eyes		Epiphoria, blepharitis, cataracts.

Reference

1. Alter BP. Fanconi's anemia and malignancies. Am J Hematol 1996; 53:99–110.

Anemia, Hemolytic

Synonyms and Related Terms: Acquired hemolytic anemia; extracorpuscular hemolytic anemia; hereditary hemolytic anemia (hereditary elliptocytosis, pyropoikilocytosis, stomatocytosis. spherocytosis); immunohemolytic anemia; intra-cor-puscular hemolytic anemia; microangiopathic hemolytic anemia; spur cell anemia.

Possible Associated Conditions: Disseminated intravascular coagulation;* eclampsia;* glucose-6-phosphatase deficiency (G6PD); hemolytic uremic syndrome;* malignant hypertension; lymphoma* and other malignancies; paroxysmal nocturnal hemo-globinuria; sickle cell disease;* thalassemia;* thrombotic thrombocytopenic purpura.* (See also below under "NOTE.")

NOTE: Hemolysis also may be caused by conditions such as poisoning with chemicals or drugs, heat injury, snake bite,* or infections or may develop as a transfusion reaction* or be secondary to adenocarcinoma, heart valve prostheses (see below), liver disease (see below), renal disease, or congenital erythropoietic porphyria.*

Organs and Tissues	Procedures	Possible or Expected Findings
External examination	Prepare skeletal roentgenograms.	Jaundice; skin ulcers over malleoli. In young patients: thickening of frontal and parietal bones with loss of outer table ("hair-on-end" appearance); paravertebral masses caused by extramedullary hematopoiesis; deformities of metacarpals, metatarsals, and phalanges. Osteonecrosis* of femoral heads.

Organs and Tissues	Procedures	Possible or Expected Findings
		Osteoporosis.*
Blood	In the absence of in vivo studies, submit samples for bacterial and viral cultures, or toxicologic, immunologic, or other laboratory studies, depending on the expected cause.	Bacteremia or septicemia. Viremia (e.g., parvovirus infection in hereditary spherocytosis). Chemical poisons or drugs. Beta-lipoprotein deficiency (abetalipoproteinemia*). Abnormal antibodies. Hyperbilirubinemia.
	For hemoglobin electrophoresis, autolyzed blood can be used; one can also use blood that was drained from tissues.	Abnormal hemoglobins.
Urine	See above under "Blood."	Hemoglobinuria.
Heart	Record weight. Request iron stain.	Hemosiderosis and cardiomegaly. Valvular heart disease with or without inserted prosthesis may be cause of hemolytic anemia.
Lungs	Perfuse at least one lung with formalin.	Infarcts in sickle cell disease.*
Liver	Record weight. Request iron stain.	Hemosiderosis and hepatomegaly. Extramedullary hematopoiesis. Liver diseases such as viral hepatitis* and acute fatty change may cause hemolytic anemia.
Gallbladder and common bile duct	Describe appearance of stones or request chemical analysis.	Cholelithiasis,* cholecystitis,* or choledocholithiasis associated with pigment stones (particularly in hereditary hemolytic anemia such as spherocytosis).
Spleen	See above under "Liver" and below under "Kidneys." Request iron stain.	Hemosiderosis and splenomegaly. Extramedullary hematopoiesis. Infarctions in sickle cell disease.*
Kidneys	If abnormalities are present, photograph cut sections.	Infarcts and papillary necrosis in sickle cell disease.* Renal diseases may also be cause of hemolytic anemia.
Other organs and tissues	Extensive histologic sampling is indicated, particularly if the cause of the hemolysis is not known.	See above under "Possible Associated Conditions" and under "Note." Search for fibrin deposits in microvasculature as seen in thrombotic thrombocytopenic purpura.*
Bones and bone marrow	Request Giemsa stains and Gomori's or Perl's iron stains. Consult roentgenograms for proper sampling.	Erythroid hyperplasia or, rarely, hypoplasia or normal marrow; hemosiderosis of bone marrow. Osteonecrosis* in sickle cell disease.*

Anemia, Hypochromic (See "Anemia, iron deficiency.")

Anemia, Iron Deficiency

Possible Associated Conditions: Conditions associated with blood loss (e.g., Crohn's disease;* diaphragmatic hernia,* diverticula,* malabsorption syndrome,* tumor,* ulcer of stomach or duodenum,* or ulcerative colitis); lead poisoning* in children.

Organs and Tissues	Procedures	Possible or Expected Findings
External examination	Record body weight and height. Photograph finger nails.	Manifestations of malnutrition.* Angular stomatitis; spoon nails (koilonychia).
Blood	Prepare smears.	Hypochromic and microcytic erythrocytes.
Heart		Dilatation of chambers.
Esophagus and neck organs with tongue	Remove as one specimen. Photograph web or stricture from above. Submit tissue samples of all segments for histologic study.	Glossitis; postcricoid esophageal web or stricture (Plummer-Vinson syndrome*).

Organs and Tissues	Procedures	Possible or Expected Findings
Gastrointestinal tract with anus	Search for possible source of chronic hemorrhage.	See above under "Possible Associated Conditions." Hemorrhoids.
Spleen	Record weight.	Splenomegaly.
Genitourinary system	Search for possible source of chronic hemorrhage.	Tumors or inflammatory conditions.
Other organs		Manifestations of congestive heart failure.*
Bone marrow	Request iron stain.	Hyperplasia. Reduced or absent iron in macrophages.

Anemia, Megaloblastic

Related Terms: Pernicious anemia; vitamin B_{12} deficiency.

NOTE: The condition can be caused by many disorders associated with cobalamin or folic acid deficiency (e.g., malabsorption-related); other causes include adverse drug effects, alcoholism, and rare metabolic disorders. The condition may occur in infancy or during pregnancy. Hemolytic anemia,* hypoparathyroidism,* adrenal cortical insufficiency* (Addison's disease), or scurvy may be present.

Organs and Tissues	Procedures	Possible or Expected Findings
External examination and oral cavity	Record body weight, color of skin and sclerae, and presence or absence of conditions listed in right-hand colum.	Jaundice. Manifestations of malnutrition.* Stomatitis with cheilosis and perianal ulcerations due to folic acid deficiency. Chronic exfoliative skin disorders. Vitiligo.
Blood	Prepare smears.	Macrocytosis; poikilocytosis; macroovalocytes; hypersegmentation of leukocytes; abnormal platelets.
Esophagus and neck organs with tongue	Submit tissue samples of tongue.	Atrophic glossitis with ulcers. Pharyngoesophagitis (folic acid deficiency).
Stomach	Remove and place in fixative as early as possible in order to minimize autolysis (alternatively, formalin can be injected *in situ*; see below).	Previous total or subtotal gastrectomy. Carcinoma of stomach.
	Samples should include oxyntic corpus and fundus mucosa.	Autoimmune gastritis (diffuse corporal atrophic gastritis) with intestinal metaplasia.
Intestinal tract		Crohn's disease;* sprue;* other chronic inflammatory disorders; jejunal diverticula; intestinal malignancies; fish tapeworm infestation; previous intestinal resection or blind intestinal loop; enteric fistulas.
Liver and spleen	Record weights.	Hepatosplenomegaly. Alcoholic liver disease.*
Vagina	Submit tissue samples for histologic study.	Giant epithelial cells.
Thyroid gland	Record weight of thyroid gland.	Hyperthyroid goiter; thyroiditis.
Brain, spinal cord, and peripheral nerves	For removal and specimen preparation, see Chapter 4. Request Luxol fast blue stain.	Demyelination of cerebral white matter (in advanced cases). Demyelination in posterior and lateral columns of spinal cord, most frequently in thoracic and cervical segments. Demyelination of peripheral nerves.
Eyes with optic nerves	For removal and specimen preparation, see Chapter 5. If there is a clinical diagnosis of anemia-related amblyopia, follow procedures described under "Amblyopia, nutritional."	Retinal hemorrhages; demyelination of optic nerves.
Bone marrow		Hypercellular; megaloblastic. Myeloproliferative disorder.

Anemia, Pernicious (See "Anemia, megaloblastic.")

Anemia, Sickle Cell (See "Anemia, hemolytic" and "Disease, sickle cell.")

Anencephaly

Organs and Tissues	*Procedures*	*Possible or Expected Findings*
External examination	Photograph all abnormalities.	Absence of calvarial bones; protrusion of orbits; area cerebrovasculosa (disorganized hypervascular neuroglial tissue at the base of the skull).
	Prepare full-body skeletal roentgenograms.	Delay in development of ossification centers.
Eyes	For removal and specimen preparation, see Chapter 5.	Absence of ganglion cells in retina; absence or hypoplasia of optic nerves.
Thymus, adrenals, gonads, and thyroid	Record weights. Submit tissue samples for histologic study.	Thymic and thyroid enlargement. Small adrenal glands with rudimentary fetal cortex after 20 wk gestation; small gonads.
Base of skull	Identify and record structures at base of skull.	Shallow sella turcica; small pituitary gland; hypoplastic medulla oblongata.
Lungs	Prepare histologic sections.	Aspiration of brain tissue.

Reference

1. Li WW, Lu G, Pang CP, et al. The eyes of anencephalic babies; a morphological and immunohistochemical evaluation. Int J Neurosci 2007; 117: 121–134

Anesthesia (See "Death, anesthesia-associated.")

Aneurysm, Aortic Sinus

NOTE: For general dissection techniques, see Part I, Chapter 3. Prepare sections of aorta and request Verhoeff–van Gieson stain. Rupture of aneurysm usually causes a fistula to the right ventricle or right atrium.

Possible Associated Conditions: Cystic medial degeneration of aorta; infective endocarditis;* ventricular septal defect.*

Aneurysm, Ascending Aorta

Possible Associated Conditions: History of polymyalgia rheumatica;* see also below under "Possible or Expected Findings."

Organs and Tissues	*Procedures*	*Possible or Expected Findings*
Aorta	Collect 5–6 specimens for microscopic study. Request Verhoeff–van Gieson stain.	Cystic medial degeneration; active arteritis (often giant cell type), or healed arteritis.
Muscular arteries	Collect specimens for microscopic study. Request Verhoeff–van Gieson stain.	Temporal arteritis; systemic giant cell arteritis.*

Aneurysm, Atherosclerotic Aortic

Organs and Tissues	*Procedures*	*Possible or Expected Findings*
Aorta	If aneurysm was perforated, identify location of rupture *in situ*. Record location and volume of blood in peritoneum and retroperitoneum. Transverse or longitudinal sections of aneurysms are instructive. Request Verhoeff–van Gieson stain. Decalcification may be required.	Saccular aneurysm, often inferior to origin of renal arteries. Mural thrombosis in aneurysm. Rupture into peritoneal cavity, retroperitoneum, or hollow viscus.
Kidneys	Major arteries and kidneys may be left attached to aorta.	Arterial and arteriolar nephrosclerosis. Atheromatous emboli and microinfarcts of kidneys.

Aneurysm, Atrial Septum of Heart

Synonyms: Aneurysm of valve of fossa ovalis; fossa ovalis aneurysm.

NOTE: For general dissection techniques, see Chapter 3.

Possible Associated Conditions: Patent oval foramen (patent foramen ovale).

Aneurysm, Berry (See "Aneurysm, cerebral artery.")

Aneurysm, Cerebral Artery

Related Terms: Berry aneurysm; congenital cerebral artery aneurysm.

Organs and Tissues	*Procedures*	*Possible or Expected Findings*
Brain	If mycotic aneurysms are expected and microbiologic studies are intended, follow procedures described below under "Aneurysm, mycotic aortic." Request Verhoeff–van Gieson, Gram, and Grocott's methenamine silver stains.	Mycotic aneurysms are often multiple and deep in brain substance.
	For cerebral arteriography, see Chapter 4.	
	If arteriography cannot be carried out, rinse fresh blood gently from base of brain until aneurysm can be identified. Record site of rupture and estimated amount of extravascular blood. For paraffin embedding of aneurysms, careful positioning is required.	Berry aneurysms are the most frequent types and often are multiple. Most frequent sites are the bifurcations and trifurcations of the circle of Willis. Saccular atherosclerotic aneurysms are more common than dissecting aneurysms, which are very rare.
Other organs	Expected findings depend on type of aneurysm.	With congenital cerebral artery aneurysm: coarctation of aorta;* manifestations of hypertension;* and polycystic renal disease. With mycotic aneurysm: infective endocarditis;* pulmonary suppurative processes; and pyemia.

Aneurysm, Dissecting Aortic (See "Dissection, aortic.")

Aneurysm, Membranous Septum of Heart

NOTE: For general dissection techniques, see Chapter 3. Most aneurysms of the membranous septum probably repre-sent spontaneous closure of a membranous ventricular septal defect by the septal leaflet of the tricuspid valve.

Aneurysm, Mycotic Aortic

NOTE: (1) Collect all tissues that appear to be infected. (2) Request aerobic, anaerobic, and fungal cultures. (3) Request Gram and Grocott methenamine silver stains. (4) No special precautions are indicated. (5) No serologic studies are available. (6) This is not a reportable disease.

Organs and Tissues	*Procedures*	*Possible or Expected Findings*
Chest and abdominal organs	Submit blood samples for bacterial culture. En masse removal of adjacent organs is recommended.	Septicemia and infective endocarditis.*
Aorta	Photograph all grossly identifiable lesions. Aspirate material from aneurysm or para-aortic abscess and submit for culture. Prepare sections and smears of wall of aneurysm and of aorta distant from aneurysm. Request Verhoeff–van Gieson and Gram stains.	Streptococcus, staphylococcus, spirochetes, and salmonella can be found in mycotic aneurysm. Para-aortic abscess.
Other organs		Septic emboli with infarction or abscess formation.

Aneurysm, Syphilitic Aortic

Organs and Tissues	*Procedures*	*Possible or Expected Findings*
Heart and aorta	En masse removal of organs is recommended. For coronary arteriography, see Chapter 10.	Aneurysm usually in ascending aorta. May erode adjacent bone (sternum). Syphilitic aortitis may cause intimal wrinkling, narrowing of coronary ostia, and shortening of aortic cusps.
	Request Verhoeff–van Gieson stain from sections at different levels of aorta, adjacent great vessels, and coronary arteries.	Disruption of medial elastic fibrils.
Other organs	See also under "Syphilis."	Aortic valvulitis and insufficiency;* syphilitic coronary arteritis; syphilitic myocarditis.

Aneurysm, Traumatic Aortic

Organs and Tissues	*Procedures*	*Possible or Expected Findings*
External examination		Cutaneous impact trauma.
Aorta	Prepare chest and abdominal roentgenograms. Open aorta along line of blood flow, or bisect into anterior and posterior halves. Photograph tear(s). Measure bloody effusions in body cavities. Measure or estimate amount of blood in mediastinum.	Mediastinum widened by hemorrhage in case of tamponaded dissection. A bleed into a body cavity of less-than-exsanguinating volume should point to an alternate mechanism of death such as neurogenic shock or lethal concussion; a posterior neck dissection may be required in such instances.
	Request Verhoeff–van Gieson stain.	Microscopy may show transmural rupture, false aneurysm, or localized dissection.

Angiitis (See "Arteritis, all types or type unspecified.")

Angina Pectoris

NOTE: See under "Disease, ischemic heart" and Chapter 3.

Angiokeratoma Corporis Diffusum (See "Disease, Fabry's.")

Angiomatosis, Encephalotrigeminal (See "Disease, Sturge-Weber-Dimitri.")

Angiopathy, Congophilic Cerebral

Synonyms and Related Terms: Beta amyloid angiopathy due to β-amyloid peptide deposition (β A4) (associated with Alzheimer's disease; hereditary cerebral hemorrhage with amyloid angiopathy of Dutch type; or sporadic beta amyloid angiopathy); hereditary cerebral amyloid angiopathy, due to deposition of other amyloidogenic proteins such as cystatin C (Icelandic type) and others (e.g., transthyretin, gelsolin) *(1)*.

Organs and Tissues	*Procedures*	*Possible or Expected Findings*
Brain		Multiple recent cerebral cortical infarctions or small cortical hemorrhages, or both, or massive hemispheric hemorrhages, both recent and old.
	Request stains for amyloid, particularly Congo red, and thioflavine S (examine with polarized and ultraviolet light, respectively). Request immunostain for β A4. Some tissue should be kept frozen for biochemical studies.	Amyloid deposition in leptomeninges and cortical blood vessels. Senile plaques are usually present. In some cases, angiopathy is part of Alzheimer's disease.*

Organs and Tissues	Procedures	Possible or Expected Findings
	Prepare material for electron microscopy.	Electron microscopic study permits definite confirmation of diagnosis.
Other organs		Organs and tissues may be minimally affected by amyloidosis.

Reference

1. Kalimo H, Kaste M, Haltia M. Vascular diseases. In: Greenfield's Neuropathology, vol. 1. Graham BI, Lantos PL, eds. Arnold, London, 1997, pp. 315–396.
2. Auer RN, Sutherland GR. Primary intracerebral hemorrhage: pathophysiology. Can J Neurol Sci 2005;32 Suppl 2:S3–12.

Anomaly, Coronary Artery

Possible Associated Conditions: With double outlet right ventricle; persistent truncal artery; tetralogy of Fallot;* and transposition of the great arteries.*

NOTE: Coronary artery between aorta and pulmonary artery, often with flap-valve angulated coronary ostium. Coronary artery may communicate with cardiac chamber, coronary sinus, or other cardiac veins, or with mediastinal vessel through pericardial vessel. Saccular aneurysm of coronary artery with abnor-mal flow, infective endarteritis of arteriovenous fistula, and myocardial infarction may be present. If one or both coronary arteries originate from pulmonary trunk, myocardial infarction may be present.

Organs and Tissues	Procedures	Possible or Expected Findings
Heart	Perform coronary angiography.	Ectopic origin of coronary arteries or single coronary artery.
	If infective endarteritis is suspected, submit blood sample for microbiologic study.	Sudden death. For a detailed description of possible additional findings, see above under "Note."

Anomaly, Ebstein's (See "Malformation, Ebstein's")

Anorexia Nervosa

NOTE: Sudden death from tachyarrhythmias may occur in advanced cases and thus, autopsy findings may not reveal the immediate cause of death.

Organs and Tissues	Procedures	Possible or Expected Findings
External examination	Record height and weight, and prepare photographs to show cachectic features. Record abnormalities as listed in right-hand column.	Cachexia, often with preserved breast tissue; hirsutism; dry, scaly, and yellow skin (carotenemia). Mild edema may be present. Parotid glands may be enlarged.
All organs	Follow procedures described under "Starvation." Record weight of endocrine organs and submit samples for histologic study.	Manifestations of starvation.* Ovaries tend to be atrophic; other endocrine organs should not show abnormalities.

Anthrax

Synonyms: Cutaneous anthrax; gastrointestinal anthrax; pulmonary (inhalational) anthrax.

NOTE: (1) Collect all tissues that appear to be infected. (2) Request aerobic cultures. (3) Request Gram stain. For the study of archival tissue samples, polymerase chain reaction (PCR) analysis can be attempted *(1)*. (4) Special **precautions** are indicated because the infection can be transmitted by aerosolization. (5) Serologic studies are available at the Center for Disease Control and Prevention, Atlanta, GA. (6) This is a **reportable** disease. Bioterrorism must be considered in current cases.

Organs and Tissues	Procedures	Possible or Expected Findings
External examination and skin	Photograph cutaneous papules, vesicles, and pustules. Prepare smears and histologic sections. Submit samples for bacteriologic study.	Disseminated anthrax infection may occur without skin lesions. Edema of neck and anterior chest in nasopharyngeal anthrax.
Blood	Submit sample for serologic study.	Anthrax septicemia. See above under "Note."

Organs and Tissues	Procedures	Possible or Expected Findings
Lungs	Record character and volume of effusions. After sampling for bacteriologic study (see above under "Note") perfuse one or both lungs with formalin. Extensive sampling for histologic study is indicated.	Pleural effusions;* hemorrhagic mediastinitis; anthrax pneumonia (inhalational anthrax; Woolsorter's disease). Histologic sections reveal hemorrhagic necrosis, often with minimal inflammation and gram-positive, spore-forming, encapsulated bacilli.
Gastrointestinal tracts and mesentery	Extensive sampling for histologic study is indicated.	Gastrointestinal anthrax with mucosal edema and ulcerations. Hemorrhagic mesenteric lymphadenitis.
Neck organs		Tongue, nasopharynx, and tonsils may be involved.
Brain	Photograph meningeal hemorrhage *in situ.*	Hemorrhagic meningitis (hemorrhage tends to predominate).

Reference

1. Jackson PJ, Hugh-Jones ME, Adair DM, Green G, Hill KK, Kuske CR, et al. PCR analysis of tissue samples from the 1979 Sverdlovsk anthrax victims: the presence of multiple Bacillus anthracis strains in different victims. Proc Natl Acad Sci USA 1998;95:1224–1229.

Antifreeze (See "Poisoning, ethylene glycol.")

Antimony (See "Poisoning, antimony.")

Anus, Imperforate

Related Terms: Anorectal malformation; ectopic anus.

Possible Associated Conditions: Abnormalities of sacrococcygeal vertebrae; cardiovascular malformations; esophageal and intestinal atresias,* including rectal stenosis or atresia; malformations of the urinary tract.

Organs and Tissues	Procedures	Possible or Expected Findings
External examination	Photograph perineum. Measure depth of anal pit, if any.	Absence of normally located anus; anal dimple.
Distal colon and rectum	Dissect distal colon, rectum, and perirectal pelvic organs *in situ* (as much as possible). Search for opening of fistulous tracts from lumen. Use roentgenologic study or dissection, or both, to determine course of tract.	Abnormal termination of the bowel into the trigone of the urinary bladder, the urethra distal to the verumontanum, the posterior wall of the vagina, the vulva, or the perineum.

Aortitis

NOTE: See also under "Arteritis" and "Aneurysm, ascending aortic."

Organs and Tissues	Procedures	Possible or Expected Findings
Heart and aorta	Remove heart with whole length of aorta and adjacent major arteries. Record width and circumference of aorta at different levels. Describe and photograph appearance of intima and of orifices of coronary arteries and other aortic branches.	Secondary aortic atherosclerosis or intimal fibroplasia. Widening of aorta; syphilitic aneurysm.*
	Submit multiple samples for histologic study and request Verhoeff–van Gieson stain.	Giant cell aortitis; rheumatoid aortitis; syphilitic aortitis; Takayasu's arteritis.*
Other organs and tissues	Procedures depend on expected findings or grossly identified abnormalities as listed in right-hand column.	Manifestations of rheumatoid arthritis,* syphilis,* systemic sclerosis,* Hodgkin's lymphoma, and many other diseases associated with vasculitis.

Aplasia, Thymic (See "Syndrome, primary immunodeficiency.")

Arachnoiditis, Spinal
Synonym: Chronic spinal arachnoiditis.

Organs and Tissues	*Procedures*	*Possible or Expected Findings*
External examination	Prepare roentgenogram of spine.	Signs of previous spinal surgery or lumbar puncture (myelography). Evidence of previous trauma or previous myelography.
Brain	For removal and specimen preparation, see Chapter 4.	Cerebral arachnoiditis.
Spine and spinal cord	For removal of spinal cord and specimen preparation, see Chapter 4. Expose nerve roots. Record appearance and photograph spinal cord *in situ*.	Fibrous arachnoidal adhesions and loculated cysts.
	Submit samples of spinal cord and inflamed tissue for histologic study. Request Gram, Gomori's iron, and Grocott's methenamine silver stains.	Tuberculosis;* syphilis;* fungal or parasitic infection.
Other organs	Procedures depend on expected findings or grossly identified abnormalities as listed in right-hand column.	Systemic infection (see above). Ascending urinary infection or other manifestations of paraplegia.

Arch, Aortic, Interrupted
Synonym: Severe coarctation.
NOTE: The basic anomaly is a discrete imperforate region in the aortic arch, with a patent ductal artery joining the descending thoracic aorta. Type A interruption is between the left subclavian and ductal arteries; type B between the left subclavian and left common carotid arteries; and type C (rare) between the left common carotid and brachiocephalic (innominate) arteries. For general dissection techniques, see Part I, Chapter 3.
Possible Associated Conditions: Bicuspid aortic valve (with type A); di George syndrome* with thymic and parathyroid aplasia (with type B); hypoplasia of ascending aorta (with all types); persistent truncal artery (truncus arteriosus); ventricular septal defect.

Arrhythmia, Cardiac
NOTE: See also under "Death, sudden cardiac." Toxicologic studies may be indicated, for instance, if digitalis toxicity (see "Poisoning, digitalis") is suspected. If a cardiac pacemaker had been implanted, the instrument should be tested for malfunction.

Organs and Tissues	*Procedures*	*Possible or Expected Findings*
Heart	For coronary arteriography, see Chapter 10. Dissection techniques depend on nature of expected underlying disease. Submit samples for histologic study. For study of conduction system, see Chapter 3.	Coronary atherosclerosis. Congenital heart disease. Valvular heart disease. Myocardial infarction. Myocarditis.* Cardiomyopathy.*

Arsenic (See "Poisoning, arsenic.")

Arteriosclerosis (See "Atherosclerosis.")

Arteritis, All Types or Type Unspecified
Synonyms and Related Terms: Allergic angiitis and granulomatosis (Churg-Strauss);* allergic vasculitis; anaphylactoid purpura* and its synonyms; angiitis; Buerger's disease;* cranial arteritis; giant cell arteritis;* granulomatous arteritis (angiitis); hypersensitivity angiitis; infectious angiitis; necrotizing arteritis; polyarteritis nodosa;* rheumatic arteritis; rheumatoid arteritis, syphilitic arteritis; Takayasu's arteritis;* temporal arteritis; thromboangiitis obliterans; and others (see also below under "Note").
NOTE: Autopsy procedures depend on (1) the expected type of arteritis, such as giant cell arteritis,* polyarteritis nodosa,* or thromboangiitis obliterans (Buerger's disease*); and (2) the nature of suspected associated or underlying disease, such as aortic arch syndrome,* Behçet's syndrome,* Cogan's syndrome, Degos' disease,* dermatomyositis,* erythema nodosum

and multiforme,* Goodpasture's syndrome,* polymyositis, rheumatic fever,* rheumatoid arthritis,* syphilis,* and other nonspecific infectious diseases, systemic lupus erythematosus,* systemic sclerosis (scleroderma),* or Takayasu's disease. For histologic study of blood vessels, Verhoeff–van Gieson stain or a similar stain is recommended.

Arteritis, Giant Cell

Synonyms and Related Terms: Cranial arteritis; giant cell aortitis; juvenile temporal arteritis; systemic giant cell arteritis; temporal arteritis.

Possible Associated Conditions: Polymyalgia rheumatica.

Organs and Tissues	*Procedures*	*Possible or Expected Findings*
External examination and skin	Prepare sections of skin lesions.	Skin nodules; scalp necroses.
	Record appearance of oral cavity; submit tissue samples of tongue.	Gangrene of tongue.
	Probe nasal cavity and record appearance of septum.	Perforation of nasal septum.
Heart	For coronary arteriography, see Chapter 10.	Coronary arteritis; myocardial infarction. Pericardial infiltrates.
Aorta and other elastic arteries	For angiographic procedures, see Chapter 2 and below, under "Arteritis, Takayasu's." Request Verhoeff–van Gieson stain.	Aortic dissection;* spontaneous rupture of aorta. Arteritis of aorta, aortic arch branches (carotid arteries, subclavian arteries, vertebral arteries, brachiocephalic artery) celiac, mesenteric, renal, iliac, and femoral arteries. Arteries may show aneurysms.
Lungs		Pulmonary arteritis.
Other organs		Giant cell arteritis may occur in many organs and tissues.
Brain and spinal cord	For removal and specimen preparation, see Chapter 4.	Cerebral infarctions.
Temporal and ophthalmic arteries	Expose temporal and ophthalmic arteries; prepare histologic sections.	Temporal and ophthalmic arteritis.
Eyes	For removal and specimen preparation, see Chapter 5.	Arteritis of ciliary and retinal vessels.
Skeletal muscles		Clinically, polymyalgia.
Bone marrow	For preparation of sections and smears, see Chapter 2.	Anemia.

Arteritis, Takayasu's

Synonyms: Aortic arch syndrome; pulseless disease.

Organs and Tissues	*Procedures*	*Possible or Expected Findings*
External examination		Facial muscular atrophy and pigmentation.
Heart, aorta, and adjacent great vessels	For *in situ* aortography, clamp distal descending thoracic aorta and neck vessels as distal as possible from takeoff at aortic arch.	Narrowing at origin of brachiocephalic arteries.
	Remove heart together with aorta and long sleeves of neck vessels. For coronary arteriography, see Chapter 10 (method designed to show coronary ostia).	Dilated ascending aorta. Narrowing of coronary arteries at origins. Myocardial infarction.
	Test competence of aortic valve.	Aortic insufficiency.*
	Open aortic arch anteriorly and measure (with calipers) lumen at origin of great neck vessels.	
	Photograph aorta and neck vessels and submit samples for histologic study. Request Verhoeff–van Gieson stain.	Aortic atherosclerosis. Thromboses of brachiocephalic arteries. Giant cell arteritis.*
Kidney	Submit tissue for histologic examination.	Diffuse mesangial proliferative glomeulonephritis *(1)*.
Eyes and optic nerve	For removal and specimen preparation, see Chapter 5.	Atrophy of optic nerve, retina, and iris; cataracts; retinal pigmentation.
Brain	For removal and specimen preparation, see Chapter 4.	Ischemic lesions.

Reference

1. de Pable P, Garcia-Torres R, Uribe N, et al. Kidney involvement in Takayasu arteritis. Clin Exp Rheumatol 2007;25:S10–14.

Artery, Patent Ductal

Synonym: Patent ductus arteriosus.

NOTE: The basic anomaly is persistent postnatal patency of the ductal artery, usually as an isolated finding (in 75% of cases in infants, and in 95% in adults). It is more common in premature than full-term infants and at high altitudes than at sea level. Possible complications in unoperated cases include congestive heart failure,* plexogenic pulmonary hypertension,* ductal artery aneurysm or rupture, fatal pulmonary embolism,* or sudden death. In some conditions, such as aortic atresia* or transposition with an intact ventricular septum,* ductal patency may be necessary for survival.

Possible Associated Conditions: Atrial or ventricular septal defect;* coarctation of the aorta;* conotruncal anomalies; necrotizing enterocolitis in premature infants; postrubella syndrome; and valvular or vascular obstructions.

Artery, Persistent Truncal

Synonym and Related Terms: Type 1, pulmonary arteries arise from single pulmonary trunk (in 55%); type 2, pulmonary arteries arise separately but close-by (in 35%); type 3, pulmonary arteries arise separately but distal from one another (in 10%).

NOTE: The basic anomaly is a common truncal artery, with truncal valve, giving rise to aorta, pulmonary arteries, and coronary arteries, usually with a ventricular septal defect. Interventions include complete Rastelli-type repair, with closure of ventricular septal defect, and insertion of valved extracardiac conduit between right ventricle and detached pulmonary arteries.

Possible Associated Conditions: Absent pulmonary artery (in 15%); atrial septal defect (in 15%); absent ductal artery (in 50%); coronary ostial anomalies (in 40%); Di George syndrome;* double aortic arch; extracardiac anomalies (in 25%); interrupted aortic arch* (in 15%); right aortic arch (in 30%); truncal valve insufficiency (uncommon) or stenosis (rare); trun-cal valve with three (in 70%), four (in 20%), or two (in 10%) cusps.

Organs and Tissues	*Procedures*	*Possible or Expected Findings*
Heart and great vessels	If infective endocarditis is suspected, follow culture procedures for endocardial vegetation described in Chapter 10.	Infective endocarditis,* usually of truncal valve. Late postoperative conduit obstruction. Postoperative late progressive truncal artery dilation with truncal valve insufficiency.
Lungs	Request Verhoeff–van Gieson stain.	Hypertensive pulmonary vascular disease.
Brain		Cerebral abscess,* if right-to-left-shunt was present.

Arthritis, All Types or Type Unspecified

NOTE: For extra-articular changes, see under the name of the suspected underlying conditions. Infectious diseases that may be associated with arthritis include bacillary dysentery,* brucellosis,* gonorrhea, rubella,* syphilis,* tuberculosis,* typhoid fever,* and varicella.* Noninfectious diseases in this category include acromegaly,* Behçet's syndrome,* Felty's syndrome,* gout,* rheumatoid arthritis,* and many others, too numerous to mention.

Organs and Tissues	*Procedures*	*Possible or Expected Findings*
Joints	Remove synovial fluid and prepare smears. Submit synovial fluid for microbiologic and chemical study. For removal of joints, prosthetic repair, and specimen preparation, see Chapter 2.	In suppurative arthritis, organisms most frequently involved are *Streptococcus hemolyticus*, *Staphylococcus aureus*, *Pneumococcus*, and *Meningococcus*.

Arthritis, Juvenile Rheumatoid

Synonym: Juvenile chronic arthritis; Still's disease.

NOTE: Involvement of more than five joints defines the polyarticular variant of the disease.

Possible Associated Condition: Amyloidosis.*

Organs and Tissues	*Procedures*	*Possible or Expected Findings*
External examination and skin	Submit samples of skin or subcutaneous lesions.	Rheumatoid nodules.
	Prepare skeletal roentgenograms.	Monarthritis or polyarthritis; abnormalities of bone, cartilage, and periosteal growth adjacent to inflamed joint(s). Osteoporosis.*

Organs and Tissues	Procedures	Possible or Expected Findings
		In the polyarticular variant, facial asymmetry may be noted.
Blood	Submit samples for serologic study and for microbiologic study.	Rheumatoid factor positive in some cases.
Heart		Pericarditis.*
Lungs	Perfuse at least one lung with formalin; submit one lobe for microbiologic study.	Interstitial pneumonitis; pleuritis. (See also under "Arthritis, rheumatoid.")
Lymph nodes	Submit samples for histologic study; record average size.	Lymphadenopathy.
Spleen	Record size and weight; submit samples for histologic study.	Splenomegaly.
Bones and joints	For removal, prosthetic repair, and specimen preparation, see Chapter 2. Include joints of cervical spine and sacroiliac joints.	Monarthritis or severe, erosive polyarthritis; see also under "Arthritis, rheumatoid" and above under "External examination and skin." Ankylosing spondylitis* may be present.
Eyes	For removal and specimen preparation, see Chapter 5.	Chronic iridocyclitis.
Other organs and tissues		See "Arthritis, rheumatoid."

Arthritis, Rheumatoid

Synonyms and Related Terms: Ankylosing spondylitis;* Felty's syndrome;* juvenile rheumatoid arthritis* (Still's disease); rheumatoid disease; and others.

Possible Associated Conditions: Amyloidosis;* polymyositis (dermatomyositis*); psoriasis;* Sjögren's syndrome;* systemic lupus erythematosus;* systemic vasculitis, and others.

Organs and Tissues	Procedures	Possible or Expected Findings
External examination and skin	Record character and extent of skin and nail changes. Prepare sections of normal and abnormal skin and of subcutaneous nodules.	Subcutaneous rheumatoid nodules on elbows, back, areas overlying ischial and femoral tuberosities, heads of phalangeal and metacarpal bones, and occiput.
	Prepare skeletal roentgenograms.	Deformities and subluxation of peripheral joints (see also below under "Joints"). Subaxial dislocation of cervical spine may be cause of sudden death.
Pleural cavities	Prepare chest roentgenogram.	Pneumothorax;* pleural empyema.*
Thymus	Record weight. Submit samples for histologic study.	T-cell abnormalities *(1)*.
Blood	Submit samples for microbiologic study.	Bacteremia.
	Keep frozen sample for serologic or immunologic study.	Positive rheumatoid factor.
Heart and blood vessels	Perform coronary arteriography. Open heart in direction of blood flow. Submit specimens with blood vessels from all organs and tissues.	Rheumatoid granulomas in myocardium (septum), pericardium, and at base of aortic and mitral valves; constrictive pericarditis;* aortic stenosis;* coronary arteritis. Systemic vasculitis (arteritis*).
Lungs	Record weights. Submit one lobe for microbiologic study. For pulmonary arteriography and bronchography, see Chapter 2. For perfusion-fixation, see Chapter 2.	Rheumatoid granulomas in pleura and lung (with pneumoconiosis*); bronchopleural fistula; rheumatoid pneumonia with interstitial pulmonary fibrosis and honeycombing; bronchiectasis;* bronchiolitis with cystic changes; pulmonary arteritis. Pneumoconiosis* in Caplan's syndrome.*
Esophagus	Record width of lumen.	Dilatation.
Stomach	Submit samples for histologic study.	Mucosal atrophy in Sjögren's syndrome.*
Mesentery and intestine	For mesenteric angiography, see Chapter 2.	Mesenteric vasculitis (acute necrotizing

Organs and Tissues	Procedures	Possible or Expected Findings
	Submit samples from mesenteric vessels for histologic study.	arteritis; subacute arteritis; arterial thrombosis; venulitis) and intestinal infarctions.
Spleen	Record weight.	Splenomegaly; rupture of spleen *(2)*.
Adrenals		Cortical atrophy.
Lymph nodes	Submit samples of axillary, cervical, mediastinal, and retroperitoneal lymph nodes for histologic study.	Lymphadenopathy.
Neck organs Sjögren's	In patients with suspected Sjögren's syndrome,* snap-freeze sample of salivary (submaxillary) gland for immunofluorescent study.	Atrophic sialadenitis with salivary gland atrophy and atrophy of taste buds in syndrome.*
	Search for evidence of upper airway obstruction. Submit samples of base of tongue, thyroid gland, cricoarytenoid joints, and paralaryngeal soft tissues for histologic study.	Hashimoto's struma; cricoarytenoid arthritis. Rheumatoid granulomas in paralaryngeal soft tissues.
Brain, spinal cord, and pituitary gland	For removal and specimen preparation, see Chapter 4.	Rheumatoid granulomas in dura mater and in leptomeninges of brain and spinal canal. Cerebral vasculitis and microinfarcts. Spinal cord compression after cervical subluxation (see above under "External examination and skin").
Eyes and lacrimal glands	For removal and specimen preparation, see Chapter 5.	Uveitis and scleritis. Dacryosial adenitis.
Middle ears	For removal and specimen preparation, see Chapter 4. If patient had a hearing problem, prepare sections of incudomalleal joints.	Rheumatoid arthritis of joints of middle ear ossicles.
Joints	Remove synovial fluid from affected joints for microbiologic study.	Bacterial arthritis.
	For removal, prosthetic repair, and specimen preparation, see Chapter 2. Remove peripheral diarthroidial joints together with synovia, adjacent tendons, adjacent bones, and bursae. Snap-freeze synovial tissue for fluorescent microscopic and histochemical study.	Destructive rheumatoid arthritis; rheumatoid tenosynovitis (particularly tendon of flexor digitorum profundus muscle); synovial outpouchings; subluxations; osteoporosis* with pseudocysts; bursitis with "rice bodies."
Skeletal muscles		Lymphorrhagia; perivascular nodular myositis; vasculitis.
Bone marrow		Megaloblastic changes; normoblastic hypoplasia; relative plasmacytosis; hemosiderosis.
External examination	Record and photograph all contractures.	Contractures. Facial anomalies, such as

References

1. Weyand CM, Goronzy JJ. Pathogenesis of rheumatoid arthritis. Med Clin North Am 1997;81:29–55.
2. Fishman D, Isenberg DA. Splenic involvement in rheumatic diseases. Semin Arthr Rheum 1997;27:141–155.

Arthrogryposis Multiplex Congenita

Synonyms and Related Terms: Congenital contractures; amyoplasia *(1)*; congenital muscular dystrophy; fetal akinesia/hypokinesia sequence.

NOTE:

Arthrogryposis *(2)* may be a primary muscle disease, or it may involve abnormalities of the brain, spinal cord, and/or peripheral nerves. Etiologies are numerous, as are the modes of inheritance. Critical to making the appropriate diagnosis is the collection of muscles from various sites for routine histology, muscle histochemistry, and electron microscopy. Portions of peripheral motor nerves must also be prepared for histology and electron microscopy.

Organs and Tissues	Procedures	Possible and Expected Findings
External examination	Obtain routine external measurements and body weight. Prepare full body radiographs.	Hypertelorism, telecanthus, epicanthal folds, malformed ears, small mouth, micrognathia.
Lungs	Record weights; perfuse one or both lungs with formalin and submit samples for histologic study.	Pulmonary hypoplasia.
Muscles	Snap freeze at –70°C at least four muscle groups (e.g., quadriceps, biceps, psoas, diaphragm) for histochemical study. Submit sections in glutaraldehyde and formalin for electron microscopy and histologic study, respectively. For specimen preparation see also Chapter 4.	Fiber type disproportion; myofiber hypoplasia; fatty replacement; fibrosis.
Nerves	Submit segments of peripheral motor nerves for electron microscopy and histologic study. Request Luxol fast blue stain for myelin.	Hypomyelination of nerves.
Brain and spinal cord		Polymicrogyria, cortical white matter dysplasia, variable decrease of anterior horn cells; increased numbers of abnormally small anterior horn cells.
Placenta		Short umbilical cord.

References

1. Sawark JF, MacEwen GD, Scott CI. Amyoplasia (A common form of arthrogryposis). J Bone Joint S 1990;72:465–469.
2. Banker BQ. Arthrogryposis multiplex congenita: spectrum of pathologic changes. Hum Path 1986;17:656–672.
3. Mennen U, van Heest A, Ezaki MD, et al. Arthrogryposis multiplex congenita. J Hand Surg [Br] 2005;30:468–474.

Asbestosis (See "Pneumoconiosis.")

Ascites, Chylous

Organs and Tissue	Procedures	Possible or Expected Findings
Abdominal cavity	Puncture abdominal cavity and submit fluid for microbiologic study.	
	Record volume of exudate or transudate and submit sample for determination of fat and cholesterol content.	For interpretation of chemical analysis, see "Chylothorax."
	Prior to routine dissection, lymphangiography (see below) may be indicated.	Lymphoma and other retroperitoneal neoplasms; surgical trauma; intestinal obstruction.
Intra-abdominal lymphatic system	For lymphangiography, see Chapter 2. Cannulate lymphatics as distally as possible.	Ruptured chylous cyst; intestinal lymphangiectasia and other malformations of lymph vessels. See also above under "Abdominal cavity."

Aspergillosis

Related Term: Allergic bronchopulmonary aspergillosis.

NOTE: (1) Collect all tissues that appear to be infected. (2) Request fungal cultures. (3) Request Grocott's methenamine silver stain. (4) No special precautions are indicated. (5) Serologic studies are available in local and state health department laboratories. (6) This is not a reportable disease.

Possible Associated Conditions: With pulmonary aspergillosis—bronchiectasis;* bronchocentric granulomatosis;* sarcoidosis;* tuberculosis.* With systemic aspergillosis—leukemia;* lymphoma;* and other conditions complicated by immunosuppression *(1,2)*.

Organs and Tissues	Procedures	Possible or Expected Findings
Lungs	Carefully make multiple parasagittal sections through the unperfused lungs. Culture areas of consolidation. If diagnosis was confirmed, perfuse lungs with formalin. Prepare histologic sections from walls of cavities, cavity contents, and pneumonic infiltrates.	Bronchiectasis;* tumor cavities; cysts.*(4)* Fungus ball may be present in any of these.
Other organs	Procedures depend on expected findings or grossly identified abnormalities as listed in right-hand column.	Suppuration and necrotic lesions from disseminated aspergillosis in heart *(3)*, brain *(1)*, bones *(1,2)*, and other organs *(3)*.

References

1. The W, Matti BS, Marisiddaiah H, Minamoto GY. Aspergillus sinusitis in patients with AIDS: report of three cases and review. Clin Infect Dis 1995;21:529–535.
2. Gonzales-Crespo MR, Gomes-Reino JJ. Invasive aspergillosis in systemic lupus erythematosus. Semin Arthritis Rheum 1995;24: 304–314.
3. Sergi C, Weitz J, Hofmann WJ, Sinn P, Eckart A, Otto G, et al. Aspergillus endocarditis, myocarditis and pericarditis complicating necrotizing fasciitis. Case report and subject review. Virchows Arch 1996;429:177–180.
4. Al-Alawi A, Ryan CF, Flint JD, et al. Aspergillus-related lung disease. Can Respir J 2005;12:377–387.

Asphyxia **(See "Hypoxia.")**

Aspiration **(See "Obstruction, acute airway.")**

Assault

NOTE: All procedures described under "Homicide" must be followed.

Asthma

NOTE: Spray death* may occur in asthma sufferers from pressurized aerosol bronchodilators.

Organs and Tissues	Procedures	Possible or Expected Findings
External examination and skin	Record appearance of skin and conjunctivae. Palpate subcutaneous tissue to detect evidence of crepitation.	Eczema. Conjunctival hemorrhages and subcutaneous emphysema may be present after fatal attack.
Chest	Prepare chest roentgenogram. For tests for pneumothorax, see under that heading.	Pneumothorax;* mediastinal emphysema. Low diaphragm (see below).
Blood	Submit sample for biochemical study.	Increased IgE concentrations in fatal asthma; postmortem tryptase determination is of doubtful value in this regard *(1)*.
Diaphragm	Record thickness and position.	Hypertrophy. Low position of diaphragm.
Lungs	Perfuse one lung with formalin. Because mucous plugs may block bronchial tree, attach perfusion apparatus to pulmonary artery or to bronchus and pulmonary artery. Monitor perfusion to ensure proper inflation. Prepare photograph of fixed cut section. Submit samples of pulmonary parenchyma and bronchi for histologic study. Request azure-eosin and Verhoeff–van Gieson stains.	Hyperinflated lungs. Thick-walled bronchi with prominent viscid mucous plugs. Typical microscopic inflammatory changes *(2)*. Asthmatic bronchitis with eosinophilic infiltrates. Bronchocentric granulomatosis.* Pulmonary atherosclerosis with breakup of elastic fibers. Paucity of ecosinophils in mucous *(6)*.
Heart	Record weight and thickness of walls.	Cor pulmonale.
Esophagus	Leave attached to stomach.	Reflux esophagitis *(3)*.
Stomach and duodenum		Peptic ulcer.*
Intestine	Photograph and submit samples for histologic study.	Pneumatosis of small intestine; emphysema of colon.
Liver		Centrilobular congestion and necrosis.

Organs and Tissues	*Procedures*	*Possible and Expected Findings*
Kidneys	Record weights. Submit samples of both kidneys for histologic study.	Kidneys and glomeruli may be enlarged.
Neck organs	Submit samples of larynx and trachea for histologic study. Request azure-eosin stains.	Laryngitis and tracheitis.
Brain and spinal cord		Petechial hemorrhages in hypothalamus; necrosis of cerebellar folia; anoxic changes in cortex, globus pallidus, thalamus, Sommer's sector of hippocampus, and Purkinje cells of cerebellum. Suspected changes in anterior horn cells of spinal cord in patients with asthma-associated poliomyelitis-like illness (Hopkins syndrome) *(4)*.
Nasal cavities	Submit samples of mucosa and polyps for histologic study. Request azure-eosin stains.	Allergic polyps and other allergic inflammatory changes *(5)*.
Bone marrow	Prepare sections and smears.	Increased erythropoiesis.

References

1. Salkie ML, Mitchell I, Revers CW, Karkhanis A, Butt J, Tough S, Green FH. Postmortem serum levels of tryptase and total and specific IgE in fatal asthma. Allergy Asthma Proc 1998;19:131–133.
2. Hogg JC. The pathology of asthma. APMIS 1997;105:735–745.
3. Sontag SJ. Gastroesophageal reflux and asthma. Am J Med 1997;103: 84S–90S.
4. Mizuno Y, Komori S, Shigetomo R, Kurihara E, Tamagawa K, Komiya K. Polyomyelitis-like illness after acute asthma (Hopkins syndrome): a histological study of biopsied muscle in a case. Brain Dev 1995; 17:126–129.
5. Glovsky MM. Upper airway involvement in bronchial asthma. Curr Opin Pulm Med 1998;4:54–58.
6. Halder P, Pavord ID. Noneosinophilic asthma: a distinct clinical and pathologic phenotype. J Allergy Clin Immunol 2007;119:1043–1052.

Ataxia, Friedreich's (See "Degeneration, spinocerebellar.")

Atherosclerosis

Synonyms and Related Terms: Arteriosclerosis obliterans.

Organs and Tissues	*Procedures*	*Possible or Expected Findings*
Arteries	For grading of atherosclerotic lesions, see Chapter 3. For angiographic techniques, see under affected organ in Chapter 2.	Atherosclerotic aneurysm.*
Other organs		Manifestations of vascular occlusions, such as infarctions and gangrene. Manifestations of diabetes mellitus.*

Atresia, Anal and Rectal (See "Anus, imperforate.")

Atresia, Aortic Valvular

Synonym: Aortic atresia; aortic atresia with intact ventricular septum; hypoplastic left heart syndrome.

NOTE: The basic anomaly is an imperforate aortic valve, with secondary hypoplasia of left-sided chambers and ascending aorta. For possible surgical interventions, see two-stage Norwood and modified Fontan procedures in Chapter 3.

Possible Associated Conditions: Atrial septal defect* (or patent foramen ovale, usually restrictive); dilatation of myocardial sinusoids that communicate with coronary vessels; dilatation of right atrium, right ventricle, and pulmonary trunk; fibroelastosis of left atrial and left ventricular endocardium; hypertrophy of ventricular and atrial walls; hypoplastic left atrium, mitral valve, left ventricle, and ascending aorta; mitral atresia* with minute left ventricle; patent ductal artery (ductus arteriosus); small left ventricle with hypertrophic wall; tubular hypoplasia of aortic arch, with or without discrete coarctation.

Atresia, Biliary

Synonyms and Related Terms: Congenital biliary atresia; extrahepatic biliary atresia; infantile obstructive cholangiopathy; syndromic (Alagille's syndrome) or nonsyndromic paucity of intrahepatic bile ducts ("intrahepatic" biliary atresia).

Possible Associated Conditions: Alpha$_1$-antitrypsin deficiency;* choledochal cyst;* congenital rubella syndrome;* polysplenia syndrome* *(1)*; small bowel atresia; trisomy 17–18; trisomy 21; Turner's syndrome;* viral infections (cytomegalovirus infection;* rubella*).

Organs and Tissues	*Procedures*	*Possible or Expected Findings*
External examination		Jaundice.
Blood	Submit samples for serologic or microbiologic study.	Congenital rubella and other viral infections.
	Submit sample of serum for determination of alpha$_1$-antitrypsin concentrations. Submit sample for chromosomal analysis.	Alpha$_1$-Antitrypsin deficiency;* defects in bile acid synthesis. Chromosomal abnormalities.
Extrahepatic bile ducts and liver	After removal of small and large bowel, open duodenum anteriorly. Squeeze gallbladder and record whether bile appeared at papilla. For cholangiography, see Chapter 2.	In atresia of the hepatic duct, the gallbladder will be empty. In isolated atresia of the common bile duct, the gallbladder contains bile but it cannot be squeezed into the duodenum.
	Dissect extrahepatic bile ducts *in situ* or leave hepatoduodenal ligament intact for later fixation and sectioning (see below). Record appearance and contents of gallbladder and course of cystic duct.	Atresia or hypoplasia of bile duct(s); choledochal cyst(s).
	In postoperative cases, submit sample of anastomosed hepatic hilar tissue for demonstration of microscopic bile ducts.	Biliary drainage created by Kasai operation.
	Remove liver with hepatoduodenal ligament.	
	Prepare horizontal sections through ligament and submit for histologic identification of ducts or duct remnants.	Obliterative cholangiopathy *(2)*.
	Prepare frontal slices of liver and sample for histologic study. Request PAS stain with diastase digestion.	Intrahepatic cholelithiasis; postoperative ascending cholangitis; secondary biliary cirrhosis; giant cell transformation; paucity of intrahepatic bile ducts. PAS-positive inclusions in alpha$_1$-antitrypsin deficiency.*
Other organs	Procedures depend on expected findings or grossly identified abnormalities as listed in right-hand column.	Polysplenia syndrome* *(1)* with malrotation, situs inversus, preduodenal portal vein, absent inferior vena cava, anomalous hepatic artery supply, and cardiac defects. For other abnormalities outside the biliary tree, see under "Possible Associated Conditions"). Nephromegaly *(3)*.

References

1. Vazquez J, Lopex Gutierrez JC, Gamez M, Lopez-Santamaria M, Murcia J, Larrauri J, et al. Biliary atresia and the polysplenia syndrome: its impact on final outcome. J Pediatr Surg 1995;30:485–487.
2. Lefkowitch JH. Biliary atresia. Mayo Clin Proc 1998;73:90–95.
3. Tsau YK, Chen CH, Chang MH, Teng RJ, Lu MY, Lee PI. Nephromegaly and elevated hepatocyte growth factor in children with biliary atresia. Am J Kidney Dis 1997;29:188–192.

Atresia, Cardiac Valves (See "Atresia, aortic valvular," "Atresia, mitral valvular," "Atresia pulmonary valvular, with intact ventricular septum," "Atresia, pulmonary valvular, with ventricular septal defect," and "Atresia, tricuspid valvular.")

Atresia, Duodenal

Possible Associated Conditions: With membranous obstruction of the duodenum—annular pancreas; atresia of esophagus* with tracheoesophageal fistula; congenital heart disease; cystic fibrosis;* Down's syndrome;* Hirschsprung's disease; imperforate anus* or other congenital obstructions of the intestinal tract *(1)*; intestinal malrotation; lumbosacral, rib-, and digit/limb anomalies; single umbilical artery; spinal defects; undescended testis *(1)*.

NOTE:
See also under "Atresia, small intestinal."

Organs and Tissues	*Procedures*	*Possible or Expected Findings*
Fascia lata, blood, or liver	Obtain cells for tissue culture for karyotype analysis.	Trisomy 21 and other aneuploidies.
Duodenum	Photograph and dissect organ *in situ*. Inflate duodenum with formalin; open only after fixation. For mesenteric angiography, see Chapter 2.	Fibrous membrane across lumen of intact duodenum. Septum may have orifice so that duodenal stenosis results. Rarely, fusiform narrowing.
Other organs		See above under "Possible Associated Findings."

Reference

1. Kimble RM, Harding J, Kolbe A. Additional congenital anomalies in babies with gut atresia or stenosis: when to investigate, and which investigation. Pediatr Surg Intl 1997;12:565–570.

Atresia, Esophageal

Possible Associated Condition: Congenital rubella syndrome;* VACTERL syndrome (Vertebral anomalies, Anal atresia, Cardiovascular anomalies, Tracheo-Esophageal fistula, Rib anomalies, Limb anomalies) *(1)*.

Organs and Tissues	*Procedures*	*Possible or Expected Findings*
External examination		Limb anomalies.
Chest organs	Photograph the atresia prior to opening the esophagus. Open the esophagus posteriorly or the trachea anteriorly for best visualization.	Tracheoesophageal fistula or tracheoesophageal atresia; cardiac, rib, and vertebral anomalies.
Abdominal organs	Photograph all anomalies. Procedures depend on expected findings or grossly identified abnormalities as listed in right-hand column.	Renal agenesis or dysplasia; anal atresia; duodenal or other small intestinal atresia;* lumbosacral anomalies; undescended testis *(2)*.

References

1. Perel Y, Butenandt O, Carrere A, Saura R, Fayon M, Lamireau T, Vergnes P. Oesophageal atresia, VACTERL association: Fanconi's anemia related spectrum of anomalies. Arch Dis Child 1998;78:375–376.
2. Kimble RM, Harding J, Kolbe A. Additional congenital anomalies in babies with gut atresia or stenosis: when to investigate, and which investigation. Pediatr Surg Intl 1997;12:565–570.

Atresia, Mitral Valvular

Synonym: Congenital mitral atresia.

NOTE: For general dissection techniques, see Chapter 3.

Possible Associated Conditions: Aortic valvular hypoplasia or atresia;* closed foramen ovale with anomalous venous channel (levoatriocardinal vein) connecting left atrium with left innominate vein; patent foramen ovale; transposition of great arteries associated with single functional ventricle;* ventricular septal defect(s).*

Atresia, Pulmonary Valvular, With Intact Ventricular Septum

NOTE: The basic anomaly is an imperforate pulmonary valve, with a hypoplastic right ventricle. In unoperated cases, ductal closure is the most common cause of death. For possible surgical interventions, see modified Blalock-Taussig shunt, mod-ified Fontan procedure, and pulmonary valvulotomy in Chapter 3. For general dissection techniques, see Chapter 3.

Possible Associated Conditions: Dilated myocardial sinusoids that may communicate with epicardial coronary arteries or veins; patent ductal artery (ductus arteriosus); patent oval foramen (foramen orale); tricuspid atresia with minute right ven-tricle; tricuspid stenosis with hypoplastic right ventricle (in 95%); tricuspid insufficiency with dilated right ventricle (in 5%).

Atresia, Pulmonary Valvular, With Ventricular Septal Defect

Synonym: Tetralogy of Fallot with pulmonary atresia.

NOTE: The basic anomaly is atresia of the pulmonary valve and of variable length of pulmonary artery, and ventricular septal defect (membranous or outlet type), with overriding aorta, and with pulmonary blood supply from ductal or systemic collateral arteries. For possible surgical interventions, see Rastelli-type repair and unifocalization of multiple collateral arteries in Chapter 3.

Possible Associated Conditions: Right ventricular outflow tract a short blind-ended pouch (70%) or absent (30%); atresia of pulmonary artery bifurcation, with nonconfluent pulmonary arteries; right aortic arch (40%); atrial septal defect (50%); persistent left superior vena cava; anomalous pulmonary venous connection; tricuspid stenosis or atresia; complete atrioventricular septal defect; transposed great arteries; double inlet left ventricle; asplenia, polysplenia, or velocardiofacial syndromes; dilated ascending aorta, with aortic insufficiency.

Atresia, Small Intestinal

Related Term: Jejuno-ileal atresia.

Possible Associated Findings: Esophageal atresia* with tracheoesophageal fistula; lumbosacral, rib-, or digit/limb anom-alies; undescended testes *(1)*.

NOTE: See also under "Atresia, duodenal."

Organs and Tissues	*Procedures*	*Possible or Expected Findings*
Fascia lata, blood, or liver	These specimens should be collected using aseptic technique for tissue culture for chromosome analysis (see Chapter 9).	Trisomy 21.
Intestinal tract	For mesenteric angiography, see Chapter 2. Leave mesentery attached to small bowel, particularly to the atretic portion.	Multiple atresias; proximal dilatation; volvulus; malrotation; meconium impaction; other evidence of cystic fibrosis. Anorectal malformation *(1)*.
Pancreas		Annular pancreas *(1)*.

Reference

1. Kimble RM, Harding J, Kolbe A. Additional congenital anomalies in babies with gut atresia or stenosis: when to investigate, and which investigation. Pediatr Surg Intl 1997;12:565–570.

Atresia, Tricuspid Valvular

NOTE: The basic anomaly is an absent right atrioventricular connection (85%) or imperforate tricuspid valve (15%), with a hypoplastic right ventricle (100%), muscular ventricular septal defect (90%) that is restrictive (85%), and a patent oval foramen (80%) or secundum atrial septal defect (20%). For possible surgical interventions, see modified Fontan or Glenn procedures in Chapter 3. For general dissection techniques, see Chapter 3.

Possible Associated Conditions: Juxtaposed atrial appendages; large left ventricular valvular orifice; large left ventricular chamber; persistent left superior vena cava; pulmonary atresia; transposition of the great arteries (25%), with aortic co-arctation (35% of those); anomalies of musculoskeletal or digestive systems (20%); Down's,* asplenia, or other syndromes.

Atresia, Urethral

Organs and Tissues	*Procedures*	*Possible or Expected Findings*
Pelvic organs	Prepare urogram. Leave ureters and kidneys attached to bladder. Open penile urethra (see Figs. 2-14). Search for fistulas. If there is evidence of drainage via the urachus, demonstrate this before removal of pelvic organs.	Posterior urethral valves; strictures; absence of canalization of penile urethra; dilated bladder; hypoplastic prostate; hydroureters and hydronephrosis;* renal cystic dysplasia; fistulas to rectum or via urachus to umbilicus. Ascites with attenuation of anterior abdominal wall; cryptorchidism.

Atrial Septal Defect (See "Defect, atrial septal.")

Atrium, Common (See "Defect, atrial septal.")

Atrophy, Multiple System

Synonyms and Related Terms: Olivopontocerebellar atrophy, Shy-Drager syndrome, striatonigral degeneration.

Organs and Tissues	*Procedures*	*Possible or Expected Findings*
Brain, spinal cord, and paraspinal sympathetic chain	Modified Bielschowsky, Bodian or Gallyas silver stains are necessary to highlight the characteristic glial cytoplasmic inclusions.	Cell loss and gliosis with characteristic cytoplasmic and nuclear glial and neuronal inclusions and neuropil threads in affected areas. Clinical subtype and duration of illness influence distribution of lesions. Involved

Organs and Tissues	*Procedures*	*Possible or Expected Findings*
	Record pallor of white matter tracts related to neuronal loss in affected areas. This can be seen especially in external capsule, striatopallidal fibers, cerebellar white matter, cerebellar peduncles and transverse pontine fibers. Immunostain for synuclein is positive in inclusions.	areas include: putamen, especially dorso-lateral, substantia nigra, locus coeruleus, cerebellar cortex (Purkinje's cells), basis pontis, inferior olive, dorsal motor nucleus of vagus, intermediolateral column of spinal cord.

Atrophy, Pick's Lobar (See "Disease, Pick's.")

Atrophy, Progressive Spinal Muscular (See "Disease, motor neuron.")

Atropine (See "Poisoning, atropine.")

Attack, Transient Cerebral Ischemic

Synonyms and Related Terms: Cerebrovascular disease; transient cerebral ischemia; transient stroke.

Organs and Tissues	*Procedures*	*Possible or Expected Findings*
Heart	If infective endocarditis* is suspected, culture using the method described in Chapter 7.	Vegetative endocarditis; mural cardiac thromboses.
Aorta and cervical arteries	For dissection of carotid and vertebral arteries, see Chapter 4.	Aortic, carotid, and vertebral atherosclerosis (see also under "Infarction, cerebral"). Atherosclerotic or other type of stenosis of subclavian artery proximal to takeoff of vertebral artery (subclavian steal syndrome).
Brain	For removal and specimen preparation, and cerebral anteriography, see Chapter 4.	Basilar atherosclerosis.

Avitaminosis (See "Deficiency, vitamin...")

B

Bagassosis (See "Pneumoconiosis.")

Barbiturate(s) (See "Poisoning, barbiturate(s).")

Baritosis (See "Pneumoconiosis.")

Bartonellosis

Synonyms and Related Terms: Bacillary angiomatosis *(1)*; *Bartonella bacilliformis, henselae*, or *quintana* infection; Carrión's disease; cat scratch disease *(1)*;* Oroya fever; Peruvian anemia; verruga peruana.

NOTE: (1) Collect all tissues that appear to be infected. (2) Organisms are usually demonstrated by direct stains rather than by culture. Detection by polymerase chain reaction (PCR) is possible *(2)*. (3) Request Giemsa stains. (4) No special precautions are indicated. (5) Serologic studies are available from the Center for Disease Control and Prevention, Atlanta GA. (6) This is a **reportable** disease.

Possible Associated Conditions: Acquired immunodeficiency syndrome (AIDS)* and other immunodeficiency states *(3)*; hemolytic anemia;* *Salmonella* infection.

Organs and Tissues	*Procedures*	*Possible or Expected Findings*
External examination and skin	Prepare sections of skin lesions. Request Giemsa stain.	Jaundice. Miliary and nodular skin lesions with or without ulceration. Histologically, pigmented (hemosiderin) vascular granulomas. Bacillary angiomatosis *(1)*.
Blood	Prepare smears. Request Giemsa stain.	*Bartonella* in erythrocytes.
Blood and lymphatic vessels (all organs and lesions)	Request Giemsa stain.	*Bartonella bacilliformis* in swollen reticuloendothelial cells lining blood and lymphatic vessels. Thromboses. Erythrophagocytosis.
Heart	Culture any grossly infected valve. For demonstration of fat, prepare frozen section of myocardium with Sudan IV stain.	Endocarditis *(4)* Fatty changes of myocardium in anemic patients.
Liver and spleen	Record weights. Submit samples for histologic study and request Giemsa and Gomori iron stains.	Centrilobular hepatic necrosis; bacillary peliosis hepatis and bacillary splenitis; granulomatous hepatitis *(3)*; hemosiderosis of liver and spleen. Erythrophagocytosis; thromboses; necrosis *(3)*; and infarcts of spleen.
Lymph nodes	See above under "Liver and Spleen."	Lymphadenopathy (see above under "Blood and lymphatic vessels").
Bone marrow	See above under "Liver and Spleen."	Erythroid hyperplasia.

References

1. Wong R, Tappero J, Cockerell CJ. Bacillary angiomatosis and other Bartonella species infections. Semin Cutan Med Surg 1997;16:188–199.
2. Goldenberger D, Zbinden R, Perschil I, Altwegg M. Nachweis von Bartonella (Rochalimaea) henselae/B. quintana mittels Polymerase-Kettenreaktion (PCR). Schweiz Med Wschr 1996;126:207–213.
3. Liston TE, Koehler JE. Granulomatous hepatitis and necrotizing splenitis due to Bartonella henselae in a patient with cancer: case report and review of hepatosplenic manifestations of bartonella infections. Clin Infect Dis 1996;22:951–957.
4. Fu J, Muttaiyah S, Pandey S, Thomas M. Two cases of endocarditis due to Bartonella henselae. N Z Med J 2007;120:U2258.

From: *Handbook of Autopsy Practice,* 4th Ed. Edited by: B.L. Waters

Beriberi

Synonyms and Related Terms: Thiamine deficiency; Wernicke encephalopathy (cerebral beriberi).

Possible Associated Conditions: Chronic alcoholism; chronic peritoneal dialysis; hemodialysis; Wernicke disease; Wernicke-Korsakoff syndrome.*

Organs and Tissues	*Procedures*	*Possible or Expected Findings*
External examination and oral cavity		Evidence of malnutrition;* edema. Glossitis.
Heart	Record weight and submit samples for histologic study.	Alcoholic cardiomyopathy;* cardiac hypertrophy.*
Brain and spinal cord with dorsal-root ganglia	For removal and specimen preparation, see Chapter 4. Request Luxol fast blue and Bielschowsky stains	For cerebral changes, see "Syndrome, Wernicke-Korsakoff."
Cerebral, spinal, and peripheral nerves	For sampling and specimen preparation of peripheral nerves, see Chapter 4.	Axonal degeneration with relative sparing of small myelinated and unmyelinated fibers. Proximal segmental demyelination is considered a secondary phenomenon *(1)*. Degeneration may also occur in terminal branches of vagus and phrenic nerves.

Reference

1. Windebank AJ. Polyneuropathy due to nutritional deficiency and alcoholism. In: Peripheral Neuropathy, vol. 2. Dyck PJ, Thomas PK, eds., W.B. Saunders, Philadelphia, PA, 1993, pp. 1310–1321.

Berylliosis

NOTE: Close similarities exist between berylliosis and sarcoidosis *(1)**.

Organs and Tissues	*Procedures*	*Possible or Expected Findings*
Skin	Prepare sections from various sites.	Granulomas.
Vitreous	For removal and specimen preparation, see Chapter 5.	Increased calcium concentration (associated with hypercalcemia *[1]*).
Lungs	Perfuse one lung with formalin. Freeze one lobe for possible chemical study. See also under "Pneumoconiosis."	Chronic interstitial and granulomatous pneumonia.
Other organs	Procedures depend on expected findings or grossly identified abnormalities as listed in right-hand column.	Noncaseating tuberculoid granulomas with giant cells and calcific inclusions in liver, spleen, lymph nodes, and other organs. Nephrolithiasis *(1)*.

Reference

1. Rossman MD. Chronic beryllium disease: diagnosis and management. Environm Health Perspect 1996;104:945–947.

Bilharziasis (See "Schistosomiasis.")

Bismuth (See "Poisoning, bismuth.")

Blastomycosis, European (See "Cryptococcosis.")

Blastomycosis, North American

Synonym: *Blastomyces dermatitidis* infection.

NOTE: (1) Collect all tissues that appear to be infected. (2) Request fungal cultures. (3) Request Grocott's methenamine silver stain. (4) No special precautions are indicated. (5) Serologic studies are available from the state health department laboratories. (6) This is not a reportable disease.

Organs and Tissues	Procedures	Possible or Expected Findings
External examination and skin	Prepare sections of skin and of subcutaneous lesions. Submit scrapings of skin lesion for fungal cultures.	Weeping and crusted elevated skin lesions, predominantly of face and hands. Abscesses, fistulas, and ulcers with central healing and scarring may be present.
	Request mucicarmine stain.	Organisms should *not* be stainable with mucicarmine.
	Prepare chest roentgenogram and roentgenographic survey of bones. spine, long bones of lower extremities, pelvic	Pulmonary infiltrates; osteomyelitis* and periostitis of thoracic, lumbar, and sacral bones, and ribs (in this order of frequency).
Lungs	Perfuse at least one lung with formalin. Photograph cut surface. For histologic staining, see above under "External examination and skin."	Chronic pneumonia; possibly, suppurative and granulomatous lesions; rarely, cavitation and calcification.
Other organs and tissues	Prepare cultures of grossly affected organs and tissues. Other procedures depend on expected findings or grossly identified abnormalities as listed in right-hand column.	Involvement probably secondary to hematogenous dissemination; cerebral abscess;* meningitis;* adrenalitis; endocarditis;* pericarditis;* thyroiditis.* Other organs, such as eyes and larynx may also be affected.
Genital organs		Inflammatory infiltrates—rarely with fistulas—of prostate, epididymis, and seminal vesicles.
Bones	For removal, prosthetic repair, and specimen preparation, see Chapter 2.	Osteomyelitis* or periostitis (see above under "External examination and skin"). Psoas abscess may be present.

Blastomycosis, South American (See "Paracoccidioidomycosis.")

Block (Heart) (See "Arrhythmia, cardiac.")

Bodies, Foreign

If a foreign body is discovered during a medicolegal autopsy or if the discovery of a foreign body may have medicolegal impli-cations (e.g., presence of a surgical instrument in the abdominal cavity), the rules of the chain of custody apply. For the handling of bullets or bullet fragments, see "Injury, firearm." If analysis of foreign material is required, commercial laboratories may be helpful.

Bolus (See "Obstruction, acute airway.")

Botulism

Synonym: *Clostridium botulinum* infection.

NOTE: (1) Submit sample of feces *(1)*. Best confirmation of diagnosis is demonstration of toxin in the same food that the victim ingested. (2) Cultures are usually not indicated. (3) Special stains are usually not indicated. (4) No special precautions are indicated. (5) Serologic studies and toxin assays are available from the state health department laboratories. (6) This is a **reportable** disease.

Organs and Tissues	Procedures	Possible or Expected Findings
Blood	Refrigerate a specimen until toxicologic study of serum can be done.	Toxin lethal to mice. Can be neutralized by specific antitoxin.
Other organs and tissues		No diagnostic morphologic findings. Aspiration;* bronchopneumonia; manifestations of hypoxia.*
Serum, gastric, or intestinal contents; stool return form sterile water enema; exudate from wound	Submit for toxicologic study.	*Clostridium botulinum* and its toxins may be found in feces.

Reference

1. Dezfulian M, Hatheway CL, Yolken RH, Bartlett JG. Enzyme-linked immunosorbent assay for detection of *Clostridium botulinum* type A and type B toxins in stool samples of infants with botulism. J Clin Microbiol 1984;20(3):379–383.

Bromide (See "Poisoning, bromide.")

Bronchiectasis

Possible Associated Conditions: Abnormalities of airway cartilage (Williams-Campbell syndrome; Mounier-Kahn syndrome); allergic bronchopulmonary fungal disease; alpha$_1$-antitrypsin deficiency;* amyloidosis;* cystic fibrosis;* IgA deficiency with or without deficiency of IgG subclasses; Kartagener's syndrome (situs inversus, chronic sinusitis, and bronchiectasis) and other primary ciliary dyskinesias; obstructive azoospermia (Young syndrome); panhypogammaglobulinemia; ulcerative colitis; rheumatoid arthritis;* yellow nail syndrome (hypoplastic lymphatics).

Organs and Tissues	*Procedures*	*Possible or Expected Findings*
External examination		Clubbing of fingers and toes.
	Prepare chest roentgenogram.	Pneumothorax;* pulmonary infiltrates; pleural effusion or exudate.*
Chest cavity	For tests for pneumothorax, see under that heading.	Pneumothorax;* pleural empyema.* Situs inversus in Kartagener's syndrome.
Blood	Submit sample for microbiologic study.	Septicemia.
Heart	Record weight and thickness of right and left ventricles.	Cor pulmonale.
Lungs	Submit one lobe for bacterial and fungal cultures. If only one lobe contains bronchiectases, aspirate contents for microbiologic study.	Bronchiectasis, usually in lower lobes. In cystic fibrosis,* upper lobes are more severely affected. Purulent bronchitis.* Peribronchiectatic pneumonia or abscess. Allergic bronchopulmonary aspergillosis; tuberculosis.*
	For bronchography, see Chapter 2.	Fungus ball in cavity (aspergillosis*).
	For bronchial arteriography, see Chapter 2.	Dilatation of bronchial arteries. Bronchopulmomary anastomoses.
	Slice perfused lung along probes introduced into bronchiectases for guidance.	Saccular, tubular, or varicose bronchiectases.
	Request Gram, Grocott's methenamine silver, and —if indicated because of suspected tuberculosis —Kinyoun's stains.	Evidence of bacterial *(P. aeruginosa; Staphylococcus aureus; H. influenzae; Escherichia coli),* mycobacterial, or fungal (Aspergillus sp.) infection.
	Prepare sections of tracheobronchial cartilage.	Abnormal cartilage; see above under "Possible Associated Conditions."
Kidneys		Amyloidosis;* glomerular enlargement.
Other organs	If amyloidosis is suspected, request Congo red, crystal violet, methyl violet, Sirius red, and thioflavine T stains.	Amyloidosis.*
	If cystic fibrosis is present, follow procedures described under that heading.	Cystic fibrosis.*
Brain and spinal cord; nasal cavity and sinuses	For removal and specimen preparation, see Chapter 4.	Cerebral abscess.* Nasal polyps; sinusitis.

Bronchitis, Acute Chemical

NOTE: This occurs after inhalation of toxic gases, such as sulfurous acid (H_2SO_3), sulfur dioxide (SO_2), chlorine (Cl_2), and ammonia (NH_3). See also under "Poisoning, gas" and under "Edema, chemical pulmonary."

Organs and Tissues	Procedures	Possible or Expected Findings
Upper airways and lungs	Remove lungs together with pharynx, larynx, and trachea. Open airways in posterior midline.	Acute chemical laryngotracheitis.
	Perfuse one lung with formalin under low pressure (tissue may be friable).	Necrotizing bronchitis; aspiration of acid vomitus; chemical pulmonary edema.*

Bronchitis, Chronic

Synonyms and Related Terms: Chronic asthmatic bronchitis; chronic bronchitis with obstruction; chronic chemical bronchitis; chronic mucopurulent bronchitis; infectious bronchitis.

Organs and Tissues	Procedures	Possible or Expected Findings
Heart	Record weight and thickness of right and left ventricles.	Cor pulmonale. See also under "Failure, congestive heart."
Lungs	Submit any area of consolidation for microbiologic study. Slice fresh lung in sagittal plane. After submitting samples of cross-sections of bronchi for histologic study, open remainder of bronchi longitudinally. For bronchography, see Chapter 2.	Bronchopneumonia. Bronchiectasis.* Emphysema.*
	For bronchial arteriography, see Chapter 2.	Dilatation of bronchial arteries; bronchopulmonary anastomoses.
	Perfuse one lung with formalin. For semiquantitative determination of severity of bronchitis, use the Reid index or related morphologic methods *(1)*.	Most methods of wet inflation tend to distend bronchi and to overinflate lungs. Hyperplasia of submucosal bronchial glands and smooth muscle tends to parallel severity of chronic bronchitis.
	Request Gram and Grocott's methenamine silver stains.	Bacterial or fungal infection.
Diaphragm	Record size and thickness of muscular diaphragm.	Decrease in surface area and thickness in chronic bronchitis.
Stomach and duodenum		Peptic ulcers.*
Kidneys		Glomerular enlargement.
Brain and spinal cord	For removal and specimen preparation, see Chapter 4.	Hypoxic changes.

Reference

1. Thurlbeck WM. Pathology of chronic airflow obstruction. In: Chronic Obstructive Pulmonary Disease, Chernack NS, ed. W.B. Saunders, Philadelphia, PA, 1991.
2. Janssens JP, Herman F, MacGee W, Michel SP. Cause of death in older patients with anatamo-pathological evidence of chronic bronchitis or emphysema: a case control study based on autopsy findings. J Am Geriatr Soc 2001;49:571–576.

Bronchopneumonia (See "Pneumonia, all types or type unspecified.")

Brucellosis

Synonyms: *Brucella* spp. infection; undulant fever; Mediterranean fever; Malta fever.

NOTE: (1) Collect all tissues that appear to be infected. (2) Request aerobic cultures for *Brucella*. (3) Request Gram stains. (4) Serologic studies are available from local or state health department laboratories. (5) This is a **reportable** disease.

Organs and Tissues	Procedures	Possible or Expected Findings
External examination	For exposure of joints and microbiologic specimen preparation, see Chapter 2.	Subcutaneous abscesses. Purulent arthritis (sacroiliac and hip joints) and periarticular bursitis.
	Prepare roentgenograms of skeletal system.	Osteomyelitis* of long bones and of spine.
Blood	Submit samples for culture and serum agglutination tests. See also above under "Note."	

Organs and Tissues	*Procedures*	*Possible or Expected Findings*
Lymph nodes		Generalized lymphadenopathy.
Heart	If endocarditis is suspected, submit valves or myocardium for culture.	Infective endocarditis* (particularly with pre-existing aortic stenosis); myocarditis;* pericardial effusions.
Arteries and veins	For angiography, see under specific site or organ. Submit samples for histologic study. Request Verhoeff–van Gieson stain.	Arterial aneurysms; arteriovenous fistulas. Granulomatous endophlebitis.
Lungs	Submit sample for culture.	Pleural effusions;* granulomas that may be associated with abscesses and calcification. Embolism secondary to granulomatous endophlebitis.
Liver	Record weight. Submit sample for culture.	Hepatomegaly; granulomatous hepatitis; nonspecific reactive changes.
Gallbladder		Acute cholecystitis.*
Spleen	Record weight. Submit sample for culture.	Splenomegaly with granulomas.
Kidneys and ureters	Submit samples of renal tissue for histologic study. Record appearance of renal pelvic and ureteral mucosa.	Granulomas; ulceration of mucosa of renal pelvis. See also above under "Lungs."
Urinary bladder	Photograph ulceration; submit for histologic study.	Ulceration of mucosa.
Ovaries, prostate, epididymides, and testes	Submit samples for culture (see also above under "Note.")	Abscesses.
Bones and joints	For removal, prosthetic repair, and specimen preparation, see Chapter 2.	Osteomyelitis* of long bones and of spine; arthritis *(1)*.
Brain	For removal and specimen preparation, see Chapter 4. Submit for culture. See also above under "Note." For cerebral arteriography, see Chapter 4.	Meningoencephalitis; mycotic intracerebral aneurysm* with rupture and hemorrhage.
Eyes	For removal and specimen preparation, see Chapter 5.	Iritis; choroiditis; keratitis.

Reference

1. Colmenero JD, Reguera JM, Martos F, Sanchez-De-Mora D, Delgado M, Causse M, et al. Complications associated with Brucella melitensis infection: a study of 530 cases. Medicine 1996;75:195–211.
2. Del Arco A, et al. Splenic abscess due to Brucella infection: is splenectomy necessary? Case report and literature review. Scand J Infect Dis 2007;39:379–381.

Burns

NOTE: Fatal burns should be reported to the medical examiner's or coroner's office. The questions to be answered by the pathologist depend on whether the incident was accidental, sui-cidal, or homicidal, and whether the victim survivied to be treated in the hospital. A pending death certificate should be issued if the fire and police investigators are not sure of the circumstances at the time of the autopsy. For electrical burns, see under "Injury, electrical."

For victims who were treated at the hospital, autopsy procedures should be directed toward the discovery or confirmation of the mechanism of death, such as sepsis or pulmonary embolism.* Death can be caused primarily by heart disease, with other-wise minor burns and smoke inhalation serving as the trigger that leads to lethal ventricular arrhythmia. Because carbon monoxide concentrations are halved approx every 30 min with 100% oxygen therapy, the pathologist must obtain the first clinical laboratory test results for CO-hemoglobin. Soot can be detected with the naked eye 2 or 3 d after inhalation of smoke. Ambulance records should be examined to determine whether a persistent coma might have been caused by hypoxic encephalopathy following resuscitation from cardiac arrest at the scene.

Admission blood samples should be acquired to test for CO-hemoglobin and alcohol. This may not have been done in the emergency room. Persons suffering from chronic alcoholism succumb to fire deaths more often than persons who do not drink. A very high initial serum alcohol concentration suggests a risk factor for the fire and presence of chronic alcoholism. Patients with chronic alcoholism typically are deprived of alcohol when they are in the burn unit and this can cause sudden, presumably cardiac, death, just as it occurs under similar circum-stances, not complicated by burns. Under these circumstances, the heart fails to show major abnormalities. This mode of dying seems to have no relationship to the presence or absence of liver disease.

Organs and Tissues	*Procedures*	*Possible or Expected Findings*
External examination and skin	If the body is found dead and charred at the scene, prepare whole body roentgenograms, before and after removal of remanants of clothing. See also under "Identification of the body" and "External examination" in Chapter 13). One or two fingerpads may yield sufficient ridge detail for identification. If this is not possible, ante- and postmortem somatic and dental radiographs must be compared for identification, or DNA comparison must be used.	Roentgenograms may detect bullets in cases where arson was used to mask murder. Bullets or knife blades must be secured as evidence. Objects such as hairpins, keys, jewelry, dentures, or other evidence, and demonstration of old fractures may help provisionally identify the victim. Fractures of bones and lacerations of soft tissue can all occur as heat artifacts and must be identified as such. See also above under "Note."
External examination and skin *(continued)*	Photograph burnt body and make diagrams of wounds.	
	Prepare histologic sections of blisters and of surrounding skin.	Inflammatory changes in the skin indicate a vital reaction.
Blood	If victim was found burnt, submit samples for carbon monoxide determination and toxicologic study, primarily for alcohol and illicit drugs.	Increased carbon monoxide concentration (saturation of >15–20%) is strong evidence that the victim was alive and breathing for some time during burning. CO-concentrations may not be elevated in flash-fire victims.
	If victim survived for some time, submit samples for bacterial and fungal culture.	Septicemia and bacteremia.
Vitreous	Submit sample for alcohol and other toxicologic studies, particularly if no blood is available, and also for electrolyte determination.	Water and electrolyte loss in patients who had survived burns for some time.
Serosal surfaces	Record volume and character of exudate or transudate.	Exudate indicates vital reaction. Watery transudate may develop with rigorous infusions of crystalloid during fruitless resuscitation efforts.
Neck organs and tracheobronchial tree	Remove carefully. Inspect hyoid bone; search for hemorrhages in soft tissues of neck.	Strangulation effect (fractured hyoid bone).
	Record appearance and photograph mucosal surfaces of larynx and trachea. If patient had survived for some time and had been intubated, search for intubation trauma.	Soot particles and other heat injuries indicate that the patient was breathing in fire. Absence of soot particles does not prove that the patient was already dead when fire started unless there is reasonable evidence that the fire was not a flash fire.
	Inspect supraglottic area.	Supraglottic edema may cause sudden death in patients who had survived burns—particularly of face—for some time.
	Submit samples of tracheobronchial mucosa for histologic study.	Herpes virus inclusions in tracheobronchial ulcerations of victims who had survived burns for some time.
Other organs	Follow routine autopsy procedures.	Bronchopneumonia; pulmonary emboli; heart disease in victims who survive for some time. See also above under "Note."
Pelvic organs	Examination of pelvic organs may permit sex determination in severely burnt bodies.	Sex determination.
	In female victims whose burns are less severe, a search should be made for evidence of rape.	Evidence of rape.*
Durae and brain		Epidural hematomas may occur as heat artifacts.

Bypass, aortocoronary (See "Surgery, aortocoronary bypass.")

Byssinosis (See "Pneumoconiosis.")

C

Cadmium (See "Poisoning, cadmium.")

Calcinosis, Mönckeberg's Medial

Synonyms: Medial sclerosis of arteries; Mönckeberg's arterio-sclerosis.

NOTE: This is generally considered an age-related phenomenon that is usually of little clinical consequence, with calcification of the internal elastic membrane and subjacent media. It commonly involves femoral and thyroid arteries.

Calcium (See "Disorder, electrolyte(s).")

Calculi, Renal (See "Nephrolithiasis.")

Canal, Complete Atrioventricular (See "Defect, complete atrioventricular septal.")

Candidiasis

Synonyms and Related Terms: Candidosis, moniliasis, thrush.

NOTE: Candidiasis may follow or complicate antibacterial or corticosteroid therapy, cardiac surgery,* dehydration,* diabetes mellitus,* drug (heroin) dependence,* leukemia* or other systemic malignant diseases, tuberculosis,* and other debilitating diseases.

(1) Collect all tissues that appear to be infected. (2) Request fungal cultures. (3) Request Grocott's methenamine silver or PAS stain, or both. (4) No special precautions are indicated. (5) Serologic studies are available from many reference laboratories. (6) This is not a reportable disease.

Organs and Tissues	*Procedures*	*Possible or Expected Findings*
External examination and skin	Prepare sections of skin. For special stains, see above under "Note."	Intertrigo. Nail destruction may occur without skin involvement.
Oral cavity		Creamy patches.
Blood	Submit sample for fungal culture.	*Candida* septicemia.
Heart	If endocarditis is suspected, for instance, in drug addicts or after cardiac surgery, submit tissue for culture and gram stain.	*Candida* endocarditis.
Lungs	Submit one lobe for bacterial and fungal culture. For special stains, see above under "Note."	*Candida* bronchopneumonia, often in association with other processes.
Pharynx, esophagus, and gastrointestinal tract with rectum; vagina, and cervix	Photograph all lesions. Submit samples for histologic study. For special stains, see above under "Note."	*Candida* infection with membranes, erosions, and ulcers.
Other organs	Submit samples of liver, pancreas, kidneys, adrenal glands, thyroid, and joints for histologic study. If available, sample umbilical cord.	Systemic candidiasis; multiple abscesses due to septic embolization. In the umbilical cord, necrotizing inflammation (funisitis) may be found.
Cerebrospinal fluid	Submit sample for fungal culture.	Meningitis.
Brain	For removal and specimen preparation, see Chapter 4. For special stains, see above under "Note."	Meningitis.

Carbon Monoxide (See "Poisoning, carbon monoxide.")

Carbon Tetrachloride (See "Poisoning, carbon tetrachloride.")

From: *Handbook of Autopsy Practice,* 4th Ed. Edited by: B.L. Waters

Carcinoma (See "Tumor...")

Cardiomegaly (See "Cardiomyopathy,... and "Hypertrophy, cardiac.")

Cardiomyopathy, Alcoholic

NOTE: For general dissection techniques, see Chapter 3.

Organs and Tissues	*Procedures*	*Possible or Expected Findings*
External examination, heart and lungs	See below under "Cardiomyopathy, dilated."	See below under "Cardiomyopathy, dilated."
Abdominal cavity and liver	Record volume of ascites. Record actual and expected weight of liver. Request iron stain.	Alcoholic cirrhosis and alcoholic cardiomyopathy rarely coexist. However, in genetic hemochromatosis,* cirrhosis and heart failure are common findings.

Cardiomyopathy, Dilated (Idiopathic, Familial, and Secondary Types)

NOTE: For general dissection techniques, see Chapter 3.

Organs and Tissues	*Procedures*	*Possible or Expected Findings*
External examination	Prepare chest roentgenogram.	Cardiomegaly; pleural or pericardial effusions;* pacemaker.
Chest cavity	Record volume of pleural and pericardial effusions.	Hydrothorax; hydropericardium.
Heart	Record actual and expected heart weights. Measure and record maximum internal short-axis diameter of left ventricular chamber. Record ventricular thicknesses and valvular circumferences. Note location and size of mural thrombus. Request iron stain.	Cardiomegaly; biventricular hypertrophy; four-chamber dilatation; focal left ventricular fibrosis; dilated valve annuli; relatively mild coronary atherosclerosis; possible iron in cardiac myocytes; microfocal interstitial fibrosis, particularly subendocardial; myocarditis (idiopathic or drug-related).
Lungs	Record actual and expected weights. Request Verhoeff–van Gieson and iron stains from one lower lobe.	Pulmonary congestion; pulmonary edema; changes of chronic pulmonary venous hypertension; pulmonary emboli; pulmonary infarcts; bronchopneumonia.
Abdominal cavity	Record volume of ascites.	Ascites.
Liver	Record actual and expected weights.	Chronic congestive hepatomegaly; centrilobular (zone 3) steatosis, fibrosis, or necrosis (not true cirrhosis).

Cardiomyopathy, Hypertrophic (Idiopathic, Familial, and Secondary Types)

Synonyms: Idiopathic hypertrophic subaortic stenosis (IHSS); hypertrophic obstructive cardiomyopathy (HOCM); and many others.

Possible Associated Conditions: See below under "Possible or Expected Findings."

Organs and Tissues	*Procedures*	*Possible or Expected Findings*
External examination	Sample skin lesions for histologic study. Prepare chest roentgenogram.	Lentiginosis (part of LEOPARD syndrome). Mild cardiomegaly.
Heart	Record actual and expected weights. Record ventricular thicknesses and valvular circumferences. Determine ratio between left ventricular septal and free wall thicknesses (normal, <1.3) at basal, midventricular, and apical levels. Request amyloid stain (Congo red or sulfated alcian blue).	Biventricular hypertrophy; disproportionate septal hypertrophy (>1.3 in 90%); gross and microscopic fibrosis; thickened anterior mitral leaflet; subaortic septal endocardial fibrotic patch (contact lesion from mitral valve); left atrial dilatation; focal septal myofiber disarray microscopically.
Brain and spinal cord	For removal and specimen preparation, see Chapter 4.	Friedreich's ataxia.*

Cardiomyopathy, Restrictive (Non-eosinophilic and Secondary Types)

NOTE: For general dissection techniques, see Chapter 3.

Organs and Tissues	*Procedures*	*Possible or Expected Findings*
Heart	Record actual and expected weights. Record ventricular thicknesses and valvular circumferences. Evaluate atrial size, compared to ventricular chamber size. Request amyloid stain (Congo red or sulfated alcian blue).	Prominent biatrial dilatation. Relatively normal ventricular size. Prominent biventricular interstitial fibrosis or amyloidosis, microscopically.

Cardiomyopathy, Restrictive (With Eosinophilia)

Synonyms: Eosinophilic endomyocardial disease; hypereosinophilic syndromes; Löffler's eosinophilic endomyocarditis; Davies' endomyocardial fibrosis.

NOTE: For general dissection techniques, see Chapter 3.

Organs and Tissues	*Procedures*	*Possible or Expected Findings*
Heart	Record actual and expected weights. Record ventricular thicknesses and valvular circumferences. Evaluate relative atrial and ventricular chamber sizes.	Mural thrombus along apex and inflow tract of one or both ventricles, with extensive intact or degranulated eosinophils microscopically. Ventricular dilatation only if mitral or tricuspid valve or both are regurgitant.
Other organs and tissues	Procedures depend on expected findings or grossly identified abnormalities as listed in right-hand column.	Conditions associated with eosinophilia, such as asthmatic bronchiolitis or Churg-Strauss syndrome (see also under "Syndrome, hypereosinophilic"); malignancies; parasitic disease; vasculitis.

Cardiomyopathy, Arrhythmogenic Right Ventricular

Synonyms: Arrhythmogenic right ventricular dysplasia; right ventricular cardiomyopathy.

NOTE: For general dissection techniques, see Chapter 3.

Organs and Tissues	*Procedures*	*Possible or Expected Findings*
Heart	Record actual and expected weights. Record ventricular thicknesses and valvular circumferences. Evaluate pattern and extent of epicardial fat, especially over right ventricle. Take multiple samples from right ventricle for microscopic study.	Prominent right ventricular dilatation, grossly; right ventricular hypertrophy, fibrosis, and adiposity, by microscopy (excessive for patient's age and body size). Occasional left ventricular involvement. Microfocal myocarditis or epicarditis.

Carditis (See "Myocarditis.")

Chickenpox (See "Varicella.")

Chloride (See "Disorder, electrolyte(s)" and Chapter 8.)

Chloroma

NOTE: Follow procedures described under "Leukemia, all types or type unspecified." For gross staining of chloroma, see Chapter 16.

Cholangiopathy, Infantile Obstructive (See "Atresia, biliary" and "Hepatitis, neonatal.")

Cholangitis, Chronic Nonsuppurative Destructive

Synonym: Primary bilary cirrhosis.

NOTE: Follow procedures described under "Cirrhosis, liver."

Cholangitis, Sclerosing

Synonyms: Idiopathic sclerosing cholangitis; primary sclerosing cholangitis; secondary sclerosing cholangitis.

Possible Associated Conditions: Acquired immunodeficiency syndrome;* acute or chronic pancreatitis;* ankylosing spondylitis;* autoimmune hemolytic anemia;* autoimmune hep-atitis; bronchiectasis;* chronic ulcerative colitis;* celiac disease; Crohn's disease;* eosinophilia; glomerulonephritis;* immune thrombocytopenic purpura; Peyronie's disease; pseudotumor of the orbit; retroperitoneal fibrosis;* rheumatoid arthritis;* Riedel's struma; sclerosing mediastinitis;* Sjogren's syndrome;* systemic lupus erythematosus;* systemic sclerosis;* vasculitis; and many others (the associations are not equally well documented) *(1)*.

Organs and Tissues	Procedures	Possible or Expected Findings
External examination	Record presence or absence of laparotomy scars and drains.	Jaundice.
Intestinal tract and pancreas		See above under "Possible Associated Conditions."
Hepatoduodenal ligament	For cholangiography, see Chapter 2. Open duodenum anteriorly and insert catheter into papilla of Vater. After removal of liver and hepatodudenal ligament, prepare cholangiograms. Record diameter of lumens and thickness of walls at various levels of common bile duct, hepatic duct, cystic duct, and gallbladder.	Sclerosis and narrowing of extrahepatic bile ducts. Choledocholithiasis; cholelithiasis; adenocarcinoma of bile ducts or gallbladder.
	Record appearance of portal veins and hepatic arteries.	Occlusion or narrowing of hepatic artery or its branches may cause ischemic cholangitis, which closely resembles primary sclerosing cholangitis *(2)*.
	Prepare histologic sections of extrahepatic bile ducts and hepatoduodenal lymph nodes.	Intraductal carcinoma may imitate primary sclerosing cholangitis. Lymph nodes may contain metastatic carcinoma. For possible infections, see below under "Liver."
Liver	Photograph before and after slicing. Submit samples for histologic study; include sections of perihilar intrahepatic bile ducts.	Intrahepatic sclerosing cholangitis; cholestasis; ascending cholangitis; biliary cirrhosis, fibrinoid necrosis of portal tracts *(3)*. Cholangiocarcinoma. Evidence of cytomegalovirus or cryptosporidium infection.
Other organs and tissues		See above under "Possible Associated Conditions."

References

1. Lazarides KN, Wiesner RH, Porayko MK, Ludwig J, LaRusso NF. Primary sclerosing cholangitis. In: Diseases of the Liver, 8th ed. Schiff ER, Sorrell MF, Maddray WC, eds. Lippincott-Raven, Philadelphia, PA, 1999.
2. Batts KP. Ischemic cholangitis. Mayo Clin Proc 1998;73:380–385.
3. Hano H, et al. An Autopsy case showing massive fibrinoid necrosis of the portal tracts of the liver with cholangiographic findings similar to those of primary sclerosing cholangitis. World J Gastroenterol 2007;13:639–42.

Cholangitis, Suppurative

Related Terms: Ascending cholangitis; obstructive suppurative cholangitis; (oriental) recurrent pyogenic cholangitis.

Organs and Tissues	Procedures	Possible or Expected Findings
External examination		Jaundice.
Blood	Submit sample for microbiologic study.	Septicemia.
Heart	If infective endocarditis is suspected, follow procedures described in Chapter 7.	Infective endocarditis.*
Hepatoduodenal ligament	For cholangiography, see Chapter 2. Dissect common bile duct, hepatic duct, and portal vein *in situ*.	Stricture; tumor, stones. Portal vein thrombosis; pylephlebitis.
Liver and gallbladder	Record weight of liver and photograph it. Submit portion of liver for aerobic and anaerobic bacterial culture. Submit samples for histologic study and request Gram stain.	Cholangitic abscesses; cholecystitis,* cholelithiasis.* Carcinoma or other conditions causing obstruction or compression of bile ducts.

Cholecystitis

Related Terms: Acute acalculous cholecystitis; chronic cholecystitis; gallstone cholecystitis.

Possible Associated Conditions: Brucellosis;* major trauma or operation unrelated to biliary system; polyarteritis nodosa;* *Salmonella typhosa* infection (typhoid fever*).

Organs and Tissues	Procedures	Possible or Expected Findings
External examination	Prepare roentgenogram of upper abdomen.	Jaundice. Air in biliary tract indicates biliary fistula. Gallstones
Abdominal cavity	Submit peritoneal exudate and aspirated contents of gallbladder for aerobic and anaerobic culture. Also submit exudate from subphrenic empyema* or other intraperitoneal empyemas (abscesses).	Peritonitis;* intraperitoneal empyemas (abscesses).
Blood	Submit sample for bacterial culture.	Septicemia.
Heart	If endocarditis is suspected, follow procedures described.	Infective endocarditis.*
Intestine	If biliary fistula is suspected, open stomach, duodenum, and hepatic flexure of colon *in situ*. Record location and size of fistula.	Biliary fistula, with or without gallstone ileus.
Gallbladder; hepatoduodenal ligament with extrahepatic bile ducts	For cholangiography, see Chapter 2. Open all extrahepatic bile ducts, portal vein, and hepatic artery *in situ*. Remove liver and gallbladder. Describe appearance, position, and contents of gallbladder. Record number and character of stones.	Acute or chronic cholecystitis; cholelithiasis;* cholangitis;* choledocholithiasis. Ulcers, abscesses, empyema, gangrene, or perforation of gallbladder; emphysematous cholecystitis; fistula. Hydrops or porcelain gallbladder; limey bile. Torsion of gallbladder. Portal vein thrombosis; pylephlebitis. Polyarteritis nodosa* of gallbladder. Hepatoduodenal lymphadenitis.
Liver	Record size and weight. Submit samples for histologic study.	Suppurative cholangitis;* cholangitic abscesses; pylephlebitis; pylephlebitic abscesses; venous thromboses.
Pancreas	If pancreatitis is present, record whether common bile duct and pancreatic duct have a common entry.	Pancreatitis.*

Choledocholithiasis

NOTE: Follow procedures described under "Cholecystitis."

Cholelithiasis

NOTE: Follow procedures described under "Cholecystitis." Cholelithiasis may be associated with all types of cholecystitis, with cholesterosis of the gallbladder, and with polyps of the gallbladder. The presence of "white bile" (limey bile) indi-cates obstruction of the cystic duct. Record number and character of stones.

Cholera

Synonym: *Vibrio cholerae* infection; asiatic cholera.

NOTE: The disease may complicate anemia,* chronic atrophic gastritis, vagotomy, gastrectomy, chronic intestinal disease, and malnutrition.

(1) Collect all tissues that appear to be infected. (2) Request cultures of intestinal contents for cholera. (3) Request Gram stain. (4) Special **precautions** are indicated see Chapter 6. (5) For serologic studies, see below under "Blood." (6) This is a **reportable** disease.

Organs and Tissues	Procedures	Possible or Expected Findings
External examination	Record body weight and length and extent of rigor.	Early onset and prolongation of rigor mortis. Shriveled fingers ("washer-woman's hands") and toes.
Vitreous	Submit sample for sodium, chloride, and urea nitrogen determination.	Dehydration.*
Blood	Prepare serum for tube agglutination or enzyme-linked immunosorbent assay (ELISA) test for retrospective diagnosis or epidemiologic purposes.	

Organs and Tissues	*Procedures*	*Possible or Expected Findings*
Intestinal tract	Record volume and appearance of intestinal contents. Submit samples of feces and other intestinal contents for culture and for determination of sodium, potassium, and chloride content.	Blood-stained or "rice-water type" intestinal contents. The organism may be present in pure culture.
	Submit samples of all portions of the intestinal tract for histologic study.	Intact mucosa with edema of lamina propria; dilatation of capillaries and lymphatics; mononuclear infiltrates and goblet cell hyperplasia. All changes confined to small bowel. Bacteria situated on or between epithelial cells.
Kidneys	Submit samples for histologic study.	Tubular necrosis;* focal cortical necrosis.
Adrenal glands		Lipid depletion.
Urine	Record volume and specific gravity.	Absence or minimal amount of urine suggests dehydration.*
Other organs and tissues		All tissues appear abnormally dry. Lungs are usually pale and shrunken, less frequently congested.

Chondrocalcinosis (See "Pseudogout.")

Chondrodysplasia

Synonyms and Related Terms: Achondroplasia; chondrodystrophia fetalis; Ellis-van Creveld syndrome.*

Organs and Tissues	*Procedures*	*Possible or Expected Findings*
External examination	Record body length, length of extremities, and abnormal features. Measure head, chest, and abdominal circumferences.	Dwarfism;* micromelia with pudgy fingers; bulging head with saddle nose.
	Prepare skeletal roentgenograms. All radiographs should be reviewed by a radiologist.	Chest deformities; separation of spinal ossification centers; abnormal pelvis and, in infants, ossification centers in metaphyseal ends of long bones.
Thyroid gland	Record weight and submit sample for histologic study.	Atrophy.
Other organs	Perfuse at least one lung with formalin.	Restrictive and obstructive lung disease *(1)*.
Base of skull, pituitary gland, brain, and spinal canal with cord	For removal and specimen preparation of brain and spinal cord, see Chapter 4. For removal of pituitary gland, see Chapter 4. Record appearance and photograph base of skull; record size of foramen magnum.	Growth retardation of base of skull with compression of foramen magnum. Internal hydrocephalus.* Narrow spinal canal with compression of spinal cord. (Clinically: paraplegia.) Atrophy of pituitary gland.
	Remove middle ears (see Chapter 4).	Otitis media* *(2)*.
Bones	For removal, prosthetic repair, and specimen preparation, see Chapter 2.	Dorsolumbar kyphosis and lumbosacral lordosis; short iliac wings; short and thick tubular bones; excessive size of epiphysis in long bones; elongated costal cartilage; tibial bowing.
	Submit samples (especially epiphyses, if present) for histologic study.	Decreased cartilage cell proliferation at costochondral junction and at epiphysis-diaphysis junction of long bones.

References

1. Hunter AG, Bankier A, Rogers JC, Sillence D, Scott CL Jr. Medical complications of achondroplasia: a multicenter patient review. J Med Genet 1998;35:705–712.
2. Erdincler P, Dashti R, Kaynar MY, Canbaz B, Ciplak N, Kuday C. Hydrocephalus and chronically increased intracranial pressure in achondroplasia. Childs Nerv System 1997;13:345–348.
3. Rimoin DL, Hollester DW, Lachman RS, et al. Histologic studies in the chondrodystrophies. Birth Defects Orig Artic Ser 1974;10:274–295.

Chondrosarcoma (See "Tumor of bone or cartilage.")

Chordoma (See "Tumor of bone or cartilage.")

Chorea, Acute

Related Terms: Infectious chorea (poststreptococcal; often part of rheumatic fever); St. Vitus' dance; Sydenham's chorea.

Organs and Tissues	*Procedures*	*Possible or Expected Findings*
Brain and spinal cord	For removal and specimen preparation, see Chapter 4. Submit sample of cerebral tissue for microbiologic study.	Morphologic changes largely unknown. Degenerative processes of basal ganglia.
Other organs	Procedures depend on expected findings or grossly identified abnormalities as listed in right-hand column.	Manifestations of carbon monoxide poisoning;* diphtheria;* hyperthyroidism;* idiopathic hypocalcemia; pertussis;* pregnancy; rheumatic fever;* systemic lupus erythematosus.*

Chorea, Hereditary

Synonyms: Chronic progressive chorea; Huntington's chorea; Huntington's disease.

NOTE: Huntington's disease maps to the short arm of chromosome 4. The gene is widely expressed but of unknown function; it contains a CAG repeat sequence, which is expanded (range, 37 to 86) in patients with Huntington's disease. A sensitive diag-nostic test is based on the determination of this CAG sequence, which can be done on fresh-frozen tissue or blood *(1)*. In the absence of genetic confirmation, sampling of organs and tissues cannot be excessive because a complex differential diagnosis must be resolved.

Organs and Tissues	*Procedures*	*Possible or Expected Findings*
Brain and spinal cord	For removal and specimen preparation, see Chapter 4. Freeze fresh cerebral tissue for further study. Stain for ubiquitin and N-terminal huntingtin.	Mild to severe cerebral atrophy. Atrophy of head of caudate nucleus, putamen, and globus pallidus (due to neuronal loss and gliosis). Neuronal intranuclear and neuropil inclusions *(2)*.
Other organs	Samples should include peripheral nerves, adrenal glands, skeletal muscle, and bone marrow. (See also above under "Note").	Respiratory and other intercurrent infections.

Reference

1. Lowe J, Lennox G, Leigh PN. Disorders of movement and system degenerations. In: Greenfield's Neuropathology, vol. 2. Graham BI, Lantos PL, eds. Arnold, London, 1997, pp. 281–366.
2. Maat-Schieman M, et al. Neuronal intranuclear and neuropil inclusions for pathological assessment of Huntington's disease. Brain Pathol 2007;17:31–37.

Choriomeningitis, Lymphocytic (See "Meningitis.")

Chylothorax

Related Terms: Congenital chylothorax.

Organs and Tissues	*Procedures*	*Possible or Expected Findings*
External examination	Prepare chest roentgenogram. Puncture pleural cavity and submit fluid for microbiologic study.	Pleural effusion.*
Chest cavity	Record volume of exudate or transudate and submit sample for determination of fat and cholesterol content. If infection is suspected (extremely rare in true chylothorax), submit sample for microbiologic study.	Chylous pleural effusions have high fat content. Nonchylous milky effusions—for instance, in tuberculosis* and rheumatoid arthritis*—have high cholesterol and low fat content. Tumor of pleura, lung, or chest wall; lymphangiomatosis *(1)*.

Organs and Tissues	Procedures	Possible or Expected Findings
Thoracic duct	For lymphangiography and for dissection of the thoracic duct, see Chapter 3.	Surgical or other traumatic lesions of thoracic duct. Tumor in posterior mediastinum.
Skeletal system	Prepare skeletal roentgenogram and, if abnormalities are present, sample bone for histologic study.	Massive osteolysis in Gorham's syndrome *(2)*.

References

1. Moerman P, van Geet C, Devlieger H. Lymphangiomatosis of the body wall: a report of two cases associated with chylothorax and fatal outcome. Pediatr Pathol Lab Med 1997;17:617–624.
2. Riantawan P, Tansupasawasdikul S, Subhannachart P. Bilateral chylothorax complicating massive osteolysis (Gorham's syndrome). Thorax 1996;51:1277–1278.

Cirrhosis, Liver

NOTE: All types of cirrhosis are included here (alcoholic, autoimmune, biliary, cryptogenic, pigment [hemochromatosis], cirrhosis with viral hepatitis, and other types).

If the cause or underlying condition is known, see also under the appropriate heading, such as alcoholic liver disease, a_1-antitrypsin deficiency, sclerosing cholangitis, or viral hepatitis. If the patient had undergone liver transplantation, see also under that heading.

Organs and Tissues	Procedures	Possible or Expected Findings
External examination	Record body weight and length, nutritional state, distribution of hair, type of skin pigmentation, appearance of breasts and hands, and abdominal circumference. Prepare sections of skin and breast tissue.	Jaundice; spider nevi; pectoral alopecia and loss or abnormal distribution of pubic hair; gynecomastia; white nail beds; clubbing of fingers. Diffuse or nodular (e.g., cervical) lipomatosis (Madelung collar) in alcoholism. Xanthelasmas and vitiligo in primary biliary cirrhosis. Skin pigmentation of hemochromatosis.* Bruises and hemorrhages.
	Prepare skeletal roentgenograms	Hypertrophic osteoarthropathy* of tibia and fibula; osteomalacia;* osteoporosis.*
Blood	Submit samples for bacterial culture and for biochemical or immunologic study, depending on expected underlying disease (see above under "Note").	Septicemia; hyperbilirubinemia. Viral antigens and/or antibodies.
Abdominal and chest cavity	Record volume and character of ascites. Culture exudate.	Ascites; spontaneous bacterial peritonitis.
	Record volume and character of pleural effusions.	Hydrothorax.
	For lymphangiography, see Chapter 2.	Dilatation of abdominal lymphatics and thoracic duct.
	For arteriography and for cholangiography, see Chapter 2. Record appearance and contents of extrahepatic bile ducts. If liver transplantation had taken place, see also under that heading.	Strictures, stones, or tumors in secondary biliary cirrhosis; portal or splenic vein thrombosis; thrombosis of surgical anastomosis. A peritoneovenous shunt may be in place.
	Remove esophagus together with stomach. Clamp midportion of stomach and remove together with esophagus for demonstration of varices. Record appearance of varices and preserve specimen, particularly in cases where attempts had been made to sclerose the varices.	Esophageal* or gastric varices, or both, with or without evidence of rupture and hemorrhage. Gastroesophageal mucosal tears in Mallory-Weiss syndrome. (See also below under "Gastrointestinal tract.")
Lungs	Perfuse at least one lung with formalin.	Manifestations of portopulmonary hypertension.
Diaphragm	Record defects and presence of dilated lymphatics.	
Gastrointestinal tract	Record estimated volume of blood in gastrointestinal tract.	Gastrointestinal hemorrhage.* Gastric varices.

Organs and Tissues	Procedures	Possible or Expected Findings
	Submit samples of abnormal lesions for histologic study	Peptic ulcers.* Crohn's disease* or chronic ulcerative colitis in primary sclerosing cholangitis.* Portal hypertensive gastropathy.
Liver and gallbladder	Record size and weight of liver and average size of regenerative nodules of liver. Describe appearance and contents of gallbladder. Prepare frontal or horizontal slices of liver. If there is evidence of tumor(s), see under "Tumor of the liver." For macroscopic iron stain, see Chapter 16.	Cirrhosis. Cholelithiasis.* Hepatocellular carcinoma. Hemosiderosis. An intrahepatic portal-caval shunt may be in place.
	Freeze hepatic tissue for possible biochemical or histochemical study. Request van Gieson's stain, PAS stain with diastase digestion, and Gomori's iron stain. If hepatitis B virus infection is suspected, request immunostains for B antigens. For preparation for electron microscopic study, see Chapter 15.	Hepatitis B or other viral antigens.
Spleen	Record size and weight.	Congestive splenomegaly.
Pancreas	Dissect pancreatic ducts.	Chronic pancreatitis, particularly with alcoholic cirrhosis.
Urine	Chemical study is feasible.	Urobilinuria; aminoaciduria.
Testes and prostate	Record weights of testes. Submit samples of testes and prostate for histologic study.	Atrophy of testes and prostate.
Brain	For removal and specimen preparation, see Chapter 4.	Hepatic encephalopathy. Histologic changes, primarily in cerebral cortex, putamen, globus pallidus, and cerebellum.
Eyes	For removal and specimen preparation, see Chapter 5.	Yellow sclerae. Cataracts in galactosemia.*

Clonorchiasis

Synonyms: *Clonorchis sinensis* infection; Chinese or oriental liver fluke infection; *Opisthorchis sinensis* infection *(1)*.

NOTE: (1) Collect all tissues that appear to be infected. (2) Culture methods are not generally available. However, aerobic and anaerobic cultures may be indicated in patients who die of superimposed sepsis. (3) Request Gram stain parasites can be identified with hematoxylin and eosin stain. (4) No special precautions are indicated. (5) Serologic studies are not available. (6) This is not a reportable disease.

Organs and Tissues	Procedures	Possible or Expected Findings
Blood	Submit sample for anaerobic and aerobic culture.	Septicemia.
Stool	Submit sample for study of eggs.	
Liver and extrahepatic biliary system	For postmortem cholangiography, see Chapter 2. Leave extrahepatic bile ducts and gallbladder attached to liver. Dissect as described as in Chapter 2. Submit samples of liver, gallbladder, and extrahepatic bile ducts for histologic study. Request Verhoeff–van Gieson stain.	Hyperplasia of bile duct epithelium; periductal chronic inflammation; severe portal fibrosis; cirrhosis. Acute or recurrent suppurative cholangitis;* Cholangiocarcinoma.
Abdominal organs	Weigh liver, spleen. Examine veins around esophagus and rectum carefully.	Evidence of portal hypertension.
Pancreas	Submit samples for histologic study. If roentgenographic study is intended, see Chapter 2.	Acute pancreatitis.* Parasitic invasion of pancreatic duct with fibrosis and dilatation.

Reference

1. Case Records of Massachusetts. General Hospital. Clonorchis sinensis [Opisthorchis sinensis] infection of biliary tract. N Engl J Med 1990;323: 467–475.

Coagulation (See "Coagulation, disseminated intravascular," "Disease, Christmas," "Disease, von Willebrand's," "Hemophilia," and "Purpura,...")

Coagulation, Disseminated Intravascular

Synonyms and Related Terms: Consumption coagulopathy; hypofibrinogenemia; intravascular coagulation and fibrinolysis syndrome (ICF).

NOTE: Disseminated intravascular coagulation (DIC) often is a complication of obstetrical mishaps such as abruptio placentae or amniotic fluid embolism,* or it complicates malignancies (such as adenocarcinomas or leukemia*) or bacterial, viral, and other infections. Other conditions such as aortic aneurysm* or hemolytic uremic syndrome* are known causes also. If the nature of the underlying disease is known, follow the procedures under the appropriate heading also.

Organs and Tissues	*Procedures*	*Possible or Expected Findings*
External examination and skin	Prepare sections of skin of grossly involved and of uninvolved areas.	Petechiae, purpura, hemorrhagic bullae, gangrene, and other skin lesions.
Heart		Nonbacterial thrombotic endocarditis.*
Large blood vessels		Thromboses, predominantly around indwelling catheters.
Other organs	Submit tissue samples from grossly involved and uninvolved areas. Organs involved include brain, heart, kidneys, lungs, adrenal glands, spleen, gastrointestinal tract, pancreas, and liver, approximately in this order. Skin, testes, and choroid plexus also are frequently involved.	Fibrin or hyaline thrombi in capillaries, venules, or arterioles, and occasionally in larger vessels. Hemorrhages and ischemic infarcts may occur.
	Special stains such as phosphotungstic acid hematoxylin are not particularly helpful. Postmortem determination of fibrin split products is not helpful either.	For common underlying diseases or conditions, see above under "Note."

Coarctation, Aortic

Related Term: Aortic isthmus stenosis.

Possible Associated Conditions: Anomalous origin of right subclavian artery; atresia or stenosis of left subclavian artery; biscuspid aortic valve;* congenital mitral stenosis;* double aortic arch with stenosis of the right arch and coarctation of the left; stenosis of right subclavian artery; Turner's syndrome;* ventricular septal defect;* Shone's syndrome.

Organs and Tissues	*Procedures*	*Possible or Expected Findings*
External examination	Prepare chest roentgenogram.	Pressure atrophy of ribs with enlargement of costal grooves or focal erosions at inferior and ventral aspects of main body of ribs (rib notching).
Blood	Submit sample for microbiologic study.	Septicemia associated with endocarditis* or endarteritis (see below).
Heart	If endocarditis is suspected, follow procedures described in Chapter 7. For general dissection techniques, see Chapter 3.	Infective endocarditis* (of bicuspid aortic valve); endocardial fibroelastosis. For associated malformations, see above under "Possible Associated Conditions."
	For coronary angiography, see Chapter 10.	Premature coronary atherosclerosis.
Aorta and adjacent arteries	Record size and location of coarctation (relation to ductal artery and great vessels).	Preductal coarctation (isthmus stenosis) is often classified as "infantile type of coarctation." "Adult type" is at insertion of duct or distal to it. Rarely, coarctation occurs proximal to left subclavian artery, in lower thoracic aorta, or at multiple sites.
	If bacterial aortitis is suspected, obtain sample for microbiologic study through sterilized window in wall of aorta.	Bacterial aortitis. For ductal artery, see below.
	For arteriography, clamp proximal and distal thoracic aorta before injecting contrast medium.	Dilatation of subclavian, internal mammary, intercostal, scapular, and anterior spinal arteries.

Organs and Tissues	Procedures	Possible or Expected Findings
		Among the intercostal arteries, the fourth through seventh pairs are predominantly affected.
Aorta and adjacent arteries *(continued)*	Record width of left subclavian artery and compare with contralateral vessel; record width of aorta and of vessels proximal and distal to coarctation. Request Verhoeff–van Gieson stain.	Subclavian artery is considerably dilated if proximal to coarctation. Other complications include poststenotic dilatation of aorta, mycotic or noninfectious saccular aneurysm distal to coarctation (with or without rupture), and dissecting hematoma of aorta* (with or without rupture).
Ductal artery	Probe duct and record width of lumen.	Ductal artery may be patent or closed.
Abdominal arteries		Dilatation of epigastric and lumbar arteries. Rarely, coarctation of abdominal aorta.
	After surgical correction of coarctation, search for infarcts and sample arteries for histologic study.	Abdominal hypertensive arteritis and visceral infarctions after correction of coarctation.
Other organs		Manifestation of congestive heart failure.*
Brain	For removal and specimen preparation and cerebral arteriography, see Chapter 4.	Rupture of aneurysm, circle of Willis.

Cocaine (See "Dependence, cocaine.")

Coccidioidomycosis

Synonyms and Related Terms: *Coccidioides immitis* infection; San Joaquin fever; valley fever.

NOTE: (1) Collect all tissues that appear to be infected. (2) Request fungal cultures. (3) Request Grocott methenamine silver stain. (4) Special **precautions** are indicated (see Chapter 6). (5) Serologic studies are available from many reference and state health department laboratories. (6) This is a **reportable** disease in some states.

Organs and Tissues	Procedures	Possible or Expected Findings
External examination and skin	Prepare chest roentgenogram.	Pulmonary infiltrates; pulmonary cavitations; hilar lymphadenopathy.
	Prepare histologic sections of skin lesions. For a special stain, see above under "Note."	Erythema nodosum or multiforme,* various types of skin rashes; skin ulcers.
Blood	Submit sample for serologic study.	
Lungs	Prior to sectioning lungs, culture for fungi and bacteria any areas of consolidation. Prepare smears from fresh, grossly infected pulmonary tissue. For special stain, see above under "Note."	Chronic pulmonary cavitation; pulmonary fibrosis, pneumonia *(1)*.
	Perfuse one lung with formalin. Submit samples of hilar lymph nodes for histologic study.	Bronchiectasis.*
Other organs	Submit samples of material for culture and histologic study wherever extrapulmonary lesions are suspected.	Lymphogenous and hematogenous dissemination to almost all organs may occur, causing abscesses and sinuses of skin, subcutaneous tissue, bones, and joints.
	If involvement of central nervous system is suspected, submit sample of cerebrospinal fluid for culture and serologic study.	Meningitis* and encephalitis.*

Reference

1. Dweik M, Baethge BA, Duarte AG. Coccidiomycosis pneumonia in a nonendemic area associated with infliximab. South Med J 2007;100-517-518.

Codeine (See "Dependence, drug[s], all types or type unspecified.")

Cold (See "Exposure, cold.")

Colitis, All Types or Type Unspecified (See "Enterocolitis, Other Types or Type Undetermined.")

Colitis, Chronic Ulcerative (See "Disease, inflammatory bowel.")

Colitis, Collagenous

Related Terms: Lymphocytic colitis; microscopic colitis.

NOTE: This is a cause of diarrhea. Microscopic colitis is associated with older age; collagenous colitis is associated with female sex *(1)*. The colon is grossly normal but microscopically, increased lymphocytes in the lamina propria and a subepithelial band of collagen is found. If only the lymphocytic infiltrate is found, the term "lymphocytic colitis" or "microscopic colitis" should be applied. A trichrome stain should be ordered in all instances, because the collagen band may be difficult to see without the special stain.

1. Pardi DS, et al. The epidemiology of microscopic colitis: a population based study in Olmstead County, Minnesota. Gut 2007;56:504–508.

Coma, Hepatic

NOTE: See under name of suspected underlying hepatic disease, such as "Cirrhosis, liver" or "Hepatitis, viral."

Complex, Eisenmenger's (See "Defect, ventricular septal.")

Complex, Taussig-Bing (See "Ventricle, double outlet, right.")

Craniopharyngioma (See "Tumor of the pituitary gland.")
Cretinism (See "Hypothyroidism.")

Crisis, Sickle Cell (See "Disease, sickle cell.")

Croup (See "Laryngitis.")

Cryptococcosis

Synonyms: European Blastomycosis; torulosis.

NOTE: Cryptococcosis may follow or complicate AIDS *(1)* and other immunodeficient states, bronchiectasis,* bronchitis,* diabetes mellitus,* leukemia,* lymphoma,* sarcoidosis,* and tuberculosis.* (1) Collect all tissues that appear to be infected. (2) Request fungal cultures. (3) Request Grocott's methenamine silver, periodic acid Schiff, and mucicarmine stains. (4) No special precautions are indicated. (5) Serologic studies are available from many reference laboratories and from state health department laboratories. (6) This is not a reportable disease.

Organs and Tissues	*Procedures*	*Possible or Expected Findings*
Cerebrospinal fluid	Submit sample for fungal culture. Use India ink or a nigrosin preparation for direct examination.	
Brain and spinal cord	For removal and specimen preparation, see Chapter 4. Submit material for Gram stain and fungal culture. For special stains, see above under "Note."	Meningitis;* meningoencephalitis; hydrocephalus;* cysts in cortical gray matter and basal ganglia. Note that inflammation may be minimal.
Eyes	For removal and specimen preparation, see Chapter 5.	Endophthalmitis; optic neuritis.
Other organs	See above under "Note." Procedures depend on expected findings or grossly identified abnormalities as listed in right-hand column.	Infiltrates and abscesses in skin, endocardium, pericardium, liver, kidneys, adrenal glands, prostate, bones, and joints. Other infections may coexist *(2)*. Hypereosinophilia may be noted *(3)*.

References

1. Kanjanavirojkul N, Sripa C, Puapairoj A. Cytologic diagnosis of Cryp-tococcus neoformans in HIV-positive patients. Acta Cytol 1997;41: 493–496.
2. Benard G, Gryschek RC, Duarte AJ, Shikanai-Yasuda MA. Cryptococcosis as an opportunistic infection in immunodeficiency secondary to paracoccidioidomycosis. Mycopathologia 1996;133:65–69.
3. Marwaha RK, Trehan A, Jayashree K, Vasishta RK. Hypereosinophilia in disseminated cryptococcal disease. Pediatr Inf Dis J 1995;14: 1102–1103.
4. Benesová P et al. Cryptococcosis–a review of 13 autopsy cases from a 54-year period in a large hospital. APMIS 2007;115:177–183.

Cryptosporidiosis

Synonym: *Cryptosporidium parvum* infection.

Possible Associated Conditions: AIDS *(1)* and other immunodeficient states.

NOTE: (1) Collect feces, intestinal wall tissue, bile ducts, and pancreas. (2) Cultures are not available. (3) Request Kinyoun stain. (4) No special precautions are indicated. (5) Serologic studies are unreliable. (6) This is not a reportable disease.

Organs and Tissues	*Procedures*	*Possible or Expected Findings*
External examination	Record body weight and length and extent of rigor.	Evidence of dehydration following chronic diarrhea in immunosuppressed hosts.
Vitreous	Submit sample for sodium, chloride, and urea nitrogen determination.	Dehydration.*
Lungs	Perfuse one lung with formalin and submit samples of bronchi and lung for histologic study.	Bronchopulmonary cryptosporidiosis in HIV *(2)*.

Organs and Tissues	Procedures	Possible or Expected Findings
Intestinal tract	Record volume and appearance of intestinal contents. Submit samples of feces prepared with saline or iodine solution. Submit samples for determination of sodium, potassium, and chloride content.	Cryptosporidiosis may complicate inflammatory bowel disease *(3)*.*
	Submit samples of small bowel for histologic and electron microscopic study.	Parasites attached to mucosa.
Bile ducts, gallbladder, and pancreas	For cholangiography, see Chapter 2.	Changes resembling sclerosing cholangitis in patients with AIDS or other immunodeficiency states complicated by cryptosporidiosis *(4)*.
	Submit samples for histologic study and electron microscopic study.	*Cryptosporidium parvum* may be found on mucosal surfaces.

References

1. Ramratnam B, Flanigan TP. Cryptosporidiosis in persons with HIV infection. Postgrad Med J 1997;73:713–716.
2. Poirot JL, Deluol AM, Antoine M, Heyer F, Cadranel J, Meynard JL, et al. Broncho-pulmonary cryptosporidiosis in four HIV-infected patients. J Eukaryotic Microbiol 1996;43:78S–78S.
3. Manthey MW, Ross AB, Soergel KH. Cryptosporidiosis and inflammatory bowel disease. Dig Dis Sci 1997;42:1580–1586.
4. Davis JJ, Heyman MB, Ferrell L, Kerner J, Kerlan R Jr, Thaler MM. Sclerosing cholangitis associated with chronic cryptosporidiosis in a child with a congenital immunodeficiency disorder. Am J Gastroenterol 1987;82:1196–1202.

Cyanide (See "Poisoning, cyanide.")

Cyst(s), Choledochal

Synonyms and Related Terms: Choledochocyst; congenital cystic dilatation of the common bile duct; idiopathic dilatation of the common bile duct.

Possible Associated Conditions: Biliary atresia;* Caroli's disease;* congenital hepatic fibrosis.*

Organs and Tissues	Procedures	Possible or Expected Findings
External examination and skin	Prepare sections of skin lesions.	Jaundice; xanthomas.
Abdominal cavity	Submit peritoneal exudate for culture.	Bile peritonitis.
Gallbladder and extrahepatic bile ducts	Follow procedures described under "Cholecystitis." Record size and location of cyst(s) and relationship to surrounding organs, particularly to the portal vein. Puncture cyst(s) and submit contents for aerobic and anaerobic bacterial cultures. Dissect and photograph *in situ*.	Cyst may displace stomach, duodenum, and colon. Portal vein may be compressed, which may cause portal hypertension.* Cyst may perforate or contain stones or a carcinoma. Congenital anomalies such as double gallbladder, double common bile ducts, absence of gallbladder, biliary atresia, or annular pancreas may co-exist.
Liver	Record size and weight. Submit samples for histologic study.	Abscesses. Fibropolycystic disease of the liver.* See also above under "Possible Associated Conditions."

Reference

1. Crittenden SI, McKinley MJ. Choledochal cyst—clinical features and classification. Am J Gastroenterol 1985;80:643–647.

Cyst(s), Liver (See "Disease, fibropolycystic, of the liver and biliary tract.")

Cyst(s), Pulmonary

Related Terms: Congenital cystic adenomatoid malformation; congenital pulmonary lymphangiectasis; intralobular bronchopulmonary sequestration.

Possible Associated Conditions: Polycystic kidney disease;* renal cysts* or cysts of other organs.

Organs and Tissues	Procedures	Possible or Expected Findings
External examination	Prepare chest roentgenogram.	Cyst(s) with air, fluid, or both.
Chest organs	Search—*in situ* or after en bloc removal of chest organs—for anomalous arterial supply from aorta. Prepare pulmonary (see below) and thoracic aortic arteriograms. If infection of cyst is suspected, submit cyst contents or portions of the lung for bacterial culture. For bronchial and pulmonary arteriography, see Chapter 2. Perfuse lungs with formalin.	Congenital cysts in lower lobes may have anomalous arterial supply ("intralobular bronchopulmonary sequestration"). Perifocal bronchopneumonia; hemorrhage. Cysts may represent lymphangiectasias (see above under "Related Terms").
Other organs		In rare instances, cysts may co-exist in other organs, e.g. the kidneys.

Cyst(s), Renal

Related Terms: Acquired cystic renal disease; autosomal dominant (adult) polycystic renal disease *(1)*; autosomal recessive (infantile and childhood form) polycystic renal disease *(1)*; cystic renal lymphangiectasis; familial juvenile nephronophthisis; glomerulocystic disease; medullary cystic disease; multicystic dysplasia.

NOTE: Bilateral cystic disease of the kidneys may be acquired after long-term hemodialysis.

Possible Associated Conditions: Alagille's syndrome; Caroli's disease;* cerebral artery aneurysm* (with adult polycystic disease) *(2)*; congenital hepatic fibrosis;* congenital pyloric stenosis; cysts of liver, pancreas, spleen, lungs,* and testes; Ehlers-Danlos syndrome;* hemihypertrophy, Meckel-Gruber syndrome.

Organs and Tissues	Procedures	Possible or Expected Findings
Kidneys	For renal arteriography, venography, or urography, see Chapter 2. If infection of cysts is suspected, submit cyst contents or portions of the kidney for bacteriologic study.	Infection or calcification of cysts; pyelonephritis;* perinephric abscess. Obstructive uropathy;* nephrolithiasis;* carcinoma *(3)* (see "Tumor of the kidneys"); hemorrhages, and related complications *(4)*.
Liver	Prepare photographs and sample for histologic study.	In recessive polycycstic renal disease, congenital hepatic fibrosis is present and cystic bile ducts may be present in dominant cases *(5)*.
Other organs	See above under "Possible Associated Conditions." Other procedures depend on expected findings or grossly identified abnormalities as listed in right-hand column.	See above under "Possible Associated Conditions." Manifestations of portal or systemic hypertension* and kidney failure;* polycythemia.*

References

1. Rapola J, Kaariainen H. Polycystic kidney disease. Morphological diagnosis of recessive and dominant polycystic kidney disease in infancy and childhood. APMIS 1988;96:68–76.
2. Chapman AB, Rubinstein D, Hughes R, Stears JC, Earnest MP, Johnson AM, et al. Intracranial aneurysm in autosomal dominant poly-cystic kidney disease. N Engl J Med 1992;327:916–920.
3. Banyai-Falger S, Susani M, Maier U. Renal cell carcinoma in acquired renal cystic disease 3 years after successful kidney transplantation. Two case reports and review of the literature. Eur Urol 1995;28:77–80.
4. Wilson PD, Falkenstein D. The pathology of human renal cystic disease. Curr Topics Pathol 1995;88:1–50.
5. Zerres K, Völpel MC, Weiss H. Cystic kidney: Genetics, pathologic anatomy, clinical picture, and prenatal diagnosis. Hum Genet 1984;68:104–135.

Cystinosis

Synonyms and Related Terms: Cystine storage disease; de Toni-Debré-Fanconi syndrome;* infantile Fanconi syndrome.

Organs and Tissues	Procedures	Possible or Expected Findings
External examination	Record body weight and length.	Growth retardation.
Kidneys	Freeze tissue samples or fix them in absolute alcohol or Carnoy's fixative for preservation of cystine crystals. See also under "Glomerulonephritis." For preparation	Cystine crystals in tubular epithelial cells *(1)* and foam cells in the interstitium. "Swan's neck" deformity of nephrons (not specific). Atrophy

Organs and Tissues	Procedures	Possible or Expected Findings
	for electron microscopy, see Chapter 15. (See also under "Other organs.)	with interstitial scarring and tubular degeneration.
Urine	Submit sample for chemical analysis.	Glycosuria; generalized aminoaciduria.
Other organs	Submit samples of lymph nodes for histologic study (see above under "Kidneys"). For removal and specimen preparation of eyes, see Chapter 5. Excellent views of crystals can be provided in scanning electron microscopic preparations.	Cystine crystals occur throughout the reticuloendothelial system and in many other tissues, such as liver *(2)* or corneae and conjunctivae. Phthisis bulbi and numerous electron-transparent membrane-bound polygonal spaces in cells of the cornea, retina, and choroid *(3)*. Diagnostic doubly refractive brick- or needle-shaped cystine crystals in frozen sections or in smears from spleen, liver, lymph nodes, and bone marrow.
Bone and bone marrow	For removal, prosthetic repair, and specimen preparation of bones, see Chapter 2.	Cystine crystals in bone marrow.
	For preparation of sections and smears of bone marrow, see Chapter 2. See also above under "Kidneys."	Hypophosphatemic rickets.

References

1. Thoene JG. Cystinosis. J Inherited Metabolic Dis 1995;18(4):380–386.
2. Klenn PJ, Rubin R. Hepatic fibrosis associated with hereditary cystinosis: a novel form of noncirrhotic portal hypertension. Modern Pathol 1994; 7:879–882.
3. Tsilov E, et al. Ophthalmic manifestations and histopathology of infantile nephropathic cyctinosis: report of a case and review of the literature. Surv Ophthalmol 2007;52:97–105.

Cytomegalovirus (See "Infection, cytomegalovirus.")

D

Damage, Diffuse Alveolar (See "Syndrome, Adult Respiratory Distress [ARDS].")

Death, Abortion-Associated

Related Terms: Criminal abortion; stillbirth.*

NOTE: Anesthesia-associated death* must be considered in some of these cases. If criminal abortion is suspected, notify coroner or medical examiner.

Organs and Tissues	*Procedures*	*Possible or Expected Findings*
External examination and breasts	Prepare roentgenograms of chest and abdomen.	Pulmonary air embolism.*
	Describe appearance of breasts and sample glandular tissue for histologic study.	Pregnancy changes.
	Record appearance of external genitalia.	Instrument marks on vulva.
Peritoneal cavity	Submit exudate for bacteriologic study.	Peritonitis.*
Blood vessels and heart	Inspect and puncture right atrium and right ventricle of heart under water, also retroperitoneal and pelvic veins.	Pulmonary air embolism.* Abdominal and pelvic veins may also contain air.
Blood	Submit for bacteriologic and toxicologic study.	Septicemia. Absorption of intrauterine corrosives or other chemicals.
Lungs	Submit portion for bacteriologic study.	Abscesses; bacterial pneumonia.
	Prepare sample for electron microscopy.	Thromboembolism; embolism of soap and other chemicals.
Pelvic organs	If there are vascular lacerations, identify vessel. Submit samples of placenta and fetal parts for histologic study. Submit liquid intrauterine contents for toxicologic study. Sample ovaries for histologic study.	Lacerated blood vessels; pelvic hemorrhages. Instrument marks; foreign bodies;* perforation(s). Placenta, fetus, and fetal parts. Soap or other toxic foreign intrauterine materials. Corpus luteum of pregnancy.
Fetus	Determine weight and length, and estimate age (see Tables in Part III). Culture portion of lung.	Malformations. See also under "Stillbirth." Inhalation of infected amnionic fluid

Death, Anaphylactic

Synonym: Generalized anaphylaxis.

NOTE: Autopsy should be done as soon as possible after death. Neck organs should be removed before embalming. If death is believed to be caused by drug anaphylaxis, inquire about type of drug(s), drug dose, and route of administration (intravenous, intramuscular, and oral or other). This will determine proper sampling procedures—for instance, after penicillin anaphylaxis. Allergy to bee stings, wasp stings, fire ants, and certain plants may also be responsible for anaphylaxis. However, envenomation also can be fatal in the absence of anaphylaxis.

Organs and Tissues	*Procedures*	*Possible or Expected Findings*
External examination	Search for injection sites or sting marks. If such lesions are present, photograph and excise with 5-cm margin.	Foam in front of mouth and nostrils. Swelling of involved tissue.
	Freeze excised tissue at –70°C for possible analysis. Prepare chest roentgenogram.	Antigen-antibody reaction in involved tissues.

From: *Handbook of Autopsy Practice,* 4th Ed. Edited by: B.L. Waters

Organs and Tissues	Procedures	Possible or Expected Findings
Blood	Submit sample for immunologic study and study of drug levels. For serum IgE testing (Mayo Medical Laboratories), sample must be kept refrigerated (frozen or refrigerated coolant).	Antibodies against suspected antigen.
Neck organs	Remove as soon as possible after death. Photograph rim of glottis from above, together with epiglottis. For histologic study, fix larynx and epiglottis in Zenker's or Bouin's (see Chapter 15) solution.	Laryngeal edema may recede soon after death.
Tracheobronchial tree and lungs	Record character of contents of tracheobronchial tree. Photograph lungs and record weights. In order to avoid artificial distention, do not perfuse with fixative. For proper fixation, see above under "Neck organs." Request Giemsa stain.	Foamy edema in trachea and bronchi; diffuse or focal pulmonary distention ("acute emphysema") alternating with collapse; pulmonary edema and congestion; accumulation of eosinophilic leukocytes.
Spleen		Eosinophilic leukocytes in red pulp.

Reference

1. Tester DJ, Ackerman MJ. The role of molecular autopsy in unexplained sudden cardiac death. Curr Opin Cardiol 2006;21:166–172.

Death, Anesthesia-Associated.

NOTE: There are many possible causes of anesthesia-associated death that are not drug-related, such as acute airway obstruction* by external compression, aspiration, arrhythmia of a heart not previously known to be diseased, tumor, or an inflammatory process. Some of the complications are characteristically linked to a specific phase of the anesthesia, and many are not revealed by customary morphologic techniques.

The task for the pathologist charged with investigating an anesthesia-associated death is to reconstruct the chain of physiologic events culminating in cessation of vital signs. Autopsy morphology plays a supporting role; the main investigations center around the record left by the anesthesiologist, testing of anesthesia equipment, and toxicological testing. A consulting anesthesiologist can divine much more information from the anesthesia and recovery room records than can the pathologist, and can suggest avenues of further investigation. Therefore, the most important step in these autopsies is to obtain the anesthesia-associated records and to secure the consulting services of an independent anesthesiologist. The changes in the vital signs during and after anesthesia will help to focus the investigation toward a cardiac mechanism of death or depression of brainstem function as a terminal mechanism.

When information is gathered about drugs and chemical agents that have been administered or to which the victim may have had access, the pathologist must keep in mind that some non-medical chemicals and many drugs are known to affect anesthesia. Drugs and their metabolic products, additives, stabilizers, impurities, and deterioration products (one of which can be carbon monoxide) may be present and can be identified in postmortem tissues. Therefore, all appropriate body fluids and solid tissue should be submitted for toxicological examination. If the anesthetic agent was injected into or near the spinal canal, spinal fluid should be withdrawn from above the injected site into a standard toxicologist's collection tube with fluoride preservative. If the anesthetic agent was injected locally, tissue should be excised around the needle puncture marks at a radius of 2–4 cm. Serial postmortem analysis of specimens may permit extrapolation to tissue concentration at the time of death. The time interval between drug administration and death sometimes can be calculated from the distribution and ratio of administered drugs and their metabolic products. For a review of anesthetic death investigation, see ref. *(1)*.

Halothane anesthesia and some other anesthetic agents may cause fulminant hepatitis and hepatic failure. The autopsy procedures suggested under "Hepatitis, viral" should be followed.

Reference

1. Ward RJ, Reay DT. Anesthetic death investigation. Legal Med 1989; 39-58.

Death, Bolus (See "Obstruction, acute airway.")

Death, Crib (See "Death, sudden unexpected, of infant.")

Death due to Child Abuse or Neglect (See "Infanticide.")

Death, Intrauterine (See "Stillbirth.")

Death, Postoperative.

NOTE: For special autopsy procedures in postoperative deaths, see Chapter 1. In some instances, procedures described under "Death, anesthesia-associated" may be indicated. For a review of investigational procedures and autopsy techniques in operating-room-associated deaths, see ref. (1). If the autopsy will involve anatomy or dissection techniques that are unfamiliar, the pathologist should not hesitate to invite the surgeon to the autopsy. In patients who develop a cerebral infarction after open heart surgery, arterial air embolism should be considered as a possible cause. The diagnosis often must be based on excluding other causes because the air has been absorbed prior to death. If a patient dies rapidly, the hospital records may be incomplete or scanty. For example, if a patient bleeds to death despite attempted repair of hepatic lacerations, hospital records may not suffice to reach the correct cause-of-death opinion; personal accounts from the surgeon and anesthesiologist may be needed. Autopsy data on patients dying following thoracic surgery may be found in ref (2).

Reference

1. Start RD, Cross SS. Pathological investigations of deaths following surgery, anaesthesia and medical procedures. J Clin Pathol 1999;52: 640–652.
2. Ooi A, Goodwin AT et al. Clinical outcome versus post-mortem finding in thoracic surgery: a 10-year experience. Eur J Cardiothoracic Surg 2003;23:878–81.

Death, Restaurant
(See "Obstruction, acute airway.")

Death, Sniffing and Spray

Related Terms: Glue sniffing; sudden sniffing death syndrome.

NOTE: No anatomic abnormalities will be noted at autopsy. Sudden death may occur after cardiac dysrhythmia or respiratory arrest.

Organs and Tissues	*Procedures*	*Possible or Expected Findings*
Lungs	If poison had been inhaled at the time when death occurred, tie main bronchi. Submit lungs in glass container for gas analysis.	Trichloroethane, fluorinated refrigerants, and other volatile hydrocarbons are most often involved in the "sudden sniffing death syndrome."
	Submit samples of small bronchi for histologic study.	Spray death may occur in asthma sufferers using pressurized aerosol bronchodilators. Freons and related propellants may also be responsible for sudden death.
Brain	For removal and specimen preparation, see Chapter 4. Submit samples of fresh or frozen brain for toxicologic study.	Toxic components of glue—such as toluene—accumulate in the brain of glue sniffers. Also present in various glues are acetone, aliphatic acetates, cyclohexane, hexane, isopropanol, methylethyl ketone, and methylisobutyl ketone.
Other organs	Submit samples in glass containers (not plastic) for toxicologic study.	Aerosols may occlude the airway by freezing the larynx. Carbon tetrachloride sniffing may cause hepatorenal syndrome (see also under "Poisoning, carbon tetrachloride").

Death, Sudden Unexpected, of Adult

NOTE: Medicolegal autopsies are usually indicated, and appropriate procedures should be followed. If anaphylactic death is suspected, see also under that heading. For all unexpected deaths, the pathologist should learn the circumstances of the death, in order to determine whether the mechanism of death was rapid or slow, and to guide the selection of ancillary tests. Whenever paramedics attended a person, the run sheet should be obtained to look for a history of recent drinking or of chronic alcoholism may be an important clue. The combination of a history of alcoholism, a negative test for ethanol, and absence of cardiovascular disease, should suggest alcohol withdrawal as the cause of a sudden death. The list of "Possible or Expected Findings" below is not complete. For general toxicologic sampling, see Chapter 13.

Organs and Tissues	*Procedures*	*Possible or Expected Findings*
External Examination	Measure weight and length of body.	Needed for interpretation of heart weight.
Abdomen	Submit sample of blood or exudate.	Hemoperitoneum; peritonitis.*
Chest Cavity	Record volume and character of contents of pleural and pericardial cavities.	Hemothorax may occur—for instance, after rupture of aortic aneurysm. Hemopericardium usually occurs after rupture of myocardial infarction or of aortic dissection.*
Blood	Submit samples for microbiologic, molecular and toxicologic study.	Meningococcal disease* or streptococcal septicemia, gene mutations for entities such as long QT syndrome (1).

Organs and Tissues	*Procedures*	*Possible or Expected Findings*
Heart	Weigh heart after removal of clots. Submit samples of myocardium with the conduction system for histologic study. Perform coronary angiography.	Hypertensive left ventricular hypertrophy. Coronary atherosclerosis, thrombosis, or arteritis; myocardial infarction, with or without perforation; myocarditis;* valvular heart disease, such as aortic stenosis or floppy mitral valve.* Anatomic conduction system defects may indicate presence of arrhythmia. Structurally normal hearts may be seen in the setting of long QT syndrome and other ion channel mutation syndromes.
Lungs	Dissect all pulmonary arteries. Submit samples for histologic study.	Pulmonary thromboembolism; tumor embolism. Pulmonary intravascular (arterial and arteriolar) platelet aggregates may be cause of sudden death.
Aorta	Procedures depend on grossly identified abnormalities as listed in right-hand column.	Ruptured aneurysm;* aortic dissection.*
Pancreas		Islet cell tumor.
Adrenal glands	Photograph adrenals if hemorrhages are noted.	Hemorrhage may indicate presence of meningococcal disease or septic shock from other organism.*
Neck organs	Remove carefully to avoid dislodging food or other objects from larynx.	Occlusion of larynx by bolus (see "Obstruction, acute airway"). Laryngeal edema may be cause of anaphylactic death.*
Meninges, brain and spinal cord		Subdural or epidural hemorrhage after trauma, subarachnoid hemorrhage after rupture of aneurysm or—occasionally—with no apparent reason. Changes suggestive of epilepsy* may be present.
Vitreous	Submit samples for possible chemical and toxicological study.	Increased glucose concentrations may indicate the presence of hyperglycemia in undetected diabetes mellitus.*

Death, Sudden Unexpected, of Infant

Synonyms and Related Terms: Sudden infant death syndrome; SIDS; cot death; crib death.

NOTE: The autopsy alone does not suffice as an adequate investigation of sudden death of an infant. A thorough medical history, as well as complete information regarding the scene and circumstances of death must also be conducted. It should be recorded whether the infant was found in a prone position. Photographs of the scene should be taken. The environmental and the infant's body temperature should be recorded as close to the time of death as possible. Cases of infanticide have been disguised as SIDS; a high level of suspicion should be maintained, particularly if more than one SIDS case reportedly occurred in the same family. Thus, while some of the "Possible or Expected Findings" in the table refer to typical cases of SIDS *(1)*, other refer to possible infanticide *(2)*.

Organs and Tissues	*Procedures*	*Possible or Expected Findings*
External examination	Record weight of infant; measure crown-rump and crown-heel length and head, chest and abdominal circumference. Photograph and culture any sites of infection. Test skin turgor and look for "sunken eyes" (signs of dehydration). Prepare skeletal roentgenograms.	Growth retardation. Signs of dehydration. Crusts or frothy fluid around nose and mouth. Emaciation indicates organic disease or neglect. Bruises or burns indicative of child abuse. Jaundice; edema. Old or recent fractures due to child abuse.

Organs and Tissues	Procedures	Possible or Expected Findings
Eyes	Ophthalmic examination.	Retinal hemorrhages indicative of "shaken baby syndrome." Conjunctival petechiae may be a sign of strangulation *(2)*.
Cerebrospinal fluid	If there is clinical or pathologic evidence of infection, submit sample for bacterial and viral cultures. Prepare smear.	
Vitreous	Submit sample only after the head has been opened to rule out any hemorrhages or craniocerebral trauma. If craniocerebral trauma is present, forego collection of vitreous in order to fix the globes for histologic examination of the retinas. Submit for electrolyte studies and urea nitrogen and glucose determination.	Increased glucose concentrations may indicate undiagnosed diabetes mellitus.* Manifestations of dehydration.*
Chest cavity		Petechial serosal hemorrhages.
Thymus	Record weight and submit samples for histologic study.	Accelerated involution indicates stress and/or disease, of prolonged duration. Thymic petechiae.
Blood	Submit for culture. Submit blood drops dried on filter paper for tests for inborn errors of metabolism. Refrigerate blood samples for toxicologic study.	In SIDS, blood in heart chambers tends to remain fluid.
Heart and great vessels; ductus arteriosus	Check venous return and origin and course of coronary arteries and great vessels. Submit samples for histologic study.	In rare instances, congenital heart disease, myocarditis, coronary artery aneurysm, or coronary artery arising from the pulmonary artery may explain the sudden death.
Lungs	Record weights; culture and Gram-stain areas of consolidation. Submit samples for histologic study.	Congestion; hemorrhage; edema; pleural petechiae; atelectasis. Acute pulmonary emphysema may indicate strangulation *(2)*.
Neck organs and trachea	Photograph and culture sites of infection. Submit samples for histologic study.	Laryngitis;* tracheitis. Epiglottitis. Infection affecting other neck organs and tissues.
	Dissect, weigh, and section carotid bodies.	Hypoplasia of carotid bodies (few are hyperplastic).
Stomach	Record character and amount of contents.	This may be pertinent to allegations of starvation.
Intestinal tract	Record appearance of serosal surface (exudate? discoloration?). Assess attachment of the mesenteric root, which normally runs obliquely from the left upper quadrant (ligament of Treitz) to the right lower quadrant near the inferior pole of the right kidney.	Contusions; malrotation; volvulus; infarction.
Pancreas	Submit samples for histologic study.	Degeneration of islets may indicate presence of undetected diabetes mellitus.*
Urine	Obtain two samples; one saved in preservative and the other frozen or refrigerated for toxicologic assays.	Drug intoxication, increased organic acids with medium chain acyl-coenzyme A dehyrogenase deficiency *(3)*.
Other organs	Submit portions of spleen, for culture as a double check for the blood culture. Carefully examine, weigh, and submit samples of organs, including endocrine organs, for histologic study.	Extramedullary hematopoiesis in the liver. Congenital adrenal hypoplasia.
Brain and spinal cord	For removal and specimen preparation, see Chapter 4. Submit portion of brain for microbiologic study if indicated by clinical history or pathologic findings.	Head trauma in abused child. Birth injuries; encephalitis. Astroglial proliferations in brain stem. Retarded myelination of brain stem.
Middle ears	Open middle ears and mastoid cells.	Otitis media.*

Organs and Tissues	*Procedures*	*Possible or Expected Findings*
	Submit exudate for microbiologic study. Prepare Gram-stained smears of exudate and histologic sections of middle ears.	
Bones and bone marrow	Submit samples from costochondral junctions or other epiphyses.	Bone changes of vitamin D deficiency* (rickets). Normoblastic hyperplasia of bone marrow. Retardation of the rate of enchondral ossification such that hematopoiesis abuts the transition zone.

References

1. Valdez-Dapena M, McFeeley PA, Hoffman HJ, et al., eds. Histopathology Atlas for the Sudden Infant Death Syndrome. Armed Forces Institute of Pathology Washington, DC, 1993. (Order from American Registry of Pathology Sales Office, AFIP, Room 1077, Washington, DC 20,306–26,000.)
2. Becroft DM, Lockett BK. Intra-alveolar pulmonary siderophages in sudden infant death: a marker for previous imposed suffocation. Pathology 1997;29:60–63.
3. Betz P, Hausmann R, Eisenmenger W. A contribution to a possible differentiation between SIDS and asphyxiation. For Sci Intl 1998;91: 147–152.
4. Bajanowski T, et al. Sudden infant death syndrome (SIDS)–standardized investigations and classification: recommendations. Forensic Sci Int 2007;165:129–143.
5. Landi K, et al. Investigation of the sudden deth of infants: a multicenter analysis. Pediatr Dev Pathol 2005;8:630–638.

Decompression (See "Accident, Diving. (Skin or Scuba)")

Defect, Aortopulmonary Septal

Synonyms: Aortopulmony window; aorticopulmonary window or septal defect.

NOTE: The basic anomaly is a defect between ascending aorta and main pulmonary artery. For general dissection techniques, see Chapter 3.

Possible Associated Conditions: Atrial septal defect;* bicuspid aortic valve;* coarctation,* hypoplasia, or interruption (type A) of aortic arch; coronary artery from main pulmonary artery; right atrial arch; patent ductal artery;* right pulmonary artery from ascending aorta; subaortic stenosis;* tetralogy of Fallot;* ventricular septal defect.* (In approx 50% of the cases, one or more of these associated conditions are found.)

Defect, Atrial Septal

NOTE: The basic anomaly is a defect of the atrial septum, usually at the oval fossa (in 85%). Possible complications in unoperated cases include atrial arrhythmias, congestive heart failure; paradoxic embolism; plexogenic pulmonary hypertension (<10%), and pulmonary artery aneurysm. Possible surgical interventions include surgical and transcatheter closure of defect. For general dissection techniques, see Chapter 3.

Possible Associated Conditions: *With secundum type:* Often isolated; may occur with conotruncal anomalies, patent ductal artery,* valvular atresia,* and ventricular septal defect.* *With primum type:* Cleft in anterior mitral leaflet. *With sinus venosus type*: Anomalous connection of right pulmonary veins. *With coronary sinus type* (unroofed coronary sinus): Left atrial connection of a persistent left superior vena cava. *With absent atrial septum or multiple large defects* (common atrium): Complete atrioventricular defect;* asplenia syndrome.*

Defect, Complete Atrioventricular Septal

Synonyms and Related Terms: Complete atrioventricular canal; complete AV canal; endocardial cushion defect.

NOTE: The basic anomaly is a large combined atrioventricular septal defect and a common atrioventricular valve, with displacement of the atrioventricular conduction tissues. For possible surgical interventions, see complete repair, "mitral" valve replacement in Chapter 3.

Possible Associated Conditions: Aortic coarctation; (35%); asplenia or polysplenia syndrome;* atrial septal defect;* common atrium; discrete subaortic stenosis;* double outlet right ventricle;* Down's syndrome;* patent ductal artery;* persistent left superior vena cava; pulmonary stenosis;* tetralogy of Fallot.*

Defect, Partial Atrioventricular Septal

Synonyms and Related Terms: Endocardial cushion defect; primum atrial septal defect with cleft mitral valve.

NOTE: The basic anomaly is a primum atrial septal defect and a cleft in the anterior mitral leaflet. Possible surgical interventions consist of surgical repair of both malformations. For general dissection techniques, see Chapter 3.

Possible Associated Conditions: Mitral regurgitation.

Defect, Ventricular Septal

Synonyms: Inlet (subtricuspid, AV canal type); membranous (paramembranous, perimembranous, infracristal); muscular (persistent bulboventricular foramen); and outlet (sub-arterial, supracristal, conal, doubly committed juxta-arterial).

NOTE: The basic anomaly is a defect of the ventricular sep-tum, usually at the membranous septum (in 75%). Possible sur-gical intervention consists of surgical closure of the defect. Late postoperative death may be sudden and related to residual pulmonary hypertension or ventricular arrhythmias. For general dissection techniques, see Chapter 3. If hypertensive pulmonary artery disease is suspected, perfuse one lung with formalin and request Verhoeff–van Gieson stain.

Possible Associated Conditions: With membranous type: Often isolated; may occur with atrial septal defect,* conotruncal anomalies, or patent ductal artery.* With outlet type: Conotruncal anomalies such as double outlet right ventricle,* persistent truncal artery,* or tetralogy of Fallot.* With inlet type: Atrioventricular septal defect* or atrioventricular discordance. With muscular type: Isolated or with tricuspid atresia* or double inlet left ventricle.

Deficiency, alpha$_1$-Antitrypsin

Possible Associated Conditions: See below under "Possible or Expected Findings."

Organs and Tissues	Procedures	Possible or Expected Findings
Skin and subcutaneous tissue	Sample normal and abnormal appearing areas for histologic study.	Panniculitis *(1)*.
Blood (serum)	Submit frozen sample for determination of alpha$_1$-antitrypsin concentrations (1 mL is required).	Decreased a$_1$-antitrypsin values. Many genetic alleles can be determined by starch-gel electrophoresis.
Lungs	Perfuse lungs with formalin. See also under "Emphysema."	Panlobular pulmonary emphysema,* primarily of lower lobes; chronic bronchitis and, rarely, brochiectases; interstitial pulmonary fibrosis.
Liver	If cirrhosis or tumor is present, follow procedures described under those headings. Request PAS stain, with diastase digestion.	Cirrhosis in infants and adults; cholangiocellular or hepatocellular carcinoma; paucity of intrahepatic bile ducts; neonatal (giant cell) hepatitis; periportal hepatitis or cirrhosis and hepatocellular carcinoma in adults *(2,3)*.
	Characteristic accumulations of alpha$_1$-antitrypsin can be shown in routine paraffin sections with PAS-D or immunostains.	PAS-positive, diastase-resistant globular inclusions, primarily in periportal hepatocytes or in the periphery of regenerative nodules.
Small and large intestine		Inflammatory bowel disease (rare) *(3)*.
Extrahepatic bile ducts	For cholangiography, see Chapter 2. Dissect bile ducts *in situ*.	Biliary atresia.* Generally no abnormalities in adults.
Pancreas		Chronic pancreatitis; fibrosis of pancreas.
Kidneys	See under "Glomerulonephritis."	Membranoproliferative glomerulonephritis* in childhood *(4)*.

References

1. O'Riordan K, Blei A, Rao MS, Abecassis M. Alpha 1-antitrypsin deficiency-associated panniculitis: resolution with intravenous alpha 1-antitrypsin administration and liver transplantation. Transplantation 1997;63:480–482.
2. Perlmutter DH. Clinical manifestations of alpha 1-antitrypsin deficiency. Gastroenterol Clin North Am 1995;24:27–43.
3. Elzouki AN, Eriksson S. Risk of hepatobiliary disease in adults with severe alpha 1-antitrypsin deficiency (PiZZ): is chronic viral hepatitis B or C an additional risk factor for cirrhosis and hepatocellular carcinoma? Eur J Gastroenterol 1996;8:989–994.
4. Yang P, Tremaine WJ, Meyer RL, Prakash UB. Alpha 1-antitrypsin deficiency and inflammatory bowel disease. Mayo Clin Proc 2000;75: 450–455.
5. Elzouki AN, Lindgren S, Nilsson S, Veress B, Erisksson S. Severe alpha1-antitrypsin deficiency (PiZ homozygosity) with membranoproliferative glomerulonephritis and nephrotic syndrome, reversi-bleafterorthotopiclivertransplantation.JHepatol1997;26:1403–1407.

Deficiency, alpha-Lipoprotein (See "Disease, Tangier's.")

Deficiency, beta-Lipoprotein (See "Abetalipoproteinemia.")

Deficiency, Congenital Transferrin (See "Hemochromatosis.")

Deficiency, Folic Acid (See "Anemia, megaloblastic.")

Deficiency, Myeloperoxidase (See "Disorder, inherited, of phagocyte function.")

Deficiency, Vitamin A

Synonyms and Related Terms: Hypovitaminosis A; kerato -malacia; xerophthalmia.

Organs and Tissues	Procedures	Possible or Expected Findings
External examination	Record extend and character of skin lesions and appearance of eyes; prepare sections of skin.	Sebaceous glands covered with keratin; keratomalacia; enlarged meibomian glands of eyelids.
Other organs		For conditions that may produce vitamin A deficiency, see under "Syndrome, malabsorption."
Eyes	For removal and specimen preparation, see Chapter 5.	Bitot's spots (keratinized epithelium and air bubbles at corneal rim); keratomalacia.

Deficiency, Vitamin B_1 (Thiamine) (See "Syndrome, Wernicke-Korsakoff.")

Deficiency, Vitamin B_6 (See "Beriberi.")

Deficiency, Vitamin B_{12} (See "Anemia, megaloblastic.")

Deficiency, Vitamin C

Synonyms: Hypovitaminosis C; scurvy.

Organs and Tissues	*Procedures*	*Possible or Expected Findings*
External examination and skin	Record extent and character of skin lesions; prepare sections of skin.	Hyperkeratotic hair follicles with perifollicular hemorrhages (posterior thighs, anterior forearms, abdomen); petechiae and ecchymoses (inner and posterior thighs); subcutaneous hemorrhages.
	Describe appearance of gums, and prepare sections.	Gingivitis.
Other organs	Record evidence of bleeding.	In rare instances, gastrointestinal or genitourinary hemorrhages.
Bones, joints, and soft tissues	For removal, prosthetic repair, and specimen preparation of bones and joints, see Chapter 2.	Hemorrhages into muscles and joints. Subperiosteal hemorrhages occur primarily in distal femora, proximal humeri, tibiae, and costochondral junctions (scorbutic rosary).

Deficiency, Vitamin D

Synonyms: Hypovitaminosis D; rickets.

NOTE: Features or rickets may be found in familial hypophosphatemia (vitamin D-resistent rickets; Fanconi syndrome).

Organs and Tissues	*Procedures*	*Possible or Expected Findings*
External examination	Prepare skeletal roentgenograms.	In infants, rachitic changes at costochondral junctions; in adults, osteoporosis* and osteomalacia*—with or without pseudofractures (Milkman's syndrome).
	In infants with suspected rickets, record size of anterior fontanelle and shape of head; state of dentition; and shape of costochondral junctions, wrists, long bones, and spine.	Craniotabes; delayed dentition and enamel defects; protrusion of sternum; rachitic rosary; swelling of costochondral junctions and of wrists.
Vitreous or blood (serum)	Submit samples for calcium, magnesium, and phosphate determination.	Hypocalcemia, hypomagnesemia, hypophosphatemia.
Other organs	Procedures depend on expected findings or grossly identified abnormalities as listed in right-hand column.	Possible causes of vitamin D deficiency include diseases associated with malabsorption syndrome,* biliary atresia,* and primary biliary cirrhosis.
	Weigh parathyroid glands and submit samples for histologic study.	Parathyroid hyperplasia (hyperparathyroidism*) secondary to hypocalcemia and impaired absorption of vitamin D.
	Submit samples of intestine for histologic study.	Conditions causing malabsorption.
Bones	For removal, prosthetic repair, and specimen preparation, see Chapter 2.	Osteomalacia.*
	In infantile rickets, diagnostic sites for histologic sampling are costochondral junctions, distal ends of radius and ulna, and proximal ends of tibia and humerus. For adults, see under "Osteomalacia."	Characteristic abnormalities of osteochondral growth plates in infants. Abundant osteoid in osteomalacia.*

Deformity, Klippel-Feil

Synonym: Congenital fusion of cervical vertebrae.

Organs and Tissues	*Procedures*	*Possible or Expected Findings*
External examination		Short neck; low posterior hairline. Disorders with dysraphia (see below).
	Prepare roentgenograms of chest, neck (lateral view), and head.	Fusion of cervical vertebrae. Congenital elevation of the scapula (Sprengel's deformity).
Neck organs		Malformed larynx *(1)*.
Skull, spine, brain,	For removal and specimen preparation of brain and spinal cord, see Chapter 4.	Arnold-Chiari malformation;* basilar impression; meningomyelocele; platybasia; spinal cord compression; syringomyelia.* Intracranial or spinal cord tumors *(2)*.
Heart		Aneurysm of sinus of Valsalva *(3)*.

References

1. Clarke RA, Davis PJ, Tonkin J. Klippel-Feil syndrome associated with malformed larynx. Case report. Ann Otol Rhinol Laryngol 1994; 103:201–207.
2. Diekmann-Guiroy B, Huang PS. Klippel-Feil syndrome in association with a craniocervical dermoid cyst presenting as aseptic meningitis in an adult: case report. Neurosurgery 1989;25:652–655.
3. Kawano Y, et al. Klippel-Feil syndrome accompanied by an aneurysm of the non-coronary sinus of Valsalva. Intern Med 2006;45:1191–1192.

Degeneration, Cerebellar Cortical

Synonyms and Related Terms: Alcoholic cerebellar degeneration; parenchymatous cerebellar degeneration.

Organs and Tissues	*Procedures*	*Possible or Expected Findings*
Brain and spinal cord	For removal and specimen preparation, see Chapter 4.	Cortical atrophy (predominantly loss of Purkinje cells) of dorsal vermis of cerebellum and adjacent anterior lobe.
Other organs	Procedures depend on expected findings or grossly identified abnormalities as listed in right-hand column.	Manifestations of chronic alcoholism,* amebiasis,* cirrhosis,* malnutrition, or pellagra.*

Degeneration, Cerebello-Olivary
(See "Degeneration, spinocerebellar.")

Degeneration, Hepatolenticular
(See "Disease, Wilson's.")

Degeneration, Spinocerebellar

Related Terms: Familial cortical cerebellar atrophy; Friedreich's ataxia; hereditary ataxia; Machado-Joseph disease; olivo-pontocerebellar atrophy *(1)*.

NOTE: The term spinocerebellar degeneration encompasses a variety of lesions whose classification is controversial. A new approach has come from linkage analysis and molecular biology. For instance, Friedreich's ataxia, the classic form of hereditary ataxia, is due to an intronic expansion of a GAA tri-nucleotide repeat. Other forms are also identified by their specific gene loci. Neuropathologic examination still is important and ample sampling is suggested, which should include cerebral cortex, basal ganglia (caudate nucleus, putamen, and globus pallidus), thalamus, subthalamic nucleus, midbrain (red nucleus and substantia nigra), pons (pontine nuclei), spinal cord (at cer-vical, thoracic, and lumbar levels), optic tract, optic nerves with lateral geniculate nucleus, and sensory and motor peripheral nerves.

Organs and Tissues	*Procedures*	*Possible or Expected Findings*
Blood	Obtain blood for molecular analysis.	Gene mutation on 16 q *(2)*.
Brain and spinal cord	For removal and specimen preparation, see Chapter 4.	Symmetric neuronal loss with reactive astrocytosis in the affected areas. See also above under "Note."
Peripheral nerves	For removal and specimen preparation, see Chapter 4.	

Reference

1. Koeppen AH. The hereditary ataxias. J Neuropathol Exp Neurol 1998;57:531–543.
2. Nozaki H, et al. Clinical and genetic characterizations of 16q-linked autosomal dominant spinocerebellar ataxia (AD-SCA) and frequency analysis of AD-SCA in the Japanese population. Mov Disord 2007;22:857–862.

Degeneration, Spongy, of White Matter

Synonyms and Related Terms: Bertrand-van Bogaert disease; Canavan's disease; familial leukodystrophy.

NOTE: The disease is caused by defective asparto acylase activity. The gene has been cloned and mutations found.

Organs and Tissues	*Procedures*	*Possible or Expected Findings*
External examination	Record head circumference. Prepare roentgenograms of skull.	Enlargement of head.
Brain and spinal cord	For removal and specimen preparation, see Chapter 4. Request Luxol fast blue stain.	Poor demarcation between cortex and gelatinous white matter. Extensive demyelination and vacuolation of white matter, particularly subcortically.
Eyes and optic nerves	For removal and specimen preparation, see Chapter 5.	Optic atrophy.

Degeneration, Striatonigral (See "Atrophy, multiple system.")

Dehydration

Related Term: Thirst.

NOTE: Possible underlying conditions not related to inaccessibility of water include burns, exposure to heat, gastrointestinal diseases, recent paracentesis, renal diseases, and use of diuretic drugs. See also under "Disorder, electrolyte(s)."

Organs and Tissues	*Procedures*	*Possible or Expected Findings*
External examination		Skin turgor may be decreased and eyes may be sunken.
	Prepare histologic sections of blisters, ulcers, or skin abrasions.	Microscopic changes help to decide whether skin lesions are antemortem or postmortem.
Vitreous	Submit sample for sodium, chloride, and urea nitrogen determination.	Sodium concentrations more than 155 meq/L, chloride concentrations more than 130 meq/ and urea nitrogen concentrations between 40 and 100 meq/dL indicate dehydration.
Urine	Record volume and specific gravity	Absence or minimal amount of urine.

Dementia (See "Disease, Alzheimer's.")

Drug abuse, Amphetamine(s)

NOTE: Methamphetamine abuse may be suggested by poor condition of the dentition. Methylenedioxymethamphetamine ("Ecstasy") abuse is often suggested by friends with whom the decedent was abusing drugs. Follow procedures described under "Dependence, drug(s)."

Drug abuse, Cocaine

NOTE: Cocaine is spontaneously hydrolyzed by blood esterases, even after death. However, one of its major metabolite, benzoylecgonine, is routinely identifiable by immunoassay screening tests. When cocaine is abused concurrently with heroin or other depressant drugs, it may be difficult to ascribe deth to a single agent, unless circumstances clearly point to a rapid cardiac mechanism or a slow brainstem depression mechanism.

Organs and Tissues	*Procedures*	*Possible or Expected Findings*
External examination	Record condition of nasal septum.	Chronic inflammation and perforation of nasal septum after prolonged sniffing of cocaine.
	Submit nasal swab for toxicologic study.	Remnant of cocaine.
Blood	Submit sample with NaF added for toxicologic study (see Chapter 13); request drug screen.	See above under "Note."
Heart	Record heart weight and thickness of ventricles. For dissection of the heart and coronary arteries, and for histologic sampling, see also Chapter 3.	Left ventricular hypertrophy caused by hypertension complicating or aggravated by cocainism. Cardiotoxicity with focal myocarditis and myocyte necrosis *(2)*,

Organs and Tissues	Procedures	Possible or Expected Findings
		contraction bands *(3)*, and coronary occlusion.
Stomach and colon	Save gastric contents for toxicologic study. Sample stomach and colon for histologic study.	Ischemia of gastric mucosa after ingestion of cocaine. Ischemic colitis *(4)*.
Liver and gallbladder	Save liver tissue and bile for toxicologic study. Sample liver for histologic study.	Zonal hepatic necrosis *(5)*.
Other body fluids and organs	Save vitreous, urine, kidneys, and brain for toxicologic study.	See above under "Note."

References

1. Brody SL, Slovis CM, Wrenn KD. Cocain-related medical problems. Consecutive series of 233 cases. Am J Med 1990;88:325–331.
2. Peng SK, French WJ, Pelikan PCD. Direct cocaine cardiotoxicity demonstrated by endomyocardial biopsy. Arch Pathol Lab Med 1989; 113:842–845.
3. Karch SB, Billingham ME. The pathology and etiology of cocaine-induced heart disease. Arch Pathol Lab Med 1988;112:225–230.
4. Brown DN, Rosenholtz MJ, Marshall JB. Ischemic colitis related to cocaine abuse. Gastroenterology 1994;89:1558–1561.
5. Silva MO, Roth D, Reddy KR, Fernandez JA, Albores-Saavedra J, Schiff ER. Hepatic dysfunction accompanying acute cocaine intoxication. J Hepatol 1991;12:312–315.

Drug abuse, all Types or Type Unspecified

Related Terms: Cocaine dependence;* crack dependence; heroin dependence; intravenous narcotism; morphinism.

NOTE: If narcotic paraphernalia and samples of the drug itself are found at the scene of the death, they should be submitted for analysis. Helpful information about the nature of a drug may be obtained from witnesses. State crime laboratories may provide much assistance. If name of drug is known, see also under "Poisoning,..." The slang name of a drug may be insufficient for identification because these names often are used for different compounds at different times of places.

Opoid narcotics can be injected intravenously, or subcutaneously, or snorted. Death may occur with such speed that the bodies may be found with needles and syringes in the veins or clenched in the hands. Drug abuse may be associated with a multitude of local (see below) or systemic complications, including malaria* and tetanus.*

As stated in Chapter 13, for a growing number of analytes, most notably tricyclic antidepressants, peripheral blood is preferred over central blood. Peripheral blood is aspirated by percutaneous puncture before autopsy, from the femoral vein or the subclavian vein. The authors prefer the femoral approach in order to avoid any question of artifact in the diagnosis of venous air embolism. It may be pru-dent to add NaF to some of the samples.

Possible Associated Conditions: Acquired immunodeficiency syndrome (AIDS) and many other acute and chronic infec-tions; malnutrition.*

Organs and Tissues	Procedures	Possible or Expected Findings
External examination and skin	In suspected homicides or other unusual circumstances, excise fresh needle marks with surrounding skin and underlying tissues and submit for toxicologic analysis. (In routine accidental drug-related deaths, this is not necessary.) Submit samples with needle marks for histologic study under polarized light. If victim has not been identified, follow procedures described in Chapter 13. Photograph changes that indicate addiction.	Foam may exude from nostrils. Erosions of the nasal septum occur in heroin sniffers. Needle marks may be found at any accessible site. Scars, "track hyperpigmentation," ulcers, skin abscesses, and subcutaneous hemorrhages may be abundant. Other complications are ischemic crush injuries with acute rhabdomyolysis, myositis ossificans (brachial muscle), and thrombophlebitis.
Blood	For toxicologic sampling, see above under "Note." Submit samples for bacterial, fungal, and viral cultures, study of viral antibodies (hepatitis B and C), and blood alcohol determination.	Septicemia; evidence of acute or chronic viral infection; alcohol intoxication.
Heart	If endocarditis is suspected, culture any suspected vegetation.	Infective endocarditis* that is often on the right side. Expected organisms include *Acinebacter* spp., *Staphylococcus aureus, Staphylococcus albus, Salmonella* spp., enterococci, and *Staphylococcus epidermidis.*

Organs and Tissues	Procedures	Possible or Expected Findings
Lungs	Submit portions for micro-biologic study. Submit multiple samples for histologic study. Request Verhoeff–van Gieson stain. Study sections under polarized light.	Pulmonary edema; aspiration; diffuse lobular pneumonia. Septic pulmonary abscesses. Perivascular pulmonary talc granulomas; foreign body emboli; pulmonary necrotizing angiitis; atelectases and fibrosis.
Gallbladder	Submit sample of bile for toxicologic study.	Heroin is metabolized to morphine, which accumulates in bile.
Liver	Submit samples for toxicologic and histologic study.	Nonspecific portal hepatitis; acute or chronic viral hepatitis;* alcoholic liver disease.* Foreign body granulomas may be present in the liver.
Perihilar lymph nodes		Chronic lymphadenitis.
Spleen	Record weight.	Splenomegaly with follicular hyperplasia.
Urine	Submit sample for toxicologic study.	Detects monoacetylmorphine to distinguish heroin from morphine poisoning.
Brain and spinal cord	For removal and specimen preparation, see Chapter 4.	Bilateral symmetric necrosis of globus pallidus; cerebral abscess;* meningitis;* transverse myelitis; mycotic aneurysms; subdural or epidural empyema.* Acute cerebral falciparum malaria.*
Bones and joints	Submit samples of grossly abnormal areas for histologic study.	Infectious spondylitis and sacroiliitis.

Depressant(s) (See "Dependence, drug(s),...")

Dermatomyositis

Related Term: Childhood dermatomyositis (or polymyositis) associated with vasculitis; dermatomyositis (or polymyositis) associated with neoplasia or collagen vascular disease; primary idiopathic dermatomyositis; primary idiopathic polymyositis.

Possible Associated Conditions: Carcinoma (lung, stomach, intestine, and prostate in males; breast, ovary, and uterus in females; miscellaneous sites in both sexes); lymphoma* (rare) and other malignancies *(1)*; lupus erythematosus;* mixed connective tissue disease; progressive systemic sclerosis;* rheumatoid arthritis;* Sjögren's syndrome;* and others. Vasculitis of childhood polymyositis (dermatomyositis).

Organs and Tissues	Procedures	Possible or Expected Findings
External examination and skin	Photograph grossly involved skin.	Erythema; maculopapular eruption; eczematoid or exfoliative dermatitis; ulcerations; calcification.
	Prepare sections of involved (anterior chest, knuckles, knees) and grossly uninvolved skin and subcutaneous tissue.	Microscopically, dermatitis and panniculitis with edema and fibrinoid necroses are found. Vasculitis in childhood cases. Lipodystrophy *(2)*.
	Prepare roentgenograms.	Pneumomediastinum and subcutaneous emphysema *(3)*.
Heart	Submit samples from myocardium for histologic study.	Mycarditis* (rare). Microscopic changes similar to those in skeletal muscles (see below).
Lungs	Perfuse one lung with formalin.	Lymphocytic pneumonitis; obliterating bronchiolitis; edema; interstitial pulmonary fibrosis (see "Pneumonia, interstitial").
Esophagus and gastrointestinal tract	Submit samples from all segments for histologic study.	Vasculitis; myositis, rarely with rupture *(4)*. Features of inflammatory bowel disease may be present.

Organs and Tissues	Procedures	Possible or Expected Findings
Kidneys		Arteritis* and phlebitis* with thrombosis, fibrosis, and infarctions.
Other organs	Submit samples of liver for histologic study. For sampling in diabetes mellitus, see under that heading.	Steatohepatitis and manifestations of diabetes mellitus* may be found *(2)*.
Skeletal muscles	Submit samples from deltoid, biceps, cervical, gluteal, and femoral muscles, and also from other muscles that may have been involved clinically (pharynx, tongue), for histologic study. Photograph abnormal gross specimens. For specimen preparation, see Chapter 4.	Myositis with muscular atrophy and fibrosis; vasculitis in childhood cases.
Peripheral nerves	For removal and specimen preparation, see Chapter 4.	Polyneuropathy (rare) *(5)*.
Joints	For removal, prosthetic repair, and specimen preparation, see Chapter 2.	Arthritis.

References

1. Maoz CR, Langevitz P, Livneh A, Blumstein Z, Sadeh M, Bank I, et al. High incidence of malignancies in patients with dermatomyositis and polymyositis: an 11-year analysis. Semin Arthritis Rheum 1998; 27:319–324.
2. Quecedo E, Febrer I, Serrano G, Martinez-Aparicio A, Aliaga A. Partial lipodystrophy associated with juvenile dermatomyositis: report of two cases. Pediatr Dermatol 1996;13:477–482.
3. de Toro-Santos FJ, Verea-Hernando H, Montero C, Blanco-Aparicio M, Torres Lanzas J, Pombo Felipe F. Chronic pneumomediastinum and subcutaneous emphysema: association with dermatomyositis. Respiration 1995;62:53–56.
4. Dougenis D, Papathanasopoulos PG, Paschalis C, Papapetropoulos T. Spontaneous esophageal rupture in adult dermatomyositis. Eur J Cardio-Thor Surg 1996;10:1021–1023.
5. Vogelsang AS, Gutierrez J, Klipple GL, Katona IM. Polyneuropathy in juvenile dermatomyositis. J Rheumatol 1995;22:1369–1372.

Diabetes Insipidus

Organs and Tissues	Procedures	Possible or Expected Findings
Brain and pituitary gland	For cerebral arteriography, see Chapter 4. For removal and specimen preparation of brain and pituitary gland, see Chapter 4. If infection is suspected, follow procedures described in Chapter 7. Submit samples from brain and pituitary gland for histologic study.	Head injury* (including birth trauma); Langerhans cell (eosinophilic) granulomatosis;* local infection; metastatic tumor (frequently from carcinoma of breast); neurosurgical procedures; primary neoplasm involving neurohypophyseal system; sarcoidosis.*
Vitreous	Submit sample for sodium, chloride, and urea nitrogen determination.	Changes associated with dehydration.*
Other organs	Procedures depend on expected findings or grossly identified abnormalities as listed in right-hand column.	No diagnostic findings. Nephrogenic diabetes insipidus is caused by renal tubular defect. Manifestations of histiocytosis,* sarcoidosis,* and other possible underlying conditions.

Diabetes Mellitus

Synonyms: Type I (insulin-dependent or juvenile-onset) diabetes mellitus; type II (insulin-independent or adult onset) diabetes mellitus; secondary diabetes mellitus (e.g., due to drugs or pancreatic disease).

NOTE: In infants of diabetic mothers, macrosomia and congenital malformations must be expected. Record size and weight of placenta and total weight and length, crown to rump length, and crown to heel length of infant. Compare with expected measurements (see Part III). Expected histologic finding include hyperpla-sia with relative increase of B cells of the islands of Langerhans with interstitial and peri-insular eosinophilic infiltrates, decid-ual changes of the endometrium, enhanced follicle growth in the ovaries, and Leydig cell hyperplasia.

Possible Associated Conditions: Acanthosis nigricans; acro-megaly;* amyotrophic lateral sclerosis;* ataxia telangiectasia;* Fanconi's anemia;* Friedreich's ataxia;* gout;* hemochro-matosis;*hyperlipoproteinemia;* hyperthyroidism;* obesity;* Turner's syndrome;* and many others, too numerous to mention.

Organs and Tissues	*Procedures*	*Possible or Expected Findings*
External examination and skin		Gangrene of lower extremities and other ischemic changes.
	Prepare sections of skin lesions, of grossly unaffected skin, and of subcutaneous tissue.	Xanthelasmas of eyelids. Diabetic xanthomas on forearms. Diabetic lipoatrophy. Subcutaneous atrophy at former sites of insulin injection.
	If there is evidence of mastopathy, sample tissue for histologic study.	Diabetic mastopathy.
	Prepare sections and smears of intertriginous and other skin infections. Request Gram and Grocott's methenamine silver stains.	Fungal vulvitis.
	Prepare whole-body roentgenograms.	Subcutaneous and vascular calcifications. Joint deformities (see below under "Joints").
	Submit samples of skin tissue for electron microscopic study.	Diabetic microangiopathy.
Blood	Submit sample for bacterial and fungal cultures. If diabetic coma must be ruled out or if disease is only suspected, submit samples of blood and vitreous (see below) for biochemical study. For interpretation, see Chapter 8.	Septicemia. Increased concentrations of blood glucose (unreliable for diagnosis) and serum ketones and lipids. Postmortem insulin determination may permit the diagnosis of insulin poisoning.
Heart	Record weight and thickness of walls. Submit tissue for histologic examination For coronary arteriography, see Chapter 10. If glycogen content is to be evaluated, place specimens in alcohol or Carnoy's fixative or—preferably—prepare for electron microscopic study (Chapter 15).	Cardiac hypertrophy;* coronary atherosclerosis;* myocardial infarction.
Lungs	Submit one lobe for bacterial and fungal cultures. Request Gram and Grocott's methenamine silver stain.	Bacterial or fungal (aspergillosis,* candidiasis,* cryptococcosis*) pneumonia.
Esophagus	Sample for histologic study. For special stains, see "Lungs."	Intramural pseudodiverticulosis (dilatation of submucosal gland ducts). Fungal esophagitis.
Liver	Record weight and sample for histologic study.	Hepatomegaly; fatty changes; diabetic steatohepatitis or steatohepatitic cirrhosis. Other types of cirrhosis may be a cause of secondary diabetes (Naunyn's diabetes).
Gallbladder	Record appearance of concrements.	Cholelithiasis.*
Spleen	Submit sample for histologic study.	Lipoid histiocytosis.
Stomach	Record size and shape of stomach and appearance of mucosa.	Gastric dilatation; mucosal hemorrhages.
Pancreas	Prepare soft tissue roentgenogram. Dissect pancreas and record weight. Slice organ in 2-mm sagittal sections. Place one slice in alcohol or Carnoy's fixative. Request Best's carmine, Masson's trichrome, Congo red, and Gomori's chromium hematoxylin phloxine stains. For the last stain, formalin-fixed organs should be refixed for 12–24 h in Bouin's solution. Whenever granules are to be demonstrated in beta cells, a slice of fresh tissue should be placed in Bouin's fixative.	Glycogenosis of beta cells in prolonged hyperglycemia (in type II diabetes); degranulation of islets of Langerhans; lymphocytic or eosinophilic infiltration around islets (in type I diabetes); amyloidosis or fibrosis of islets. Lesions that may have caused secondary diabetes include pancreatitis, tumors of the pancreas,* cystic fibrosis,* and hemochromatosis.* Focal or diffuse nesidioblastosis in infants of diabetic mothers (may be a cause of hyperinsulinemic hypoglycemia).

Organs and Tissues	*Procedures*	*Possible or Expected Findings*
Adrenal glands	Record weights. If abnormalities are noted, sample for histologic study.	Adrenocortical nodules or tumor or pheochromocytoma (see also under "Syndrome, Cushing's" and "Tumor of the adrenal glands").
Kidneys	Record weights of both organs. For renal arteriography, see Chapter 2. Submit samples for histologic and electron microscopic study. Request PAS-alcian blue and Grocott's methenamine silver stains. All sections should include papillae.	Diabetic nephropathy and microangiopathy. Arteriolonephrosclerosis; diabetic intercapillary glomerulosclerosis; tubular atrophy and interstitial fibrosis; pyelonephritis* and necrotizing papillitis.
	Submit fresh material for immunofluorescence study.	Glomerular capillary and tubular basement membranes stain for IgG and albumin.
Urine	Prepare sediment and submit sample for protein, glucose, and acetone determination.	Abnormal sediment. Proteinuria, glycosuria, and acetonuria.
Urinary bladder		Urocystitis.
Seminal vesicles, spermatic cords, and testes	Submit samples for histologic study.	Submucosal granular deposits in seminal vesicles; calcification of vas deferens; tubular atrophy of testes.
Ovaries	Submit samples for histologic study.	Stromal hyperthecosis.
Lower extremities	For arteriography, see Chapter 2. Submit samples from smaller arteries for histologic study. For decalcification procedures, see Chapter 2.	Gangrene. Obliterating arteriosclerosis of anterior and posterior tibial arteries, peroneal arteries, and dorsal artery of the foot.
	Request von Kossa's and Verhoeff–van Gieson stains.	Mönckeberg's sclerosis* of muscular arteries.
Calvarium	Record color of bone.	Calvarium often strikingly yellow (carotene deposition).
Brain and spinal cord	For removal and specimen preparation, see Chapter 4.	Degeneration of spinal tracts and micro-infarctions.
	If cerebral infection is suspected, submit sample for bacterial and fungal cultures.	Cerebral mucormycosis.*
	For cerebral arteriography, see Chapter 4.	Cerebral infarctions *(2)*.*
Pituitary gland	For removal and specimen preparation, see Chapter 4.	Infarctions.
Eyes	For removal and specimen preparation, see Chapter 5.	Diabetic retinopathy with capillary micro-aneurysms; cataracts; microaneurysms of
	conjunctival vessels. Nutritional amblyopia.*	
Vitreous	If diabetic coma or ketoacidosis must be ruled out, submit sample of vitreous from one eye for determination of glucose and ketone concentrations.	Glucose values less than 2 h after death or combined glucose and lactate values several days after death can be used for the diagnosis of hyperglycemia *(1)*.
Peripheral nerves	Include anterior tibial and sciatic nerves. Request Luxol fast blue stain for myelin.	Diabetic neuropathy. Patchy demyelinization.
Skeletal muscles	For sampling and specimen preparation, see Chapter 4.	Diabetic myopathy.
Breast tissue	Submit sample for histologic study.	Hyalinization around mammary ducts.
Joints	For removal, prosthetic repair, and specimen preparation, see Chapter 4.	Deformation (Charcot joints) of tarsal and metatarsal joints or—less commonly—of ankle and knee joints. Such deformations occur after diabetic neuropathy.

Reference

1. Sippel H, Möttönen M. Combined glucose and lactate values in vitreous humor for postmortem diagnosis of diabetes mellitus. Forens Sci Internat 1982;19:217–222.
2. Arvanitakis Z, Schneider JA, et al. Diabetes is related to cerebral infarction but not to AD pathology in older persons. Neurology 2006;67:1960–1965.

Dialysis (for Chronic Renal Failure)

NOTE: Body fluids and tissues may be infectious (e.g., hepatitis C).

Organs and Tissues	*Procedures*	*Possible or Expected Findings*
External examination	Expose intraperitoneal catheters or arteriovenous shunts with as little contamination as possible. Submit material for aerobic and anaerobic bacterial and fungal cultures. Remove vessel from shunt site for histologic study.	Infection of catheters and shunts. Infectious vasculitis.
Blood	Submit sample for aerobic and anaerobic bacterial and for fungal cultures.	Septicemia.
Heart	If endocarditis is suspected, follow procedures described under that heading in Chapter 7.	Infective endocarditis.*
Peritoneal cavity	If peritoneal dialysis had been used, culture contents of peritoneal cavity (see above under "Blood"). Submit samples of peritoneum for histologic study.	Peritonitis.*
Liver	Submit samples for histologic study.	Chronic hepatitis B or C.* Hepatic granulomas *(1)*.
Kidneys and other organs	Procedures depend on expected findings or grossly identified abnormalities as listed in right-hand column.	Chronic renal disease (e.g., glomerulonephritis) and systemic manifestations of kidney failure.*

Reference

1. Kurumaya H, Kono N, Nakanuma Y, Tomoda F, Takazahura E. Hepatic granulomata in long-term hemodialysis patients with hyperalbuminemia. Arch Pathol Lab Med 1989;113:1132–1134.

Diathesis, Bleeding (See "Coagulation, disseminated intravascular," "Disease, Christmas," "Disease, von Willebrand's," and "Hemophilia.")

Digitalis (See "Poisoning, digitalis.")

Diphtheria

Synonyms: *Corynebacterium diphtheriae* infection; diphtheric fever.

NOTE: The disease has been nearly eliminated in the USA but not in many other countries.

(1) Collect all tissues that appear to be infected. (2) Request aerobic bacterial cultures. (3) Request Gram stain. (4) Special **precautions** are indicated. (5) Serologic studies are not helpful, but the organism may be typed for epidemiologic purposes. Toxin assays are also available. (6) This is a **reportable** disease.

Organs and Tissues	*Procedures*	*Possible or Expected Findings*
Head and neck	Remove neck organs with oropharynx, tongue, tonsils, soft palate, and uvula. Record degree of laryngeal obstruction. Photograph larynx and pharynx before and after opening.	Diphtheric pharyngitis.
	Submit sample of pharyngeal pseudomembranes for culture; prepare smears of membranes.	Gram-positive pleomorphic bacilli.
Heart	Photograph. Record weight and submit samples for histologic study.	Diphtheric myocarditis.
Kidneys	Submit samples for histologic study.	Nonsuppurative interstitial nephritis. Renal tubular necrosis.*
Brain and peripheral nerves	For removal and specimen preparation, see Chapter 4. Request Luxol fast blue stain.	Myelin degeneration and destruction of myelin sheaths.
Nasal cavities, sinuses, and middle ears	For exposure of epipharynx, nasal cavities, sinuses, and middle ears, see Chapter 4. Prepare smears and swab cultures of these spaces. Photograph, prepare histologic sections, and request Gram stain.	Diphtheritic pseudomembranes.

Disease,... (See subsequent entries and under "Sickness,..." and "Syndrome,...")

Disease, Addison's (See "Insufficiency, adrenal.")

Disease, Albers-Schönberg (See "Osteopetrosis.")

Disease, Alcoholic Liver

Related Terms: Alcoholic cirrhosis; alcoholic fatty liver; alcoholic hepatitis.

NOTE: Several conditions such as obesity-related steatohepatitis may be histologically indistinguishable from alcoholic liver disease *(1)*. Thus, the diagnosis should not be based on liver histology alone.

Organs and Tissues	*Procedures*	*Possible or Expected Findings*
External examination	Record presence or absence of features listed in right-hand column.	Jaundice; clubbing of fingers; Dupuytren's contractures; decreased body hair and gynecomastia in men.
Serosal cavities	Record volume of effusions.	Ascites; pleural effusions.*
Blood and urine	Submit samples for alcohol determination and other toxicologic studies.	Alcoholic cardiomyopathy* *(2)*.
Heart		Record weight. Alcoholic cardiomyopathy* *(2)*.
Lungs	Prepare frozen sections for fat stains.	Fat embolism* (if severe, systemic circulation may be involved—for instance, kidneys and brain).
Esophagus	For demonstration of varices, see Chapter 2.	Esophageal varices.
Liver	Record weight and sample for histologic study.	Micro- or macronodular alcoholic cirrhosis; alcoholic hepatitis (steatohepatitis); alcoholic fatty liver. Hepatocellular carcinoma. Typical groundglass changes in some patients who were treated with disulfiram or cyanamide *(3)*.
Portal vein system		See "Hypertension, portal."
Spleen	Record weight.	Congestive splenomegaly.
Pancreas		Alcoholic pancreatitis.*
Brain, peripheral nerves, skeletal muscles, and other organs	For removal of muscles, peripheral nerves, and brain, see Chapter 4.	Myopathy; neuropathy;* see also under "Alcoholism and alcohol intoxication" and "Syndrome, Wernicke-Korsakoff."
	For removal of lacrimal glands, see Chapter 5. Remove parotid tissue from scalp incision with biopsy needle.	Parotid and lacrimal gland enlargement with increased glandular secretions.
Testes	Record weights.	Testicular atrophy.

Reference

1. Kanel GC. Hepatic lesions resembling alcoholic liver disease. Pathology 1994;3:77–104.
2. Estruch R, Fernandez-Sola J, Sacanella E, Pare C, Rubin E, Urbano-Marquez A. Relationship between cardiomyopathy and liver disease in chronic alcoholism. Hepatology 1995;22:532–538.
3. Yokoyama A, Sato S, Maruyama K, Nakano M, Takahashi H, Okuyama K, et al. Cyanamide-associated alcoholic liver disease: a sequential histologic evaluation. Alcohol Clin Exp Res 1995;19:1307–1311.

Disease, alpha-Chain (See "Disease, heavy-chain.")

Disease, Alzheimer's

Synonyms and Related Terms: Alzheimer's dementia; presbyophrenic dementia; presenile dementia syndrome.

NOTE: For pathogenesis and criteria for staging, see refs. *(1–3)*.

Organs and Tissues	*Procedures*	*Possible or Expected Findings*
Brain and spinal cord	For removal and specimen preparation, see Chapter 4. Record brain weight. Histologic sections should include frontal, temporal, occipital, cingulate, enthorinal, and amygdala, hippocampus, deep nuclei and thalamus, substantia nigra, and occipital cortex and hippocampus. For silver impregnation of paraffin sections, request Bielchowsky silver stain. Immunostain for βA4 and tau protein are available for plaques and tangles. Some tissue samples should be kept frozen for biochemical studies.	Cortical atrophy, particularly of frontal and temporal lobes, with dilatation of ventricles. Neuronal loss and reactive astrocytosis; characteristic senile plaques (argentophilic neuritic plaques) and Alzheimer's neurofibrillary tangles. In some cases, cerebral meningeal and cortical blood vessels show amyloid angiopathy.

Reference

1. Esiri MM, Hyman BT, Beyreuther K, Masters CL. Aging and dementia in Greenfield's Neuropathology, vol. 2. Graham BI, Lantos PL, eds. Arnold, London, 1997, pp. 153–233.
2. The National Institute on Aging, and Reagan Institute Working Group on Diagnostic Criteria for the Neuropathological Assessment of Alz-heimer's Disease. Consensus recommendations for the postmortem diag-nosis of Alzheimer's disease. Neurobiol Aging 1997;Jul-Aug;18(4 Suppl):S1-2.
3. The Ronald and Nancy Reagan Research Institute of the Alzheimer's Association and the National Institute on Aging Working Group. Con-sensus report of the Working Group on: Molecular and Biochemical Markers of Alzheimer's Disease. Neurobiol Aging 1998;Mar-Apr;19 (2):109–116. (Published erratum appears in Neurobiol Aging 1998; May-Jun;19(3):285.)

Disease, Atherosclerotic Heart (See "Disease, ischemic heart.")

Disease, Bornholm (See "Pleurodynia, epidemic.")

Disease, Bourneville's (See "Sclerosis, tuberous.")

Disease, Buerger's

Synonyms: Thromboangitis obliterans; Winiwater-Buerger syndrome.

Organs and Tissues	*Procedures*	*Possible or Expected Findings*
External examination	Record presence or absence of abnormalities listed in right-hand column.	Ischemic ulcers of digits; gangrene; amputations; elevated skin lesions accompanying thrombophlebitis.*
Extremities	If permitted, submit samples from dorsal artery of the foot, and tibial, anterior fibular, popliteal, and femoral arteries. Include specimens of accompanying veins. Section arteries and veins crosswise at different levels. Request Verhoeff–van Gieson stain. Section veins that have gross evidence of thrombosis* or thrombophlebitis.*	Arterial lesions are often segmental. Digital arteries are involved more often than are ulnar and radial arteries. Thrombophlebitis* is part of the disease. Thrombi in small and medium-sized vessels contain mixed inflammatory cells, giant cells, and sterile microabscesses. Later stages of the process are characterized by hypercellular intraluminal granulation tissues without medial scarring.
Abdominal and visceral vasculature	Dissect abdominal aorta with iliac, mesenteric, and renal arteries. Dissect coronary arteries. Submit samples for histologic study, including Verhoeff–van Gieson stain.	Thromboses in mesenteric, renal, and coronary arteries are rare. Aortoiliac disease is also rare. Manifestations of the Budd-Chiari syndrome* may be present.
Brain	For removal and specimen preparation, and cerebral arteriography, see Chapter 4.	Cerebral artery involvement may be present and may be associated with cortical ischemic lesions.

Disease, Caisson (See "Sickness, decompression.")

Disease, Canavan's (See "Degeneration, spongy, of white matter.")

Disease, Caroli's

Synonyms and Related Terms: Caroli's syndrome; fibropolycystic liver disease; idiopathic dilatation of intrahepatic bile ducts.

NOTE: The term "Caroli's syndrome" often is used for cases that also show histologic features of congenital hepatic fibrosis or other manifestations of fibropolycystic liver disease,* whereas the name "Caroli's disease" refers to idiopathic dilatation of intrahepatic bile ducts, without associated abnormalities.

Possible Associated Conditions: Choledochal cyst* and related extrahepatic biliary abnormalities *(1)*; congenital hepatic fibrosis;* cysts of kidneys (renal tubular ectasia or medullary sponge kidney; autosomal-recessive polycystic kidney disease, and rarely, autosomal-dominant polycystic kidney disease *[2]*)* and of pancreas.

Organs and Tissues	*Procedures*	*Possible or Expected Findings*
Blood	Submit samples for aerobic and anaerobic bacterial cultures.	Septicemia.
Liver and extrahepatic bile ducts	If there are superficial abscesses or easily accessible cysts, sterilize capsule of liver and aspirate contents for aerobic and anaerobic	Dilatation of the hepatic and common bile ducts (may not involve entire liver *[1]*); choledochal-type cyst;* hepatolithiasis;

Organs and Tissues	Procedures	Possible or Expected Findings
	cultures. Remove small and large bowel, and open duodenum *in situ*. Aspirate bile from gallbladder or dilated ducts for bacterial culture. For cholangiography, see Chapter 2. Open extra-hepatic bile ducts *in situ* and record width. Slice liver in frontal or horizontal plane and submit samples for histologic study.	cholelithiasis;* choledocholithiasis; rupture of bile duct *(3)*; suppurative cholangitis;* hepatic abscesses. Adenocarcinoma of bile ducts.
Kidneys	If abnormalities are present, prepare photographs prior to histologic sampling.	See above under "Possible Associated Conditions."
Other organs		Manifestations of portal hypertension.*

References

1. Dagli U, Atalay F, Sasmaz N, Bostanoglu S, Temucin G, Sahin B. Caroli's disease: 1977–1995 experiences. Eur J Gastroenterol Hepatol 1998;10:109–112.
2. Mousson C, Rabec M, Cercueil JP, Virot JS, Hillon P, Rifle G. Caroli's disease and autosomal dominant polycystic kidney disease: a rare asso-ciation? Nephrol Dialysis Transplant 1997;12:1481–1483.
3. Chalasani N, Nguyen CC, Gitlin N. Spontaneous rupture of a bile duct and its endoscopic management in a patient with Caroli's syndrome. Am J Gastroenterol 1997;92:1062–1063.

Disease, Cat Scratch

Possible Associated Conditions: AIDS and other immuno-deficient conditions.

Organs and Tissues	Procedures	Possible or Expected Findings
External examination and skin		Cat-scratch mark and lymphadenopathy.
Heart	If endocarditis is suspected, submit tissue for culture.	Endocarditis *(1)*.
Liver	Sample for histologic study.	Granulomatous hepatitis; bacillary peliosis hepatis *(2)* (see also below under "Other organs").
Other organs	Photograph lesions that might have been caused by the infection. Sample material for microbiologic and histologic study; prepare Gram stains.	Infection caused by *Bartonella hensleae* or *Afipia felis*. In patients with AIDS, bacillary (epithelioid) angiomatosis and bacillary peliosis hepatis are associated with *B. hensleae (1)* infection.
Skeletal system	If osteomyelitis is suspected, follow procedures described under that heading.	Osteomyelitis.*
Brain and spinal cord	For removal and specimen preparation, see Chapter 4.	Encephalitis; meningitis; transverse myelitis.

References

1. Holmes AH, Greenough TC, Balady GJ, Regnery RL, Anderson BE, O'Keane JC, et al. Bartonella henselae endocarditis in an immunocom-petent adult. Clin Inf Dis 1995;21:1004–1007.
2. Chomel BB. Cat-scratch disease and bacillary angiomatosis. Rev Sci-entifique Technique 1996;15:1061–1073.

Disease, Celiac (See "Sprue, celiac.")

Disease, Cerebrovascular (See "Attack, transient cerebral ischemic" and "Infarction, cerebral.")

Disease, Chagas'

Synonyms and Related Terms: American trypanosomiasis; Chagas' syndrome; *Trypanosoma cruzi* infection.

NOTE: (1) Collect all tissues that appear to be infected. (2) Request cultures for trypanosomiasis. (3) Request Giemsa stain. (4) Special **precautions** are indicated. (5) Sero-logic studies are available from the Centers for Disease Control and Prevention, Atlanta, GA. (6) Usually, this is not a report-able disease.

Possible Associated Conditions: AIDS *(1)* and other condi-tions associated with immunosuppression.

Organs and Tissues	Procedures	Possible or Expected Findings
External examination and skin	Record and photograph the findings listed in right-hand column. Prepare sections of skin lesions.	In acute disease, unilateral bipalpebral edema, chemosis, and swelling of preauricular lymph nodes (Romaña's sign); skin nodules showing histiocytic and granulomatous inflammation; regional lymphadenitis, primarily in uncovered regions (chagoma), and subcutaneous edema. Hypopigmentation.
Body cavities	Record volume of effusions.	Effusions in congestive cardiac failure.*
Blood	Prepare smears of fresh blood or of buffy coat, or make thick-drop preparation.	In acute Chagas' disease, trypanosomes in blood.
	Submit sample for xenodiagnosis or animal inoculation and for serologic study.	In acute cases, positive hemagglutination and precipitin tests; in chronic cases, positive complement-fixation tests.
Heart	Record weight. In chronic Chagas' disease, perfuse intact heart with formalin (Chapter 3) and slice fixed heart in a frontal plane so as to create anterior and posterior halves. Prepare photographs. Histologic samples should include conduction system.	In chronic Chagas' disease, cardiac hypertrophy and dilatation; fibrous epicarditis, myocardial cell hypertrophy; apical aneurysm; endomyocardial fibrosis, intracardiac thrombi *(4)*, and atrial and apical ventricular mural thrombi. Valves and coronary arteries are normal.
	Include several sections of atrial (auricular) walls for histologic study of autonomous ganglia.	There may be parasitic pseudocysts or granulomas, fibrosis, myocytolysis, and degeneration and fibrous replacement of ganglion cells. In acute Chagas' disease, heart shows acute or subacute myocarditis* with dilatation. Intracellular parasites (i.e., pseudocysts with amastigote forms); necrosis of ganglion cells in atrial walls.
Lungs	Perfuse at least one lung with formalin.	In chronic Chagas' disease, emboli with infarctions, bronchiectasis,* fibrosis, hemosiderosis, and, rarely, acute hemorrhage.
Esophagus and gastrointestinal tract	Leave affected hollow viscera intact and fill with formalin. Cut fixed organs in half, photograph, and cut histologic sections on edge.	Megaesophagus is frequent, with or without carcinoma. Stomach, duodenum, colon *(2)*, and appendix (rarely) may be enlarged; diminution in number of ganglion cells in Auerbach plexus.
Liver and biliary system	Record liver weight and submit samples for histologic study.	In acute Chagas' disease, hepatomegaly may be present. Rarely, in chronic cases, the gallbladder and bile ducts may be enlarged.
Spleen	Record weight.	Infarctions. In acute Chagas' disease, splenomegaly.
Kidneys, ureters, and urinary bladder	Prepare photographs of abnormalities.	Renal infarctions. Rarely, in chronic Chagas' disease, the ureters and urinary bladder may be enlarged.
Placenta	Weigh and examine. Prepare histologic sections.	Pale, enlarged placenta; chronic villitis; increased perivillous fibrin; amastigotes in Hofbauer cells, amniotic epithelium and syncytiotrophoblasts.*
Brain and spinal cord	For removal and specimen preparation, see Chapter 4.	Cerebral infarctions.* Meningoencephalitis (particularly in reactivated forms in immunodeficient patients *[3]*) with or without involvement of spinal cord; cerebral atrophy with pressure atrophy of frontal gyri. Histologically, ruptured pseudocysts with

Organs and Tissues	Procedures	Possible or Expected Findings
		spread of amastigote forms.
Skeletal muscles, peripheral nerves, and other tissues	For sampling of skeletal muscles, see Chapter 4. For sampling of peripheral nerves, see Chapter 4.	There is a predilection for muscle and nerve tissue, but all organs and tissues can be involved.

Reference

1. Sartori AM, Shikanai-Yasuda MA, Amato Neto V, Lopes MH. Follow-up of 18 patients with human immunodeficiency virus infection and chronic Chagas' disease, with reactivation of Chagas' disease causing cardiac disease in three patients. Clin Inf Dis 1998;26:177–179.
2. Oliveira EC, Lette MS, Ostermayer AL, Almeida AC, Moreira H. Chagasic megacolon associated with colon cancer. Am J Trop Med Hyg 1997;56:596–598.
3. Chimelli L, Scaravilli F. Trypanosomiasis. Brain Pathol 1997;7:599–611.
4. Nunes, Mdo C, et al., Pecular aspects of cardiogenic embolism in patients with Chagasic cardiomyopathy: a transthoracic and transespophageal echocardiograpic study. J Am Soc Echocardiogr 2005;18:761–767.

Disease, Cholesteryl Ester Storage

Related Terms: Lysosomal acid lipase deficiency; Wolman's disease.*

Organs and Tissues	Procedures	Possible or Expected Findings
Fascia lata	Specimens should be collected using aseptic technique for tissue culture for biochemical studies.	The lysosomal acid lipase deficiency can be demonstrated in cultured fibroblasts.
Blood		Hyperbetalipoproteinemia; hypercholesterolemia.
Liver and spleen	Accumulation of cholesteryl esters may be demonstrated by thin-layer chromatography of lipid extracts of liver tissue. Lipid is PAS and aldehyde-fuchsin positive.	Hepatosplenomegaly. Hepatic fibrosis or cirrhosis with fatty changes in hepatocytes, cholangiocytes, portal macrophages, and Kupffer cells; deposition of cholesteryl crystals and triglycerides in Kupffer cells *(1)*.
Other organs and tissues		Atherosclerosis and its manifestations may be more severe than expected for the age of the patient *(2)*.

Reference

1. Di Bisceglie AM, Ishak KG, Rabin L, Hoeg JM. Cholesteryl ester storage disease: Hepatopathology and effects of therapy with lovestatin. Hepatology 1990;11:764–772.
2. Tylki-Szymanska A, Rujner J, Lugowska A, Sawnor-Korsznska D, Wozniewicz B, Czarnowska E. Clinical, biochemical and histological analysis of seven patients with cholesterol ester storage disease. Acta Paediatr Japan 1997;39:643–646.

Disease, Christmas

Synonyms: Christmas factor deficiency; Factor IX deficiency.

NOTE: Follow procedures described under "Hemophilia." The expected findings are the same as for hemophilia.

Disease, Chronic Granulomatous

Synonyms and Related Terms: Autosomal recessive chronic granulomatous disease; chronic granulomatous disease of child-hood; X-linked chronic granulomatous disease.

NOTE: The condition occurs not only in children but also in adults. Infections with catalase-positive microorganisms such as *S. aureus, Pseudomonas sp.* or *Aspergillus sp.*, predominate. The disease is part of a family of inherited disorders of phagocyte function (neutrophil dysfunction syndrome); other disorders in this family include the Chediak-Higashi syndrome,* myeloperoxidase deficiency, and other rare disorders.

Organs and Tissues	Procedures	Possible or Expected Findings
External examination, skin, and oral cavity	Record extend and character of skin lesions, particularly those around body orifices. Photograph skin lesions and prepare sections.	Seborrheic dermatitis, mainly around eyes (with conjunctivitis), around mouth (with stomatitis), and around nose and anus. Aphthous ulcers; gingivitis. Bacterial or fungal perianal and perineal abscesses and fistulas; wound infections. Skin granulomas with pigmented macrophages *(1)*.

Organs and Tissues	Procedures	Possible or Expected Findings
	Prepare chest and skeletal roentgenograms.	Pulmonary infiltrates. Osteomyelitis,* particularly of hands and feet.
Abdominal cavity	Submit sample of exudate for microbiologic study (see below under "Lymph nodes").	Subphrenic empyema.*
Chest cavity	Submit sample of exudate for microbiologic study (see below under "Lymph nodes"). Record volume of contents.	Pleural effusions;* empyema.
Blood	Submit sample for bacterial and fungal cultures.	Septicemia (staphylococci, gram-negative organisms, or fungi, such as *Aspergillus* and *Candida*).
Lymph nodes	Submit samples of inguinal, axillary, mediastinal, mesenteric, and other grossly involved lymph nodes for microbiologic and histologic study. Request Gram and Grocott methenamine silver stains for fungi and Sudan black-stained frozen sections for lipid.	Lymphadenitis with abscesses and lipid-filled macrophages; granulomas with central necrosis. For suspected organisms, see above under "Blood."
Heart		Pericarditis and, rarely, endocarditis* *(2)*.
Lungs	Submit any consolidated area for microbiologic study; perfuse one lung with formalin.	Bacterial and fungal bronchopneumonia and abscesses; hilar lymphadenitis.
Esophagus and gastrointestinal tract	Prepare photographs of abnormal lesions. Submit samples of normal and abnormal appearing areas for histologic study.	Involvement by granulomatous disease may occur from mouth to anus. Colon lesions may resemble chronic ulcerative colitis *(3)*.
Liver and spleen	Record weights; photograph. Submit samples for microbiologic and histologic study (see above under "Lymph nodes").	Hepatosplenomegaly with bacterial and fungal abscesses and granulomas.
Other organs	Submit samples of abnormal appearing areas for histologic study.	Abscesses and granulomas may occur in all organs and tissues.
Brain, spinal cord, and eyes	For removal and specimen preparation, see Chapter 4.	Granulomatous lesions in central nervous system *(4)* and eyes *(5)*.
Bones and bone marrow	For removal, prosthetic repair, and specimen preparation of bones, see Chapter 2. For microbiologic sampling, see Chapter 7. For preparation of sections and smears of bone marrow, see Chapter 2.	Fungal osteomyelitis* that may be multifocal, including sites such as metacarpals and metatarsals.

References

1. Dohil M, Prendiville JS, Crawford RI, Speert DP. Cutaneous manifestations of chronic granulomatous disease. A report of four cases and review of the literature. J Am Acad Dermatol 1997;36:899–907.
2. Casson DH, Riordan FA, Ladusens EJ. Aspergillus endocarditis in chronic granulomatous disease. Acta Pediatr 1996;85:758–759.
3. Sloan JM, Cameron CH, Maxwell RJ, McCluskey DR, Collins JS. Colitis complicating chronic granulomatous disease. A clinicopathological case report. Gut 1996;38:619–622.
4. Adachi M, Hayashi A, Ohkoshi N, Nagata H, Mizusawa H, Shoji S, et al. Hypertrophic cranial pachymeningitis with spinal epidural granulomatous lesion. Intern Med 1995;34:806–810.
5. Valluri S, Chu FC, Smith ME. Ocular pathologic findings of chronic granulomatous disease of childhood. Am J Ophthalmol 1995;120: 120–123.

Disease, Chronic Obstructive Pulmonary (See "Bronchitis, chronic" and "Emphysema.")

Disease, Collagen

Synonym: Connective tissue disease.

NOTE: See under specific name, such as "Arthritis, rheumatoid," "Dermatomyositis," "Lupus erythematosus, systemic," "Polyarteritis nodosa," "Sclerosis, systemic," and "Syndrome, Sjögren's."

Disease, Congenital Heart (See under specific name of malformation.)

Disease, Creutzfeldt-Jakob

Synonyms and Related Terms: Creutzfeldt-Jakob disease (CJD), "new variant"; iatrogenic Creutzfeldt-Jakob disease; familial Creutzfeldt-Jakob disease; fatal familial insomnia; Gerstmann-Straussler-Scheinker syndrome; Kuru; Prion disease; sporadic spongiforme encephalopathy; subacute spongiforme encephalopathy; transmissible spongiforme encephalopathy; variant Creutzfeldt-Jakob disease.

NOTE:

Autopsy is desirable in suspected cases because the diagnosis can only be firmly established after neuropathologic examination. Serologic studies are not available. Unfortunately, all tissues (not just the brain and spinal cord) may remain infectious even after prolonged fixation and histologic processing. Thus, the autopsy recommendations for most other infectious diseases do not apply here. This is a **reportable** disease in some states. Special **precautions** are indicated and therefore, the procedures described here should be followed strictly *(1–4)*:

All persons in the autopsy room must wear disposable long-sleeved gowns, gloves, and masks. Contamination of the autopsy table should be prevented by covering it with a disposable, non-permeable plastic sheet. Autopsy generally should be restricted to the brain. If organs in the chest or abdomen need to be examined, this is best done *in situ*. To prevent aerosolization of potentially infectious bone dust, a hood or other protective device should be used while opening the skull with a Stryker saw. After completing the autopsy, instruments and other potentially contaminated objects should be autoclaved in a steam autoclave (1 h at 134°C). Porous load is considered more effective than gravity displacement autoclaves. Immerse autopsy instruments in distilled water before and during autoclaving, in order to protect them from corrosion. If no autoclave is available, chemical disinfection (see below) is a satisfactory alternative. Disposable items should be put in a container for infectious hospital waste and ultimately incinerated. Contaminated objects not suitable for autoclaving (such as the Stryker saw) should be soaked with a 2 *N* NaOH solution for 1 h (alternatively, 1 *N* NaOH may be used for 2 h). Contaminated surfaces should be thoroughly washed with the same solution. Aluminum should be treated for 2 h with a fresh 5% NaOCl (sodium hypochlorite) solution with at least 20,000 ppm free chloride. Wash waters should be collected; if no autoclave is available, 2 *N* NaOH or >4 volumes of 5% sodium hypochlorite bleach should be added to the water and left for a minimum of 2 h before being discarded. Before removing the body from the autopsy room, it should be sponged with 5% sodium hypochlorite.

To deactivate CJD infectivity, tissue blocks, 5 mm or less in thickness, should be fixed in formalin in a formalin-to-tissue ratio of at least 20:1 for at least 48 h and then soaked in concentrated formic acid (95–100%) for 1 h, followed by another 48 h of formalin fixation. The fixation fluid should be collected and decontaminated, as described earlier for wash water. Glassware and tissue carriers should also be decontaminated as previously described. After this deactivation, the tissue blocks can be processed in a routine fashion. At any stage of these procedures, special care must be taken to avoid cuts with potentially contaminated glassware, blades, or other objects. Parenteral exposure to potentially contaminated material also should be avoided.

Remains of patients who have died of the disease should not be accepted for anatomy teaching for students. If specimens are prepared for pathology collections, they should be handled with great caution. Morticians and mortuary workers should be warned of possible hazards posed by tissues of patients with transmissible spongiforme encephalopathies; they should be advised about proper use of disinfectants. Clinical laboratories that receive autopsy tissues or fluids must be warned about the infectious nature of the material. If possible, decontamination should be done at the site where the autopsy was done. For the shipping of potentially infected material, see Chapter 15.

Organs and Tissues	*Procedures*	*Organs and Tissues*
Cerebrospinal fluid	Submit sample for neuron-specific enolase (NSE).	Increased concentrations of NSE *(5)*.
Brain	For removal and specimen preparation, see Chapter 4 and above under "Note." Submit fresh-frozen material for confirmation of diagnosis by histoblot technique on protease K-digested frozen tissue or Western blot preparations on brain homogenates. Immunohistochemical localization of PrP and HLA-DR protein on paraffin-embedded tissue is possible.	Spongiforme changes, astrocytosis, neuronal loss, amyloid plaque formation, PrP deposition, and proliferation of activated microglia *(6)*.

Reference

1. Ironside JW. Review: Creutzfeldt-Jakob disease. Brain Pathol 1996;6:379–388.
2. Gajdusek DC, Gibbs CJ Jr. Survival of Creutzfeldt-Jakob disease virus in formol-fixed brain tissue. N Engl J Med 1976;294:553.
3. Brown P. Guidelines for high risk autopsy cases: special precautions for Creutzfeldt-Jakob disease. In: (Hutchins GM, ed.) Autopsy Performance and Reporting. College of American Pathologists, Northfield, IL, 1990, pp. 68–74.
4. Budka H, Aguzzi A, Brown P, Brucher JM, Bugiani O, Collinge J, et al. Tissue handling in suspected Creutzfeldt-Jakob disease and other human spongiforme encephalopathies (prion diseases). Brain Pathol 1995;5:319–322.
5. Zerr I, Bodemer M, Racker S, Grosche S, Poser S, Kretzschmar HA, Weber T. Cerebrospinal fluid concentration of neuron-specific enolase in diagnosis of Creutzfeldt-Jakob disease. Lancet 1995;345:1609–1610.
6. Iwasaki Y, et al. Autopsy case of sporadic Creutzfeldt-Jakob disease presenting with signs suggestive of brainstem and spinal cord involvement. Neuropathology 2006;26:550–556.

Disease, Crohn's

Synonyms and Related Terms: Inflammatory bowel disease;* regional enteritis.

NOTE: If the distinction between Crohn's disease and chronic ulcerative colitis cannot be made clearly, see under "Disease, inflammatory bowel."

Possible Associated Conditions: Amyloidosis;* ankylosing spondylitis;* polyarthritis; Sjögren's syndrome.*

Organs and Tissues	*Procedures*	*Possible or Expected Findings*
External examination and skin	Record character and extent of skin lesions. Submit samples for histologic study.	Orbital edema and lid edema; ulcerative oral lesions; cutaneous fistulas after laparotomies; clubbing of fingers; perianal fistulas; vulval abscesses; cutaneous polyarteritis nodosa; erythema multiforme; erythema nodosum; pyoderma gangrenosum. Granulomatous inflammatory changes in mucosal/skin lesions *(1)*.
	Prepare skeletal roentgenograms.	See below under "Bones and joints."
Vitreous	If dehydration or other electrolyte disturbances are expected, request determination of sodium, chloride, potassium, and urea nitrogen concentrations.	Dehydration;* electrolyte disorders.*
Blood	Submit sample for culture and for determination of immunoglobulin concentrations.	Septicemia; selective IgA deficiency.
Heart	See "Stenosis, acquired valvular aortic."	Aortic stenosis.*
Lung	Submit at least one sample from each lobe for histologic study.	Noncaseating granulomas in rare instances *(2)*.
Esophagus	Leave specimen attached to stomach; submit tissue samples for histologic study.	Esophagus may be affected by the disease.
Gastrointestinal tract	In some instances, adhesions may be so severe that the intestines must be removed and sliced en bloc. Dissect fistulas *in situ*, or inject for roentgenographic study.	All segments of the gastrointestinal tract (appendix included) may be affected. Complications include adenocarcinoma, lymphoma,* or other tumors (rare), pneumatosis coli, fistulas (enterovaginal, perirectal, and others), and perirectal abscess. Acute toxic dilatation of the colon may be present.
	Submit samples of stomach and of all portions of intestinal tract for histologic study.	Mucosal abnormalities also may be present in grossly normal portions of colon and rectum.
Mesentery	Submit lymph nodes for histologic study.	Granulomatous lymphadenitis. Mesenteric fibromatosis *(3)*.
Liver	Record weight. For postmortem cholangiography, see Chapter 2. Submit multiple samples for histologic study.	Primary sclerosing cholangitis,* with or without cholangiocarcinoma* *(4)*; biliary cirrhosis;* fatty changes; granulomas.
Gallbladder	Record nature of concrements.	Cholelithiasis.*
Retroperitoneal tissues with pancreas	Submit abscess contents for microbiologic study.	Psoas abscess; para-aortic lymphadenopathy. Granulomatous pancreatitis *(5)*.
Kidneys with ureters	Submit stones for chemical analysis. Photograph kidneys with renal pelves and ureters. Sample for histologic study.	Nephrolithiasis* (uric acid and calcium stones); hydronephrosis.* Hydroureters; periureteral fibrosis and ureteral obstruction.
Internal genital organs	Submit purulent material for microbiologic study.	Pyosalpinx.
Eyes	For removal and specimen preparation, see Chapter 5.	Conjunctivitis; marginal corneal ulcers; keratitis; scleritis; episcleritis; retinitis; neuroretinitis; optic neuritis.
Skeletal muscles	For sampling and specimen preparation, see Chapter 4.	Myositis; in rare instances, dermatomyositis* *(6)*.
Bones and joints	For removal, prosthetic repair, and specimen preparation, see Chapter 2.	Aseptic necrosis of bone; ossifying periostitis; granulomatous bone disease; ankylosing spondylitis;* polyarthritis; nonspecific or granulomatous synovitis.
Brain and spinal cord		Manifestations of disseminated intravascular coagulation.*

Reference

1. Kafity A, Pellegrini A, Fromkes J. Metastatic Crohn's disease: a rare cutaneous manifestation. J Clin Gastroenterol 1993;17:300–303.
2. Calder CJ, Lacy D, Raafat F, Weller PH, Booth IW. Crohn's disease with pulmonary involvement in a 3 year old boy. Gut 1993;34:1636–1638.
3. DiGiacomo JC, Lasenby AJ, Salloum LJ. Mesenteric fibromatosis asso-ciated with Crohn's disease. Am J Gastroenterol 1994;89:1103–1105.
4. Choi PM, Nugent FW, Zelig MP, Munson JL, Schoetz DJ Jr. Cholangiocarcinoma and Crohn's disease. Dig Dis Sci 1994;39:667–670.
5. Gschwantler M, Kogelbauer G, Klose W, Bibus B, Tscholakoff D, Weiss W. The pancreas as a site of granulomatous inflammation in Crohn's disease. Gastroenterology 1995;108:1246–1249.
6. Leibowitz G, Eliakim R, Amir G, Rachmilewitz D. Dermatomyositis associated with Crohn's disease 1994;18:48–52.

Disease, Cushing's (See "Syndrome, Cushing's.")

Disease, Cytomegalic Inclusion (See "Infection, cytomegalovirus.")

Disease, Demyelinating
(See "Degeneration, spongy, of white matter," "Encephalomyelitis, all types or type unspecified," "Leukodystrophy, globoid cell," "Leukodystrophy, sudanophilic," "Sclerosis, multiple," and "Sclerosis, Schilder's cerebral.")

Disease, Diffuse Alveolar

Synonym: Diffuse pulmonary disease.

NOTE: Autopsy procedures are listed under the more specific diagnoses, such as "Hemosiderosis, idiopathic pulmonary," "Lipoproteinosis, pulmonary alveolar," "Microlithiasis, pulmonary alveolar," "Pneumonia, lipoid," and "Syndrome, Goodpasture's."

Disease, Eosinophilic Endomyocardial
(See "Cardiomyopathy, restrictive [eosinophilic type].")

Disease, Fabry's

Synonyms: Alpha-galactosidase deficiency; Anderson-Fabry disease; angiokeratoma corporis diffusum; glycosphingolipid lipidosis.

Organs and Tissues	*Procedures*	*Possible or Expected Findings*
External examination and skin	Prepare skin sections from multiple sites. Request Sudan black, PAS, and toluidine blue O stains.	Telangiectatic lesions. Glycolipid storage (PAS-positive, Sudan black-positive, metachromatic, and double refractile with toluidine blue) in arrectores pilorum muscles, vascular endothelium, and sweat glands.
Blood		Leukocyte alpha-galactosidase deficiency.
Heart	For recommended special stains, see above under "External examination and skin."	Glycolipid storage with nonobstructive hypertrophic cardiomyopathy* (this may be the only manifestation *[1,2]*). Myocardial infarction.
Lungs	For recommended special stains, see above under "External examination and skin."	Narrowing of airways by glycosphingolipid in patients with clinical features of obstructive lung disease *(3)*.
Urine	Examine sediment.	"Mulberry cells" in sediment.
Kidneys	For recommended special stains, see above under "External examination and skin."	Glycosphingolipids in glomeruli and distal convoluted tubules. If applicable, see also under "Failure, kidney."
Other organs	Procedures depend on expected findings or grossly identified abnormalities as listed in right-hand column.	Glycosphingolipid storage in liver, spleen, small and large bowel, lymph nodes, and bone marrow.
Brain and spinal cord	For removal and specimen preparation, see Chapter 4. For cerebral angiography and dissection of vertebral arteries, see Chapter 4. For recommended special stains, see above under "External examination and skin."	Elongated tortuous and ectatic vertebral and basilar arteries *(4)*, sometimes with thrombosis *(5)*. Glycosphingolipid storage. Cerebral infarction(s)* or hemorrhages.
Eyes	For removal and specimen preparation, see Chapter 5. For recommended special stains, see above under "External examination and skin."	Glycosphingolipid storage in cornea; lens opacities; dilated vessels in conjunctiva and lens; thrombi in blood vessels *(5)*.

References

1. Elleder M, Bradová V, Smid F, Budesinsky M, Harzer K, Kustermann-Kuhn B, et al. Cardiocyte storage and hypertrophy as a sole manifestation of Fabry's disease. Report on a case simulating hypertrophic non-obstructive cardiomyopathy. Virchows Arch [Pathol Anat] 1990;417:449–455.
2. Von Scheidt W, Eng CM, Fitzmaurice TF, Erdmann E, Hubner G, Olsen EG, et al. An atypical variant of Fabry's disease with manifestations confined to the myocardium. N Engl J Med 1991;324:395–399.
3. Brown LK, Miller A, Bhuptani A, Sloane MF, Zimmerman MI, Schilero G, et al. Pulmonary involvement in Fabry disease. Am J Respir Crit Care Med 1997;155:1004–1110.
4. Mitsias P, Levine SR. Cerebrovascular complications of Fabry's disease. Ann Neurol 1996;40:8–17.
5. Utsumi K, Yamamoto N, Kase R, Takata T, Okumiya T, Saito H, et al. High incidence of thrombosis in Fabry's disease. Intern Med 1997;36:327–329.

Disease, Fibropolycystic, of the Liver and Biliary Tract

NOTE: "Fibropolycystic disease of the liver and biliary tract" comprises a group of well defined conditions, which may occur together and hence need a collective designation. The conditions include autosomal-recessive (infantile) and auto-somal dominant (adult) polycystic disease of the liver; Caroli's disease or syndrome;* choledochal cyst,* congenital hepatic fibro-sis,* multiple biliary microhamartomas, and related disorders. For autopsy procedures, see also under more specific designations.

Organs and Tissues	*Procedures*	*Possible or Expected Findings*
External examination	Record and photograph abnormalities.	Polydactyly; spina bifida.
Lungs	If cysts can be identified, prepare arteriograms (Chapter 2) and perfuse with formalin. See also below under "Liver and hepatoduodenal ligament."	Cysts of lungs.*
Esophagus	For demonstration of esophageal varices, see Chapter 2.	Esophageal varices.*
Gastrointestinal tract	Estimate and record volume of blood in lumen.	Gastrointestinal hemorrhage* after rupture of varices.
Spleen	Record weight.	Splenomegaly in presence of portal hypertension.*
Liver and hepatoduodenal ligament	Dissect common bile duct *in situ* (see also under "Cyst(s), choledochal"). Record weight of liver; photograph surface of liver. For cholangiography, venography, or arteriography, see Chapter 2. Aspirate contents of infected cysts or abscesses and submit samples for microbiologic study. Prepare smears of exudate. Inject large cysts with warm, freshly prepared, 5% gelatin solution dissolved in 10% formalin. Slice with large knife after solution has hardened. Photograph cut surface; record size and distribution of cysts; submit tissue samples for histologic study.	Microcysts associated with ductal plate malformations *(1)*. Large intra-hepatic cysts may be calcified *(2)*. Choledochal cyst.* Hepatomegaly. Hepatic fibrosis, Abscesses.
Other organs	Procedures depend on expected findings or grossly identified abnormalities as listed in right-hand column.	Cysts of kidneys,* pancreas, and ovaries. Polycystic kidney disease (autosomal-recessive or autosomal-dominant) may be the main finding at autopsy.

Reference

1. Shedda S, Robertson A. Carolis syndrome and aadult polycystic kidney disease. ANZ J Surg 2007;77:292–294.
2. Coffin B, Hadengue A, Degos F, Benhamou JP. Calcified hepatic and renal cysts in adult dominant polycystic kidney disease. Dig Dis Sci 1990; 35:1172–1175.

Disease, Gaucher's

Synonyms and Related Terms: Adult, infantile, or juvenile Gaucher's disease; glucosylceramide lipidosis; acute neuronopathic (infantile) Gaucher's disease; chronic non-neuronopathic (adult) Gaucher's disease.

Possible Associated Conditions: Leukemia,* lymphoma,* and other malignant neoplasms.

Organs and Tissues	Procedures	Possible or Expected Findings
External examination and skin	Record and photograph skin changes. Prepare histologic sections of skin. Request Gomori's iron stain.	Yellowish brown skin pigmentation; pingueculae near cornea. Sinus tracts.
	Prepare skeletal roentgenograms.	Lytic defects and osteonecrosis may occur in long bones, phalanges, ribs, spine, pelvis, and skull. Aseptic necrosis of femoral head. Fractures of long bones may be present.
Blood	Submit sample for biochemical and molecular study.	Increased plasma glucosylceramide concentrations. Recomination within the glucocerebrosidase gene locus *(1)*.
Heart		Cor pulmonale.
Lungs	Perfuse one lung with formalin. Submit consolidated area for bacterial culture.	Pulmonary involvement in severe cases of Gaucher's disease *(2)*; manifestations of pulmonary hypertension* in adults. Pulmonary infections in children.
Spleen	Record weight. Photograph cut surface. Submit samples of fresh material for biochemical study, and snap-freeze specimens for histochemical analysis. Prepare unstained smears for phase-contrast microscopy. Request PAS and Masson's trichrome stains. Prepare material for electron microscopy.	Splenomegaly caused by accumulation of glucocerebroside-containing Gaucher cells. Increased acid phosphatase in Gaucher cells.
Other organs	Submit tissue samples of liver, pancreas, kidneys, gastrointestinal tract, intrathoracic and intra-abdominal lymph nodes, thymus, tonsils, thyroid, and adrenal glands. For processing, see above under "Spleen."	Hepatomegaly; manifestations of portal hypertension; lymphadenopathy. Infiltration of organs (listed in middle column) by Gaucher cells; hemosiderosis.
Brain and spinal cord	For removal and specimen preparation, see Chapter 4. See also above under "Spleen."	Acute nerve cell degeneration. Accumulation of glucocerebrosides and—in children with acute neuronopathic disease—gangliosides.
Bones and bone marrow	Submit specimens of involved bones, as indicated on skeletal roentgenograms; include femur in all instances. Photograph saw section of femur. For prosthetic repair and for decalcification, see Chapter 2. For preparation of bone marrow sections and smears, see Chapter 2.	See above under "External examination and skin."

Reference

1. Sidransky E. Gaucher disease: complexity in a "simple disorder. Mol Genet Metab 2004;83:6–15.
2. Cox TM, Schofield JP. Gaucher's disease: clinical features and natural history. Baillieres Clin Haematol 1997;10:657–689.

Disease, Glycogen Storage

Synonyms: Andersen's disease or brancher deficiency (glycogenosis, type IV); Cori's or Forbes' disease (glycogenosis, type III); cyclic AMP dependent kinase (type X); glycogen synthetase deficiency (type O); Hers' disease (glycogenosis, type VI); McArdle's disease (glycogenosis type V); phosphorylase B kinase deficiency (types IXa, b, and c); Pompe's disease (glycogenosis, type II); Tarui disease (glycogenosis type VII); von Gierke's disease (glycogenosis, type Ia); X-linked glycogenosis (type VIII).

NOTE: If the diagnosis had not been confirmed prior to death, samples of liver, skeletal muscle, blood, and fascia (for fibroblast culture, see below) should be snap-frozen for enzyme assay, which will determine the specific deficiency. Types Ia and b, III, VI, and hepatic phosphorylase B kinase deficiency (types IXa, b and c) are hepatic-hypoglycemic disorders, whereas types V and VII affect muscle energy processes. Type II also affects the musculature, whereas type IV may cause cirrhosis and death in infancy from extreme hypotonia.

Determination of type of glycogenosis usually can be based on (1) pattern of glycogen storage in liver, (2) presence or absence of nuclear hyperglycogenation in liver, (3) cytoplasmic lipid in liver, (4) presence or absence of liver cirrhosis, and (5) presence or absence of glycogen and basophilic deposits in skeletal muscles.

Possible Associated Conditions: Fanconi syndrome* or gout* with type Ia glycogenosis; neutropenia, recurrent infections, and Crohn's disease with types Ib or Ic.

Organs and Tissues	*Procedures*	*Possible or Expected Findings*
External examination and skin	Record body weight and length. Submit tissue samples of skin lesions. Record size of tongue and submit specimens for histologic study (may be easier to do after removal with neck organs). For specimen preparation, see below under "Heart...."	Growth retardation. Xanthomas in von Gierke's disease. Macroglossia.
Blood	Submit sample for uric acid and ketone determination. If blood is to be used for tissue culture, follow procedures described in Chapter 9 (see also "Fascia lata" below).	Hyperuricemia in gout.* Ketoacidosis may be associated with sudden death. Hypoglycemia* and hyperlipidemia occur in von Gierke's disease.
Fascia lata	Specimens should be collected using aseptic technique for tissue culture for biochemical studies (see Chapter 9).	For enzyme deficiencies, see above under "Note."
Liver	For recommended fixatives and special stains, see below. Frozen sections protected with celloidin and then stained with PAS allows an accurate determination of the glycogen content.	Enlarged hepatocytes with glycogen storage in types I, III, and IV. Fatty changes most common in types 0, I and III. Periportal fibrosis in types III and IV and, rarely, cirrhosis in type IV.
	Prepare samples for electron microscopic study, particularly in glycogenosis types II and IV.	Adenomas and, rarely, hepatocellular carcinomas may be found in type Ia. No abnormalities in types V and VII. See also above under "Note."
Heart, blood vessels, lungs, skeletal muscles, esophagus, intestine, pancreas, spleen, kidneys, adrenal glands, urinary bladder, lymph nodes, bone marrow.	Photograph enlarged or discolored organs and obtain samples for histologic study. Recommended fixatives for glycogen include alcohol, Bouin's or Carnoy's fixative and formalin alcohol. Glycogen may still be dissolved during exposure to watery staining solutions. Request van Gieson's stain, PAS stain with and without diastase digestion, and Best's stain for glycogen. Request Sudan-stained frozen sections of myocardium, liver, and skeletal muscles. For use of frozen sections for study of glycogen, see above under "Liver." Embed tissue samples for electron microscopic study.	Uric acid nephropathy and glomerulo-sclerosis in type Ia. Distribution of glycogen storage and other abnormalities varies with subtype of disease. Glycogen depositis may be found in myocardium (cardiomegaly), small and large arteries, skeletal muscle (for instance, of diaphragm, neck, trunk, and extremities), bronchial mucosa, and all other organs listed in left-hand column. See also above under "Note."
Eyes	For removal and specimen preparation, see Chapter 5. Use formalin solution for fixation.	Glycogen primarily in retinal ganglion cells and ciliary muscle.
Brain and spinal cord	For removal and specimen preparation, see Chapter 4. Submit specimens of sympathetic nerve ganglia for histologic study.	Glycogen in sympathetic nerve ganglia and neurons of cranial nerves in type VII.
Joints	For removal, prosthetic repair, and specimen preparation, see Chapter 2.	Gouty arthritis.

Disease, Graft-Versus-Host

NOTE: This disease occurs most commonly after bone marrow transplantation. The disease has also occurred after transfusion of viable lymphocytes, for example, to patients with cancer or leukemia.*

In patients with graft-versus-host disease (GVHD), autopsy also may reveal recurrence of the underlying disease such as leukemia.

Organs and Tissues	*Procedures*	*Possible or Expected Findings*
External examination and skin; oral cavity	Record and photograph skin lesions and prepare histologic sections of normal and abnormal skin.	Generalized erythroderma and jaundice. Microscopic examination shows irregular epidermal-dermal junctions with basal cell vacuolation, spongiosis, and eosinophilic bodies associated with infiltrates of aggressor lymphocytes.
	Small biopsies of labial salivary glands and buccal mucosa may be useful to evaluate chronic GVHD *(1)*.	Buccal mucositis; lichenoid lesions in chronic GVHD *(1)*.
Heart	Record volume of pericardial fluid.	Pericardial effusion (in rare cases with features of polyserositis in chronic GVHD) *(2)*.
Lungs	Perfuse at least one lung with formalin. Submit areas of consolidated lung for microbiologic study.	Diffuse alveolar damage; lymphocytic bronchitis/bronchiolitis obliterans; organizing pneumonia *(3)*. Bronchiectases in rare instances *(4)*.
Liver	Record weight. Submit samples for histologic study.	Hepatomegaly. Portal and periportal hepatitis with destruction of interlobular ducts; oncocytic metaplasia of bile duct epithelium *(5)*; endotheliitis; cholestasis.
Esophagus	Prepare photographs of mucosa and sample for histologic study.	Infectious esophagitis or chronic GVHD with vesicobullous lesions or, in late stages, strictures.
Small and large intestine	Submit samples for histologic study.	Enteritis with cellular debris in crypts, atypical epithelial lining of crypts, and inflammatory infiltrates.
Other organs	Procedures depend on expected findings or grossly identified abnormalities as listed in right-hand column.	Inflammatory infiltrates. Hemorrhagic necroses in lymph nodes and spleen. Immune-mediated myelopathy *(6)*.
Eyes	For removal and specimen preparation, see Chapter 5.	Keratoconjunctivitis. Optic neuropathy *(6)*.
Bone marrow	For preparation of sections and smears, see Chapter 2.	Evidence of proliferating graft cells.

References

1. Nakamura S, Hiroki A, Shinohara M, Gondo H, Ohyama Y, Mouri T, et al. Oral involvement in chronic graft versus host disease after allogenic bone marrow transplantation. Oral Surg Oral Med Oral Pathol 1996;82:556–563.
2. Toren A, Nagler A. Massive pericardial effusion complicating the course of chronic graft-versus-host disease (cGVHD) in a child with acute lymphoblastic leukemia following allogeneic bone marrow transplantation. Bone Marrow Transplant 1997;20:805–807.
3. Yousem AS. The histological spectrum of pulmonary graft-versus-host disease in bone marrow transplant recipients. Hum Pathol 1995; 26:668–675.
4. Morehead RS. Bronchiectasis in bone marow transplantation. Thorax 1997;52:392–393.
5. Bligh J, Morton J, Durrant S, Walker N. Oncocytic metaplasia of bile duct epithelium in hepatic GVHD. Bone Marrow Transplant 1995; 16:317–319.
6. Openshaw H, Slatkin NE, Parker PM, Forman SJ. Immune-mediated myelopathy after allogeneic marrow transplantation. Bone Marrow Transplant 1995;15:633–636.

Disease, Graves' (See "Hyperthyroidism.")

Disease, Günther's (See "Porphyria, congenital erythropoietic.")

Disease, Heavy-Chain

Synonyms and Related Terms: Gamma heavy-chain disease (Franklin's disease); alpha heavy-chain disease (Seligmann's disease); μ heavy-chain disease.

NOTE: Alpha heavy-chain disease is related to Mediterranean lymphoma and μ heavy-chain disease occurs in rare patients with chronic lymphocytic leukemia.* Infections generally are the cause of death in gamma heavy-chain disease. Evidence of malabsorption* may be observed in alpha heavy-chain disease.

Organs and Tissues	*Procedures*	*Possible or Expected Findings*
External examination and oral cavity	Record body weight and length.	Profound wasting in alpha-chain disease. For oral changes, see under "Neck organs."
Blood	Submit samples for microbiologic study and for protein electrophoresis.	Septicemia. See also above under "Note." Anomalous serum M component in gamma heavy-chain disease.
Lungs	Submit consolidated area for microbiologic study.	Pneumonia in gamma heavy-chain disease. Rarely lymphoplasmacytoid infiltrates in alpha heavy-chain disease.
Urine	Submit sample for protein electrophoresis.	Anomalous serum M component in gamma heavy-chain disease.
Lymph nodes	Prepare Wright stains of touch preparations. Fix tissue in B-Plus™ (BBC Biochemical, Stanwood, WA).	Mesenteric and para-aortic lymphadenopathy with infiltrates of lymphocytes and plasma cells.
Small bowel and mesentery	For microscopic study, submit samples of all segments of gastrointestinal tract and portions of mesentery with lymph nodes.	Infiltrates of lymphocytes and plasma cells in lamina propria of small bowel in alpha heavy-chain disease. See also under "Syndrome, malabsorption."
Neck organs	Remove together with pharynx.	Palatal edema (Waldeyer ring lymphadenopathy) in gamma heavy-chain disease.
Bone marrow	For preparation of sections and smears, see Chapter 2.	Infiltrates of lymphocytes and plasma cells; eosinophilia.
Bones	For removal, prosthetic repair, and specimen preparations, see Chapter 2.	Osteoporosis* in alpha heavy-chain disease.

Disease, Hippel-Lindau (See "Disease, von Hippel-Lindau.")

Disease, Hirschsprung's (See "Megacolon, congenital.")

Disease, Hodgkin's (See "Lymphoma.")

Disease, Hookworm (See "Ancylostomiasis.")

Disease, Huntington's (See "Chorea, hereditary.")

Disease, Hydatid (See "Echinococcosis.")

Disease, Inflammatory Bowel

Synonyms and Related Terms: Chronic ulcerative colitis; Crohn's disease;* idiopathic proctocolitis.

Possible Associated Conditions: Alpha$_1$-antitrypsin deficiency;* amyloidosis;* ankylosing spondylitis;* primary sclerosing cholangitis;* Sjögren's syndrome.* See also below under "Possible or Expected Findings."

NOTE: In many instances, either chronic ulcerative colitis or Crohn's disease* had been diagnosed clinically, but sometimes, the distinction is difficult to make, even at autopsy. Many features described below occur in chronic ulcerative colitis but some manifestations of Crohn's disease or conditions that may occur in all types of inflammatory bowel disease also are listed so that both positive and negative findings can be recorded properly.

Organs and Tissues	*Procedures*	*Possible or Expected Findings*
External examination, skin, and oral cavity	Record nature and extent of skin lesions, photograph, and submit specimens of accessible lesions for histologic study.	Aphthous stomatitis; pyoderma gangrenosum; erythema nodosum and multiforme; papular or pustular dermatitis; ulcerating erythematous plaques; neurodermatitis; herpes zoster; anal fissures.
	Record appearance of hands and feet.	Clubbing of fingers and toes. Emaciation.
	Prepare roentgenograms of fistulas after injection of contrast medium.	Perianal abscesses and fistulas.
	Prepare skeletal roentgenograms.	See below under "Bones and joints."
Synovial fluid	If arthritis is suspected, submit sample of	Arthritis.*

Organs and Tissues	Procedures	Possible or Expected Findings
	synovial fluid for microbiologic study, cell counts, and smears.	
Blood	Submit sample for microbiologic study.	Septicemia.
Heart	If pericarditis or endocarditis are expected, follow procedures described under these headings.	Endocarditis;* pericarditis.*
Lungs	Dissect pulmonary arteries; sample all lobes for histologic study. Request Verhoeff–van Gieson stain.	Thromboemboli; pulmonary vasculitis.
Abdominal cavity with retroperitoneum and pelvic organs	If peritonitis is present, submit exudate for aerobic and anaerobic bacteriologic study. Aspirate contents of abscesses and record their size and location. Record volume of exudate and prepare smears.	Peritonitis.* Perianal, presacral, and ischio-rectal abscesses; fistulas and anal fissures. Dilatation of colon ("toxic megacolon"). Fournier's gangrene (necrotizing fasciitis of the genitalia) in Crohn's disease.
Small and large intestine	For *in situ* fixation, see Chapter 2. If fistulas are present, dissect affected areas *in situ*. Opened colon and affected portions of small bowel should be pinned on corkboard and fixed with formalin. Submit samples of all types of lesions for histologic study.	Segmental (skip areas), transmural and granulomatous inflammation in Crohn's disease. Toxic megacolon more common in chronic ulcerative colitis. Retroperitoneal and rectovaginal fistulas; mucosal ulcers and pseudopolyps; multicentric lymphoma; dysplasia; carcinoma(s); hemorrhage. Rectal stricture. "Backwash ileitis." Colonic cytomegalovirus inclusions, associated with toxic dilatations. See ref. *(1, 4)*.
Bile ducts	For cholangiography, see Chapter 2. Dissect extra-hepatic bile ducts *in situ* (see also under "Tumor of the bile ducts").	Sclerosing cholangitis;* adenocarcinoma of bile ducts.
Liver	Record weight; submit samples for histologic study.	Biliary cirrhosis.* Cholangiocarcinoma.
Stomach and duodenum		Ulcerative gastritis and duodenitis in Crohn's disease.
Pancreas	Submit samples for histologic study.	Pancreatitis.
Kidneys, ureters, and urinary bladder	Submit samples for histologic and bacterio-logic study. If glomerulitis is suspected, follow procedures described under "Glomerulonephritis."	Glomerulonephritis;* pyelonephritis;* tubular degeneration; nephrocalcinosis. Renovascular disease *(2)*.
	Describe size and contents of urinary bladder, ureters, and renal pelves.	Cystopyelitis; urolithiasis; nephrolithiasis (oxalate stones).
Veins and arteries		Thrombophlebitis; arteritis *(2)* and arterial thromboses.
Eyes	For removal and specimen preparation, see Chapter 5. If there is evidence of Sjögren's syndrome,* remove lacrimal glands (Chapter 5).	Blepharitis; conjunctivitis; corneal ulcers; iritis; keratitis; neuroretinitis; retrobulbar neuritis; uveitis.
Brain and cerebral venous sinuses	For removal and specimen preparation, see Chapter 4.	Cerebral venous sinus thrombosis* *(3)*.
Bones and joints	For removal, prosthetic repair, and specimen preparation, see Chapter 2.	Osteoporosis;* ankylosing spondylitis;* arthritis of peripheral joints; periarthritis; hypertrophic osteoarthropathy;* tendinitis (particularly of ankle and Achilles tendons).

References

1. Podolsky D. Inflammatory bowel disease (first of two parts). N Engl J Med 1991;325:928–937 (part 1) and 1008–1016 (part 2).
2. Sakhuja V, Gupta KL, Bhasin DK, Malik N, Chugh KS. Takayasu's arteritis associated with idiopathic ulcerative colitis. Gut 1990;31:831–833.
3. Johns D. Cerebrovascular complications of inflammatory bowel disease. Am J Gastroenterol 1991;86:367–370.
4. Gramlich T, Petras RE. Pathology of inflammatory bowel disease. Semin Pediatr Surg 2007;16:154–163.

Disease, Iron Storage (See "Hemochromatosis.")

Disease, Ischemic Heart

Related Terms: Atherosclerotic heart disease.

NOTE: The most common anatomic finding at autopsy in subjects older than 30 yr is coronary atherosclerosis. Unusual under-lying or associated conditions include chronic aortic stenosis or regurgitation; coronary artery anomalies; coronary artery dissection; coronary embolism; coronary ostial stenosis (due to calcification of aortic sinotubular junction or, rarely, to syphilitic aortitis); coronary vasculitis (for instance, in polyarteritis nodosa* or acute hypersensitivity arteritis); hyperthyroidism,* gastrointestinal hemorrhage;* hypothyroidism,* idiopathic arterial calcification of infancy; intramural coronary amyloidosis; pheochromocytoma, polycythemia vera;* pseudoxanthoma elasticum,* radiation-induced coronary stenosis; severe pulmonary hypertension (with *right* ventricular ischemia); sickle cell disease;* and others. If bypass surgery had been performed, see "Surgery, coronary bypass."

Organs and Tissues	*Procedures*	*Possible or Expected Findings*
External examination		Cyanosis; edema of legs; venous congestion. Gangrene of toes. Diabetic ulcers.
	Prepare chest roentgenogram.	Cardiomegaly; pleural effusions.*
Blood	If underlying metabolic disease is suspected, submit sample for biochemical study.	See above under "Note."
Heart	For coronary arteriography, see Chapter 3. For specimen preparation and grading of coronary arteries, see Chapter 3. Request Verhoeff–van Gieson stain.	Coronary atherosclerosis; coronary thrombosis or embolism; congenital malformation(s) of coronary arteries; accidental operative coronary ligation; coronary arteritis (see above under "Note.")
	For dissection technique of the heart and for histologic sampling, see Chapter 3. For detection of early myocardial infarction, see Chapter 3. Record actual and expected heart weight, ventricular wall thicknesses, and valvular annular circumferences. Record appearance, extent, and location of infarcts, mural thrombus, and aneurysms.	Myocardial infarction, old or acute. Mural thrombus. Ventricular aneurysm, true or false. Ventricular rupture (free wall, septum, or papillary muscles). Aortic insufficiency;* aortic stenosis.*
Aorta		Acute aortic dissection.*
Other organs		Manifestations of congestive heart failure* and of possible underlying conditions (see above under "Note"), such as diabetes mellitus.*

Disease, Jakob-Creutzfeldt (See "Disease, Creutzfeldt-Jakob.")

Disease, Kawasaki (See "Syndrome, mucocutaneous lymph node.")

Disease, Krabbe's (See "Leukodystrophy, globoid cell.")

Disease, Legionnaires'

Synonyms and Related Terms: *Legionella pneumophila* infection; Pontiac fever.

NOTE: (1) Collect lung specimens, serum, and other tissues that appear to be infected. These should be inoculated on a nonselective medium, such as BCYE agar supplemented with α-ketoglutaric acid. A good selective agar is BCYE supplemented with antibiotics. (2) Request aerobic and anaerobic cul-tures for exclusion of other bacterial diseases. (3) Request Gram, Kinyoun, and Grocott's methenamine silver stains for exclusion of other bacterial or fungal diseases. The Dieterle silver impregnation procedure is recommended for demonstration of the organism in paraffin-embedded sections *(1–3)*. (4) No special precautions are indicated. (5) Serologic immunofluorescent studies are available from the Centers for Disease Control and Prevention, Atlanta, GA. (6) This is a **reportable** disease.

Organs and Tissues	Procedures	Possible or Expected Findings
Skin	Photograph any rashes.	Macular rash *(4)*.
Blood, pleural fluid	Submit sample for culture.	
Lungs	Culture any areas of consolidation. Perfuse at least one lung with formalin. Slice in the parasagittal plane. Submit affected areas for histological study.	Multifocal fibrinopurulent pneumonia with sparing of the bronchi and bronchioles. Exudate is rich in phagocytes, fibrin, and karyorrhectic debris.

References

1. Edelstein PH. Legionnaires' disease. Clin Infect Dis 1993;16(6):741–747.
2. Stout JE, Yu VL. Legionellosis. NEJM 1997;337(10):682–687.
3. Bhopal R. Source of infection for sporadic Legionnaires' disease: a review. J Infect 1995;30:9–12.
4. Calza L, Briganti E, Casolari S, et al. Legionnaire's disease associated with macular rash; two cases. Acta Derm Venereol 2005;85:342–344.

Disease, Lyme

Synonym: Lyme arthritis

NOTE: This infection is caused by the spirochete, *Borrelia burgdorferi*, which is transmitted from rodents to human by the hard deer ticks, *Ixodes dammini, I. ricinus*, and others.

Organs and Tissues	Procedures	Possible and Expected Findings
External examination and skin	Photograph skin lesions. Record presence of enlarged lymph nodes. Submit sections of affected skin for histologic study.	Erythema chronicum migrans; skin vesicles; annular skin lesions; lymphadenopathy; conjunctivitis.
Cerebrospinal fluid	Submit for IgG study and prepare smear.	Antispirochete IgG; lymphocytes and plasma cells *(1)*.
Blood	Obtain blood for chemical and serologic analysis.	Elevated liver enzymes; elevated IgM early in illness; normal or elevated C3 and C4; rheumatoid factor usually absent.
Joints	Aspirate fluid from joint effusions. Submit synovium of affected joints for histologic study.	Neutrophils in synovial fluid; synovitis resembling early rheumatoid arthritis with a distinctive arteritis with onionskin-like lesions; later in the disease, cartilage destruction.
Heart	Submit sections for histologic study.	Myocarditis; spirochetes may be demonstrable.
Liver	Submit sections for histologic study.	Dense portal infiltrates *(2)*.
Brain and spinal cord	For removal and specimen preparation, see Chapter 4. Include meninges in histologic sections.	Mononuclear meningitis and meningoradiculitis.

Reference

1. Sindern E, Malin JP. Phenotypic analysis of cerebrospinal fluid cells over the course of Lyme meningoradiculitis. Acta Cytol 1995;39:73–75.
2. Zaidi SA, Singer C. Gastrointestinal and hepatic manifestations of tick-born diseases in the United States. Clin Infect Dis 2002;34:1206–1212.

Disease, Lymphatic

NOTE: In all diseases of the thoracic duct and its major tributaries and also in cases of lymphedema or other peripheral lymphovascular diseases, postmortem lymphangiography may be an effective method of study.

Disease, Maple Syrup Urine

Synonyms and Related Terms: Branched-chain hyperaminoacidemia (various types); classic maple syrup urine disease; hyperleucinemia; hypervalinemia. See also aminoaciduria.*

NOTE: Collect all obtainable urine and freeze at –20°C; this should be done as soon as possible.

Organs and Tissues	Procedures	Possible or Expected Findings
Blood and urine	Submit samples for biochemical study.	Increased amino acids and urinary organic acids. The urine may have a "maple syrup" odor.
Fascia lata (or skin)	Submit sample for karyotype and biochemical analysis. Use sterile technique.	Enzyme deficiency can be demonstrated in cultured fibroblasts, leukocytes, or amniocytes.

Organs and Tissues	Procedures	Possible or Expected Findings
Other organs		Bronchopneumonia. Steatosis or increased glycogen deposition in liver.
Brain and spinal cord	For removal and specimen preparation, see Chapter 4.	Spongiosis; gliosis; edema; defective myelinization.

Disease, Marble Bone (See "Osteopetrosis.")

Disease, Marchiafava-Bignami

NOTE: Patients with this disease suffer from chronic alcoholism. Malnutrition, nutritional amblyopia,* and Wernicke-Korsakoff syndrome* may be present.

Organs and Tissues	Procedures	Possible or Expected Findings
Brain and spinal cord	For removal and specimen preparation, see Chapter 4. Request Luxol fast blue stain for myelin.	Symmetric and zonal demyelination in corpus callosum, anterior commissure, optic chiasm, optic tracts, and white matter of frontal lobes.

Disease, Mast Cell (See "Mastocytosis, systemic.")

Disease, Medullary Cystic Renal (See "Cyst(s), renal.")

Disease, Meningococcal

Synonyms: Meningococcemia; *Neisseria meningitidis* infec-tion; Waterhouse-Friderichsen syndrome (fulminant meningococcemia).

NOTE: (1) Submit all tissues that appear to be infected (2). Request aerobic bacterial cultures. (3) Request Gram stain. (4) Special **precautions** are indicated. (5) Usually, serologic studies are not available. However, isolates should be segregated by seroagglutination into serogroups, i.e., A,B,C,D,X,Y,Z. (6) This is a **reportable** disease.

Possible Associated Conditions: Disseminated intravascular coagulation* is a common component of the disease.

Organs and Tissues	Procedures	Possible or Expected Findings
External examination and skin	Record extent of skin lesions and prepare photographs; submit tissue samples of skin for histologic study.	Cutaneous or subcutaneous hemorrhages (purpura fulminans, with or without skin loss and deep muscle damage *(1)*); herpes labialis; rarely, jaundice.
	Prepare skeletal roentgenograms if bone lesions are expected.	Osteomyelitis and osteonecrosis (see below) *(2)*.
Cerebrospinal fluid	Submit sample for aerobic bacterial culture.	
Blood	Submit sample for microbiologic study and determination of serum cortisol concentration.	Meningococcal septicemia. Low serum cortisol level.
Heart and pericardial fluid	Submit samples of pericardium, pericardial fluid, and myocardium or any valvular vegetations for aerobic bacterial cultures and Gram stain.	Pericarditis.* Infective endocarditis.*
Lungs	Submit consolidated areas for culture.	Primary or secondary pneumonia; pleuritis.
Spleen	Record weight and submit tissue specimens for histologic study.	Splenitis.
Adrenal glands	Photograph; record weights; request Gram stain for histologic sections.	Acute hemorrhage and necrosis.
Genital organs	Submit tissue samples for histologic study.	Urethritis; orchitis; epididymitis; endometritis.

Organs and Tissues	Procedures	Possible or Expected Findings
Brain and spinal cord	Any infectious material should be obtained for culture. For removal and specimen preparation of brain and spinal cord, see Chapter 4. Request Bodian stain.	Scant exudate with numerous bacteria in the hyperacute form; In the acute form, abundant pus surrounds the entire brain, vertex, and base and may extend to the ventricular system. In the chronic form, communicating hydrocephalus and cortical infarction are common complications.
Middle and inner ears	For removal and specimen preparation, see Chapter 4.	Otitis media.*
Nasopharynx	For exposure, see Chapter 4. Prepare smears and submit tissue samples for histologic study.	Posterior nasopharyngeal meningococcal infection.
Eyes	For removal and specimen preparation, see Chapter 5.	Conjunctivitis; panophthalmitis.
Bones, joints, and soft tissues	Remove synovial fluid and submit sample for bacteriologic study. For removal of bones and joints, prosthetic repair, and specimen preparation, see Chapter 2, respectively. Prepare histologic sections of synovia and skeletal muscle.	Necrosis and hemorrhage of synovia. Osteonecrosis (rare in adults *[2]*) and osteomyelitis; rhabdomyolysis *(3)*. Purulent arthritis *(4)*.

Reference

1. Huang S, Clarke JA. Severe skin loss after meningococcal septicemia: complications in treatment. Acta Paediatr 1997;86:1263–1266.
2. Campbell WN, Joshi M, Sileo D. Osteonecrosis following meningococcemia and disseminated intravascular coagulation in an adult: case report and review. Clin Infect Dis 1997;24:452–455.
3. Van Deuren M, Neeleman C, Assmann KJ, Wetzels JF, van der Meer JW. Rhabdomyolysis during the subacute stage of meningococcal sepsis. Clin Infect Dis 1998;26:214–215.
4. Bilavasky E, et al. Primary meningococcal arthritis in a child: case report and literature review. Scan J Infect Dis 2006;38:396–399.

Disease, Motor Neuron

Synonyms and Related Terms: Infantile spinal muscular atrophy; progressive spinal muscular atrophy, Werdnig-Hoffman disease.

Organs and Tissues	Procedures	Possible or Expected Findings
External examination		Congenital fixation of multiple joints of extremities.
Brain and spinal cord	For removal and specimen preparation, see Chapter 4.	Degeneration and loss of motor neurons from anterior horn and brainstem motor nuclei (particularly hypoglossal and facial) and thalamus (posteroventral nucleus).
Skeletal muscles	For sampling and specimen preparation, see Chapter 2.	Neurogenic atrophy.

Disease, Multicystic Renal (See "Cyst(s), renal.")

Disease, Niemann-Pick

Synonyms and Related Terms: Sphingomyelinase deficiency; sphingomyelin lipidosis; Niemann-Pick disease, types A, B, C, or D.

NOTE: For further details on specimen preparation, see ref. *(1)*.

Organs and Tissues	Procedures	Possible or Expected Findings
External examination and fascia lata	If diagnosis must be confirmed, prepare fibroblast culture for assay of sphingomyelinase.	Growth retardation.
Skin and conjunctiva	Prepare samples for electron microscopic study (see Chapter 15).	Membrane-bound lamellar cytoplasmic inclusions.
Heart		Endocardial fibroelastosis.
Lungs	In infants, snap-freeze portion of fresh lung and perfuse one lung with formalin. Submit consolidated areas for microbiologic study.	Vacuolated histiocytes (foam cells) containing sphingomyelin, cholesterol, and ganglioside within alveoli and interstitium. Acute or organizing bronchopneumonia.
Liver and spleen	Record sizes and weights; snap-freeze tissue for biochemical sphingomyelin determination. Special stains of frozen sections for phospholipids and cholesterol are positive but not diagnostic. Submit sample for electron microscopic study.	Hepatosplenomegaly; foam cell transformation of Kupffer cells and hepatocytes; cholestasis; intra-acinar fibrosis and, rarely, cirrhosis. Hepatocellular giant cells may be present. Abundant foam cells in spleen. Laminated inclusions in the cytoplasm of affected cells.
Other organs		Transformation of reticuloendothelial cells to autofluorescent foam cells.
Bone marrow	For preparation of sections and smears, see Chapter 2. Prepare sample for electron microscopic study. Prepare unstained smears for phase-contrast microscopy.	"Sea-blue" histiocytes may be present in variant forms of the disease. Lipid-laden cells have membrane-bound lamellar cytoplasmic inclusions.
Brain and spinal cord	For removal and specimen preparation, see Chapter 4. See also under "Liver and spleen."	In the infantile form but not in the childhood form of the disease, neurons are distended with lipid. Eventually, neuronal loss, gliosis, and demyelination occur. Cerebral atrophy; neurons with inclusion; neuronal loss; gliosis and demyelination.
Eyes	For removal and specimen preparation, see Chapter 5.	In the infantile form of the disease, retinal degeneration.

Reference

1. Jevon GP, Dimmick JE. Histopathologic approach to metabolic liver disease. Persp Pediatr Pathol 1998;1:179–199.

Disease, Ollier's (See "Dyschondroplasia, Ollier's.")

Disease, Osler-Rendu-Weber

Synonyms: Hereditary familial angiomatosis; hereditary hemorrhagic telangiectasia.

Organs and Tissues	Procedures	Possible or Expected Findings
External examination and skin; oral cavity	Record distribution of skin lesions and submit tissue samples for histologic study.	Telangiectatic (often papular) lesions most commonly found in cheeks, scalp, nasal orifices, oral cavity, ears, neck, shoulders, fingers, toes, and nail beds. Cyanosis and clubbing may be prominent.
Lungs	For preparation of angiograms of the pulmonary arterial and venous vasculature, see Chapter 2.	Arteriovenous malformations/fistulas.
Aorta	If aneurysm or dissection is present, follow procedures described under those headings.	Aneurysm;* aortic dissection.*

Organs and Tissues	Procedures	Possible or Expected Findings
Mesenteric vasculature	Prepare mesenteric angiograms.	Mesenteric arteriovenous fistulas; aneurysms of the splenic and hepatic arteries; arteriovenous malformations of the colon.
Gastrointestinal tract	For demonstration of esophageal varices, see Chapter 2.	Telangiectasias in stomach and intestinal tract; see also above under "Mesenteric vasculature." Gastrointestinal hemorrhage.*
Liver	If cirrhosis is present, prepare angiograms of hepatic arteries and veins (Chapter 2). Photograph and prepare sections of angiomatous lesions.	Hepatohepatic or hepatoportal arteriovenous malformations/fistulas with cirrhosis-like changes. Cavernous hemangiomas.
Urinary bladder and internal sex organs		Telangiectatic lesions.
Brain and spinal cord	For removal and specimen preparation, see Chapter 4. For preparation of cerebral arteriograms, see Chapter 4.	Arteriovenous malformations; aneurysms of cerebral arteries.* Brain abscess.*
Eyes	For removal and specimen preparation, see Chapter 5.	Retinal arteriovenous malformations.
Nasal cavities	For exposure, see Chapter 4.	Telangiectatic lesions.
Bone marrow		Hyperplasia (in patients with polycythemia).

Disease, Paget's, of Bone

Synonym: Osteitis deformans.

Organs and Tissues	Procedures	Possible or Expected Findings
External examination	Prepare skeletal roentgenograms.	Most commonly involved are sacrum, pelvic bones, tibia, and femur. Skull and other parts of the skeleton may also be affected.
Bones	For removal, prosthetic repair, and specimen preparation, see Chapter 2. If there is a history of cranial nerve palsies, measure diameter of corresponding bony apertures. If there were symptoms of paraplegia, expose and measure diameter of vertebral foramina.	Kyphosis; deformities of long bones; osteosarcomas and other malignant tumors *(1,2)*. See also under "Tumor of bone or cartilage." Thickening of calvarium. Accelerated osteoarthritis of joints in the vicinity of Paget's disease of bone *(3)*.
Heart		Cardiac hypertrophy.*
Other organs		Manifestations of congestive heart failure.*
Parathyroid glands	Record weights and submit samples for histologic study.	Normal size and histologic appearance.

Reference

1. Brandolini F, Bacchini P, Moscato M, Bertoni F. Chondrosarcoma as a complicating factor in Paget's disease of bone. Skeletal Radiol 1997;26:497–500.
2. Yu T, Squires F, Mammone J, DiMarcangelo M. Lymphoma arising in Paget's disease. Skeletal Radiol 1997;26:729–731.
3. Helliwell PS. Osteoarthritis and Paget's disease. Br J Rheumatol 1995; 34:1061–1063.

Disease, Parainfluenza Viral
(See "Laryngitis.")

Disease, Parkinson's

Synonyms and Related Terms: Idiopathic Parkinson's disease; paralysis agitans.

NOTE: Parkinson's syndrome is caused by conditions that may simulate Parkinson's disease; these include carbon monoxide* and manganese poisoning, corticobasal degeneration, drug-induced parkinsonism, Huntington's disease, multiple system atrophy,* progressive supranuclear palsy* (Steele-Richardson-Olszewski syndrome), space-occupying lesions (rare), trauma (dementia pugilistica), and causes related to tumors and vascular diseases.

Organs and Tissues	Procedures	Possible or Expected Findings
Brain	For removal and specimen preparation, see Chapter 4. Histologic sections should include midbrain (substantia nigra), upper pons (locus ceruleus), medulla, nucleus basalis (substantia innominata), and basal ganglia. If Parkinsonian syndrome was diagnosed, follow procedures described under the name of the suspected underlying condition (see above under "Note").	Depigmentation of substantia nigra and locus coeruleus; neuronal loss and reactive gliosis; eosinophilic intracytoplasmic inclusion bodies (Lewy bodies) in some of the surviving neurons; no significant changes in basal ganglia.

Disease, Pelizaeus-Merzbacher

Synonyms: Sudanophilic (orthochromatic) leukodystrophy.

Organs and Tissues	Procedures	Possible or Expected Findings
Brain and spinal cord	For removal and specimen preparation, see Chapter 4. Request Luxol fast blue/PAS stain for myelin and Bielschowsky's stain for axons. Prepare frozen sections for Sudan stain.	Brain generally atrophic. Myelin loss in centrum ovale, cerebellum, and part of brain stem, with a tigroid pattern of residual myelin near vessels. Axons are preserved. Diffuse gliosis with relatively few lipoid-containing macrophages, compared to the myelin loss. Lipoid material stains with Sudan.

Disease, Periodic (See "Fever, familial Mediterranean.")

Disease, Perthes' (See "Osteonecrosis.")

Disease, Pick's

Synonym: Pick's lobar atrophy.

Organs and Tissues	Procedures	Possible or Expected Findings
Brain and spinal cord	For removal and specimen preparation, see Chapter 4. Request silver stains (Bielchowsky or Bodian stain). Histochemical stains in Pick's cells and bodies reveal phosphorylated neurofilaments, ubiquitin, and tubulin. Some tissue should be kept frozen for biochemical studies.	Severe cerebral atrophy, involving primarily frontal and anterior temporal lobes (knife-blade atrophy; walnut brain). Microscopically, severe neuronal loss accompanied by astrocytosis. Characteristic argyrophilic, intracytoplasmic inclusions (Pick's bodies), particularly in hippocampus and swollen, distended "ballooned" neurons (Pick's cells). These changes are not always present.

Disease, Polycystic Kidney (See "Cyst(s), renal.")

Disease, Polycystic Liver (See "Disease, fibropolycystic, of the liver and biliary tract.")

Disease, Prion (See "Disease, Creutzfeldt-Jakob.")

Disease, Pulmonary Veno-Occlusive (See "Obstruction, pulmonary venous.")

Disease, Pulseless (See "Arteritis, Takayasu's.")

Disease, Raynaud's

Related Term: Raynaud's phenomenon.

Organs and Tissues	Procedures	Possible or Expected Findings
External examination	Record extent of ischemic lesions.	Sclerodactyly; necrosis of fingertips; rarely, ischemic necroses on toes, ears, nose, cheeks, and chin.
Chest cavity and upper extremity	Dissect upper mediastinal, supraclavicular, and axillary soft tissues. Subclavian or axillar arteriograms can be prepared at this time. Tissue samples of brachial, ulnar, radial, and digital arteries can be submitted after embalming (consult with funeral director first).	Thoracic outlet compression by tumor or other lesions; thromboangiitis obliterans (Buerger's disease*); arteriosclerosis obliterans; arterial emboli; mural thrombosis of heart.
Abdominal cavity and lower extremity	Submit tissue samples for histologic study of aorta and other elastic arteries, muscular arteries, and veins. For removal of femoral vessels, see Chapter 3.	Thromboangiitis and arteriosclerosis obliterans.
Other organs		Systemic sclerosis* or other immune connective tissue diseases may be present.
Brain and spinal cord	For removal and specimen preparation, see Chapter 4.	Poliomyelitis;* syringomyelia.*

Disease, Recklinghausen's (See "Hyperparathyroidism" and "Neurofibromatosis.")

Disease, Refsum

Synonym: Phytanoyl-coenzyme A hydroxylase deficiency.

NOTE: This peroxisomal disorder may occur in adults but also in an infantile form where it may be a cause of neonatal cholestatic jaundice. For a current review, see ref. *(1)*.

Organs and Tissues	Procedures	Possible or Expected Findings
External examination, skin, and adipose tissue		Ichthyosis. Phytanic acid accumulation in adipose tissues.
Blood	Submit sample for determinaion of phytanic acid concentration and for molecular studies.	Phytanic acidemia, mutation of PHYH or PEX 7 *(2)*.
Cerebrospinal fluid	For obtaining a sample, see Chapter 7.	Increased protein concentrations.
Heart		Cardiomyopathy.*
Liver and kidneys	Sample for histologic study.	Phytanic acid accumulation.
Brain, spinal cord, and peripheral nerves	For removal and specimen preparation, see Chapter 4.	Axonal neuropathy.
Eyes	For removal and specimen preparation, see Chapter 5.	Retinitis pigmentosa.

Reference

1. Pareyson D. Diagnosis of hereditary neuropathies in adult patients. J Neurol 2003;250:148–160.
2. Jansen GA, Waterham HR, Wanders RJ. Molecular basis of Refsum disease: sequence variations in phytanoyl-CoA hydroxylase (PHYH) and PTS2 receptor (PEX7). Hum Mutat. 2004;23:209–218.

Disease, Schilder's (See "Sclerosis, Schilder's cerebral.")

Disease, Schüller-Christian (See "Histiocytosis, Langerhans cell.")

Disease, Sheehan's (See "Insufficiency, pituitary.")

Disease, Sickle Cell

Synonyms and Related Terms: Hemolytic anemia;* sickle cell anemia; sickle cell crisis.

NOTE: See also under "Anemia, hemolytic" and—if applicable—under "Exposure, cold," "Hypoxia," or the name of the infection that may have precipitated a fatal sickle cell crisis. Sickling of erythrocytes may be produced by formalin fixation, in the absence of sickle cell disease. If complications of transfusions or bone marrow transplantation *(1)* are expected, see under those headings.

Organs and Tissues	*Procedures*	*Possible or Expected Findings*
External examination	Record body weight, length, and habitus.	Asthenic habitus; jaundice; skin ulcers over malleoli.
	Prepare skeletal roentgenograms.	Abnormal trabeculations and infarctions of bone; osteonecrosis* of heads of femora or humeri; deformities of metacarpals, metatarsals, and phalanges; elevation of periosteum; widening of marrow cavities.
Blood	Submit sample for culture, toxicologic study, hemoglobin electrophoresis, and determination of bilirubin level. Prepare smears.	Bacteremia; septicemia; presence of hemoglobin S; hyperbilirubinemia.
Heart		Cardiomegaly; cor pulmonale.
Lungs	Submit consolidated area for microbiologic study.	Pneumonia (various types) thrombo or fat embolism,* infarctions, edema, microvasular occlusive thrombi *(2)*.
Liver	Record weight. Request Gomori's iron stain.	Hepatocellular ischemic necrosis caused by accumulation of erythrocytes in sinusoids; sinusoidal dilatation *(3)*.
Gallbladder and common bile duct	Describe appearance of stones or request chemical analysis.	Cholelithiasis;* cholecystitis;* choledocholithiasis.
Spleen	Record weight.	In infants, splenomegaly; in adults, infarctions and fibrosis.
Kidneys, renal veins, ureters, and urinary bladder	Open renal veins *in situ*; section kidneys in frontal plane and prepare photographs.	Infarctions; papillary necroses; renal vein thrombosis;* renal failure;* urinary tract infection.
Penis	Submit tissue samples for histologic study of corpora cavernosa.	Priapism.
Other organs		Manifestations of congestive heart failure* and of hemolytic anemia.*
Bones and bone marrow	For removal, prosthetic repair, and specimen preparation of bone, see Chapter 2. For preparation of sections and smears of bone marrow, see Chapter 2.	Hyperplastic bone marrow; megaloblastic changes.
	For microbiologic study of osteomyelitis, see Chapter 7. Consult roentgenograms for proper sampling.	*Salmonella* osteomyelitis.*
Eyes	For removal and specimen preparation, see Chapter 5.	Angioid streaks; anterior segment necrosis; inferior conjunctival capillary abnormalities; retinopathy; central vitreous hemorrhage.

References

1. Lane PA. Sickle cell disease. Pediatr Clin North Am 1996;43:639–664.
2. Graham JK, Mosunjac M, Hauzlick RL, et al. Sickle cell disease and sudden death: a retrospective/prospective study of 21 autopsy cases and literature review. Am J Forensic Med Pathol 2007;28:168–172.
3. Charlotte F, Bachir D, Nenert M, et al. Vascular lesions of the liver in sickle cell disease. A clinicopathologic study in 26 living patients. Arch Pathol Lab Med 1995;119:46–52.

Disease, Silo-Filler's (See "Edema, chemical pulmonary.")

Disease, Still's (See "Arthritis, juvenile rheumatoid.")

Disease, Sturge-Weber-Dimitri

Synonym: Encephalotrigeminal angiomatosis; encephalofacial angiomatosis.

Organs and Tissues	Procedures	Possible or Expected Findings
External examination	Descibe extent of facial angioma, and photograph. Prepare roentgenogram of skull. Record appearance of limbs.	Facial angioma; unilateral exophthalmos; hemiatrophy of skull; linear cortical cerebral calcifications. Hypoplasia of limb.
Brain and spinal cord	For removal and specimen preparation, see Chapter 4. Photograph surface and coronal slices of brain. Prepare roentgenograms of whole brain and of slices to demonstrate calcifications. Submit tissue samples for histologic study of vascular lesions.	Excessive unilateral capillary and venous-type vessels in leptomeninges; calcification within underlying cortex of one hemisphere that may be atrophic (ipsilateral to facial angioma) *(1)*.
Eyes	For removal and specimen preparation, see Chapter 5.	Choroidal hemangioma; manifestations of congenital glaucoma.

Reference

1. Harding B, Copp AJ. Pathology of Malformations. In: Greenfield's Neuropathology, vol. I. Graham BI, Lantos BL, eds. Arnold, London, 1997, pp. 397–507.

Disease, Takayasu's (See "Arteritis, Takayasu's.")

Disease, Tangier

Synonyms: Alpha-lipoprotein deficiency; familial high-density lipoprotein deficiency.

Organs and Tissues	Procedures	Possible or Expected Findings
Blood	Submit sample for electrophoretic and immunochemical analysis.	Hypoalphalipoproteinemia.
Lymph nodes	Submit samples for histologic study; snap-freeze samples for histochemical study and prepare specimens for electron microscopy.	Lymphadenopathy with diffuse deposition of cholesterol esters.
Heart; elastic and muscular arteries		Premature atherosclerotic cardiovascular disease *(1)*.
Liver and spleen	Record weights. For preparation of specimens, see above under "Lymph nodes."	Hepatosplenomegaly with foam cells.
Neck organs and pharynx	If pharyngeal tonsils cannot be removed with neck organs, attempts should be made to take samples perorally. For preparation of specimens, see above under "Lymph nodes."	Enlarged tonsils with characteristic orange discoloration.
Peripheral nerves	For removal and specimen preparation, see Chapter 4.	Polyneuropathy *(2)*.
Eyes	For removal and specimen preparation, see Chapter 5.	In adults, corneal infiltrates.
Bone marrow	Prepare sections and smears (Chapter 2).	Foam cells.

Reference

1. Vega GL, Grundy SM. Hypoalphalipoproteinemia (low density lipoprotein) as a risk factor for coronary heart disease. Curr Opin Lipidol 1996;7:209–216.
2. Case Rec Mass Gen Hosp. Case 16-1996. A 36-year-old woman with bilateral facial and hand weakness and impaired truncal sensation [clinical conference]. N Engl J Med 1996;334:1389–1394.

Disease, Tay-Sachs (See "Gangliosidosis.")

Disease, Thomsen's (See "Myotonia congenita [Thomsen's disease].")

Disease, Valvular Heart (See "Insufficiency,..." and "Stenosis,..." For congenital valvular diseases, see also under "Valve, congenitally...and name of specific malformation.)

Disease, Veno-Occlusive, of Liver

NOTE: Follow procedures described under "Syndrome, Budd-Chiari." Most cases of fatal veno-occlusive disease in the USA are drug-induced *(1)*.

Reference

1. Culic S, de Kraker J, Kuljis D, Kuzmic I, Saraga M, Culic V, et al. Fatal hepatic veno-occlusive disease with fibrinolysis as the cause of death during preoperative chemotherapy for nephroblastoma. Med Pediatr Oncol 1998;31:175–176.

Disease, Veno-occlusive, of Lung (See "Hypertension, pulmonary.")

Disease, von Gierke's (See "Disease, glycogen storage.")

Disease, von Hippel-Lindau

NOTE: The gene for the disease has been identified. Type I VHL-disease without pheochromocytoma and type II VHL-disease with pheochromocytoma result from different mutations.

Organs and Tissues	*Procedures*	*Possible or Expected Findings*
Pancreas and kidneys; other organs		Cysts;* renal cell carcinoma; papillary cystadenoma of the epidydimis.
Adrenal glands	See "Tumor of the adrenal glands."	Pheochromocytoma.
Brain and spinal cord	For removal and specimen preparation, see Chapter 4. For cerebral arteriography, see Chapter 4.	Hemangioblastoma in cerebellum, medulla, and spinal cord, very rarely involving supratentorial area or peripheral nerve.
Eyes	For removal and specimen preparation, see Chapter 5.	Retinal angiomatosis.

Disease, von Recklinghausen's (See "Hyperparathyroidism" and "Neurofibromatosis.")

Disease, von Willebrand's

Synonyms: Factor VIII deficiency; vascular hemophilia.

NOTE: Follow procedures described under "Hemophilia." The expected findings are essentially the same as in classic hemo-philia. However, hemarthrosis is rare in von Willebrand's disease.

Disease, Vrolik's (See "Osteogenesis imperfecta.")

Disease, Waldenström's (See "Macroglobulinemia, Waldenström's.")

Disease, Weber-Christian

NOTE: This probably is not a specific entity but represents panniculitis, which may be an incidental finding or part of a systemic disease. For further details, see under "Panniculitis."

Disease, Werdnig-Hoffmann (See "Disease, motor neuron.")

Disease, Whipple's

Organs and Tissues	*Procedures*	*Possible or Expected Findings*
External examination and skin	Record body weight and length and extent and character of pigmentation and edema. Submit skin samples for histologic study.	Emaciation. Hyperpigmentation, particularly of exposed skin and in scars. Hyperkeratosis.
Joints	If joints are swollen, remove synovial fluid for cell counts and smears. See also below under "Other organs and tissues."	Arthritis involving ankles, knees, shoulders, and wrists.
Abdominal cavity	Record character and volume of fluid, submit sample for microbiologic study, and prepare smears of sediment. Prepare sections of small intestinal serosa and of parietal peritoneum. Request PAS stain. In granulomas, bacilli are not always PAS positive *(2)*.	Ascites; fibrinous peritonitis.* Nodules in peritoneum containing sickle-form particle-containing cells (SPC cells). For a classification of the bacillus, see ref. *(1)* *Tropheryma whippelii.*
Heart	Section all grossly involved tissues for histologic examination. Submit section for electron microscopy.	Pancarditis; SPC cells in cardiac valves, interstitium of ventricles and atria, and pericardium. Fibrous-adhesive pericarditis;

Organs and Tissues	Procedures	Possible or Expected Findings
	Request PAS stain of paraffin sections.	myocardial fibrosis; endocarditis with valvular fibrosis.
Lungs	Perfuse at least one lung with formalin.	SPC cells in parenchymal stroma and visceral pleura.
Intestine and mesentery	For *in situ* fixation and preparation for study in dissecting microscope, see Chapter 2. Submit tissue samples of various segments of intestinal wall; request PAS stain. Submit portions of mucosa and of mesenteric lymph nodes for electron microscopy. If immunofluorescent studies are intended, snap-freeze tissue samples.	SPC cells, primarily in lamina propria of villi; villous atrophy; thickening of intestinal wall. Rod-shaped bacillary bodies and serpiginous membranes in cytoplasm of SPC cells or extracellularly. Mesenteric lymphadenitis with SPC cells, granulomas, and giant cells.
Other organs and tissues	Submit tissue samples for histologic study of all gross lesions and—even in the absence of macroscopic changes—of esophagus, stomach, colon, spleen, pancreas, retroperitoneal soft tissues, kidneys, adrenal glands, urinary bladder, peripheral and other extramesenteric lymph nodes, brain, spinal cord, synovium with joint capsules, bone marrow, and skeletal muscles. For histologic techniques, see above under "Intestine and mesentery."	Characteristic SPC cells can occur in practically all organs and tissues, particularly in capsule and portal areas of spleen, interstitium of pancreas, stomach, retroperitoneal organs and tissues, lymph nodes, and central nervous system *(3)*. Myopathy may occur.

References

1. Dutly F, Altwegg M. Whipple's disease and "Tropheryma whippelii." Clin Microbiol Rev 2001;14:561–583.
2. Wilcox GM, Tronic BS, Schecter DJ, Arron MJ, Righi DF, Weiner NJ. Periodic acid-Schiff-negative granulomatous lymphadenopathy in patient with Whipple's disease. Localization of the Whipple bacillus to noncaseating granulomas by electron microscopy. Am J Med 1987;83:165–170.
3. Yu C, Jiang A, Yu Y. Serial imaging studies of cerebral Whipple's disease: from onset to end. J Neuroimaging 2007;17:81–83.

Disease, Willebrand's (See "Disease, von Willebrand's.")

Disease, Wilson's

Synonym: Hepatolenticular degeneration.

NOTE: For the gene defect, see ref. *(1)*.

Organs and Tissues	Procedures	Possible or Expected Findings
External examination and skin	Record character and extent of pigmentation; submit skin samples for histologic study.	Jaundice; hyperpigmentation of anterior aspects of lower legs; blue lunulae of nails; increased fingerprint "whorl" pattern.
	Prepare skeletal roentgenograms.	See below under "Bones and joints."
Blood	Submit sample for biochemical study and for hemoglobin electrophoresis.	Low ceruloplasmin concentration (<20 mg/dL); normal or decreased serum copper concentrations. Hemolytic anemia and increase in hemoglobin A_2.
Urine		Increased copper (>100 µg Cu in 24 h) excretion, but single specimen of little use.
Liver	Record weight and photograph. Tissue copper concentrations can be determined from sample in paraffin block *(2)*. Request rhodanine stain for copper.	Fatty changes, periportal hepatitis or cirrhosis,* depending on stage of disease. Rarely massive hepatic necrosis. Stainable copper in many but not all specimens. Tissue copper concentrations >250 µg/g dry wt.
Kidneys	See above under "Liver."	Copper in proximal tubules; tubular fatty changes.
Other organs and tissues		Increased copper in skeletal muscles.
Brain and spinal cord	For removal and specimen preparation,	Symmetrical dilatation of lateral ventricles;

Organs and Tissues	Procedures	Possible or Expected Findings
	see Chapter 4. If biochemical copper determination is intended, see above under "Liver."	discoloration of striatum, often with cavitation of putamen. Thalamic and cortical involvement is common. Microscopically, neuronal loss and gliosis, among other possible abnormalities *(3)*. Alzheimer's type 2 cells increased. Copper deposition primarily perivascular.
Eyes	For removal and specimen preparation, see Chapter 5. For copper staining, use rhodanine method.	Copper of Kayser-Fleischer ring lies in Descemet's membrane. Copper-containing foreign bodies are found in posterior layer of lens capsule.
Bones and joints	For removal, prosthetic repair, and specimen preparation, see Chapter 2.	Osteoarthritis;* bone fragmentation; osteochrondritis of the vertebral column; osteochondritis dissecans of knees and ankles.

References

1. Bull PC, Thomas GR, Rommens JM, Forbes JR, Cox DW. The Wilson's disease gene is a putative copper transporting P-type ATPase similar to Menke's gene. Nature Genet 1993;5:327–337.
2. Ludwig J, Moyer TP, Rakela J. The liver biopsy diagnosis of Wilson's disease. Methods in pathology. Am J Clin Pathol 1994;102:443–446.
3. Harper C, Butterworth R. Hepatolenticular degeneration (Wilson's disease). In: Greenfield's Neuropathology, vol. 1. Graham BI, Lantos PL, eds. Arnold, London, 1997, pp. 632–633.

Disorder, Coagulation (See "Coagulation, disseminated intravascular," "Disease, Christmas," "Disease, von Willebrand's," "Hemophilia," and "Purpura,...")

Disorder, Electrolyte(s)

Organs and Tissues	Procedures	Possible or Expected Findings
Vitreous	Submit sample for determination of sodium, potassium, chloride, glucose, urea nitrogen, and creatinine concentrations. Calcium and phosphate concentrations can also be tested. If sample is small, indicate priority for testing.	Considerably increased or decreased values for sodium (more than 155 meq/L or less than 130 meq/L) and chloride (more than 135 meq/L or less than 105 meq/L) indicate that changes were present before death. For further interpretation, see Chapter 8.
Blood		Postmortem electrolyte concentrations are quite unreliable.
Urine	If indicated, submit sample for chemical study.	May be useful for calcium determination.
Kidneys	Submit tissue samples for histologic study.	Vacuolar nephropathy (vacuolar changes in proximal convoluted tubules) in potassium deficiency (may also occur after infusion of hypertonic solutions).

Disorder, Hemorrhagic
(See "Coagulation, disseminated intravascular," "Disease, Christmas," "Disease, von Willebrand's," "Hemophilia," and "Purpura,...")

Disorder, Inherited, of Phagocyte Function

NOTE: Several conditions represent phagocyte function disorders. Autopsy procedures for one of these disorders can be found under "Disease, chronic granulomatous." Consult this entry for other phagocyte function disorders.

Disorder, Lysosomal Storage

Synonyms and Related Terms: Fabry's disease* (angiokeratoma corporis diffusum); gangliosidosis;* Gaucher's disease;* glycogenosis,* type II; leukodystrophies (Krabbe's or globoid cell,* metachromatic leukoencephalopathy*); mucopolysaccharidoses* (Hunter, Hurler, Morquio, and Sanfilippo disease); mucolipidosis; Niemann Pick disease* (type A, B, C, or sphingomyelinase deficiency); neuraminidase deficiency; neuronal ceroid lipofuscinosis (Batten's disease or Kufs' disease).

Organs and Tissues	Procedures	Possible or Expected Findings
External examination	Obtain routine body measurements and weights. Photograph all abnormalities Prepare skeletal roentgenograms.	Coarse facial features are frequently present. Corneal clouding. Skeletal abnormalities may be present.
Fascia lata	Prepare specimen for fibroblast culture, for enzyme assay, and for electron microscopy.	See entries listed under "Synonyms and Related Terms."
Other organs and tissues (including bone marrow)	Record weights. See also below under "Brain and spinal cord."	Storage deposits in histiocytes ("sea-blue histiocytes" in Niemann-Pick disease); heart, liver, spleen (with hepatosplenomegaly), and kidneys may be involved.
Brain and spinal cord	For removal and specimen preparation, see Chapter 4. Request LFB/PAS stain. Submit samples for electron microscopy. Store fresh/frozen tissue for enzyme assay or molecular genetic studies.	Atrophy. Cellular storage in neurons, histiocytes, and other cells. For possible storage sites, see under name of specific disorder.

Reference

1. Lake B. Lysosomal and peroxisomal disorders. In: Greenfield's Neuropathology, vol. 1. Graham BI, Lantos PL, eds. Arnold, London, 1997, pp. 658–753.

Disorder, Myeloproliferative (See "Leukemia, all types or type unspecified," "Myelofibrosis with myeloid metaplasia," and "Polycythemia.")

Disorder, Plasma Cell (See "Amyloidosis," "Disease, heavy chain," "Macroglobulinemia, Waldenström's," and "Myeloma, multiple.")

Dissection, Aortic

Synonym: Dissecting aortic aneurysm; dissecting aortic hematoma.

Organs and Tissues	Procedures	Possible or Expected Findings
External examination	Record and photograph abnormal features (see right-hand column). Prepare chest roentgenogram.	Features of Marfan's syndrome* or Turner's syndrome.* Widened aorta or mediastinum.
Pericardium	Record appearance and volume of contents.	Hemopericardium.
Aorta	Remove heart and major arteries attached to intact aorta. Open aorta along posterior midline. Photograph intimal tears and record their location and size. Record external rupture site, if possible, and extent of mediastinal or retroperitoneal hemorrhage. Record location and volume of blood in "false" lumen and presence or absence of intramural hematoma, not connected to lumen. Record location and size of re-entry tear, if present.	Coarctation of the aorta.* Dissection may involve major branches of aorta. Blood may be present in periaortic tissues and pericardium (see above). Intimal tear is most commonly located in ascending thoracic aorta. False lumen occurs with or without tear of reentry. The aorta may be atherosclerotic. In the descending thoracic or abdominal aorta, an intimal tear may involve an ulcerated plaque (penetrating ulcer).
	Request Verhoeff–van Gieson and PAS-alcian blue stains. Sections should include grossly involved and uninvolved portions of aortic wall and of adjacent elastic arteries.	Cystic medial degeneration of aorta. Rarely, giant cell aortitis.
Heart	Procedures depend on expected findings or grossly identified abnormalities as listed in right-hand column.	Congenitally bicuspid aortic valve.* Concentric left ventricular hypertrophy. Myxomatous mitral valve.
Other organs		Manifestations of hypertension* or of third-trimester pregnancy.
Brain and spinal cord	For removal and specimen preparation of brain and spinal cord, see Chapter 4.	Ischemic lesions in brain and spinal cord and in other organs.

Diverticula

Related Terms: Diverticular disease; diverticulitis; diverticulosis; Meckel's diverticulum; pulsion diverticulum; traction diverticulum; Zenker's diverticulum.

Organs and Tissues	*Procedures*	*Possible or Expected Findings*
Esophagus	Dissect diverticulum *in situ* and photograph. Fix specimen in formalin before opening.	Hypopharyngeal pulsion diverticulum (Zenker's diverticulum) at lower margin of inferior constrictor muscle of pharynx. Traction diverticulum at midesophagus after an inflammatory process—for instance, tuberculous lymphadenitis. Epiphrenic diverticulum may also occur.
Stomach		Juxtacardiac or juxtapyloric diverticulum.
Small bowel	Prepare histologic sections of Meckel's diverticulum.	Heterotopic tissue in Meckel's diverticulum, with or without peptic ulceration.
Colon	Rinse carefully; openings of diverticula may be difficult to identify. Record thickness of colonic wall and extent, approximate number, and location of diverticula.	Colonic muscular hypertrophy and stenosis, usually in sigmoid colon. Diverticulitis with perforation, fistulas, or peritonitis.*

Diverticulitis (See "Diverticula.")

Diving (See "Accident, diving (skin or scuba).")

Drowning

Related Terms: Dry drowning; fresh-water drowning; near-drowning; salt (sea)-water drowning (see the following table).

Deaths from Drowning

Primary Drowning ("Immediate Drowning")	*Secondary Drowning ("Near-Drowning")*
Deaths occurring within minutes after immersion, before or without resuscitative measures	Deaths occurring from within 30 min to several weeks after resuscitation, because of metabolic acidosis, pulmonary edema, or infective or chemical pneumonitis
Type I ("Dry Drowning")	*Type II ("Wet Drowning")*
Deaths from hypoxia and acidosis caused by glottal spasm on breath holding. There may be no evidence of water entering stomach or lungs and no appreciable morphologic changes at autopsy.	Deaths from hypoxia and acidosis caused by obstruction of airway by water related to: Hypervolemia Hemolysis Hyponatremia Hypochloremia Hyperkalemia

NOTE: The diagnosis is one of exclusion. The pathologist should help the police to determine: 1) How did the person (or dead body) get in the water, and 2) why could that person not get out of the water? It is not enough to ask if a person could swim but investigators should find out how well (what strokes did the victim know?) and how far he or she could swim. The inquiry must include the depth of the water and must address hazards such as undertow or underwater debris, and the behavior of the victim immediately before submerging. Deaths of adults in bathtubs and swimming pools are usually from natural, cardiac causes, or they are suicides, unless the victim was drunk.

Diatom tests *(1)* have not proven useful in the United States but there is enthusiasm for such tests among European pathologists. The distinction between hyponatremic deaths in fresh water and hypernatremic deaths in salt water derives from experimental studies; in practice, one cannot reliably predict the salinity of the immersion medium from autopsy studies. Because many bodies of drowning victims are recovered only after the body floats to the surface, decomposition will often obscure even the nondiagnostic findings such as pleural effusions, which are often associated with drowning.

Organs and Tissues	*Procedures*	*Possible or Expected Findings*
External examination and skin (wounds)	If identity of drowning victim is not known, record identifying features as described in Chapter 13. Prepare dental and whole-body roentgenograms. Submit tissue samples for histologic study of wounds.	There may be wounds that were inflicted before drowning occurred—for instance, in shipwrecks or vehicular and diving accidents. Other wounds may be inflicted after death—for instance, from ship propellers or marine animals. Sometimes, premortem and postmortem wounds can be distinguished histologically.
	Inspect inside of hands.	Object (hair?) held by hands in cadaveric spasm. Cutis anserina and "washerwoman" changes of hands and feet are of no diagnostic help.
	Collect fingernail scrapings.	
	Record appearance and contents of body orifices.	Foreign bodies; semen (see also under "Rape").
	Record features indicative of drowning.	Foam cap over mouth and nose. In the autopsy room, water running from nose and mouth is usually pulmonary edema or water from the stomach.
	Photograph face from front and in profile. Take pictures of all injuries, with and without scale and autopsy number.	
	Remove vitreous for analysis.	High concentrations of alcohol indicate intoxication (see under "Alcoholism and alcohol intoxication").
	If diatom search is intended, clean body thoroughly before dissection to avoid contamination of organs and body fluids with algae and diatoms (see below).	
Blood	Submit sample for toxicologic study.	Evidence of alcohol intoxication may be found.
Organ samples for diatom search	Sample early during autopsy, before carrying out other dissections. Use fresh instruments for removal of specimens to avoid contamination. Submit subpleural portion of lung: subcapsular portions of liver, spleen, and kidneys; bone marrow; and brain. Store samples in clean glass jars. For technique of diatom detection, see below.	Diatoms may occur in the liver and in other organs of persons who have died from causes other than drowning. Comparison with diatoms in water sample from area of drowning may be helpful.
Serosal surfaces and cavities	Record volume of fluid in pleural spaces. Photograph petechial hemorrhages.	Penny-sized or smaller hemorrhages may indicate violent respiratory efforts or merely intense lividity. Presence of pleural fluid suggests drowning.
Neck organs and lungs	Photograph layerwise neck dissection if strangulation* is suspected. Open airways posteriorly, and photograph, remove and save mud, algae, and any other material in tracheobronchial tree. Record size and weight of lungs.	

Organs and Tissues	*Procedures*	*Possible or Expected Findings*
	Request frozen sections for Sudan fat stain.	Fat emboli and bone marrow emboli indicate fractures during life.
Heart		Coronary atherosclerosis and coronary thrombosis.*
Intestinal tract and stomach	Save stomach contents and record volume. Record character of intestinal contents and submit for toxicologic study. Record appearance of serosal and mesenteric lymphatics.	Gastric and intestinal contents indicate type and occasionally time of last meal. Intestinal lymphatics ("lacteals") dilated and quite conspicuous during resorptive state. Tablet residues may be present.
Other organs		Evidence of disseminated intravascular coagulation* may be found after fresh-water submersion.
Genital organs	Search for evidence of rape,* pregnancy,* or both.	
Brain	For removal and specimen preparation, see Chapter 4.	Anoxic changes.
Middle ears, paranasal sinuses, and mastoid spaces	Expose with chisel, and record presence or absence of hemorrhages; photograph hemorrhages; inspect eardrums for presence of perforation. If perforated, prepare histologic sections.	Hemorrhages in middle ears or mastoid air spaces are strong evidence of drowning. Middle ear or mastoid hemorrhages can be documented histologically. Watery liquid in sphenoid sinuses.

Technique of Diatom Detection

For diatom detection *(1)*, boil 2–5 g of tissue for 10–15 min in 10 mL of concentrated nitric acid and 0.5 mL of concentrated sulfuric acid. Then, add sodium nitrate in small quantities until the black color of the charred organic matter has been dispelled. It may be necessary to warm the acid-digested material with weak sodium hydroxide, but the material must soon be washed free from alkali to avoid dissolving the diatoms. The diatoms should be washed, concentrated, and stored in distilled water. For examination, allow a drop of the concentrate to evaporate on a slide, and then mount it in a resin of high refractive index. All equipment must be well-cleaned, and distilled water must be used for all solutions. There are several variations and adaptations of this method.

Reference

1. Camps FE. Immersion in fluids. In: Recent Advances in Forensic Pathology. J & A Churchill, London, 1969, pp. 70–79.

Drugs (See "Abuse,...," "Dependence,...," and "Poisoning,...")

Drug Abuse, Amphetamine(s)

NOTE: Methamphetamine abuse may be suggested by poor condition of the dentition. Methylenedioxymethamphetamine ("Ecstasy") abuse is often suggested by friends with whom the decedent was abusing drugs. Follow procedures described under "Dependence, drug(s)."

Ductus Arteriosus, Patent (See "Artery, patent ductal.")

Dwarfism

Synonyms and Related Terms. Achondroplastic dwarf; asexual dwarf; ateliotic dwarf; micromelic dwarf; normal dwarf; pituitary dwarf; true dwarf; and many other terms, too numerous to mention.

Organs and Tissues	*Procedures*	*Possible or Expected Findings*
External examination	Record lengths of extremities and length of rump (calculate ratio), head circumference, and other suspected abnormal dimensions. Prepare skeletal roentgenograms.	Short or deformed extremities, deformed head, and other deformities. Abnormalities of primary and secondary sex characteristics. Osseous and cartilaginous deformities; skeletal tumor (adamantinoma).
Endocrine organs	Record weights and prepare histologic sections of all endocrine organs.	Tumor; infection; posttraumatic lesions; infiltrates of Langerhans cell histiocytosis.*

Organs and Tissues	Procedures	Possible or Expected Findings
Other organs	Follow procedures described under suspected underlying disease (see right-hand column). In true or primordial dwarfism, no associated abnormalities can be suspected.	Achondroplasia;* congenital heart disease;* Hurler's syndrome (see "Mucopolysaccharidosis"); hypothyroidism;* malabsorption syndrome;* pituitary insufficiency;* renal failure* (chronic); sexual precocity with premature fusion of epiphyses; other systemic diseases.

Dysbetalipoproteinemia, Familial (See "Hyperlipoproteinemia.")

Dyschondroplasia, Ollier's

Synonyms and Related Terms: Multiple enchondromatosis; Ollier's disease; osteochondrodysplasia.

Organs and Tissues	Procedures	Possible or Expected Findings
External examination	Record height and weight. Prepare skeletal roentgenograms.	Growth retardation. Abnormal growth of epiphyseal cartilage with enlargement of metaphysis. Long bones and pelvis most commonly affected.
Skin and soft tissues		Cavernous hemangiomas (Maffucci's syndrome).
Bones and joints	For removal, prosthetic repair, and specimen preparation, see Chapter 2.	See above under "External examination." Chondrosarcoma.

Dyscrasia, Plasma Cell

NOTE: These conditions are characterized by abnormally proliferated B-immunocytes that produce a monoclonal immunoglobulin. Multiple myeloma,* plasma cell leukemia, plasma-cytoma, and Waldenström's macroglobulinemia* as well as heavy-chain diseases and monoclonal gammopathies of unknown type belong to this disease family. Amyloidosis* is closely related to these conditions. For autopsy procedures, see under "amyloidosis," "macroglobulinemia," or "multiple myeloma" and under name of condition that may have caused the plasma cell dyscrasia. Such conditions include carcinoma (colon, breast, or biliary tract), Gaucher's disease,* hyperlipoproteinemia,* infectious or noninfectious chronic inflammatory diseases, and previous cardiac surgery.

Dysentery, Bacillary

Synonym: *Shigella* dysentery.

NOTE: (1) Collect all tissues that appear to be infected. (2) Request aerobic bacterial cultures. (3) Request Gram stain. (4) Special **precautions** are indicated (see Chapter 6). (5) Serologic studies are available from local and state health department laboratories. (6) This is a **reportable** disease.

Organs and Tissues	Procedures	Possible or Expected Findings
Blood	Submit sample for culture and for serologic study.	*Escherichia coli* septicemia.
Bowel	Submit sample of feces or preferably blood-tinged mucus for culture. If bacteriologic diagnosis has already been confirmed, pin colon on corkboard, photograph, and fix in formalin for histologic study.	Colitis with microabscesses; transverse shallow ulcers and hemorrhages, most often in terminal ileum and colon.
Eyes	Submit sample of vitreous for study of sodium, potassium, chloride, and urea nitrogen concentrations.	Dehydration* pattern of electrolytes and urea nitrogen.
	For removal and specimen preparation of eyes, see Chapter 5.	Conjunctivitis, iritis.
Joints	For removal, prosthetic repair, and specimen preparation, see Chapter 2.	Serous arthritis* of knee joints is a late complication.

Dysfibrinogenemia

NOTE: Bleeding and thromboembolism* may be noted at autopsy. Clotting studies with postmortem blood are not indicated. AIDS,* liver disease, and lymphoproliferative disorders are possible underlying conditions.

Dysgenesis, Gonadal (Ovarian) (See "Syndrome, Turner's.")

Dysgenesis, Seminiferous Tubule (See "Syndrome, Klinefelter's.")

Dyskinesia, Ciliary

Synonyms and Related Terms: Immotile cilia syndrome; Kartagener's triad.

NOTE: Multiple conditions belong into this disease category, all characterized by a hereditary defect of the axoneme (the "motor" of the cilia).

Organs and Tissues	*Procedures*	*Possible or Expected Findings*
Blood	Submit blood for molecular analysis.	TXNDC3 gene mutation *(1)*.
Chest cavity	If situs inversus is present, photograph chest organs *in situ*.	Situs inversus in Kartagener's triad (with sinusitis and bronchiectases—see below).
Lungs	Submit samples from one lung for microbiologic study. Perfuse on lung with formalin.	Bronchiectases and bronchopneumonia.
Nasal cavities, sinuses, and middle ears	For exposure and specimen preparation, see Chapter 4.	Nasal polyps; sinusitis, and otitis media.*
	Prepare samples of mucosa for electron microscopic study of cilia (see Chapter 15).	Missing dynein arms.

Reference

1. Duriez B, et al. A common variant in combination with a nonsense mutation in a member of the thioredoxin family causes primary ciliary dyskinesia. Proc Natl Acad Sci USA 2007;104:3336–3341.

Dysphagia, Sideropenic (See "Syndrome, Plummer-Vinson.")

Dysplasia, Chrondroectodermal (See "Syndrome, Ellis-van Creveld.")

Dysplasia, Fibrous, of Bone

Related Term: McCune-Albright syndrome.

Possible Associated Conditions: Acromegaly;* Cushing's syndrome;* hyperthyroidism.*

Organs and Tissues	*Procedures*	*Possible or Expected Findings*
External examination	Record extent of pigmentation, facial features, and primary and secondary sex characteristics.	Unilateral skin pigmentation and precocious puberty in females (Albright's syndrome), less commonly in males. Abnormal facial features caused by distortion of facial bones.
	Prepare skeletal roentgenograms.	Cystlike lesions in metaphyses and shafts of bone; fractures; deformities.
Soft tissues		Myxomas.
Bones	For removal, prosthetic repair, and specimen preparation, see Chapter 2.	See above under "External examination."
	Record size of apertures of cranial nerves in base of skull.	Encroachment of cranial nerves.

Dysplasia, Renal (See "Cyst(s), renal.")

Dysplasia, Thymic (See "Syndrome, primary immunodeficiency.")

Dystonia, Torsion (See "Syndrome, Dystonia.")

Dystrophy, Duchenne's Progressive muscular (See "Dystrophy, muscular.")

Dystrophy, Muscular

Synonyms and Related Terms: Becker's muscular dystrophy; congenital muscular dystrophy; Duchenne's progressive muscular dystrophy; dystrophinopathy; Emery-Dreifuss mucular dystrophy; facioscapulohumeral dystrophy; limb girdle dystrophy; myotonic muscular dystrophy.

Organs and Tissues	*Procedures*	*Possible or Expected Findings*
External examination	Record pattern of scalp hair.	Frontal baldness (in myotonic muscular dystrophy).
	Record status of skeletal musculature.	Atrophy and wasting of muscles (generalized or local: predominantly distal in myotonic muscular dystrophy). Pseudohypertrophy of calf muscles in Duchenne's muscular dystrophy.
Skeletal muscle	Obtain sections for histologic examination. Dystrophin staining of the sarcolemma is absent in Duchenne's muscular dystrophy and patchy in Becker's dystrophy.	Dystrophic changes include variations in fiber size, fiber degeneration and regeneration, peri- and endomysial fibrosis, and fatty replacement of muscle.

Reference

1. Engel AG, Yamamoto M, Fischbeck KH. Dystrophinopathies. In: Myology, 2nd ed., vol. 2. Engel AG, Franzini-Armstrong C, eds. MacGraw-Hill, New York, 1994, pp. 1130–1187.

Dystrophy, Myotonic Muscular (See "Dystrophy, muscular.")

E

Echinococcosis

Synonym: Hydatid disease.

NOTE: (1) Collect all tissues that appear to be infected. (2) Usually, cultures are not required, only direct examination for parasites. (3) Request Giemsa stain for parasites. (4) Special **precautions** should be exercised in removing the cysts, as the contents are highly infectious. (5) Serologic studies are available from the Center for Disease Control and Prevention, Atlanta, GA. (6) This is not a reportable disease.

Organs and Tissues	*Procedures*	*Possible or Expected Findings*
Liver	If the liver is the site of involvement, prepare roentgenogram. Prepare cholangiogram if *Echinococcus multilocularis* organisms are present. Photograph intact cysts and cut sections. Cysts should be placed in formalin before processing.	The liver, especially the right lobe, is the most common site of involvement. Secondary infection or calcification may be present.
Lungs	If the lung is the site of involvement, prepare roentgenogram. Photograph cysts. For further processing, the lung should be perfused with formalin (see Chapter 2).	The lung is the second most common site of involvement. Fluid and air may be visible on the roentgenogram.
Other organs	Procedures depend on expected findings or grossly identified abnormalities as listed in right-hand column.	Cysts may be present in the abdominal cavity, muscles, kidneys, spleen, bones, heart, and brain.
Blood and bone marrow	For preparation of sections and smears, see Chapter 2. Request Giemsa stain.	Eosinophilia.

Eclampsia (See "Toxemia of pregnancy.")

Edema, Angioneurotic

Synonym: Angioedema.

NOTE: Possible causes and suggested autopsy procedures are described under "Death, anaphylactic."

Edema, Chemical Pulmonary

Related Term: Silo-filler's disease.

NOTE: This condition is caused by inhalation of toxic gases, such as oxides of nitrogen (silo-filler's disease) and phosgene ($COCl_2$). See also "Bronchitis, acute chemical" and "Poisoning, gas."

Organs and Tissues	*Procedures*	*Possible or Expected Findings*
Upper airways and lungs	Remove lungs together with pharynx, larynx, and trachea. Open airways posteriorly. Record lung weights. Submit a sample of lung for microbiologic study. Perfuse at least one lung with formalin.	Acute chemical laryngotracheitis; acute pulmonary edema. Obliterating fibrous bronchiolitis and diffuse, progressive pulmonary fibrosis may be present after prolonged survival.

From: *Handbook of Autopsy Practice,* 4th Ed. Edited by: B.L. Waters

Effusion(s) and Exudate(s), Pleural

Organs and Tissues	*Procedures*	*Possible or Expected Findings*
External examination	Prepare chest roentgenogram.	300–500 mL of fluid must be present before it becomes visible.
Chest cavities and chest organs	Submit samples of pleural fluid for microbiologic study. These samples should be obtained before the chest is opened because laceration of the subclavian veins renders clear exudates or transudates hemorrhagic. In true hemorrhagic exudates, determination of the hematocrit value may be useful. For cytologic study, spin down pleural fluid and prepare smears and histologic sections of pellet. Record volume of pleural fluid; remove fluid with vacuum suction apparatus. If the fluid is milky-white, dissect and record appearance of thoracic duct system (see Chapter 3).	Myocardial infarction or other cardiac abnormalities that may have caused congestive heart failure;* pneumonia; pulmonary infarction; tumor(s); bacterial, fungal, or viral infection; immune connective tissue disease; amebiasis;* trauma to thoracic duct system; other causes.
Other organs		Pancreatitis;* subphrenic empyema;* other intra-abdominal disease, with or without ascites.

Electricity (See "Injury, electrical.")

Electrocution (See "Injury, electrical.")

Electrolyte(s) (See "Disorder, electrolyte(s).")

Elliptocytosis, Hereditary (See "Anemia, hemolytic.")

Embolism, Air

NOTE: Possible causes of venous air embolism include: (1) gunshot and shotgun wounds of the head involving dural sinuses; (2) injury to large veins, particularly cranial sinuses (during neurosurgical procedures) and veins of the neck (knife wounds, surgery) or uterus (criminal abortion); (3) insufflation of fallopian tubes (particularly in pregnancy or during menstrual period); (4) infusion of blood components or crystalloid; (5) malfunctioning of dialysis machines; (6) subclavian vein catheterization in the semi-Fowler position; and (7) fracture in the hub of a central venous catheter used for parenteral nutrition.

Possible causes of arterial air embolism include: (1) open heart surgery involving the aorta, left atrium, or left ventricle; (2) positive-pressure ventilation in newborn infants; and (3) underwater ascent with closed glottis (see *Accident, Diving*)

Autopsy Procedure and Diagnosis

If air embolism is suspected, the autopsy should be performed as soon after death as possible. Decomposition gases may be produced within a few hours. Roentgenography of the whole body may detect large quantities of air, and the roentgenograms may serve as a guide to the most advantageous way of dissection.

The postmortem diagnosis of arterial air embolism is made largely on the basis of medical history and circumstances. The autopsy serves to rule out competing conditions.

The diagnosis of venous air embolism is made by chest roentgenography before the autopsy (1). The air in the right chambers of the heart can be confirmed at autopsy by aspiration into a syringe. The formerly recommended procedure of clamping the internal mammary vessels below the sternoclavicular joints, and then cutting across the sternum distal to these clamped vessels so that the sternoclavicular joint area remains intact, is designed to prevent the production of a vacuum that pulls air into the veins. The procedure is not necessary if the air is well-documented by roentgenography before autopsy. At autopsy, a large fatal pulmonary air embolism is readily apparent. The right atrium and ventricle are distended with fine, frothy, bright-red blood, which also may distend the pulmonary arteries and superior vena cava.

Microbiologic examination of blood and pericardial sac contents may help to rule out the presence of gas-forming bacteria that may simulate air embolism (Fig. II-1). However, the presence of putrefactive emphysema in any part of the body points toward a bacterial origin of the gas. Differentiation of air and decomposition gases at the autopsy table with the pyrogallol test is described below.

A 2% pyrogallol solution is prepared (it should be water-clear). Two 10-mL syringes (syringe A and syringe B) are loaded with 4 mL of the pyrogallol solution in each, without permitting any air to enter the system. Immediately before the solution is used, 4 drops of 0.5 *N* NaOH is aspirated through the needle of syringe A to adjust the pH to about 8 (1 drop per 1 mL of solution); the mixture will turn faint yellow. Six mL of gas is then aspirated from the heart or blood vessels. The needle is immediately sealed with a cork or replaced by a cap, and the syringe is vigorously shaken for about 1 min. In the presence of air, the pyrogallol solution will turn brown. If the solution remains clear, decomposition gases were present. In the latter instance, 4 drops of 0.5 *N* NaOH and 6 mL of room air should be aspirated into syringe B, which is then also sealed and shaken for 1 min. The mixture should turn brown, thus serving as a

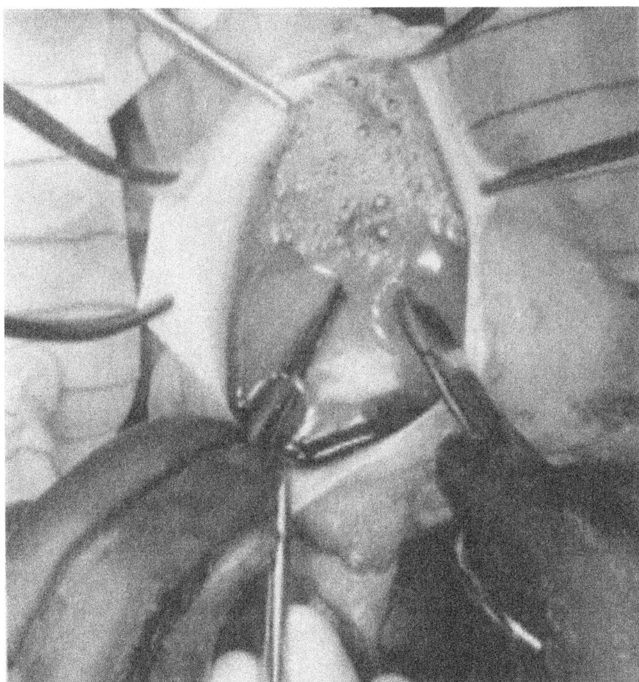

Fig. II-1. Gas-forming bacteria simulating air embolism. The pericardial sac is opened and filled with water. The heart is kept submerged with a pair of scissors. The coronary arteries have been incised with a scalpel. Note gas bubbles and foam on the water surface. No discoloration of 2% pyrogallol was noted. Blood cultures were positive for *Enterococcus* organisms. Microscopically, gram-negative rods were found in most tissues.

control that the pyrogallol solution had been properly prepared. Syringe B may also serve as a reserve. If only one syringe is used, the decomposition gas can be expelled and room air can be aspirated for the control test.

If only small amounts of gas can be aspirated, the volume of the pyrogallol solution should be decreased so that the gas-fluid volume ratio is at least 3:2.

If no bacterial gas formation is present, the edges of the pericardial incision are elevated and the pericardial sac is filled with water. Clamping of the ascending aorta and venae cavae prevents the escape of gas into these vessels. The heart is held under water while the coronary arteries are incised, and the escape of bubbles is recorded. When the right coronary artery is opened, care must be taken that the right atrium is not incised. Air in the coronary arteries indicates systemic embolism. The heart chambers are then incised.

When there is gas in any of the arteries or heart chambers, gas bubbles rise to the surface of the water in the pericardial sac ("bubble test"). Sometimes the vessels have to be somewhat compressed in order to cause the gas to escape. Because large amounts of air or other gases cause the heart to float, it must be kept submerged before the vessels and chambers are incised. Basically the same procedure is used for demonstrating the presence of gas in the superior or inferior vena cava and the pelvic veins (for example, in cases of criminal abortion). In this situation, the abdominal cavity is filled with water and the inferior vena cava and its tributaries are incised.

In support of the diagnosis of systemic arterial air embolism, the skull vault may be removed without puncturing the meninges, so that the cerebral arteries can be inspected for gas bubbles. The demonstration of gas bubbles in the meningeal vessels and in the circle of Willis is meaningful only when the neck vessels are still intact and the internal carotid artery and basilar artery have been clamped before the brain is removed. In acute cases, gas bubbles will be visible within the cerebral vessels. They are released under water when the clamps are removed and the vessels are slightly compressed.

For the collection of gas from blood vessels or cavities, a system of little quantitative reliability is an air-tight, water-filled glass syringe with a needle. The needle is inserted into the vessel or cavity in question and gas is carefully aspirated.

A combined qualitative and quantitative method has been described by Kulka *(2,3)* (see Fig. II-2). He devised an apparatus for gas collection and described it as shown in Fig. II-2 and caption.

The entire system is filled with mineral oil so that, when the funnel is level with the upright bottle, the oil fills only about half of the funnel. In operation, the funnel is first raised to a position 30–40 cm above the level of the upright bottle. All the cocks are opened and the position is held until every trace of gas has been driven from the system through the needle, which is thereby coated on the inside by a film of oil. After all air has been expelled, the cocks are closed and the funnel is lowered to its original position.

As a precautionary measure and control, the air-tightness of the whole system should be tested before operation. This is done by inserting the needle into musculature or skin and attempting aspiration in the manner described in the next paragraph.

To make the test, the bottle is inverted and the needle is inserted into the cavity in question. When the needle is in position, all cocks are opened. The funnel is lowered about 70–90 cm, or until adequate suction is created. This aspirates the contents of the cavity, which may consist of air or other gases, either pure or mixed with blood or other liquid. Any gas or liquid entering this system may be observed through the wall of the short bent glass tubing. In a positive test, gas bubbles will collect in the bottle above the level of the oil. If desired, this gas can be saved for further examination by closing all the cocks and returning the bottle to its upright position *(4)*.

Interpretation of Findings

The volume of intravenous air needed to cause death in adults depends of the cross sectional area of the cardiac cavity or great vessel that is the site of the gas lock, which in turn depends on the position of the decedent at the time of the embolism (5). 100 mL of gas can pass through an intravenous hub in just a few seconds. Small amounts of air entering the systemic circulation may cause death within minutes. Delayed air embolism with fatal outcome may also occur.

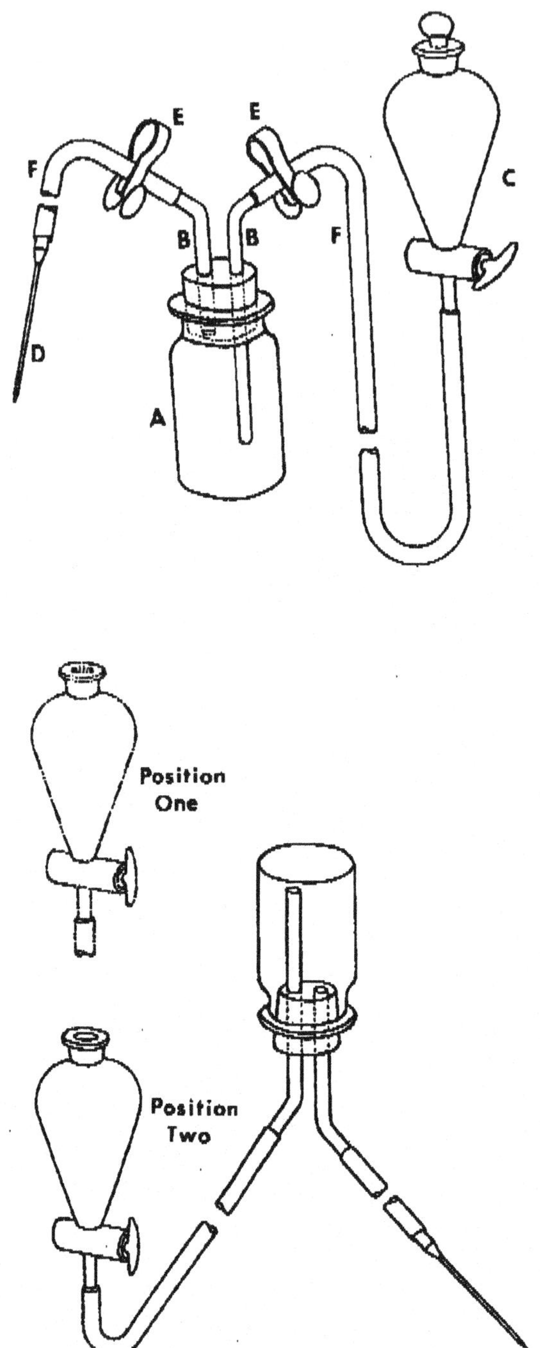

Fig. II-2. Apparatus for demonstration of air embolism. *Top*, Apparatus. *Bottom*, Position of separatory funnel during test. (**A**) One wide-mouth glass bottle (2–3 ounces; 60–90 mL) fitted tightly with a two-hole rubber stopper. (**B**) Two sections of glass tubing, approx 3 mm inside diameter, each bent at an angle of 120°. One of these sections should be longer than the other. The shorter one should reach just through and be even with the inner surface of the stopper. The longer one should reach to within 1 or 1.5 cm of the bottom of the bottle. Both tubes should fit tightly into the holes of the stopper. (**C**) One separatory funnel (60–100 mL, pear-shaped) connected to the longer section of bent glass tubing by rubber tubing 100 cm in length (**F**). An amber, pure gum rubber tubing, such as is used on blood-diluting pipets, has proved satisfactory. (**D**) One transfusion needle, 14- or 15-gauge and 4–5 cm long, connected to the shorter glass tube by a short (<5 cm) section of rubber tubing (F). (**E**) Two pinchcocks, one for each length of tubing. They may be of the spring type or of the household syringe type. The latter will prove advantageous if the gas collected is to be transported for analysis. Adapted with permission from ref. *(3)*.

References

1. Adams V, Guidi C. Venous air embolism in homicidal blunt impact head trauma: Case reports. Am J Forensic Med Pathol 2001;22:322–326.
2. Kulka W. A practical device for demonstrating air embolism. J Forens Med 1965; 12:3–7.
3. Kulka W. Laboratory methods and technical notes: a practical device for demonstrating air embolism. Arch Pathol 1949; 48:366–369.
4. Bajanowski T, West A, Brinkmann B. Proof of fatal air embolism. Int J legal Med 1998;111:208–211.
5. Adams VI, Hirsch CS. Venous air embolism from head and neck wounds. Arch Pathol Lab Med 1989;113:498–502.

Embolism, Amniotic Fluid

Organs and Tissues	*Procedures*	*Possible or Expected Findings*
External examination	If purpura is present, prepare photographs and record extent.	Skin purpura.
Blood	Submit sample (from right atrium) for microbiologic study. Collect blood from right atrium and right ventricle. After the heart has been removed, allow blood in pulmonary vessels to pool in the pericardial sac. Centrifuge this blood and submit sample of flocculent layer above buffy coat for microscopic study *(1)*.	Vernix, lanugo hairs, and meconium can be found in pericardial blood pool.
Lungs	Submit a section of lung for bacteriologic study. Dissect pulmonary arteries; prepare histologic sections of all lobes; request mucicarmine stain and the alcian blue and phloxine-tartrazine stain of Lendrum. Also request Sudan stain on frozen sections.	Meconium-type material in blood vessels. In histologic sections, squamous epithelium, meconium, and fat from vernix caseosa.
Uterus and placenta		Complete or incomplete lower uterine tear; chorioamnionitis.
Other organs		Manifestations of disseminated intravascular coagulation* and fibrinolysis.
Lungs of stillborn		Intrauterine pneumonia.

Interpretation of Findings

Large amounts of debris in the blood vessels of all sections of the lungs may be considered to be lethal if there is no other cause of death. Small amounts in one or more blocks of pulmonary tissue are more likely incidental *(1)*. A small uterine tear is more likely followed by a fatal amniotic fluid embolization than is a large tear, which may result in fatal hemorrhage or fibrinogen depletion. Chorioamnionitis, intrauterine pneumonia, and positive lung cultures of the mother indicate infection of the amniotic fluid.

Reference

1. Attwood HD. Amniotic fluid embolism. In: Pathology Annual 1972. Sommers SC, Rosen PP, eds. Appleton-Century-Crofts, New York, 1972, pp. 145–172.

Embolism, Arterial

Synonyms and Related Terms: Arterial thromboembolism; atheroembolism; bone marrow embolism; embolic syndrome; foreign body embolism; paradoxic embolism; tumor embolism.

NOTE: A history of urinary eosinophilia may have been obtained in patients with renal atheroembolism.

Organs and Tissues	*Procedures*	*Possible or Expected Findings*
External examination		Gangrene of extremities.
Heart	Record patency and size of oval foramen, or presence of septal defect(s).*	In presence of intracardiac right-to-left communication, paradoxic embolism may occur.
	If infective endocarditis is suspected, culture valves and/or any vegetations.	Infective endocarditis.*
	For general dissection techniques, see Chapter 3.	Myocardial infarction; mural or valvular thrombi in left atrium or in left ventricle; atrial dilatation in patients who had atrial fibrillation; mitral or aortic valve prostheses.

Organs and Tissues	Procedures	Possible or Expected Findings
Aorta and elastic artery branches		Thrombi on atheromatous ulcers; thrombi in aneurysms.
	For celiac or mesenteric arteriography, see Chapter 2.	Embolism to celiac or mesenteric artery system.
Other organs		Multiple infarctions may be present. See also above under "Note."
Peripheral arteries	For arteriography and removal of vessels of the lower extremities, see Chapter 3. Submit samples of arteries and veins for histologic study. Request Verhoeff–van Gieson stain.	Localized arterial disease may simulate embolism. This includes infectious arteritis, such as bacterial arteritis after infective endocarditis* or syphilitic or tuberculous arteritis.

Embolism, Cerebral (See "Infarction, cerebral.")

Embolism, Fat

NOTE: Formalin-fixed tissues can be postfixed with osmium tetroxide, embedded in epoxy or paraffin, and stained with tolui -dine blue, hematoxylin, or Oil red O. Fat emboli are more easily recognized than in frozen tissue after Oil Red O staining *(1)*.

Organs and Tissues	Procedures	Possible or Expected Findings
External extermination		Petechial hemorrhages of skin (chest, neck, and face).
	Record evidence of trauma.	Wounds; other traumatic lesions.
	Prepare skeletal roentgenograms.	Bone fractures.
Eyes	For ophthalmoscopic examination, see Chapter 5.	Petechiae of conjunctivas and retinas.
Blood	Pool blood from pulmonary arteries.	Fat may accumulate on surface of blood pool. No useful technique is available for estimating the amount of fat globules in the blood.
Urine	Record presence of fat droplets.	
Lungs, myocardium, spleen, adrenal glands, kidneys	Record weights. Prepare frozen sections of fresh or formalin-fixed material. Request Sudan IV or oil red O stain.	Fat emboli in lumen of small vessels and in pulmonary air spaces.
Liver	Record weight and sample for histologic study.	Severe fatty changes may be the cause of fat embolism.
Bones		Fractures are the most common cause of fat embolism.
Brain and spinal cord	For removal and specimen preparation, see Chapter 4. Photograph horizontal sections through brain, brain stem, and spinal cord.	Petechial hemorrhages, fat emboli *(2)*.
	Prepare frozen sections and request Sudan stain.	Fat emboli.
Pituitary gland	Prepare frozen sections of one-half of gland and paraffin sections of the other half.	Fat emboli and hemorrhages are common in posterior lobe.

Reference

1. Davison PR, Cohle SD. Histologic detection of fat emboli. J Forensic Sci 1987;32:1426–1430.
2. Nastauski F, Gordon WL, Lekawa ME. Posttraumatic paradoxical fat embolism to the brain: a case report. J Trauma 2005;58:372–4.

Embolism, Pulmonary

Synonyms and Related Terms: Bone marrow embolism; foreign body embolism; pulmonary thromboembolism; tumor embolism.

NOTE: If air embolism, amniotic fluid embolism, or fat embolism is suspected, see under those headings. See also under "Phlebitis" and "Thrombosis, venous."

Organs and Tissues	*Procedures*	*Possible or Expected Findings*
External examination	Record circumference of legs, 20 cm above and below patella.	Leg edema accompanying venous thrombosis.
	Prepare chest roentgenogram.	Infarction; pneumothorax* complicating perforated pulmonary infarction.
Pleural cavities	Record volume and character of pleural contents.	Effusion(s);* serofibrinous pleuritis; empyema.*
Heart	In the presence of systemic embolism, record patency of oval foramen or presence of septal defect(s).* Open pulmonary arteries *in situ*.	Paradoxic embolism. Mural thrombi in right atrium or right ventricle. Thrombi on pacing leads or indwelling central catheters.
Lungs	Inspect lumens of hilar pulmonary arteries to detect emboli. Perfuse lungs for a brief period during autopsy and then inspect slices to detect peripheral emboli.	Bland infarcts are more common in lower lobes; infarct abscesses are more common in upper lobes.
Veins	Remove and dissect femoral veins (after embalming) and pelvic veins.	Phlebothrombosis or thrombophlebitis. See also above under "Note."

Emphysema

Synonyms and Related Terms: Chronic obstructive lung disease; pulmonary emphysema; vanishing lung disease.

Possible Associated Conditions: Alpha$_1$-antitrypsin deficiency; chronic bronchitis.*

Organs and Tissues	*Procedures*	*Possible or Expected Findings*
External examination		Cyanosis; clubbing of fingers.
	Prepare chest roentgenogram (roentgenograms are of limited value for detecting or assessing severity of emphysema).	Low diaphragm; pneumothorax.* Unilateral emphysema (congenital lobar emphysema) in infants. Incidental unilateral emphysema in adults (Macleod's syndrome).
Heart	Record weight of heart and thickness of ventricles. For separate weighing of right and left ventricles, see Chapter 3.	Cor pulmonale.
Pulmonary artery	Record width of artery and appearance of intima. For histologic sections, request Verhoeff–van Gieson stain.	Pulmonary atherosclerosis; broken-up elastic membranes.
Lungs	For pulmonary arteriography and bronchography, see Chapter 2. For gaseous or perfusion fixation, slicing, barium impregnation, preparation of paper-mounted sections, see Chapter 2.	Rarefaction of pulmonary artery tree. Chronic bronchitis;* bronchial obstruction; pneumoconiosis.* Emphysema may be centriacinar (centrilobular), focal, giant bullous, irregular, panacinar (panlobular), or paraseptal (distal acinar), or it may be related to scars (para-cicratical airspace enlargement).
	Submit areas of consolidation for microbiologic study.	*Haemophilus influenzae* and *Streptococcus pneumoniae* or other infections.
Diaphragm	Record thickness; submit specimens for histologic study.	Muscular hypertrophy.
Stomach and duodenum		Peptic ulcer(s).*
Liver	For histologic sections, request PAS stain with diastase digestion.	Centrilobular congestion. In alpha$_1$-antitrypsin deficiency,* PAS-positive, diastase-resistant hepatocellular intracytoplasmic globules.

Organs and Tissues	*Procedures*	*Possible or Expected Findings*
Kidneys		Glomerular enlargement.
Bone marrow	For preparation of sections and smears, see Chapter 2.	Increased erythropoiesis.
Brain	For removal and specimen preparation, see Chapter 4.	Anoxic changes in cortex, corpus striatum, globus pallidus, thalamus, Sommer's sector of hippocampus, and Purkinje cells of cerebellum. Petechial hemorrhages of hypothalamus and necrosis of cerebellar folia may be present.

Empyema, Epidural

Synonym: Epidural abscess.

Organs and Tissues	*Procedures*	*Possible or Expected Findings*
External examination		Infected surgical wound(s).
	Prepare roentgenogram of skull.	Skull fracture(s).
Cerebrospinal fluid	Submit sample for microbiologic study.	
Skull	In order to avoid contamination, aspirate infectious material for microbiologic study as soon as calvarium is removed. For exposure of sinuses, middle ears, and adjacent structures, see Chapter 4.	Mastoiditis; osteomyelitis* of parietal, mastoid, and other cranial bones; purulent sinusitis; skull fracture(s); postoperative state.

Empyema, Pleural

Synonym: Pyothorax.

Organs and Tissues	*Procedures*	*Possible or Expected Findings*
External examination	Prepare chest roentgenogram.	Pneumothorax.*
Pleural cavities	Record volume and appearance of empyema fluid. Submit sample of empyema fluid for microbiologic study. Prepare smears and request Gram, Kinyoun's, and Grocott's methenamine silver stains. Submit tissue samples of visceral and parietal pleura for histologic study.	Seropurulent or purulent empyema fluid with evidence of bacteria or fungi. Rarely other infectious agents.
Lungs	Submit any consolidated areas for microbiologic study.	Emboli; infarcts; abscesses; pneumonia (various types); tuberculosis;* lung abscess;* tumor;* surgical or other trauma.
Other organs and tissues		Subphrenic empyema* and other intra-abdominal inflammatory diseases.

Empyema, Subdural

Synonym: Subdural abscess.

NOTE: Autopsy procedures and possible or expected findings are essentially the same as those described under "Empyema, epidural."

Empyema, Subphrenic

Synonyms: Subdiaphragmatic abscess; subphrenic abscess.

Organs and Tissues	*Procedures*	*Possible or Expected Findings*
Abdominal cavity	Submit sample of subphrenic exudate for gram stain and cultures. Record location and volume of subphrenic exudate.	Possible causes of subphrenic empyema include appendicitis, cholecystitis,* diverticulitis, intrahepatic abscess, pancreatitis,* ruptured viscus; penetrating abdominal wound(s), perforated ulcer of stomach or duodenum,* and other conditions.

Organs and Tissues	Procedures	Possible or Expected Findings
Pleural cavities and lungs	Record volume of effusion or exudate in pleural space.	Basal pleuritis and pneumonia, adjacent to empyema.

Encephalitis, All Types or Type Unspecified

Synonyms and Related Terms: Acute disseminated encephalomyelitis;* acute hemorrhagic encephalitis; acute infective encephalitis or encephalomyelitis; acute poliovirus encephalitis or encephalomyelitis; amoebic encephalitis; Arbovirus encephalitis (Japanese encephalitis; eastern encephalitis, western encephalitis, venezuelan equine encephalitis, St. Louis encep-halitis); bulbar encephalitis;* brain stem encephalitis;* herpes encephalitis (cytomegalovirus encephalits, Epstein-Barr virus encephalitis, varicella-zoster encephalitis); herpes simplex ence-phalitis; HIV encephalitis; measles encephalitis; measles inclusion body encephalitis; postinfectious encephalitis; postvaccinal encephalitis; progressive multifocal leukoencephalitis or leukoencephalopathy; rabies* encephalitis; subacute encephalitis; subacute sclerosing panencephalitis; viral encephalitis, west nile encephalitis and other terms *(1)*, too numerous to mention. See also under "Note" and under "Possible or expected findings."

NOTE: If the condition that caused the encephalitis is known, see also under that heading. If the cause of the encephalitis is unknown, submit samples of tissue for microbiologic and toxicologic study, particularly if there is a suspicion of lead poisoning.* See also under "Encephalitis, brain stem," "Encephalomyelitis,...," "Encephalopathy" and "Myelopathy, Myelitis."

Organs and Tissues	Procedures	Possible or Expected Findings
Cerebrospinal fluid	Submit sample for microbiologic study. Prepare cytospin.	
Blood	Submit sample for microbiologic or toxicologic study, or both. Freeze serum sample for possible serologic study.	
Brain and spinal cord; anterior and posterior spinal roots; sensory ganglia	For microbiologic study, submit sample of fresh cerebral tissue. If infectious agent is known and need not be confirmed, fix intact brain in formalin. For toxicologic sampling, see Chapter 13.	Bacterial, fungal, rickettsial, viral, protozoal, or other infection, including amebiasis, cysticercosis, echinococcosis,* leptospirosis,* malaria* (falciparum), schistosomiasis,* syphilis,* toxoplasmosis,* trichinosis,* and trypanosomiasis.* Inclusion bodies may be present in various viral diseases or conditions. Neuronal loss, gliosis, neurofibrillary tangles with West Nile virus *(4)*.
Other organs	Microbiologic, toxicologic, and histologic studies may be indicated, depending on the expected underlying disease.	

References

1. Esiri MM, Kennedy PGE. Viral diseases. In: Greenfield's Neuropathology, vol. 2. Graham BI, Lantos PL, eds. Arnold, London, 1997, pp. 3–64.
2. Scaravilli F, Cook GC. Parasitic and fungal infections. In: Greenfield's Neuropathology, vol. 2. Graham BI, Lantos PL, eds. Arnold, London, 1997, pp. 65–112.
3. Gray F, Nordmann P. Bacterial infections. In: Greenfield's Neuropathology, vol. 2. Graham BI, Lantos PL, eds. Arnold, London, 1997, pp. 113–152.
4. Schafernak KT, Biqio EH. West Nile encephalomyelitis with polio-like paralysis and nigral degeneration. Can J Neurol Sci 2006:33:407–410.

Encephalitis, Brain Stem

Synonyms and Related Terms: Brain stem abscess; infectious brain stem encephalitis; Listeria monocytogenes brain stem encephalitis; viral brain stem encephalitis.

NOTE: See also under "Encephalitis, limbic."

Organs and Tissues	Procedures	Possible or Expected Findings
Brain	For removal and specimen preparation, see Chapter 4.	Necrotizing encephalitis, with or without abscess formation *(1)*.

Reference

1. Hall WA. Infectious lesions of the brain stem. Neurosurg Clin North Am 1993;4:543–551.

Encephalitis, Herpes Simplex (See "Infection, herpes simplex.")

Encephalitis, Limbic

Synonyms and Related Terms: Brain stem encephalitis; limbic encephalopathy; paraneoplastic encephalomyelitis; paraneoplastic sensory neuropathy.

Organs and Tissues	*Procedures*	*Possible or Expected Findings*
Blood and cerebrospinal fluid		Commonly high titers of antibodies anti-Hu (anti neuronal nuclear antibodies, type 1 or ANNA 1) *(1)*.
Brain, spinal cord, and dorsal root ganglia	For removal and specimen preparation, see Chapter 4.	Neuronal degeneration; neuronophagia; microglial nodules; gliosis in hippocampus, brain stem, and dorsal root ganglia; perivascular lymphoid infiltrates, especially in nerve roots.
Other organs	See also under "Tumor...," depending on expected primary site. Search for a thymoma.	Carcinoma (bronchogenic small cell carcinoma in most instances; other primary tumors include non-small cell lung cancer or cancers of breast, ovary, uterus, and stomach). Thymoma *(2)*.

Reference

1. Moll JWB, Vecht CH. Immune diagnosis of paraneoplastic neurological disease. Clin Neurol Neurosurg 1995;97:71–81.
2. Evoli A, et al. Paraneoplastic diseases associated with thymoma. J Neurol 2007;254:756–762.

Encephalomyelitis, Acute Disseminated

Synonyms and Related Terms: Acute hemorrhagic necrotizing encephalomyelitis; acute perivascular myelinoclasis; allergic encephalomyelitis; perivenous encephalomyelitis; postinfectious or parainfectious encephalomyelitis; postrabies vaccinal encephalomyelitis; postvaccinal encephalomyelitis.

Organs and Tissues	*Procedures*	*Possible or Expected Findings*
Brain and spinal cord; anterior and posterior spinal roots; sensory ganglia	Submit multiple sections for histologic examination. Microscopic findings vary and depend on the phase of the disease.	In acute phase, swelling and congestion of brain. Scattered perivenous demyelination with histiocytic and lymphocytic infiltrates, predominantly in white matter. Small perivascular hemorrhages may be present. In the hyperacute form of the condition (acute hemorrhagic necrotizing encephalopathy), swelling and congestion of the brain with signs of herniation. Petechial hemorrhages in the centrum semiovale white matter. Neutrophilic perivascular infiltrates with venule necrosis and fibrinous exudate.

Encephalomyopathy (See "Myopathy.")

Encephalopathy, Hepatic

Synonyms and Related Terms: Acute hepatic encephalopathy; portal-systemic encephalopathy; Reye's syndrome.*

Organs and Tissues	Procedures	Possible or Expected Findings
Brain and spinal cord	For removal and specimen preparation, see Chapter 4.	In fulminant hepatic failure, cytotoxic brain swelling with herniation and Duret's hemorrhages. In portal systemic encephalopathy, brain may be grossly normal. Alzheimer type 2 astrocytes, with pale watery nuclei (common in globus pallidus, thalamus, and deep layers of cortex). Emperipolesis by astrocytes *(1)*.
Liver	Procedures depend on suspected underlying conditions as listed in right-hand column.	Alcoholic liver disease;* cirrhosis;* massive or submassive hepatic necrosis; microvesicular fatty changes in Reye's syndrome,* fatty liver of pregnancy, and other conditions; poisoning with hepatotoxic substances (e.g., mushroom poisoning with *Amanita phalloides*).

Reference

1. Nishie M, et al. Oligodendrocytes within astrocytes ("emperipolesis") with cerebral white matter in hepatic and hypoglycemic encephalopathy. Neuropathol 2006;26:62–5.

Encephalopathy, Hypertensive

Synonyms and Related Terms: Acute hypertensive encephalopathy; Binswanger's disease; progressive subcortical encephalopathy; subcortical dementia.

NOTE: See also under "Hypertension (systemic arterial), all types or type unspecified."

Organs and Tissues	Procedures	Possible or Expected Findings
Brain	Request Luxol fast blue-PAS stains.	Edema in sudden malignant hypertension. Focal ischemic changes; intracerebral hemorrhages. In Binswanger's disease, multiple small old infarctions or patchy or diffuse demyelination of the cerebral white matter is present, associated with sclerosis of small arteries. Demyelination and infarctions may occur together. Infarctions may be present in other portions of the brain.
Heart, kidneys, vascular system, and other organs		Causes (e.g., chronic renal disease) and manifestations of acute or chronic hypertension.

Encephalopathy, Type Unspecified

Related Term: Toxic encephalopathy.

NOTE: If a specific toxic exposure is expected—for example, lead poisoning, see under that heading.

Enchondromatosis, Multiple (See "Dyschondroplasia, Ollier's.")

Endocarditis, Infective

Synonyms and Related Terms: Acute endocarditis; bacterial endocarditis; prosthetic valve endocarditis; subacute endocarditis.

Possible Associated Conditions: See below under "Possible or Expected Findings."

Organs and Tissues	Procedures	Possible or Expected Findings
External examination and skin; peripheral veins	If jaundice is present, search for evidence of gonococcal infection. Record skin changes and prepare photographs.	Manifestations of malnutrition; jaundice; clubbing of fingers and toes; petechial hemorrhages of skin and mucous membranes; splinter hemorrhages of nail beds. Needle marks, furuncles, and other skin infections or scars may indicate dependence on intravenous drug(s).*

Organs and Tissues	Procedures	Possible or Expected Findings
External examination and skin; peripheral veins *(continued)*	If intravenous catheter is present, leave in place, tie vessel proximally and distally from tip, and submit for microbiologic study. If this is not possible, prepare smears and sections of thrombus at tip of catheter. Request Gram and Grocott's methenamine silver stains.	Infected surgical arteriovenous shunts; infected intravenous catheters, including devices in surgically treated patients with hydrocephalus.*
	Submit tip for culture, even if it is contaminated.	
	Record appearance of oral cavity.	Dental infection; petechial hemorrhages.
	Prepare chest roentgenogram.	
Eyes	For removal and specimen preparation, see Chapter 5.	Petechial hemorrhages of conjunctivas; Roth's spots.
Blood	If cultures had not been prepared antemortem, submit samples for bacterial and fungal cultures. Request aerobic and anaerobic bacterial cultures. Freeze serum sample for serologic study.	Septicemia.
Heart	Photograph valvular lesions before submitting tissue for culture. Prepare sections of vegetations; request Gram and Grocott's methenamine silver stains.	Rheumatic valvulitis; congenital cardiac malformations; prosthetic valve(s) with valvular ring abscesses; mycotic aneurysms of ascending aorta; valvular perforations.
	For coronary arteriography, see Chapter 10.	Coronary arterial emboli.
	For collection of nonvalvular tissue for histologic study, see Chapter 3.	Myocardial infarction; myocardial abscesses.
Arteries and veins	For histologic sections, request Verhoeff–van Gieson stain.	Mycotic aneurysms; septic thrombophlebitis.
Lungs		Metastatic abscesses—for instance, after right-sided endocarditis in heroin addicts.
Intestinal tract and mesentery	Dissect mesenteric arteries. Other procedures depend on expected findings or grossly identified abnormalities as listed in right-hand column.	Mesenteric emboli; intestinal infarction. Adenocarcinoma of colon may be associated with *Strep. bovis* endocarditis.
Spleen	Record size and weight.	Infarctions or abscesses, or both.
Liver		Alcoholic liver disease.
Kidneys	For histologic sections, request 4-μm sections, stained with PAS and with methenamine silver for glomerular lesions.	Glomerulitis. Macroscopically, minute hemorrhages, infarctions, and abscesses may be present.
Internal genital organs		Complications of abortion;* gonococcal infection.
Bones	For removal; prosthetic repair, and specimen preparation, see Chapter 2.	Osteomyelitis.*
Brain	If cerebral involvement is suspected, submit sample for microbiologic study.	Infarctions, abscesses, or hemorrhages; mycotic aneurysms.

Endocarditis, Löffler's (See "Cardiomyopathy, restrictive [with eosinophilia].")

Endocarditis, Nonbacterial Thrombotic (NBTE)

Synonyms and Related Terms: Libman-Sacks verrucous nonbacterial endocarditis; marantic endocarditis; verrucous endocarditis.

NOTE: A history of multiple miscarriages may have been obtained.

Possible Associated Conditions: Disseminated intravascular coagulation;* antiphospholipid antibody syndrome; lupus anticoagulant.

Organs and Tissues	Procedures	Possible or Expected Findings
Heart	If the diagnosis is suspected, photograph and remove vegetations, as described for infective endocarditis, and submit portions for microbiologic and histologic study.	The mitral valve is usually affected, without other valvular abnormalities.

Organs and Tissues	Procedures	Possible or Expected Findings
Heart (continued)	Prepare histologic sections of vegetations and of affected valve(s). If microorganisms appear to be present, request Gram stain.	
Other organs	Procedures depend on expected findings or grossly identified abnormalities as listed in right-hand column.	Emboli and infarctions. Possible underlying conditions include carcinoma of the lung, pancreas, stomach, and other, primarily mucus-producing adenocarcinomas, systemic systemic lupus erythematosus,* antiphospholipid syndrome, and chronic debilitating diseases.

Enteritis, All Types or Type Unspecified (See "Enterocolitis,...," "Enteropathy,...," "Gastroenteritis, eosinophilic," and names of specific infectious diseases, such as "Fever, typhoid," or possible noninfectious underlying conditions, such as "Shock.")

Enteritis, Eosinophilic (See "Gastroenteritis, eosinophilic.")

Enteritis, Granulomatous (See "Disease, Crohn's.")

Enteritis, Necrotizing

Synonyms and Related Terms: Clostridial gastroenteritis; Darmbrand; enteritis necroticans.

NOTE: Follow procedures described under "Enterocolitis, pseudomembranous." Clostridial enterotoxemia (*C. perfringens)* seems to be the cause of necrotizing enteritis. Hemorrhagic necrosis of the small bowel mucosa with pseudomembranes, ulcers, and peritonitis is the main finding at autopsy.

Enteritis, Other Types or Type Undetermined (See "Enterocolitis, Other types or Type Undetermined.)

Enteritis, Regional (See "Disease, Crohn's.")

Enterocolitis, Ischemic

Synonyms and Related Terms: Hemorrhagic enteropathy; hemorrhagic necrosis (gangrene; infarction) of intestine; necrotizing enterocolitis; ischemic colitis; pseudomembranous enterocolitis.*

NOTE: It is assumed here that the intestinal changes are clearly ischemic. In ischemic enterocolitis, superinfection should be ruled out and therefore, appropriate studies may be needed also: (1) Collect all tissues that appear to be infected. (2) Request aerobic and anaerobic bacterial cultures. (3) Request Gram stain. (4) No special precautions are indicated. (5) Serologic studies are not available. (6) This is not a reportable disease.

Organs and Tissues	Procedures	Possible or Expected Findings
Intestinal tract and mesentery	For mesenteric arteriography, see Chapter 2. Dissect mesenteric vessels. If infection is expected as a cause, submit portions of intestine for cultures.	Emboli, atherosclerosis, or other conditions that may cause obstruction of mesenteric arteries. Primary or secondary thrombosis of mesenteric veins. Fibrinous ischemic membranes or pseudomembranes and ulcers may be present in small and large intestine. Air in the mucosa or muscularis.
Other organs		Manifestations of hypotension and shock.*

Enterocolitis, Neutropenic

Synonyms and Related Terms: *C. septicum* enterocolitis; necrotizing cecitis or typhlitis.

NOTE: (1) Collect all tissues that appear to be infected. (2) Request aerobic and anaerobic bacterial cultures. (3) Request Gram stain. (4) No special precautions are indicated. (5) Serologic studies are not available. (6) This is not a reportable disease.

Organs and Tissues	Procedures	Possible or Expected Findings
Intestinal tract	Collect material from lesions in cecum for aerobic and anaerobic culture. Sample for histologic study.	*C. septicum* infection (or infection with other Clostridiae) with ulcers, hemorrhages, and pseudomembranes, primarily in cecum and ascending colon.
Other organs and tissues		Malignancies that required chemotherapy or other conditions associated with neutropenia and treatment with antibiotics.

Enterocolitis, Other Types or Type Undetermined

NOTE: A multitude of infectious and noninfectious agents may cause inflammation of the small bowel, large bowel, or both. If the condition is not listed under "Colitis," "Enteritis," or "Enterocolitis" or under another specific heading such as "Dysentery, bacillary," obtain sufficient material for microbio-logic and histologic study to identify organisms such as *Clos-tridium, Chlamydia, Shigella, Salmonella, Yersinia, Helicobacter, vero-toxic E. coli,* and others. If lymphogranuloma venereum,* or tuberculosis* are suspected, see also under these headings. See also under "Disease, inflammatory bowel" and "Disease, Crohn's."

Enterocolitis, Pseudomembranous

Synonyms and Related Terms: *C. difficile* colitis; Darmbrand; hemorrhagic necrosis (gangrene; infarction) of intestine; ischemic enteritis or enterocolitis;* neutropenic enterocolitis;* pseudomembranous colitis.

NOTE: The name "Pseudomembranous enterocolitis" is descriptive; the condition may be infectious, ischemic, or both. If the intestinal changes are clearly ischemic, see above under "Enterocolitis, ischemic." If the cause is in doubt and if pseudomembranes can be identified, follow the procedures described here.

(1) Collect all tissues that appear to be infected. (2) Request aerobic and anaerobic bacterial cultures. (3) Request Gram stain. (4) No special precautions are indicated. (5) Serologic studies are not available. (6) This is not a reportable disease.

For other infectious intestinal diseases, see under specific names, such as "Enterocolitis, neutropenic" or "Enterocolitis, staphylococcal."

Organs and Tissues	*Procedures*	*Possible or Expected Findings*
Intestinal tract and mesentery	Collect material from pseudomembranes for culture and for *C. difficile* toxin assay.	Bacterial growth (*C. difficile* or verocyto-toxin producing *E. coli* or other organisms such as *Shigella dysenteriae*). Generally, the condition is confined to the colon.
	Sample intestinal wall with pseudomembranes for histologic study.	Lamellated pseudomembranes with much mucin and layers of neutrophils and necrotic epithelial cells. Mucous glands distended with mucin. Gram-positive bacilli in exudate.
	If the condition is suspected to be caused by ischemia, follow procedures described above under "Enterocolitis, ischemic."	Occlusive vascular lesions or other conditions causing impaired intestinal perfusion.
Other organs		Manifestations of hypotension and shock.* Conditions that were treated with antibiotics (which in turn allowed the selective proliferation of the intestinal pathogens).

Enterocolitis, Staphylococcal

Related Term: Staphylococcal diarrhea.

NOTE: (1) Collect all tissues that appear to be infected. (2) Request aerobic bacterial cultures. (3) Request Gram stain. (4) No special precautions are indicated. (5) Usually, serologic studies are not helpful. (6) This is not a reportable disease.

Organs and Tissues	*Procedures*	*Possible or Expected Findings*
External examination		Dehydration.*
Gastrointestinal tract	Culture contents of stomach, small intestine, and large intestine. Prepare sections and Gram-stained smears of mucus on intestinal wall.	*Staphylococcus aureus.*
Other organs	Procedures depend on expected findings as listed in right-hand column.	Conditions that may have required administration of antibiotics. Previous surgery.

Enteropathy, Gluten-Sensitive (See "Sprue, celiac.")

Enteropathy, Hemorrhagic (See "Enterocolitis, pseudomembranous.")

Enteropathy, Protein-Losing

NOTE: This a collective name for a diverse group of diseases and conditions that cause gastrointestinal protein loss. Carcinoma of the esophagus, heart diseases,* nephrosis, and primary immunodeficiency syndrome also may be causes of this condition.

Organs and Tissues	Procedures	Possible or Expected Findings
Heart	Dissection procedures depend on the specific type of heart disease.	Atrial septal defect;* primary cardiomyopathy;* constrictive pericarditis.* Other conditions associated with congestive heart failure.*
Esophagus	If a carcinoma is present, see also under "Tumor of the esophagus."	Carcinoma.*
Stomach	Dissect and immerse in fixative as soon as possible. If a carcinoma is present, see also under "Tumor of the stomach."	Allergic gastroenteropathy; carcinoma; giant hypertrophy of mucosa (Ménétrier's disease); atrophic gastritis. Status post gastrectomy.
Small intestine	For postmortem lymphangiography, see Chapter 2. For *in situ* fixation and for preparation of intestinal mucosa for study under the dissecting microscope, see Chapter 2. For histologic sections, request PAS and azure-eosin stains. If infectious intestinal disease is suspected, submit portions of intestine for microbiologic study.	Allergic gastroenteropathy; celiac* or tropical sprue;* Crohn's disease; intestinal lymphangiectasia; jejunal diverticulosis; lymphenteric fistula; lymphoma* and other malignancies; primary tuberculosis;* other infectious intestinal diseases (see also under "Enterocolitis,..."); Whipple's disease.*
Colon	Procedures depend on expected findings or grossly identified abnormalities as listed in right-hand column.	Carcinoma and other malignancies; chronic ulcerative colitis or Crohn's disease;* megacolon.
Other organs	Procedures depend on expected findings or grossly identified abnormalities as listed in right-hand column.	Manifestations of malabsorption syndrome* with osteomalacia;* manifestations of congestive heart failure.* Conditions associated with nephrotic syndrome;* systemic sclerosis* (sclerodema) in cases with involvement of small intestine.

Eosinophilia, Tropical Pulmonary (See "Syndrome, eosinophilic pulmonary.")

Epiglottiditis (See "Laryngitis.")

Epilepsy, Idiopathic (Cryptogenic)

Related Term: Status epilepticus.

Organs and Tissues	Procedures	Possible or Expected Findings
Brain	Histologic sections should include (as a minimum) both hippocampi, cerebellar cortex, cerebral cortex, and thalami.	By definition, no gross changes or histologic lesions are demonstrable that could be responsible for seizures. In chronic epilepsy, secondary tissue changes, attributable to repeated anoxic episodes, are found. These include hippocampal sclerosis and Purkinje cell loss in cerebellum and changes attributable to closed head injury,* such as superficial contusions in frontal or temporal lobes.
Other organs		For possible side effects of therapy, see "Epilepsy, symptomatic."

Epilepsy, Myoclonus

Synonyms and Related Terms: Baltic myoclonus; Lafora's disease; Lafora body disease; progressive myoclonus epilepsy with Lafora bodies; progressive myoclonus epilepsy without Lafora bodies; Unverricht-Lundborg disease.

NOTE: Myoclonic seizures also have been described in a number of progressive encephalopathies with complex neurological symptoms, such as GM1 and GM2 gangliosidosis,* and Niemann-Pick* and Krabbe's disease but also acquired disorders, including Alzheimer's disease,* Creutzfeldt-Jakob

Epilepsy, Myoclonus *(continued)*

disease,* posthypoxic encephalopathy, and subacute sclerosing panencephalitis. Mitochondrial encephalomyopathy also can present with myoclonus epilepsy and a mitochondrial myopathy with ragged red fibers (MERRF syndrome) in skeletal muscles.

Organs and Tissues	*Procedures*	*Possible or Expected Findings*
Brain	For histologic sections, request methyl violet or toluidine blue, Alcian blue, and PAS stains, with and without diastase digestion.	Mild cortical atrophy. Diffuse neuronal loss with mild astrocytosis. In Lafora's disease, basophilic, metachromatic, PAS-positive, diastase-resistant, single or multiple (1–30 μm diameter) intracytoplasmic neuronal inclusion bodies (Lafora bodies), primarily in cerebral cortex (central region and prefrontal motor cortex), thalamus, globus pallidus, substantia nigra, cerebellar cortex, and dentate nuclei. Cerebellar atrophy (Dilantin).
Other organs and tissues, including eyes and peripheral nerves	For removal and specimen preparation of eyes, see Chapter 5. For sampling and specimen preparation of peripheral nerves, see Chapter 4. For histologic sections, request methyl violet or toluidine blue stain and PAS stain with and without diastase digestion.	Lafora-body-type material in the heart, liver, retinas, peripheral nerves, skeletal muscles, and sweat gland ducts (especially axillary).
Skeletal muscles	For removal and specimen preparation, see Chapter 2. Request modified Gomori's trichrome stain.	Ragged red fibers in mitochondrial myopathies.

Epilepsy, Symptomatic

NOTE: Possible causes or underlying conditions include cerebrovascular diseases, congenital malformations of the brain, degenerative and demyelinating diseases of the brain, head injury,* intracranial and cerebral infections, toxic or metabolic disorders (alcoholism,* barbiturate,* carbon monoxide,* and lead poisoning,* hemodilution, hypocalcemia, or hypoglycemia),* and tumors of the brain.*

Organs and Tissues	*Procedures*	*Possible or Expected Findings*
External examination	If gum hypertrophy or hirsutism are present, record and prepare photographs. Record skin changes and presence or absence of lymphadenopathy.	Gum hypertrophy, hirsutism (in young women), and lymphadenopathy may be found in patients who received phenytoin (Dilantin); drug-related dermatitis may be found also.
Brain	For histologic sampling, see under "Epilepsy, idiopathic (cryptogenic)."	See above under "Note."
	For cerebral arteriography, see Chapter 4.	Cerebrovascular abnormalities.
	Culture any suspected sites of infection.	Intracranial and cerebral infections.
Other organs	If a toxic or metabolic disorder is suspected, submit samples of body fluids and tissues for toxicologic study.	Complications of anticonvulsive therapy: agranulocytosis (carbamazepine), megaloblastic anemia* (barbiturates) or liver damage (dilantin, valproic acid).

Erythema Multiforme

Synonyms and Related Terms: Erythema exudativum multiforme major; Stevens-Johnson syndrome; toxic epidermal necrolysis.

NOTE: The histologic changes of erythema multiforme, Stevens-Johnson syndrome, and toxic epidermal necrolysis may be quite similar *(1)*.

Organs and Tissues	Procedures	Possible or Expected Findings
External examination and skin	Record extent and character of skin lesions. Submit samples of affected and of unaffected skin for histologic study. Record extent and character of lesions in oral cavity.	Macules; papules; vesicles; bullae; hemorrhages. Vulvitis may be present. Ulcers, fissures, and hemorrhagic lesions of oral cavity.
Pleural cavities		Effusion(s).*
Lungs	Submit consolidated areas for microbiologic study. Perfuse at least one lung with formalin.	Bronchitis;* bronchopneumonia.
Heart		Pericarditis.*
Other organs	Record appearance of all mucosal surfaces. Submit samples for histologic study. Other procedures depend on expected findings or grossly identified abnormalities as listed in right-hand column.	Laryngitis;* pharyngitis; esophagitis; colitis; vaginitis; urethritis; hepatitis *(2)*. Possible underlying diseases include nephritis, infectious disease, collagen disease, and malignant tumor. Radiation treatment may have been given also.
Eyes	For removal and specimen preparation, see Chapter 5.	Conjunctivitis; iritis, iridocyclitis; panophthalmitis.
Other organs and tissues		Lymphoma* (with erythema multiforme as paraneoplastic syndrome) *(3)*.

References

1. Rzany B, Hering O, Mockenhaupt M, Schroder W, Goerttler E, Ring J, Schopf E. Histopathological and epidemiological characteristics of patients with erythema exudativum multiforme major, Stevens Johnson syndrome and toxic epidermal necrolysis. Br J Dermatol 1996;135:6–11.
2. Carrera C et al. Erythema multiforme presenting as cholestatic acute hepatitis caused by Epstein-Barr virus. J Eur Acad Dermatol Venereol 2006;20:1350–1352.
3. Kreutzer B, Stubiger N, Thiel HJ, Zierhut M. Oculomucocutaneous changes as paraneoplastic syndrome. Ger J Ophthalmol 1996;5:176–181.

Erythroblastosis Fetalis

Related Terms: Bilirubin encephalopathy; fetal hydrops; hemolytic anemia of the newborn; kernicterus.

NOTE: *Cytomegalovirus, Parvovirus,* syphilis, and *Toxoplasma* infections can cause erythroblastosis fetalis. These may be sought with routine histological as well as immunohistochemical methods on tissue sections. Immune-mediated destruction of fetal red cells or platelets, causing fetal hemorrhages and erythroblastosis. Serologic tests are also available.

Organs and Tissues	Procedures	Possible or Expected Findings
Blood (maternal and fetal)	Perform a direct Coombs test on fetal cells and antibody screen on fetal or maternal cells. Determine the hematocrit on the fetal blood.	Alloantibody-mediated hemolysis; anemia.
External examination and oral cavity	Record body weight and length.	Generalized, severe edema (fetal hydrops); jaundice; purpuric rash. In long-term survivors, discolored deciduous teeth with hypoplastic enamel.
Thymus	Record weight.	Accelerated maturation.
Heart and lungs	Submit samples for histologic study.	Erythroblasts in vessels of myocardium and of lungs. Look for intranuclear inclusions typical of *Parvovirus*.
Liver	Submit tissue for viral culture. Record weight. Submit samples for histologic study. Request Gomori's stain for iron. Use immunohistochemical stains to confirm the presence of *Parvovirus*.	Hepatomegaly with increased extramedullary hematopoiesis and hemosiderosis.
Spleen	Record weight. See also above under "Liver."	Splenomegaly with increased extramedullary hematopoiesis; hemosiderosis; small or absent Malpighian corpuscles.
Pancreas	Submit sample for histologic study.	Increased extramedullary hematopoiesis.
Retroperitoneal tissues with adrenal glands and kidneys	Submit samples for histologic study.	Extramedullary hematopoiesis in adrenal glands and in retroperitoneal (peripelvic and renal) soft tissues.

Organs and Tissues	Procedures	Possible or Expected Findings
Lymph nodes		Hypoplasia with hemosiderosis.
Bone marrow		Erythroblastic hyperplasia.
Fascia lata	Establish a cell culture.	Rule out aneuploidy. The cells may be used to identify a metabolic cause.
Brain and spinal cord	Prepare photographs of stained areas of brain.	Diffuse cerebral icterus or selective staining of subthalamic nuclei, globus pallidus, hippocampus, pontine nuclei, medullary nuclei in the floor of the fourth ventricle, thalamus, and cerebellar nuclei. Cortical and spinal gray matter is rarely involved.
Placenta	Weigh and submit samples for histologic study.	Villous edema; erythroblasts in vessels; inclusions consistent with *Cytomegalovirus* or *Parvovirus* infection; chronic plasma cell villitis.

Esophagus, Barrett's

Organs and Tissues	Procedures	Possible or Expected Findings
Lungs	Perfuse at least one lung with formalin.	Aspiration (reflux) pneumonitis with fibrosis.
Diaphragm	Record size of diaphragmatic hernia.	Diaphragmatic hernia.*
Esophagus and stomach	Remove whole length of esophagus, together with stomach and portion of diaphragm with hiatus. Record diameter of esophageal stricture (a glass cone or wooden cone can be used) before opening narrowed portion of esophagus. After opening, pin esophagus and stomach on corkboard, photograph, and fix in formalin (in this position).	The esophagus (most commonly the distal portions) is lined by columnar epithelium that causes a brownish red discoloration of the mucosa. Chronic reflux esophagitis is present, and an ulcer and a stricture often are found at the squamocolumnar junction. Dysplasia and adenocarcinoma are common complications and arise in the areas of intestinal metaplasia.
Neck organs		Laryngitis and pharyngitis in cases of severe chronic reflux.

Ethanol (Ethyl Alcohol) (See "Alcoholism and alcohol intoxication," "Cardiomyopathy, alcoholic," "Disease, alcoholic liver," "Syndrome, fetal alcoholic," and "Syndrome, Wernicke-Korsakoff.")

Exposure, Cold

NOTE: In all instances, the blood alcohol level should be determined and a drug screen should be done. The tissues tend to be well preserved.

Possible Associated Conditions: Age-related increased susceptibility to cold (in infancy and senility); alcohol intoxication;* myxedema; pituitary insufficiency;* poisoning by depressants, narcotics, or other drugs; stroke.

Organs and Tissues	Procedures	Possible or Expected Findings
External examination, skin, and subcutaneous tissues	Prepare photographs of abnormalities, as listed in right-hand column.	Red discoloration of the face and extremities; generalized edema; erythematous patches on trunk and limbs.
	Submit samples of skin and of subcutaneous tissue for histologic study.	Frostbite; bullae; gangrene. Subcutaneous tissue usually contains little blood.
Blood and vitreous	Submit samples for toxicologic study.	Blood is fluid and bright red.
Lungs	Record weights and sample for histologic study.	Pulmonary hemorrhages.
Gastrointestinal tract	Record sites of lesions and submit samples for histologic study.	Small mucosal hemorrhages or—if patient had survived exposure for some time—ulcers. Rarely, perforation of ulcers.
Pancreas	Prepare photographs and sample for histologic study.	Peripancreatic fat tissue necroses, with or without pancreatitis.*
Other organs		Fatty changes of myocardium, liver, and kidneys; congestion of viscera; sludging of blood in small vessels.
Brain		Perivascular hemorrhages around third ventricle.

F

Failure, Congestive Heart

NOTE: Coronary atherosclerosis and manifestations of ischemic heart disease,* valvular heart disease, congenital cardio-vascular diseases, and manifestations of systemic or pulmonary hypertension are the most frequent findings in patients dying of or with congestive cardiac failure. Other causes include cardiomyopathies* and secondary myocardial disease (such as amyloid or pericardial constriction). If the cause of the congestive cardiac failure is unknown or not immediately evident after dissection of the heart and of the great vessels, myocardium and other appropriate tissues may be submitted for microbiologic study—including viral cultures—and for electron microscopy. Specimens can also be snap-frozen for possible immunofluorescent, biochemical, or histochemical studies, particularly of the myocardium.

Organs and Tissues	*Procedures*	*Possible or Expected Findings*
External examination	Record body weight and length. Prepare roentgenogram of chest.	Cyanosis; edema of legs; dilatation of veins. Cardiomegaly; pleural effusion(s).*
Chest and abdominal cavities	Record volume and character of effusion(s).	Hydrothorax; ascites.
Heart and great vessels	See above under "Note." Record weight of heart, valve circumferences, and ventricular wall thickness. Estimate extent of dilatation of each cardiac chamber. Note consistency of myocardium.	Possible causes of congestive cardiac failure are too numerous to mention. Dilatation of heart, with or without mural thrombosis. Myocardium may be soft, normal, or firm.
Other organs	Organs mentioned in right-hand column should be described and, if appropriate, weighed and measured. Submit samples for histologic study.	Pulmonary congestion, with or without hemosiderosis; congestion of viscera with organomegaly. Other organ manifestations include bowel edema or hemorrhagic enteropathy (without mechanical vascular occlusion) and zonal hepatic steatosis, fibrosis, or necrosis, with or without evidence of liver failure. Acute renal tubular necrosis may be present also.

Failure, Kidney

Synonyms and Related Terms: Acute kidney failure; chronic kidney failure; renal failure; uremia.

NOTE: If acute kidney failure had been diagnosed, the autopsy procedures will depend on the expected causes, such as poisoning with ethylene glycol,* lead,* mercury,* or methyl alcohol;* disseminated intravascular coagulation* and its various underlying conditions; glomerulonephritis* and its various underlying conditions; diabetes mellitus;* or multiple myeloma.* The procedures described below deal primarily with chronic renal failure. If the patient had had dialysis, see also under "Dialysis (for chronic renal failure)." If transplantation had been carried out, see also under "Transplantation, kidney."

Organs and Tissues	*Procedures*	*Possible or Expected Findings*
External examination and skin	Submit samples of skin for histologic study. Record position of shunts. Prepare skeletal roentgenograms and roentgenograms of soft tissues.	"Uremic frost." Uremic skin discoloration. Teflon-Silastic shunts. Bone deformities and fractures. (See also below under "Bones and joints.") Metastatic calcifications in soft tissues and bursae.

From: *Handbook of Autopsy Practice,* 4th Ed. Edited by: B.L. Waters

Organs and Tissues	Procedures	Possible or Expected Findings
Vitreous	Submit sample for determination of urea nitrogen, creatinine, sodium, and chloride concentrations.	Markedly elevated urea nitrogen and creatinine; near normal sodium, and chloride.
Blood	Submit sample for microbiologic study. Retain frozen serum for serologic or immunologic study. Submit sample for determination of urea nitrogen and creatinine concentrations.	Elevated urea nitrogen and creatinine.
Heart		Myocarditis;* pericarditis.*
Blood vessels	If infection or clotting of shunt is suspected, remove shunt together with ligated vessels and submit for culture.	Infected shunts; manifestations of hypertension;* metastatic calcification.
Lungs	Submit any consolidated area for bacterial, fungal, and viral cultures; prepare smear of fresh cut section for the demonstration of *Pneumocystis carinii*.* Collect fresh lung samples and freeze for possible immunofluorescent study. Perfuse at least one lung with formalin.	Bacterial, fungal, viral, and/or uremic pneumonitis; pulmonary edema.
Esophagus		*Candida* esophagitis.
Gastrointestinal tract	Record character of contents; submit tissue samples for histologic study.	Hemorrhages; gastroenteritis.
Liver	For gross iron staining, see Chapter 16.	Transfusion hemosiderosis. Chronic hepatitis C.
Pancreas	Submit samples for histologic study.	Inspissation of pancreatic ducts.
Kidneys	For renal arteriography, renal venography, and retrograde urography, see Chapter 2. For other procedures, see under name of specific renal disease. Dissect and fix kidneys as soon as possible.	See under name of specific renal disease, such as "Glomerulonephritis." Acquired cystic disease may occur after long-term intermittent maintenance hemodialysis.
Urine	Collect and submit sample for urinalysis.	
Testes	Submit samples for histologic study or rete testis.	Cystic transformation of rete testis *(1)*.
Parathyroid glands	Record weights; submit samples for histologic study.	Hyperplasia, with or without adenoma(s).
Brain and spinal cord	For removal and specimen preparation, see Chapter 4. If the choroid plexus is to be used for immunologic study, dissect fresh brain and snap-freeze plexus.	Edema and petechiae. Neuronal damage.
Eyes	For removal and specimen preparation, see Chapter 5.	Hypertensive retinopathy; steroid cataracts.
Skeletal muscles		Myopathy.
Bones and joints	Obtain strip of vertebral column.	Renal osteodystrophy (osteoporosis;* osteomalacia*). Gout.*

Reference

1. Nistal M, Santamaria L, Paniagua R. Acquired cystic transformation of the rete testis secondary to renal failure. Hum Pathol 1989;20:1065–1070.

Failure, Liver

NOTE: See under name of suspected underlying disease, such as "Cirrhosis, liver" or "Hepatitis, viral."

Failure, Lung

NOTE: See under name of suspected underlying conditions such as "Pneumonia,...," "Syndrome, adult respiratory distress (ARDS)," or "Syndrome, respiratory distress, of infant."

Fascioliasis (See "Clonorchiasis.")

Feminization, Testicular

Related Term: Hereditary male pseudohermaphroditism.

NOTE: This x-linked recessive condition is characterized by impairment of male phenotypic differentiation or virilization; it occurs in a complete and an incomplete (see below) form. Together with Reifenstein's syndrome* and the infertile male syndrome, these conditions represent androgen receptor disorders.

Organs and Tissues	Procedures	Possible or Expected Findings
External examination and breasts	Record body weight and length. Record appearance of breasts and submit samples of breast tissue for histologic study.	Female appearance with female external genitalia; sparse axillary and pubic hair.
Blood or fascia lata	Specimens should be collected using aseptic technique for tissue culture for chromosome analysis (see Chapter 9). Record presence of sex chromatin.	Karyotype is 46,XY.
Gonads and vagina	Record weights of testes and prepare histologic sections of both. Prepare histologic sections of vaginal mucosa.	Blind-ending vagina; absent internal genitalia except for testes, which may have descended to inguinae or labia. No spermatogenesis (but Leydig cells and seminiferous tubules are present). In incomplete testicular feminization, partial fusion of labioscrotal folds, clitoromegaly, and normal pubic hair are found.

Fever, Colorado Tick

Related Term: Orbivirus infection.

NOTE: (1) Collect all tissues that appear to be infected. (2) Request cultures for orbiviruses (*Reoviridae* family). This requires animal inoculation, and not all laboratories have the capability of isolating orbiviruses. (3) Special stains are not indicated. (4) Special **precautions** are indicated (see Chapter 6). (5) Serologic studies are available from local or state health department laboratories. The virus also can be detected by reverse tran-scription PCR of whole blood and serum *(1, 2)*. (6) This is not a reportable disease.

Organs and Tissues	Procedures	Possible or Expected Findings
External examination		Skin rash; thrombocytopenic hemorrhages.
Cerebrospinal fluid	If meningitis or encephalitis is suspected, submit samples for viral culture and for cytologic study.	Increased leukocyte counts and positive viral culture.
Blood	Submit samples for viral culture and for serologic study or study by PCR (see above under "Note.").	
Other organs and tissues		Thrombocytopenic hemorrhages; focal necrosis in multiple organs.
Brain and spinal cord	For removal and specimen preparation, see Chapter 4. Submit fresh cerebral tissue for viral culture.	Meningitis* and encephalitis.*

Reference

1. Johnson AJ, Karabatsos N, Lanciotti RS. Detection of Colorado tick fever virus by using reverse transcription PCR and application of the technique in laboratory diagnosis. J Clin Microbiol 1997;35:1203–1208.
2. Lambert AJ et al. Detection of colorado Tick Fever viral RNA in acute human serum samples by a quantitative real-time RT-PCR assay. J Virol Methods 2007;140:43–48.

Fever, Familial Mediterranean

Synonyms: Familial paroxysmal polyserositis; periodic fever; periodic polyserositis; recurrent polyserositis.

Organs and Tissues	Procedures	Possible or Expected Findings
Chest and abdomen	Record volume of pericardial, pleural, and peritoneal exudates. Submit samples for microbiologic study. Prepare smears or sections of spun-down sediment. Submit samples of serosal surfaces for histologic study.	Exudate should be sterile, with many neutrophils. Acute serositis.

Organs and Tissues	*Procedures*	*Possible or Expected Findings*
Other organs	Request Congo red or other amyloid stains. For further details on staining procedures, see under "Amyloidosis." Other procedures depend on expected findings or grossly identified abnormalities as listed in right-hand column.	Amyloidosis *(1)* (common cause of death) involving arterioles, venules, glomeruli, and spleen. Heart and liver show only small-vessel amyloidosis. Acalculous cholecystitis* is a common complication. Acute orchitis *(2)*.
Joints	For removal, prosthetic repair, and specimen preparation, see Chapter 2. Submit samples of synovium for histologic study.	Arthritis,* mostly of large joints.

Reference

1. Yonem O, Bayraktar Y. Secondary amyloidosis due to FMF. Hepatogastro 2007;54:1061–1065.
2. Moskovitz B, Bolkier M, Nativ O. Acute orchitis in recurrent polyserositis. J Pediatr Surg 1995;30:1517–1518.

Fever, Hemorrhagic, with Renal Syndrome

Related Terms: Balkan hemorrhagic fever with renal syndrome; Bunyaviridae infection; endemic or epidemic nephrosonephritis; Far Eastern hemorrhagic fever; Hantaan virus infection *(1)*; Korean hemorrhagic fever; Manchurian epidemic hemorrhagic fever; nephropathia epidemica.

NOTE: (1) Collect all tissues that appear to be infected. (2) Viral cultures are not available. (3) Special stains are not indicated. (4) Special **precautions** are indicated (see Chapter 6). (5) Serologic studies are available from the Centers for Disease Control and Prevention, Atlanta, GA. (6) This is a **reportable** disease. Bioterrorism must be considered in current cases.

Organs and Tissues	*Procedures*	*Possible or Expected Findings*
External examination	Record presence and location of petechiae.	Conjunctival petechiae; subconjunctival hemorrhages. Widespread petechiae.
Vitreous		Increased potassium and phosphate concentrations, calcium concentrations decreased.
Blood	Submit sample for demonstration of specific IgM antibodies by ELISA and for determination of immune adherence hemagglutination titers.	See also above under "Note."
Gastrointestinal tract	Open bowel and fix samples of mucosa as early in the autopsy procedure as possible. Measure volume of blood in lumens. (If contents are fluid, one can attempt to obtain a hematocrit value.)	Intraluminal hemorrhages.
Liver	Submit samples for histologic study.	Midzonal necrosis *(2)*.
Kidneys, ureters and urinary bladder	Remove kidneys, ureters, and urinary bladder en block. Photograph cut surfaces of kidneys with renal pelves and ureters; submit samples for histologic study.	Parenchymal hemorrhages; tubular necrosis. Blood in renal pelves, ureters, and urinary bladder.
Other organs and tissues	Submit samples for histologic study.	Manifestations of hemorrhagic shock and hypotension;* retroperitoneal edema.
Brain and spinal cord		Hemorrhages.

References

1. Duchin JS, Koster FT, Peters CJ, Simpson GL, Tempest B, Zaki SR, et al. Hantavirus pulmonary syndrome: a clinical description of 17 patients with a newly recognized disease. N Engl J Med 1994;330:949–955.
2. Elisaf M, Stefanaki S, Repanti M, Korakis H, Tsianos E, Siamopoulos KC. Liver involvement in hemorrhagic fever with renal syndrome. J Clin Gastroenterol 1993;17:33–37.
3. Saggioro FP, et al. Hantavirus infection induces a typical myocarditis that may be responsible for myocardial depression and shock in hanta virus pulmonary syndrome. J Infec Dis 2007;195:1541.

Fever, Lassa

Related Terms: Arenavirus infection; Argentine or Bolivian hemorrhagic fever.

NOTE:

Lassa fever is a **highly communicable** disease and **autopsy studies are not recommended** in the usually available surround-ings. If Lassa fever is suspected, contact the state health department and the Centers for Disease Control and Prevention, Atlanta, GA, for disposition and further studies *(1)*. If an autopsy is done, disinfection can be accomplished by washing instruments with 0.5% phenol in detergent (i.e., Lysol), 0.5% hypochlorite solution, formalin, or paracetic acid. For shipping procedures, see Chapter 15. This is not a reportable disease.

Organs and Tissues	Procedures	Possible or Expected Findings
All organs	Experience is quite limited with cases of Lassa fever *(2)*. If an autopsy is done, it should be regarded as a research procedure. Prepare photographs. Submit samples of many organs and tissues for viral and other microbiologic studies and for histologic study. Prepare material for electron microscopic study.	Gastrointestinal and cerebral hemorrhages; intercurrent infection; foci of necrosis.
Blood	Collect serum for serologic testing and for culture of the virus. An early diagnosis can be made from serum samples by reverse transcription PCR *(3)*.	Fourfold rise in antibody titer; high IgG titer or virus-specific IgM. Detection of Lassa virus RNA.
Other body fluids (e.g., urine, cerebrospinal fluid, breast milk, or joint fluid)	Freeze fluids at –70°C for arenavirus isolation.	

References

1. Holmes GP, McCormick JB, Trock SC, Chase RA, Lewis SM, Mason CA, et al. Lassa fever in the United States. Investigation of a case and new guidelines for management. N Engl J Med 1990;323:1120–1123.
2. Nzerue MC. Lassa fever: review of virology, immunopathogenesis, and algorithms for control and therapy. Centr Afr J Med 1992;38:247–252.
3. Demby AH, Chamberlain J, Brown DW, Clegg CS. Early diagnosis of Lassa fever by reverse transcription-PCR. J Clin Microbiol 1994; 32:2898–2903.

Fever, Periodic
(See "Fever, familial Mediterranian.")

Fever, Q

Synonyms: Acute Q fever; chronic Q fever; *Coxiella burnetii* infection.

NOTE: (1) Collect blood, urine, and all tissues that appear to be infected. (2) For the definite diagnosis of this rickettsial disease, inoculation into animals or embryonated eggs is required, which cannot be done safely in the usual clinical laboratory. (3) Special stains are not indicated. (4) This is a **highly communicable** disease, and special precautions are indicated (see Chapter 6). (5) Serologic studies are available from local and state health department laboratories. (6) This is a **reportable** disease.

Organs and Tissues	Procedures	Possible or Expected Findings
Blood	Submit blood sample for microbiologic study and serum for complement-fixation or agglutination tests.	
Heart	If endocarditis is suspected, follow procedures described in Chapter 7.	Bacterial suppurative vegetative endocarditis* may be present, and this is a likely cause of death. Pericarditis* and pericardial effusion.
Lungs	Submit consolidated areas for microbiologic study. Perfuse at least one lung with formalin.	Patchy hemorrhagic, necrotizing pneumonia; necrotizing bronchitis *(1)* and bronchiolitis.
Liver	Record weight and submit samples for histologic study.	Hepatomegaly; granulomas with fibrin ring and central lipid vacuole (not specific for the disease).
Spleen and bone marrow	Record weight and submit samples for histologic study.	Splenomegaly; splenitis with large granulomas.
Kidneys		Glomerulonephritis *(2)*.
Veins	Examine femoral veins.	Thrombophlebitis.
Brain	For removal and specimen preparation, see Chapter 4.	Meningitis.*
Eyes	For removal and specimen preparation, see Chapter 5.	Uveitis; optic neuritis.
Bones, joints, and skeletal muscles	For removal and specimen preparation, see Chapter 2.	Osteoarticular infection *(3)*; rhabdomyolysis *(4)*, Osteomyelitis *(5)*.

References

1. Kayser K, Wiebel M, Schulz V, Gabius HJ. Necrotizing bronchitis, angiitis, and amyloidosis associated with chronic Q fever. Respir 1995; 62:114–116.
2. Korman TM, Spelman DW, Perry GJ, Dowling JP. Acute glomerulonephritis associated with acute Q fever: case report and review of the renal complications of Coxiella burnetii infection. Clin Inf Dis 1998;26:359–364.

3. Cottalorda J, Jouve JL, Bollini G, Touzet P, Poujol A, Kelberine F, Raoult D. Osteoarticular infection due to Coxiella burnetii in children. J Pediatr Orthopaed 1995;4:219–221.
4. Carrascosa M, Pascual F, Borobio MV, Gonzales Z, Napal J. Rhabdomyolysis associated with acute Q fever. Clin Inf Dis 1997;25:1243–1244.
5. Nourse C et al. Three cases of Q fever osteomyelitis in children and a review of the literature. Clin Infec Dis 2004;39:e61–e66.

Fever, Relapsing

Synonyms: Borreliosis; louseborne (epidemic) relapsing fever; tickborne (endemic) relapsing fever.

NOTE: (1) Collect all tissues that appear to be infected. (2) Rat/mouse inoculation with infected blood is the most sensitive method for the detection of the organism. Consult the state health department. (3) Before the autopsy, consultation with the microbiology laboratory is advised. (4) Request direct dark-field examination and Giemsa or Wright stain. (4) No special precautions are indicated. (5) Serologic studies are of questionable value due to the antigenic variability of the organism. (6) This is not a reportable disease.

Organs and Tissues	*Procedures*	*Possible or Expected Findings*
Blood	Prepare smears and request Giemsa or Wright stain.	Species of spirochetes of the genus *Borrelia*.
Spleen	Record weight. Stain touch preparations and paraffin sections with Giemsa or Wright stain.	Organisms abundant in reticulum cells of white pulp.
Other organs	See above under "Note" and under "Spleen." Sample for histologic study as suggested in right-hand column.	Organisms in biliary epithelium, gastrointestinal tract, convoluted tubules of kidneys, brain, and meninges, with lymphocytic meningitis *(1)*

Reference

1. Cadavid D, Barbour AG. Neuroborreliosis during relapsing fever: a review of the clinical manifestations, pathology, and treatment of infections in humans and experimental animals. Clin Inf Dis 1998;26:151–164.

Fever, Rheumatic

NOTE: In young children, arthritis may be less conspicuous. Cardiac and other visceral manifestations may predominate in this age group.

Organs and Tissues	*Procedures*	*Possible or Expected Findings*
External examination, skin, and throat	Prepare histologic sections of subcutaneous nodules and other skin lesions and of grossly unaffected skin.	Rheumatic nodules (over bony prominences, such as elbow or occiput); erythema marginatum (annulare); cutaneous rheumatic arteritis.
	Submit swabs for throat culture.	Group A streptococci.
Pericardium	Submit fluid from pericardial sac for culture. Record volume of pericardial contents.	Pericardial effusion or pericarditis.*
Blood	Submit samples for microbiologic and serologic studies (C-reactive protein, immunoglobulin, serum haptoglobin).	
Heart and ascending aorta	If infective endocarditis is suspected, follow procedures described in Chapter 7.	In chronic cases, infective endocarditis.*
	Record weight of heart; use inflow-outflow method for dissection (see Chapter 3) and submit samples for histologic study. Histologic samples should include posterior wall of the left atrium and chordae tendineae with papillary muscles. For histochemical and immunologic studies, freeze samples of epicardium and myocardium and of valves. Submit samples of coronary arteries and of ascending aorta for histologic study. Request Verhoeff–van Gieson stain.	Rheumatic myocarditis; Aschoff bodies, predominantly beneath endocardium of left-sided heart chambers and within valves. Rheumatic valvular aseptic vegetative endocarditis. Coronary arteritis; intimal hyperplasia of ascending aorta, just above aortic valve.
Lungs	Submit any consolidated areas for microbiologic study. Perfuse one lung with formalin. For pulmonary arteriography, see Chapter 2. Request Verhoeff–van Gieson stain.	Rheumatic pneumonitis *(1)*; pulmonary vasculitis (arteritis). Chronic rheumatic mitral valvulitis may be complicated by hypertensive pulmonary vascular disease and—in rare instances—intra-alveolar ossification.

Organs and Tissues	Procedures	Possible or Expected Findings
Kidneys	Prepare thin (4-µm) paraffin sections; submit tissue samples for immunofluorescent study and for electron microscopy.	Glomerulonephritis *(2)*; rheumatic arteritis.
Other organs	Prepare histologic sections of all organs and tissues, including skeletal muscles and cerebrospinal tissue. Request Verhoeff–van Gieson stain.	Rheumatic arteritis with lesions distributed as in polyarteritis nodosa.* Thrombotic microangiopathy.
Eyes	For removal and specimen preparation, see Chapter 5.	Scleritis; uveitis *(3)*.
Brain		Sydenham's chorea.*
Joints	Submit samples of synovial fluid from swollen joints for microbiologic study and prepare smears for cytologic study. For joint removal, prosthetic repair, and specimen preparation, see Chapter 2. Histologic samples should include synovia and periarticular tissue.	Rheumatic arthritis. Knees, ankles, hands, and wrists are primarily involved. In adults, large joints of lower extremities are usually affected.

References

1. Burgert SJ, Classen DC, Burke JP, Veasy LG. Rheumatic pneumonia: reappearance of a previously recognized complication of rheumatic fever. Clin Inf Dis 1995;21:1020–1022.
2. Imanaka H, Eto S, Takei S, Yoshinaga M, Hokonohara M, Miyata K. Acute rheumatic fever and poststreptococcal acute glomerulonephritis caused by T serotype 12 Streptococcus. Acta Paediatr Jap 1995;37: 381–383.
3. Ortiz JM, Kamerling JM, Fischer D, Baxter J. Scleritis, uveitis, and glaucoma in a patient with rheumatic fever. Am J Ophthalmol 1995; 120:538–539.

Fever, Rocky Mountain Spotted

Related Terms: *Rickettsia rickettsii* infection; tick typhus.

NOTE: (1) Collect all tissues that appear to be infected. (2) Request cultures for *Rickettsia*. This requires a special laboratory, and previous consultation with such a laboratory is recommended. Specimens for culture must be processed immediately or frozen at –60°C to ensure viability. (3) Request Giemsa stain for rickettsiae. (4) Special **precautions** are indicated. See Chapter 6. Laboratory infections have occurred. *(1)*. Gloves should be worn when handling blood specimens. 5) Serologic studies are available from local and state health department laboratories. Direct fluorescent antibody tests are available for formalin-fixed paraffin-embedded tissue *(2)*. (6) This is a **reportable** disease.

Organs and Tissues	Procedures	Possible or Expected Findings
External examination and skin	Submit samples of skin lesions.	Maculopapular and petechial skin lesions.
Blood	Collect serum for serologic diagnosis.	Indirect immunofluorescence positivity; ELISA positivity.
Lungs	Submit consolidated areas for microbiologic study.	Bronchopneumonia.
Liver and spleen	Submit samples for microbiologic and histologic study.	Hepatitis and splenitis.
Other organs and tissues	Submit tissue samples with hemorrhages and other gross lesions for microbiologic and histologic study.	Manifestations of disseminated intravascular coagulation* and of kidney failure.* (These conditions are the most frequent causes of death.) Arteriolar thromboses and necrosis with hemorrhage.
Brain and middle ears	For removal and specimen preparation, see Chapter 4.	Otitis media.*
Skeletal muscles		Necrosis.

References

1. Oster CN, Burke DS, Kenyon RH, Ascher MS, Harber P, Pedersen CE Jr. Laboratory-acquired Rocky Mountain spotted fever: the hazard of aerosol transmission. N Engl J Med 1977;297:859–863.
2. Walker DH, Cain BG. A method for specific diagnosis of Rocky Mountain Spotted Fever on fixed paraffin-embedded tissue by immunofluorescence. J Inf Dis 1978;137:206-209.

Fever, Scarlet

NOTE: Usually, this disease is a nonfatal group A streptococcal tonsillitis and pharyngitis with skin rash. Potentially fatal complications include suppurative otitis media,* mastoiditis, and pharyngeal abscess *(1)*, with or without septicemia.

(1) Collect all tissues that appear to be infected. (2) Request aerobic bacterial cultures. (3) Request Gram stain. (4) Usually, no special precautions are indicated. (5) Serologic studies are available from local and state health department laboratories. (6) This is not a reportable disease.

Reference

1. Chan TC, Hayden S. Early retropharyngeal abscess formation after treatment of scarlet fever. J Emerg Med 1996;14:377.

Fever, Tick
(See "Fever, relapsing" and "Fever, Rocky Mountain spotted.")

Fever, Typhoid

Synonym: *Salmonella typhi* infection.

NOTE: (1) Collect all tissues that appear to be infected. (2) Request aerobic bacterial cultures especially of blood. (3) Request Gram stain. (4) Special **precautions** are indicated (Chapter 6). (5) Serologic studies are available from local and state health department laboratories. (6) This is a **reportable** disease.

Organs and Tissues	*Procedures*	*Possible or Expected Findings*
External examination and skin	Prepare sections of skin lesions.	Maculopapular lesions; rose spots.
Cerebrospinal fluid	If meningitis or other intracranial abnormalities are suspected, submit sample of cerebrospinal fluid for culture and cell count.	
Abdominal cavity	If peritonitis is present, record volume of exudate and submit sample for aerobic bacterial culture; prepare sections of peritoneum.	Peritonitis* *(1)*.
Intestine	Inspect intestine *in situ* and record site(s) of perforation. For *in situ* fixation of small bowel, see Chapter 2. If intestinal hemorrhage is suspected, collect bowel contents and record volume of blood. Submit feces for aerobic bacterial culture.	Perforation of ileum *(1)*; inflammation and ulceration of Peyer's plaques. Intestinal hemorrhage. Between third and fifth weeks of the disease, feces most often positive for *Salmonella typhi*.
Mesentery	Submit lymph nodes for histologic study.	Mesenteric lymphadenitis.
Blood	Submit samples for aerobic bacterial culture and for serologic study.	See above under "Note."
Heart	If endocarditis is suspected, follow procedures described in Chapter 7. Submit sample of myocardium for aerobic bacterial culture.	Endocarditis;* myocarditis.*
Lungs	Submit areas of consolidation for aerobic bacterial culture.	Bronchitis and bronchopneumonia; diffuse alveolar damage *(1)*.
Liver and extrahepatic biliary system	Submit bile for aerobic bacterial culture. Submit samples of extrahepatic bile ducts, gallbladder, and liver for histologic study.	Cultures of bile may be positive for *Salmonella typhi*, particularly in chronic carriers. Acute acalculous cholecystitis;* cholelithiasis;* hepatitis *(2)* with focal necroses.
Spleen	Record weight. Submit sample for histologic study.	Splenitis; abscess.
Urine	Submit sample for aerobic bacterial culture.	During third and fourth weeks of the disease, urine cultures most often positive for *Salmonella typhi*.
Veins	For removal of femoral veins, see Chapter 3.	Thrombophlebitis.
Brain and spinal cord		Meningitis;* thrombosis of intracranial vessels; hydrocephalus.*
Bone, joints, and bone marrow	Submit samples of bone marrow for aerobic bacterial culture. For removal, prosthetic repair, and specimen preparation of bones, see Chapter 2. For preparation of sections and smears of bone marrow, see Chapter 2. If osteomyelitis is present, submit sample for aerobic bacterial culture. Aspirate joint fluid at sites of joint effusion.	Bone marrow may still harbor *Salmonella typhi* when blood cultures have become negative. Megakaryocytosis may be present *(1)*. Osteomyelitis;* arthritis. Hemophagocytosis and granulomas in bone marrow *(3)*

References

1. Azad AK, Islam R, Salam MA, Alam AN, Islam M, Butler T. Comparison of clinical features and pathologic findings in fatal cases of typhoid fever during the initial and later stages of the disease. Am J Trop Med Hyg 1997;56:490–493.
2. Khan M, Coovadia Y, Sturm AW. Typhoid fever complicated by acute renal failure and hepatitis: case reports and review. Am J Gastroenterol 1998;93:1001–1003.
3. Sakhalkar VS et al. Hemophagocytosis and granulomas in the bone marrow of a child with Down syndrome. J Pediatr Hematol Oncol 2001;23:623–625.

Fever, Typhus

Synonyms and Related Terms: Brill-Zinsser disease; classic typhus; endemic typhus; louse-borne typhus; murine typhus; primary epidemic typhus; recrudescent typhus; *Rickettsia mooseri* infection; *Rickettsia prowazekii* infection.

NOTE: (1) Collect all tissues that appear to be infected. (2) Request cultures for *Rickettsia*. This requires a special laboratory, and previous consultation with such a laboratory is recommended. (3) Request Giemsa stain for rickettsiae. (4) Special **precautions** are indicated (see Chapter 6). (5) Serologic studies are available from local and state health department laboratories. Indirect fluorescent antibody tests are available for use with formalin fixed paraffin-embedded tissue. (6) This is not a reportable disease.

Organs and Tissues	*Procedures*	*Possible or Expected Findings*
External examination and skin	Submit skin lesions for histologic study.	Macular and maculopapular rash; infectious vasculitis of small vessels. Rarely furunculosis.
	If gangrene of extremities is present, submit samples of necrotic tissues for histologic study.	Gangrene due to small vessel thrombosis.
Blood	See above under "Note." Specimens with viable organisms can be stored for a few days at 5°C.	Indirect immunofluorescence positivity; ELISA positivity.
Heart	Submit samples of myocardium for histologic study.	Infectious vasculitis of small myocardial vessels; myocarditis.
Kidneys	Submit samples for histologic study.	Infectious vasculitis. Renal failure* may be the cause of death.
Veins	Examine femoral veins (Chapter 3).	Thrombophlebitis.
Brain and spinal cord	For removal and specimen preparation, see Chapter 4.	Infectious vasculitis and meningitis;* inflammatory nodules within grey matter.
Middle ears	If otitis media is suspected, remove middle ears for histologic study.	Otitis media.*

Fever, Yellow

Synonyms and Related Terms: Flavivirus (Group B arbovirus) infection; hemorrhagic fever syndrome; yellow fever virus infection.

NOTE: (1) Collect all tissues that appear to be infected. (2) After consultation with microbiology laboratory, request viral cul-ture. (3) Usually, special stains are not helpful. (4) Special **precautions** are indicated (Chapter 6). (5) Serologic studies are available from the Center for Disease Control and Prevention, Atlanta, GA. (6) This is a **reportable** disease.

Organs and Tissues	*Procedures*	*Possible or Expected Findings*
External examination		Jaundice; bleeding from nose and gums; rash; "black vomit."
Blood	Submit sample for serologic and microbiologic study. Store blood at 4°C to maintain viral viability.	
Heart	Submit samples of myocardium for histologic study. Request Sudan stain for frozen sections of myocardium.	Myocardial degeneration.
Liver	Record weight and submit tissue for virologic study. Submit samples for histologic study. Request Sudan stain for frozen sections.	Mild hepatitis with confluent focal and midzonal hepatic necrosis; Councilman bodies. Rarely, intranuclear Torres bodies. Fatty changes may be prominent.
Kidneys	See above under "Heart."	Fatty changes of renal tubular epithelium.
Other organs	Procedures depend on expected findings or grossly identified abnormalities as listed in right-hand column.	Disseminated intravascular coagulation* seems to be a frequent cause of death. Gastrointestinal hemorrhage* also may occur.
Brain	For removal and specimen preparation, see Chapter 4.	Focal hemorrhages.

Fibrillation and Flutter, Atrial (See "Arrhythmia, cardiac.")

Fibroelastosis, Endocardial (EFE)

Note: Many cases of EFE are associated with left ventricular outflow obstruction, such as hypoplastic left heart, aortic stenosis/atresia, but may also be seen with viral myocarditis, type II glycogen storage disease (Pompe disease) and carnitine deficiency. Thus, a metabolic disorder must be considered. It is ideal to perform the autopsy as soon after death as possible *(1)*.

Organs and Tissues	*Procedures*	*Possible or Expected Findings*
Urine	Assay for organic acids. Freeze for possible. biochemical analysis	May be normal and may rule out other mitochondiopathies.
Plasma	Assay for carnitine. Freeze for possible biochemical analysis.	Low levels of carnitine.
Skin fibroblasts	Establish cell culture.	Biochemical profile of carnitine metabolism.
Heart	Careful gross and microscopic examination. Submit myocardium for viral culture. Submit frozen section for oil red O stain. Submit portion for EM.	Calcified coronary arteries and papillary muscles; aortic stenosis or atresia; hypoplastic left ventricle; viral myocarditis, ventricular dilation; fat infiltration with carnitine deficiency. Clear, glycogen-rich myofibers with Pompe disease.
Skeletal muscle	Snap freeze for biochemical assay of carnitine. Submit frozen section for oil red O stain.	Low levels of total, free and esterified carnitine.
Liver, placenta, other viscera	Snap freeze portions for biochemical and DNA analysis. Examine with H&E and submit frozen section for oil red O stain. Stain liver with PAS.	Hepatic steatosis, in the form of fine vacuolization in carnitine deficiency. PAS positivity with type II glycogen storage disease.

Reference

1. Applegarth DA, Dimmick JE, Hall JG, eds. Organelle Diseases. London: Chapman and Hall, 1997.

Fibrosis, Congenital Hepatic

Related Terms: Ductal plate malformation *(1)*; fibropolycystic disease of the liver and biliary tract.*

Possible Associated Conditions: Autosomal-recessive (rarely autosomal-dominant) polycystic kidney disease.* Caroli's syndrome;* choledochal cyst(s);* medullary cystic renal disease (medullary tubular ectasia)* or nephronophthisis; multiple biliary microhamartomas.

Organs and Tissues	*Procedures*	*Possible or Expected Findings*
Portal vein system	Examine portal vein. Record status of shunt if present.	Shunt for relief of portal hypertension.*
Liver	Record size and weight. For portal venous and hepatic arterial angiography and cholangiography, see Chapter 2. Photograph cut surface of liver.	Hepatomegaly; portal fibrosis; hypoplasia of portal veins. Cysts may be the site of hemorrhages. In rare instances, carcinoma of bile duct may occur. Ductal plate malformation, cholangitis (*2*).
Spleen	Record size and weight.	Congestive splenomegaly.
Esophagus and gastrointestinal tract	For demonstration of esophageal varices, see Chapter 2. Record volume of blood in lumen of gastrointestinal tract.	Esophageal varices.* Gastrointestinal hemorrhage.*
Kidneys	See under "Cyst(s), renal."	Cysts (see above under "Possible Associated Conditions").
Urine	Assay for organic acids. Freeze for possible. biochemical analysis	May be normal and may rule out other mitochondiopathies.
Plasma	Assay for carnitine. Freeze for possible biochemical analysis.	Low levels of carnitine.
Skin fibroblasts	Establish cell culture.	Biochemical profile of carnitine metabolism.
Heart	Careful gross and microscopic examination. Submit myocardium for viral culture. Submit frozen section for oil red O stain. Submit portion for EM.	Calcified coronary arteries and papillary muscles; aortic stenosis or atresia; hypoplastic left ventricle; viral myocarditis, ventricular dilation; fat infiltration with carnitine deficiency. Clear, glycogen-rich myofibers with Pompe disease.
Skeletal muscle	Snap freeze for biochemical assay of carnitine. Submit frozen section for oil red O stain.	Low levels of total, free and esterified carnitine.
Liver, placenta, other viscera	Snap freeze portions for biochemical and DNA analysis. Examine with H&E and submit frozen section for oil red O stain. Stain liver with PAS.	Hepatic steatosis, in the form of fine vacuolization in carnitine deficiency. PAS positivity with type II glycogen storage disease.

Reference

1. Applegarth DA, Dimmick JE, Hall JG, eds. Organelle Diseases. London: Chapman and Hall, 1997.
2. Waters BL, Blaszyk H. Diseases involving intrahepatic bile ducts. Curr Diagn Path 2005;11:7–18.

Fibrosis, Cystic
Synonym: Mucoviscidosis.

Organs and Tissues	*Procedures*	*Possible or Expected Findings*
External examination	Record body weight and length.	Malnutrition *(1)* with growth retardation; clubbing of fingers.
	Prepare roentgenogram or do other tests for pneumothorax.*	Pneumothorax. Hypertrophic osteoarthropathy.
Mediastinum		Mediastinal emphysema.
Blood	Submit sample for microbiologic study.	Septicemia (see also under "Lungs").
Heart	Record weight and thickness of ventricles.	Cor pulmonale.
Lungs	Submit consolidated areas for microbiologic study. Request Gram stain.	Infections most frequently caused by *Hemophilus influenzae*, *Pseudomonas aeruginosa*, *Staphylococcus aureus*, and *Streptococcus pyogenes*.
	For postmortem bronchography and pulmonary angiography, see Chapter 2. If the bronchi are obstructed by tenacious secretions, formalin perfusion may be possible through pulmonary artery only. Photograph cut surface. Submit samples of bronchi and parenchyma of all lobes for microscopic study.	Chronis bronchitis.* Bronchiectasis* and bronchiolectases; abscesses; bronchopneumonia; atelectases.
Esophagus and gastrointestinal tract	Submit samples of upper, middle, and lower esophagus; stomach, duodenum; jejunum; ileum; and colon for histologic study. If malabsorption was present, see under "Syndrome, malabsorption."	Esophageal varices (see below under "Liver"). Abnormal esophageal glands. Peptic esophagitis *(2)* and ulcers.* Meconium ileus* in small infants or meconium ileus equivalent in children and young adults. Fibrosing (submucosal) colonopathy *(2)*.
Liver	Record weight, measure, and photograph cut section. Submit sample for histologic study.	Cirrhosis* ("focal or multilobular biliary cirrhosis"); fatty changes.
Gallbladder	Record volume and character of contents. Submit sample for histologic study.	Cholecystitis;* cholelithiasis;* decreased amount of bile.
Pancreas	Record weight of dissected organ and photograph frontal section. Submit samples of head, body, and tail for histologic study.	Parenchymal atrophy with cystic fibrosis. Islets of Langerhans often preserved (manifestations of diabetes mellitus* increasingly prevalent with age *[3]*).
Male sex organs	Submit samples of testes, prostate, seminal vesicles, and spermatic ducts for histologic study.	Occlusion of vasa deferentia and associated changes, including absence or atrophy of body of epididymis.
Bones and joints	For removal, prosthetic repair, and specimen preparation, see Chapter 2.	Hypertrophic osteoarthropathy in adults. Joint abnormalities may be present also *(4)*.

References

1. Reilly JJ, Edwards CA, Weaver LT. Malnutrition in children with cystic fibrosis: the energy-balance equation. J Pediatr Gastroenterol Nutr 1997; 25:127–136.
2. Eggermont E. Gastrointestinal manifestations in cystic fibrosis. Eur J Gastroenterol Hepatol 1996;8:731–738.
3. Lanng S. Diabetes mellitus in cystic fibrosis. Eur J Gastroenterol Hepatol 1996;8:744–747.
4. Turner MA, Baildam E, Patel L, David TJ. Joint disorders in cystic fibrosis. J Roy Soc Med 1997;31:13–20.

Fibrosis, Endomyocardial (See "Cardiomyopathy restrictive [with eosinophilia].")

Fibrosis, Interstitial Pulmonary (See "Pneumonia, interstitial.")

Fibrosis, Mediastinal (See "Mediastinitis, chronic.")

Fibrosis, Pulmonary (See "Pneumonia, interstitial.")

Fibrosis, Retroperitoneal

Synonyms and Related Terms: Idiopathic retroperitoneal fibrosis; multifocal fibrosclerosis;* periureteral fibrosis; systemic idiopathic fibrosis.

Possible Associated Conditions: Immune complex glom-erulonephritis; Peyronie's disease; pseudotumor of the orbit *(1)*; Riedel's fibrosing thyroiditis (Riedel's struma); sclerosing cholangitis;* sclerosing mediastinitis (mediastinal fibrosis).

Organs and Tissues	*Procedures*	*Possible or Expected Findings*
Retroperitoneal and pelvic tissues	For retrograde urography, see Chapter 2. Remove retroperitoneal and pelvic organs en bloc. Record character of dislocation and of obstruction of ureter(s), of inferior vena cava, and of other affected organs or tissues. This is best demonstrated in horizontal slices through the fibrosed areas. Submit samples for histologic study.	Hydronephrosis;* pyelonephritis;* renal amyloidosis. Fibrosis adjacent to kidneys, duodenum, descending colon, and urinary bladder or surrounding ureter(s), inferior vena cava, or pelvic organs. Lymphoma,* scirrhous adenocarcinoma, severe atherosclerosis of aorta *(2)* with or without abdominal aortic aneurysm,* or pelvic and retroperitoneal inflammatory diseases may imitate or be associated with retroperitoneal fibrosis.
Abdominal wall		Fibrosis of abdominal subcutaneous adipose tissue.
Other organs	See under "Failure, kidney" and above under "Possible Associated Conditions."	See above under "Possible Associated Conditions." Renal failure* is the most frequent cause of death.
Orbitae	For exposure, see Chapter 5.	Pseudotumor *(1)*.

References

1. Aylward GW, Sullivan TJ, Garner A, Moseley I, Wright JE. Orbital involvement in multifocal fibrosclerosis. Br J Ophthalmol 1995;79:246–249.
2. Gilkeson GS, Allen NB. Retroperitnoneal fibrosis. A true connective tissue disease. Rheum Dis Clin North Am 1996;22:23–38.

Fire (See "Burns.")

Flukes, Hepatic (Biliary) (See "Clonorchiasis.")

Fluorosis

Organs and Tissues	*Procedures*	*Possible or Expected Findings*
External examination		Kyphosis; flexion contractures; enamel changes.
	Prepare skeletal roentgenograms.	Osteosclerosis; formation of osteophytes; ossification of tendons and ligaments.
Bones and teeth	For removal, prosthetic repair, and specimen preparation of bones, see Chapter 2. Snap-freeze fresh bone tissue for possible chemical analysis. Submit samples of tendons and ligaments for histologic study.	Osteomalacia* and osteosclerosis with periosteal new bone formation. Abnormal dental enamel. See also above under "External examination."
Spinal cord		Bone changes may have caused compression of spinal cord.

Fructose (See "Intolerance, fructose.")

Fusion, Congenital, of Cervical Vertebrae (See "Impression, basilar.")

G

Galactosemia

Organs and Tissues	*Procedures*	*Possible or Expected Findings*
External examination	Record body weight and length and head circumference.	Manifestations of malnutrition; dehydration;* jaundice; microcephaly.
Vitreous	Submit sample for determination of glucose; galactose, lactic acid, and ketone concentrations.	
Blood	Submit sample for determination of galactose-1-phosphate uridyl transferase activity in erythrocytes. Compare with values in blood of controls.	Galactose-1-phosphate uridyl transferase deficiency.
Urine	Refrigerate immediately.	Reducing substances; glucosuria; aminoaciduria; phosphaturia.
Abdomen	Record volume of fluid.	Ascites.
Kidney	Submit sections for histologic study.	Tubular dilatation.
Liver	Record size and weight; photograph cut section; submit samples for histologic and electron microscopic study. If histochemical study *(1)* is intended, snap-freeze tissue. Request frozen sections for Sudan stain.	Giant cell transformation; ductular proliferation; acinar transformation of hepatocytes; cholestasis; regenerative nodules; macrovesicular steatosis; fibrosis; cirrhosis* *(2)*.
Pancreas	Submit samples of head, body, and tail for histologic study.	Hyperplasia of islets of Langerhans.
Brain and spinal cord	For removal and specimen preparation, see Chapter 4.	Fibrillary astrocytosis of white matter; loss of Purkinje cells; lipofuscin overload in large neurons.
Eyes	For removal and specimen preparation, see Chapter 5.	Cataracts.

References

1. Landing BH, Ang SM, Villarreal-Engelhardt G, Donnell GN. Galactosemia: clinical and pathologic features, tissue staining patterns with labeled galactose- and galactosamine-binding lectins, and possible loci of nonenzymatic galactosylation. Persp Pediatr Pathol 1993;17:99–124.
2. Jevon GP, Dimmick JE. Histopathologic approach to metabolic liver disease: Part 2. Pediatr Dev Pathol 1998;1:261–269.

Ganglioneuroma (See "Tumor of the peripheral nerves.")

Gangliosidosis

Synonyms and Related Terms: Activator protein deficiency (type AB); beta galactosidase deficiency; GM_1 gangliosidosis, infantile, type 1 (with visceral involvement); late infantile, type 2; adult, type 3; GM2 gangliosidosis with infantile, late infantile, and adult forms; hexosaminidase A deficiency (type B); hexosamine A and B deficiency (type 0); lysosomal disorder *(1)*; Tay Sachs disease; Sandhoff's disease.

From: *Handbook of Autopsy Practice,* 4th Ed. Edited by: B.L. Waters

Organs and Tissues	Procedures	Possible or Expected Findings
External examination	Obtain routine body measurements and weight. Photograph all abnormalities.	Hydrops fetalis; coarse facies; macroglossia; depressed, broad nose; large ears; frontal bossing; gingival hypertrophy; squat hands and feet; flexor contractures; ascites; hernias.
Fascia lata (see also "Liver and spleen")	Fascia lata should be collected using aseptic technique for tissue culture for biochemical studies and electron microscopic examination.	Cultured fibroblasts can be used for enzyme assay. "Empty" vacuoles in lymphocytes by EM.
Liver and spleen	Record weights. See also below under "Brain and spinal cord." Obtain tissue for tissue culture for assay of enzyme deficiency. Enzyme assay can be performed on fresh or frozen liver tissue.	Hepatosplenomegaly; accumulation of PAS and Sudan Black positive material (ganglioside) in histiocytes *(1)*.
Other organs	If evidence of other organ involvement (heart, kidney) is present, follow procedures described below under "Brain and spinal cord."	
Brain and spinal cord	Request LFB/PAS and/or Sudan Black (on frozen tissue) stains. Submit samples for electron microscopic study. Enzyme assay can be performed on fresh or frozen brain tissue. If analysis of lipids is intended, place fresh tissue in liquid nitrogen and store at –90°C until lipids can be extracted and analyzed—for instance, by thin-layer chromatography.	Cerebral atrophy; neurons distended by lipid (ganglioside); disintegration of neurons and reactive phagocytosis and astrocytosis; fibrillogranular inclusions in fibroblasts and endothelial cells *(2–4)*.
Placenta	Weigh, snap-freeze a portion, and submit portion for histologic study.	Vacuolated syncytiotrophoblast.

References

1. Jevon GP, Dimmick JE. Histopathologic approach to metabolic liver disease: Part 2. Pediatr Dev Pathol 1998;1:261–269.
2. Lake B. Lysosomal and peroxisomal disorders. In: Greenfield's Neuropathology, vol. 1. Graham BI, Lantos PL, eds. Arnold, New York, 1997, pp. 658–668.
3. Rapola J, Lysosomal storage diseases in adults. Pathol Res Pract 1994; 190:759–766.
4. Suzuki K. Neuropathology of late onset gangliosidosis. A review. Dev Neurosci 1991;13:205–210.

Gangrene, Gas

Synonym: Clostridial infection.

NOTE: (1) Collect all tissues that appear to be infected. (2) Request aerobic and anaerobic bacterial cultures. (3) Request Gram stain. Inflammation may be minimal or absent. (4) No special precautions are indicated. (5) Serologic studies are not indicated. (6) This is not a reportable disease.

Organs and Tissues	Procedures	Possible or Expected Findings
External examination	Record appearance of wounds or of other possibly infected lesions. If foreign bodies are present, record their nature and location (roentgenograms may be helpful). Prepare smears of wounds and request Gram stain.	Edema surrounding wound; gas bubbles in a discharge; foul odor of the wound; loose blebs containing serosanguinous fluid.
Skeletal muscles	Prepare roentgenograms of suspected areas; palpate abnormal areas and record extent of crepitation; submit samples of grossly involved and of uninvolved skeletal muscle for bacteriologic and histologic study (see above under "Note").	Muscle necrosis (Clostridial myonecrosis) and accumulation of gas; little leukocytic infiltration.

Organs and Tissues	Procedures	Possible or Expected Findings
Other organs	Procedures depend on expected findings or grossly identified abnormalities as listed in right-hand column. See also above under "Note" and under "Skeletal muscles."	Pneumonia;* empyema;* cholecystitis;* uterine infection (postabortal or postpartum).

Gastroenteritis, Eosinophilic

Organs and Tissues	Procedures	Possible or Expected Findings
Abdomen	Record volume of peritoneal exudate and prepare smears of sediment.	Chronic peritonitis and ascites in cases with serosal involvement of the affected stomach or gut segments.
Esophagus and gastrointestinal tract	Record location of and photograph involved segments; state distance of these areas from anatomic landmarks. Leave esophagus attached to stomach. For *in situ* fixation of small bowel, see Chapter 2. Record thickness of wall, width of lumen, and length of involved segments. Submit samples of all grossly involved and of grossly uninvolved segments for histologic study. Request azure-eosin or Giemsa stain.	Eosinophilic esophagitis may occur *(1)*. Presence of infiltrates most common in antrum of stomach with thickening of the pylorus. Ulcers may be found in antrum or duodenum. Various portions of small bowel also may be involved, with or without intestinal obstruction. Colonic involvement *(2)* is rare. Eosinophilic infiltrates may be found in all layers of the affected hollow viscera. There should be no evidence of parasite infestation.
Pancreas and bile ducts	Submit samples for histologic study. Request azure-eosin or Giemsa stain.	Pancreatitis *(3)* and cholangitis *(2)* in rare instances.
Other organs	Procedures depend on expected findings or grossly identified abnormalities as listed in right-hand column.	Manifestations of malabsorption syndrome* and of protein-losing enteropathy.* There should be no evidence systemic eosinophilic disease.

References

1. Mahajan L, Wyllie R, Petras R, Steffen R, Kay M. Idiopathic eosinophilic esophagitis with stricture formation in a patient with longstanding eosinophilic gastroenteritis. Gastrointest Endosc 1997;46: 557–560.
2. Schoonbroodt D, Horsmans Y, Laka A, Geubel AP, Hoang P. Eosinophilic gastroenteritis presenting with colitis and cholangitis. Dig Dis Sci 1995; 40:308–314.
3. Maeshima A, Murakami H, Sadakata H, Saitoh T, Matsushima T, Tamura J, et al. Eosinophilic gastroenteritis presenting with acute pancreatitis. J Med 1997;28:265–272.

Gastroenteropathy, Hemorrhagic
(See "Enterocolitis, pseudomembranous" and "Shock.")

Gigantism, Hyperpituitary
(See "Acromegaly.")

Glomerulonephritis

Synonyms and Related Terms: Acute postinfectious glomerulonephritis (nonstreptococcal postinfectious glomerulonephritis;* minimal change disease; mesangial proliferative glomerulonephritis;* focal and segmental glomerulosclerosis with hyalinosis (focal sclerosis); poststreptococcal glomerulonephritis; idiopathic nephrotic syndrome; IgA nephropathy (Berger's disease); membranous glomerulonephritis; membranoproliferative glomerulonephritis; mesangial proliferative glomerulonephritis; rapidly progressive glomerulonephritis (associated with systemic infectious or immunologic multisystem diseases; drug idiosyncrasy; or as primary crescentic glomerulonephritis or superimposed on another primary glomerular disease).

Possible Associated Conditions: Acquired immunodeficiency syndrome (AIDS);* Alport's syndrome;* amyloidosis; anaphylactoid purpura; bee stings; chronic allograft rejection; dermatomyositis;* dermatitis herpetiformis; diabetes mellitus;* drug dependence;* Fabry's disease;* Goodpasture's syndrome;* Guillain-Barré syndrome;* Henoch-Schönlein purpura;* hemolytic uremic syndrome;* infective endocarditis;* leprosy;* malig-nancies; mixed connective tissue disease; myxedema; polyarteritis nodosa;* rheumatoid arthritis;* preeclamptic toxemia; renovascular hypertension; sarcoidosis;* serum sickness;* Sjögren's syndrome;* syphilis;* systemic lupus erythematosus;* systemic sclerosis;* thrombotic thrombocytopenic purpura;* thyroiditis;* vasculitis; viral hepatitis;* Wegener's granulomatosis;* and many other conditions.

Organs and Tissues	*Procedures*	*Possible or Expected Findings*
Blood	Refrigerate sample for possible serologic study —for instance, of basement membrane antibodies.	
Urine	Submit sample for urinalysis.	Cylindruria; hematuria; proteinuria.
Kidneys	Examine as soon as possible to minimize autolysis. Record weights; photograph surfaces and cut sections. Submit sample for immunofluorescent study, and electron microscopic study. Request 3-μm paraffin sections stained with PAS, methenamine silver, and Masson's trichrome stains.	For specific types of glomerulonephritis, see above under "Synonyms and Related Terms." For further information, appropriate nephropathological texts should be consulted.
Other organs	Procedures depend on expected underlying, associated, or complicating conditions. If leg ulcers, wounds, or other acute infections are present, or if possibly nephritogenic chronic infections are found, submit material for appropriate bacterial cultures—for instance, from pharynx or middle ears.	See above under "Possible Associated Conditions." See also under "Failure, kidney" and, if applicable, under "Dialysis (for chronic renal failure)."
Eyes	For removal and specimen preparation, see Chapter 5.	Hypertensive retinopathy; in Alport's syndrome,* cataracts and other abnormalities.

Glycogenosis (See "Disease, glycogen storage.")

Gout

Related Term: Hyperuricemia.

Possible Associated Conditions: Alcoholism;* berylliosis;* chronic renal failure with long-term renal dialysis; diabetes insipidus;* Down's syndrome;* drug toxicity; glycogenosis (III, V, and VII); hemolysis; hyperparathyroidism;* hypertension;* hypothyroidism;* lead poisoning;* obesity;* Paget's disease; polycystic renal disease; polycythemia vera;* previous chemotherapy or radiation therapy of myeloproliferative disease; psoriasis;* pyelonephritis;* Reiter's syndrome;* rheumatoid arthri-tis;* sarcoidosis;* status post renal transplantation; toxemia of pregnancy,* and others.

Organs and Tissues	*Procedures*	*Possible or Expected Findings*
External examination and subcutaneous tissues	Photograph and record location of tophi. For fixation for histologic study, place tophi in alcohol, formalin-alcohol, or Carnoy's fixative. For murexide test for the macroscopic diagnosis of urates, see Chapter 16.	In tophaceous gout, tophi at helices of ears and on elbows, knees, hands, and feet.
	Prepare skeletal roentgenograms.	Acute or chronic gouty arthritis with punched-out bone lesions.
Blood	Submit sample for determination of uric acid concentration.	Hyperuricemia. For interpretation of postmortem findings, see Chapter 8.
Heart and blood vessels	Submit samples of myocardium and of elastic and muscular arteries for histologic study. For fixation procedures, see above under "External examination and subcutaneous tissues."	Sodium urate deposits (uncommon in heart but may be responsible for cardiac dysrhythmia*).
Trachea and major bronchi	Submit samples for histologic study.	
Kidneys	Prepare roentgenogram of soft tissues; photograph surfaces and cut sections. For fixation procedures, see above under "External examination and subcutaneous tissues."	Nephrolithiasis;* urate nephropathy; uric acid nephropathy.
Other organs	In cases of secondary gout, procedures depend on suspected underlying disease, as listed above under "Possible Associated Conditions."	See above under "Possible Associated Conditions."
Bones, joints, bursae, and tendons	Place a small drop of synovial fluid on a slide; coverslip; seal the cover slip with nail polish and examine under polarized light.	In rare instances, pseudogout* or pyarthrosis may occur. Monosodium urate in synovial neutrophils.
	For removal, prosthetic repair, and specimen preparation of bones and joints, see Chapter 2.	

Organs and Tissues	Procedures	Possible or Expected Findings
Bones, joints, bursae, and tendons *(continued)*	Use brush to clean frontal saw section of spine, and photograph. Photograph joint surfaces and other synovial surfaces that show white deposits. Submit samples of all involved tissues for histologic study. For fixation procedures and murexide test, see above under "External examination and subcutaneous tissues." For proper sampling of joints, consult roentgenograms. For preparation of museum specimens, see Chapter 16.	Urate deposits in intervertebral disks and on synovial surfaces; gouty and tophaceous arthritis.
Eyes	For removal and specimen preparation, see Chapter 5. For fixation procedures, see above.	Urate deposits in scleras and corneas.

Granulocytopenia (See "Pancytopenia.")

Granuloma, All Types or Type Unspecified (See "Disease, chronic granulomatous," "Granuloma,...," "Granulomatosis,...," and "Pneumoconiosis." See also under name of specific granulomatous disease, such as "Sarcoidosis" and "Tuberculosis.")

Granuloma, Eosinophilic (See "Histiocytosis, Langerhans cell.")

Granuloma, Midline

Synonyms: Idiopathic midline granuloma; lethal midline granuloma; granuloma gangrenescens. (The last two names are obsolete.)

NOTE: Midline granulomas may belong to the angiocentric immunoproliferative lesions, which are related to lymphomatoid granulomatosis* and malignant lymphoma. The name "idiopathic midline granuloma" should be reserved for the few cases without evidence of malignant lymphoma or Wegener's granulomatosis* *(1)*. The diagnosis of *idiopathic* midline granuloma also can be ruled out if studies reveal fungal organisms or features of leishmaniasis;* leprosy,* rhinoscleroma, pseudotumor of the orbit or tuberculosis.* Complications of nasal cocaine abuse also may mimic midline granuloma *(2)*.

Organs and Tissues	Procedures	Possible or Expected Findings
External examination	Record extent of necrosis, and photograph facial lesions.	Necrosis of skin of nose and eyelids.
Nasal cavities and paranasal sinuses	For exposure of nasal cavities and sinuses, see Chapter 4. Submit material for bacterial and fungal cultures. Prepare smears and histologic sections of affected tissues. Request Verhoeff–van Gieson, Gram, and Grocott's methenamine silver stains. Submit lesional tissue for flow cytometry.	Necrosis with perforation of nasal septum, hard and soft palate, paranasal sinuses, and orbital cavities. Noncaseating granulomas with intense inflammatory reaction. NK/T cell lymphoma *(3)*
Neck organs	Submit lymph nodes for microbiologic and histologic study.	See above under "Nasal cavities and paranasal sinuses."
Other organs		For manifestations of diseases that may produce features of midline granuloma, see above under "Note."

References

1. Barker TH, Hosni AA. Idiopathic midline destructive disease: does it exist? J Laryngol Otol 1998;112:307–309.
2. Sevinsky LD, Woscoff A, Jaimovich L, Terzian A. Nasal cocain abuse mimicking midline granuloma. J Am Acad Dermatol 1995;32:286–287.
3. Menden hall WM et al. Lethal midline granoloma-nasal natural killer/T-cell lymphoma. Am J Clin Oncol 2006;29:202–206.

Granulomatosis, Allergic, and Angiitis (Churg-Strauss Syndrome)

Related Term: Pulmonary granulomatous vasculitis *(1)*.

Possible Associated Condition: Asthma.*

Organs and Tissues	Procedures	Possible or Expected Findings
External examination	Record extent of skin lesions and prepare photographs.	Purpura; cutaneous and subcutaneous nodules (see below under "Other organs").
Blood	Serologic analysis	Anti-phospholipid antibodies *(5)*.

Organs and Tissues	Procedures	Possible or Expected Findings
Lungs	Perfuse lungs with formalin and sample for histologic study.	Eosinophilic pneumonitis (degenerating eosinophils with Charcot-Leyden crystals) and granulomas. Angiitis (mostly arteritis), typically with giant cells in tunica media *(1)*.
Other organs and soft tissues	Procedures depend on expected findings or grossly identified abnormalities as listed in right-hand column. Techniques are similar to those described under "Polyarteritis nodosa."	Findings resemble those in polyarteritis nodosa.* Heart *(2)*, grastrointestinal tract *(3)*, skin, muscles, and joints are commonly involved. However, renal disease is often (but not always) mild or absent.
	Histologic sampling should include cutaneous and subcutaneous nodules.	Necrotizing vasculitis of small arteries and veins is present, with extravascular granulomas and eosinophilic infiltration of vessels and perivascular tissues.
Eyes	For removal and specimen preparation, see Chapter 5.	Optic neuritis may be found *(4)*.
Brain, spinal cord, and peripheral nerves	For removal and specimen preparation, see Chapter 4.	May be affected by the vasculitis *(4)*.

References

1. Travis WD. Pathology of pulmonary granulomatous vasculitis. Sarcoid Vasculit Diff Lung Dis 1996;13:14–27.
2. Terasaki F, Hayashi T, Hirota Y, Okabe M, Suwa M, Deguchi H, et al. Evolution of dilated cardiomyopathy from acute eosinophilic pancarditis in Churg-Strauss syndrome. Heart Vessels 1997;12:43–48.
3. Matsuo K, Tomioka T, Tajima Y, Takayama K, Tamura H, Higami Y, et al. Allergic granulomatous angiitis (Churg-Strauss syndrome) with multiple intestinal fistulas. Am J Gastroenterol 1997;92:1937–1938.
4. Sehgal M, Swanson JW, DeRemmee RA, Colby TV. Neurologic manifestations of Churg-Straus syndrome. Mayo Clin Proc 1995;70:337–341.
5. Ferenczi K et al. A case of Churg-strauss syndrome associated with antiphospholipid antibodies. J Am Acad Dermatol 2007;56:101–104.

Granulomatosis, Bronchocentric

Synonyms and Related Terms: Allergic bronchopulmonary aspergillosis *(1)*; eosinophilic pneumonia (eosinophilic pulmonary syndrome*); extrinsic allergic alveolitis; idiopathic bronchocentric granulomatosis; microgranulomatous hypersensitivity reaction of lungs; mucoid impaction of bronchi.

Possible Associated Conditions: Asthma;* cystic fibrosis.*

Organs and Tissues	Procedures	Possible or Expected Findings
Lungs	Submit a section for bacterial and fungal cultures. Prepare smears of fresh cut sections. For pulmonary arteriography and bronchography, see Chapter 2. Perfuse one lung through bronchi and also through pulmonary arteries (plugged bronchi may prevent proper perfusion).	*Aspergillus* (usually *Aspergillus fumigatus*) in dilated bronchi *(2)*, with or without inspissation of mucus or fungus ball; necrotizing granulomatous pneumonia or bronchitis *(2)* with bronchial chondritis; eosinophilic pneumonia; obstructive (cholesterol-type) pneumonia; atelectases; emphysema.* Secondary arteritis may be present.

References

1. Bosken C, Myers J, Greenberger P, Katzenstein A-L. Pathologic features of allergic bronchopulmonary aspergillosis. Am J Surg Pathol 1988;12: 216–222.
2. Yousem SA. The histological spectrum of chronic necrotizing forms of pulmonary aspergillosis. Hum Pathol 1997;28:650–656.

Granulomatosis, Lymphomatoid

Related Term: Angiocentric immunoproliferative lesion; angiocentric malignant lymphoma.

Possible Associated Conditions: AIDS* *(1)* and other immunodeficiency states such as Wiskott-Aldrich syndrome or post-transplant immunosuppression.

Organs and Tissues	Procedures	Possible or Expected Findings
External examination and skin	Record extent of skin lesions; photograph skin lesions; prepare histologic sections of involved skin and of grossly uninvolved skin.	Lymphoreticular infiltrates, primarily in dermis but also in subcutis. See also under "Lungs."

Organs and Tissues	Procedures	Possible or Expected Findings
External examination and skin *(continued)*	Prepare chest roentgenogram.	Multiple nodules, with or without cavitation; cavitation; rarely pneumothorax *(2)*.
Blood	Submit sample for bacterial, fungal, and viral cultures. Snap-freeze sample for possible biochemical and immunologic study.	
Lungs	Record weights; submit samples of fresh tissue for B- and T-cell gene derangement studies, frozen-section immunostains, and other investigations (see refs. *3* and *4*). Submit consolidated areas for microbiologic study. Touch preparations of cut surfaces of lungs for cytologic study may be helpful.	PCR studies on paraffin sections via RNA *in situ* hybridization may confirm presence of Epstein-Barr virus-positive B-cell proliferations combined with dense T-cell accumulations *(3–5)*. The condition closely resembles angiocentric T-/NK cell lymphoma *(3)*.
	For pulmonary arteriography, see Chapter 2. Perfuse one lung with formalin. Photograph cut sections of lungs. Submit samples of all lobes and of hilar lymph nodes for histologic study. Request Verhoeff–van Gieson, Gram, and Gridley's fungal stains. Prepare specimens for electron microscopy.	Infiltration of lymphocytoid cells, plasma cells, and macrophages with necroses and granulomatous features, which are found primarily in the vicinity of blood vessels. Special stains may reveal evidence of infection.
Liver	Record weight and sample for histologic studies.	Lymphoreticular and granulomatous infiltrates (see "Lung").
Kidneys	Follow procedures described under "Glomerulonephritis."	Lymphoreticular and granulomatous infiltrates (see "Lung").
Other organs and tissues	Samples for histologic study should include heart, pancreas, spleen, adrenal glands, urinary bladder, prostate, neck organs (with nasopharynx and tongue), salivary glands, lymph nodes, thymus, bone marrow, and all other tissues with grossly identifiable lesions.	Characteristic infiltrates may be present in all organs and tissues. Involvement of spleen, lymph nodes, and bone marrow is uncommon. In rare instances, the disease is confined to the abdomen.
Brain and spinal cord		In most instances, characteristic infiltrates are present *(6)*.

References

1. Haque AK, Myers JL, Hudnall SD, Gelman BB, Lloyd RV, Payne D, et al. Pulmonary lymphomatoid granulomatosis in acquired immunodeficiency syndrome: lesions with Epstein-Barr virus infection. Mod Pathol 1998;11:347–356.
2. Morris MJ, Peacock MD, Lloyd WC III, Johnson JE. Recurrent bilateral spontaneous pneumothoraces associated with pulmonary angiocentric immunoproliferative lesion. South Med J 1995;88: 771–775.
3. Jaffe ES, Wilson WH. Lymphomatoid granulomatosis: pathogenesis, pathology and clinical implications. Canc Surv 1997;30:233–248.
4. McNiff JM, Cooper D, Howe G, Crotty PL, Tallini G, Crouch J, et al. Lymphomatoid granulomatosis of the skin and lung. An angiocentric T-cell-rich B-cell lymphoproliferative disorder. Arch Dermatol 1996; 132:1464–1470.
5. Myers J, Kurtin P, Katzenstein A-L, Tazelaar H, Colby T, Strickler J, et al. Lymphomatoid granulomatosis. Evidence of immunophenotypic diversity and relationship to Epstein-Barr virus infection. Am J Surg Pathol 1995;19:1300–1312.
6. Patsalides AD, et al. Lymphomatoid granulomatosis: abnormalities of the brain at MR imaging. Radiol 2005;237:265–273.

Granulomatosis, Wegener's

Related Terms: Angiocentric granulomatosis; granulomatous angiitis; pulmonary angiitis and granulomatosis *(1)*.

Organs and Tissues	Procedures	Possible or Expected Findings
External examination and skin; oral cavity; breasts	Prepare histologic sections of skin lesions and of grossly uninvolved skin.	Skin papules, vesicles, ulcers. Subcutaneous nodules (vasculitis and granulomas). Granulomatous infiltrates of breast *(2)*. Gangrene of digits *(2,3)*.
	Prepare histologic sections of accessible mucosal lesions in mouth.	Necrotizing and ulcerative stomatitis.

Organs and Tissues	*Procedures*	*Possible or Expected Findings*
Blood	Submit samples for microbiologic and for immunologic study.	Septicemia; circulating immunoglobulin complexes, and antiendothelial antibodies *(7)*.
Lungs	Submit any areas of consolidation for microbiologic study. Perfuse at least one lung with formalin. Request Verhoeff–van Gieson stain.	Angiocentric granulomatosis *(4)*; necrotizing arteritis with infarctions; granulomatous bronchitis; pleuritis.
Spleen	Record weight; submit samples for histologic study.	Necrotizing arteritis. Infarctions *(5)*.
Kidneys	Follow procedures described under "Glomerulonephritis."	Focal necrotizing glomerulitis; necrotizing arteritis *(1)*.
Neck organs with larynx and trachea	Remove neck organs together with oropharynx and soft palate. Photograph lesions. For histologic study, submit samples with gross lesions and samples of grossly uninvolved tissue.	Necrotizing granulomatous inflammation and ulcers of soft palate, larynx, and trachea. Subglottic stenosis. Acute obstruction may be a cause of death *(6)*.
Other organs and tissues	Procedures depend on expected findings or grossly identified abnormalities as listed in right-hand column.	Necrotizing arteritis and granulomatous inflammation—for example in heart, gastrointestinal tract, and urogenital organs *(1)*.
Paranasal sinuses; ear, nose	Specimens should include surrounding bone; submit samples for histologic study (for decalcification procedures, see Chapter 2). For exposure of middle ear, see Chapter 4.	Necrotizing and ulcerative sinusitis with perifocal osteomyelitis. Necrotizing lesions in nasal cavities. Otitis media.
Brain and spinal cord	For removal and specimen preparation, see Chapter 4.	Angiocentric granulomatous lesions may be present *(1)*.
Eyes and orbitae	For removal and specimen preparation, see Chapter 5.	Pseudotumor of the orbit; other ocular lesions *(1)*, such as conjunctivitis, dacryocystitis, scleritis, and episcleritis, granulomatous sclerouveitis; ciliary vasculitis.
Bones and joints		Arthritis.*

References

1. Lie JT. Wegener's granulomatosis: histological documentation of common and uncommon manifestations in 216 patients. VASA 1997; 26:261–270.
2. Trueb RM, Pericin M, Kohler E, Barandun J, Burg G. Necrotizing granulomatosis of the breast. Br J Dermatol 1997;137:799–803.
3. Handa R, Wali JP. Wegener's granulomatosis with gangrene of toes. Scand J Rheumatol 1996;25:103–104.
4. Travis WD. Pathology of pulmonary granulomatous vasculitis. Sarcoidosis, Vascul Diff Lung Dis 1996;13:14–27.
5. Fishman D, Isenberg DA. Splenic involvement in rheumatic diseases. Semin Arthritis Rheum 1997;27:141–155.
6. Matt BH. Wegener's granulomatosis, acute laryngotracheal airway obstruction and death in a 17-year-old female: case report and review of the literature. Int J Pediatr Otolaryngol 1996;37:163–172.
7. Sebastian JK et al. Antiendothelial antibodies in patients with Wegener's granulomatosis: prevalence and correlation with disease activity and manifestations. J Rheumatol 2007;34:1027–1031.

Gunshot (See "Injury, firearm.")

H

Hallucinogen(s) (See "Abuse, hallucinogen(s).")

Halothane (See "Death, anesthesia-associated.")

Hanging

NOTE: Most hangings in the United States are suicides with short drops producing no cervical derangements, in contrast to the now uncommon judical hangings. A few hanging deaths are industrial accidents, and a few are consequences of asphyxia, self-induced for the purpose of sexual pleasure. Clues to autoerotic asphyxia are nudity, cross dressing, bondage paraphernalia, pornography, remotely operated video cameras, escape mechanisms, and a history or evidence of prior such acts.

Organs and Tissues	*Procedures*	*Possible or Expected Findings*
External examination and skin	Photograph the neck and head with and without the ligature in place, from anterior, left, right, and posterior aspects, and the ligature after removal.	Corresponding patterns of ligature and furrow; presence or absence of cyanosis and factial petecchiae; protrusion of tongue.
	Record and photograph liver mortis.	Shift from lower extremities to back; Tardieau spots (petecchiae caused by pooling).
	Measure diameter of the ligature and the depth and width of the furrow.	Size and pattern of ligature should match size and pattern of furrow.
	Measure the circumference of both the ligature and the neck. Measure the vertical distance of the furrow from the ear lobe.	Circumference of ligature will be less than circumference of neck.
Neck organs	Use layerwise anterior dissection and photograph all abnormalities.	Dessicated tan compressed subcutaneous facia; fractures of superior laryngeal cornua or hyoid in the elderly are consistent with hanging and can occur after prolonged suspension.

Hashish (See "Abuse, marihuana.")

Heart Disease, Congenital

NOTE: See under individual malformations, such as "Defect, ventricular septal." see, also, Chapter 3. For a listing of Latin terms and their Anglicized equivalents, see Chapter 3

Heat (See "Burns" and "Heatstroke.")

Heatstroke

Synonyms and Related Terms: Heat exhaustion; heat syncope; hyperthermia.

NOTE: Possible complications include disseminated intravascular coagulation* and fibrinolysis syndrome and Gram-negative septicemia.

From: *Handbook of Autopsy Practice,* 4th Ed. Edited by: B.L. Waters

Organs and Tissues	*Procedures*	*Possible or Expected Findings*
External examination	Inquire about ambient and body temperature.	Hyperthermia when body was discovered.
Vitreous	Submit sample for determination of chloride, sodium, and urea nitrogen concentrations.	Frequently, evidence of hypertonic dehydration.* See also Table 8-2.
Blood	Submit sample for toxicologic study, particularly for alcohol and drug screen.	Alcohol intoxication.
Urine	Record volume; determine specific gravity; record appearance of sediment.	High specific gravity; casts.
Thyroid gland	Sample for histologic study, particularly in unusual cases of heatstroke.	Thyroid disease such as Hashimoto's thyroiditis may predispose to heatstroke *(2)*.
Other organs	Submit samples for toxicologic and histologic study.	There may be no macroscopic changes *(2)*. Hemorrhages may be present, particularly in central nervous system, kidneys, and liver. Small parenchymal necroses with or without microthrombi may be found.

References

1. Donoghue ER, Graham MA, Jentzen JM, Lifschultz BD, Luke JL, Mirchandani HG. Criteria for the diagnosis of heat-related deaths: National Association of Medical Examiners. Position paper. National Association of Medical Examiners Ad Hoc Committee on the Definition of Heat-Related Fatalities. Am J Forens Med Pathol 1997;18:11–14.
2. Siegler RW. Fatal heatstroke in a young woman with previously undiagnosed Hashimoto's thyroiditis. J Forens Sci 1998;43:1237–1240.

Hematoma, Dissecting Aortic (See "Dissection, aortic.")

Hematoma, Spinal Epidural

Organs and Tissues	*Procedures*	*Possible or Expected Findings*
Spinal cord		Traumatic lesions; vascular malformations.
Other organs		Manifestations of hypertension.*

Hematoma, Subdural

Synonym: Subdural hemorrhage.

Organs and Tissues	*Procedures*	*Possible or Expected Findings*
External examination	Record evidence of trauma.	Abrasions; lacerations; subcutaneous hematomas.
	Prepare roentgenogram of skull.	Fractures.
Skull, meninges, and brain	For opening of skull and removal of calvarium, see Chapter 4.	Fractures may be identifiable only after stripping of dura.
	Record site, thickness, and volume of subdural hematoma and relation of hematoma to burr holes (if present).	Compression of cerebral hemispheres, with or without edema, and secondary compression of rostral brain stem.
	Remove vitreous—particularly if subdural hematoma appears to be nontraumatic—and determine sodium, potassium, and chloride concentrations.	Nontraumatic subdural hematoma rarely may be caused by hypernatremia and other hyperosmolar conditions. For interpretation of electrolyte values, see Table 8-1.

Hemochromatosis

Synonyms and Related Terms: Genetic hemochromatosis; pigment cirrhosis; primary hemochromatosis; secondary hemochromatosis.

NOTE: Secondary iron overload in other types of cirrhosis (e.g., alcoholic cirrhosis; alpha$_1$-antitrypsin deficiency, chronic viral hepatitis) may be severe enough to suggest genetic hemochromatosis. In such cases, quantitative iron studies (see below under "Liver") and calculation of the iron index are indicated *(1)*.

Organs and Tissues	*Procedures*	*Possible or Expected Findings*
External examination and skin and oral cavity	Record character and extent of pigmentation. Prepare histologic sections of pigmented areas and request Gomori's iron and Fontana-Masson silver stains.	Melanin hyperpigmentation of skin in face, neck, dorsal aspect of forearms and hands, genital area and scars; pigmentation of oral mucosa in some instances. A positive Fontana-Masson stain is not specific for the presence of melanin. Some hemosiderin may be present also.
	Prepare skeletal roentgenograms, which should include major joints, wrists, and hands, as listed in right-hand column.	Osteoporosis* and osteoarthritis* of hands and wrists, with chondrocalcinosis, subarticular cysts (second and third metacarpophalangeal joints), or osteophytes; osteoarthritis of hip, knee, and other major joints. Calcification of synovium.
Heart	Record weight. For gross staining for iron, see Chapter 16. For dissection of the conduction system, see Chapter 3. Submit samples of myocardium for histologic study and request Gomori's iron stain.	Cardiomyopathy with hemosiderosis and fibrosis of cardiac musculature.
Liver	Record weight and photograph. For gross staining for iron, see Chapter 16. For microscopic sections, request Gomori's iron stain. For quantitative iron studies, submit sample (this can be dug out from a paraffin block) for atomic absorption spectrophotometry *(1)*.	Pigment cirrhosis (see also above under "Note" and under "Cirrhosis, liver"). Hepatocellular carcinoma (see under "Tumor of the liver"), even in the absence of cirrhosis *(2)*.
Pancreas	Record color and weight. Submit samples for histologic study, particularly of tail. See also above under "Liver."	Hemosiderosis of exocrine and endocrine parenchyma; interstitial fibrosis.
Other organs and tissues	Histologic samples should include oral mucosa, tongue, stomach, intestinal tract, spleen, adrenal glands, kidneys, thyroid gland, parathyroid glands, lymph nodes, pituitary gland, and bone marrow. For gross and microscopic staining procedures, see above under "Liver."	Manifestations of diabetes mellitus;* features of congestive heart failure,* particularly in patients with hemochromatotic cardio-myopathy. Generalized hemosiderosis with fibrosis of adrenal glands and pituitary gland. Secondary hemochromatosis may be caused by various conditions, such as spherocytosis, thalassemia,* and other types of anemia (see "Anemia, hemolytic"), treated or untreated by transfusions. See also above under "Note."
Testes	Record weights and submit samples for histologic study.	Tubular atrophy.
Bones and joints	For removal, prosthetic repair, and specimen preparation, see Chapter 2.	Osteoporosis* and osteoarthritis.* Hemosiderosis of joints and synovial mem branes. Calcium pyrophosphate crystals in synovium. See also above under "External examination and skin and oral cavity."
Eyes	For removal and specimen preparation, see Chapter 5. Request Gomori's iron stain.	Hemosiderosis of margin of retinal disk, ciliary body, and corneal epithelium.

Reference

1. Ludwig J, Hashimoto E, Porayko MK, Moyer T, Baldus WP. Hemosiderosis in cirrhosis: a study of 447 native livers. Gastroenterology 1997; 112: 882–888.
2. Britto MR et al. Hepatocellular carcinoma arising in non-cirrhotic liver in genetic haemochromatosis. Scand J Gastroenterol 2000;35:889–893.

Hemoglobinuria, Paroxysmal Nocturnal (See "Anemia, hemolytic.")

Hemophilia

Synonyms: Hemophilia A (factor VIII coagulant protein deficiency); hemophilia B (Factor IX deficiency; Christmas disease).

NOTE: Rare hereditary deficiencies of other blood coagulation factors (II, V, VII, X, XI) may cause some symptoms of hemophilia. A reliable postmortem diagnosis is not possible; postmortem blood coagulation studies do not yield useful results.

Possible Associated Conditions: Acquired immunodeficiency syndrome (AIDS)* *(1)*, chronic viral hepatitis* with or without cirrhosis, and other infections from contaminated plasma products.

Organs and Tissues	*Procedures*	*Possible or Expected Findings*
External examination	Record character and extent of skin changes.	Cutaneous ecchymoses; soft tissue hematoma; blood in body orifices.
	Prepare skeletal roentgenograms.	Joint deformities (ankle, knee, elbow); erosions of bones by pseudotumors; soft tissue calcifications.
Blood	If infectious complications are expected, submit samples for culture and serologic study.	For common infections in hemophilic patients, see above under "Note."
Liver	Record weight and sample for histologic study.	Viral hepatitis C is very common but hepatitis B also may be encountered *(2)*. (See also under "Hepatitis, chronic.")
Other organs	Record sites and sizes of hematomas and hemorrhages, and photograph.	Hematomas and hemorrhages in soft tissues of floor of mouth, neck, subdural space, retroperitoneum, mesentery, renal pelves, gastrointestinal tract, and other sites. Polyarteritis nodosa *(4)*.
Brain and spinal cord	For removal and specimen preparation, see Chapter 4.	Hemorrhage *(1)*; microinfarctions, possibly related to treatment with large amounts of antihemophilic factor.
Joints	For removal, specimen preparation, and prosthetic repair, see Chapter 2. Photograph joint lesions.	Arthropathy with severe degenerative changes *(3)*; hemarthrosis.

References

1. Cahill MR, Colvin BT. Haemophilia. Postgrad Med J 1997;73: 201–206.
2. Lee CA. Transfusion-transmitted disease. Baillieres Clin Haematol 1996;9:369–394.
3. Lan HH, Eustace SJ, Dorfman D. Hemophilic arthropathy. Radiol Clin North Am 1996;34:446–450.
4. Matsushita T, et al. Classic polyarteritis nodosa presenting rare clinical manifestations in a patient with hemophilia A. Int J Hematol 2006;83:420–425.

Hemorrhage, Cerebral (See under name of suspected underlying condition, such as "Aneurysm, cerebral artery," "Infarction, cerebral," "Injury, head," and "Tumor of the brain."

Hemorrhage, Gastrointestinal

Organs and Tissues	*Procedures*	*Possible or Expected Findings*
Abdomen		Diaphragmatic hernia.*
Esophagus and stomach	For demonstration of esophageal varices, see Chapter 2. Record appearance of mucosa; record volume of blood in lumen.	Reflux esophagitis; varices;* strictures with erosions; tumor;* mucosal erosions and peptic ulcer(s);* petechial mucosal hemorrhages.
Duodenum		Peptic ulcer(s).*
Small bowel and large bowel	If infectious enteritis is suspected, submit material for microbiologic study. Submit samples of all segments for histologic study. If free blood is present, record volume.	Infectious—for instance, in typhoid fever*—and noninfectious enteritis; circulatory or neoplastic intestinal disease; other diseases, such as diverticulitis.
Other organs	Procedures depend on expected findings or grossly identified abnormalities as listed in right-hand column.	Cerebral space-occupying lesions; manifestations of coagulation disorder, including leukemia* or other neoplastic disease; pancreatitis;* manifestations of portal hypertension* or of kidney failure.*

Hemorrhage, Intracranial (See under "Hematoma, subdural" and under name of suspected underlying condition, such as "Aneurysm, cerebral artery," "Infarction, cerebral," "Injury, head," and "Tumor of the brain."

Hemorrhage, Subarachnoid (See under name of suspected underlying condition, such as "Aneurysm, cerebral artery," "Infarction, cerebral," "Injury, head," and "Tumor of the brain."

Hemosiderosis, Idiopathic Pulmonary

NOTE: This diagnosis is made by exclusion; involvement of organs other than the lungs (see below under "Kidneys") suggests another disease.

Organs and Tissues	*Procedures*	*Possible or Expected Findings*
Heart		Cor pulmonale.
Lungs	Photograph fresh lungs (side by side with normal lung). Perfuse lungs with formalin; for iron staining of gross specimens, see Chapter 16; for microscopic sections, request Gomori's iron stain. For quantitation of iron in paraffin blocks, see "Hemochromatosis."	Hemorrhages into alveolar spaces. Hemosiderin in pulmonary septa and macrophages; interstitial pulmonary fibrosis; degeneration, shedding, and hyperplasia of alveolar epithelial cells.
	Immunofluorescent and electron microscopic studies (see below) also may be of value.	Goodpasture's syndrome and immune-complex mediated vasculitis need to be ruled out.
Kidneys	Prepare tissue for immunofluorescent study. Submit samples for electron microscopic study.	Kidneys should not be involved; if they are, Goodpasture's syndrome* must be considered as a cause.
Bone marrow		Secondary hyperplasia caused by anemia.

Hepatitis, Alcoholic (See "Disease, alcoholic liver.")

Hepatitis, Chronic

Synonyms and Related Terms: Autoimmune hepatitis; chronic viral hepatitis B (with or without D) and C.

NOTE: The term "chronic hepatitis" is not a complete etiologic diagnosis and related names such as chronic active (aggressive) hepatitis, chronic active liver disease, and chronic per-sistent hepatitis are obsolete. Most cases in these categories represent autoimmune hepatitis or chronic viral hepatitis B or C. Many other liver diseases, including drug-induced hepatitis, inborn errors of metabolism (e.g., alpha$_1$-antitrypsin deficiency* or Wilson's disease*), developmental disorders, and chronic biliary diseases such as primary biliary cirrhosis or primary sclerosing cholangitis also may present as chronic hepatitis.

If chronic hepatitis was the cause of death, submassive hepatic necrosis or cirrhosis* is usually present, often with manifestations of portal hypertension,* hepatic encephalopathy, hepatorenal syndrome,* and with ascites or spontaneous bacterial peritonitis.

Possible Associated Conditions: See also below under "Possible or Expected Findings." Conditions that may be associated with hepatitis C include *(1)*: autoimmune hepatitis; Behcet's disease; diabetes mellitus (type 2);* glomerulonephritis;* Guillain-Barré syndrome;* idiopathic pulmonary fibrosis; idiopathic thrombocytopenic purpura; IgA deficiency; lichen planus; mixed essential cryoglobulinemia; Mooren's corneal ulcers; polyarthritis; porphyria cutanea tarda;* thyroiditis.*

Organs and Tissues	*Procedures*	*Possible or Expected Findings*
External examination and skin	Record body weight and length, habitus, and extent and character of skin changes. Prepare histologic sections of skin lesions.	Hirsutism; cushingoid face; acne; maculopapular rash; erythema nodosum; lupus erythematosus-like changes in face; localized scleroderma; purpura; vitiligo; cutaneous small-vessel vasculitis and porphyria cutanea tarda in chronic hepatitis C *(2)*.
Blood	Submit sample for serologic studies if type of viral hepatitis (B, D, or C) or of autoimmune hepatitis is in question.	Viral antigens or antibodies; autoantibodies (ANA, SMA, and others) in autoimmune hepatitis. Essential mixed cryoglobulinemia in chronic hepatitis C *(2)*.
Heart		Pericarditis.
Arteries		Polyarteritis nodosa*
Liver	Record weight and photograph surface and cut	Chronic viral or autoimmune hepatitis, with

Organs and Tissues	Procedures	Possible or Expected Findings
Liver *(continued)*	sections. If chronic hepatitis B is suspected, order immunostains for B surface and core antigen. Request PAS stain with diastase digestion. If Wilson's disease must be ruled out, order rhodanine stain and quantitative copper study. Request Gomori's iron stain.	or without cirrhosis;* hepatocellular carcinoma. Alpha$_1$-antitrypsin deficiency.* High hepatic tissue copper concentrations in Wilson's disease.* Hemosiderosis common in hepatitis C.
Gallbladder	Describe concrements.	Cholelithiasis
Pancreas	Submit samples for histologic study.	Changes associated with diabetes mellitus.*
Intestinal tract	Procedures depend on expected findings or grossly identified abnormalities as in conditions listed in right-hand column.	Crohn's disease* or chronic ulcerative colitis often associated with primary sclerosing cholangitis.* (See above under "Note.")
Kidneys	Follow procedures described under "Glomerulonephritis."	Membranous and membranoproliferative glomerulitis and nephrotic syndrome.
Thyroid gland	Record weight, photograph, and submit samples for histologic study.	Hashimoto's thyroiditis. Thyroid dysfunction in interferon-treated chronic hepatitis B and C *(3)*.
Brain and spinal cord	For removal and specimen preparation, see Chapter 4.	Cerebritis and peripheral neuropathy in chronic hepatitis C *(2)*.
Eyes and lacrimal glands	For removal and specimen preparation, see Chapter 5.	Keratoconjunctivitis; fibrosis and inflammation of lacrimal glands; manifestations of Sjögren's syndrome.*
Parotid and submandibular glands	Samples can be biopsied from scalp incision and removed with floor of the mouth respectively.	Fibrosis and inflammation.
Nose, pharynx, and larynx	Submit samples of mucosa for histologic study.	Atrophy of mucosal glands.
Bone, bone marrow, and joints		Osteoporosis* (particularly after steroid treatment); hypocellular bone marrow (aplastic anemia).

References

1. Gordon SC. Extrahepatic manifestations of Hepatitis C. Dig Dis 1996; 14:157–168.
2. Gross JB Jr. Clinician's guide to hepatitis C. Mayo Clinic Proc 1998; 73:355–361.
3. Deutsch M, Dourakis S, Manesis EK, Gioustozi A, Hess G, Horsch A, Hadziyannis S. Thyroid abnormalities in chronic viral hepatitis and their relationship to interferon alpha therapy. Hepatology 1997;26: 206–210.

Hepatitis, Fulminant (See "Hepatitis, viral.")

Hepatitis, Neonatal

Synonyms and Related Terms: Giant cell hepatitis; idiopathic neonatal hepatitis (familial or nonfamilial); infantile obstructive cholangiopathy; neonatal cholestasis.

NOTE: Neonatal hepatitis may have been a biopsy diagnosis in an earlier stage of paucity of intrahepatic bile ducts; at autopsy, biliary cirrhosis with ductopenia would be the main finding. For other conditions that may present clinically as neonatal hepatitis or jaundice, see below.

Organs and Tissues	Procedures	Possible or Expected Findings
External examination		Jaundice. Lymphedema in one form of hereditary neonatal hepatitis *(1)*.
Blood	Submit samples for microbiologic and serologic study. If chromosome abnormalities are suspected, submit sample for chromosome analysis.	Hepatitis virus antigens or antibodies, including hepatitis B or C, cytomegalovirus, coxsackievirus, herpes simplex, rubeola, and varicella virus. Toxoplasmosis,* congenital syphilis,* and *Listeria monocytogenes* infection may also cause neonatal hepatitis.
Extrahepatic bile ducts	For postmortem cholangiography, see Chapter 2. If no roentgenologic studies can be carried out, open duodenum *in situ*, squeeze gallbladder, and record whether bile emerged from papilla.	Biliary atresia;* paucity of intrahepatic bile ducts (syndromic [Alagille's syndrome] or nonsyndromic); choledochal cyst.*

Organs and Tissues	Procedures	Possible or Expected Findings
Liver	Record size and weight; photograph surface and cut section; submit sample of fresh liver for viral culture; submit samples for histologic study; request PAS stain with diastase digestion.	Giant cell transformation of liver, with or without biliary atresia or paucity of intrahepatic bile ducts. Cholestasis and cirrhosis may be present *(4)*. Alpha$_1$-antitrypsin deficiency. Fatty livers also may be found *(2)*.
Other organs and tissues	Procedures depend on expected findings or grossly identified abnormalities as listed in right-hand column.	Manifestations of conditions that may present clinically as neonatal hepatitis or jaundice, e.g., cystic fibrosis *(3)*;* erythroblastosis fetalis;* congenital rubella syndrome;* galactosemia;* Niemann-Pick disease;* trisomy 17-18; Turner's syndrome.*

References

1. Sharp HL, Krivit W. Hereditary lymphedema and obstructive jaundice. J Pediatr 1971;78:491–496.
2. Nishinomiya F, Abukawa D, Takada G, Tazawa Y. Relationships between clinical and histological profiles of non-familial idiopathic neonatal hepatitis. Acta Paediatr Japn 1996;38:242–247.
3. Lykavieris P, Bernard O, Hadchouel M. Neonatal cholestasis as the presenting feature in cystic fibrosis. Arch Dis Child 1996;75:67–70.
4. Okçu-Heper A, et al. Nonobstructive neonatal cholestasis: clinical outcome and scoring of the histopathological changes in liver biopsies. Pediatr Dev Pathol 2006;9:44–51.

Hepatitis, Viral

Synonyms: Acute (or subacute) viral hepatitis; fulminant viral hepatitis; hepatitis virus hepatitis; viral hepatitis A, B, B with D, C, E, F, G, or type undetermined.

NOTE: Coinfection with other hepatitis viruses (e.g., C and G) and/or systemic viruses such as the immunodeficiency virus are common, particularly in drug addicts *(1,2)*. In many cases of fulminant hepatitis, tests for known hepatitis viruses are negative *(3,4)*. If the hepatitis was caused by a systemic virus, see under the specific disease name, for example, "Infection, cytomegalovirus." For chronic viral hepatitis, see under "Hepatitis, chronic." If the patients underwent liver transplantation *(3)* or bone marrow transplantation for complicating aplastic anemia *(4)*, see also under "Transplantation,..."

(1) Collect all tissues that appear to be infected. (2) Request viral cultures if systemic disease such as cytomegalovirus infection* is expected. (3) Stains for hepatitis B core and surface antigen may be helpful. (4) Special **precautions** are indicated, particularly in suspected hepatitis B and D infection. (5) Serologic studies are essential in undiagnosed cases and can be obtained from most clinical laboratories. (6) Hepatitis virus hepatitis is not a reportable disease.

Possible Associated Conditions: See "Hepatitis, chronic."

Organs and Tissues	Procedures	Possible or Expected Findings
External examination	If patient was on dialysis for chronic renal failure, see also under that heading.	Jaundice; skin rash or hemorrhages and other abnormalities. Needle marks may indicate intravenous substance abuse.
Blood	Submit sample for serologic studies for viral antigens or antibodies.	Viral antigens or antibodies may or may not be positive.
Heart	Procure at least six sections for histologic. examination.	Myocarditis;* necrosis of fibers in bundle of His.
Lungs	Perfuse at least one lung with formalin. Sample for histologic study and request Verhoeff–van Gieson stain.	Manifestations of pulmonary hypertension.*
Liver	Record weight and photograph surface and cut sections. If hepatitis B is suspected, order immunostains for B surface and core antigen. Immunostains for hepatitis D are also available.	Lobular inflammation with bridging necrosis or multilobular collapse; massive necrosis with complete loss of parenchyma. Stains for viral antigens often are negative.
Gallbladder	Record appearance and volume of bile.	Bile may be absent.
Pancreas	Submit samples for histologic study.	Pancreatitis.*
Spleen	Record weight; request Gomori's stain for iron.	Pulpal hyperplasia; hemosiderosis; congestive splenomegaly.
Esophagus	Leave attached to stomach; submit sample for histologic study.	Ulcerations or erosions of distal esophagus; varices.
Stomach	Submit sample for histologic study.	Gastritis.

Organs and Tissues	Procedures	Possible or Expected Findings
Small intestine	Fix bowel as soon as possible. Submit samples for histologic study.	Flattening, broadening, and possible fusion of villi. Phlegmonous inflammation and edema, mainly in ileocecal region.
Kidneys	Follow procedures described under "Glomerulonephritis."	Glomerular changes; bile casts in tubules; interstitial edema.
Lymph nodes	Submit cervical and mediastinal lymph nodes for histologic study.	Lymphadenitis.
Thyroid	Sample for histologic study.	See "Hepatitis, chronic."
Brain and spinal cord	For removal and specimen preparation, see Chapter 4.	Encephalitis.*
Bone marrow	For preparation of sections and smears, see Chapter 2.	Leukopenia; thrombocytopenia; aplastic anemia *(4)* (pancytopenia*).
Joints	For removal, prosthetic repair, and specimen preparation, see Chapter 2. Submit samples of synovia for histologic study.	Synovitis (arthritis*).

References

1. Thiers V, Pol S, Persico T, Carnot F, Zylberberg H, Berthelot P, et al. Hepatitis G virus infection in hepatitis C virus-positive patients co-infected or not with hepatitis B virus and/or human immunodeficiency virus. J Viral Hep 1998;5:123–130.
2. Bortolotti F, Tagger A, Giacchino R, Zuccoti GV, Crivellaro C, Balli F, et al. Hepatitis G and C coinfection in children. J Pediatr 1997;131: 639–640.
3. Ferraz ML, Silva AE, Macdonald GA, Tsarev AS, Di Bisceglie AM, Lucey MR. Fulminant hepatitis in patients undergoing liver transplantation: evidence for a non-A, non-B, non-C, non-D, and non-E syndrome. Liv Transpl Surg 1996;2:60–66.
4. Kiem HP, McDonald GB, Myerson D, Spurgeon CL, Deeg HJ, Sanders JE, et al. Marrow transplantation for hepatitis-associated aplastic anemia: a follow up of long-term survivors. Biol Blood Bone Marrow Transpl 1996;2:93–99.

Hepatoma (See "Tumor of the liver.")

Hernia, Diaphragmatic

Related Terms: Congenital diaphragmatic hernia; hiatal hernia; sliding hiatus hernia.

NOTE: Congenital diaphragmatic hernia is right-sided or more commonly, left-sided and may be associated with cardiac anomalies, such as the hypoplastic heart syndrome (with left-sided diaphragmatic hernia) *(1)* or anomalies of lungs or upper airways *(2)*.

Organs and Tissues	Procedures	Possible or Expected Findings
Thoracic and abdominal cavity	Record extent of hernia by palpation from abdominal cavity, before organ removal. Remove esophagus and stomach as one specimen; photograph opened esophagus and stomach, and pin on corkboard for fixation and histologic study.	Reflux esophagitis; esophageal ulcer(s) and stricture(s), Barrett's esophagus,* with or without adenocarcinoma.
	In infants or newborns, search for associated malformations in the chest cavity (see above under "Note"). Weigh lungs to evaluate degree of pulmonary hypoplasia. In teenagers or adults with repaired congenital diaphragmatic hernias, prepare chest roentgenograms. Perfuse lungs with formalin.	In long-term survivors of repaired congenital diaphragmatic hernias, thoracic deformities, and restrictive or obstructive lung disease may be found *(3)*. Cardiovascular malformations *(4)*.

References

1. Losty PD, Vanamo K, Rintala RJ, Donahoe PK, Schnitzer JJ, Lloyd DA. Congenital diaphragmatic hernia: does the side of the defect influence the incidence of associated malformations? J Pediatr Surg 1998;33:507–510.
2. Ryan CA, Finer NN, Etches PC, Tierney AJ, Peliowski A. Congenital diaphragmatic hernia: associated malformations: cystic adenomatoid malformation, extralobular sequestration, and laryngotracheoesophageal cleft: two case reports. J Pediatr Surg 1995;30:883–885.
3. Vanamo K, Rintala R, Sovijarvi A, Jaaskelainen J, Turpeinen M, Lindahl H, Louhimo I. Long-term pulmonary sequelae in survivors of congenital diaphragmatic defects. J Pediatr Surg 1996;31:1096–1099.
4. Lin AE, Pober BR, Adatia I. Congenital diaphragmatic hernia and associated cardiovascular malformations: type, frequency, and impact on management. Am J Med Genet C Semin Med Genet 2000;145:201–216.

Heroin
(See "Dependence, drug(s), all types or type unspecified.")

Herpes Simplex
(See "Infection, herpes simplex.")

Herpes Zoster
(See "Infection, herpes zoster.")

Histiocytosis, Langerhans Cell

Synonym and Related Terms: Abt-Letterer-Siwe disease; eosinophilic granuloma of bone; Hand-Schüller-Christian disease; histiocytosis X (use of these names is no longer recommended *[1]*).

NOTE: Langerhans cell histiocytosis is a monoclonal disorder and thus a true neoplasm *(2)*. The disease most commonly is found in pediatric patients and is rare in adults *(3)*.

Possible Associated Conditions: Diabetes insipidus;* malignant lymphoma.*

Organs and Tissues	*Procedures*	*Possible or Expected Findings*
External examination, skin, and oral cavity	Prepare photograph of gross lesions as listed in right-hand column.	Exophthalmos ("Hand-Schüller-Christian disease." see below under "Eyes"). Nodules in scalp. Vulvar lesions. Hyperplasia and ulcerations of gums.
	Prepare skeletal roentgenograms.	Monostotic or polyostotic destructive bone lesions (lesions most common is skull); pathological fractures.
	Sample skin lesions for histologic study (see below under "Lymph nodes").	Papular, eczema-like eruptions; xanthomas; erythematous, purpuric, and ecchymotic lesions. Histiocytic and eosinophilic infiltrates (see lymph nodes).
Blood	Submit sample for microbiologic study.	Septicemia.
Lymph nodes	Sample grossly involved and uninvolved lymph nodes and perform immunohistochemistry for langerin and CD1a *(6)*.	Typical mononuclear cells and eosinophils in sinuses, with or without microabscess formation.
	Prepare material for electron microscopy.	Mononuclear cells with Langerhans' or Birbeck granules.
Heart	Record weight and thickness of walls.	Cor pulmonale.
Lungs	Dissect one fresh lung and sample for histologic study (see above under "Lymph nodes). Submit sample for microbiologic study. Perfuse one lung with formalin.	Destructive granulomas centered around distal bronchioles *(4)*. Pneumonia of various types.
Other organs and tissues	Sample grossly involved and uninvolved tissue for histologic study (see "Lymph nodes"), including liver, spleen, gastrointestinal tract, kidneys, and perirenal fat.	Histiocytosis with hepatosplenomegaly ("Letterer-Siwe disease"). Many other organs and tissues may be involved.
	Submit tissue samples for biochemical study (total cholesterol) and for electron microscopic study.	Increased tissue concentrations of total cholesterol.
Brain and spinal cord	Histologic samples must include hypothalamus, pituitary gland, and cerebellum.	Langerhans cell infiltrates, most commonly in hypothalamic-pituitary area *(5)*; infiltrates arise from bone lesions, meninges, or choroid plexus.
Eyes	For removal and specimen preparation, see Chapter 5.	Orbital histiocytic infiltrates.
Middle ears	For removal and specimen preparation, see Chapter 4.	Otitis media* (in "Hand-Schüller-Christian disease").
Bones	Review roentgenograms. For removal and specimen preparation, see Chapter 2.	Monostotic lesions may be found ("eosinophilic granuloma").

References

1. Nezelof C, Basset F. Langerhans cell histiocytosis research. Past, present, and future. Hematol Oncol Clin North Am 1998;12: 385–406.
2. Willman CL, McClain KL. An update on clonality, cytokines, and viral etiology in Langerhans cell histiocytosis. Hematol Oncol Clin North Am 1998;12:407–416.
3. Malpas JS. Langerhans cell histiocytosis in adults. Hematol Oncol Clin North Am 1998; 12:259–268.
4. Soler P, Tazi A, Hance AJ. Pulmonary Langerhans cell granulomatosis. Curr Opin Pulm Med 1995;1:406–416.
5. Grois NG, Favara BE, Mostbeck GH, Prayer D. Central nervous system disease in Langerhans cell histiocytosis. Hematol Oncol Clin North Am 1998;12:287–305.
6. Sholl LM et al. Immunohistochemical analysis of langerin in langerhans cell histocytosis and pulmonary inflammatory and infectious diseases. Am J Surg Path 2007;31:947–952.

Histoplasmosis

Synonyms: Darling's disease; *Histoplasma capsulatum* infection.

NOTE: (1) Collect all tissues that appear to be infected. (2) Request fungal cultures. (3) Request Grocott's stain for fungi. (4) Usually, no special precautions are indicated. (5) Serologic studies are available from local and state health department laboratories. (6) This is not a reportable disease.

Possible Associated Conditions: Histoplasmosis may be a complication of the acquired immunodeficiency syndrome* *(1)* and this possibility should be ruled out in all instances.

Organs and Tissues	*Procedures*	*Possible or Expected Findings*
Cerebrospinal fluid	If there is suspicion of cerebral involvement, submit for culture.	
Oral cavity	Prepare histologic sections of ulcers. Submit specimens for fungal culture.	Ulcerations of tongue and palate.
Blood and urine	Submit samples for fungal culture. Obtain sample for serologic study.	
Heart	If endocarditis is suspected, follow procedures described in Chapter 7.	Infective endocarditis;* pericarditis.*
Mediastinum and lungs (see also below under "Neck organs").	Perfuse one lung with formalin. Brief decalcification may be necessary in chronic cases (Chapter 2).	Miliary granulomas, with or without calcification; cavitating pneumonia; mediastinal fibrosis; obstruction of bronchi by lymphadenopathy.
Esophagus	Leave esophagus attached to fundus of stomach.	Obstruction by enlarged mediastinal lymph nodes; traction diverticula of esophagus.
Liver	Record weight	Hepatomegaly; granulomatous hepatitis.
Spleen	Record weight; decalcification may be necessary.	Splenomegaly; granulomatous splenitis.
Adrenal glands	Dissect glands, record weights, and photograph (if there is evidence of involvement).	Severe destruction in systemic histoplasmosis; may be the cause of Adrenal insufficiency.*
Neck organs	After fixation, sample ulcers for histologic study.	Ulcers of epiglottis and larynx.
Lymph nodes		Granulomatous lymphadenopathy.
Eyes	For removal and specimen preparation, see Chapter 5.	Ocular histoplasmosis *(3)*.
Brain, Spinal cord	For removal and specimen preparation, see Chapter 4. See also above under "Note"	*Histoplasma* meningitis.*, isolated spinal cord lesion *(4)*.
Bone marrow	For preparation of sections and smears, see Chapter 2.	*Histoplasma* granulomas. Hemophagocytic histiocytosis in patients with reactive hemophagocytic syndrome *(2)*.

References

1. Raza J, Harris MT, Bauer JJ. Gastrointestinal histoplasmosis in a patient with acquired immune deficiency syndrome. Mt Sinai J Med 1996;63:136–140.
2. Koduri PR, Chundi V, DeMarais P, Mizock BA, Patel AR, Weinstein RA. Reactive hemophagocytic syndrome: a new presentation of disseminated histoplasmosis in patients with AIDS. Clin Inf Dis 1995;21:1463–1465.
3. Callanan D, Fish GE, Anand R. Reactivation of inflammatory lesions in ocular histoplasmosis. Arch Ophthalmol 1998;116:470–474.
4. Bollyky PL, et al. Histoplasmosis presenting as an isolated spinal cord lesion. Arch Neurol 2006;63:1802–1803.

Homicide

NOTE: Not all of the following procedures can be carried out or will be required in all cases, nor will this checklist be sufficient in all instances. Consult also the entries indicating the cause of death, such as "Injury, firearm" or "Injury, stabbing." If the victim is an infant, see all under "Infanticide."

Before the body arrives or before autopsy is begun:

1. Investigate the scene where the body was found and where the crime may have been committed (these may be two separate locations). If this is not possible, study the report and photographs submitted by the investigator or the police. Study all available information. Request previous medical records and roentgenograms of the victim.
2. Emphasize to first responders and autopsy personnel that the body of the victim should not be undressed, washed, or otherwise disturbed until it has been inspected by the pathologist. Embalming is not permitted before completion of the autopsy. Advise first responders or transporters to put paper bags over the hands of the victim. This will protect possible evidence, such as hair from the assailant.
3. Prepare record sheets to document the time of arrival and release of the body; chain of custody for the body and specimens; the name, age, sex, and other information about the victim; the names of the technician, pathologist and guests; and the specimens taken.
4. Prepare roentgenographic and photographic equipment.

After Body Arrives but Before Autopsy Is Begun:

1. If the body is left unguarded—for instance, overnight—a lock should be placed on the refrigerator or cool room where the deceased is kept, and the key should be retained by the technician.
2. If the pathologist is not accustomed to a busy autopsy room, he or she should feel free to ask all persons other than the pathologist(s), technicians, and law enforcement personnel who are not immediately involved in the actual performance of the autopsy to leave the morgue.
3. The body temperature of the victim can be recorded at the autopsy facility, but this is rarely useful, particularly if the victim seems to have been dead for longer than a day or two or if the body had previously been stored in a refrigerator or cool room. Insert thermometer deep into the anus (about 7–8 cm). Record temperature and manner and time of procedure.
4. Aspirate vitreous from one or both eyes and store the specimen in a refrigerator.
5. Prepare roentgenograms. In each case, a decision must be made whether roentgenograms should be made of the entire body or only of parts of it—or not at all—and whether they should be made before the victim is undressed, after the victim is undressed, or at both times.

Photographs:

1. Take overall survey photographs that depict the anterior surfaces of the body as it is on arrival to the facility, before any undressing, manipulation for roentgenographs, or cleaning.
2. Take close-up photographs of any trace evidence such as fibers or flakes of gunpowder before undressing or cleaning.
3. Photograph the face of the victim for identification purposes after it has been cleaned of any blood and foreign matter. To avoid perspective distortion from wide angle lenses, the lens should be about 4 ft from the face.
4. Photograph all injuries and other forensically significant findings after blood and foreign matter have been cleaned off the body. A moist towel is useful; brushes are too abrasive. Two photographs should be taken of each finding. One should include the autopsy number and a scale. A second photograph should be taken without any extraneous objects.

Collection and Documentation of Evidence:

1. Fingerprinting can be done before or after the autopsy but should be done in all homicide cases. In cases involving close contact between assailant and victim, fingernail scrapings or clippings (use a new clipper) and hair with roots should be collected , and its source should be identified (hair pulled from scalp, axillae, and pubis is identified as that of the victim; hair in hands or under fingernails or on clothing of victim may be from the assailant). Hair exemplars can be collected in cases of homicide by firearm but are rarely of use.
2. If the body is decomposed or mutilated or for any other reason has not been identified, prepare roentgenograms of the head, neck, and torso before the autopsy (the radiographic appearance is altered by the autopsy). These can be used for comparison purposes if antemortem films are located. If films of the extremities are needed they can be prepared after the autopsy. Dental roentgeno¬grams are taken, usually after the autopsy, when investigators have located antemortem dental records. Detailed descriptions and sizes of clothing, with photographs of clothing, can be useful then there is no putative identity.
3. In cases in which sexual assault may have been involved, collect pieces of clothing that may contain seminal fluid stains. Follow procedures described under "Rape."
4. Preserve clothing or part of clothing as evidence. Wet clothing should be dried before it is stored in labeled and sealed bags.

The Autopsy:

1. The measured length and weight, extent of rigor, and color and distribution of livor should be recorded, along with the state of preservation, nutrition, and hydration. Do not omit examination of the hands, particularly of the volar surfaces.
2. If air embolism is suspected, see procedure described under Part II "Embolism, Air". If pneumothorax is suspected, see procedure described under Part II "Pneumothorax". If there is evidence of strangulation or other neck injury, perform a layerwise dissection of the neck that includes the hyoid bone and tongue.
3. Prepare diagrams of wounds and identify their location by anatomic region. For wounds of the torso, state the distance from the soles of a foot and the distance laterally from to the right or left of the midline.
4. Submit samples of wounds for histologic study when there is any question of the age of the wounds.
5. The records should show when body fluids and tissues were collected for laboratory analysis, the volume and appearance of such specimens, and what was done with them. If most of the toxicology specimens are collected immediately after the internal examination has commenced, the time of the internal examination serves as the collection time. In all instances, the following items should be collected: blood of victim for DNA comparison and toxicologic study (determination of alcohol, carbon monoxide, and drug concentrations will be requested most frequently); vitreous; urine; gastric contents; at least one solid organ specimen for toxicologic study (liver and brain have the most comparison data). For appropriate methods of sampling for toxicologic study, use of preservatives, methods of storage, type of containers, labeling, shipping, and chain of custody, see Chapters 13 and 15. Obtain receipts of specimens that were forwarded to the Forensic Physical Evidence Laboratory.
6. Bullets or other foreign bodies should be handled with gloved fingers or non-metallic forceps.

7. Most of the important observations relevant to the paths of gunshot wounds and stab wounds are made at the autopsy table, during inspection of the open body cavities, before the organs are removed, regardless of whether the pathologist removes the organs en bloc or one by one. The pathologist should not be in a rush to remove the organs in such cases because removal of the organs destroys relationships.
8. For general forensic autopsy protocols and procedures, see Chapter 13.

Homocystinuria

Related Terms: Aminoaciduria;* cystathionine β synthase deficiency; cystathioninuria; sulfuraminoacidemia.

NOTE: For autopsy procedures and expected findings, see under "aminoaciduria*" and "Syndrome, Marfan's." Lax ligaments, lengthened extremities, and fine sparse hair may be present. Ocular abnormalities include dislocated lens, retracted zonular fibers, retinal degeneration with loss of pigmented epithelium and presence of pigment-laden macrophages, and cataracts. Ocular, vascular, and skeletal changes in older patients also may resemble those present in Marfan's syndrome.* Thromboembolism is a frequent cause of death. Submit sample of urine for determination of homocystine concentration (in homocystinuria, values should be increased).

Hydrocephalus

Synonyms and Related Terms: Active or progressive hydro -cephalus; arrested hydrocephalus; communicating or malresorptive hydrocephalus; high pressure (or normal pressure or intermittent or occult) hydrocephalus; hydrocephalus ex vacuo; obstructive or noncommunicating hydrocephalus.

Organs and Tissues	*Procedures*	*Possible or Expected Findings*
External examination	If size or shape of head is abnormal, record head circumference. Prepare skull roentgenogram.	Enlarged head in presence of hydrocephalus that was acquired early. Enlargement of skull with distended sutures.
Head	If an extracerebral congenital malformation is suspected, follow procedures described under "Malformation, Arnold-Chiari." If cerebrospinal fluid is aspirated with a syringe, record volume.	Arnold-Chiari malformation* and related abnormalities; tentorial bleeding at time of birth; communicating or noncommunicating hydrocephalus.
Brain	Record weight of brain; record size of brain in relation to inner dimensions of skull. Describe size of ventricles.	In obstructive hydrocephalus, only one lateral ventricle may be enlarged or lateral and third ventricles may be involved (three-ventricular hydrocephalus); in communicating hydrocephalus, all ventricular cavities are enlarged.
	Other procedures depend on expected findings or grossly identified abnormalities as listed in right-hand column. If a surgical shunt is present, its location should be recorded and both ends of the implanted specimen that was used for shunting may be submitted for microbiologic study. If the shunt is not patent, record site and nature of obstruction.	Traumatic subarachnoid hemorrhage; rupture of congenital cerebral artery aneurysm;* adhesions after bacterial meningitis* or toxoplasmosis* in infancy or after tuberculosis,* mycotic basal meningitis, sarcoidosis,* or cysticercosis in adulthood; intracranial tumor of third and fourth ventricles; meningeal carcinomatosis.
Spine		Lipomeningocele, diastematomyelia, tethered cord *(2)*.

References

1. Squier MV. Pathological approach to the diagnosis of hydrocephalus. J Clin Pathol 1997;50:181–186.
2. Pettorini BL, et al. Thoracic lipomeningocele associated with diastematomyelia, tethered spinal cord, and hydrocephalus. Case report, J Neurosurg 2007;106:394–397.

Hydronephrosis

Related Term: Obstructive uropathy.

Organs and Tissues	*Procedures*	*Possible or Expected Findings*
External examination	Prepare abdominal roentgenogram.	Stone; foreign bodies.
Blood	Submit sample for bacterial culture.	Septicemia.
Retroperitoneal space	Record size of urinary bladder, width of ureters, and size of kidneys and renal pelves. Dissect *in situ*: ureters, abdominal aorta, and inferior vena cava and the major branches of these vessels. Prepare photographs of dissected retroperitoneal structures, showing the site of obstruction.	Tumor (lymphoma, carcinoma), cysts, fibrous band, or aberrant renal artery. Other possible causes include retroperitoneal fibrosis* and related extrinsic obstructive processes—for instance, radiation fibrosis, trauma, or accidental surgical ligation of ureter.

Kidneys, ureters, and pelvic organs	Record volume of urine in the three compartments. For postmortem angiography and urography, see Chapter 2. Leave kidneys, abdominal aorta, ureters, urinary bladder, and—in male infants—entire urethra in one specimen.	Pyelonephritis;* ureteritis; intraluminal tumor, clot, sloughed papillae, or foreign body; congenital narrowing or obstruction of ureterovesical junction, ureterocele, retrocaval ureter, and anterior or posterior urethral valves.
	Procedures depend on expected findings or grossly identified abnormalities as listed in right-hand column.	Meatal urethral stenosis or phimosis. Acquired strictures, tumors, calculi. Angulation or ptosis; diverticula; Endometriosis; malakoplakia; benign
	prostatic hyperplasia with median bar.	
Spinal cord and peripheral nerves	For dissection and specimen preparation, see Chapter 4.	Spinal cord disease; diabetic neuropathy, and other causes of neurogenic obstructive uropathy.

Hydrops Fetalis

Related Terms: Antibody-mediated hydrops fetalis; erythroblastosis fetalis;* nonimmune hydrops fetalis.

NOTE: The classic example of antibody mediated (Rh incompatibility) hydrops fetalis is hemolytic disease of the newborn (erythroblastosis fetalis*). However, nonimmune hydrops fetalis also may be caused by hematologic disorders, e.g., alpha-thalassemia* *(1)* or it may have no known cause. Infections, e.g., with human parvovirus B19 *(2)*, cytomegalovirus, or syphilis;* heart and vascular diseases *(3)* (cardiac tumors, cardi-omyopathy,* myocarditis,* arterial calcification, and others); storage disease *(4)*; tumors (including neonatal leukemia*); and many other fetal (e.g., congenital chylothorax* or lymphatic dysplasia; pulmonary sequestration and cystic adenomatoid malformation) or maternal conditions, e.g., maternal thyrotoxicosis, also may cause nonimmune hydrops fetalis.

Organs and Tissues	*Procedures*	*Possible or Expected Findings*
Placenta	Record weight, size, and gross appearance. Sample for histologic study.	Placental hydrops; chorangioma and other vascular abnormalities; erythroblastosis.*
Blood	Submit sample if there is no autolysis.	Anemia; alpha-thalassemia.*
External examination	Record weight, size and gross appearance of neonate.	Fetal hydrops; sacrococcygeal teratoma; cystic hygroma.
	Photograph all external abnormalities.	
	Obtain fascia lata or liver sample for karyotype analysis.	Monosomy X (Turner's syndrome*); Trisomy 21 (Down's syndrome*); Trisomy 18 (Edward's syndrome).
	Obtain radiograph of fetus.	Chondrodysplasia* (many types). Chest and
abdominal cavities	Record volume and color of effusions.	Pleural effusions that may be chylous; ascites. (Effusions become serosanguinous with intrauterine retention following fetal death.)
Heart and great vessels	Ascertain venous and arterial connections before separating the heart from the organ block.	Left or right ventricular hypoplasia;* atrioventricular septal defect;* rhabdomyoma.
Lungs	Note positioning of lungs *in situ*.	Right-sided diaphragmatic hernia with impingement on the inferior vena cava.
Genitourinary system	Ascertain patency of entire urinary system, from renal pelvis to urethra, including entire length of penis.	Urethral obstruction due to urethral valves or lack of canalization of distal penile urethra; cloacal malformations. Cystic renal disease *(5)*.
Other organs and tissues	Conduct complete autopsy with extensive histologic sampling; procedures depend on suspected underlying conditions *(6)*. Examine erythropoietic cells closely, looking for Parvovinas inclusions *(2)*.	See above under "Note" and also under the heading "Erythroblastosis fetalis."

References

1. Barron SD, Pass RF. Infectious causes of hydrops fetalis. Semin Perinatol 1995;19:493–501.
2. Cameron AD, Swain S, Patrick WJ. Human parvovirus B19 infection associated with hydrops fetalis. Aust NZ J Obstet Gynaecol 1997;37:316–319.
3. Knilans TK. Cardiac abnormalities associated with hydrops fetalis. Semin Perinatol 1995;19:483–492.
4. Tasso MJ, Martinez-Gutierrez A, Carrascosa C, Vazquez S, Tebar R. GM1-gangliosidosis presenting as nonimmune hydrops fetalis: a case report. J Perinat Med 1996;24:445–449.
5. Kim CK, Kim SK, Yang YH, Lee MS, Yoon JH, Park CI. A case of recurrent infantile polycystic kidney associated with hydrops fetalis. Yonsei Med J 1989;30:95–103.
6. Knisely AS. The pathologist and the hydropic placenta, fetus, or infant. Semin Perinatol 1995;19:525–531.

Hyoscyamine (See "Poisoning, alkaloid" and "Poisoning, atropine.")

Hyperaminoaciduria (See "Aminoaciduria.")

Hyperbetalipoproteinemia (See "Hyperlipoproteinemia.")
Hypercalcemia (See "Disorder, electrolyte(s).")

Hypercholesterolemia (See "Hyperlipoproteinemia.")

Hypercorticism (See "Hyperplasia, congenital adrenal" and "Syndrome, Cushing's.")

Hyperglycemia (See "Diabetes mellitus" and p. 114.)
Hyperkalemia (See "Disorder, electrolyte(s)" and p. 114.)

Hyperlipemia (See "Hyperlipoproteinemia.")

Hyperlipoproteinemia

Synonyms and Related Terms: Primary hyperlipoproteinemia (familial forms of apoprotein CII deficiency, hyperalphalipoproteinemia; hypercholesterolemia, hypertriglyceridemia, lipoprotein lipase deficiency, multiple lipoprotein-type hyperlipidemia, and type 3 hyperlipoproteinemia; polygenic hypercholesterolemia).

Organs and Tissues	*Procedures*	*Possible or Expected Findings*
External examination and skin	Record body weight and length. Record extent and nature of skin changes, including evidence of gangrene. Prepare photographs and histologic sections of skin tumors and other cutaneous lesions.	Obesity* is a common finding. Eruptive xanthomas (palms, elbows, knees) in some but not all types of hyperlipoproteinemia. Most prominent in apoprotein CII deficiency. Xanthomas of tendons (knees, elbows, dorsum of hands), xanthelasmas, and arcus corneae in familial hypercholesterolemia. Gangrene of lower extremities (see below under "Arteries").
Blood	Submit sample of serum for biochemical study.	
Heart	Photograph valvular lesions; freeze involved tissue for biochemical and histochemical study. Submit samples of involved tissue for electron microscopic study. If valvular leaflets contain calcific deposits, decalcification may be required. Request Verhoeff–van Gieson stain and frozen sections for Sudan stain. If coronary insufficiency or myocardial infarction is suspected, follow procedures described under "Disease, ischemic heart." For coronary arteriography, see Chapter 10.	Severe coronary atherosclerosis and myocardial infarcts in type 3 hyperlipoproteinemia and multiple lipoprotein-type hyperlipidemia.
Arteries	Record distribution of atherosclerotic lesions in aorta. Samples for histologic study should include aorta, coronary arteries, and peripheral arteries. See also above under "Heart."	Atherosclerosis of abdominal aorta and its branches and of carotid arteries. Coronary atherosclerosis (see above).
Pancreas	Submit samples of head, corpus, and tail for histologic study. If applicable, see also under "Diabetes mellitus."	Pancreatitis* in familial apoprotein CII deficiency.
Other organs	For special procedures and stains, see above under "Heart." Other procedures depend on expected findings or grossly identified abnormalities as listed in right-hand column.	Foam cells with triglycerides in liver, spleen, and bone marrow in familial lipoprotein lipase deficiency. Manifestations of diabetes mellitus* and hypothyroidism* in some cases of type 3 hyperlipoproteinemia.
Brain	For removal and specimen preparation, see Chapter 4.	Cerebral infarct (stroke*) in type 3 hyperlipoproteinemia.

Hypernatremia (See "Disorder, electrolyte(s).")

Hyperoxaluria

Synonyms and Related Terms: Oxalosis; primary hyperoxaluria type I (alanineglyoxylate aminotransferase deficiency); primary hyperoxaluria type II (D-glyceric acid dehydrogenase deficiency); secondary hyperoxaluria (see under "Note").

NOTE: In ethylene glycol poisoning,* oxalate crystals in media of small arteries, with associated ischemic lesions. Similar deposits may occur after long-term hemodialysis *(1)*. These conditions must be distinguished from the genetic disease. Also, oxa-late nephropathy may be a complication of short bowel syndrome.

If patient with congenital hyperoxaluria underwent liver or combined liver/kidney transplantation *(2)*, see also under these headings.

Organs and Tissues	*Procedures*	*Possible or Expected Findings*
External examination and skin	Submit samples of skin for histologic study. Prepare skeletal roentgenograms.	Oxalates in skin. Osteosclerosis, periosteal changes; calcifications of vessels and soft tissues.
Liver	Record weight and submit samples for histologic study.	Grossly normal but site of peroxisomal enzyme deficiency in type I hyperoxaluria (see "Synonyms and Related Terms").
Kidneys	Record weights, photograph surfaces and cut surfaces with renal pelves. Submit samples for histologic study.	Calcium oxalate nephrolithiasis;* nephrocalcinosis.
Other organs and tissues	Procedures depend on expected findings or grossly identified abnormalities as listed in right-hand column.	Oxalosis. Manifestations of kidney failure (uremia).* For oxalate deposits unrelated to congenital hyperoxaluria, see above under "Note."
Urine	Submit sample for biochemical study (see right-hand column).	Excess oxalate and glycolate in type I hyperoxaluria. In type II disease, L-glyceric acid and oxalate are found in excess.
Peripheral nerves		Oxaluria-associated polyneuropathy *(3)*.
Bones		Osteosclerosis, periosteal changes.

References

1. Elmstahl B, Rausing A. A case of hyperoxaluria. Radiological aspects. Acta Radiol 1997;38:1031–1034.
2. Watts RWE, Morgan SH, Danpure CJ, Purkiss P, Calne RY, Rolles K, et al. Combined hepatic and renal transplantation in primary hyperoxaluria type I: clinical report of nine cases. Am J Med 1991;90:179–188.
3. Galloway G, Giuliani MJ, Burns DK, Lacomis D. Neuropathy associated with hyperoxaluria: improvement after combined renal and liver trans-plantation. Brain Pathol 1998;8:247–251.

Hyperparathyroidism

Synonyms and Related Terms: Primary hyperparathyroidism; secondary hyperparathyroidism (see below under "Kidneys").

Possible Associated Conditions: Multiple endocrine neoplasia, type 1 (Wermer's syndrome): Hyperparathyroidism, tumors of the pituitary gland* and tumors of pancreatic islet cells, often with peptic ulcers; Multiple endocrine neoplasia, type 2a (Sipple's syndrome): Hyperparathyroidism, pheochromocytoma, and medullary carcinoma of the thyroid.

Organs and Tissues	*Procedures*	*Possible or Expected Findings*
External examination and skin	Record location of scars of previous operations in neck area.	
	If skin gangrene is present, prepare photographs and sample for histologic study.	Cutaneous skin gangrene in hyperparathyroidism due to chronic renal failure *(1)*, calcinosis cutis *(3)*.
	Prepare skeletal roentgenograms (include calvarium, distal clavicles, phalanges, and lamina dura of tooth sockets).	In severe cases, generalized osteitis fibrosa cystica (osteoclastic osteoporosis) may be present.
Vitreous	Submit specimen for calcium and phosphate determination.	Increased calcium concentrations.
Blood	Submit sample of serum for determination of calcium concentration.	Hypercalcemia occurs in primary hyperparathyroidism. Phosphate and phosphatase determinations are not reliable in postmortem blood. Calcium values may also increase after death.

Organs and Tissues	*Procedures*	*Possible or Expected Findings*
Urine		Hypercalciuria.
Neck organs	Photograph neck organs with parathyroid glands or tumor(s) *in situ*. Dissect all 4 (or more) glands, trim carefully, and record weight of each gland. Snap-freeze adenomatous, hyperplastic, or carcinomatous parathyroid tissue for biochemical study. Prepare tissue sample for electron microscopic study. Embed all glands in paraffin for histologic study. If metastases are suspected or identified, dissect all cervical lymph nodes and embed for histologic study. Dissect and record weight of thyroid gland. Prepare thin slices of gland and record presence and location of tumor(s) or intrathyroid parathyroid tissue.	Solitary adenoma; double or multiple adenomas; chief cell hyperplasia; carcinoma(s). Adenomas usually in the inferior glands. Aberrant glands in thymus, thyroid gland, pericardium, or behind esophagus. Cervical lymph node metastases from thyroid (medullary carcinoma of the thyroid gland) or parathyroid carcinoma.
Lungs	Submit samples for histologic study and request von Kossa's stain.	Metastatic calcification. Metastatic carcinoma.
Stomach and duodenum	Submit samples of stomach for histologic study.	Peptic ulcer(s);* metastatic calcification.
Gallbladder		Cholelithiasis.*
Pancreas	Submit samples of head, body, and tail for histologic study.	Pancreatitis* *(2)*, with or without calcifications.
Kidneys	Photograph cut surfaces with renal pelves. For histologic specimens, decalcification may be required. Request von Kossa's stain.	Nephrocalcinosis; nephrolithiasis* with calcium oxalate or calcium phosphate stones; pyelonephritis;* chronic glomerulonephritis* or other chronic renal disease causing secondary hyperparathyroidism.
Other endocrine glands	Dissect all endocrine glands. If endocrine tumors or other abnormalities are present, follow procedures described above under "Neck organs."	See above under "Possible Associated Conditions."
Bones	For removal, prosthetic repair, and specimen preparation, see Chapter 2; consult also roentgenograms.	Osteitis fibrosa generalisata (osteoclastic osteoporosis); osteoclastomas.
Joints	For study of synovial fluid, see under "Gout." For removal, prosthetic repair, and specimen preparation, see Chapter 2.	Chondrocalcinosis; pseudogout.*
Eyes	For removal and specimen preparation, see Chapter 5.	Band keratopathy; cataracts.

References

1. Torok L, Kozepessy L. Cutaneous gangrene due to hyperparathyroidism secondary to chronic renal failure (uremic gangrene syndrome). Clin Exp Dermatol 1996;21:75–77.
2. Inabnet WB, Baldwin D, Daniel RO, Staren ED. Hyperparathyroidism and pancreatitis during pregnancy. Surgery 1996;119:710–713.
3. Dubois LA. et al. Surgical images: soft tissue. Calcinosis cutis. Can J Surg 2007;50:217–218.

Hyperpituitarism (See "Acromegaly.")

Hyperplasia, Congenital Adrenal

Synonyms and Related Terms: Adrenocortical hyperplasia; deficiency of 17α-hydroxylase, 20α-hydroxylase, or 11β-hydrox-ylase *(1)*; deficiency of 21-hydroxylase *(1,2)*; deficiency of 3β-hydroxysteroid dehydrogenase *(1)*; deficiency of 18-hydroxylase/hydroxysteroid dehydrogenase; deficiency of 20,22 desmolase; female pseudohermaphroditism.

Organs and Tissues	*Procedures*	*Possible or Expected Findings*
External examination	Record body weight and length. Describe and photograph primary and secondary sex characteristics.	Ambiguous, incompletely differentiated external genitalia; virilism in female infants and teenagers; precocious puberty in male patients; premature pubic hair *(3)*.
Adrenal glands	Record sizes and weights. Snap-freeze material	Cortical hyperplasia with elevated weight.

Organs and Tissues	Procedures	Possible or Expected Findings
	for biochemical, DNA or histochemical study.	
Gonads		Polycystic ovaries, testicular adrenal rests *(4)*.
Other organs and body fluids, including urine	Submit samples for histologic study.	Manifestations of hypertension.*
	Submit urine sample for biochemical study.	Increased concentration of urinary pregnanetriol and 17-ketosteroids.
	Remove vitreous for biochemical evalvation.	Electrolyte abnormalities in vitreous, related to dehydration,* hyperkalemia, and hyponatremia. Hypoglycemia* may have been present but usually cannot be demonstrated after death.
	Submit tissue (i.e., fascia lata) for karyotype analysis.	

References

1. Pang S. Congenital adrenal hyperplasia. Baillieres Clin Obstet Gynaecol 1997;11:281–306.
2. Cutler GB Jr, Lave L. Congenital adrenal hyperplasia due to 21-hydroxylase deficiency. N Engl J Med 1990;323:1806–1813.
3. Rosenfield RL. Hyperandrogenism in peripubertal girls. Ped Clin North Am 1990;37:1333–1358.
4. Fitoz S, et al. Testicular adrenal rests in a patient with congenital adrenal hyperplasia: US and MRI features. Comput Med Imaging Graph 2006;30:465–468.

Hypertension (Systemic Arterial), All Types or Type Unspecified

Synonyms and Related Terms: Arterial hypertension; benign hypertension; essential hypertension; idiopathic hypertension; malignant hypertension; paroxysmal hypertension.

NOTE: If underlying disease is known—for instance, coarctation of the aorta, pheochromocytoma, or toxemia of pregnancy—see also under that entry.

Organs and Tissues	Procedures	Possible or Expected Findings
External examination	Record body weight and length. Prepare chest roentgenogram.	Obesity;* cushingoid features.
Blood and urine	Submit samples for biochemical and toxicologic study.	Lead poisoning;* porphyria.*
Heart	Record actual and expected weights (see Part III tables). For coronary arteriography, see Chapter 10. Submit samples for histologic examination.	Hypertrophy of the heart, primarily of the left ventricle; coronary atherosclerosis; ischemic myocardial changes; catecholamine cardiomyopathy (see below under "Adrenal glands").
Arteries	For carotid and cerebral arteriography, see Chapter 4. For arteriography of lower extremities, see Chapter 10. Request Verhoeff–van Gieson stain for histologic sections of elastic and muscular arteries.	Atherosclerosis and arteriolosclerosis. Renal artery stenosis* or fibromuscular dysplasia. Coarctation of the aorta.* Polyarteritis nodosa.*
Pancreas	Submit samples for histologic study.	Arteriolar necrosis with hemorrhages and infarctions (in malignant hypertension).
Kidneys	Record appearance of renal ostia and arteries. If parenchymal renal disease is suspected, follow procedures described under "Glomerulonephritis."	Renal artery stenosis* or dysplasia. Diabetic nephropathy. Renal involvement in immune connective tissue disease; chronic or acute glomerulonephritis;* pyelonephritis.*
Adrenal glands	Freeze tissue for possible biochemical study (indicated only if a tumor is present or evidence is obtained of adrenocortical hyperfunction). "See also under "Tumor, of the adrenal glands."	Pheochromocytoma; congenital adrenal hyperplasia.* (See also under "Aldosteronism.")
Ovaries	If a tumor is present, snap-freeze tissue for possible biochemical study.	Hypertension-producing ovarian tumor.
Parathyroid glands	See under "Hyperparathyroidism."	Hyperplasia or adenoma with hyperparathyroidism.*

Organs and Tissues	*Procedures*	*Possible or Expected Findings*
Brain	For removal and specimen preparation, see Chapter 4.	Subarachnoid or intraparenchymal hemorrhage; infarction* or other condition causing increased intracranial pressure.
Eyes	For removal and specimen preparation, see Chapter 5.	Hypertensive retinopathy.

Hypertension, Intracranial (See "Pseudotumor cerebri.")

Hypertension, Portal

Related Terms: Idiopathic portal hypertension; postsinusoidal portal hypertension; presinusoidal portal hypertension.

Organs and Tissues	*Procedures*	*Possible or Expected Findings*
External examination	Record circumference of abdomen.	Periumbilical veins that were distended during life (caput medusae; Cruveilhier-Baumgarten syndrome) usually collapse after death.
Abdominal cavity	Submit fluid for bacterial culture; record volume; submit samples of peritoneum for histologic study.	Ascites; peritonitis;* carcinomatosis.
Heart, inferior vena cava, and hepatic veins	If portal hypertension is suspected to have been caused by cardiac or other postsinusoidal venous disease, follow procedures described under "Syndrome, Budd-Chiari."	Manifestations of Budd-Chiari syndrome.*
Lungs	Submit samples for histologic evaluation of pulmonary vasculature. Request Verhoeff-van Gieson stain.	Coexistent pulmonary hypertension; hepatopulmonary syndrome.
Abdominal wall	If presence of portal vein thrombosis is suspected in a neonate, submit samples of umbilicus and umbilical vein for histologic study.	Umbilical sepsis in neonate.
	In adults with caput medusae, submit samples of ductus venosus and of umbilical vein for determination of luminal width.	Caput medusae.
Portal vein system	Open portal, splenic, and mesenteric veins *in situ* or after en bloc removal of abdominal organs. If site of obstruction is unknown, prepare portal angiogram from splenic or mesenteric vein.	Portal vein thrombosis; pylephlebitis. Developmental obliteration or valve formation of portal vein is rare. Splenic arteriovenous fistula, tumor, or abscess may be present.
	If cavernous transformation of portal vein is suspected, prepare horizontal sections through hepatoduodenal ligament.	Cavernous transformation of portal vein.
Thoracic duct	For dissection of the thoracic duct, see Chapter 3.	Dilatation of thoracic duct.
Esophagus, stomach, and intestinal tract (with anus)	For demonstration of varices, see Chapter 2. Record volume of blood in lumen.	Esophageal varices;* gastric varices; gastritis *(1)*. gastrointestinal hemorrhage;* hemorrhoids.
Liver	Record weight and photograph. Slice liver in frontal planes and leave hepatoduodenal ligament attached to slice in hilar plane. Submit samples for histologic study. Other procedures depend on expected findings or grossly identified abnormalities as listed in right-hand column.	Cirrhosis;* tumor of the liver;* congenital hepatic fibrosis;* chronic alcoholic or nonalcoholic steatohepatitis; nodular regenerative hyperplasia, associated with conditions such as Felty's syndrome* or rheumatoid arthritis.* Schistosomiasis,* vascular malformation, and other hepatic conditions also may cause portal hypertension.

Organs and Tissues	Procedures	Possible or Expected Findings
Spleen	Record weight and size. Submit samples for histologic study.	Congestive splenomegaly; extramedullary hematopoiesis (see above under "Liver").
Pancreas		Pancreatitis.*
Other organs	If pylephlebitis is suspected, record site and character of suspected source of infection.	Appendicitis; other suppurative abdominal infection; malignant tumor; manifestations of polycythemia* or of other hematologic disorder. See also above under "Liver."
Brain		Hepatic encephalopathy.*

Reference

1. El-Rifai N, et al. Gastropathy and gastritis in children with portal hypertension. J Pediatr Gastroenterol Nutr 2007;45:137–140.

Hypertension, Pulmonary

Synonyms and Related Terms: Chronic pulmonary venous hypertension; coexistent portal and pulmonary hypertension; cor pulmonale; hypoxic pulmonary hypertension; neoplastic embolic pulmonary hypertension; primary pulmonary hypertension; plexogenic pulmonary hypertension; pulmonary heart disease; pulmonary veno-occlusive disease; thromboembolic pulmonary hypertension.

Organs and Tissues	Procedures	Possible or Expected Findings
External examination	Prepare chest roentgenogram.	Enlarged right atrium and pulmonary arteries.
Heart	Record heart weight and dimensions.	Hypertrophy and dilatation of right ventricle and right atrium. Straightened septum with D-shaped ventricles. Dilated tricuspid and pulmonary valves.
Lungs	Record weights of lungs. For pulmonary arteriography and venography, see Chapter 2. Perfuse lungs with formalin. Prepare slides from each lobe, both centrally and peripherally. Request Verhoeff–van Gieson stain on all blocks.	Obstructive pulmonary arterial and/or pulmonary venous lesions (most commonly plexogenic or thrombotic type). Interstitial pneumonia;* bronchiectases;* pulmonary emphysema;* pulmonary artery aneurysm; pulmonary artery rupture; pulmonary capillary hemangiomatosis. See also above under "Synonyms and Related Terms."
Abdominal viscera	Record actual and expected weights of liver and spleen.	Congestive hepatosplenomegaly. Pre-existing cirrhosis with portal and pulmonary hypertension.

Hyperthermia (See "Heatstroke.")

Hyperthyroidism

Synonyms and Related Terms: Basedow's disease; Graves' disease; thyrotoxicosis.

Organs and Tissues	Procedures	Possible or Expected Findings
External examination, skin, and breasts	Record body weight and length; photograph face and neck; record neck circumference. Prepare histologic sections of skin lesions and of breast tissue.	Emaciation; exophthalmos; hyperpigmentation and vitiligo, particularly of hands and feet; fingernail (ring finger) abnormalities; pretibial myxedema above level of lateral malleolus; gynecomastia.
	Prepare skeletal roentgenograms.	Osteoporosis.*
Blood and urine	If hormone assay or preparation of a drug screen is intended, store samples in deepfreeze. Determination of serum calcium concentration is unreliable (use vitreous).	Postmortem concentrations of thyroxine or thyroid-stimulating hormone appear to reflect antemortem values. Hypercalcemia may be present.
Thymus	Dissect and record weight. Submit samples for histologic study.	Hyperplasia of thymus.
Heart	Record weight of heart and size of heart chambers. Submit sections for histologic study.	Atrial dilatation indicates previous episodes of atrial fibrillation *(1)*.

Organs and Tissues	Procedures	Possible or Expected Findings
Neck organs	Remove neck organs together with goiter and and tongue; record weights of thyroid and parathyroid glands. If thyroid tumor is present, photograph together with scale. If carcinoma of the thyroid gland is suspected, dissect regional lymph nodes and submit for histologic study.	Nodular (colloid) goiter; diffuse thyroid hyperplasia; thyroid adenoma(s) or carcinoma(s); subacute thyroiditis.*
Lymph nodes; other endocrine glands	Record average size of lymph nodes. In addition to thyroid weight, record weights of all other endocrine glands and submit samples for histologic study. See also below under "Pituitary gland."	Lymphadenopathy.
Tumor with possible endocrine activity	Submit samples for hormone assay, light microscopic study, and electron microscopy.	Choriocarcinoma of uterus or testis; hydatidiform mole may cause thyrotoxicosis without thyroid abnormalities. See also below under "Pituitary gland".
Other organs		Manifestations of congestive heart failure.*
Pituitary gland	For removal and specimen preparation, see Chapter 4. If a pituitary tumor is present, it should be weighed, measured, split in half, photographed, and one-half placed in deep-freeze for hormone assay. From the other half, a small sample should be prepared for electron microscopic study and the remainder for light microscopy.	Pituitary adenoma with secretion of thyroid-stimulating hormone may cause thyrotoxicosis without thyroid abnormalities. Acromegaly* (see above) may be present.
Vitreous	If electrolyte abnormalities are suspected, submit sample of vitreous.	Manifestations of electrolyte disorder.*
Eyes and their adnexae	For removal and specimen preparation of eyes, see Chapter 5. Submit samples of retrobulbar tissue, extraocular muscles, and lacrimal glands.	Exophthalmos with puffy lids, chemosis, and eye infection.
Bones		Osteoporosis.*

Reference

1. Aronow WS. The heart and thyroid disease. Clin Geriatr Med 1995;11:219–229.

Hypertrophy, Cardiac

Organs and Tissues	Procedures	Possible or Expected Findings
Heart	Record actual and expected weights. If determination of myocardial mass is needed, record specific gravity of heart. For coronary arteriography, see Chapter 10. Record ventricular wall thicknesses and appearance and annular circumferences of valves. If cardiomyopathy is suspected, electron microscopic study may be indicated.	Coronary atherosclerosis; myocardial infarction; pericarditis;* congenital or acquired valvular heart disease; other congenital heart disease. Most abnormal conditions of the heart are associated with hypertrophy (or increased mass), with or without chamber dilatation Cardiomyopathy.*
Other organs	Procedures depend on expected findings or grossly identified abnormalities as listed in right-hand column.	Manifestations of systemic hypertension;* pulmonary vascular disease with hypertension, including pulmonary embolism;* amyloidosis,* hemochromatosis,* Fabry's disease,* or glycogen storage disease.*

Hypervitaminosis A

Related Term: Vitamin A toxicity.

NOTE: The findings listed below refer to chronically increased vitamin A ingestion.

Organs and Tissues	*Procedures*	*Possible or Expected Findings*
External examination	Record extent and character of skin lesions; photograph skin lesions. Submit specimens of affected and unaffected skin for histologic study. Prepare skeletal roentgenograms.	Yellow or orange skin *(2)*. Brittle hair; desquamation of skin, particularly of palms and soles; nail abnormalities. Clubbing of fingers (in children). Osteoporosis;* fractures; periosteal proliferation, particularly of ulnae, clavicles, and metatarsal bones; tumefaction of midshafts of long bones. Osteoarthritis *(1)*.
Liver	Record weight and size; photograph surface and cut section; submit fresh tissue for demonstration of vitamin A fluorescence in frozen sections or for chemical analysis. Request frozen sections for Sudan stain. For paraffin sections, request van Gieson's stain.	Fatty changes in liver with characteristic quick-fading green fluorescence. Hepatic fibrosis or cirrhosis.*
Other organs	Submit samples of spleen, kidneys, and parathyroid glands for histologic study.	
Brain	For removal and specimen preparation, see Chapter 4.	Pseudotumor cerebri;* hydrocephalus,* particularly in infants.
Bones and joints	For optimal sites for histologic study, see above under "External examination and skin." For removal, prosthetic repair, and specimen preparation, see Chapter 2.	Calcification of cartilage, osteoporosis *(3)*. and periosteal proliferations. Hyperostotic and destructive osteoarthritis *(1)*. See also above under "External examination and skin."

Reference

1. Romero JB, Schreiber A, von Hochstetter AR, Wagenhauser FJ, Michel BA, Theiler R. Hyperostotic and destructive osteoarthritis in a patient with vitamin A intoxication syndrome: a case report. Bull Hosp Joint Dis 1996;54:169–174.
2. Miesen W. Yellow or orange hands as presenting signs of carotenaemia. Neth J Med 2006;64:56–57.
3. Penniston KL, Tanumihardio SA. The acute and chronic toxic effects of vitamin A. Am J Clin Nutr 2006;83:191–201.

Hypervitaminosis D

Related Term: Vitamin D toxicity.

Organs and Tissues	*Procedures*	*Possible or Expected Findings*
External examination and skin	Prepare skeletal roentgenograms.	Osteoporosis;* para-articular calcifications; other metastatic calcifications. In infants, radiopacity may be found—primarily at epiphyseal ends of the shafts of long tubular bones.
	Submit specimens of skin and of subcutaneous tissue for histologic study.	Metastatic calcification.
Vitreous	Submit sample for determination of calcium and phosphate concentrations. If histologic study of eyes is intended, remove vitreous from only one eye.	Increased calcium concentrations.
Blood	Postmortem calcium values are unreliable.	Hypercalcemia.
Lungs	Inflate one fresh lung with carbon dioxide and prepare roentgenogram for demonstration of calcium deposits. Then, perfuse lung with formalin. For histologic sections, request von Kossa's stain for calcium. Decalcification of tissue may be required.	Metastatic calcification.

Organs and Tissues	Procedures	Possible or Expected Findings
Kidneys	Prepare soft tissue roentgenograms. Request von Kossa's stain. Decalcification of tissue may be required.	Metastatic calcification.
Parathyroid glands	Record weights of all parathyroid glands and submit samples for histologic study.	Normal parathyroid glands.
Other organs	Histologic samples should include heart, pancreas, fundus and body of stomach, elastic and muscular arteries, and lymph nodes. See also above under "Kidneys."	Metastatic calcification. If applicable, see also under "Failure, kidney."
Brain and spinal cord	Submit samples of tentorium and falx cerebri for histologic study.	Metastatic calcification of tentorium and falx cerebri.
Eyes	For removal and specimen preparation, see Chapter 5. See also above under "Vitreous."	Metastatic calcium deposits in corneas and conjunctivas.
Bones and joints	For removal, prosthetic repair, and specimen preparation, see Chapter 2. For optimal sampling, consult roentgenograms.	Metastatic calcification in synovial tissue and in bone marrow. See also above under "External examination and skin."

Hypnotic(s) (See "Dependence, drug(s), all types or type unspecified" and "Poisoning, barbiturate(s).")

Hypocalcemia (See "Disorder, electrolyte(s).")

Hypofibrinogenemia (See "Coagulation, disseminated intravascular.")

Hypogammaglobulinemia

Synonyms and Related Terms: Acquired hypogammaglobulinemia; agammaglobulinemia; congenital hypogammaglobulinemia; Good's syndrome (thymoma and hypogammaglobulinemia) *(1)*.

Possible Associated Conditions: Campylobacter, meningococcal, pneumococcal and other infections, including infections by *S. pneumoniae* and *H. influenzae*. Malabsorption syndrome;* multiple myeloma,* and systemic amyloidosis* *(2)*. (See also under "Syndrome, primary immunodeficiency.")

Organs and Tissues	Procedures	Possible or Expected Findings
Chest cavity		Thymoma *(1)*.
Intestinal tract	Open and fix the intestine as soon as possible.	Sprue-type changes of intestinal mucosa with malabsorption syndrome.* *Giardia lamblia* infection.
Liver		Chronic hepatitis C *(3)*.
Brain and spinal cord	For removal and specimen preparation, see Chapter 4.	Encephalomyelitis *(4)*.
Bones and joints	For removal, prosthetic repair, and specimen preparation, see Chapter 2.	Arthritis (with features of rheumatoid arthritis*)
Eye		Retinitis pigmentosa *(5)*.

References

1. Verne GN, Amann ST, Cosgrove C, Cerda JJ. Chronic diarrhea associated with thymoma and hypogammaglobulinemia (Good's syndrome). South Med J 1997;90:444–446.
2. Kotilainen P, Vuori K, Kainulainen L, Aho H, Saario R, Asola M, et al. Systemic amyloidosis in a patient with hypogammaglobulinemia. J Intern Med 1996;240:103–106.
3. Quinti I, Pandolfi F, Paganelli R, el Salman D, Giovannetti A, Rosso R, et al. HCV infection in patients with primary defects of immunoglobulin production. Clin Exp Immunol 1995;102:11–16.
4. Rudge P, Webster AD, Revesz T, Warner T, Espanol T, Cunningham-Rundles C, et al. Encepahomyelitis in primary hypogammaglobulinemia. Brain 1996;119:1–15.
5. Starr JC, et al. Retinitis pigmentosa and hypogammaglobulinemia. South Med J 2006;99:989–991.

Hypoglycemia

NOTE: Currently, no reliable diagnostic tests are available for the postmortem diagnosis of hypoglycemia.

Organs and Tissues	Procedures	Possible or Expected Findings
Vitreous	Submit sample of vitreous for determination of glucose and ketone levels.	Postmortem glycolysis by the retinal cells may be very rapid. Thus, an elevated vitreous glucose level establishes the presence of hyperglycemia. For interpretation of findings, see Table 8-1.
Blood		Glucose concentrations are totally unreliable.
Brain	Request Luxol fast blue stain.	Petechial or larger hemorrhages; ganglion cell degeneration, gliosis, and demyelinization, all of which are non-specific.

Hypokalemia (See "Disorder, electrolyte(s)" and p. 114.)

Hypolipoproteinemia (See "Abetalipoproteinemia" and "Disease, Tangier's.")

Hyponatremia (See "Disorder, electrolyte(s)")

Hypoparathyroidism

Synonyms: Acquired hypoparathyroidism; hereditary hypoparathyroidism; idiopathic hypoparathyroidism.

Possible Associated Conditions: Autoimmune polyglandular deficiency (often with alopecia, megaloblastic anemia;* mucocutaneous candidiasis, and vitiligo); DiGeorge syndrome* (defective development of thymus, parathyroid glands, and other organs).

Organs and Tissues	Procedures	Possible or Expected Findings
External examination and skin; teeth	Record location of scars of previous neck surgery and abnormalities of skin, hair, nails, and teeth. Submit samples of normal and abnormal skin for histologic study.	Scars of previous neck surgery; coarse skin, with or without subcutaneous calcifications; malformed nails; dysplasia of enamel; alopecia.
	Prepare skeletal roentgenograms.	Dense bones; thickening of calvarium.
Urine and vitreous	Submit samples for determination of calcium concentrations. Postmortem calcium values in blood are unreliable.	Hypocalcemia; hypocalciuria.
Parathyroid glands	Record weights of all parathyroid glands. Submit samples for histologic study.	Parathyroid glands may not be present (after intentional or unintentional surgical removal).
Other organs	Procedures depend on expected findings or grossly identified abnormalities as listed in right-hand column. If an infection is suspected, submit material for microbiologic study.	Cardiomyopathy* *(1)*; manifestations of Addison's disease; candidiasis;* ovarian failure, or megaloblastic anemia *(2)**. Malabsorption with steatorrhea and myopathy with muscular atrophy may occur.
Brain and spinal cord		Calcification in basal ganglia.
Eyes	For removal and specimen preparation, see Chapter 5.	Cataracts.
Bones	For removal, prosthetic repair, and specimen preparation, see Chapter 2. Consult roentgenograms.	See above under "External examination and skin."

References

1. Suzuki T, Ikeda U, Fujikawa H, Saito K, Shimada K. Hypocalcemic heart failure: a reversible form of heart muscle disease. Clin Cardiol 1998;21: 227–228.
2. Abramowicz MJ, Cochaux P, Cohen LH, Vamos E. Pernicious anaemia and hypoparathyroidism in a patient with Kearns-Sayre syndrome with mitochondrial DNA duplication. J Inherit Metabol Dis 1996;19:109–111.

Hypophosphatasia (See "Deficiency, vitamin D" and "Osteomalacia.")

Hypophosphatemia, Familial (See "Syndrome, Fanconi.")
Hypopituitarism (See "Insufficiency, pituitary.")

Hypoplasia, Left Ventricular
Possible Associated Conditions: Congenital aortic valvular stenosis* or atresia (hypoplastic left heart syndrome); coarctation of the aorta;* hypoplasia of ascending aorta; left ventricular endocardial fibroelastosis;* mitral atresia.*

Hypoplasia, Right Ventricular
Possible Associated Conditions: Congenital pulmonary stenosis* or atresia with intact ventricular septum;* congenital tricuspid stenosis or atresia;* restrictive ventricular septal defect;* transposition of the great arteries.

Hypoplasia, Tubular, of Aortic Arch
Possible Associated Conditions: Coarctation of the aorta;* malaligned ventricular septal defect; patent ductal artery;* subaortic stenosis.

Hypothermia (See "Exposure, cold.")

Hypothyroidism
Synonyms: Cretinism; goitrous hypothyroidism; myxedema; primary hypothyroidism; secondary hypothyroidism.

Organs and Tissues	*Procedures*	*Possible or Expected Findings*
External examination, skin, and breasts	Record body weight and length and facial features; record location of scars of previous neck surgery.	In cretinism, body is small for age and head is large with coarse facial features and protruding tongue. In adults, brittle hair, sparse eyebrows, and puffiness of face are present. Surgical scars of neck.
	Prepare histologic sections of skin and of breast tissue.	Perifollicular keratosis of skin; thickened nails; galactorrhea.
	Prepare roentgenograms of chest and of joints.	Pleural* and pericardial effusions; joint effusions; degenerative joint disease involving knees, hips, hands, and other joints *(1)*; thicke ing of joint capsules; bursitis.
Vitreous	Submit for determination of sodium concentration.	Low sodium concentration.
Abdomen	Record volume of effusion.	Ascites.
Pleural and pericardial cavities	Record volume of effusion(s).	Hydrothorax and hydropericardium, with or without cardiac tamponade.
Blood	Submit sample for microbiologic study. If hormone assay is intended, snap-freeze sample.	Septicemia; hypercholesterolemia.
Thymus	Record weight and submit samples for histologic study.	
Heart	Record weight; photograph; submit samples for histologic study.	Dilatation of the heart.* See also under "Failure, congestive heart."
Arteries	Record degree of atherosclerosis of aorta, coronary arteries, cerebral arteries, and other muscular arteries.	Increased atherosclerosis.
Neck organs	Remove neck organ together with tongue. Prepare histologic sections of tongue with papillae. Record weight of thyroid gland; photograph and submit samples for histologic study. Record weights of parathyroid glands. If patient was recently treated with radionuclides, see Chapter 11.	Macroglossia; Hashimoto's thyroiditis; Riedel's struma; subacute thyroiditis (see also under "Thyroiditis"); colloid goiter; tumor of the thyroid gland after treatment with radioactive iodine; surgically removed thyroid gland; thyroid aplasia (in cretinism).
Lymph nodes	Record average size and submit samples of histologic study.	
Intestinal tract		Ileus; megacolon.

Organs and Tissues	Procedures	Possible or Expected Findings
Urine	Submit sample for determination of glucose and ketone concentrations.	In presence of hypoglycemia,* urine contains no glucose or ketone.
Other organs	Submit samples of adrenal glands, gonads, and tail of pancreas (for islets of Langerhans) for histologic study.	
Brain, spinal cord, and pituitary gland	For removal and specimen preparation, see Chapter 4.	Hypothalamic congenital defects, infections, tumor, or sarcoidosis* may cause trophoprivi chypothyroidsim. For other causes, see "Insufficiency, pituitary."
Skeletal muscles	For sampling and specimen preparation, see Chapter 2.	
Joints and bursae	For removal, prosthetic repair, and specimen preparation of joints, see Chapter 2.	See above under "External examination, skin, and breasts."

Reference

1. McLean RM, Podell DN. Bone and joint manifestations of hypothyroidism. Semin Arthritis Rheum 1995;24:282–290.

Hypovitaminosis A (See "Deficiency, vitamin A.")

Hypovitaminosis D (See "Deficiency, vitamin D.")

Hypoxemia (See "Hypoxia.")

Hypoxia

Related Terms: Asphyxia; hypoxemia; suffocation.

NOTE: There are no diagnostic autopsy findings for hypoxia. Possible causes of acute hypoxia include anesthesia-associated death,* compression of the torso by a vehicle, diving accident,* exposure to toxic gases—for instance, carbon monoxide poisoning;* mechanical failure of an oxygen supply system, as in an airplane; and sudden mechanical airway obstruction,* as in aspiration of a foreign body or strangulation. Causes of chronic asphyxia include prolonged exposure to high altitude and chronic pulmonary disease.

Organs and Tissues	Procedures	Possible or Expected Findings
External examination	Record appearance of head, oral cavity, and neck area.	Cyanosis is found in any congested body; but red lividity may indicate carbon monoxide poisoning. Foreign body in mouth or pharynx. Ligature or fingernail marks.
Skin, sclerae, mucosal surfaces, and serosal surfaces		Petechiae and Tardieu spots are non-specific manifestations of increased venous pressure including that caused by lividity but may help point the investigation toward mechanical asphyxia.
Blood	Submit sample for toxicologic study, for instance, for determination of carbon monoxide concentration.	Blood is often liquid. Clotted blood does not rule out asphyxia because death by asphyxia may be hastened by ventricular arrhythmia in a subject with heart disease.
Heart	Record weight. Determine ventricular wall thickness.	Right ventricular hypertrophy.
Lungs	Record weights. Perfuse at least one lung with formalin. Request Verhoeff–van Gieson stain.	Profound medial hypertrophy of small pulmonary arteries and of pulmonary veins from chronic exposure to hypoxia. Acute pulmonary edema may also occur in chronic hypoxia.

Organs and Tissues	*Procedures*	*Possible or Expected Findings*
Neck organs	Dissection and removal should be done by the pathologist, not a technician. Remove carefully to avoid dislodging foreign body.	
Brain	For removal and specimen preparation, see. Chapter 4	Cerebral edema in acute mountain sickness.
Middle ears	For removal and specimen preparation, see Chapter 4.	Mucosal hemorrhages and congestion are non-specific manifestations of increased vascular pressure, including that caused by lividity.

I

Ileus, Meconium

Possible Associated Conditions: Congenital megacolon;* cystic fibrosis;* syphilis.* *(1)*.

Organs and Tissues	*Procedures*	*Possible or Expected Findings*
External examination	Record height, weight, and abdominal circumference.	Malnutrition.
Abdominal cavity and intestinal tract	Examine and sample the bowel early in the procedure to minimize autolysis. Record location and character of meconium and of liquid contents, and determine thickness of intestinal wall. Record location of stenosis, atresia, or dilatation. Submit samples of all portions of intestinal tract for histologic study.	Empty and collapsed colon; small amounts of gray and dry meconium in terminal ileum; meconium masses in dilated and hypertrophied mid-ileum; liquid contents in proximal intestine *(1)*; appendicitis; bowel perforation. Glandular inspissation and atrophy of intestinal mucosa. Volvulus, infarction, necrosis, perforation, peritonitis, and acquired intestinal atresia may be present. Absence of neural plexuses in congential megacolon* (Hirschsprung's disease).
Other organs	Procedures depend on expected findings or grossly identified abnormalities as listed in right-hand column.	Manifestations of cystic fibrosis, with or without cirrhosis;* biliary atresia* *(3)*.

References

1. Siplovich L, Davies MR, Kaschula RO, Cywes S. Intestinal obstruction in the newborn with congenital syphilis. J Pediatr Surg 1988;23:810–813.
2. Maurage C, Lenaerts C, Weber A, Brochu P, Yousef I, Roy CC. Meconium ileus and its equivalent as a risk factor for the development of cirrhosis: an autopsy study in cystic fibrosis. J Ped Gastroenterol Nutr 1989;9:17–20.
3. Adam G, Brereton RJ, Agrawal M, Lake BD. Biliary atresia and meconium ileus associated with Nieman-Pick disease. J Ped Gastroenterol Nutr 1988;7:128–131.

Immunodeficiency (See "Syndrome, acquired immunodeficiency" and "Syndrome, primary immunodeficiency.")

Impression, Basilar

NOTE: Basilar impression constitutes an upward bulging of the margins of the foramen magnum. When occipital condyles are displaced above the plane of the foramen magnum, basilar invagination is present.

Possible Associated Conditions: Klippel-Feil syndrome;* osteogenesis imperfecta;* osteomalacia;* Paget's disease of bone;* rheumatoid arthritis; rickets; syringobulbia; syringomylia.*

Organs and Tissues	*Procedures*	*Possible or Expected Findings*
External examination		Shortness of neck.
Skull and spine	Prepare roentgenograms. For dissection of cervical spine, see Chapter 4.	Arnold-Chiari malformation;* fusion of atlas to base of skull; malpositioning of odontoid process; platybasia.*

From: *Handbook of Autopsy Practice,* 4th Ed. Edited by: B.L. Waters

Organs and Tissues	Procedures	Possible or Expected Findings
Brain and spinal cord	For removal and specimen preparation, see Chapter 4.	Compression and secondary ischemic injury to lower brain stem and spinal cord. See also above under "Skull and spine" and under "Possible Associated Conditions."

Incompetence,... (See "Insufficiency,...")

Infanticide

Related Terms: Battered-child syndrome; child-abuse or child-neglect death.

NOTE: Vitreous should *not* be aspirated until the skull has been opened and trauma ruled out, because there is a risk of artifactual damage to the retina. In the presence of craniocerebral trauma the pathologist can opt to examine the eyes by removal, fixation, and histologic study; or retinal photography.

Follow general procedures described under "Homicide" and, if necessary,. the procedures described under "Rape."

Organs and Tissues	Procedures	Possible or Expected Findings
External examination	See above under "Note." Prepare roentgenograms of entire body.	In the abused child, bruises, hematomas, burn marks, or other patterned injuries. In any child, diaper rash, Mongolian spots, self-inflicted fingernail scratches, skin infections, and emaciation. In the previously battered child, fractures in various states of healing.
Vitreous	See above under "Note." In other situations, or after study of the fundus, submit sample of vitreous for chemical and possible toxicologic study.	In hypertonic dehydration,* sodium concentrations more than 150 meq/L. This may be caused by organic disease, improper medical treatment, or physical neglect.
Umbilical cord attachment	Prepare histologic sections of umbilicus. and end of umbilical cord	If infant was born alive, inflammatory changes may be found, depending on survival interval.
Blood	Submit sample for toxicologic study. Consider retaining dried blood on filter paper for possible DNA testing for paternity investigation.	
Lungs	If there is a possibility that the cadaver represents a stillbirth, see Part II, "Stillbirth".	For the hydrostatic lung test, see "Stillbirth." The test is unreliable. Extraneous material in air passages indicates that child was alive.
Gastrointestinal tract	If infant is thought to have died shortly after birth, determine the location of air in the intestinal tract; roentgenograms may be helpful.	Air reaches the stomach after 15 min, the small intestine after 1–2 h, the colon after 5–6 h, and the rectum after 12 h. There is no difference in the speed of gas propulsion between full-term and premature infants. Bacterial gas production and previous resuscitation attempts are potential sources of errors.
	Save stomach contents and record amount.	In questionable stillbirth, presence of milk proves that infant was alive and had been nursed.
Other organs	See also under "Homicide."	Traumatic lesions and signs of neglect may be present.

Reference

1. Hart BL, Dudley MH, Zumwalt RE. Postmortem cranial MRI and autopsy correlation in suspected child abuse. Am J Forens Med Pathol 1996;17:217–224.

Infarction, Cerebral
Related Term: Stroke

Organs and Tissues	Procedures	Possible or Expected Findings
Heart	If infective endocarditis is suspected, culture any possible vegetation. Record presence or absence of patent oval foramen or other septal defects.	Myocardial infarction or other cardiac lesions that may cause systemic circulatory failure. Valvular vegetations and mural thrombi may be source of cerebral emboli; paradoxic embolism.
Aorta	Procedures depend on expected findings or grossly identified abnormalities as listed in right-hand column.	Aortic dissection. atherosclerosis with or without mural thrombi; atheromas.
Cervical arteries	For dissection and roentgenologic demonstration of carotid and vertebral arteries, see Chapter 4.	Dissecting hematoma of cervical arteries; atherosclerosis with or without thrombosis; atheromas of cervical arteries, particularly in carotid bulb.
Femoral and other systemic veins	For removal of femoral veins, see Chapter 3.	Thromboses as source of paradoxic cerebral embolism.
Brain	For cerebral arteriography, see Chapter 10. For removal and specimen preparation, see Chapter 4.	Atherosclerosis of intracranial arteries. Cerebral infarcts (white or red) of different size, age, and distribution. Watershed (boundary) zones are most frequently affected in global ischemia caused by systemic circulatory failure.
Cerebral venous sinuses	For exposure of venous sinuses, see Chapter 4.	Cerebral venous sinus thrombosis;* thrombosis of tributaries of venous sinuses. Parasagittal, bilateral, and hemorrhagic infarcts after sagittal sinus thrombosis.

Infarction, Myocardial (See "Disease, ischemic heart.")

Infarction, Pulmonary (See "Embolism, pulmonary.")

Infection, Cytomegalovirus

Synonyms: Cytomegalic inclusion disease; salivary gland virus disease.

NOTE: Cytomegalovirus infection may complicate any chronic debilitating disease, and may follow treatment with immunosuppressive and cytotoxic drugs.

(1) Collect all tissues that appear to be infected. (2) Request viral cultures. (3) Immunohistochemical stains on paraffin-embedded sections are available in many laboratories. (4) No special precautions are indicated. (5) Serologic studies are avail-able from many reference laboratories, but these are not necessary to make the diagnosis. (6) This is not a reportable disease.

Possible Associated Conditions: *Pneumocystis carinii* infection.* Bacterial, fungal, protozoal, and other viral infections.

Organs and Tissues	Procedures	Possible or Expected Findings
Placenta	Record weight.	In congenital cytomegalovirus infection, mononuclear plasma cell villitis with villous edema and intranuclear and cytoplasmic inclusions.
External examination	Record changes as listed in right-hand column.	In congenital cytomegalovirus infection, microcephaly, jaundice, and a petechial rash may be found.
Urine	Submit sample for viral culture. Prepare smears of sediment.	
Lungs	Culture consolidated areas of lung or random sites if the clinical suspicion is high.	Focal interstitial pneumonia. See also above under "Possible Associated Conditions."
Esophagus and gastrointestinal tract	Submit samples for histologic study.	Ulcers or grossly normal mucosa with cytomegalic inclusions in epithelial and endothelial cells.
Liver	Record weight and submit samples for	Hepatitis with hepatomegaly.

Organs and Tissues	Procedures	Possible or Expected Findings
	histologic study and viral culture.	
Other organs	Submit samples of myocardium, pancreas, spleen, kidneys, adrenal glands, and eyes for histologic study and, if indicated, viral culture. For special stains, see above under "Note." If accessible, prepare sections of salivary glands [e.g., submandibular gland in floor of mouth].	Myocarditis; pancreatitis; splenitis; and adrenalitis. Pseudotumor in stomach *(1)*. In adult and in congenital infections, focal necrotizing nephritis; chorioretinitis. Virtually all organs may be affected and have cytomegalic cells with viral inclusions.
Brain	For removal and specimen preparation, see Chapter 4.	Meningoencephalitis with subependymal calcifications of lateral ventricles.
Bone marrow		Fibrin ring granulomas in rare instances *(2)*.

References

1. Mohan H, et al. Cytomegalovirus-associated pseudotumor simulating gastric malignancy in acquired immuno-deficiency syndrome: a case report with review of literature. Jpn J Infect Dis 2007;60:134–136.
2. Young J, Goulian M. Bone marrow fibrin ring granulomas and cytomegalovirus infection. Am J Clin Pathol 1993;99:65–68.

Infection, Hantavirus (See "Fever, hemorrhagic, with renal syndrome.")

Infection, Herpes simplex

Synonyms and Related Terms: Herpes simplex, type I; herpes simplex, type II; sporadic acute herpes simplex type I (rarely type II) encephalitis. For other names and manifestations, see below under "Possible or Expected Findings."

Organs and Tissues	Procedures	Possible or Expected Findings
Mouth, esophagus, distal colon, liver, adrenal glands, and other organs and tissues	Multiple organs and tissues may be involved, including oral cavity, esophagus, colon, liver, and adrenal glands. Sample tissue from these sites.	Herpetic gingivostomatitis, esophagitis, distal colitis, and proctitis (mostly type II infection); herpetic hepatitis with or without extensive necrosis, and adrenalitis with cortical necrosis.
Brain	Nuclear virus antigens can be identified immunohistochemically. Viral nucleic acid may persist years after the acute phase and be identified by *in situ* hybridization. In the acute phase, submit tissue for culture.	In the acute phase, generalized swelling. Bilateral, often asymmetrical necrosis, involving particularly the temporal lobes. Neocortex, white matter, hippocampus, amygdaloid nucleus, and putamen may be involved and lesions may extend to the insular cortex *(1)*. Typically, diffuse necrotizing herpetic meningoencephalitis; intranuclear inclusions may be difficult to detect. In the chronic phase, shrunken tissue with marked neuronal loss, gliosis, and frequently cystic degeneration.
Eyes	For removal and specimen preparation, see Chapter 5. Electron microscopy, immunocytochemistry, *in situ* hybridization, and the polymerase chain reaction may be needed to confirm the diagnosis.	Herpes simplex keratitis and retinal necrosis. Corneal perforation.

Reference

1. Naito K, et al. Herpes simplex virus type-1 meningoencephalitis showing disseminated cortical lesions. Intern Med 2007;46:761–763.

Infection, Herpes Zoster

Synonyms and Related Terms: Herpes zoster oticus (Ramsay Hunt syndrome); postherpetic neuralgia; shingles; zona; zoster encephalomyelitis; zoster encephalopathy; zoster ophthalmicus.

NOTE: (1) Collect all tissues that appear to be infected. (2) Request viral cultures. (3) Stain for inclusion bodies (Lendrum's method). Electron microscopy, labeled-antibody techniques, and *in situ* hybridization also can be useful in identifying viral particles. (4) Usually, no special precautions are indicated. (5) Serologic studies are available from the state health department laboratories. (6) This is not a reportable disease.

Possible Associated Conditions: Heavy metal poisoning; leukemia;* lymphoma;* multiple myeloma;* other malignant tumors (particularly when the spine is involved or when the patient had been treated with immunosuppressive agents or irradiation); trauma; tuberculosis;* other chronic debilitating diseases.

Organs and Tissues	Procedures	Possible or Expected Findings
External examination	Record distribution of lesions. Prepare histologic sections of affected areas. For virus culture, aspirate vesicles aseptically.	Unilateral groups of skin vesicles, pustules, and crusts in thoracic, cervical, facial, lumbar, or sacral distribution. Eruptions may be bullous or gangrenous. Vesicles may be present on tip of nose. Generalized infections may occur. Granuloma annulare-like lesions following herpes zoster infection *(1)*.
Lymph nodes	Prepare histologic sections of lymph nodes that drained the region of the zoster lesions.	Lymphadenitis.
Blood	Submit sample for serologic study.	
Pleural and peritoneal cavities	Record appearance and volume of effusions	Effusions in presence of visceral herpes zoster.
Gastrointestinal tract	Submit samples from areas with gross lesions for histologic study.	Inflammatory lesions in visceral zoster.
Urinary bladder	Submit samples from areas with gross lesions for histologic study.	Unilateral ulcers in visceral zoster.
Brain and spinal cord	For removal and specimen preparation, see Chapter 4. Submit fresh material for virologic study.	In rare instances, diffuse meningo-encephalitis may occur. Limited necrotic and inflammatory lesions in the cord or brain stem at the level of the affected ganglion are common. Posterior horn myelitis *(3)*.
Sensory ganglia	For exposure of posterior root ganglia, see Chapter 4. If the face is involved, study trigeminal ganglia.	Ganglion cell necrosis; lymphocytic infiltration, hemorrhage, and, later, fibrosis. As a rule, only one ganglion is severely involved, but less severe lesions may occur in the ganglia that are immediately adjacent.
Peripheral nerves	For sampling and specimen preparation, see Chapter 4. Request Luxol fast blue stain.	Diffuse lymphocytic infiltration; demyelination; axonal destruction; fibrosis.
Eyes	For removal and specimen preparation; see Chapter 5. Indicated only if there is clinical evidence of zoster ophthalmitis. If eye is affected, study also trigeminal nerve and ganglia.	Conjunctivitis; keratitis; iridocyclitis; retrobulbar neuritis; neuroretinitis; occlusion of retinal vessels.
Ears	Record appearance of pinna. If there was clinical evidence of herpes zoster oticus, remove tympanic membrane, middle ear, and inner ear (Chapter 4).	Herpes zoster otitis.
Other organs	Procedures depend on expected findings as listed in right-hand column and above under "Note."	Evidence of hematologic malignancies *(2)* or other conditions, as listed above under "Note."

References

1. Gibney MD, Nahass GT, Leonardi CL. Cutaneous reactions following herpes zoster infections: report of three cases and a review of the literature. Br J Dermatol 1996;134:504–509.
2. Smith JB, Fenske NA. Herpes zoster and internal malignancy. South Med J 1995;88:1089–1092.
3. Toledano R, et al. Posterior horn varicella-zoster virus myelitis. J Neurol 2007;254:400–401.

Infection, Middle Ear (See "Otitis media.")

Infection, *Pneumocystis carinii*

Synonym: Pneumocystosis.

NOTE: (1) Collect all tissues that appear to be infected. (2) This organism cannot be cultured at present but is frequently associated with viral, bacterial, or fungal infections that can be diagnosed by culture. (3) For rapid staining of aspirates, use Gram-Weigert stain, which will stain cysts of *Pneumocystis carinii* and also fungi and bacteria. *Pneumocystis carinii* is best demonstrated with Grocott's methenamine silver stain. (4) No special precautions are indicated. (5) Usually, no serologic studies are available. (6) This is not a reportable disease.

Organs and Tissues	Procedures	Possible or Expected Findings
Lungs	Prepare smears of fresh cut sections. For special stains for smears and paraffin sections, see above under "Note."	Pneumonia with foamy intra-alveolar exudate containing cysts of *Pneumocystis carinii*.
Other organs	Procedures depend on expected findings or grossly identified abnormalities as listed in right-hand column.	Manifestations of conditions requiring high-dose immunosuppressive therapy; AIDS;* hypogammaglobulinemia, leukemia,* lymphoma,* and prematurity.

Infection, Respiratory Syncytial Virus (See "Pneumonia, all types or type unspecified.")

Infection, Spinal Epidural

Organs and Tissues	Procedures	Possible or Expected Findings
External examination	If skin infections are presence, record character and extent; prepare photographs.	Pyogenic skin infections which may be trivial (*S. aureus*).
Cerebrospinal fluid	Submit sample for microbiologic study prepare smears.	Protein concentrations increased; WBC < 150/mm^3 (findings compatible with parameningeal infection).
Spinal canal and epidural space	Local removal of uncontaminated infectious material may not be possible. Prepare sections and smears. Prepare saw sections through adjacent bone. Submit samples of epidural granulomas or from walls of abscesses for histologic study.	Trauma or osteomyelitis* (or both) of vertebrae. Occasionally, pleural, sub-diaphragmatic, or perirenal infections may be present. Tuberculous abscesses may also occur.
Other organs	Procedures depend on expected findings or grossly identified abnormalities as listed in right-hand column.	Manifestations of cirrhosis;* diabetes mellitus;* intravenous drug abuse; malignancy; obstructive uropathy; or steroid-treated degenerative joint disease.

Influenza

Related Terms: Influenza A and B.

NOTE: (1) Collect all tissues that appear to be infected. (2) Request viral and aerobic bacterial cultures. (3) Request Gram stain. (4) Special **precautions** are indicated. (5) Serologic studies are available from the state health department laboratories. (6) This is not a reportable disease.

Organs and Tissues	Procedures	Possible or Expected Findings
Larynx, trachea, and lungs	Remove en bloc; open extrapulmonary airways posteriorly and photograph mucosa.	Necrosis of respiratory tract epithelium.
	Submit samples of trachea for histologic study. Record weight of each lung. Submit consolidated or hemorrhagic/edematous areas for viral and bacterial culture.	Primary influenzal pneumonia; super-infection with *Pneumococcus*, *Staphylococcus*, *Hemophilus influenzae*, and *Streptoccocus*.
	Perfuse at least one lung with formalin.	Emphysema; interstitial pulmonary fibrosis; chronic bronchitis.
Nasal cavities and sinuses	For exposure, see Chapter 4.	Coryza.
Other organs	Procedures depend on expected findings or grossly identified abnormalities as listed in right-hand column.	Myositis; myocarditis;* Reye's syndrome;* transverse myelitis (rare).

Injury, Electrical

Synonyms and Related Terms: Electric burns; electric shock.

NOTE: Immediate scene investigation with an experienced electrical engineer may be crucial for reconstruction of the fatal events and for prevention of similar injuries to others (the expertise of electricians may not suffice; many erroneously believe that 110 volt alternating current cannot kill a human). Search for evidence of wetness that might have precipitated the fatal circuit through the victim. See also ref. *(1)*.

Organs and Tissues	*Procedures*	*Possible or Expected Findings*
Power lines and power tools	Examination of street power lines is done by technicians from the power company. Examination of unplugged electrical appliances and tools may be done by the pathologist using an ohmmeter, or by an electrical or electronic engineer. Testing of household outlets for faulty wiring can be accomplished with a simple device.	Downed power line or ladder or bucket truck touching intact power line. Ground fault in the wiring of a tool. Hot line wired to ground plug in outlet.
External examination and skin	Record appearance of shoes and clothing, and retain burned areas with surrounding clothing for possible spectrographic and chemical tests. Photograph and record appearance and location of electrical burns; record appearance of hair around such lesions. Prepare histologic sections of electrical injuries.	Electric burns of shoes and clothing may be obvious when cutaneous burns are subtle. Metal particles may be found near the burned areas. Small, multiple, craterlike defects or massive fourth-degree burns of hands or other areas of contact; arborescent skin markings; characteristic defects on surface of hair. Degeneration of epithelium and collagen with typical microblisters in epidermis. Gangrene may occur after electrically induced vascular thrombosis.
Blood	Record presence or absence of blood clots. Submit sample for alcohol determination. (Alcohol concentrations are important in compensation cases.)	Fluid blood or thrombi.
Blood vessels	Submit portions of suspected lesions for histologic study. Request Verhoeff–van Gieson stain.	Intimal degeneration and tearing of elastic fibers, with or without thrombosis.
Heart	Record weight. Examine for coronary, valvular and myocardial disease, and sample for histologic study.	Electrically induced myocardial hemorrhagic necroses *(2)*. Disease capable of causing sudden ventricular arrhythmia. Often, with sudden death scenarios involving household current, the differential is natural heart disease versus electrocution.
Kidneys	Prepare histologic sections.	Congestion; lower nephron nephrosis in cases with extensive muscle destruction.
Urine		Hemoglobinuria.
Skeletal muscles	Prepare histologic sections of traumatized portions.	Tears after tetanic convulsions.

References

1. Wright RK. Death or injury caused by electrocution. In: Clinics of Laboratory Medicine, vol. 3, No. 2. Symposium on Forensic Pathology, DiMaio JM, ed. W.B. Saunders, Philadelphia, PA, 1983, pp. 343–353.
2. Colonna M, Caruso G, Nardulli F, Altamura B. Myocardial hemorrhagic necrosis in delayed death from electrocution. Acta Medicinae Legaliset Socialis 1989;39:145–147.

Injury, Fire (See "Burns.")

Injury, Firearm

NOTE: Protect all drains of autopsy table, which will prevent accidental loss of bullets or bullet fragments. Recovery of bullet fragments and pellets can also be improved by passing tissue fragments, blood, and other appropriate materials through a fine nonmetallic sieve. Caution must be exercised because sharp edges and jagged projections of bullets and bullet fragments may cause injury *(1)*. This applies particularly to the Black Talon bullet. Bullets and bullet fragments should not be touched with forceps or other metal instruments that may produce artifactual markings; they must be placed in properly labeled evidence containers, and the chain of custody must be preserved. From a birdshot wound, at least 10 pellets should be recovered. The firearms examiner will divide the total pellet weight by 10 and derive median pellet weight. From a buckshot wound, all pellets should be recovered. In many of these cases, procedures described under "Homicide" must also be followed.

Do not excise wounds before completion of autopsy (see below). As an academic exercise, excised firearm wounds may be used later for analysis of metal traces by neutron activation or for tests for carboxyhemoglobin. In practice, however, a high quality photograph is adequate to establish the presence or absence of gunpowder stippling or soot deposition toward the end of establishing the range of fire. The dimensions of the stippled areas and soot deposits should be recorded.

After completion of external examination, dry the wet clothing and keep as evidence. Clothing may also be used for possible test firing or for stain, powder, or particle analysis.

Organs and Tissues	*Procedures*	*Possible or Expected Findings*
External examination	If identity of victim is unknown, follow procedures described in Chapter 13.	
	Prepare initial roentgenograms of the body regions that have been shot, before disrobing of body, and then lateral films of body regions with bullets. Follow up with films of other body regions as needed in the course of autopsy. If the body is decomposed to the extent that the external examination cannot be relied upon to determine cutaneous gunshot perforations, prepare roentgenograms of the entire body before autopsy.	Additional roentgenograms during the autopsy may be needed to find bullets embolized to the femoral veins or down the spinal canal. Systemic roentgenograms may reveal bullets from obscure entrance wounds, particularly in decomposed bodies, old bullets, bullets in the skin flaps reflected at autopsy, or bullets external to the body in clothing.
	Record location and number of bullet holes in all layers of garments, indicating whether the involved area is bloodstained or shows gunpowder or soot.	Bullet(s) may have been arrested in hollow viscus or blood vessel and may have been transported to distant sites by peristalsis or bloodstream ("bullet embolus"). Bullets may be deflected in unexpected directions from bony surfaces.
	If there are several cutaneous perforations, number or letter each consecutively and refer to these numbers in all records. Location of bullet holes should be described by recording distance from soles of feet or top of head, and from midline of body. Prepare diagrams and photograph holes, with and without labels.	Soot ("smudging") and gunpowder stippling may occur around entrance wound, depending on the muzzle-to-skin distance. There may also be an impression from a recoiling handgun or from a power piston.
	Photographs should show surrounding garments and extent of blood stains. In hairy areas, shave around bullet wounds for better photographic documentation.	Wounds may be stellate, round, jagged, or slit-like, with or without wide margins of abrasion.
	For evaluation of distance from where a shot had been fired, see Fig. II–3.	
	Inspect hands for powder marks. Skin swabs or adhesive lifts can be used for primer residue testing.	Primer residues on hand of suicide victim after use of a handgun.
Internal examination	Describe wound track(s) in anatomic order and in complete separate paragraphs, with summarizing description of course of bullet with respect to the standard anatomical position (e.g., front to back, left to right, somewhat down). Avoid using numerical angular measurements.	Fatal secondary injuries, particularly hemorrhages.
	For toxicologic sampling of body fluids and tissues, see Chapter 8.	Alcohol intoxication is a frequent finding.

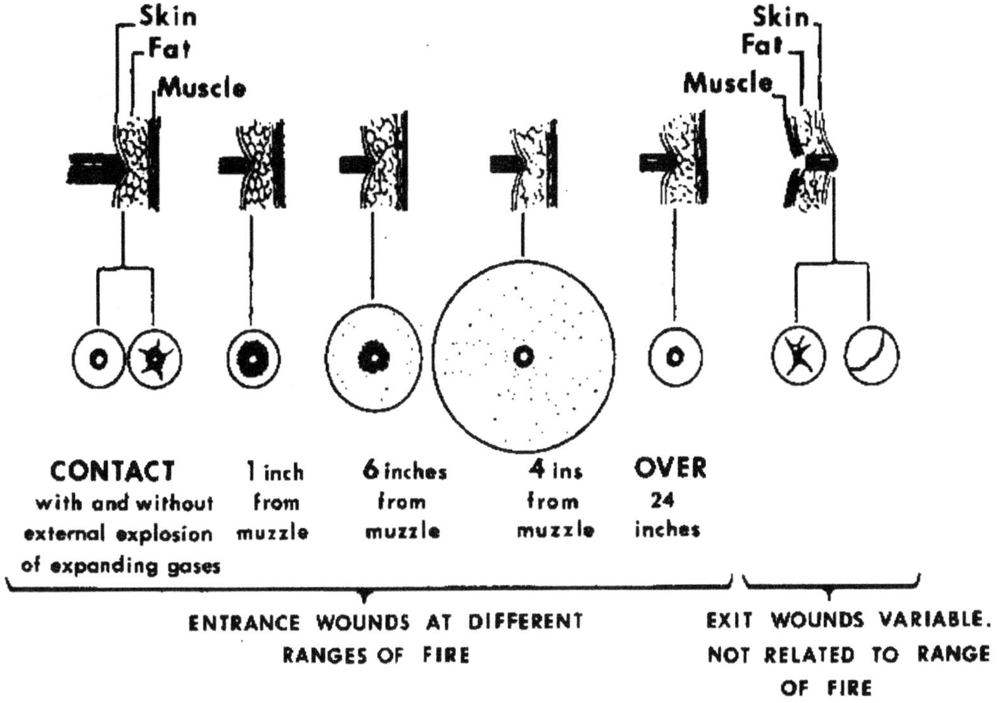

Fig. II-3. Bullet wounds. Differences in the appearance of cutaneous wounds of entrance and of exit and differences in wounds of entrance according to the distance between muzzle and skin at the moment of fire. Entrance wounds often differ from exit wounds in that the former are usually surrounded by a narrow zone of abrasion. If the muzzle of a gun is in close contact with the skin at the moment of fire, the combustion products will be blown into the wound and will not be visible on the surface. For close-range wounds, the stippling of the skin around the wound, produced by particles of burned and unburned powder, becomes progressively more dispersed as the range of fire increases and is ordinarily not perceptible if the range has been greater than 24 inches (61 cm) (with permission from Moritz AR, Morris CR. Handbook of Legal Medicine. Third edition, 1970. CV Mosby Company, St. Louis, MO.) Exit wounds usually have no marginal abrasion *(1)* and have no apparent tissue deficit.

Reference

1. Russell MA, Atkinson RD, Klatt EC, Noguchi TT. Safety in bullet recovery procedures: a study of the Black Talon bullet. Am J Forens Med 1995;16:120–123.

Injury, Head

Synonyms and Related Terms: Contact injury; impact trauma, craniocerebral trauma, diffuse axonal damage; shearing injury; head motion injury.

NOTE: The brain may have focal injury manifest by contrecoup contusions and localized swelling; or may have diffuse white matter (axonal) injury manifested by microscopic evidence of axonal degeneration in cerebral white matter, corpus callosum, and upper brainstem; and small hemorrhages in frontal white matter, corpus callosum, dorsolateral midbrain, and rostral pons. With survival, macrophages infiltrate sites of injury, followed by microglial clusters and gliosis.

In cases of gunshot injury to the head, see under "Injury–Firearm".

Organs and Tissues	*Procedures*	*Possible or Expected Findings*
External examination	Record extent and character of soft tissue and scalp wounds. Prepare roentgenogram of skull and, in case of possible skull fracture, roentgenogram of the chest.	Face and scalp contusions, abrasions, and lacerations. Firearm injury.* Linear, radiating, depressed, bursting, diastatic, and other skull fracture(s). Venous air embolism.*
Neck organs	In obscure cases of coma it may be necessary to consider occlusion of arteries normally reserved for the undertaker. For carotid and vertebral arteriography, see Chapter 4. Expose, remove, embed and study histologic sections of carotid and vertebral arteries after embalming.	Traumatic dissection of vertebral or carotid artery with or without thrombosis.

Organs and Tissues	Procedures	Possible or Expected Findings
Skull (see also below under "Brain")	Record sites, pattern, and distribution of fractures. For detection of hairline fractures, strip dura from the base of skull and vault.	Character of fractures may indicate site of impact.
	Record separations or lacerations of dura. Open dural sinuses. Locate air embolus ingress. If osteomyelitis is suspected, submit material for bacterial culture and smears.	Dural trauma indicates severe force. Superior longitudinal sinus thrombosis. Ingress of air embolus. Osteomyelitis* of skull bones.
	Record thickness, volume, clotting, and adherence of subdural blood.	Fresh or chronic subdural hematoma.
Brain	Observe brain in-situ.	Swelling, herniation, or shift of brain.
	Record site of subarachnoid hemorrhage, and whether it is thin or thick.	For gross and microscopic findings, see above under "Note." Thick subarachnoid hematomas suggest arterial bleed (a ruptured aneurysm can precipitate a fall). Subdural bleeds with gunshot wounds point to penetration of cerebral arteries. Epidural or subdural hematomas;* subarachnoid hemorrhage. Cerebral abscess;* meningitis.*
Lungs	Examine H & E stained section. Optionally prepare frozen, Sudan-stained sections.	Fat embolism* is easily recognized on H & E sections.

Injury, Intubation

Organs and Tissues	Procedures	Possible or Expected Findings
External examination and neck organs	Intubation tube should be left in place until position is verified. Prepare roentgenograms.	Intubation tube in wrong place; soft tissue emphysema.
	Pathologist personally examines neck organs in-situ and personally removes and examines. Open trachea posteriorly or opposite perforation or fistula. Photograph lesions and submit samples for histologic study.	Ulcers; erosions; chondromalacia; perforation; fistula; herpetic infection.

Injury, Lightning

Organs and Tissues	Procedures	Possible or Expected Findings
External examination and skin		Electrical burns (head and legs) *(1)* or explosive tearing of clothing; mechanical damage from blast effects. See also under "Burns" and "Injury, electrical."
	Photograph erythema, electric burns, and injuries. Prepare histologic sections.	Fernlike distribution of electrically induced erythema is characteristic for lightning injury.
Other organs	For procedures involving the heart, see "Disease, ischemic heart."	See under "Injury, electrical." The most severe visceral manifestations of lightning injury generally affect the cardiovascular and central nervous system (see below) *(2)*. Sequelae of attempted resuscitation from cardiac or respiratory arrest are commonly noted.
Brain and spinal cord		Cerebral edema with brain stem herniation; epidural hemorrhage.
Middle ear	For exposure of the middle ear, see Chapter 4.	Rupture of eardrums.
Eyes	For removal and specimen preparation, see Chapter 5.	Cataracts; interstitial keratitis; iridocyclitis; chorioretinal atrophy; hemorrhages *(2)*.
Skeletal muscle	Sample for histologic study, particularly if myoglobinuria had been observed.	Muscle necroses.

References

1. Cooper MA. Lightning injuries: Prognostic signs of death. Ann Emerg Med 1980;9:134–138.
2. Tribble CG, Persing JA, Morgan RF, Kenney JG, Edlich RF. Lightning injuries. Comprehensive Ther 1985;11:32–40.

Injury, Radiation

Synonyms and Related Terms: Acute radiation syndrome; chronic (delayed) radiation injury; radiation enterocolitis; radiation nephritis; radiation pneumonitis.

NOTE: Procedures and expected findings depend on type of radiation damage, whether acute or chronic, localized or whole-body irradiation. If suspected radiation injury was associated with the administration of radionuclides such as ^{32}P, ^{131}I, or ^{198}Au, follow procedures suggested in Chapter 11. In fatal whole-body irradiation, findings are most likely related to bone marrow injury, and the suggested procedures and expected findings are those described under "Pancytopenia." Record extent of oropharyngeal and intestinal ulcerations and hemorrhages. Late complications include malignant tumors (carcinoma, leukemia,* lymphoma*), manifestations of hypothyroidism,* and cataracts. Organ changes in localized radiation injury depend on site of irradiation (lung, brain, kidney, intestine). The skin is involved in both acute (erythema) and chronic (atrophy, epilation) radiation injury.

Injury, Stabbing

Related Terms: Cutting injury; knife injury.

NOTE: In many of these cases, procedures described under "Homicide" must also be followed.

Organs and Tissues	*Procedures*	*Possible or Expected Findings*
External examination and skin (wounds)	Prepare diagrams and photographs of all wounds. Each wound can be labeled with identifying number or letter that can also appear on photographs and histologic sections.	Defense wounds occur on hands and arms.
	Examine edges of wounds on clothing and skin with hand lens, if necessary; record appearance of edges. Record location of wounds by stating distance from top of head or from sole of foot, distance from midline, location at front or back, and relation to fixed anatomic landmarks.	Serrations of skin tags along incised wound margins are caused by dragging action of knife. If contusions or abrasions are present, wounds are more likely caused by laceration. Undivided nerves, hair bulbs, and vessels in depth of wounds indicate laceration. (Knives or other sharp-edged instruments tend to cut these structures.)
	Record the dimensions of the wounds and state whether the measurement is taken with the wound margins approximated (pushed together) or unapproximated. Keep clothing as evidence.	
	Submit samples from edges of wounds for histologic study, if necessary.	Inflammatory changes indicate vital response (absent in wounds received after death).
	Prepare roentgenograms of areas around wounds.	Metallic parts may have broken off weapon.
	If wounds were not immediately fatal or if tetanus* was present, cultures from wounds may be indicated.	Wound infection.
Wound tracks	Dissect layer by layer and follow tracks of cutting or stabbing instrument. Do not probe. Record lacerated vessels and organs penetrated.	
Body cavities	Record volume of accumulated blood.	Hematomas; hemothorax; hemoperitoneum.
Heart	Submit blood samples for alcohol determination and other toxicologic studies.	
Lungs	Request Sudan stain of frozen sections.	Pulmonary fat embolism.
Other organs	For toxicologic sampling, see Chapter 13.	

Insecticides (See "Poisoning, organophosphate(s).")

Insuffiency, Adrenal

Synonyms and Related Terms: Adrenocortical insufficiency; polyglandular autoimmune syndrome (type I, usually in childhood, with parathyroid insufficiency and chronic mucocutaneous moniliasis; type II, usually in adults, with two or more autoimmune endocrine disorders such as thyroiditis and diabetes mellitus*); primary adrenal insufficiency (Addison's disease); secondary adrenal insufficiency (in hypothalamic-pituitary disease or steroid induced); X-linked adrenal hypoplasia.

NOTE: Primary adrenal insufficiency (Addison's disease) is caused by anatomic changes (see below under "Adrenal glands"), drugs (enzyme inhibitors or cytotoxic drugs), or ACTH-blocking antibodies.

Possible Associated Conditions: AIDS with systemic infections *(1)*; antiphospholipid antibody syndrome *(2)*; autoimmune hepatitis; chronic lymphocytic thyroiditis; type I diabetes mellitus;* hypoparathyroidism;* hypothyroidism;* megaloblastic anemia;* surgical procedures, such as heart surgery or orthopedic procedures. Large cell lymphoma *(5)*.

Organs and Tissues	*Procedures*	*Possible or Expected Findings*
External examination and skin	Prepare sections of pigmented areas of skin. Prepare photographs of pigmented abnormalities.	Decreased axillary and pubic hair in women; diffuse brown hyperpigmentation; bluish-black spots on mucous surfaces of lips and cheeks.
Vitreous	Submit sample for sodium, potassium, chloride, and urea nitrogen analysis.	Electrolyte changes associated with dehydration.* Decreased sodium and chloride in primary adrenal insufficiency.
Blood	Submit sample for microbiologic and chemical study.	Septicemia, including systemic fungal infections. Low plasma cortisol concentration.
Adrenal glands	Record weights; photograph; prepare roentgenograms; submit portion for microbiologic study; submit samples for histologic study. Decalcification may be necessary. Request acid fast, Gram, and Grocott's methenamine silver stains.	Idiopathic (autoimmune?) atrophy of adrenal cortex; tuberculosis* (also *Mycobacterium avium intracellulare* infection in AIDS); coccidioidomycosis;* cryptococcosis* or nocardiosis* *(1)* (in AIDS); cytomegalovirus infection* (in AIDS); histoplasmosis;* rarely amyloidosis;* hemorrhages *(3)*; widespread lymphoma* *(4)* or metastases of malignant tumors.
Other endocrine glands	Describe and weigh all endocrine glands and sample for histologic study.	Abnormalities of pituitary gland (in secondary adrenal insufficiency), thyroid, parathroid glands, gonades, or islets of Langerhans (see under "Possible Associated Conditions.")
Other organs	Search for conditions that may have caused adrenal insufficiency.	See above under "Adrenal glands" and under "Possible Associated Conditions."

References

1. Arabi Y, Fairfax MR, Szuba MJ, Crane L, Schuman P. Adrenal insufficiency, recurrent bacteremia, and disseminated abscesses caused by Nocardia asteroides in a patient with acquired immunodficiency syndrome. Diagn Microbiol Inf Dis 1996;24:47–51.
2. Argento A, DiBenedetto RJ. ARDS and adrenal insufficiency associated with the antiphospholipid antibody syndrome. Chest 1998;113:1136–1138.
3. Cozzolino D, Peerzada J, Heaney JA. Adrenal insufficiency from bilateral adrenal hemorrhage after total knee replacement surgery. Urology 1997;50:125–127.
4. Nasu M, Aruga M, Itami J, Fujimoto H, Matsubara O. Non-Hodgkin's lymphoma presenting with adrenal insufficiency and hypothyroidism: an autopsy case report. Pathol Internat 1998;48:138–143.
5. Zhang L, Talwalker SS, Shaheen SP. A case of primary unilateral adrenal Burkitt-like large cell lymphoma presenting as adrenal insufficiency. Ann Diagn Pathol 2007;11:127–131.

Insufficiency, Aortic

Synonyms: Aortic incompetence; aortic regurgitation.

NOTE: For general dissection techniques in valvular heart disease, see Chapter 3. For procedures in infective endocarditis, see Chapter 7.

Possible Associated Conditions: Acute aortic dissection* with or without Marfan's syndrome;* ankylosing spondylitis;* aortitis; congenitally bicuspid aortic valve;* cystic medial degeneration of aorta; giant cell aortitis;* hypertension;* late postoperative conotruncal anomalies (e.g., tetralogy); rheumatic aortic valve disease; syphilitic aortitis; Takayasu's arteritis;* trauma; ventricular septal defect.*

Organs and Tissues	*Procedures*	*Possible or Expected Findings*
External examination	Prepare chest roentgenogram.	Cardiomegaly; dilated ascending aorta.
Blood	If infective endocarditis is suspected, submit sample for microbiologic study (Chapter 7).	Septicemia.
Heart and great vessels		See above under "Possible Associated Conditions."
	If infective endocarditis is suspected, follow procedures described in Chapter 7.	Infective endocarditis.*
	Record weight and measurements of heart. For dissection, tests for valvular insufficiency, and measurement of valve size, see Chapter 3.	Cardiomegaly; acute or old myocardial infarction.
Other organs		See above under "Possible Associated Conditions."

Insufficiency, Coronary (See "Disease, ischemic heart.")

Insufficiency, Mitral (Chronic or Acute)

Synonyms and Related Terms: Acquired mitral insufficiency; mitral incompetence; mitral regurgitation; congenital mitral insufficiency; floppy valve syndrome; mitral annular calcification; mitral valve prolapse; mitral regurgitation; myxomatous mitral valve disease; rheumatic mitral valve disease.

Possible Associated Conditions: Autoimmune connective tissue disorders; bicuspid aortic valve;* cardiomyopathy* (dilated, hypertrophic, or restrictive); infective endocarditis;* Marfan's syndrome;* metabolic/storage diseases, such as mucopolysaccharidoses;* ischemic heart disease;* rheumatic heart disease.*

Organs and Tissues	*Procedures*	*Possible or Expected Findings*
External examination	Prepare chest roentgenogram.	Cardiomegaly; calcification in and around mitral valve.
Blood	If infective endocarditis is suspected, submit sample for microbiologic study.	Septicemia.
Heart and great vessels	For general dissection techniques in valvular and congenital heart disease, see Chapter 3.	See above under "Possible Associated Conditions."
	If infective endocarditis is suspected, follow procedures described in Chapter 7.	Infective endocarditis.*
	Record weight and measurements of heart.	Cardiomegaly; acute myocardial infarction, with or without rupture of papillary muscles; fibrosis of papillary muscles; myxomatous (floppy) mitral valve; rheumatic valvulitis; rupture of tendinous cords; other coexistent valve disease.
Other organs		See above under "Possible Associated Conditions."

Insufficiency, Pituitary

Synonym: Hypopituitarism.

Possible Associated Conditions: Diabetes mellitus;* pregnancy;* and other conditions listed below under "Brain, spinal cord, and pituitary gland."

Organs and Tissues	*Procedures*	*Possible or Expected Findings*
External examination	Record weight and length of body and distribution and intensity of hair growth.	Dwarfism in childhood cases.
	Prepare roentgenogram of skull.	Evidence of skull fractures or tumor.
Blood	Freeze sample for possible biochemical study.	
Extrapituitary endocrine organs	Dissect and record weights of all endocrine organs. Submit samples for histologic study.	Polyglandular atrophy.
Other organs	Procedures depend on expected findings or grossly identified abnormalities as listed in right-hand column.	Fatty changes of liver *(1)*. Manifestations of diabetes mellitus.* Systemic amyloidosis* or genetic hemochromatosis* with secondary infiltration of pituitary gland region.
Urine	Freeze sample for possible biochemical study.	
Brain, spinal cord, and pituitary gland	For removal and specimen preparation, see Chapter 4. For cerebral arteriography, see Chapter 4. Record weight of pituitary gland.	Developmental anomalies (pituitary aplasia or basal encephalocele). Postpartum necrosis of pituitary gland (Sheehan's syndrome*); lymphocytic hypophysitis; granulomatous inflammation (in sarcoidosis*); chromophobe pituitary adenoma; craniopharyngioma in childhood; other benign or malignant pituitary tumors; extrasellar cysts; effects of trauma or irradiation. Pituitary abscess *(3)*.
Base of skull	Expose venous sinuses. Strip dura for inspection of bone.	Skull fractures; cavernous sinus thrombosis; primary or metastatic tumors.

Organs and Tissues	Procedures	Possible or Expected Findings
Skeletal system		Bone fractures *(2)*.
Vitreous	Refrigerate sample for possible glucose and electrolyte determination.	

References

1. Takano S, Kanzaki S, Sato M, Kubo T, Seino Y. Effect of growth hormone on fatty liver in panhypopituitarism. Arch Dis Childhood 1997;76:537–538.
2. Rosen T, Wilhelmsen L, Landin-Wilhelmsen K, Lappas G, Bengtsson BA. Increased fracture frequency in adult patients with hypopituitarism and GH deficiency. Eur J Endocrinol 1997;137:240–245.
3. Su YH, Chen Y, Tseng SH. Pituitary abscess. J Clin Neurosci 2006;13:1038–1041.

Insufficiency, Pulmonary

Synonyms: Pulmonary incompetence; pulmonary regurgitation.

NOTE: Infective endocarditis due to *Strept. bovis*, especially when it involves the pulmonary valve, is often associated with an underlying adenocarcinoma of the colon.

Possible Associated Conditions: Carcinoid heart disease; congestive heart failure;* infective endocarditis;* pulmonary hypertension;* tetralogy of Fallot* with absent pulmonary valve (*not* the same as pulmonary atresia).

Organs and Tissues	Procedures	Possible or Expected Findings
External examination		Cyanosis; edema.
Heart	If infective endocarditis is suspected, follow procedures described in Chapter 7. For dissection and histologic sampling, see Chapter 4.	Infective endocarditis.* Carcinoid heart disease; Epstein's anomaly; rheumatic valve disease.
Lungs	Perfuse both lungs with formalin. Request Verhoeff–van Gieson stain.	Hypertensive pulmonary vascular changes (see "Hypertension, pulmonary").
Other organs		See "Failure, congestive heart."*

Insufficiency, Tricuspid (Chronic or Acute)

Synonyms: Tricuspid incompetence; tricuspid regurgitation.

Possible Associated Conditions: Cardiomyopathy* (dilated or restrictive); chronic congestive heart failure (any cause); chronic pulmonary hypertension (any cause)*. See also below under "Possible or Expected Findings."

Interruption of Aortic Arch (See "Coarctation, aortic.")

Intolerance, Fructose

Synonyms: Hereditary fructose intolerance; hereditary fructosemia, deficiency of fructose-1-phosphate aldolase.

Organs and Tissues	Procedures	Possible or Expected Findings
External examination	Record body weight and length.	Signs of extreme weight loss; evidence of coagulopathy.
Eyes	Submit sample of vitreous for sodium, potassium, chloride, urea nitrogen, and glucose determination.	Evidence of dehydration.* There is no reliable test for hypoglycemia.*
Blood	Submit plasma/serum for chemical study (see right-hand column).	Increased fructose and bilirubin concentrations.
Abdomen	Record volume of fluid.	Ascites.
Urine	Submit sample for chemical study.	Aminoaciduria;* fructosuria; proteinuria; urobilinuria.
Liver	Record weight. Snap-freeze tissue for histochemical or biochemical study. Submit samples for light microscopic and electron microscopic study.	Hepatomegaly; steatosis; cholestasis; necrosis; fibrosis; cirrhosis; negative aldolase activity; "fructose holes" by electron microscopy *(1)*.
Spleen		Splenomegaly.
Other organs	Submit samples for histologic and histochemical study.	Evidence of coagulopathy.
Brain and spinal cord		Cerebral edema.
Bone	Submit samples of epiphysis, if available, for histologic study.	Rickets.

Reference

1. Phillips MJ, Poucell S, Patterson J, Valencia P. The Liver: An Atlas and Text of Ultrastructural Pathology, Raven Press, New York, 1987.

Intubation (See "Injury, intubation.")

Iodine (See "Poisoning, iodine.")

Ischemia, Cerebral (See "Attack, transient cerebral ischemic" and "Infarction, cerebral.")

Ischemia, Heart (See "Disease, ischemic heart.")

Isomorism (See "Syndrome, polysplenia and asplenia.")

K

Kala-Azar

Synonyms and Related Terms: *Leishmania donovani* infection; Dumdum fever; visceral leishmaniasis; infantile kala-azar.

NOTE: (1) Collect all tissues that appear to be infected. (2) Usually, cultures are not required, but direct examination for para-sites is indicated. (3) Request Giemsa or Wright's stain. (4) Usually, no special precautions are indicated. (5) Serologic studies are available from the Centers for Disease Control and Prevention, Atlanta, GA. (6) This is not a reportable disease in the United States.

Organs and Tissues	*Procedures*	*Possible or Expected Findings*
External examination and skin	Photograph skin lesions; prepare histologic sections of normal and abnormal skin; request Giemsa or Wright's stain.	Emaciation; jaundice or skin pigmentation from melanin accumulation; subcutaneous edema; petechiae; macular or nodular dermal leishmaniasis. Manifestations of vitamin C deficiency.*
Blood	Submit sample for bacterial culture.	Superimposed bacteremia.
Oral cavity and other mucosal surfaces		Petechial hemorrhages and ulcers; noma.
Abdominal and pleural cavities	Record volume of effusions; centrifuge and prepare smears of sediment; request Giemsa or Wright's stain.	Leishmanial infection or bacterial infection; pleural adhesions; intraperitoneal hemorrhages.
Heart	For histologic examination, request Giemsa or Wright's stain.	Infiltrates of lymphocytes and plasma cells with some eosinophils and mononuclear cells filled with *Leishmania* amastigotes.
Lungs	Submit a section for bacterial culture. Prepare smears; request Giemsa and Gram stains.	Bacterial or leishmanial pneumonia, or both.
Liver	Record size and weight; photograph; submit samples for histologic study.	Hepatomegaly; diffuse leishmanial hepatitis, with or without cholestasis.
Spleen	Record size and weight; photograph; prepare smears of cut section; submit samples for histologic study.	Splenomegaly, often extreme, with possible hemorrhage from diagnostic puncture; infarctions; leishmanial splenitis.
Lymph nodes	Submit samples for histologic study.	Lymphadenopathy; see also above under "Heart."
Other organs	Procedures depend on expected findings or grossly identified abnormalities as listed in right-hand column.	See above under "Heart." Manifestations of anemia, agranulocytosis, or thrombocytopenia.
Bone marrow	For preparation of sections and smears, see Chapter 2.	Osteomyelitis with amastigotes present *(1)*.
Brain and skeletal muscles		Not involved.

Reference

1. Kumar PV et al. Visceral leishmaniasis: bone marrow findings. J Pediatr Hematol Oncol 2007;29:77–80.

Ketoacidosis (See "Disorder, electrolyte(s)" and Table 8-2.)

From: *Handbook of Autopsy Practice,* 4th Ed. Edited by: B.L. Waters

Knife Wounds (See "Injury, stabbing.")

Kwashiorkor (See "Malnutrition...")

L

Laryngitis

Synonyms and Related Terms: Acute infectious airway obstruction; croup; obstructive laryngitis with epiglottitis of infants.

NOTE: (1) Collect all tissues that appear to be infected. (2) Request aerobic bacterial and viral cultures. (3) Request Gram stain. (4) Usually, no special precautions are indicated. (5) Serologic studies may be helpful in determining the etiologic agent. (6) This may be a reportable disease, depending on the etiologic agent.

Organs and Tissues	*Procedures*	*Possible or Expected Findings*
Blood and lungs	Submit for bacterial and viral cultures. If diphtheria is suspected, see also under that heading.	*Hemophilus influenzae* (cannot always be isolated from larynx). Measles virus, myxovirus, parainfluenza virus, and other respiratory viruses that may affect infants and children.
Larynx and pharynx	Should be removed as soon as possible (before embalming), either from cervical midline incision or from chest (neck of cadaver must be well-extended). Photograph obstruction before larynx is opened, and inside of larynx and epiglottis after larynx is is opened in posterior midline.	Airway obstruction.*
	Make Gram-stained touch preparations.	*Hemophilus influenzae* (small, pleomorphic, Gram-negative bacilli) in smear.
	Make histologic sections of larynx and epiglottis.	Other pathogenic and nonpathogenic microorganisms may be present. Acute laryngitis, often with ulcerations.

Lead (See "Poisoning, lead.")

Leishmaniasis (See "Kala-azar.")

Leprosy

Synonyms: Hansen's disease; lepromatous leprosy; *Mycobacterium leprae* infection; tuberculoid leprosy.

NOTE: (1) Collect all tissues that appear to be infected and submit for direct examination. (2) Cultivation of leprosy bacilli is not yet available for routine use. (3) Request Gram, Ziehl-Neelsen, Kinyoun, or fluorochrome stains. (4) Usually, no special precautions are indicated. (5) Serologic studies are now available in some laboratories *(1)*. PCR assays are also available *(2)*. (6) This is a **reportable** disease.

Possible Associated Conditions: Amyloidosis;* tuberculosis.*

Organs and Tissues	*Procedures*	*Possible or Expected Findings*
External examination and skin	Photograph lesions, and record extent of skin involvement.	Hyperpigmented macules; annular plaques; nodules; erythematous lesions. In lepromatous leprosy, leonine face with enlarged earlobes and loss of eyebrows. Other mutilations and plantar ulcerations.

From: *Handbook of Autopsy Practice,* 4th Ed. Edited by: B.L. Waters

Organs and Tissues	*Procedures*	*Possible or Expected Findings*
External examination and skin	Prepare sections of skin. For special stains, see above under "Note." Make touch preparations of skin specimens.	Skin and dermal nerves may be involved histologically.
Other organs	Submit samples of liver, spleen, kidneys, and bone marrow for histologic study.	Visceral involvement usually mild; amyloidosis;* tuberculosis;* erythema nodosum leprosum.
Lymph nodes	Submit samples for histologic study, particularly from drainage area of skin lesions.	Lepromatous lymphadenitis.
Peripheral nerves	For sampling and specimen preparation, see Chapter 4. Include ulnar, radial, median, and popliteal nerves.	Dermal nerves may be involved (see "External examination and skin"). Nerves may be thickened and fibrotic and may show obliteration of normal architecture. Nerve abscesses.
Eyes and extraglobal orbital tissues	For removal and specimen preparation, see Chapter 5. Include ciliary nerves.	Iritis and keratitis; granulomas of anterior segment (in lepromatous leprosy) *(3)*; extraglobal granulomas, particularly in ciliary nerves (in tuberculoid leprosy).
Nasal cavity	For exposure, see Chapter 4. Submit tissue for histologic study.	Blockage of nasal cavity by lepromatous rhinitis.

References

1. Parkash O, Chaturvedi V, Girdhar BK, Sengupta U. A study on performance of two serological assays for diagnosis of leprosy. Leprosy Rev 1995;66:26–30.
2. Wichitwechkarn J, Karnjan S, Shuntawuttisettee S, Sornprasit C. Detection of *Mycobacterium leprae* infection by PCR. J Clin Micro 1995;33:45–49.
3. Job CK, Ebenezer GJ, Thompson K, Daniel E. Pathology of eye in leprosy. Ind J Leprosy 1998;70:79–91.

Leptospirosis

Synonyms: Canicola fever; Weil's disease; Fort Bragg Fever.

NOTE:

(1) Collect all tissues that appear to be infected. (2) Special culture media are required to cultivate the organisms. We recommend consultation with the microbiology laboratory before the postmortem examination is begun. (3) Direct dark-field examination by an experienced technologist is recommended for demonstrating the *Leptospira* organisms. Silver impregnation techniques are also useful. (4) Special **precautions** may be indicated, as this is a communicable disease (see Chapter 6). (5) Serologic studies can be obtained from the state health department laboratories. (5) This is not a reportable disease.

Organs and Tissues	*Procedures*	*Possible or Expected Findings*
External examination		Jaundice; skin hemorrhages.
Blood, urine, and cerebrospinal fluid	Submit samples for bacteriologic and serologic study.	Pleocytosis of CSF early in the course.
Heart	Submit samples for histologic study.	Myocarditis;* endocarditis;* hemorrhages.
Lungs	Submit samples for histologic study.	Hemorrhages *(1)*; pneumonia.
Liver and spleen	Record sizes and weights; submit samples for histologic study.	Cholestatic hepatitis; hemorrhages; hepatomegaly and splenomegaly.
Stomach		Mucosal hemorrhages.
Kidneys	Submit samples for histologic and electron microscopic study.	Hemorrhages; tubular degeneration and necrosis; hyaline and bile casts; interstitial nephritis; fusion of foot processes by electron microscopy.
Skeletal muscles	For sampling and specimen preparation, see Chapter 4.	Hemorrhages; necrosis.
Brain	For removal and specimen preparation, see Chapter 4.	Aseptic meningitis;* subarachnoid hemorrhages.*
Eyes	For removal and specimen preparation, see Chapter 5.	Optic neuritis; iridocyclitis; conjunctivitis; uveitis.

Reference

1. Dolhnikoff M et al. Pathology and pathophysiology of pulmonary manifestations in leptospirosis. Braz J Infect Dis 2007;11:142–148.

Leukemia, All Types or Type Unspecified

Synonyms and Related Terms: Acute or chronic lymphocytic leukemia, acute or chronic myelogenous leukemia, and hairy cell leukemia. Multiple subtypes have been identified; they are characterized by cell surface markers, chromosomal abnormalities, staining reactions, and morphologic features.

NOTE: At the time of autopsy, most leukemias have been properly classified and often treated. In these cases, the goal of the autopsy is to document the extent of the disease and the presence of complications. If the leukemia had not been classified or if the features might have changed from the time of the last work-up (e.g., in suspected cases of superimposed diffuse large cell lymphoma [Richter's syndrome]), material should be snap-frozen and studied in more detail. If the patient was treated by bone marrow transplantation,* see also under that heading.

Possible Associated Conditions: Agnogenic myeloid metaplasia with myelofibrosis; Bloom's syndrome;* cutaneous mastocytosis; Down's syndrome;* immunodeficiency syndromes* (Bruton's disease; Louis-Bar syndrome; Wiskott-Aldrich syndrome); infantile genetic agranulocytosis; Klinefelter's syndrome;* lymphoma;* multiple myeloma;* polycythemia;* and many others.

Organs and Tissues	*Procedures*	*Possible or Expected Findings*
External examination, oral cavity, and skin	Record extent and character of skin lesions; photograph lesions and prepare histologic sections. Record appearance of oral cavity and eyes (see also below under "Eyes" and "Lacrimal glands; parotid and other salivary glands").	Nonspecific skin reactions; petechial and other types of hemorrhages; leukemic infiltrates; perianal ulcerations and abscesses; exophthalmos and salivary gland enlargement (Mikulicz's syndrome); gingival hemorrhages; mucosal ulcerations of mouth and nose; alopecia.
Blood and fascia lata	If chromosome study is intended, see Chapter 9.	Trisomy 21; Philadelphia chromosome; Christchurch chromosome; 47,XXY and less common variants of Klinefelter's syndrome.
	Submit sample of blood for bacterial, fungal, and viral studies.	Septicemia. Blood most commonly positive for *Escherichia coli*, *Pseudomonas aeruginosa*, *Klebsiella pneumoniae*, *Staphylococcus aureus*, *Candida* spp., and *Aspergillus*.
Thymus	Record weight. See also below under "Lymph nodes."	Leukemic infiltrates.
Lungs	Submit consolidated areas for bacterial, fungal, and viral studies. Make touch preparation from cut sections and request Gram stain and Grocott's methenamine silver stain for demonstration of fungi and *Pneumocystis carinii*. Perfuse at least one lung with formalin.	Bacterial and fungal pneumonia; viral pneumonitis; hemorrhages and leukemic infiltrates. *Pneumocystis carinii* pneumonitis.
Gastrointestinal tract	Estimate volume of blood in lumen. If there are mucosal lesions, submit samples for histologic study.	Gastrointestinal hemorrhages; mucosal hemorrhagic necroses; leukemic infiltrates.
Liver and spleen	Record weight and size. Request Gomori's iron stain.	Hepatosplenomegaly. Enlarged liver may be free of leukemic infiltrates.
Kidneys	Fix specimen in alcohol for preservation of urates.	Urate deposits.
Lymph nodes	Record average size. Fix specimens in B-Plus® fixative (see Chapter 15). Make touch preparations. Request Giemsa or Wright stain.	Leukemic lymphadenopathy; lymphadenitis.
Brain and spinal cord	For removal and specimen preparation, see Chapter 4. Make touch preparations from meningeal lesions; request Gram and Grocott's methenamine silver stains for histologic sections.	Meningeal leukemic infiltrates, particularly around brain stem; hydrocephalus; hemorrhages; meningitis* or meningoencephalitis.

Organs and Tissues	Procedures	Possible or Expected Findings
Middle and inner ears	For removal and specimen preparation, see Chapter 4.	Otitis media;* hemorrhages; leukemic infiltrates, particularly along eighth cranial nerve.
Eyes	For removal and specimen preparation, see Chapter 5. Include extrabulbar orbital tissue.	Hemorrhages in conjunctiva and retina; leukemic infiltrate in uvea.
Lacrimal glands; parotid and other salivary glands	Remove for histologic study. Parotid gland can be biopsied from scalp incision (see Chapter 4). Submaxillary gland can be removed with floor of mouth.	Leukemic infiltrates (Mikulicz's syndrome).
Bone marrow	Expell rib marrow and take marrow from vertebrae and iliac bones.	Leukemic infiltrates. Nonneoplastic proliferation of hematopoietic cells after bone marrow transplantation.
Joints	Remove synovial fluid for identification of crystals in secondary gout. For removal, prosthetic repair, and specimen preparation of joints, see Chapter 2. If gout is suspected, fix tissue specimen in alcohol.	Leukemic infiltrates; gout.*
Other organs and tissues	Use Bouin's fixative; request Wright stain. For color preservation of chloroma, see Chapter 16.	Leukemic infiltrates, thromboses, infections, and hemorrhages may occur in all organs or tissues.

Leukemia, Eosinophilic ("Leukemia, all types or type unspecified.")

Leukemia, Mast Cell (See "Leukemia, all types or type unspecified" and "Mastocytosis, systemic.")

Leukodystrophy, All Types or Type Unspecified

NOTE: This term describes a group of diseases characterized by widespread and often symmetric bilateral demyelination or failure of myelin formation, or both, in the central nervous system. These conditions are thought to be caused by inborn errors of metabolism and enzymatic defects, which have been identified in at least two instances—namely, metachromatic leukoencephalopathy* and globoid cell leukodystrophy.* See also under "Degeneration, spongy, of white matter" and "Leukodystrophy, sudanophilic."

Leukodystrophy, Globoid Cell

Synonyms: Galactocerebroside lipidosis; Krabbe's disease.

Organs and Tissues	Procedures	Possible or Expected Findings
Cerebrospinal fluid	Submit sample for determination of protein concentration.	Increased protein concentration.
Brain, spinal cord, and peripheral nerves	For removal and specimen preparation, see Chapter 4. Place samples of cerebral tissue into liquid nitrogen and submit for biochemical and histochemical studies. Submit tissue for electron microscopy. Request Luxol fast blue stain for myelin.	Areas of myelin loss in the central nervous system. Globoid cells containing cerebrosides in areas of demyelination. Segmental demyelination of peripheral nerves. Optic nerve enlargement *(1)*.

Reference

1. Bussièr M, et al. Optic nerve enlargement associated with globoid cell leukodystrophy. Can J Neurol Sci 2006;33:235–236.

Leukodystrophy, Sudanophilic

Synonym: Pelizaeus-Merzbacher disease.

Organs and Tissues	Procedures	Possible or Expected Findings
Brain and spinal cord	For removal and specimen preparation, see Chapter 4. Request Luxol fast blue stain for myelin. Prepare frozen sections for Sudan stain.	Demyelination in centrum ovale, cerebellum, and part of brain stem. Diffuse gliosis and perivascular sudanophilic lipid in white matter.

Leukoencephalopathy, Metachromatic

Synonyms: Sulfatide lipidosis; sulfatidosis.

Organs and Tissues	*Procedures*	*Possible or Expected Findings*
Cerebrospinal fluid	Submit sample for determination of protein concentration.	Increased protein concentration.
Urine	Collect and stain sediment with toluidine blue.	Material in sediment stains red with toluidine blue.
Other organs	Stain sections of liver, gallbladder, spleen, kidneys, lymph nodes, adrenal glands, and ovaries for metachromasia. Submit fascia for establishment of cell line for biochemical assay.	Metachromatic material. Arylsulfatase-A deficiency.
Brain and spinal cord	For removal and specimen preparation, see Chapter 4. Request Luxol fast blue and cresyl violet stain.	Excessive loss of myelin with large amounts of metachromatic material (see above under "Urine") in white matter and also in some neurons.
Peripheral nerves	For sampling and specimen preparation, see Chapter 4.	Demyelination with metachromatic material (see above under "Urine").

Leukoencephalopathy, Progressive Multifocal

Possible Associated Conditions: AIDS* and other immunosuppressed states; carcinoma; malignant myeloproliferative or lymphoproliferative disorder; sarcoidosis;* tuberculosis.*

Organs and Tissues	*Procedures*	*Possible or Expected Findings*
Brain and spinal cord	Submit portion of fresh brain for viral culture. Fix remainder of brain and spinal cord in formalin and submit samples for histologic study. *In situ* hybridization for JC virus is available on paraffin-embedded tissue.	Small patches of demyelination with tendency to form confluent areas in the cerebral white matter. White matter necrosis may be present. Eosinophilic intranuclear inclusions occur in affected oligodendroglia cells. Subsequently, large, bizarre astrocytes develop. No inflammatory (lymphocyte) cell reaction is present.

Lightning (See "Injury, lightning.")

Lipoproteinemia (See "Hyperlipoproteinemia.")

Lipoproteinosis, Pulmonary Alveolar

Synonym: Idiopathic alveolar lipoproteinosis.

NOTE: The condition has been described in allografts *(1)*; in such cases, see also under "Transplantation, lung."

Organs and Tissues	*Procedures*	*Possible or Expected Findings*
External examination	Prepare chest roentgenogram.	"Butterfly" shadow on chest roentgenogram.
Lungs	Submit one lobe for bacterial, fungal, and viral cultures. Prepare smears for identification of *Pneumocystis carinii.* Record weight of lungs; photograph. Request PAS, toluidine blue, Gram, and Grocott's methenamine silver stains and fresh frozen sections for Sudan stain. Prepare samples for electron microscopic study. Snap-freeze tissue for histochemical study.	Superinfection with fungi (nocardiosis;* cryptococcosis*), viruses (cytomegalovirus infection*), or *Pneumocystis carinii.** Increased lung weights. Alveolar contents PAS-positive, metachromatic, and positive for lipids. Microorganisms may be present. Osmiophilic densities; myelin figures.

Reference

1. Yousem AS. Alveolar lipoproteinosis in lung allograft recipients. Hum Pathol 1997;28:1383–1386.

Listeriosis

Synonyms: *Listeria monocytogenes* infection; listerosis.

NOTE: (1) Collect all tissues that appear to be infected. (2) Request aerobic bacterial cultures. Alert the laboratory that *Listeria* is suspected. (3) Request Gram stain. (4) Usually, no special precautions are indicated. (5) Usually, serologic studies are not helpful. (6) This is not a reportable disease.

Possible Associated Conditions: Cirrhosis* of the liver; malignant neoplasms and other debilitating diseases, including human immunodeficiency virus infection *(1)*; previous steroid therapy.

Organs and Tissues	*Procedures*	*Possible or Expected Findings*
Placenta	Record weight and size; photograph. Prepare histologic sections.	Intervillous abscesses containing gram-positive, non-acid-fast bacilli.
External examination and skin	Record extent of skin lesions; prepare histologic sections of skin.	
Heart	If infective endocarditis is suspected, sample tissue for culture.	Infective endocarditis* and, rarely, pericarditis *(2)*.
Lungs and trachea	Culture consolidated areas. Then, perfuse both lungs.	Tracheobronchitis and bronchopneumonia.
Liver and spleen	Record weights and submit samples for histologic study.	Hepatosplenomegaly; necrosis; granulomas; abscesses *(3)*. Bacteria are predominantly intracellular.
Intestine	Submit sample of meconium for culture.	Enterocolitis. *Listeria monocytogenes* can be cultured from meconium.
Lymph nodes	Prepare samples for histologic study.	Generalized lymphadenitis.
Other organs and tissues, including pharynx	Procedures depend on expected findings or grossly identified abnormalities as listed in right-hand column.	Disseminated abscesses and/or granulomas, particularly after transplacental infection; purulent conjunctivitis; uveitis; arthritis; osteomyelitis; peritonitis; cholecystitis.
Brain and spinal cord	For removal and specimen preparation, see Chapter 4.	Meningitis;* brain abscess *(4)*; meningo encephalitis. The organism may appear coccoid in CSF.
Middle ears	Remove for histologic study.	Otitis media.*

References

1. Marron A, Roson B, Mascaro J, Carratala J. Listeria monocytogenes empyema in an HIV infected patient. Thorax 1997;52:745–746.
2. Manso C, Rivas I, Peraire J, Vidal F, Richart C. Fatal Listeria meningitis, endocarditis and pericarditis in a patient with haemochromatosis. Scand J Inf Dis 1997;29:308–309.
3. Marino P, Maggioni M, Preatoni A, Cantoni A, Invernizzi F. Liver abscesses due to Listeria monocytogenes. Liver 1996;16:67–69.
4. Turner D, Fried M, Hoffman M, Paleacu D, Reider I, Yust I. Brainstem abscess and meningitis due to Listeria monocytogenes in an adult with juvenile chronic arthritis. Neurology 1995;45:1020–1021.

LSD (d-Lysergic Acid Diethylamide) (See "Abuse, hallucinogen(s).")

Lung, Farmer's (See "Pneumoconiosis.")

Lung, Honeycomb (See "Pneumonia, interstitial.")

Lupus Erythematosus, Systemic

Related Terms: Immune complex disease; immune connective tissue disease.

Possible Associated Conditions: Rheumatoid arthritis;* Sjögren's syndrome.*

Organs and Tissues	Procedures	Possible or Expected Findings
External examination and skin; oral cavity		Malar, discoid, maculopapular, and other rashes; oral ulcers; lichenoid mucositis; alopecia.
	Prepare histologic sections of grossly abnormal and of unaffected skin.	Hyperkeratotic dermatitis with liquefaction necrosis. Vasculitis and panniculitis.
	Prepare histologic sections of subcutaneous nodules. If joints appear swollen, withdraw synovial fluid for cell count, and culture.	Erosions and ulcers (including leg ulcers); ischemic changes of fingers. Rheumatoid granulomas (elbows, hands).
	Prepare skeletal roentgenograms.	Arthritis (see below under "Joints"); osteoporosis* and osteonecrosis* in steroid-treated patients.
Serosal cavities	Record volume of pericardial, pleural, or peritoneal exudates or effusions, and submit samples for culture. Submit samples of serosal surfaces for histologic study.	Pleuritis; pericarditis;* ascites.
Blood	Submit sample for microbiologic and serologic study.	Septicemia; circulating anticoagulant.
Heart	If infective endocarditis is suspected, remove vegetations for microbiologic study.	Infective endocarditis.*
	Photograph valvular lesions and submit samples for histologic study. Include chordae tendineae, papillary muscles, and endocardium (where it borders on valves).	Libman-Sacks endocarditis (lupus endocarditis), with small vegetations on all valves and adjacent structures; myocarditis;* pericarditis.*
	For coronary arteriography, see Chapter 10. Submit samples of all coronary arteries for histologic study.	Coronary occlusion; coronary arteritis. Myocardial infarction. Cor pulmonale in cases with pulmonary hypertension *(1)*.
Lymph nodes	Submit axillary, tracheobronchial, and inguinal lymph nodes for histologic study.	Lymphadenitis.
Lungs	Submit consolidated areas for microbiologic study. Snap-freeze sample for possible special studies. Perfuse at least one lung with formalin.	Interstitial pneumonitis and fibrosis; bronchopneumonia. Adult respiratory distress syndrome and pulmonary hemorrhages. Arterial and arteriolar thrombi and plexiform lesions *(1)*.
Gastrointestinal tract and mesentery	For mesenteric arteriography, see Chapter 2. Submit samples of all segments of gastrointestinal tract for histologic study. Dissect mesenteric vessels and submit sample, together with mesenteric lymph nodes, for histologic study.	Hemorrhagic necroses; ulcers; gastro intestinal vasculitis; mesenteric vasculitis.
Spleen, liver, and pancreas	Record weights; submit samples for histologic study.	Splenitis; nonspecific hepatic changes; rarely arteritis, infarctions, or nodular regenerative hyperplasia *(2)*. Chronic pancreatitis *(3)*.
Kidneys	Follow procedures described under "Glomerulonephritis."	Lupus glomerulonephritis. Kidney failure* is a common cause of death.
Neck organs	Submit thyroid, parathyroid, and submandibular glands and cervical lymph nodes for histologic study.	Manifestations of Sjögren's syndrome.*
Brain, spinal cord, and peripheral nerves		Subarachnoid hemorrhage; aseptic meningitis; perivascular necroses *(4)*; transverse myelitis; optic neuritis. Peripheral neuropathy.
Eyes and lacrimal glands	For removal and specimen preparation, see Chapter 5.	Conjunctivitis; episcleritis; Retinal and choroidal hemorrhages. Dacryoadenitis in Sjögren's syndrome.*
Blood vessels	For removal of femoral vessels, see Chapter 3. Submit samples of small blood vessels of	Peripheral arteritis *(8)*; arterial occlusions; thrombophlebitis.

Organs and Tissues	Procedures	Possible or Expected Findings
	extremities for histologic study.	
Skeletal muscles	For sampling and specimen preparation, see Chapter 4. Refer to neurologic findings for proper sampling sites.	Myositis and vascultis *(5)*.
Joints	Remove affected diarthrodial joints, together with synovia, periarticular tissues, and tendon sheaths.	Arthritis, in decreasing order of frequency, in knees, small joints of hands, wrists, shoulders, ankles, elbows, and hips.
Bones and bone marrow		Osteoporosis* and osteonecrosis.* (Ischemic necroses in hip joints *(6)*, femoral condyles, and small bones of hands.) These are complications of steroid therapy.
	Sample bone marrow for histologic study.	Storage and hemophagocytic histiocytes *(7)*.

References

1. Yokoi T, Tomita Y, Fukaya M, Ichihara S, Kakudo K, Takahashi Y. Pulmonary hypertension associated with systemic lupus erythematosus: predominantly thrombotic arteriopathy accompanied by plexiform lesions. Arch Pathol Lab Med 1998;122:467–470.
2. Matsumoto T, Yoshimine T, Shimouchi K, Shiotu H, Kuwabara N, Fukuda V, Hoshi T. The liver in systemic lupus erythematosus: pathologic analysis of 52 cases and review of Japanese autopsy registry data. Hum Pathol 1992;23:1151–1158.
3. Borum M, Steinberg W, Steer M, Freedman S, White P. Chronic pancreatitis: a complication of systemic lupus erythematosus. Gastroenterology 1993;104:613–615.
4. Shintaku M, Matsumoto R. Disseminated perivenous necrotizing encephalomyelitis in systemic lupus erythematosus: report of an autopsy case. Acta Neuropathol 1998;95:313–317.
5. Lim KL, Lowe J, Powell RJ. Skeletal muscle lymphocytic vasculitis in systemic lupus erythematosus: relation to disease activity. Lupus 1995;4:148–151.
6. Aranow C, Zelicof S, Leslie D, Solomon S, Barland P, Norman A, Klein R, et al. Clinically occult avascular necrosis of the hip in systemic lupus erythematosus. J Rheumatol 1997;24:2318–2322.
7. Morales-Polanco M, Jimenez-Balderas FJ, Yanez P. Storage histiocytes and hemophagocytosis: a common finding in the bone marrow of patients with active systemic lupus erythematosus. Arch Med Res 1996;27:57–62.
8. Kumar N et al. Extensive medium vessel vasculitis with SLE: an unsual association. J Clin Rheumatol 2007;13:140–142.

Lye (See "Poisoning, lye.")

Lymphatics (See "Disease, lymphatic vascular.")

Lymphogranuloma Venereum

Synonym: Lymphogranuloma venereum *Chlamydia* infection.

NOTE: (1) Collect all tissues that appear to be infected. (2) Culture of tissues can be performed but requires special laboratory tests. Request consultation with a microbiology laboratory before a specimen is submitted. (3) Usually, special stains are not helpful. (4) Usually, no special precautions are indicated. (5) Serologic tests are available from the state health department laboratories. (6) This is a **reportable** disease.

Organs and Tissues	Procedures	Possible or Expected Findings
External examination and skin	Record skin changes and prepare sections of affected skin. Record presence of perianal fistulas (see also below under "Pelvic organs and lymph nodes").	Elephantiasis of penis, scrotum, or vulva (in chronic cases); skin rash *(1)* and conjunctivitis (in acute cases); genital ulcers.
Blood	Submit serum for complement-fixation test.	
Pelvic organs and lymph nodes	If there are perirectal or lymphocutaneous fistulas, injection of dyes or contrast media may help for dissection.	Suppurative or fibrosing inguinal, iliac, or pelvic lymphadenitis, with or without sinus tracts. Rectal strictures and fistulas in chronic cases *(2)*.
	Prepare histologic sections of affected lymph nodes.	
Other organs	Procedures depend on expected findings or grossly identified abnormalities as listed in right-hand column.	Systemic involvement in the acute stage with pericarditis,* and arthritis,* and meningitis,* proctitis *(3)*

References

1. Rosen T, Brown TJ. Cutaneous manifestations of sexually transmitted diseases. Med Clin North Am 1998;82:1081–1104.
2. Papagrigoriadis S, Rennie JA. Lymphogranuloma venereum as a cause of rectal strictures. Postgrad Med J 1998;74:168–169.
3. Richardson D, Goldmeier D. Lymphogranuloma venereum: an emerging cause of proctitis in men who have sex with men. Int J STD AIDS 2007;18:11–14.

Lymphoma

Synonyms and Related Terms: AIDS-related lymphoma; adult T-cell leukemia/lymphoma; angioimmunoblastic lymphadenopathy; B-cell lymphoma; Burkitt's lymphoma; cutaneous T-cell lymphoma (includes mycosis fungoides and Sézary syndrome); Hodgkin's disease; non-Hodgkin's lymphoma (low grade, intermediate grade, high grade, all with multiple subtypes too numerous to list, which vary in natural history); natural killer cell neoplasms; post-transplant lymphoproliferative disorders (PTLD); T-cell lymphoma.

NOTE: At the time of autopsy, most lymphomas have been properly classified and often treated. In these cases, the goal of the autopsy is to document the extent of the disease and the presence of complications. If the lymphoma had not been classified or if the features might have changed from the time of the last work-up, material should be snap-frozen and studied in more detail. If the patient was treated by bone marrow transplantation,* see also under that heading.

For current terminologies of Hodgkin's disease and non-Hodgkin lymphomas as well as for staging criteria, appropriate hematologic textbooks should be consulted.

Possible Associated Conditions: Acquired immunodeficiency diseases (e.g., after organ transplantation; human immunodeficiency virus-1 infection); autoimmune disease (e.g., celiac sprue,* rheumatoid arthritis,* systemic lupus erythematosus,* or Sjögren's syndrome*); chemotherapy with or without radiation treatment; Epstein-Barr virus infection; human T-cell leukemia virus infection; inherited diseases with immunodeficiency (e.g., Klinefelter syndrome;* common variable immunodeficiency disease, Wiskott-Aldrich syndrome); radiation.

Organs and Tissues	*Procedures*	*Possible or Expected Findings*
External examination, skin, and oral cavity	Record distribution of hair; record facial features and character and extent of skin lesions and of pigmentations. Record appearance of oral and nasal mucosa. Prepare histologic sections of skin.	Alopecia; disfigurement of face in Burkitt's lymphoma. Exophthalmos and salivary gland enlargement (Mikulicz's syndrome). Lymphomatous infiltrates of skin with or without ulcerations; herpes zoster;* jaundice.
	Prepare skeletal and chest roentgenograms.	Lymphomatous bone changes—for instance, skull defects in Burkitt's lymphoma. Calcifying lymphomatous tumors. Pulmonary infiltrates.
Blood and fascia lata	Submit sample of blood for bacterial, fungal, and viral cultures.	Septicemia. Blood most commonly positive for *Escherichia coli*, *Pseudomonas aeruginosa*, *Klebsiella pneumoniae*, *Staphyloccus aureus*, *Candida* spp., and *Aspergillus*.
	If chromosomal abnormalities are suspected, submit sample of blood or fascia lata for chromosome analysis.	Chromosomal abnormalities.
	Collect serum for study of antibodies and of immunoglobulins.	Antibodies against reovirus type 3 or Epstein-Barr virus in Burkitt's lymphoma. Dysgammaglobulinemia.
Thymus	Record weight and submit samples for histologic study. See also below under "Lymph nodes."	Lymphomatous infiltrates.
Lungs	Submit one lobe for bacterial, fungal, and viral cultures. Prepare smears of cut surface and request Grocott's methenamine silver stain for demonstration of fungi and *Pneumocystis carinii*.	Bacterial, fungal, and viral pneumonia. *Pneumocystis carinii* infection.*
	Perfuse one lung with formalin (see Chapter 2).	Lymphomatous infiltrates.
Lymph nodes	Record average size. Fix specimens in B-Plus® (see Chapter 15). Make touch preparations and request Giemsa or Wright stain. Snap-freeze lymphomatous tissue if immunophenotype studies are intended or for identification of surface markers for B- and T-lymphocytes and other lymphoreticular cells.	Lymphoma. Lymph nodes often unaffected in Burkitt's lymphoma.
Liver and spleen	Record size and weight. Submit samples for histologic study.	Spleen often unaffected in Burkitt's lymphoma; hepatosplenomegaly in most lymphomas.

Organs and Tissues	*Procedures*	*Possible or Expected Findings*
Other organs	Submit samples of all grossly abnormal tissues for histologic study. If systemic infection is suspected, collect appropriate specimens for microbiologic study.	All organs and tissues can be involved by lymphoma and by complicating infections. Retroperitoneal lymphoma with renal and ovarian involvement is common in Burkitt's lymphoma. Complications of radiation or cytostatic therapy also may be present.
Cerebrospinal fluid	Refrigerate sample for possible microbiologic study, depending on cerebral changes. Prepare smear of sediment.	Lymphoma cells.
Brain and spinal cord	Make touch preparations of meningeal lesions. Request Giemsa, Gram, and Grocott's methenamine silver stains.	Meningeal lymphomatous infiltrates. Hydrocephalus.* Meningitis* or meningoencephalitis.
Eyes and lacrimal glands	For removal and specimen preparation, see Chapter 5. Include lacrimal glands and orbital soft tissue.	Burkitt's lymphoma may involve orbitae. Lacrimal lymphoma is found in Mikulicz's syndrome.
Middle and inner ears	For removal and specimen preparation, see Chapter 4.	
Salivary glands (parotid, submandibular)	Submit samples for histologic study. Parotid gland can be biopsied from scalp incision. Submaxillary gland can be removed with floor of mouth.	Lymphomatous infiltrates in Burkitt's lymphoma and in Mikulicz's syndrome.
Thyroid gland		Often involved in Burkitt's lymphoma.
Bones and bone marrow		Lymphomatous infiltrates. Involvement of maxilla and mandible in Burkitt's lymphoma.

M

Macroglobulinemia, Waldenström's

Synonyms and Related Terms: Dysproteinemia; monoclonal gammopathy; paraproteinemia; plasma cell dyscrasia.*

Organs and Tissues	*Procedures*	*Possible or Expected Findings*
External examination and oral cavity	Record extent of skin and oral mucosal lesions. Prepare histologic sections of affected tissues.	Vascular purpura. Gangrene after cold exposure.
Blood	Submit samples for microbiologic study and for protein electrophoresis.	Increased IgM concentration. No evidence of hypercalcemia.
Lymph nodes	Record appearance and average size of lymph nodes. Snap-freeze tissue for immunophenotype study. Make touch preparations and request Wright stain. Tissue for paraffin sections should be fixed in B-Plus™ fixative.	Lymphadenopathy. Follicular hyperplasia with proliferation of lymphocytes and plasma cells that exhibit IgM immunofluorescence.
Liver and spleen	Record size and weight; sample for histologic study.	Hepatosplenomegaly. Proliferation of lymphocytes and plasma cells that exhibit IgM immunofluorescence.
Other organs and tissues	Record size and weight of all parenchymatous organs. Fix bowel as soon as possible. For further procedures, see above under "Lymph nodes." Request PAS and amyloid stains (see under "Amyloidosis"). Submit samples of all grossly abnormal tissues for histologic study.	Infiltrates of lymphocytes and plasma cells. Evidence of recurrent infections. Intestinal lymphangiectasia *(1)*. If features of other plasma cell disorders (amyloidosis,* heavy chain disease,* multiple myeloma*) are found, see under those headings.
Brain, spinal cord, and peripheral nerves		Cerebral hemorrhages. Peripheral neuropathy.*
Eyes	For removal and specimen preparation, see Chapter 5.	Retinal hemorrhages and exudates. Cyst of pars plana.
Skeletal muscles	For sampling and specimen preparation, see Chapter 4.	Myopathy.*
Bone marrow	For preparation of sections and smears, see Chapter 2.	Proliferation of lymphocytes and plasma cells with clasmacytosis, eosinophilia, and mast cell proliferation. No osteolytic lesions as in multiple myeloma.*

Reference

1. Pratz KW, et al. Intestinal lymphangiectasia with protein-losing enteropathy in Waldenstrom macroglobulinemia. Med 2007;86:210–214.

Malakoplakia

NOTE: Malakoplakia is a chronic inflammatory lesion with foamy macrophages, intracellular bacteria, and laminated, calcium-containg inclusions (Michaelis-Gutmann bodies). The lesions are found most commonly in the urinary bladder and other parts of the urinary tract, but may also occur at many other sites, including skin *(1)* and upper respiratory tract *(2)*.

From: *Handbook of Autopsy Practice,* 4th Ed. Edited by: B.L. Waters

Organs and Tissues	*Procedures*	*Possible or Expected Findings*
Urinary tract, colon, or other tissues	Photograph gross lesions; record size and location. Submit samples for histologic and electron microscopic study. Request PAS and von Kossa stains.	Grayish nodular lesions with or without ulceration. Microscopic Michaelis-Gutmann bodies. Adenocarcinoma of the colon may be associated with malakoplakia *(3)*.

References

1. Barnard M, Chalvardjian A. Cutaneous malakoplakia in a patient with acquired immunodeficiency syndrome (AIDS). Am J Dermatol 1998;20:185–188.
2. Salins PC, Trivedi P. Extensive malakoplakia of the nasopharynx: management of a rare disease. J Oral Maxillofac Surg 1998;56:483–487.
3. Bates AW, Dev S, Baithun SI. Malakoplakia and colorectal adenocarcinoma. Postgrad Med J 1997;73:171–173.

Malaria

Synonyms and Related Terms: *Plasmodium falciparum* infection; *Plasmodium malariae* infection; *Plasmodium ovale* infection; *Plasmodium vivax* infection; malignant pernicious malaria; blackwater fever.

NOTE: (1) Collect all tissues that appear to be infected. (2) Usually, cultures are not indicated. (3) Request Giemsa or Wright stain. Tissue blocks should be rinsed of blood and be as thin as possible before fixation in refrigerated buffered and neutral 10% formalin solution. This is to avoid precipitation of formalin pigment that may be confused with malaria pigment. The formalin solution should be used in a ratio of 100 parts formalin to one part tissue and should be agitated every few hours. If one is dealing with tissues that contain formalin pigment, this pigment may be removed with a bleaching solution. (4) Usually, no special precautions are indicated. (5) Serologic studies may be helpful and are available from the Cen-ters for Disease Control and Prevention, Atlanta, GA. (6) This is a **reportable** disease.

Organs and Tissues	*Procedures*	*Possible or Expected Findings*
Blood	Prepare "thick" and "thin" films.	Parasites; malaria pigment in erythrocytes.
Spleen	Record size and weight. Photograph cut section. For preparation of samples for histologic study, see above under "Note."	Splenomegaly with brown to gray discoloration because of malaria pigment; diffuse cellular hyperplasia and congestion; black opaque globules in histiocytes and in erythrocytes; parasitized red cells in sinusoids.
Liver	Record size and weight. Photograph cut section. For preparation of samples for histologic study, see above under "Note."	Hepatomegaly with congestion and centrilobular necrosis; malaria pigment in histiocytes; parasitized red cells in sinusoids.
Kidneys	For preparation of samples for histologic study, see above under "Note."	Ischemic cortex; congested medullary vessels; hemoglobin casts.
Other organs	Histologic sampling will depend on gross findings and clinical diagnosis of associated conditions. If placenta is present, prepare sections and smears. See also above under "Note."	Manifestations of disseminated intravascular coagulation;* parasitized red cells in any organ. Placenta may appear black; parasitized maternal cells; fetal cells rarely infected.
Brain, eye and spinal cord	For removal and specimen preparation, see Chapter 4 & Chapter 5.	Edema; "ring" hemorrhages; focal necrosis (acute cerebral malaria). Parasitized red cells in small vessels; reactive gliosis and malarial granulomas ("Dürck's" glial nodules); malarial retinopathy *(1)*.
Bone marrow	For preparation of sections and smears, see Chapter 2.	Erythroid and myeloid hyperplasia; parasitized red cells.

Reference

1. Beare NA, et al. Malarial retinopathy: a newly established diagnostic sign in severe malaria. Am J Trop Med Hyg 2006;75:790–797.

Malformation(s), Aortic Arch System (See "Artery, patent ductal," "Coarctation, aortic," and "Hypoplasia, tubular, of aortic arch.")

Malformation, Arnold-Chiari

Synonyms: Arnold-Chiari malformation, type I, adult form; Arnold-Chiari malformation, type II, infantile form; Arnold-Chiari malformation, type III (see below under "Note").

NOTE: In type I, relative frequent craniocervical bony malformations (platybasia,* basilar impression,* suboccipital dysplasia, Klippel-Feil syndrome*). For type II cases, see below. In type III, occipitocervical bony defect with cerebellar herniation into the encephalocele.

Possible Associated Conditions: Syringomyelia* (in 50% of type I cases); myelomeningocele, hydrocephalus,* and often craniolacunia in type II cases.

Organs and Tissues	Procedures	Possible or Expected Findings
External examination	Prepare roentgenograms of skull and cervix.	For bony malformations, see above under "Note."
Brain and spinal cord; base of skull and cervical spine	For removal of spinal cord, use combined approach (Chapter 4). If possible, prepare photographs to show bony malformations. If possible, especially with fetuses or neonates, try to access the brain and spinal cord by the posterior approach, so as to obtain in situ photographs. See description of the combined, ie posterior approach in Chapter 4.	Downward displacement of cerebellar tonsils and vermis through foramen magnum; elongation and caudal displacement of brain stem (medulla and 4th ventricle). Herniated cerebellar tissue shows neuronal loss and gliosis. Beak-like deformity of quadrigeminal plate; upwards direction of the upper 4 to 6 cervical spinal roots. Aqueduct abnormalities may be present. Hydrocephalus* may occur in all forms of the disease.

Malformation, Arteriovenous, Cerebral or Spinal (or Both)

Synonyms and Related Terms: Arteriovenous aneurysm; arteriovenous anomaly; Foix-Alajouanine syndrome; hemangioma of brain or spinal cord; vascular malformation of brain or spinal cord.

NOTE: A group of abnormal vessels is fed by one or more arteries without intermediate capillary channels and emptying directly into one or more large veins; this anomaly is associated with compressive atrophy of intervening and adjacent nervous tissue or with evidence of recent or old hemorrhage, or with both. In the Foix-Alajouanine syndrome, enlarged, tortuous subarachnoid veins cover the cord, especially posteriorly, and are associated with patchy necrosis of the spinal cord tissue and small blood vessels with thickened collagenous walls, not clearly distinguishable as arteries or veins.

Organs and Tissues	Procedures	Possible or Expected Findings
Brain and spinal cord	For cerebral arteriography, see Chapter 4.	For expected findings, see above under "Note."
Spine and spinal canal		Vertebral hemangioma. Calcification of spinal canal.

Malformation(s), Biliary System (See "Atresia, biliary," "Cyst(s), choledochal," "Disease, Caroli's," "Disease, fibropolycystic, of the liver and biliary tract," and "Fibrosis, congenital hepatic.")

Malformation(s), Congenital, Cardiac and Vascular

NOTE: See under specific name of malformation.

Malformation(s), Coronary Artery (See "Anomaly, coronary artery.")

Malformation(s), Coronary Sinus

NOTE: See also "Defect, atrial septal, coronary sinus type."

Possible Associated Conditions: *Unroofed* coronary sinus with atrial septal defect* at site normally occupied by coronary sinus and with left superior vena cava terminating in the left atrium. *Absent* coronary sinus associated with asplenia syndrome or right isomerism.

Malformation, Ebstein's

Synonym: Ebstein's anomaly of tricuspid valve.

NOTE: The basic anomaly is a downward placement of func-tional tricuspid annulus, with adherent septal and posterior leaflets, and with redundant deformed anterior leaflet. Sudden death may occur in this condition. It may become symptomatic at any age and is often associated with cardiomegaly due to marked right atrial and right ventricular dilatation.

Possible Associated Conditions: Congenitally corrected transposition of the great arteries; interatrial communication; pulmonary atresia;* tricuspid insufficiency;* Wolff-Parkinson-White ventricular preexcitation syndrome.*

Malformation(s), Pulmonary Artery

Related Terms: Absence of one pulmonary artery; aortic origin of one pulmonary artery; connection of pulmonary artery with left atrium; ductal origin of one or both pulmonary arteries; idiopathic dilatation of pulmonary trunk; discrete pulmonary artery stenosis; supravalvular pulmonary stenosis.*

Possible Associated Conditions: Post-rubella syndrome; pul-monary atresia with a ventricular septal defect;* tetralogy of Fal-lot;* supravalvular aortic stenosis;* Williams-Beuren syndrome.

Malformation(s), Thoracic Vein

Related Terms: Atresia of common pulmonary vein; azygos continuation of inferior vena cava; connection of a vena cava or hepatic vein with left atrium; continuity of inferior vena cava with left atrium; levoatriocardinal vein; partial anomalous pulmonary venous connection; persistent left superior vena cava; polysplenia syndrome;* pulmonary arteriovenous fistula; stenosis of common pulmonary vein (triatrial heart); scimitar syndrome; stenosis of individual pulmonary vein; total anomalous pulmonary venous connection.

NOTE: Type of venous malformation usually must be determined before separartion of thoracoabdominal viscera, particularly the course and connections of the inferior vena cava, hepatic veins, and azygos and hemiazygos veins. En masse removal of organs is recommended. Venography may be helpful.

Possible Associated Conditions: With anomalies of the pulmonary veins: asplenia syndrome (right isomerism), anomalous connections to the systemic veins, common atrium; complete atrioventricular septal defect;* polysplenia syndrome;* Scimitar syndrome. With connection of the inferior vena cava with the vena azygos: anomalous pulmonary venous return and polysplenia syndrome* (left isomerism). With intrapulmonary arteriovenous fistula: Osler-Weber-Rendu disease* or previous Glenn cavopulmonary venous anastomosis. With levoatriocardinal vein between left atrium or left pulmonary vein and left innominate vein; stenotic oval foramen, or mitral or aortic stenosis* or atresia* or both. With persistent left superior vena cava: isolated or with various malformations of the heart and great vessels.

Malnutrition

Synonyms and Related Terms: Hypoproteinemic malnutrition (kwashiorkor); marasmus; protein-energy malnutrition; starvation.*

Possible Associated Conditions: Anemia, iron deficiency, and vitamin deficiencies are common complications of malnutrition. Gastrointestinal, infectious, renal, and other diseases, including malignancies of all types, are found in many cases and represent the likely causes of the malnutrition.

Organs and Tissues	*Procedures*	*Possible or Expected Findings*
External examination and skin	Record body weight and length to calculate body mass index (BMI). See Part III for BMI formula.	Weight loss (may be compensated by edema and ascites).
	Photograph and record extent of skin lesions; prepare histologic sections of skin.	Generalized pitting edema; pigmented, pellagra-type skin lesions, particularly of extremities and face; brittle hair. Atrophy of epidermis with hyperkeratosis and parakeratosis.
Vitreous	Submit sample for sodium, potassium, chloride, and urea nitrogen determination.	Dehydration* and other electrolyte disorders.*
Abdomen	Record volume and character of fluid.	Ascites.
Liver	Record weight; request frozen sections for Sudan stain.	Fatty changes, predominantly periportal.
Intestinal tract	Fix the bowel as soon as possible. Submit samples for histologic study.	Mucosal atrophy.
Other organs	Procedures depend on expected findings or grossly identified abnormalities as listed in right-hand column and above under "Note."	Atrophy, particularly of pancreas and endocrine glands. For possible underlying conditions, see also above under "Note."

Marasmus (See "Malnutrition" and "Starvation.")

Marihuana (See "Abuse, marihuana.")

Mast Cells (See "Mastocytosis, systemic.")

Mastocytosis, Systemic

Synonyms and Related Terms: Mast cell disease; mastocytic leukemia; urticaria pigmentosa of childhood.

Possible Associated Conditions: Myelodysplastic or myeloproliferative disorders.

Organs and Tissues	*Procedures*	*Possible or Expected Findings*
External examination and skin	Record extent and character of skin lesions; photograph skin lesions. Fix skin specimens in formalin or alcohol and request Giemsa or toluidine blue stains for mast cells.	Macules with telangiectasias, papules, and nodules. Cachexia. Accumulation of mast cells in dermis.
	Prepare skeletal roentgenograms.	Multiple lytic bone lesions or new bone formation.

Organs and Tissues	Procedures	Possible or Expected Findings
Abdominal cavity		Ascites.
Gastrointestinal tract	Submit samples from all segments for histologic study.	Peptic ulcer* with perforation; gastroenteritis. See also under "Syndrome, malabsorption."
Liver, spleen, and lymph nodes	Record sizes and weights of liver and spleen and average size of lymph nodes. Submit tissue samples for histologic study (see above under "External examination and skin").	Hepatosplenomegaly; hepatic fibrosis; lymphadenopathy; mast cell infiltrates. Manifestations of portal hypertension *(1)*.*
Other organs	If infection is suspected, submit appropriate material for microbiologic study. For staining of histologic sections, see above under "External examination and skin."	Hemorrhages and infections may complicate mast cell disease. Mast cell infiltrates may be leukemic (see "Leukemia, all types or type unspecified").
Bone and bone marrow	For removal, prosthetic repair, and specimen preparation of bone, see Chapter 2. Consult roentgenograms. For preparation of sections and smears of bone marrow, see p. 96.	Mast cell infiltrates with osteolysis and new bone formation. Eosinophils, lymphocytes, plasma cells and fibroblasts may be prominent. Osteomalacia* in patients with malabsorption syndrome.*

Reference

1. Ghandur-Mnaymneh L, Gould E. Systemic mastocytosis with portal hypertension. Autopsy findings and ultra-structural study of the liver. Arch Pathol Lab Med 1985;109:76–78.

Measles

Synonyms: Morbilli; rubeola (the term rubeola is also used by some for "rubella").

NOTE: Various types of debilitating conditions may be complicated by measles—for instance, leukemia,* other neoplastic diseases and tuberculosis.*

(1) Collect all tissues that appear to be infected. (2) Request viral and aerobic bacterial cultures. (3) Request Gram stain. Electron microscopy may demonstrate the virus. (4) Special **precautions** are indicated (see Chapter 6). (5) Serologic studies may be helpful. (6) This is a **reportable** disease.

Possible Associated Diseases: Adenovirus, parainfluenza virus, and other viral infections *(1)*.

Organs and Tissues	Procedures	Possible or Expected Findings
External examination and skin	If skin or oral lesions can be identified, submit samples for histologic study.	Maculopapular rash, Koplik spots; congestion; edema; perivascular lymphocytic infiltrates; thrombosis; red cell extravasation; multinucleated giant cells.
Thymus	Record weight; submit sample for histologic study.	Hyperplasia (see below under "Intestinal tract").
Urine	Submit sample for virologic culture.	
Heart		Myocarditis* (very rare).
Lungs	Submit areas of consolidation for bacterial and viral cultures. Perfuse at least one lung. with formalin. Obtain areas of infected tissue for electron microscopy and place in suitable fixative.	Bacterial pneumonia *(1) (Pneumococcus, Streptococcus pyogenes, Staphylococcus aureus, Hemophilus influenzae);* giant cells lining alveoli. Interstitial pneumonia* or giant cell pneumonia *(2)* and inclusion bodies in children with leukemia.*
Intestinal tract	Prepare histologic sections of Peyer's patches and appendix.	Lymphoid hyperplasia with Warthin-Finkeldey giant cells.
Kidneys, ureters, urinary bladder	Submit samples for histologic study.	Mononuclear cells with cytoplasmic inclusions; giant cells.
Neck organs	Remove together with palatine tonsils and pharyngeal lymphatic tissue. Prepare sections of lymphatic tissue and and larynx.	See above under "Intestinal tract."
Other organs and tissues		Thrombocytopenic hemorrhages at various sites.
Brain and spinal cord	For removal and specimen preparation, see Chapter 4.	Subacute sclerosing panencephalitis with inclusion bodies.

Organs and Tissues	*Procedures*	*Possible or Expected Findings*
Middle ears	For removal and specimen preparation, see Chapter 4.	Otitis media;* mastoiditis.
Eyes	For removal and specimen preparation, see Chapter 5.	Optic neuritis; viral retinitis *(3)*; keratoconjunctivitis.

References

1. Quiambao BP, Gatchalian SR, Halonen P, Lucero M, Sombrero L, Paladin FJ, et al. Coinfection is common in measles associated pneumonia. Ped Inf Dis J 1998;17:89–93.
2. Rahman SM, Eto H, Morshed AS, Itakura H. Giant cell pneumonia: light microscopy, immunohistochemical, and ultrastructural study of an autopsy case. Ultrastr Pathol 1996;20:585–591.
3. Park DW, Boldt HC, Massicotte SJ, Akang EE, Roos KL, Bodnar A, et al. Subacute sclerosing panencephalitis manifesting as viral retinitis: clinical and histopathologic findings. Am J Ophthalmol 1997;123:533–542.

Measles, German (See "Rubella.")

Mediastinitis, Chronic

Synonyms and Related Terms: Fibrosing mediastinitis; granulomatous mediastinitis; idiopathic sclerosing mediastinitis.

Possible Associated Conditions: Histoplasmosis* and other chronic fungal infections; immune connective tissue diseases such as rheumatoid arthritis* *(1)*; malignancies *(1)*; sarcoidosis;* silicosis;* tuberculosis* *(1)*.

NOTE: In rare instances, fibrosing mediastinitis appears to be associated with other chronic fibrosing conditions such as retroperitoneal fibrosis,* Riedel's thyroiditis (Riedel's struma), or sclerosing cholangitis.*

Organs and Tissues	*Procedures*	*Possible or Expected Findings*
Chest cavity and mediastinum	Dissect superior vena cava system, aorta, and trachea, either *in situ* or after en bloc removal of mediastinal organs. Horizontal slices may be informative.	Superior vena cava obstruction.
	Prepare histologic sections from sclerosing process around great vessels, right atrium, trachea, and pericardium and from mediastinal lymph nodes. Submit tissue sample for fungal culture, and request Grocott's methenamine silver stain.	See above under "Possible Associated Conditions."
Other organs and tissues		See above under "Possible Associated Conditions."

Reference

1. Mole TM, Glover J, Sheppard MN. Sclerosing mediastinitis: a report of 18 cases. Thorax 1995;50:280–283.

Megacolon, Congenital

Synonyms: Hirschsprung's disease; idiopathic megacolon; megacolon.

Possible Associated Conditions: Atrial septal defect;* Down's syndrome;* meconium ileus;* megalobladder; megaloureter; ventricular septal defect.*

Organs and Tissues	*Procedures*	*Possible or Expected Findings*
External examination	Record weight, length, and abdominal circumference of body.	Manifestations of malnutrition;* abdominal distention; growth retardation.
Intestinal tract	Photograph *in situ*. Remove colon with rectum and anus; photograph colon before and after opening.	Necrotizing enterocolitis* and perforation of the colon or appendix (in neonates and infants). Narrow segment in distal colon.
	Submit transmural samples for histologic study from all portions of intestinal tract, particularly from several portions of narrowed segment. Cut sections on edge, and prepare frozen sections for acetylcholine esterase assay *(2)*.	Aganglionosis of narrow distal segment; intestinal neuronal dysplasia *(1)*.

References

1. Puri P, Wester T. Intestinal neuronal dysplasia. Sem Ped Surg 1998;7:181–186.
2. Kobayashi H, O'Brian DS, Hirakawa H, Wang Y, Puri P. A rapid technique of acetylcholinesterase staining. Arch Pathol Lab Med 1994;118:1127–1129.

Melioidosis

Synonyms and Related Terms: Glanders; *Pseudomonas mallei* infection; *Pseudomonas pseudomallei* infection.

NOTE: (1) Collect all tissues that appear to be infected. (2) Request aerobic bacterial cultures. (3) Request Gram stain. Polyclonal antibodies can be used for the diagnosis. Formalin-fixed, paraffin embedded autopsy tissues can be stained with a modified immunoperoxidase technique *(1)*. (4) Usually, no special precautions are indicated. (5) Serologic studies are available through state and local health departments. (6) This is not a reportable disease.

Organs and Tissues	*Procedures*	*Possible or Expected Findings*
Blood	Submit sample for aerobic bacterial culture.	Septicemia.
Lungs	Submit consolidated areas for microbiologic study. Perfuse at least one lung with formalin.	Pneumonia, sometimes with cavitation and calcification, resembling tuberculosis.
Other organs	Procedures depend on expected findings or grossly identified abnormalities as listed in right-hand column.	Abscesses may occur in skin, lymph nodes, liver, lungs, heart, spleen, kidneys, and bones *(2)*.

Reference

1. Wong KT, Vadivelu J, Puthucheary SD, Tan KL. An immunohistochemical method for the diagnosis of melioidosis. Pathology 1996;28:188–191.
2. Wong KT, Puthucheary SD, Vadivelu J. The histopathology of human melioidosis. Histopath 1995;26:51–55.

Meningitis

Related Terms: Meningoencephalitis; meningoencephalomyelitis.

NOTE: If the infectious agent is known, follow procedures described under the name of the corresponding infectious disease. Meningitis may complicate many noninfectious diseases, such as carcinoma, lymphoproliferative or myeloproliferative disorders, sarcoidosis,* and other conditions, particularly if they require treatment with immunosuppressive agents.

Organs and Tissues	*Procedures*	*Possible or Expected Findings*
External examination	Prepare chest roentgenogram.	Pulmonary infiltrates—for example, in fungal pneumonia or tuberculosis.*
Cerebrospinal fluid	Submit sample for microbiologic study, cell count, and chemical analysis.	
Brain and spinal cord	Submit samples for viral, fungal, and bacterial cultures. Record distribution of exudate; photograph, and make smears, touch preparations, and sections. Request Gram, acid fast (see "Tuberculosis"), and Grocott's methenamine silver stains. Make India ink preparations.	Bacterial (including tuberculous), fungal, and viral meningitis. Aseptic nonsuppurative inflammatory conditions. Uncal and cerebellar herniation; subdural effusion.
Blood	Submit sample for microbiologic study.	Septicemia.
Other organs	Search for possible sites of primary infection. Procedures depend on expected findings or grossly identified abnormalities as listed in right-hand column.	Infective endocarditis,* with or without congenital heart disease; pulmonary infection (origin of infection in tuberculous meningitis in infancy); pulmonary fungal infection, with or without bronchiectasis and cavitation; purulent arthritis. Manifestations of disseminated intravascular coagulation.* Adrenal hemorrhages.

Meningocele

Related Terms: Complete rachischisis; meningomyelocele; spina bifida aperta; spina bifida occulta.

Possible Associated Conditions: Arnold-Chiari malformation;* diastematomyelia; diplomyelia; hydrocephalus;* hydromyelia; syringomyelia;* tethered cord.

Organs and Tissues	*Procedures*	*Possible or Expected Findings*
External examination	Record location and extent of skin changes or skin defects on back. Prepare skeletal roentgenograms. If meningitis is suspected, submit sample of cerebrospinal fluid for culture.	Atrophic skin over meningocele, lacking rete pegs and skin appendages; skin defect in complete rachischisis. Bony defects of spine.
Brain and spinal cord	Use the posterior approach to remove the spinal cord.	In meningocele and spina bifida occulta, arachnoid and dura herniate through the vertebral defect. Spinal cord and roots are generally not involved. Lumbosacral mass in meningomyelocele, with a highly vascular mass (area medullovasculosa) in spina bifida aperta. Neural defects in complete rachischisis. Diastematomyelia, hydrocephalus *(1)*.
Other organs		Pyelonephritis;* enlarged urinary bladder ("neurogenic bladder").

Reference

1. Pettorini BL et al. Thoracic lipomeningocele associated with diastematomyelia, tethered spinal cord, and hydrocephalus. Case report. J Neurosurg 2007;106:394–397.

Meningococcemia (See "Disease, meningococcal.")

Meningoencephalitis (See "Encephalitis, all types or type unspecified" and "Meningitis.")

Mercury (See "Poisoning, mercury.")

Metaplasia, Agnogenic Myeloid, With Myelofibrosis

Synonym: Idiopathic myelofibrosis.

Organs and Tissues	*Procedures*	*Possible or Expected Findings*
External examination	Prepare skeletal roentgenograms.	Osteosclerosis of vertebrae, ribs, clavicles, pelvic bones, scapulae, skull, and metaphyseal ends of femur and humerus.
Bones and bone marrow	For removal, prosthetic repair, and specimen preparation of bone, see Chapter 2. For preparation of sections and smears of bone marrow, see Chapter 2. See above (under "External examination) for selection of bones.	Osteomyelofibrosis or osteoreticulosis; rarely, panhyperplasia of bone marrow; increase of megakaryocytes.
	Request Giemsa, Masson's trichrome, and reticulum stains for bone marrow sections. See also under "Leukemia."	Changes associated with chronic granulocytic leukemia* or with polycythemia vera* may imitate idiopathic myelofibrosis.
Other organs	Record weights of liver and spleen.	Widespread extramedullary hematopoiesis *(1)* with splenomegaly.
	Other procedures depend on expected findings or grossly identified abnormalities as listed in right-hand column.	Infectious diseases, including tuberculosis;* gouty arthritis; ascites and other manifestations of portal hypertension;* or hepatic vein thrombosis (Budd-Chiari syndrome*). Cardiac tamponade *(1)*.

Reference

1. Imam TH, Doll DC. Acute cardiac tamponade associated with pericardial extramedullary hematopoiesis in agnogenic myeloid metaplasia. Acta Haematol 1997;98:42–43.

Methanol (Methyl Alcohol) (See "Poisoning, methanol (methyl alcohol).")
Microangiopathy, Thrombotic Thrombocytopenic (See "Purpura, thrombotic thrombocytopenic.")

Microlithiasis, Pulmonary Alveolar

Organs and Tissues	*Procedures*	*Possible or Expected Findings*
External examination	Prepare chest roentgenogram.	Miliary mottling in lower lung fields.
Heart	Procedures depend on expected findings or grossly identified abnormalities as listed in right-hand column.	Mitral stenosis* may be a cause of microlithiasis (mostly intra-alveolar ossification).* Cor pulmonale and heart failure *(1)* may complicate chronic microlithiasis.
Lungs	Record weights. Prepare photographs and roentgenograms of fresh and fixed lung specimens. Perfuse one lung with formalin. For preparation of paper-mounted sections, see Chapter 2.	Increased weights and hardness. Miliary mottling, mainly in lower lobes. Pleural fibrosis and calcification *(2)*.
	Submit one lobe for microbiologic and chemical study. Decalcify tissue for histologic study.	Calcospherites containing calcium, phosphate, iron, and magnesium. Reactive pulmonary fibrosis.
	Request van Gieson's, Hale's colloidal iron, PAS, and Sudan stains.	Center of calcospherites strongly positive with PAS and colloidal iron stains. Sudanophilic and doubly refractile fatty material in calcospherites.

Reference

1. Mariotta S, Guidi L, Mattia P, Torrelli L, Pallone G, Pedicelli G, Bisetti A. Pulmonary microlithiasis. Report of two cases. Respiration 1997;64: 165–169.
2. Kacmaz E et al. A case of pulmonary alveolar microlithiasis with cardiac constriction secondary to severe adjacent pleural involvement. Cardiol 2007;107:213–216.

Mongolism (See "Syndrome, Down's.")
Mononucleosis, Infectious

Related Terms: *Cytomegalovirus* infection; *Epstein-Barr virus* (EBV) infection.

NOTE: If the EBV infection occurred after organ transplantation *(1)*, see also under that heading.

(1) Collect all tissues that appear to be infected. (2) Viral isolation, especially with EBV, is not diagnostically useful, due to long incubation periods. (3) No special precautions are indicated. (4) Serologic studies are the method of choice and are available from local or state health department laboratories. (6) This is not a reportable disease.

Organs and Tissues	*Procedures*	*Possible or Expected Findings*
External examination		Jaundice; petechial rash.
Blood	Submit samples for bacterial and viral cultures and for serologic study.	Septicemia. High Epstein-Barr virus antibody and heterophil titers.
	Prepare Giemsa-stained smear.	Atypical lymphocytes.
Heart	Record weight and submit samples for histologic study.	Myocarditis.*
Lungs	Submit consolidated areas for bacterial culture.	Edema and bacterial pneumonia.
Gastrointestinal tract		Hemorrhage.*
Spleen	Record size and weight. Submit sample for histologic study and make touch preparations. Request Giemsa stain.	Splenomegaly; hematomas and rupture. Extensive hyperplasia of red pulp. See below, under "Lymph Nodes."
Liver	Record size and weight. Submit sample for histologic study.	Massive EBV necrosis *(2)*; granulomatous hepatitis; cytomegalovirus inclusions within hepatocytes and endothelial cells.
Lymph nodes	Submit samples for histologic study and make	Generalized lymphadenopathy; abundant

Organs and Tissues	Procedures	Possible or Expected Findings
	touch preparations. Request azure-eosin stain.	immunoblasts resembling Reed-Sternberg cells.
Neck organs	Make touch preparations and request sections of lingual, palatine, and pharyngeal lymphoid tissue. Request azure-eosin stain.	Nasopharyngeal hemorrhage. Glottis edema. Lymphoid hyperplasia (see also above under "Spleen" and "Lymph nodes").
Other organs	Procedures depend on grossly identified abnormalities as listed in right-hand column.	Manifestations of bleeding due to thrombocytopenia; lymphoid infiltrates in any organ.
Brain, spinal cord, and spinal ganglia		Meningoencephalitis; lymphocytic or serous meningitis;* polyradiculitis (clinically, Guillain-Barré syndrome*).
Peripheral nerves	For sampling and specimen preparation, see Chapter 4.	Peripheral neuritis.
Bone marrow	For preparation of sections and smears, see Chapter 2.	Agranulocytosis.

References

1. Hubscher SG, Williams A, Davison SM, Young LS, Niedobitek G. Epstein-Barr virus in inflammatory diseases of the liver and liver allografts: an in situ hybridization study. Hepatology 1994;20:899–907.
2. Papatheodoridis GV, Delladetsima JK, Kavallierou L, Kapranos N, Tassopoulos NC. Fulminant hepatitis due to Epstein-Barr virus infection. J Hepatol 1995;23:348–350.

Morphine (See "Dependence, drug(s), all types or type unspecified.")

Mucopolysaccharidosis

Synonyms and Related Terms: Mucopolysaccharidosis I H (gargoylism, Hurler's disease or syndrome, α-L-iduronidase deficiency, MPS I H); mucopolysaccharidosis I S (Scheie's syn -drome, α-L-iduronidase deficiency, MPS I S, MP V); mucopolysaccharidosis II (Hunter's disease or syndrome, MPS II); mucopolysaccharidosis III (heparitinuria, MPS III, polydystrophic oligophrenia, Sanfilippo's syndrome); mucopolysaccharidosis IV (Morquio's syndrome, keratosulfaturia, MPS IV); mucopolysaccharidosis VI (Maroteaux-Lamy syndrome, MPS VI, polydystrophic dwarfism); mucopolysaccharidosis VII (β-glucuronidase deficiency, MPS VII).

NOTE: These diseases are characterized by a deficiency of a variety of hydrolases, resulting in accumulation of glycosaminoglycans (mucopolysaccharides) and glycolipids within lysosomes of fibroblasts, macrophages, white cells, and parenchymal cells of many organs *(1,2)*. Mucopolysaccharides are also excreted in the urine. The general approach is similar in all types. Formalin may dissolve all of the stored material and leave empty vacuoles in the involved cells. Therefore, frozen sections should be utilized or tissues should be fixed in absolute alcohol. The accumulated material will show intense metachromasia if stained with toluidine blue. It will also stain with PAS, alcian blue, and colloidal iron. Oil red O will also stain the material from frozen sections. For specimen preparation for elec-tron microscopy, see Chapter 15.

Characteristic external features include dwarfism; thickened long bones; coarse facial features; coarse hair; macrocephaly; prognathism; hypertelorism; malformed teeth, and scaphocephalic skull with hyperostosis of sagittal suture; short neck; chest deformity; umbilical and inguinal hernias; lower thoracic and lumbar gibbus; genu valgum and coxa valga; pes planus and other joint deformities; wide hands (clawhands) and feet. Coarse thickened skin, covered with lanugo-like hair. Hyperlordosis; ovoid deformities of vertebrae; odontoid hypoplasia; large, shoe-shaped sella turcica; kyphosis; hypoplasia of femoral heads; osteoporosis.*

If patient underwent bone marrow transplantation *(3)*, see also under that heading.

Organs and Tissues	Procedures	Possible or Expected Findings
External examination and extent and skin	Record body weight and length and type of deformities. Photograph head and deformities. Prepare sections of skin. Prepare skeletal roentgenograms.	Characteristic external features and possible roentgenographic features are listed above under "Note."
Placenta	Submit sections for histologic study.	Storage of material in Hofbauer cells and stromal cells.
Fascia lata	Submit sample for fibroblast tissue culture for enzyme assay.	Increased intracellular mucopolysaccharides. Cultures are well-suited for special studies.
Blood	Prepare smears (see below under "Bone marrow"). Submit sample for microbiologic study.	

Organs and Tissues	*Procedures*	*Possible or Expected Findings*
Urine	Submit sample for biochemical study.	Increased mucopolysaccharides.
Heart	Record weight. Prepare coronary arteriogram (see Chapter 10).	Diffuse coronary narrowing because of the presence of intimal gargoyle cells (smooth muscle cells), elastic fiber proliferation, and other deformities. (Heart disease is a frequent cause of death.)
	Test competence of valves (Chapter 3).	Nodular thickening of mitral *(4)*, aortic *(4)*, tricuspid, and pulmonary valves (in this order of involvement).
	Prepare histologic sections of all valves and chordae tendineae.	Gargoyle cells in valves and chordae tendineae.
	Record thickness of ventricles and extent of myocardial necroses or scarring.	Hypertrophy of the heart. Myocardial infarction.
	Photograph valves and myocardium.	Endocardial fibroelastosis.
	Submit samples of epicardium, myocardium, coronary arteries, and conduction system for histologic study.	Mucopolysaccharide deposits in epicardium and endocardium.
Aorta, pulmonary arteries, other great vessels, and peripheral muscular arteries	Request Verhoeff–van Gieson stain.	Extensive intimal deposits, as in coronary arteries.
Tracheobronchial tree and lungs	For pulmonary arteriography, see Chapter 2.	Pulmonary vascular changes (see above).
	Submit consolidated areas for microbiologic study.	Purulent bronchitis and bronchopneumonia. (Respiratory infection is a frequent cause of death).
	Perfuse one lung with formalin. Submit samples of tracheal and bronchial cartilage for histologic study.	Gargoyle cells in cartilage.
Spleen	Record weight. Submit specimen for tissue culture. Submit sample for histologic study.	Splenomegaly; gargoyle cells.
Liver	Record weight and submit samples for histologic study.	Hepatomegaly;* enlarged vacuolated hepatocytes with mucopolysaccharides; fibrosis.
Kidneys	Record weight and submit samples for histologic study.	Vacuolated cells in Bowman's capsule.
Endocrine organs	Record weight of all endocrine organs and submit samples for histologic study.	Gargoyle cells.
Brain, spinal cord, and peripheral ganglia	For removal and specimen preparation, see Chapter 4.	Hydrocephalus; cerebral cortical atrophy; storage of mucopolysaccharides in ganglion cells. Mucopolysaccharides may stain well with PAS reagent.
Eyes	For removal and specimen preparation, see Chapter 5.	Corneal clouding and retinal degeneration associated with storage of mucopolysaccharides in nuclear layer of retina.
Middle and inner ears	For removal and specimen preparation, see Chapter 4. (Study particularly indicated if patient was deaf.)	Chronic infections.
Sinuses and nasal cavities	Expose from base of skull, and submit samples of mucosa for histologic study.	Chronic upper respiratory infections.
Bone marrow	For preparation of sections and smears. Prepare air-dried smears (without formalin fixation) for demonstration of metachromatic granules.	Large cytoplasmic granules in neutrophils.
Bones and joints, periosteum, tendons, and fasciae		Storage of mucopolysaccharides in osteocytes, chondrocytes, and fibroblasts of periosteum, tendons, fasciae, and other connective tissues; dysostosis multiplex.

Organs and Tissues	*Procedures*	*Possible or Expected Findings*
Other tissues	Histologic sampling cannot be excessive.	Storage of mucopolysaccharides may occur anywhere.

References

1. Wraith JE. The mucopolysaccharidoses: a clinical review and guide to management. Arch Dis Child 1995;72(3):263–267.
2. Di Natale P, Annella T, Daniele A, De Luca T, Morabito E, Pallini R, et al. Biochemical diagnosis of mucopolysaccharidoses: experience of 297 diagnoses in a 15-year period (1997-1991). J Inher Metabolic Dis 1993;16(2):473–483.
3. Gatzoulis MA, Vellodi A, Redington AN. Cardiac involvement in mucopolysaccharidosis: effects of allogeneic bone marrow transplantation. Arch Dis Childhood 1995;73:259–260.
4. Wippermann CF, Beck M, Schranz D, Huth R, Michel-Behnke I, Jungst BK. Mitral and aortic regurgitation in 84 patients with mucopolysaccharidosis. Eur J Pediatr 1995;154:98–101.

Mucormycosis

Synonym: Phycomycosis; zygomycosis.

NOTE: Diseases that may be complicated by mucormycosis include burns,* diabetes mellitus,* leukemia,* lymphoma,* and tuberculosis.*

(1) Collect all tissues that appear to be infected. (2) Request fungal culture. (3) Request Grocott's methenamine silver stain. (4) No special precautions are indicated. (5) Serologic studies are not available. (6) This is not a reportable disease.

Organs and Tissues	*Procedures*	*Possible or Expected Findings*
External examination and skin	Photograph all lesions attributable to this infection.	Skin ulcerations.
Lungs	Submit consolidated areas for fungal and bacterial culture. Make touch preparation of fresh lung. Perfuse both lungs with formalin.	Necrotizing bronchopneumonia.
Gastrointestinal tract		Mucosal ulcers.
Other organs	Culture all tissues with gross evidence of thrombosis or infarction. Other procedures depend on expected findings or grossly identified abnormalities as listed in right-hand column.	Disseminated fungal arteritis with secondary thromboses and infarctions in heart, kidneys, and many other organs.
Skull with brain	For removal of brain and exposure of orbitae and paranasal sinuses, see Chapter 4. Prepare sections of abnormal tissues.	Primary infection in sinuses or orbitae; orbital cellulitis; fungal arteritis with cerebral infection; thrombosis of cavernous sinus and internal carotid artery.

Mucoviscidosis (See "Fibrosis, cystic.")

Mumps

NOTE: (1) Collect all tissues that appear to be infected. (2) Request viral cultures. (3) Usually, special stains are not helpful. (4) Special **precautions** are indicated. (5) Serologic studies are available from state health department laboratories. (6) This is not a reportable disease.

Organs and Tissues	*Procedures*	*Possible or Expected Findings*
External examination and skin	Prepare sections of skin.	Thrombocytopenic purpura.
Breasts	Submit tissue sample for histologic study.	Mastitis.
Blood	Submit samples for biochemical (serum amylase) and serologic study.	Complement-fixing antibodies.
Urine	Submit sample for viral cultures.	
Heart	Submit samples for histologic study.	Myocarditis* may be cause of death. Pericarditis* and endocardial fibroelastosis.*
Liver and pancreas	Record weights and submit samples for histologic study.	Hepatitis* and pancreatitis.*

Organs and Tissues	Procedures	Possible or Expected Findings
Spleen	Record weight and size.	Splenomegaly.
Kidneys	Record weights and submit samples for histologic study.	Nephritis.*
Male sex organs	Record weights of testes and epididymides; prepare histologic sections of testes, epididymides, seminal vesicles, and prostate, especially in postpubertal males.	Orchitis; epididymitis; seminal vesiculitis; prostatitis.
Female sex organs	Submit samples of ovaries and Bartholin's glands for histologic study.	Ovaritis (oophoritis); bartholinitis.
Neck organs	Prepare histologic sections of pharynx, submaxillary and sublingual glands, and thyroid.	Sialadenitis; thyroiditis.
Brain, spinal cord, and spinal roots	For removal and specimen preparation, see Chapter 4. Prepare sections of cranial nerves and spinal nerve roots.	Meningitis or postinfectious encephalitis;* perivenous demyelination and mononuclear inflammation; neuritis of cranial nerves II, III, VI, VII, and VIII. Polyneuritis; meningoradiculitis. Myelitis.
Eyes and lacrimal glands	For removal and specimen preparation, see Chapter 5.	Conjunctivitis; keratitis; uveitis; retinitis; dacryoadenitis.
Middle and inner ears	For removal and specimen preparation, see Chapter 4.	Labyrinthitis.
Parotid glands	Remove tissue from scalp incision with biopsy needle.	Parotitis.
Joints		Arthritis.*

Murder (See "Homicide.")

Mushroom (See "Poisoning, mushroom.")

Myasthenia Gravis

Synonyms and Related Term: Acquired autoimmune myasthenic (due to anti-acetylcholine receptor antibodies, anti-AchR); myasthenic syndromes, acquired (Eaton-Lambert syndrome) or congenital.

NOTE: The acquired myasthenic syndrome is associated in 40–50% of cases with bronchogenic carcinoma.

Organs and Tissues	Procedures	Possible or Expected Findings
Thymus	Record size and weight. Submit sample for histologic studies. If a thymoma is present, prepare sections of tumor and of uninvolved thymus.	In early onset myasthenia (55% of cases), thymus shows hyperplasia with lymphoid follicles with germinal centers. In late onset myasthenia, thymus is atrophic. 10% of cases are associated with thymoma.
Blood	Submit sample for serologic study.	Serum concentrations of Anti Ach R (anti-acetylcholine receptor) autoantibodies are high in myasthenia. 85% of patients with myasthenia and thymoma have high anti-
	striated muscle autoantibodies.	
Other organs	Search for tumors of any site (primarily lung small cell carcinoma) in acquired myasthenia syndrome (Eaton-Lambert); search for manifestations of "autoimmune" systemic diseases.	Manifestations of diabetes mellitus,* hyperthyroidism,* and rheumatoid arthritis* or other immune connective tissue diseases in myasthenia gravis. Thyroid abnormalities other than hyperplasia in myasthenia gravis. Tumors of lungs (small cell carcinoma), breast, and other sites in myasthenia syndrome (Eaton-Lambert).
Skeletal muscles	For sampling and specimen preparation, see Chapter 4. Respiratory musculature should always be included. Submit tissue samples for electron microscopic study.	Abnormalities of postsynaptic membrane in myasthenia gravis.

Reference

1. Engel AG. Myasthenic syndromes. In: Myology, 2nd ed., vol. 2. Engel AG, Franzini-Armstrong C, eds. MacGraw-Hill, New York, 1994, pp. 1798–1835.

Mycosis (See under specific disease designation, such as "Candidiasis.")

Mycosis Fungoides

Related Terms: Lymphoma;* Sézary syndrome.

NOTE: If mycosis fungoides was the cause of death, the patient probably was in the tumor stage of the disease with lymph node and general organ involvement. Follow procedures described under "Lymphoma." Viscera most commonly involved in late mycosis fungoides are, in order of frequency, lungs, spleen, liver, kidneys, thyroid gland, pancreas, bone marrow, and heart. Almost all organs and tissues of the body may be involved.

Myelinosis, Central Pontine

Organs and Tissues	*Procedures*	*Possible or Expected Findings*
External examination		Malnutrition* or severe burns* may be causes of central pontine myelinosis.
Cerebrospinal fluid	Submit sample for microbiologic study.	Sample should be sterile.
Brain and spinal cord	For removal and specimen preparation, see Chapter 4. Request Luxol fast blue/PAS and Bielschowsky stains.	Demyelination involving paramedian portion of the base of the pons, from just below the midbrain through the upper two-thirds of the pons. Myelin is lost and some axons may be fragmented while neurons in the nuclei pontis are preserved (unlike in centrale pontine infarct). Histiocytes may abound *(1)*.
Other organs	Procedures depend on expected findings or grossly identified abnormalities as listed in right-hand column.	Manifestations of alcoholism;* electrolyte disorders* (including too rapid correction of hyponatremia); severe infections; liver disease (especially after liver transplantation*); neoplastic conditions; renal diseases.

Reference

1. Kumar S, et al. Central pontine myelinolysis, an update. Neurol Res 2006;28:360–366.

Myelofibrosis with Myeloid Metaplasia (See "Metaplasia, agnogenic myeloid, with myelofibrosis.")

Myeloma, Multiple

Synonyms: Myeloma; osteosclerotic myeloma *(1)* POEMS syndrome; plasma cell myeloma.

Possible Associated Condition: Acute myeloblastic or monocytic leukemia;* amyloidosis;* chronic myelogenous leukemia *(2)*; hyperviscosity syndrome.

Organs and Tissues	*Procedures*	*Possible or Expected Findings*
External examination, skin, and tongue	Record extent of skin lesions and size of tongue (may be accessible only after removal of neck organs). Take sections of skin lesions and tongue. Request amyloid stains (see "Amyloidosis").	Vascular purpura. Skin tumors. Macroglossia secondary to amyloid deposition.
	Prepare skeletal roentgenograms.	Osteolytic skeletal tumors. Calvarium may be involved. Tumors are rarely osteoblastic (osteosclerotic *[1]*). Generally, no lymphadenopathy.
Vitreous	Submit sample for sodium, potassium, chloride, urea nitrogen, and calcium determination.	Evidence of electrolyte and other disorders (see under "Blood").*
Blood	Submit samples for bacterial and fungal cultures for serum electrophoresis, and for determination of calcium (post-mortem values not reliable) and uric acid concentrations.	Septicemia. Anemia (may be megaloblastic*). Hyperglobulinemia with hypogammaglobulinemia Hypercalcemia; hyperuricemia. Hyperviscosity of serum.
Urine	Submit sample for determination of Bence Jones protein.	Bence Jones protein. Light-chain proteinuria.

Organs and Tissues	Procedures	Possible or Expected Findings
Heart	Record weight. Request amyloid stains (see "Amyloidosis").	Cardiac amyloidosis.
Lungs	Submit one lobe for bacterial and fungal cultures.	Various types of pneumonia.
	Make touch preparations of cut surface and request Grocott's methenamine silver stain.	*Pneumocystis carinii* pneumonia.
	Perfuse one lung with formalin.	
	Histologic sections may need decalcification.	Metastatic calcification.
Spleen and gastrointestinal tract	Request amyloid stains (see "Amyloidosis").	Amyloidosis.* Metastatic calcification in stomach. Tumor infiltrates generally are inconspicuous.
Kidneys	Submit sample for histologic study. Fix at least one specimen in alcohol. Decalcify, if necessary.	Pyelonephritis.* Metastatic calcification; calcium and urate casts.
	Request amyloid stains (see "Amyloidosis").	Amyloidosis.*
Other organs	Submit samples of liver, pancreas, adrenal glands, thyroid, lymph nodes, and all grossly involved tissues for histologic study.	Amyloidosis;* myeloma infiltrates; evidence of infection. Lymph nodes are rarely involved.
Brain, spinal cord, and peripheral nerves		Cord compression after vertebral collapse.
	Request amyloid stains of peripheral nerves (see "Amyloidosis").	Amyloidosis of peripheral nerves. Demyelinating polyneuropathy in osteosclerotic myeloma *(1)*.
Bones and bone marrow	For removal, prosthetic repair, and specimen preparation of bone, see Chapter 2. For decalcification, see Chapter 2.	Osteolytic tumors
	Also consult roentgenograms. For preparation of sections and smears of bone marrow, see Chapter 2. Snap-freeze bone marrow if immuno-phenotype study of immunoglobulin-producing cells is intended.	Plasmacellular bone marrow.

References

1. Lacy MQ, Gertz MA, Hanson CA, Inwards DJ, Kyle RA. Multiple myeloma associated with diffuse osteosclerotic bone lesions: a clinical entity distinct from osteosclerotic myeloma (POEMS syndrome). Am J Hematol 1997;56:288–293.
2. Tanaka M, Kimura R, Matsutani A, Zaitsu K, Oka Y, Oizumi K. Coexistence of chronic myelogenous leukemia and multiple myeloma. Case report and review of the literature. Acta Haematol 1998;99:221–223.

Myelomeningocele (See "Meningocele.")

Myelopathy/Myelitis

Synonyms and Related Terms: Acute transverse myelitis; acute or subacute necrotizing myelopathy; angiodysgenetic necrotizing myelopathy; compression myelopathy; encephalomyelitis;* infectious myelitis; ischemic myelopathy; traumatic myelopathy; postvaccinal/postinfectious myelitis.

Possible Associated or Underlying Conditions: Angiodysgenetic (subacute) necrotizing myelopathy results from arteriovenous malformations* (Foix-Alajouanine syndrome); com-pression myelopathy may complicate degenerative vertebral disease, rheumatoid arthritis* or ankylosing spondylitis,* bony abnormalities at the foramen magnum (basilar impression,* platybasia*), or infections (spinal epidural, tuberculous osteomyelitis), or neoplastic processes involving the vertebrae and meninges; subacute necrotizing myelopathy may be a manifestation of multiple sclerosis* or it may be a paraneoplastic condition, primarily associated with small cell carcinoma; traumatic myelopathy occurs with or without penetrating injury. Myelitis due to intramedullary infections may include bacterial or mycobacterial abscess, fungal or parasitic infections and viral infections, in particular, cytomegalovirus infection,* Herpes zoster,* poliomyelitis,* and human immunodeficiency virus (HIV) infection (acquired immunodeficiency syndrome*).

Organs and Tissues	Procedures	Possible or Expected Findings
Cerebrospinal fluid	Submit sample for microbiologic study.	Bacterial, fungal, or viral infection.
Chest and abdominal organs; blood; spine	If the myelitis is thought to be infectious, submit samples of blood and appropriate tissues for microbiologic study. Procedures depend on expected findings and grossly identified abnormalities as listed in right-hand column.	Tuberculous osteomyelitis.* Cervical spondylitis in acute transverse myelitis. Rarely, parasitic disease. Neoplasm. Manifestations of nutritional deficiencies or vascular disease.
Brain, spinal cord, spinal roots, and sensory ganglia	If there are abscesses or other acute infectious lesions, submit material for culture, prepare smears, and request Gram and Grocott's methenamine silver stains. Request Luxol fast blue stain for myelin and Bielschowsky's stain for axons.	Bacterial or fungal epidural or subdural empyema or granuloma.

Myocardiopathy (See "Cardiomyopathy,...")

Myocarditis

Synonyms and Related Terms: Bacterial myocarditis; drug-induced myocarditis; fungal myocarditis; giant cell myocarditis; human immunodeficiency virus myocarditis; infectious myocarditis; interstitial myocarditis; Lyme carditis; protozoal myocarditis; rheumatic myocarditis; viral myocarditis.

Possible Associated Conditions: Bacterial, fungal, protozoal (toxoplasmosis) or viral infections (particularly coxsackievirus B); human immunodeficiency virus infection; hypersensitivity states (e.g., acute rheumatic fever); idiosyncratic or toxic reaction to drugs; irradiation; Lyme disease.

Organs and Tissues	Procedures	Possible or Expected Findings
Blood	Submit sample for microbiologic and, if, indicated, toxicologic and biochemical study.	Septicemia; viremia; toxemia.
Pericardial sac	Submit sample of pericardial exudate for microbiologic study. Record volume of exudate; centrifuge; prepare smear of pellet. Request Gram and Grocott's methenamine silver stains.	Pericarditis.*
Heart	Record heart weight. Excise apical portion of myocardium and submit for microbiologic study. If infective endocarditis is suspected, follow procedures described in Chapter 7.	Infectious myocarditis (for possible infectious agents, see above under "Possible Associated Conditions). Infective endocarditis.* Giant cell myocarditis *(1)*.
Other organs, tissues, and body fluids	Depending on clinical findings, submit samples of cerebrospinal fluid, serosal exudates or transudates, intestinal contents, pulmonary tissue, liver, spleen, kidneys, and cerebral tissue for bacterial, fungal, and viral cultures.	Bacterial, mycotic, protozoal, or viral diseases. Postinfectious states. Manifestations of drug toxicity or hypersensitivity; Pheochromocytoma. Burns.* Manifestations of congestive heart failure.*

Reference

1. Regnante R, Poppas A. Giant cell myocarditis presenting as isolated right ventricular dysfunction. Med Health RI 2007;90:50–51.

Myonecrosis, Clostridial (See "Gangrene, gas.")

Myopathy

Synonyms and Related Terms: Congenital myopathy (central core disease, centronuclear myopathy, mitochondrial myopathy (see also "Epilepsy, myoclonus"); myotubular myopathy, nemaline or rod myopathy); familial myoglobinuria; familial periodic paralysis; myositis ossificans; myotonia congenita (Thomsen's disease).

NOTE: Muscular dystrophy and motor neuron disease are listed separately.

Organs and Tissues	Procedures	Possible or Expected Findings
External examination		Kyphoscoliosis, pigeon breast, and pes cavus in congenital myopathy.
	Prepare soft tissue roentgenograms.	Myositis ossificans.
Heart	Submit samples for light microscopic and electron microscopic study. For study of the conduction system, see Chapter 3.	Cardiomyopathy;* conduction system abnormalities.
Skeletal muscles	For sampling and specimen preparation, see Chapter 4. Refer also to clinical findings. Prepare specimens for electron microscopic study.	Variable changes, depending on disease entities.
Brain, spinal cord, and spinal ganglia	For removal and specimen preparation, see Chapter 4.	Should be normal in primary myopathies (important for differentiation from Werdnig-Hoffmann and other primarily (central) neurological disorders).
Eyes and gonads	If diagnosis is uncertain, prepare sections of eyes and gonads.	No cataracts and no gonadal atrophy (important for differentiation from muscular dystrophy).

Myotonia Congenita (Thomsen's Disease) (See "Myopathy.")

Myxedema (See "Hypothyroidism.")

Myxoma, Heart (See "Tumor of the heart.")

N

Narcotic(s) (See "Dependence, drug(s), all types or type unspecified.")

Necrolysis, Toxic Epidermal

Synonyms: Lyell's disease; scalded skin syndrome.

NOTE: Toxic epidermal necrolysis usually represent an adverse reaction to drugs or, rarely, other chemicals. If it appears linked to hyperacute graft-versus-host disease after allogeneic bone marrow transplantation *(1)*, see also under that heading.

Organs and Tissues	*Procedures*	*Possible or Expected Findings*
External examination and skin	Record extent of skin lesions and prepare photographs; prepare sections of affected and unaffected skin. Request Gram stain of sections and smears.	Extensive epidermal necrosis. Shedding of granular and horny layers of epidermis.
Blood; other organs and tissues	Submit samples of blood and grossly affected organs or tissues for microbiologic study. Other procedures depend on expected findings or grossly identified abnormalities as listed in right-hand column.	Septicemia; staphylococcal infection of nose, throat, ears, eyes, heart valves, urogenital tract, and other sites. Bronchial epithelial detachment and bacterial pneumonia *(2)*.

References

1. Takeda H, Mitsuhashi Y, Kondo S, Kato Y, Tajima K. Toxic epidermal necrolysis possibly linked to hyperacute graft-versus-host disease after allogeneic bone marrow transplantation. J Dermatol 1997;24:635–641.
2. Lebargy F, Wokenstein P, Gisselbrecht M, Lange F, Fleury-Feith J, Delclaux C, et al. Pulmonary complications in toxic epidermal necro-lysis: a prospective clinical study. Intensive Care Med 1997;23:1237–1244.

Necrosis, Aseptic, of Bone (See "Osteonecrosis.")

Necrosis, Bilateral Renal Cortical (See "Coagulation, disseminated intravascular.")

Necrosis, Renal Tubular

Synonyms and Related Terms: Acute kidney failure;* acute tubular necrosis; lower nephron nephrosis.

NOTE: The morphologic diagnosis of this condition may be difficult to discern from autolysis. The features that suggest tubular necrosis are: tubular dilation with epithelial flattening, intertubular edema and necrotic epithelial cells in the collecting ducts. The autopsy should be performed as soon as possible. Needle specimens of the kidneys obtained in the immediate postmortem period may yield acceptable material. If nephrotoxic drugs or chemicals are thought to be responsible for tubular necrosis, submit samples for toxicologic study (see also under "Poisoning,..." and under name of suspected drug or poison). If tubular necrosis occurred after transfusion of incompatible blood, see under "Reaction to transfusion." Autopsy procedures depend on suspected underlying condition, such as trauma or infection.

Neoplasia, Multiple Endocrine

Synonyms and Related Terms: Multiple endocrine neoplasia (MEN), **type 1** (parathyroid hyperplasia or adenoma; pancreatic islet cell hyperplasia, adenoma, or carcinoma; pituitary hyperplasia or adenoma); or **type 2A** (medullary thyroid carcinoma, parathyroid hyperplasia or adenoma; and pheochromocytoma); or **type 2B** (medullary thyroid carcinoma, pheochromocytoma, mucosal and gastrointestinal neuromas, and marfanoid features).

NOTE: In MEN, type 1, foregut carcinoids and subcutaneous and visceral lipomas also may be found. In type 2A, cutaneous lichen amyloidosis may be observed. Mixed syndromes include (1) familial pheochromocytoma and islet cell tumor, (2) von Hippel-Lindau syndrome, pheochromocytoma and islet cell tumor, (3) neurofibromatosis* with features of MEN1 or 2, and myxomas, spotty skin pigmentation, and generalized endocrine overactivity (Carney complex).

In all instances, the autopsy should be done as soon as possible so that tissues for biochemical study can be frozen without delay.

From: *Handbook of Autopsy Practice,* 4th Ed. Edited by: B.L. Waters

Organs and Tissues	*Procedures*	*Possible or Expected Findings*
External examination	Record height, weight, habitus, and abnormal external features.	Marfanoid habitus; cushingoid features, features of acromegaly.*
	Record appearance of skin and oral cavity.	Spotty skin pigmentation. Thickened lips; nodules in anterior third of tongue. Cleft palate.
	Prepare skeletal roentgenograms. Studies should include long bones of extremities, bones of hands, feet, skull with calvarium, base of skull, and jaws.	Osteoporosis with osteoclastic cysts. Acromegalic features.
Blood	Snap-freeze specimen for hormone assay. Submit sample for determination of calcium concentration.	Hypercalcemia.
	If chromosome studies are intended, see Chapter 9.	Normal karyotype.
Urine	Snap-freeze specimen for hormone assays.	
	If pheochromocytoma is suspected, request catecholamine determination.	Increased catecholamine concentrations associated with pheochromocytoma.
Mediastinum	If a tumor is present, photograph *in situ* and after removal. See also under "Neck organs."	Thymoma and other mediastinal tumors or cysts. Cardiac myxoma.
Neck organs	Dissect, photograph, and weigh thyroid and all parathyroid glands. Snap-freeze tumor tissue for histochemical and biochemical study. Prepare tumor tissue samples for electron microscopy. Submit samples of normal and abnormal endocrine tissue and cervical lymph nodes for histologic study.	Nodular (toxic) goiter; lymphocytic thyroiditis; multifocal hyperplasia of C cells of thyroid gland. Medullary carcinoma of thyroid with amyloid stroma. Chief cell hyperplasia of parathyroids. Parathyroid adenomas.
	Also submit samples of cervical sympathetic chain and vagus nerves.	Ganglioneuromatosis.
Small and large bowel	If tumors are present, prepare tissue for biochemical, histochemical, electron microscopic, and routine light microscopic study. See also above under "Neck organs."	Carcinoid tumors in small bowel. Diffuse ganglioneuromatosis of small and large bowel. Megacolon. Diffuse diverticulosis.
Stomach and duodenum	See above under "Small and large bowel."	Carcinoid tumors. Ganglioneuromatosis. Diffuse gastric polyposis. Peptic ulcer of stomach or duodenum.*
Pancreas	Prepare 2-mm sagittal slices throughout entire pancreas. If tumor is present, follow procedures suggested above under "Neck organs." Submit samples of parapancreatic lymph nodes for histologic study.	Islet cell adenomas or carcinomas, usually of non-beta cell type.
Adrenal glands	Record weights and photograph. If tumors are present, follow procedures described under "Tumor of the adrenal glands" and above under "Neck organs."	Nodular hyperplasia of adrenal medulla; pheochromocytoms, frequently bilateral; primary pigmented nodular adrenal disease.
Ovaries	Submit samples for histologic study. Record size and contents of cysts.	Ovarian cysts.
Testes	Record number and size of tumors. Submit samples for histologic study.	Large-cell calcifying Sertoli cell tumor.
Other organs and tissues	Procedures depend on expected findings or grossly identified abnormalities.	See under "Synonyms and Related Terms" and under "Note."
Brain, spinal cord, and pituitary gland	For removal and specimen preparation, see Chapter 4.	Pinealoma.
	If tumor tissue is present, follow procedures suggested above under "Neck organs."	Pituitary hyperplasia or adenoma, usually chromophobe type.
Bones	For removal, prosthetic repair, and specimen preparation, see Chapter 2.	Osteoclastic osteoporosis secondary to hyperparathyroidism.* Benign cysts.

Nephritis

NOTE: See under specific designation, such as "Glomerulonephritis" and "Pyelonephritis," or under name of suspected underlying condition, such as "Gout" or "Lupus erythematosus, systemic."

Nephroblastoma (See "Tumor of the kidney(s).")

Nephrolithiasis

Synonyms and Related Terms: Renal stones; urolithiasis.

Possible Associated Conditions: Carcinomatosis; Cushing's syndrome;* Cystinuria;* Fanconi syndrome;* hyperoxaluria;* hypervitaminosis D;* gout;* multiple myeloma;* osteoporosis;* polycystic renal disease;* primary hyperparathyroidism;* rheumatoid arthritis* *(1)*; sarcoidosis* *(2)*.

Organs and Tissues	*Procedures*	*Possible or Expected Findings*
Kidneys	Remove kidneys, ureters, and urinary bladder en bloc. Excise and bivalve kidneys to reveal renal pelves. Open ureters. Record size, number, and appearance of stones, and save for chemical analysis *(4)*.	Pyelonephritis;* nephrocalcinosis; granulomas; tumor infiltrates; manifestations of the conditions listed below under "Other organs." Calcium, cystine, struvite, and uric acid stones may form staghorn calculi.
Ureters, urinary bladder, and urethra		Obstructive uropathy with foreign bodies, stones, strictures, valves, or other lesions.
Other organs	Record heart weight. Dissect and record weights of all parathyroid glands. Other procedures depend on suspected underlying conditions, as listed above under "Possible Associated Conditions."	Manifestations of hypertension *(3)*. Parathyroid hyperplasia.

References

1. Ito S, Nozawa S, Ishikawa H, Tohyama C, Nakazono K, Murasawa A, et al. Renal stones in patients with rheumatoid arthritis. J Rheumatol 1997;24:2123–2128.
2. Rizzato G, Colombo P. Nephrolithiasis as a presenting feature of chronic sarcoidosis: a prospective study. Sarcoidosis Vasculitis Diff Lung Dis 1996;13:167–172.
3. Madore F, Stampfer MJ, Rimm EB, Curhan GC. Nephrolithiasis and risk of hypertension. Am J Hypertension 1998;11:46–53.
4. Kasidas GP et al. Renal stone analysis: why and how? Ann Clin Biochem 2004;41:91–97.

Nephropathy

NOTE: See under name of suspected underlying condition, such as "Diabetes mellitus," "Disorder, electrolyte(s)" (hypercalcemia, potassium depletion), "Gout," "Hypertension (arterial), all types or type unspecified," or "Poisoning,..." (heavy metal). If kidney failure was present, procedures under that heading should also be followed. Renal tissue may need decalcification or fixation in water-free solution.

Nephrosis, Lipoid (See "Glomerulonephritis.")

Neuroblastoma (See "Tumor of the peripheral nerves.")

Neurofibromatosis

Synonyms and Related Terms: Neurofibromatosis type 1 (peripheral neurofibromatosis; von Recklinghausen's disease; von Recklinghausen's neurofibromatosis); neurofibromatosis, type 2 (bilateral acoustic neurofibromatosis).

NOTE: The term "von Recklinghausen's disease" should not be used for neurofibromatosis type 2. Because of the different manifestations, autopsy procedures for neurofibromatosis type 1 and type 2 are presented here separately.

Neurofibromatosis, type 1 *(1)*

Organs and Tissues	*Procedures*	*Possible or Expected Findings*
External examination, skin, soft tissues, and skeletal system	Sample skin tumors, pigmented areas of skin, and soft tissue tumors for microscopic study. Prepare roentgenograms of skeletal abnormalities.	Short stature; bone deformities (see below). Café au lait spots; axillary and/or inguinal freckling; dermal neurofibromas; rhabdomyosarcoma. Kyphoskoliosis; macrocephaly with asymmetry of facial and skull bones; sphenoid wing dysplasia; thinning, bending and pseudarthrosis of long bones (tibia).
Arteries	Prepare longitudinal sections and request Verhoeff-van Gieson stains.	Fibromuscular dysplasia or renal and cervical arteries.

Organs and Tissues	*Procedures*	*Possible or Expected Findings*
Gastrointestinal tract	Search for tumors.	Duodenal carcinoid.
Adrenal glands	Record weights. If a tumor is present, see also under "Tumor of the adrenal gland(s)").	Pheochromocytoma (more common on the left).
Brain, spinal cord, and spinal roots; base of skull	For removal and specimen preparation, see Chapter 4. Dissect cranial nerves.	Optic nerve gliomas; pilocytic astrocytomas; glioblastomas; nerve sheath tumors *(3)*. Hydrocephalus* (due to aqueduct stenosis).
Eyes and orbitae	For removal and specimen preparation, see Chapter 5.	Pigmented hamartomas, elevated on the surface of the iris (Lisch nodules). Neurofibromatosis of ciliary nerves; optic nerve gliomas.
Peripheral nerves, trunks, and plexuses	For removal and specimen preparation, see Chapter 4.	Benign neurofibromas and malignant peripheral nerve sheath tumors, including MPNST with divergent differentiation (malignant triton tumor). Peripheral neuropathy.
Other organs and tissues; bones and bone marrow	For removal of bones and prosthetic repair, and bone marrow preparations, see Chapter 2. If leukemia is expected, see also under that heading.	Neurofibromas rarely in other organs such as the liver. For skeletal abnormalitis, see above under "External examination, skin, soft tissues, and skeletal system." Bone marrow and other tissues may show features of juvenile chronic myeloid leukemia.*

Neurofibromatosis, type 2 *(2)*

NOTE: In this condition, lesions in the brain and cranial nerves, spinal cord, and spinal roots may be schwannomas (including bilateral vestibular schwannomas); multiple meningiomas; gliomas (generally of spinal cord), mostly ependymomas (75%) and pilocytic astrocytomas; or schwannosis of spinal dorsal root entry zones. Intracortical meningioangiomatosis; glial hamartia (intracortical, basal ganglia, thalamus, cerebellum, and dorsal horns of spinal cord) and cerebral calcifications also may be found.

Organs and Tissues	*Procedures*	*Possible or Expected Findings*
External examination and skin	Sample skin tumors for histologic study.	Schwannomas of skin.
Brain with cranial nerves, spinal cord, and spinal roots	For removal and specimen preparation, see Chapter 4.	A multitude of tumors or tumor-like lesions may be found, as listed above under "Note."
Eyes	For removal and specimen preparation, see Chapter 5.	Posterior lens opacities; retinal hamartomas.
Peripheral nerves	For removal and specimen preparation, see Chapter 4.	Peripheral neuropathy with focal schwannomatous changes or onion-bulb-like Schwann cell or perineural cell proliferation.

References

1. Von Deimling A, Krone W. Neurofibromatosis type 1. In: Pathology and Genetics of Tumours of the Nervous System. Kleihues P, Cavenee WK, eds. IARC, Lyon, 1997, pp. 172–174.
2. Louis DN, Wiestler OD. Neurofibromatosis type 2. In: Pathology and Genetics of Tumours of the Nervous System. Kleihues P, Cavenee WK, eds. IARC, Lyon, 1997, pp. 175–178.
3. Hsieh HY, et al. Neurological complications involving the central nervous system in neurofibromatosis type I. Acta Neurol Taiwan 2007;16:68–73.

Neuropathy

Synonyms and Related Terms: Multiple neuropathy; peripheral neuropathy; polyneuropathy; polyradiculoneuropathy; retrobulbar neuropathy (nutritional amblyopia).

Organs and Tissues	*Procedures*	*Possible or Expected Findings*
Spinal cord, dorsal root ganglia, and peripheral nerves	For removal and specimen preparation, see Chapter 4.	Fiber loss; segmental demyelination or wallerian degeneration, or both.

Organs and Tissues	Procedures	Possible or Expected Findings
Spinal cord, dorsal root ganglia, and peripheral nerves *(continued)*	Sural nerve is commonly used for peripheral nerve study. Stains for paraffin sections may include trichrome, LFB/PAS, methyl violet, and Congo red. Stain semithin sections with toluidin blue.	Distribution of lesions depends on type of neuropathy. Vasculitis; amyloid deposition or other manifestations of the underlying condition may be present.
Other organs	Procedures depend on expected findings or grossly identified abnormalities as listed in right-hand column.	Manifestations of underlying conditions, such as alcoholism,* celiac sprue;* diabetes mellitus,* hormonal disorder, immune connective tissue disease, malignant tumor, malnutrition, pellagra,* peripheral vascular disease, megaloblastic anemia,* poisoning (with heavy metals, organophosphates, or drugs), post-gastrectomy syndrome, or uremia.

Neurosyphilis, Adult (See "Syphilis, acquired.")

Neurosyphilis, Congenital

NOTE: See also "Syphilis, congenital."

Organs and Tissues	Procedures	Possible or Expected Findings
External examination	Record presence or absence of abnormal external features, as listed in right-hand column. Prepare photographs.	Hydrocephalus;* dental deformities (Hutchinson's teeth); saddle nose; frontal bossing of skull; saber shins; nasal septal perforation; rhagades; ulnar deviation of fingers.
Cerebrospinal fluid	Submit samples for biochemical, cytologic, and microbiologic study.	See below under "Brain and spinal cord."
Blood	Submit sample for serologic study.	
Brain and spinal cord	For removal and specimen preparation, see Chapter 4. For histologic sections, request Warthin-Starry stain for spirochetes.	Chronic syphilitic meningitis, encephalitis, and myelitis.
Eyes	For removal and specimen preparations, see Chapter 5.	Interstitial keratitis; chorioretinitis.

Nitrogen Oxide (See "Poisoning, gas.")

Nocardiosis

Synonym: *Nocardia* spp. infection.

NOTE: (1) Collect all tissues that appear to be infected. (2) Request culture for nocardiosis. (3) Request Gram and Ziehl-Neelsen stains. (4) Usually, no special precautions are indicated. (5) Generally, serologic studies are not available. (6) This is not a reportable disease.

Possible Associated Conditions: Acquired immunodeficiency syndrome (AIDS);* alveolar lipoproteinosis of lungs;* anthracosilicosis; asthma;* chronic obstructive pulmonary disease; leukemia,* post-transplantation, and other immunosuppressed or dysproteinemic states; systemic lupus erythematosus.*

Organs and Tissues	Procedures	Possible or Expected Findings
External examination	Sample involved skin for culture and histologic study.	Cutaneous abscess *(1)*.
Pleural cavities, pericardium, and lungs	Record presence (and sites) of pleural, pericardial, and chest-wall fistulas. Prepare smears from exudate or from caseating material. Culture consolidated areas. If diagnosis has already been confirmed, perfuse lungs with formalin.	Acute necrotizing nocardial pneumonia with abscesses or sinus formation into surrounding tissues; empyema.

Organs and Tissues	Procedures	Possible or Expected Findings
Pulmonary and mediastinal lymph nodes	Submit samples for culture and histologic study.	Regional lymphadenitis.
Other organs	Submit samples from all organs and tissues with suspicious gross lesions for culture and histologic study.	Poorly encapsulated abscesses of any organ; endocarditis *(2)*.

References

1. Merigou D, Beylot-Barry M, Ly S, Deutre MS, Texier-Maugein J, Billes P, Beylot C. Primary cutaneous *Nocardia asteroides* infection after heart transplantation. Dermatol 1998;196:246–247.
2. Dhawan VK, Gadgil VG, Paliwal YK, Chavroshiya PS, Trivedi RR. Native valve endocarditis due to *Nocardia*-like organisms. Clin Inf Dis 1998;27:902–904.

Nutrition, Parenteral

Related Term: Total parenteral nutrition.

NOTE: Air embolism* or blood loss may have occurred if line became detached from the catheter hub. Metabolic complications such as fluid overload or disturbances of acid-base and electrolyte balance often cannot be diagnosed reliably at autopsy.

The disease(s) that may have necessitated parenteral nutrition therapy are not considered here; they include the acquired immunodeficiency syndrome (AIDS);* cancer cachexia; inflammatory bowel disease; liver or kidney failure;* severe pancreatitis;* short bowel syndrome, and others.

Organs and Tissues	Procedures	Possible or Expected Findings
External examination	Inspect skin site where catheter enters tunnel to venous access (e.g., subclavian or jugular vein; femoral vein).	Infection at any site along the catheter. Displacement of intravenous catheter; fractures or tears in catheter.
	Inspect gastrostomy or jejunostomy sites, if present.	Enteral nutrition may have been combined with parenteral nutrition. Infection and displacement of tube may occur.
	Prepare chest roentgenogram.	Pneumothorax.*
Vitreous		Electrolyte disorders.*
Blood	Submit sample for culture.	Septicemia (*Staphylococcus* or *Candida*).
Internal examination of major veins	Follow catheter from access site to its open end, generally in the superior vena cava. If clots are found, particularly at the catheter tip, submit material for culture and prepare sections and smears (order Gram stain).	Infection at any site along the catheter. Displacement of catheter with perforation of wall of vein; hemothorax; pneumothorax.*
Urine		Hypercalciuria
Trachea and lungs	If an enteral feeding tube is in place, search for feeding fluid in tracheobronchial tree and lungs.	Aspiration* and aspiration bronchopneumonia.
Gallbladder	Record nature of contens.	Cholelithiasis*
Liver	Record weight. Submit samples for histologic study.	Chronic liver disease with cholestasis and cirrhosis, particularly in children *(1,2)*.
Gastrointestinal tract	If feeding tube is in place, determine location.	Nasogastric, nasoduodenal, nasojejunal, and other tubes (see also above under "External examination").
Skeletal system		Osteoporosis.

References

1. Fein B, Holt P. Hepatobiliary complications of total parenteral nutrition. J Clin Gastroenterol 1994;18:62–66.
2. Mullock FG, Ishak KG. Total parenteral nutrition: a histopathologic analysis of the liver changes in 20 children. Mod Pathol 1994;7:190–194.

O

Obesity

Related Term: Morbid obesity; primary obesity; secondary obesity.

Organs and Tissues	*Procedures*	*Possible or Expected Findings*
External examination and subcutaneous tissue	Record body weight and length (for calculation of body mass index), distribution of fat, and thickness of subcutaneous fat layers.	Decubital ulcers; intertriginous infections.
Breast		Breast cancer *(1)*.
Blood		Hyperlipoproteinemia.
Heart and arteries	Record weight of heart and thickness of ventricular walls.	Obesity cardiomyopathy *(3)* caused by pulmonaryor systemic hypertension.* Cor pulmonale in Pickwickian syndrome. Atherosclerosis.
Liver	Record weight. Submit samples for histologic study. Request trichrome stain.	Hepatomegaly and fatty changes; steatohepatitis with or without cirrhosis *(2)*.
Stomach	Record features of surgical procedures.	Weight-reducing surgery (gastroplasty or gastric bypass).
Pancreas	Cut in thin, sagittal slices.	Insulinoma (rare).
Other organs	Procedures depend on expected findings or grossly identified abnormalities as listed in right-hand column.	Manifestations of Cushing's syndrome,* type II diabetes mellitus,* hypothyroidism,* hypothalamic disorders (Laurence-Moon-Biedl syndrome* or Prader-Willi syndrome) and systemic hypertension.* Nephrotic syndrome* is a rare complication of obesity.

References

1. Pujol P, Galtier-Dereure F, Bringer J. Obesity and breast cancer risk. Hum Reprod 1997;12:116–125.
2. Ludwig J, McGill DB, Lindor KD. Nonalcoholic steatohepatitis. J Gastroenterol Hepatol 1997;12:398–403.
3. Wong C, Marwick TH. Obesity cardiomyopathy: pathogenesis and pathophysiology. Nat Clin Pract Cardiovasc Med 2007;4:436–443.

Obstruction, Acute Airway

Synonyms and Related Terms: Aspiration; bolus death; "café coronary"; croup; restaurant death.

NOTE: If permission has been obtained, remove neck organs through straight incision from chest to chin to avoid dislodging a foreign body. If dissection has to be accomplished from chest, neck of unembalmed cadaver should remain well extended during procedure. Inspect larynx and trachea from above and below, respectively, before opening them carefully along the posterior midline.

Organs and Tissues	*Procedures*	*Possible or Expected Findings*
Oral cavity		Edentulous mouth; malfitting dentures; food or other foreign body in oral cavity.
Blood	Submit sample for alcohol and other toxicologic studies. If infectious airway obstruction is suspected, submit sample for microbiologic study.	Evidence of alcohol intoxication.*

From: *Handbook of Autopsy Practice*, 4th Ed. Edited by: B.L. Waters

Organs and Tissues	Procedures	Possible or Expected Findings
Larynx and pharynx	For dissection procedures, see above under "Note."	
	Photograph larynx with foreign body or tumor.	Foreign body (food bolus; denture); malignant tumor of pharynx or larynx.
	If infectious obstructive laryngitis is expected, follow procedures described under "Laryngitis."	Obstructive laryngitis* with epiglottiditis in infants.
Lungs	Record weights.	Acute pulmonary edema.
Brain and spinal cord	For removal and specimen preparation, see Chapter 4.	Chronic neurologic disorder.

Obstruction, Arteriomesenteric

Organs and Tissues	Procedures	Possible or Expected Findings
External examination		Lax abdominal musculature.
Intestinal tract and mesentery	For mesenteric arteriography, see Chapter 2. Photograph obstruction *in situ*.	Superior mesenteric artery or abnormal arterial branch crosses and obstructs third portion of duodenum; dilatation of duodenum proximal to obstruction.

Obstruction, Biliary (See "Atresia, biliary," "Cholelithiasis," and "Tumor of the bile ducts (extrahepatic or hilar or of papilla of Vater.")

Obstruction, Chronic Airway (See "Asthma," "Bronchitis, chronic," and "Emphysema.")

Obstruction, Hepatic Vein (See "Syndrome, Budd-Chiari.")

Obstruction, Inferior Vena Cava

Organs and Tissues	Procedures	Possible or Expected Findings
Chest organs and abdominal organs	Remove thoracoabdominal viscera en masse (Letulle technique.) and dissect inferior vena cava from posterior aspect. Phlebography from lower extremities requires much contrast medium and interferes with clean dissection.	Adhesions; aortic aneurysm;* congenital malformation; enlargement of pancreas; annular pancreas; cirrhosis* and other conditions that may cause hepatomegaly (see also under "Syndrome, hepatorenal"); IVC filter with entrapped thromboembolus; surgical ligation; thrombosis; tumor (especially renal cell or hepatocellular carcinoma).

Obstruction, Portal Vein (See "Hypertension, portal.")

Obstruction, Pulmonary Venous

Synonyms and Related Terms: Congenital stenosis or atresia of pulmonary veins; pulmonary veno-occlusive disease; pulmonary venous hypertension.

Organs and Tissues	Procedures	Possible or Expected Findings
External examination	Prepare chest roentgenogram.	Mediastinal fibrosis or tumor.
Chest cavity	Record appearance of mediastinum and hilum of lungs. Remove chest organs en bloc. If an infectious process is suspected, submit samples for microbiologic study.	Idiopathic mediastinal or pulmonary hilar fibrosis; mediastinal radiation fibrosis; sclerosing mediastinitis;* mediastinal neoplasm; granulomas (histoplasma, sarcoid).

Organs and Tissues	Procedures	Possible or Expected Findings
Lungs	For pulmonary venography, see Chapter 2. Perfuse lungs with formalin. Submit samples of tissues from periphery of lungs and from perihilar areas. Record sites from where tissues were sampled. Request Verhoeff–van Gieson stain.	Congenital stenosis or atresia of pulmonary veins. Pulmonary veno-occlusive disease with old thrombi. Pulmonary venous hypertensive changes, most prominent in lower lobes.
Heart	Procedures depend on expected findings or grossly identified abnormalities as listed in right-hand column.	Thrombus or myxoma of left atrium; mitral or aortic stenosis;* chronic heart failure.*

Obstruction, Superior Mesenteric Artery (or Vein)

Organs and Tissues	Procedures	Possible or Expected Findings
Superior mesenteric artery system	For mesenteric arteriography, see Chapter 2. For dissection, en masse removal is recommended. Open aorta posteriorly and record appearance of celiac and mesenteric artery orifices.	Atherosclerosis; emboli.
Superior mesenteric vein system	Dissect portal, splenic, and superior mesenteric vein branches *in situ*.	Thrombosis; migratory thrombophlebitis.
Intestine	Locate and photograph abnormalities *in situ*.	Infarction; strangulation; volvulus; intussusception.
Other organs	Procedures depend on expected findings or grossly identified abnormalities as listed in right-hand column.	Thromboembolic disease; atherosclerosis or vasculitis complicated by arterial occlusion; peritonitis;* tumor; previous operations or cirrhosis* complicated by venous thromboses.

Occlusion (See "Obstruction,...")

Ochronosis (See "Alkaptonuria.")

Onchocerciasis

Synonyms and Related Terms: Disseminated microfilariasis; *Onchocerca volvulus* infection; river blindness.

NOTE: (1) Collect cerebrospinal fluid, blood, urine, and all tissues that appear to be infected. (2) Request parasitologic examination. (3) Request Giemsa and PAS stains. (4) No special precautions are indicated. (5) No serologic studies are available. (6) This is not a reportable disease.

Organs and Tissues	Procedures	Possible or Expected Findings
External examination, skin, subcutaneous tissue, and lymph nodes	Submit samples for histologic study.	Granulomatous inflammation with fibrosis; cutaneous lymphedema with leathery, depigmented, thickened skin; pendulous sacs of inguinal or femoral lymph nodes.
Cerebrospinal fluid	Submit sample for parasitologic study. See also above under "Note."	Microfilariae may be present.
Abdomen	If ascitic fluid is present, record volume and submit sample for parasitologic study.	Microfilariae may be present.
Blood and urine	Prepare smears. Centrifuge urine prior to smear preparation.	Microfilariae may be present.
Other organs	Procedures depend on expected findings or grossly identified abnormalities as listed in	Microfilariae or, in rare instances, adult *Onchocerca volvulus* may be found in

Organs and Tissues	Procedures	Possible or Expected Findings
	right-hand column. Submit samples for histologic study.	internal organs, such as lungs, liver, spleen, pancreas, and kidneys.
Eyes	For removal and specimen preparation, see Chapter 5.	Microfilariae, in anterior chamber and cornea of eyes as seen with a slit lamp; punctate keratitis; uveitis.

Opiate(s) (See "Dependence, drug(s), all types or type unspecified.")

Organophosphate(s) (See "Poisoning, organophosphate(s).")

Origin of Both Great Arteries from Right Ventricle (See "Ventricle, double outlet right.")

Ornithosis

Synonyms and Related Terms: *Chlamydia* infection; psittacosis; parrot fever.

NOTE: (1) Collect all tissues that appear to be infected. (2) Request cultures for ornithosis. Consult with microbiology laboratory before obtaining postmortem specimens. (3) Stains are not helpful in demonstrating the organism. (4) Special **precautions** are indicated. (5) Serologic studies are available from the state health department laboratories. (6) This is a **reportable** disease.

Organs and Tissues	Procedures	Possible or Expected Findings
External examination and skin	Photograph lesion.	Pale macular rash (Horder's spots); jaundice.
Chest	Record volume of effusions; submit samples for microbiologic and cytologic study.	Pleural effusions.*
Blood	Submit sample for serologic study.	
Heart	Submit samples for histologic study.	Pericarditis* and myocarditis.*
Lungs	Perfuse at least one lung with formalin. Submit multiple samples for histologic study.	Lymphocytic pneumonitis, which may be focally hemorrhagic and necrotizing; inclusion bodies.
Liver and spleen	Record weights and sample for histologic study.	Inclusion bodies in Kupffer cells; hepatosplenomegaly.
Other organs	Extensive histologic sampling is indicated.	Inclusion bodies may occur in kidneys, adrenal glands, brain and meninges, and other organs.

Osteitis Deformans (See "Disease, Paget's, of bone.")

Osteoarthritis

Related Term: Degenerative joint disease.

Possible Associated Conditions: Acromegaly;* acute and chronic trauma; alkaptonuria;* congenital or developmental bone diseases (e.g., congenital hip dislocation); diabetes mellitus;* Gaucher's disease;* hemochromatosis;* hyperparathyroidism;* hypothyroidism;* obesity;* Wilson's disease.*

Organs and Tissues	Procedures	Possible or Expected Findings
External examination		Heberden's nodes at interphalangeal joints of fingers.
	Prepare skeletal roentgenograms.	Degenerative changes, primarily of spine, hip joints, and knee joints.
Joints	For removal, prosthetic repair, and specimen preparation, see Chapter 2. Submit samples of osteocartilaginous and synovial tissues for histologic study; sagittal or frontal saw section through spine provides for best routine evaluation.	Histologic and macroscopic degeneration of cartilage; exposure of subchrondral bone; formation of marginal osteophytes; bone cysts; synovial fibrosis; hypertrophic synovitis.

Organs and Tissues	Procedures	Possible or Expected Findings
	If artificial joints (e.g., hip or knee) had been implanted, record state of implant site.	Loose joint prostheses.

Osteoarthropathy, Hypertrophic

Synonyms: Hypertrophic pulmonary osteoarthropathy; pac-hydermoperiostosis (idiopathic hypertrophic osteoarthropathy *[1]*).

NOTE: In all instances, an underlying disease must be identified; they include cardiac disease (cyanotic congenital heart dis-ease with right-to-left shunt; infective endocarditis*); gastroeso-phageal reflux *(3)*; neoplasms of lungs, esophagus, intestine, and liver; chronic liver disease; inflammatory bowel disease;* pulmonary disease (e.g., abscess;* bronchiectasis;* cystic fibrosis;* emp-yema;* emphysema;* lipoid pneumonia* *(4)*; *Pneumocystis* pneumonia; sarcoidosis;* tuberculosis*); hyperthyroidism.*

Organs and Tissues	Procedures	Possible or Expected Findings
External examination		Clubbing of fingers or toes (see below under "Elastic arteries"); swelling of extremities.
	Prepare roentgenograms of extremities.	Periosteal new bone formation in distal shafts of bones of forearms and legs. All bones of extremities may be involved.
Bones	For removal, prosthetic repair, and specimen preparation, see Chapter 2.	See above under "External examination."
Elastic arteries	Record presence of aneurysms (thoracic aorta, subclavian) or arteriovenous fistula of brachial vessels.	Unilateral clubbing.
	If abdominal aortic aneurysm had been surgically repaired, search for evidence of graft infection *(2)*.	Clubbing of toes but not of fingers.
Other organs	Procedures depend on expected findings or grossly identified abnormalities as listed above under "Note."	See above under "Note."

References

1. Sinha GP, Curtis P, Haigh D, Lealman GT, Dodds W, Bennett CP. Pachydermoperiostitis in childhood. Br J Rheum 1997;36:1224–1247.
2. Stevens M, Helms C, El-Khoury G, Chow S. Unilateral hypertrophic osteoarthropathy associated with aortofemoral graft infection. Am J Roentgenol 1998;170:1584–1586.
3. Greenwald M, Couper R, Laxer R, Durie P, Silverman E. Gastroesophageal reflux and esophagitis-associated hypertrophic osteoarthropathy. J Pediatr Gastroenterol Nutr 1996;23:178–181.
4. Hugosson C, Bahabri S, Rifai A, al-Dalaan A. Hypertrophic osteoarthropathy caused by lipoid pneumonia. Pediatr Radiol 1995;25:482–483.

Osteochondrodysplasia (See "Achondroplasia" and Dyschondroplasia, Ollier's.")

Osteodystrophy, Renal (See "Failure, kidney.")

Osteogenesis Imperfecta

Synonyms and Related Terms: Lobstein's syndrome; Osteogenesis imperfecta congenita; OI type I, II, and III; osteogenesis imperfecta cystica; osteogenesis imperfecta tarda; osteopsathyrosis; van der Hoeve's syndrome; Vrolik's disease (infantile form of OI).

NOTE: Contact the Osteogenesis Imperfecta Foundation, 804 W. Diamond Avenue, Suite 210, Gaithersburg, MD 20878, phone: 800-981-2663 (website: www.oif.org).

Organs and Tissues	Procedures	Possible or Expected Findings
External examination and skin	Record body weight and length, shape of skull, shape of extremities, and appearance of eyes and teeth.	Soft skull bones (caput membranaceum); short and deformed long bones; blue sclerae (Lobstein's syndrome); abnormal teeth.
	Prepare sections of skin for histologic study.	Thin skin.
	Prepare skeletal roentgenograms. Submit fascia lata for tissue culture to reference laboratory for classification of collagen metabolism defect.	Narrow bones with multiple fractures in various phases of healing; exuberant callus formation; compression of vertebrae with weight bearing.

Organs and Tissues	*Procedures*	*Possible or Expected Findings*
Blood	Obtain serum to assay for alkaline phosphatase activity. Postmortem and determination of calcium concentration is unreliable.	Normal values rule out hypophosphatasia. Hypercalcemia *(1)*.
Urine	Submit urine for determination of phospho-ethanolamine concentration.	
Gastrointestinal tract	Photograph abnormalities *in situ.*	Fecal impaction due to pelvic deformity in OI, type III *(2)*.
Bones	For removal, prosthetic repair, and specimen preparation, see Chapter 2. Samples for histologic study should include areas of endochondral and periosteal bone formation.	Normal epiphysis; deficient ossification of metaphysis, diaphysis and cortex; multiple fractures with fibrosis and callus formation.
Tendons and ligaments	Submit samples for histologic study.	Thin, translucent structures that may have ruptured.
Eyes	For removal and specimen preparation, see Chapter 5.	Thin sclerae *(3)*.
Parathyroid glands	Record weights and submit samples for histologic study.	Normal parathyroid glands.
Middle ears	For exposure of middle ears, see Chapter 4. This procedure is particularly indicated if patient had been deaf.	Otosclerosis (van der Hoeve's syndrome).

References

1. Williams CJ, Smith RA, Ball RJ, Wilkinson H. Hypercalcemia in osteogenesis imperfecta treated with pamidronate. Arch Dis Child 1997;76: 169–170.
2. Lee JH, Gamble JG, Moore RE, Rinsky LA. Gastrointestinal problems in patients who have type-III osteogenesis imperfecta. J Bone Joint Surg 1995;77:1352–1356.
3. Mietz H, Kasner L, Green WR. Histopathologic and electron-microscopic features of corneal and scleral collagen fibers in osteogenesis imperfecta type III. Graefes Arch Clin Exp Ophthalmol 1997;235: 405–410.

Osteomalacia

Related Terms: Osteoporosis;* renal osteodystrophy; rickets.

NOTE: Many possible causes of osteomalacia may not be apparent at autopsy, e.g., sodium fluoride or diphosphonate toxicity or use of anticonvulsant drugs.

Possible Associated Conditions: Neurofibromatosis;* hypo -phosphatasia (inborn error of metabolism) and hypophosphatemic states *(1)*; parenteral nutrition;* vitamin D deficiency.* (See also below under "Other organs and tissues.")

Organs and Tissues	*Procedures*	*Possible or Expected Findings*
External examination	Prepare skeletal roentgenograms.	Pseudofractures (Looser's zones), most common at axillary borders of scapulae, ischial and pubic rami, femoral necks, and ribs.
Bones	Consult roentgenograms. Request cyanuric chloride stain.	Abundant osteoid. May be associated with fibro-osteoclastic osteoporosis (renal osteodystrophy). Kyphoscoliosis *(2)*.
Other organs and tissues	Procedures depend on expected findings or grossly identified abnormalities as listed in right-hand column.	Changes secondary to chronic kidney failure* with phosphate depletion,* generalized renal tubular disorders (Fanconi syndrome*), vitamin D deficiency,* and chronic gastrointestinal, pancreatic or hepatobiliary diseases. Benign or malignant giant cell and other mesenchymal tumors or carcinoma of the prostate may cause (oncogenous) osteomalacia.
Parathyroid glands	Record weights and submit samples for histologic study.	If chronic renal disease was present, secondary parathyroid hyperplasia can be expected.

Reference

1. Clarke BL, Wynne AG, Wilson DM, Fitzpatrick LA. Osteomalacia associated with adult Fanconi syndrome: clinical and diagnostic features. Clin Endocrinol 1995;43:479–490.
2. Motosuneya T, et al. Severe kyphoscoliosis associated with osteomalacia. Spine J 2006;6:587–590.

Osteomyelitis

Organs and Tissues	*Procedures*	*Possible or Expected Findings*
External examination		Swelling; fistulas.
	Prepare skeletal roentgenograms.	Bone defect(s) and focal osteosclerosis.
Bones	For submission of material for microbiologic study, see Chapter 7. Record presence of contiguous infections.	Bacterial or fungal infections, most common in metaphyseal region of bones; paravertebral or psoas abscess in osteomyelitis of spine.
	Submit samples for histologic study. Request Gram stain and Grocott's methenamine silver stain for fungi.	Bacterial or fungal osteomyelitis, with or without cavitation and fistulas.
Other organs	Procedures depend on expected findings or grossly identified abnormalities as listed in right-hand column.	Trauma, surgery, insertion of prosthesis, generalized *(1)* or contiguous infection, inflammatory bowel disease *(2)*, diabetes mellitus,* and peripheral vascular diseases, deep vein thrombosis *(3)*.

References

1. Copie-Bergmann C, Niedobitek G, Mangham DC, Selves J, Baloch K, Diss TC, et al. Epstein-Barr virus in B-cell lymphomas associated with chronic suppurative inflammation. J Pathol 1997;183:287–292.
2. Freeman HJ. Osteomyelitis and osteonecrosis in inflammatory bowel disease. Can J Gastroenterol 1997;11:601–606.
3. Hollmig ST, et al. Deep vein thrombosis associated with osteomyelitis in children. J Bone Joint Surg Am 2007;89:1517–1523.

Osteonecrosis

Synonyms and Related Terms: Aseptic necrosis of bone; avascular necrosis of bone; idiopathic osteonecrosis; Perthes' dis-ease; postfracture osteonecrosis; renal transplant associated osteonecrosis.

NOTE: Possible underlying conditions include chronic alcoholism,* decompression sickness,* diseases that have been treated with high doses of corticosteroids *(1)*, Gaucher's disease,* human immunodeficiency virus infection* *(2)*, tuberculosis* *(1)*, sickle cell disease,* systemic lupus erythematosus,* tuberculosis* *(2)*, and bisphosphonate therapy *(3)*.

Organs and Tissues	*Procedures*	*Possible or Expected Findings*
Blood	Submit sample for biochemical study.	Hyperlipidemia; hyperuricemia.
Bones and joints	For removal, prosthetic repair, and specimen preparation, see Chapter 2. If osteonecrosis is suspected because one of the possible underlying conditions (see above) is present, prepare saw sections through femoral heads, medial femoral condyles, and heads of humeri.	Fracture or traumatic dislocation of hip, causing avascular necrosis of bone.
Other organs	Procedures depend on suspected underlying conditions, as listed above under "Note."	See above under "Note."

References

1. Freeman HJ. Osteomyelitis and osteonecrosis in inflammatory bowel disease. Can J Gastroenterol 1997;11:601–606.
2. Rademaker J, Dobro JS, Solomon G. Osteonecrosis and human immunodeficiency virus infection. J Rheumatol 1997;24:601–604.
3. Heras Rincón I, et al. Osteonecrosis of the jaws and bisphosphonates. Report of fifteen cases. Therapeutic recommendations. Med Oral Patol Oral Cir Bucal 2007;12:E267–271.

Osteopetrosis

Synonyms and Related Terms: Albers-Schönberg disease; autosomal-dominant osteopetrosis; carbonic anhydrase-II deficiency; malignant infantile osteopetrosis *(1)*; marble bone disease.

NOTE: Manifestations of renal tubular acidosis may have been a clinical complication.

Possible Associated Conditions: Bone marrow transplantation* (for infantile osteopetrosis). Anemia, recurrent infections, bleeding, and bruises may have resulted from myelophthisis associated with osteopetrosis. Upper airway obstruction in malignant infantile osteopetrosis may have necessitated tracheostomy *(1)*.

Organs and Tissues	*Procedures*	*Possible or Expected Findings*
External examination	Record weight and height.	Growth failure in infants; hypoplastic dentition.
	Prepare skeletal roentgenograms.	Increased density of all bones; bone deformities; narrowing of marrow spaces; malformation of the mastoid and paranasal sinuses; osteomyelitis* of jaws with facial fistulas. Exophthalmos.
Liver and spleen	Record weights and sizes; submit samples for histologic study.	Hepatosplenomegaly; extramedullary hematopoiesis.
Kidneys	Record weights and sizes; submit samples for histologic study.	Renal tubular acidosis in carbonic anhydrase II deficiency *(2)*.
Parathyroid glands	Record weights and submit samples for histologic study.	Normal parathyroid glands.
Brain	For removal and specimen preparation, see Chapter 4.	Hydrocephalus;* cerebral calcification. Arnold-Chiari malformation *(4)*. See also under "Skeletal system and skull."
Eyes	Remove for study in patients with visual disturbances.	Retinal degeneration.
Skeletal system with skull	For removal, prosthetic repair, and specimen preparation of bones, see Chapter 2. Expose base of skull and record size of nerve foramina (optic, acoustic, and other cranial nerves). If there is evidence of infection, expose nasal cavities and prepare histologic sections. Histologic samples should include bone and bone marrow.	Spondylolysis in children *(3)*. Rhinogenic osteomyelitis; atrophy of cranial nerves after compression at foramina. (This may have caused optic atrophy or deafness, or both. See also above under "External examination.") Otitis media* *(1)*; osteomalacia* or rickets may complicate osteopetrosis. Myelophthisis secondary to osteopetrosis.

References

1. Stocks RM, Wang WC, Thompson JW, Stocks MC 2nd, Horwitz EM. Malignant infantile osteopetrosis: otolaryngological complications and management. Arch Otolaryngol Head Neck Surg 1998;124:689–694.
2. Nagai R, Kooh SW, Balfe JW, Fenton T, Halperin ML. Renal tubular acidosis and osteopetrosis with carbonic anhydrase II deficiency: pathogenesis of impaired acidification. Pediatr Nephrol 1997;11:633–636.
3. Martin RP, Deane RH, Collett V. Spondylolysis in children who have osteopetrosis. J Bone Joint Surg 1997;79:1685–1689.
4. Kulkarni ML, et al. Osteopetrosis with Arnold chiari malformation type 1 and brain stem compression. Indian J Pediatr 2007;74:412–415.

Osteoporosis

Synonym and Related Terms: Drug-induced osteoporosis; idiopathic osteoporosis; juvenile osteoporosis; osteopenia; type I or type II osteoporosis; postmenopausal osteoporosis.

NOTE:

In heritable osteoporotic disorders of connective tissue (osteogenesis imperfecta,* Marfan's syndrome,* and others) are pre-sented separately. For "osteomalacia," see above. For "osteodystrophy," see under "Failure, kidney."

Possible Associated Conditions: Acromegaly;* chronic alco-holism;* chronic obstructive pulmonary disease; chronic kidney failure* *(1)*; Cushing's syndrome;* debilitating disease (various kinds, often with immobilization); diabetes mellitus* *(2)*; epilepsy;* hyperthyroidism *(2)*;* hypogonadism; malabsorption syndrome;* malnutrition;* primary biliary cirrhosis;* rheu-matoid arthritis;* scurvy;* steroid therapy or anticonvulsant medication.

Organs and Tissues	*Procedures*	*Possible or Expected Findings*
External examination	Record body length and shape of spine.	Kyphosis or kyphoscoliosis.
	Prepare skeletal roentgenograms.	Gross deformities of bones; alveolar bone loss; fractures of vertebrae, wrist, hip, humerus, or tibia. Calvarium uninvolved in most uncomplicated cases. Malnutrition* and senility.
Other organs	Procedures depend on expected underlying conditions, as listed in right-hand column and above under "Possible Associated Conditions."	In acute cases, metastatic calcifications with nephrocalcinosis. For other findings, see above under "Possible Associated Conditions."

Organs and Tissues	Procedures	Possible or Expected Findings
Parathyroid glands	Record weights and submit samples for histologic study.	Normal parathyroid glands in uncomplicated cases. Hyperparathyroidism* *(1)* (without osteitis fibrosa) may be present, however.
Bones	For removal, prosthetic repair, and specimen preparation, see Chapter 2. Record appearance of saw sections of vertebral column, calvarium, and femur. Submit samples for histologic study.	Features of osteitis fibrosa (osteoclastic osteoporosis; see "Hyperparathyroidism") or osteomalacia* exclude the diagnosis of uncomplicated osteoporosis. Osteoporosis, which may be localized, occurs in various neoplastic (e.g., mastocytosis) and inflammatory diseases.

References

1. Nishizawa Y, Morii H. Osteoporosis and atherosclerosis in chronic renal failure. Osteoporos Int 1997;7 Suppl 3:S188–S192.
2. Rosen CJ. Endocrine disorders and osteoporosis. Curr Opin Rheumatol 1997;9:355–361.

Otitis Media

Organs and Tissues	Procedures	Possible or Expected Findings
External examination	Examine external ear canal.	Draining, foul-smelling greasy material associated with acquired cholesteatoma.
Brain and base of skull with middle ears	For removal and specimen preparation, see Chapter 4. Culture any lesion appearing to be infectious.	Bacterial or viral infection, with or without mastoid osteitis. Neck abscess, sinus thrombosis *(1)* and brain abscess* and meningitis* may complicate otitis media.

Reference

1. Garcia RD, Baker AS, Cunningham MJ, Weber AL. Lateral sinus thrombosis associated with otitis media and mastoiditis in children. Pediatr Inf Dis J 1995;14:617–623.

Otosclerosis *(1, 3)*

NOTE: Otosclerosis may be a measles-virus-associated disease *(1)* and therefore, studies to rule out a past infection may be indicated.

Organs and Tissues	Procedures	Possible or Expected Findings
Middle and inner ears	For removal and specimen preparation, see Chapter 4. For current methods of temporal bone studies, see ref. *(2)*.	Spongy bone in the capsule of the labyrinth. Trabeculae of woven bone show pagetoid changes. If stapedectomy had been done, a prosthesis may be in place.

References

1. Niedermeyer HP, Arnold W. Otosclerosis: a measles virus associated inflammatory disease. Acta Oto-Laryngol 1995;115:300–303.
2. Cherukupally SR, Merchant SM, Rosowski JJ. Correlations between pathologic changes in the stapes and conductive hearing loss in otosclerosis. Ann Otyol Rhinol Laryngol 1998;107:319–326.
3. Menger DJ, Tange RA. The aetiology of otosclerosis: a review of the literature. Clin Otolaryngol Allied Sci 2003;28:112–120.

Oxaluria (see "Hyperoxaluria.")

P

Palsy, Progressive Bulbar (See "Disease, motor neuron.")

Palsy, Progressive Supranuclear

Synonyms: Steele-Richardson-Olszewski syndrome.

Organs and Tissues	*Procedures*	*Possible or Expected Findings*
Brain	For removal and specimen preparation, see Chapter 4. Histologic samples should include all sites listed in right-hand column. Request Bielschowsky stain for paraffin sections and histochemical stains with ubiquitin and tau proteins.	Brain is externally normal or mildly atrophic. Characteristic is midbrain atrophy with aqueduct dilatation and depigmentation of the substantia nigra. Neuronal loss with reactive gliosis, associated with neurofibrillary tangles (globose tangles). Primarily affected are globus pallidus, subthalamic nucleus, red nucleus, substantia nigra, tectum, periaqueductal gray matter, and dentate nucleus (grumose degeneration).

Palsy, Pseudobulbar (See "Disease, motor neuron.")

Pancreatitis

Related Terms: Acute pancreatitis; alcoholic pancreatitis; chronic (or chronic fibrosing) pancreatitis; interstitial pancreatitis.

NOTE: Some causes of pancreatitis such as adverse drug reactions (e.g., due to azathioprine, furosemide, or estrogens) cannot be diagnosed at autopsy.

Possible Associated Conditions: Acute fatty liver of pregnancy; apolipoprotein CII deficiency; cystic fibrosis;* hyperparathyroidism;* kidney transplantation.* Status post endoscopic retrograde cholangiopancreatography.

Organs and Tissues	*Procedures*	*Possible or Expected Findings*
External examination and skin	Record appearance of subcutaneous fat tissue and prepare histologic sections.	Fat tissue necroses.
	Prepare skeletal roentgenograms.	Intraosseous calcification (femur and tibia).
Vitreous	Submit sample for determination of calcium, potassium, and sodium concentrations.	Increased calcium concentration.
Abdominal cavity	If there are abscesses or other inflammatory changes, aspirate pus or exudate and submit sample for microbiologic study.	Exudate or abscesses in lesser sac or other peritoneal pockets; ascites.
Chest cavity	Record volume of effusions. Submit sample for lipase and amylase determination.	Pleural effusions.*
Blood	Submit sample for microbiologic study. Postmortem determination of calcium level is unreliable. Study of viral antibodies may be indicated.	Hypercalcemia or hypertriglyceridemia. Cultures or serologic studies may be positive for cytomegalovirus infection,* infectious mononucleosis,* mumps,* scarlet fever,* typhoid fever,* or viral hepatitis.

From: *Handbook of Autopsy Practice,* 4th Ed. Edited by: B.L. Waters

Organs and Tissues	Procedures	Possible or Expected Findings
Heart and coronary arteries		Coronary thrombosis.
Lungs		Pulmomary embolism.*
Liver, gallbladder, extrahepatic bile ducts, and pancreas; splenic and portal veins	After removal of pancreas, open pancreatic ducts. Record type of entry of pancreatic ducts in relationship to common bile duct. Open common bile duct (including papilla of Vater) and splenic and portal veins *in situ*. For cholangiography and pancreatography, see Chapter 2. Remove liver and gallbladder, and record contents of gall-bladder. Sample pancreas, liver, and grossly identifiable abnormalities for histologic study.	Pancreatic and peripancreatic fat tissue necroses; abscesses; hemorrhages; pseudocysts; calcification. Pancreatolithiasis. Carcinoma of pancreas *(1)*. Stenosis of intrapancreatic common bile duct in chronic pancreatitis. Obstruction of ampulla by ulcer in Crohn's disease* or duodenal diverticulum. Ascariasis. Choledocholithiasis. Splenic vein thrombosis; may also involve portal vein. Cholecystitis* and cholelithiasis.* Alcoholic liver disease.
Other organs and tissues	Procedures depend on expected findings or grossly identified abnormalities as listed in right-hand column. If polyarteritis nodosa is suspected, study arteries of lower extremities. For possible systemic infections, see above under "Blood."	Extrahepatic manifestations of chronic alcoholism,* chronic renal failure; hyper-parathyroidism* *(2)*, multiple myeloma,* polyarteritis nodosa,* thrombotic thrombo-cytopenic purpura *(3)*; sarcoidosis,* surgical and other types of trauma, systemic lupus erythematosus,* and other conditions.
Peripheral veins		Venous thromboses and thrombophlebitis.
Bones and bone marrow	For removal, prosthetic repair, and specimen preparation of bones, see Chapter 2. For preparation of sections and smears of bone marrow, Chapter 2.	Necroses. Multilacunar osteolysis.
Eyes	For removal and specimen preparation, see chapter 5.	Retinopathy (rare) *(4)*.

References

1. Andren-Sandberg A, Dervenis C, Lowenfels B. Etiologic links between chronic pancreatitis and pancreatic cancer. Scand J Gastroenterol 1997; 32:97–103.
2. Inabnet WB, Baldwin D, Daniel RO, Staren ED. Hyperparathyroidism and pancreatitis during pregnancy. Surgery 1996;119:710–713.
3. Silva VA. Thrombotic thrombocytopenic purpura/hemolytic uremic syndrome secondary to pancreatitis. Am J Hematol 1995;50:53–56.
4. Soledad Donoso Flores M, Narvaez Rodriguez I, Lopez Bernal I, del Mar Alcalde Rubio M, Galvan Ledesma A, et al. Retinopathy as a sys-temic com-plication of acute pancreatitis. Am J Gastroenterol 1995;90:321–324.

Pancytopenia

Related Terms: Agranulocytosis;* aplastic anemia; Fanconi's anemia.*

NOTE: Some causes of pancytopenia such as adverse drug reactions (e.g., due to antimetabolites, sulfa drugs, or gold com -pounds) cannot be diagnosed at autopsy.

Possible Associated Conditions: Acquired immunodeficiency syndrome;* diffuse eosinophilic fasciitis; paroxysmal nocturnal hemoglobinuria;* pregnancy;* radiation injury;* systemic lupus erythematosus;* systemic viral infections and viral hepatitis; transfusion-related graft-versus-host disease.*

Organs and Tissues	Procedures	Possible or Expected Findings
External examination	Record skin abnormalities and prepare photographs.	Jaundice; ulcers of skin. Thrombocytopenic hemorrhages.
Other organs and blood	If toxicity of drugs or chemicals is suspected, submit appropriate tissue samples for toxicologic study. If viral infection is suspected as a cause, submit material for serologic or other diagnostic studies.	Manifestations of leukopenia or thrombo-cytopenia (infections, including septicemia; hemorrhages; various types of pneumonia*). Systemic viral infection; viral hepatitis.* Radiation injury.*
Neck organs with oropharynx, tongue,	Request Gram and Grocott's methenamine silver stains for bacteria and fungi, respectively;	Ulcers in mouth and pharynx.

Organs and Tissues	Procedures	Possible or Expected Findings
tonsils, and soft palate	photograph lesions.	
Lymph nodes and spleen	Record weight of spleen.	Reactive lymphadenitis and splenitis.
Rectum and vagina	See above under "Neck organs").	Rectal and vaginal ulcers.
Bone marrow	For specimen preparation, see Chapter 2.	Bone marrow may be hypocellular, normal, or hypercellular. Hematologic malignancies (myelodysplastic syndromes) or metastases may be present. Agnogenic myeloid metaplasia,* osteopetrosis,* or storage diseases are rare findings.

Panencephalitis, Subacute Sclerosing
(See "Encephalitis, all types or type unspecified.")

Panhypopituitarism (See "Insufficiency, pituitary.")

Panniculitis

Synonyms and Related Terms: Calcifying panniculitis; histiocytic cytophagic panniculitis; mesenteric panniculitis (mes-enteric lipodystrophy); "sclerema neonatorum."

NOTE: The term Weber-Christian disease described systemic panniculitis with fever, bleeding, pulmonary and pancreatic lesions, and other abnormalities also involving lungs and pancreas, among others. However, this condition is not a specific entity and thus, the name has become obsolete. The term histiocytic cytophagic panniculitis is more descriptive and preferred.

Leukemia* and subcutaneous T-cell lymphoma* may closely simulate panniculitis.

Possible Associated Conditions: $Alpha_1$-antitrypsin deficiency;* dermatomyositis;* rheumatoid arthritis;* scleroderma and morphea; Sjögren's syndrome;* systemic lupus erythematosus.*

Organs and Tissues	Procedures	Possible or Expected Findings
External examination, skin, subcutaneous tissue, and breasts	Record extent and character of skin lesions. Record size, location, and gross appearance of subcutaneous nodules. Submit tissue samples for histologic study of grossly unaffected skin, skin lesions, and subcutaneous nodules. Request Verhoeff–van Gieson, Gram, and Grocott's methenamine silver stains.	Dimpling of skin; necroses; fistulas. Panniculitis with subcutaneous nodules in trunk, breasts, and thighs *(5)*. Calcification may occur in breast tissue but also at other sites (e.g., in kidney failure*). Pancreatic enzyme-induced fat necroses associated with severe pancreatitis. Widespread hardening of fat tissue with rupture of fat cells and crystal formation in "sclerema neonatorum." Focal traumatic panniculitis also may occur in newborns.
	Request S-100 protein stain. Ascertain that cell infiltrates are not leukemic or lymphomatous *(1)*.	S-100 stain negative in panniculitis but positive in Rosai-Dorfman disease (sinus histiocytosis with massive lymphadenopathy).
Chest	Submit tissue samples for histologic study of pretracheal and pericardial fat tissue.	Mediastinal panniculitis.
Heart	Record weight. Submit multiple sections for histologic analysis.	Pericarditis;* interstitial myocarditis.*
Lungs	Submit any consolidated areas for microbiologic study. Perfuse one lung with formalin. Prepare frozen sections and request Sudan stain.	Pneumonia;* pleuritis. Fat embolism.*
Liver and spleen	Record weights and submit samples for histologic study. Request PAS/diastase stain of liver.	Features of $alpha_1$-antitrypsin deficiency* *(2)*. Fatty changes of liver; splenitis.
Mesentery and intestine	For mesenteric arteriography, see Chapter 2. Submit tissue samples for histologic study of mucosal lesions and grossly uninvolved portions of intestine.	Intestinal mucosal erosions and ulcers, with or without perforation. Massive gastro-intestinal hemorrhage in histiocytic cytophagic panniculitis. Blind intestinal loop *(3)*.

Organs and Tissues	Procedures	Possible or Expected Findings
Mesentery and intestine *(continued)*	Prepare thin slices of mesentery. Record size of nodules and appearance of vessels. Submit tissue samples for histologic study of nodules and vessels.	Mesenteric panniculitis.
Retroperitoneum with pancreas	Submit tissue samples for histologic study.	Retroperitoneal panniculitis. Necrotizing pancreatitis.*
Kidneys and adrenal glands	Dissect renal and adrenal vessels *in situ*. Record weights, prepare photographs, and sample for histologic study.	Vasculitis with thrombi; adrenocortical infarctions.
Other organs and tissues	Submit tissue samples for histologic study of large and small peripheral vessels. Request Verhoeff–van Gieson stain. Samples should include all organs and tissues with gross lesions and also lymph nodes and bone marrow.	Vasculitis with thrombi and infarctions. Relapsing polychondritis *(4)*. See also above under "Possible Associated Conditions."

References

1. Kumar S, Krenacs L, Medeiros J, Elenitoba-Johnson KS, Greiner TC, Sorbara L, et al. Subcutaneous panniculitic T-cell lymphoma is a tumor of cytotoxic T lymphocytes. Hum Pathol 1998;29:397–403.
2. O'Riordan K, Blei A, Rao MS, Abecassis M. Alpha 1-antitrypsin defi-ciency-associated panniculitis: resolution with intravenous alpha 1-anti-trypsin administration and liver transplantation. Transplant 1997;63: 480–482.
3. Caux F, Halimi C, Kevorkian JP, Pinquier L, Dubertret L, Segrestaa JM. Blind loop syndrome: an unusual cause of panniculitis. J Am Acad Dermatol 1997;37:824–827.
4. Disdier P, Andrac L, Swiader L, Veit V, Fuzibet JG, Weiller-Merli C, et al. Cutaneous panniculitis and relapsing polychondritis: two cases. Dermatology 1996;193:266–268.
5. Reguena L. Normal subcutaneous fat, necrosis of adipocytes and classification of the panniculitides. Semin Cutan Med Surg 2007;26:66–70.

Paracoccidioidomycosis

Synonyms: *Paracoccidioides brasiliensis* infection; South American blastomycosis.

NOTE: (1) Collect all tissues that appear to be infected. (2) Request fungal cultures. (3) Request Grocott's methenamine silver stain for fungi. A simple KOH mount of exudate or pus will demonstrate the organism in a majority of cases. (4) No special precautions are indicated. (5) Serologic studies are available from the Centers for Disease Control and Prevention, Atlanta, GA. (6) This is not a reportable disease.

Organs and Tissues	Procedures	Possible or Expected Findings
External examination with mouth and nose; lymph nodes	Record and photograph skin lesions. Submit sample of exudate for fungal culture, and prepare smears. Record appearance of mouth, nose and conjunctivas; record site of primary lesion. Excise regional lymph nodes and submit for histologic study.	Mucosal ulcerations (mulberry-like) of mouth and nose; cutaneous verrucous or ulcerated lesions; regional lymph-adenopathy. See below under "Other organs..."
Lungs	Submit samples of consolidated lung tissue for culture.	Consolidation; cavitation; fibrosis; bullae.
Gastrointestinal tract	Submit samples of all segments for histologic study; include sample of anorectal mucosa.	Stomach and intestines are common sites of primary infection. Suppurative, ulcerative, and granulomatous lesions may occur.
Other organs and tissues; nasal cavities	Sample the nasal cavities.	Nasal cavities may be the site of the primary infection; hematogenous dissemination to any organ, including the central nervous system.

Paralysis Agitans (See "Disease, Parkinson's.")

Paralysis, Familial Periodic

Synonyms and Related Terms: Hyperkalemic (hypokalemic, normokalemic) periodic paralysis *(1)*; myotonia, paramyotonia congenita.

Organs and Tissues	*Procedures*	*Possible or Expected Findings*
Skeletal muscles	For sampling and specimen preparation, see Chapter 4. Prepare samples for electron microscopy.	Vacuolar myopathy.

Reference

1. Lanzi R et al. Hypokalemic periodic paralysis in a patient with acquired growth hormone deficiency. J Endocrinol Invest 2007;30:341–345.

Paralysis, Landry's Ascending (See "Syndrome, Guillain-Barré.")

Paralysis, Spinal (See name of suspected underlying condition, such as "Poliomyelitis" and "Sclerosis, multiple.")

Paresis, General (See "Syphilis, acquired.")

Parkinsonism, All Types or Type Unspecified (See "Disease, Parkinson's.")

Parotitis, Epidemic (See "Mumps.")

Patent ductus arteriosus (See "Artery, patent ductal.")

Pellagra

Related Terms: Niacin deficiency; tryptophan deficiency.

Possible Associated Conditions: Chronic alcoholism;* chronic peritoneal dialysis;* hemodialysis; other vitamin deficiencies; refeeding after starvation.*

Organs and Tissues	*Procedures*	*Possible or Expected Findings*
External examination, skin, oral cavity, and tongue	Record extent of skin and mucosal lesions, photograph, and prepare histologic sections of skin and tongue.	Dermatitis with dark pigmentation; cheilosis (angular stomatitis); stomatitis; glossitis; necrotizing ulcerative gingivitis with Vincent's organisms.
Esophagus	Photograph and sample for histologic study.	Esophagitis *(1)*.
Liver	Record weight and submit samples for histologic study.	Alcoholic cirrhosis.*
Gastrointestinal tract	Submit samples of all segments (with and without ulcers) for histologic study.	Proctocolitis with or without ulcers and perianal excoriations *(2)*.
Urethra and vagina	Submit samples for histologic study.	Urethritis and vaginitis.
Brain and spinal cord	For removal and specimen preparation, see Chapter 4. Request Luxol fast blue stain for myelin.	Degeneration of large pyramidal cells (Betz's cells) of motor cortex. Demyelination in posterior and lateral columns of spinal cord.

References

1. Segal I, Hale M, Demetriou A, Mohamed AE. Pathological effects of pellagra on the esophagus. Nutr Canc 1990;14: 233–238.
2. Segal I, Ou Tim L, Demetriou A, Paterson A, Hale M, Lerios M. Rectal manifestations of pellagra. Int J Colorect Dis 1986;1:238–243.

Pemphigus

Synonyms: Paraneoplastic pemphigus; pemphigus erythematosus; pemphigus foliaceus; pemphigus neonatorum; pemphigus vegetans; pemphigus vulgaris.

Possible Associated Conditions: Leukemia,* lymphoma,* and other neoplastic disorders associated with paraneoplastic pemphigus *(1)*.

Organs and Tissues	*Procedures*	*Possible or Expected Findings*
External examination, skin, and mouth	Record extent of skin lesions; photograph; submit multiple samples for histologic study, preferably of areas that are free of secondary infection.	Bullous and other lesions of scalp, eyelids, nose, axillae, umbilicus, inframammary areas, back, hands, groins, genitalia, anus, knees, and feet. Similar lesions may occur in the mouth. Acantholysis is suprabasal or near granular layer.
	Prepare sections for immunofluorescent staining.	IgG deposits on the surfaces of keratinocytes.

Organs and Tissues	*Procedures*	*Possible or Expected Findings*
Blood	Submit sample for culture.	Septicemia.
Heart		Focal myocarditis.
Lungs	Submit any consolidated areas for microbiologic study.	Bronchopneumonia; thromboemboli after steroid therapy.
Esophagus	Sample for histologic study.	May be involved in pemphigus vulgaris *(2)*.
Kidneys and urinary bladder		Urinary tract infection.
Adrenal glands	Record weights; record appearance of cortex.	Cortical lipid depletion.
Neck organs	Sample for histologic study.	Pemphigus lesions of mucosa of pharynx and larynx.
Bones	For removal, prosthetic repair, and specimen preparation, see Chapter 2.	Osteoporosis* after steroid therapy.
Brain, spinal cord, and spinal ganglia	For removal and specimen preparation, see Chapter 4.	Degenerative changes in brain, spinal cord, and spinal ganglia.
Eyes	For removal and specimen preparation, see Chapter 5.	Pemphigus lesions of conjunctivas. Invasion of conjunctivas by connective tissue; possible conjunctival shrinkage.

References

1. Anhalt GJ. Paraneoplastic pemphigus. Adv Dermatol 1997;12:77–96.
2. Amichai B, Grunwald MH, Gasper N, Finkelstein E, Halevy S. A case of pemphigus vulgaris with esophageal involvement. J Dermatol 1996;23: 214–215.

Periarteritis Nodosa (See "Polyarteritis nodosa.")

Pericarditis

Organs and Tissues	*Procedures*	*Possible or Expected Findings*
External examination	Prepare chest roentgenogram.	Pericardial calcification; effusion.
Pleural cavities	If there are pleural exudates, follow procedures described below.	Pleuritis.
Pericardial sac	Aspirate exudate and submit for microbiologic study. Record volume of pericardial fluid. Centrifuge fluid and prepare smear or section of pellet. Request Gram, Grocott's methenamine silver, and auramine-rhodamine stains.	Infective pericarditis (pyogenic, tuberculous, or other bacterial infection; fungal or viral infection). (Gram-negative bacilli, *Staphylococcus aureus*, *Streptococcus*, and *Pneumococcus*.)
	If there is extensive calcification, see under "Syndrome, Budd-Chiari."	Constrictive pericarditis (idiopathic; irradiation; tuberculous; postoperative).
Blood	Submit sample for microbiologic study.	Septicemia.
Heart	Histologic samples should include epicardium, pericardium, and myocardium.	Old or recent heart surgery; myocardial infarction.
	For coronary arteriography, see Chapter 10.	Coronary atherosclerosis with stenosis.
Other organs	Procedures depend on expected findings or grossly identified abnormalities as listed in right-hand column.	Neoplasm; trauma; manifestations of kidney failure* with uremia or of rheumatic fever;* sternal osteomyelitis (postoperative wound infection); rheumatoid arthritis* *(1)*; lupus erythematosus,* and other autoimmune diseases.

Reference

1. McRorie ER, Wright RA, Errington ML, Lugmani RA. Rheumatoid constrictive pericarditis (clinical conference). Br J Rheumatol 1997;36:100–103.

Peritonitis, Benign Paroxysmal (See "Fever, familial Mediterranean.")

Peritonitis, Infectious

NOTE: (1) Collect all tissues that appear to be infected. (2) Request aerobic, anaerobic, acid-fast, and fungal cultures. (3) Request Gram, Grocott's methenamine silver, and Kinyoun's stains. (4) No special precautions are indicated. (5) Serologic studies are not available. (6) This is not a reportable disease.

Organs and Tissues	*Procedures*	*Possible or Expected Findings*
External examination	Prepare chest and abdominal roentgenograms.	Extraintestinal gas after perforation of hollow viscus; foreign body.
Vitreous	Request determination of sodium, chloride, and urea nitrogen concentrations.	Manifestations of severe dehydration.*
Abdominal cavity	Aspirate fluid and submit for culture, particularly if cloudy.	Acute bacterial peritonitis (rarely, other infective agents); bile or chemical peritonitis.
	If cause of acute peritonitis is unknown, inspect *in situ* all intraperitoneal, pelvic, and extraperitoneal organs. If abscess is present, record location, size, and volume. Submit portion for culture.	Possible causes include appendicitis, colitis, diverticulitis, enteritis, infarction, peptic ulcer, trauma, tumor, surgical complication and pelvic disease (for instance, after attempted abortion).
	Absence of causative lesions must be documented.	Primary peritonitis, most commonly in female children.
	If exudate is milky, lymphangiography may be indicated (Chapter 2).	Chylous ascites.
Blood	Submit sample for aerobic, anaerobic, and fungal cultures.	Septicemia.

Pertussis

Synonyms: *Bordatella pertussis* infection; whooping cough.

NOTE: (1) Collect all tissues that appear to be infected. (2) Request culture for *Bordatella*, as well as aerobic and anaerobic cultures. Special medium is required (see below) (3) Request Gram stain. (4) No special precautions are indicated. (5) Serologic studies are not available in most institutions. (6) This is a **reportable** disease.

Organs and Tissues	*Procedures*	*Possible or Expected Findings*
External examination	Record body weight and length. If diagnosis had not been confirmed, prepare nasopharyngeal swabs, and culture immediately on Bordet-Gengou medium.	Manifestations of malnutrition;* petechiae, especially on face; scleral hemorrhages.
	Prepare chest roentgenogram.	Pneumothorax.*
Cerebrospinal fluid	Culture on Bordet-Gengou medium.	Infectious meningitis.*
Blood	Submit sample for culture (see above under "Note").	Septicemia.
Lungs	Submit any consolidated area for culture. Prepare Gram-stained smears from fresh cut section; perfuse one lung with formalin.	Localized or interstitial pulmonary emphysema; atelectasis.
	Prepare histologic sections of bronchi, bronchioli, and pulmonary parenchyma.	Bronchitis; bronchiolitis; bronchopneumonia.
Neck organs and trachea	Prepare histologic sections of pharynx, larynx, and trachea.	Aspiration of vomitus; pharyngitis; laryngitis;* tracheitis.
Brain		Serous meningitis;* anoxic encephalopathy; epidural hematoma; petechial hemorrhages.
Middle ears	For removal and specimen preparation, see Chapter 4.	Bacterial otitis media.*

Pesticide (See "Poisoning, organophosphate(s).")

Phenylketonuria

NOTE: See also under "Aminoaciduria."

Organs and Tissues	*Procedures*	*Possible or Expected Findings*
Blood	If diagnosis had not been confirmed, submit plasma from a heparinized blood sample for ion-exchange test.	Hyperphenylalaninemia.
Urine	See above under "Blood."	Phenylketonuria. Urine may have a"mousy" odor.
Brain and spinal cord	For removal and specimen preparation, see Chapter 4. Record brain weight. Request Luxol fast blue stain for myelin. Fresh material should be used for Sudan stain for fat.	Microcephaly; delayed neuronal and myelin maturation; demyelinization with sudanophilic gitter cells; normal grey matter.

Pheochromocytoma (See "Tumor of the adrenal gland(s).")

Phlebitis

Related Terms: Migratory phlebitis; phlebothrombosis; phlegmasia alba dolens; phlegmasia cerulea dolens; thrombophlebitis migrans,* Trousseau's syndrome; venous thrombosis.*

NOTE: A clear distinction between phlebothrombosis and thrombophlebitis generally cannot be made.

Organs and Tissues	*Procedures*	*Possible or Expected Findings*
External examination	Describe discoloration of extremities, swelling or palpable venous lesions. Compare leg circumferences (measure above and below knees).	Stasis dermatitis of legs; varicous veins; gangrene of toes.
Lungs		Pulmonary embolism.*
Other organs	If systemic emboli and infarctions are present, record whether oval foramen was patent and whether there were other lesions with possible right-to-left shunt.	Paradoxic embolism. Carcinoma of pancreas, lung, stomach, colon, kidney, or other organs. Arteritis. Nonbacterial thrombotic endocarditis.*
Veins and arteries	For postmortem phlebography and ateriography, see Chapter 2. For removal of femoral vessels, see Chapter 3. If gangrene is present, demonstrate absence of concomitant arterial occlusion.	Thromboses are likely to be found (in decreasing order of frequency) in small saphenous veins, deep veins of calves, iliofemoral veins, great saphenous veins, superficial veins and varices of legs, and veins of arms. Other sites are rarely involved.

Phlegmasia Alba (or Cerulea) Dolens (See "Phlebitis.")

Phosgene ($COCl_2$) (See "Poisoning, gas.")

Phosphate Ester (Insecticide) (See "Poisoning, organophosphate(s).")

Phosphorus (See "Disorder, electrolyte(s)" or "Poisoning, phosphorus.")

Phycomycosis (See "Mucormycosis.")

Plague

Synonym: *Yersinia (Pasteurella) pestis* infection; Black Death; bubonic plague.

NOTE: (1) Collect all tissues that appear to be infected. (2) Request aerobic bacterial cultures. (3) Request Gram stain. (4) Special **precautions** are indicated, as this is a highly communicable disease. (5) Serologic studies are available from the Centers for Disease Control and Prevention, Atlanta, GA. (6) This is a **reportable** disease.

Organs and Tissues	*Procedures*	*Possible or Expected Findings*
External examination and skin	Photograph and record extent of hemorrhages. Prepare histologic sections of skin.	Petechial and other types of hemorrhages in skin and subcutaneous tissues.
Blood	Submit sample for microbiologic (see above under "Note") and serologic study. Prepare smear and stain with Wright-Giemsa.	Septicemia; bipolar staining rods.

Organs and Tissues	Procedures	Possible or Expected Findings
Lymph nodes	Collect inguinal, popliteal, axillary, and supraclavicular lymph nodes for aerobic culture. Photograph enlarged lymph nodes, and prepare smears of fresh cut surfaces.	Hemorrhagic necrosis; variable suppuration.
Lungs	Submit consolidated areas for microbiologic study (see above under "Note"). Perfuse both lungs with formalin. Submit samples of pulmonary tissue and bronchial lymph nodes for histologic study.	Severe hemorrhagic edema; pneumonia with lobular to lobar features.
Other organs	Submit samples of grossly abnormal organs, exudates, or drainage fluids for culture and Gram stain.	Large areas of necrosis teeming with organisms and minimal to suppurative inflammation.

Plasmacytoma (See "Myeloma, multiple.")

Platybasia

NOTE: Possible causes or associated conditions include Arnold-Chiari malformation;* basilar impression* or invagination; fusion of atlas to the foramen magnum; Klippel-Feil syndrome;* malpositioning of odontoid process; osteitis deformans (Paget's disease of bone*); osteogenesis imperfecta;* osteomalacia;* rickets; syringobulbia, syringomyelia.*

Organs and Tissues	Procedures	Possible or Expected Findings
Skull and spine	Prepare roentgenograms of skull and cervical spine.	Flattening of the base of the skull (angle formed by the plane of the clivus and the plane of the anterior fossa exceeds 135°).

Pleuritis (See "Effusion(s) and exudate(s), pleural.")

Pleurodynia, epidemic

Synonyms: Bornholm disease; devil's grip; epidemic myalgia; epidemic myositis.

Organs and Tissues	Procedures	Possible or Expected Findings
Blood	Submit samples for viral culture.	Coxsackie B virus infection.
Heart and pericardium	Sample for histologic study and for viral cultures (Coxsackievirus A and B; echoviruses). If pericardial fluid can be obtained, submit for viral culture also. Cultures may be negative and search for viral RNA by *in situ* hybridization may be indicated.	Myocarditis* may be associated with Coxsackievirus B infection; may be rapidly fatal in infants.

Pneumatosis Cystoides Intestinalis

NOTE: Some potential causes such as steroid, chemo- or immunosuppressive therapy may not be apparent at autopsy.

Possible Associated Conditions: Acquired immunodeficiency syndrome* (AIDS) *(1)*; amyloidosis* *(2)*; primary combined immunodeficiency *(3)*; progressive systemic sclerosis;* organ or bone marrow *(4)* transplantation.*

Organs and Tissues	Procedures	Possible or Expected Findings
Abdomen	Expose serosal surfaces. Record location and size of cysts.	Gas cysts in stomach, small bowel, colon, mesentery, omentum, gastrohepatic ligament, gallbladder, retroperitoneal tissues, and renal capsule.

Organs and Tissues	*Procedures*	*Possible or Expected Findings*
Chest organs	Dissect thoracic duct and its tributaries (see Chapter 3). Perfuse one or both lungs with formalin.	Gas in thoracic duct. Emphysema* of lungs.
Gastrointestinal tract	Procedures depend on expected findings or grossly identified abnormalities as listed in right-hand column.	Necrotizing enterocolitis in premature infants. Pyloric stenosis, colitis *(5)*, redundant sigmoid colon, ischemic bowel disease. Mucosal pseudolipomatosis *(6)*.
	Submit samples of cystic lesions for histologic study.	Usually, cysts are subserosal in adults and located between muscularis mucosae and muscularis propria in infants and children. Mucosa may be inflamed.
Other organs	Submit samples of cystic lesions for histologic study.	Extraintestinal cysts, as listed above under "Abdomen." Cysts may also occur in vaginal mucosa.

References

1. Cunnion KM. Pneumatosis intestinalis in pediatric acquired immunodeficiency syndrome. Pediatr Inf Dis J 1998;17:355–356.
2. Pearson DC, Price LM, Urbanski S. Pneumatosis cystoides intestinalis: an unusual complication of systemic amyloidosis. J Clin Gastro-enterol 1996;22:74–76.
3. Tang ML, Williams LW. Pneumatosis intestinalis in children with primary combined immunodeficiency. J Pediatr 1998;132:546–549.
4. Takanashi M, Hibi S, Todo S, Sawada T, Tsunamoto K, Imashaku S. Pneumatosis cystoides intestinalis with abdominal free air in a 2-year-old girl after allogeneic bone marrow transplantation. Pediatr Hematol Oncol 1998;15:81–84.
5. Pear BL. Pneumatosis intestinalis: a review. Radiol 1998;207:13–19.
6. Gagliardi G, Thompson IW, Hershman MJ, Forbes A, Hawley PR, Talbot IC. Pneumatosis coli: a proposed pathogenesis based on study of 25 cases and review of the literature. Intl J Colorect Dis 1996;11: 111–118.

Pneumoconiosis

Etiologic Types of Pneumoconiosis (With typical Examples): Collagenous inorganic dust pneumoconiosis, diffuse type: Aluminosis; asbestosis; chronic pulmonary berylliosis; talcosis; Collagenous inorganic dust pneumoconiosis, nodular type: Silicosis; Noncollagenous inorganic dust pneumoconiosis (includes mixed-dust fibrosis): Baritosis; China clay pneumoconiosis; chromite pneumoconiosis; coal worker's pneumoconiosis; fuller's earth pneumoconiosis; hematite or magnetite miner's lung; siderosis or welder's lung; stannosis; Organic dust pneumoconiosis: Byssinosis.

NOTE: In addition to the aforementioned classic forms of pneumoconiosis, many other airborne substances have been impli-cated in recent years, for example, cerium, manmade vitreous fibers, polyvinyl chloride, silicon carbide, and titanium *(1)*.

Chemical analysis of large samples of digested tissue is best suited for quantitative studies, particularly of trace substances. If only small tissue samples are available and if individual par-ticles are to be analyzed and correlated with histologic lesions, *in situ* microanalysis must be done. Methods used include bright-field and polarized light microscopy, transmission electron microscopy, scanning or transmission electron microscopy with energy dispersive X-ray analysis *(2)*, ion beam instrumentation, and secondary ion mass spectrometry. The last three methods are time-consuming, requirc much skill and expensive equipment, and do not lend themselves well to quantitation. Ideally, bulk analysis and *in situ* microanalysis should be used in combination.

Analyses can be conducted in specialized laboratories at the following centers (for charges and other information, consult the appropriate laboratories):

Meixa Tech and Forensic
Science Consultants Group
Box 844
Cardiff-by-the-sea, CA
92007-0844

Environmental and
Occupational Pathology
Division
Department of Pathology
College of Medicine
SUNY Upstate Medical
University
Syracuse, NY 13210

Organs and Tissues	Procedures	Possible or Expected Findings
External examination	Prepare chest roentgenogram.	Clubbing of fingers. Diffuse or nodular pulmonary infiltrates.
Blood	Submit sample for microbiologic study. Refrigerate sample for possible immunologic study.	Rheumatoid factor in Caplan's syndrome.* Positive in vitro lymphocyte transformation test in berylliosis *(3)*.
Lungs	Submit one lobe or samples of all lobes for bulk analysis and for in situ microanalysis (see above under "Note"). Microincineration may permit preliminary dust analysis. For demonstration of asbestos fibers, see Chapter 2 and ref. *(4)*.	Large amounts of dust (up to 20 g) in coal worker's pneumoconiosis and other noncollagenous inorganic dust pneumoconioses. Small amounts of dust in silicosis (5–6 g).
	Submit one lobe or segment for microbiologic study.	Tuberculosis* (including infection with atypical mycobacteria *[5]*).
	For pulmonary arteriography and bronchography, see Chapter 2.	
	Prepare roentgenograms of entire lungs and slices. Perfuse one lung (or both, if only routine studies are intended) with formalin. Submit samples for histologic study of nodular dust lesions, diffuse fibrotic lesions, grossly uninvolved areas, bronchi, and bronchopulmonary lymph nodes.	Asbestosis may be associated with pleural mesothelioma (see "Tumor of the pleural") and carcinoma of lung (see "Tumor of the lung or bronchus"). In silicotic lungs, squamous cell or small cell carcinomas are rather common *(6)*.
	For preparation of paper-mounted sections, see Chapter 2.	Chronic bronchitis.* Coniosis of lymph nodes.
	Prepare samples for transmission and scanning electron microscopic study.	Particle identification.
Joints	For removal, prosthetic repair, and specimen preparation, see Chapter 2.	Arthritis in Caplan's syndrome.*

References

1. Gong H Jr. Uncommon causes of occupational interstitial lung diseases. Curr Opin Pulm Med 1996;2:405–411.
2. McDonald JW, Ghio AJ, Sheehan CE, Bernhardt PF, Roggli VL. Rare earth (cerium oxide) pneumoconiosis: analytical scanning electron microscopy and literature review. Mod Pathol 1995;8: 859–865.
3. Williams WJ. Diagnostic criteria for chronic beryllium disease (CBD) based on the UK registry 1945–1991. Sarcoidosis 1993;10:41–43.
4. King JA, Wong SW. Autopsy evaluation of asbestos exposure: retrospective study of 135 cases with quantitation of ferruginous bodies in digested lung tissue. South Med J 1996;89:380–385.
5. De Coster C, Verstraeten JM, Dumortier P, De Vuyst P. Atypical mycobacteriosis as a complication of talc pneumoconiosis. Eur Respir J 1996;9:1757–1759.
6. Honma K, Chiyotani K, Kimura K. Silicosis, mixed dust pneumoconiosis, and lung cancer. Am J Ind Med 1997;32:595–599.

Pneumocystis Carinii (See "Infection, Pneumocystis carinii.")

Pneumomediastinum

NOTE: This condition is diagnosed by inspection, palpation, and roentgenography. Tension pneumomediastinum may compromise venous return to the heart and may compress major bronchi. The condition is rapidly fatal and occurs after alveolar rupture with dissection of air into the mediastinum in neonates with respiratory distress (see "Syndrome, respiratory distress, of infant") and in adult patients ventilated on volume respirators.

Organs and Tissues	Procedures	Possible or Expected Findings
External examination	Prepare chest roentgenogram.	Roentgenograms provide the best permanent record of a pneumomediastinum.
Chest cavity	Photograph mediastinum. Explore major veins and record compression in cases of tension pneumomediatinum.	Air bubbles in mediastinal soft tissues.

Organs and Tissues	*Procedures*	*Possible or Expected Findings*
Lungs and mediastinum	Perfuse one lung with formalin. Other procedures depend on expected findings or grossly identified abnormalities as listed in right-hand column.	Intubation injury *(1)*; perforation or rupture of major bronchus, trachea, or esophagus. Alveolar rupture, e.g., in asthma* *(2)*, may not be discernible. Bronchiolitis obliterans *(3)*, interstitial pneumonia* *(4)* and other lung conditions also may lead to pneumomediastinum.
Abdomen and neck organs	Search for evidence of trauma of other lesions that may have allowed air to enter soft tissues.	Dissection of air from lesions in abdomen (e.g., retroperitoneal colonic perforation*[5]*) or in neck area.

References

1. Vezina D, Lessard MR, Bussieres J, Topping C, Trepanier CA. Complications associated with the use of the Esophageal-Tracheal Combitube. Can J Anaesth 1998;45:76–80.
2. Van der Klooster JM, Grootendorst AF, Ophof PJ, Brouwers JW. Pneumomediastinum: an unusual complication of asthma in a young man. Netherl J Med 1998;52:150–154.
3. Galanis E, Litzow MR, Tefferi A, Scott JP. Spontaneous pneumomediastinum in a patient with bronchiolitis obliterans after bone marrow transplantation. Bone Marrow Transpl 1997;20:695–696.
4. Nagai Y, Ishikawa O, Miyachi Y. Pneumomediastinum and subcutaneous emphysema associated with fatal interstitial pneumonia in dermatomyositis. J Dermatol 1997;24:484–484.
5. Alvares JF, Dhawan PS, Tibrewala S, Shankaran K, Kulkarni SG, Rananavare R, et al. Retroperitoneal perforation in ulcerative colitis with mediastinal and subcutaneous emphysema. J Clin Gastroenterol 1997;453–455.

Pneumonia, All Types or Type Unspecified

NOTE: If the type of underlying infection is known, follow procedures suggested under the name of the infectious disease. If the etiologic agent of the pneumonia is unknown, proceed as follows: (1) Collect all tissues that appear to be infected. (2) Request aerobic, anaerobic, acid-fast, fungal, and viral cultures. (3) Request Gram, Kinyoun's acid-fast, and Grocott's methenamine silver stains. (4) Special **precautions may be required** (see Chapter 6). (5) Serologic studies may be helpful once a specific etiologic agent is suspected. Thus, collect serum at the time of autopsy or procure serum that was collected prior to death. (6) This **may be a reportable** disease.

Organs and Tissues	*Procedures*	*Possible or Expected Findings*
External examination		Herpes labialis; pyoderma; jaundice.
	Prepare chest roentgenogram.	Pneumothorax* or pneumatocele (in staphylococcal pneumonia of infancy); pleural effusions;* pulmonary infiltrates; abscesses.
Abdomen	Photograph abnormalities *in situ.*	Gastric dilatation and ileus; rarely, peritonitis.*
Pleural cavities	Puncture; submit samples of fluid for culture.	Fibrinous pleuritis; pleural effusions and exudates.*
Blood	Submit sample for culture.	Septicemia.
Heart		Infective endocarditis;* pericarditis.*
Lungs	Record weights. Submit consolidated areas for culture. Prepare touch preps of fresh cut sections. Perfuse lungs with formalin. For special stains, see above under "Note."	Bacterial, fungal, viral, or protozoal pneumonia; abscesses (*Staphylococcus aureus*) or hemorrhages (influenza, infection with *Pseudomonas* spp., and others). See also under name of suspected underlying infectious disease or underlying noninfectious disorder, such as rheumatoid arthritis.* Perifocal pneumonia around tumors. Bronchiectasis;* bronchial obstruction.
Mediastinum and neck organs	Submit samples of larynx, trachea, and major bronchi for histologic study.	Laryngotracheitis and tracheobronchitis.
Arteries and veins	For removal of femoral veins and arteries, see Chapter 3.	Infective vasculitis and thrombosis.

Organs and Tissues	Procedures	Possible or Expected Findings
Brain and spinal cord	For appropriate microbiologic study, see Chapter 7.	Meningitis.*
Joints	For removal, prosthetic repair, and specimen preparation, see Chapter 2.	Rarely, septic arthritis.

Pneumonia, Eosinophilic
(See "Syndrome, eosinophilic pulmonary.")

Pneumonia, Interstitial

Related Terms: Acute interstitial pneumonia (Hamman-Rich syndrome); desquamative interstitial pneumonia (DIP); idiopathic organizing pneumonia (or "bronchiolitis obliterans with patchy organizing pneumonia [BOOP]" or "cryptogenic organizing pneumonitis"); idiopathic pulmonary fibrosis; lymphoid interstitial pneumonitis (LIP); nonspecific interstitial pneumonia (NSIP) (or "cellular interstitial pneumonia" [CIP]); usual interstitial pneumonia (UIP); fibrosing alveolitis; pulmonary alveolitis; and many others.

NOTE: The conditions listed under "Related Terms" are histologic variants of idiopathic interstitial pneumonia. UIP is synonymous with idiopathic pulmonary fibrosis (IPF) *(1)*. Diffuse alveolar damage is the histologic finding in patients with the adult respiratory distress syndrome* (ARDS) causing interstitial and intra-alveolar fibrosis. This is an acute condition, referred to as acute interstitial pneumonia when it occurs as an idiopathic form of rapidly progressive interstitial pneumonia.

Possible Associated Conditions: Acquired immunodeficiency syndrome* (AIDS) in patients with with LIP or nonspecific interstitial pneumonia *(2,3)*; trauma and shock in ARDS. Secondary pulmonary fibrosis from inhalants (extrinsic allergic alveolitis or pneumonia; pneumoconiosis*), in drug-induced pneumonia, hypersensitivity pneumonitis (microgranulomatous hypersensitivity reaction of lung), rheumatoid arthritis,* Sjögren's syndrome,* and other collagen-vascular diseases; primary biliary cirrhosis in patients with nonspecific interstitial pneumonia *(2)*.

Organs and Tissues	Procedures	Possible or Expected Findings
External examination	Prepare chest roentgenogram.	Clubbing of fingers. Distribution of densities may be important for determining the specific type of the condition. Pleural effusions.
Blood	Submit sample for bacterial, fungal, and viral cultures and protein electrophoresis. Snap-freeze sample for possible serologic studies.	Underlying or superimposed infections. Dysproteinemia in LIP *(2)*.
Lungs with hilar lymph nodes	Record weights and photograph both lungs. Submit any consolidated areas for viral, bacterial, and fungal cultures. Make touch preparations from cut surfaces. Perfuse lungs with formalin. Request Gram and Grocott's methenamine silver for micro-organisms, and Verhoeff–van Gieson or other special stains to identify collagen and smooth muscle fibers.	Interstitial pulmonary fibrosis, often with interstitial inflammatory infiltrates, alveolar edema, Masson bodies, and bronchiolitis obliterans. Minute noncaseating granulomas in extrinsic allergic alveolitis *(4)* and large granulomas in sarcoidosis.* Diffuse aggregates of lightly pigmented macrophages in DIP. Hyaline membranes in diffuse alveolar damage. LIP may be difficult to separate from lymphoma, with or without evidence of Epstein-Barr virus DNA *(2)*.
	Prepare samples of fresh lung for electron microscopy.	Tubuloreticular structures and electron-dense deposits in systemic lupus erythematosus;* identification of viruses, *Pneumocystis,* or particles in pneumoconiosis *(5)*.
	Prepare sections of hilar lymph nodes.	Granulomas in sarcoidosis.*
Other organs		Manifestations of conditions listed above under Possible Associated Conditions."

References

1. Katzenstein A-L, Myers J. Idiopathic pulmonary fibrosis: clinical relevance of pathologic classification. Am J Respir Crit Care Med 1998; 157:1301–1315.
2. Fishback N, Koss M. Update on lymphoid interstitial pneumonitis. Curr Opin Pulm Med 1996;2:429–433.
3. Schneider RF. Lymphocytic interstitial pneumonitis and nonspecific interstitial pneumonitis. Clin Chest Med 1996;17:763–766.
4. Coleman A, Colby TV: Histologic diagnosis of extrinsic allergic alveolitis. Am J Surg Pathol 1988;12:514–518.
5. Panchal A, Koss MN. Role of electron microscopy in interstitial lung disease. Curr Opin Pulm Med 1997;3:341–347.

Pneumonia, Lipoid

Related Terms: Exogenous lipoid pneumonia; inhalation lipoid pneumonia; lipid pneumonia; mineral oil pneumonia.

Organs and Tissues	*Procedures*	*Possible or Expected Findings*
Lungs	Submit one lobe for microbiologic study. For bronchography, see Chapter 2. Dissect bronchial tree to demonstrate absence of bronchial obstruction. For formalin perfusion of lung, see Chapter 2. Request Verhoeff–van Gieson, Gram, and Kinyoun's stains.	Saprophytic growth of acid-fast mycobacteria or, rarely, fungi *(1)*. Lipoid or liquid paraffin granulomas; foreign-body granulomas; endarteritis obliterans; pulmonary fibrosis. In rare instances, evidence of hemoptysis *(2)*.
Other organs	Procedures depend on expected findings or grossly identified abnormalities as listed in right-hand column.	Achalasia of esophagus* and other chronic esophageal or laryngopharyngeal diseases, including carcinoma. Hypertrophic pyloric stenosis. Parkinson's disease* or other chronic cerebrovascular and neurologic diseases.
Bones and joints		Rheumatoid arthritis.* Hypertrophic osteoarthropathy* may be a rare complication *(3)*.

References

1. Jouannic I, Desrues B, Lena H, Quinquenel ML, Donnio PY, Delaval P. Exogenous lipoid pneumonia complicated by Mycobacterium fortuitum and Aspergillus fumigatus infection. Eur Respir J 1996;9:172–174.
2. Haro M, Murcia I, Nunez A, Julia E, Valer J. Massive haemoptysis complicating exogenous lipid pneumonia. Eur Respir J 1998;11:507–508.
3. Hugosson C, Bahabri S, Rifai A, al-Dalaan A. Hypertrophic osteoarthropathy caused by lipoid pneumonia. Pediatr Radiol 1995;25: 482–483.

Pneumothorax

Postmortem chest roentgenograms provide the only reliable and permanent record of a pneumothorax and its main complication, mediastinal shift due to a tension pneumothorax (Fig. II-4). If roentgenograms cannot be prepared, a reasonably reliable diagnosis still can be made if the prosector inserts a needle through the lateral chest wall. The needle should be connected to a water-filled flask. If a pneumothorax is present, gas bubbles appear in the flask as shown in Fig. II-5. One can also expose the intact parietal pleura and observe if the lung tissue is separated from the parietal pleura by gas. Incising the thorax at the base of a water-filled skin pocket is the least reliable method.

Infants can be totally submerged under water before the chest cavity is incised. However, care must be taken not to make an accidental incision into the underlying lung tissue.

Poisoning, All Types or Type Unspecified

NOTE: If a specific substance is suspected—for instance, arsenic or ethylene glycol—follow procedures described under the appropriate entry. Similar entries can be found for poisons whose general character or source is known—for instance, gas or mushroom poisoning. For some substances, the appropriate entry can be found under "Abuse,...," "Death,...," or "Dependence,..." In all instances, routine sampling of toxicologic material should be done as described in Chapter 13. If no specific substances can be incriminated, the toxicologist must be provided with all available clinical information, as shown in Chapter 13.

In most cases of fatal poisoning, the coroner or medical examiner must be notified.

Poisoning, Alkaloid

NOTE: See under specific name of alkaloid—for instance, "Dependence, cocaine," "Poisoning, atropine," "Poisoning, digitalis," or "Poisoning, strychnine." Only a fraction of this large group of plant poisons has been listed. Whether the specific name of the alkaloid is known or unknown, complete toxicologic sampling is recommended.

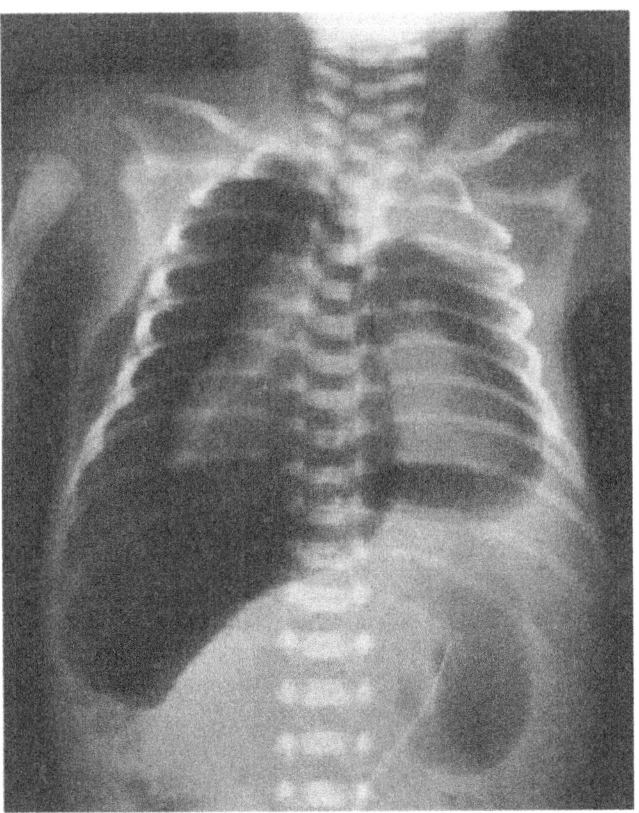

Fig. II-4. Tension pneumothorax. This premature newborn (26 wk gestation) had been intubated but died suddenly because of a pneumothorax on the left and a tension pneumothorax on the right. Pneumomediastinum was also present. These complications had not been recognized prior to death.

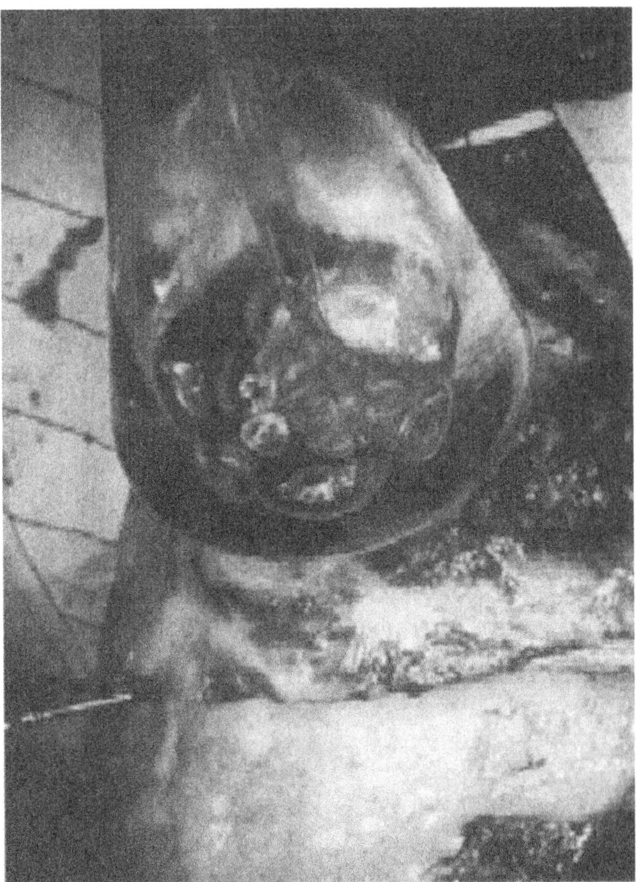

Fig. II-5. Tension pneumothorax. Skin has been dissected off right side of chest, and needle is inserted into chest wall. Rubber hose connects needle with glass tube. Note gas bubbles emerging from tip of glass tube at bottom of water-filled flask.

Poisoning, Ammonia

NOTE: The appropriate autopsy procedures are described under "Bronchitis, acute chemical" and under "Poisoning, gas." Blood ammonia concentrations are markedly increased. Formalin perfusion of lungs is not recommended; it may cause artifactual ballooning and internal ruptures of organ.

Poisoning, Antifreeze (See "Poisoning, ethylene glycol.")

Poisoning, Antimony

NOTE: Toxicologic material should be submitted for analysis, as suggested under "Poisoning, arsenic." Iatrogenic antimony toxicity may occur after treatment with antimony compounds for conditions such as filariasis, fungal infections, and schistosomiasis.*

Organs and Tissues	*Procedures*	*Possible or Expected Findings*
External examination and eyes	Record skin changes and eye abnormalities.	If exposure was from dust in smelting work, dermatitis and conjunctivitis may be present.
Pharynx and gastrointestinal tract	For toxicologic sampling of contents, see Chapter 13. Submit tissue samples for histologic study.	Severe gastroenteritis in acute poisoning. If victim drank antimony trichloride, ulcerative pharyngitis and gastritis may be present.
Heart, liver, and kidneys	Request frozen sections for Sudan stain.	Fatty changes of myocardium and hepatic and renal parenchyma.

Poisoning, Arsenic

NOTE: Toxicologic material will be contaminated by bringing it in contact with fluids. Keratinized tissues take up arsenic from solutions. Put plastic bags over hands of victim.

If exhumed bodies are investigated for arsenic poisoning, include material from surrounding soil and coffin along with tissues submitted for chemical analysis.

Interpretation of toxicologic findings: After fatal poisoning, arsenic concentrations in the liver tend to exceed 0.5–1.0 mg/100 g wet tissue. In acute poisoning, arsenic concentrations in hair may reach 3 μg/g *(1)* and in nails 8 μg/g.

Organs and Tissues	*Procedures*	*Possible or Expected Findings*
External examination and skin	Pull (do not cut) 10 g of hair from scalp and tie in locks with cotton. The ends with the hair roots should be identified. Collect some whole fingernails and toenails. Collect skin for toxicologic study. Record findings as listed in right-hand column; prepare photographs.	In chronic poisoning—manifestations of malnutrition,* alopecia, hyperpigmentation, eczematoid skin changes, hyperkeratosis of plantar and palmar surfaces, and white streaks (Mee's lines) on fingernails.
Blood	Submit sample for toxicologic study. Prepare smear.	Basophilic stippling; immature cells.
Heart	For histologic sampling. Prepare frozen section of myocardium and request Sudan stain for fat.	Subendocardial ventricular hemorrhages; fatty changes and round cell infiltrates of myocardium; myocardial infarction.
Arteries	Request Verhoeff–van Gieson stain of samples from skin, heart, stomach, intestine, mesentery, liver, pancreas, spleen, and kidney.	Intimal thickening in chronic poisoning of infants.
Stomach	Submit all contents for toxicologic analysis. Inspect wall with magnifying glass for identification of crystals.	Acute gastritis (in acute poisoning) with arsenous sulfide crystals in mucus coating wall of stomach.
Intestinal tract	Submit contents (feces) for toxicologic study.	Congestion and inflammation of mucous membranes.
Liver	Record weight. Submit (together with bile) for toxicologic study. Submit samples for histolgic study.	Cirrhosis. Fatty changes.
Kidneys	Submit samples for histologic study.	Fatty changes. Tubulo-interstitial nephritis *(2)*.
Urine	Submit sample for toxicologic and chemical study.	Test for coproporphyrin positive.
Pharynx and larynx		Inflamed mucous membranes.
Bone	Submit sample for toxicologic study.	
Bone marrow		Toxic changes.

References

1. Pazirandeh A, Brati AH, Marageh MG. Determination of arsenic in hair using neutron activation. Appl Radiat Isot 1998;49:753–759.

2. Prasad GV, Rossi NF. Arsenic intoxication associated with tubulointerstitial nephritis. Am J Kidney Dis 1995;26:373–376.

Poisoning, Atropine

Synonyms and Related Terms: Belladonna; hyoscine (scopolamine); hyoscyamine; hyoscyamus; stramonium.

Organs and Tissues	*Procedures*	*Possible or Expected Findings*
External examination		Body dry and warm after death.
Eyes	Record diameter of pupils.	Mydriasis.
Blood and liver	Submit samples for toxicologic study.	
Heart		Iatrogenic atrioventricular block *(1)*.
Gastrointestinal tract	Collect all contents, particularly in accidental poisoning in children.	Fruits of *Atropa belladonna* or seeds of *Datura stramonium* may be found.
Other organs		No characteristic findings.

Reference

1. Brunner-La Rocca HP, Kiowski W, Bracht C, Weilenmann D, Follath F. Atrioventricular block after administration of atropine in patients follow-ing cardiac transplantation. Transplant 1997;63:1838–1839.

Poisoning, Barbiturate(s)

NOTE: This type of poisoning has become uncommon. Barbiturates may cause sudden death. In all instances, concomitant alcohol intoxication* must be ruled out. Standard toxicologic sampling is sufficient.

Organs and Tissues	*Procedures*	*Possible or Expected Findings*
Blood	Submit samples of blood from portal vein and peripheral veins or heart for toxicologic study.	Evidence of alcohol intoxication.* Poisoning by other addictive drugs.
Bile	Refrigerate for possible toxicologic study.	
Urine	Record total volume and pH value. Request tests for protein, glucose, and ketones; request drug screen.	
Esophagus and stomach	Submit all contents and record their character. Analyze for barbiturates and alcohol.	Gritty residues of unabsorbed tablets, powder, or capsules. Mucosal corrosion, ulceration, and discoloration from capsules may occur.
Liver and brain	Submit samples for toxicologic study.	Concentration of barbiturate in parenchyma important for interpretation.

Poisoning, Bismuth

NOTE: Accidental poisoning is common (industrial exposure or drugs with soluble bismuth compounds). Search also for other heavy metals. Acute kidney failure* may be the cause of death.

Organs and Tissues	*Procedures*	*Possible or Expected Findings*
External examination and oral cavity	Record abnormalities as listed in right-hand column.	Stomatitis with bluish black discoloration of gums; loose teeth; sticky white membranous patches in mouth and throat. Jaundice.
Blood	Submit sample for toxicologic study.	
Urine	Submit sample for toxicologic study. Use one sample for preparation of sediment.	Protein casts and tubular epithelial cells in sediment.
Gastrointestinal tract	Submit contents for toxicologic study. Record appearance of mucosa. Submit samples for histologic study.	Gray or black mucosal membranes; swelling of mucosa; intestinal ulcers that may be perforated. Hemosiderosis.
Liver	Submit samples for toxicologic and histologic study. Request Gomori's iron stain.	Fatty changes; hemosiderosis.
Spleen	Submit samples for toxicologic and histologic study.	Hemosiderosis.
Kidneys	Submit samples for toxicologic and histologic study.	Fatty changes; renal tubular degeneration with amorphic basophilic deposits in epithelium of convoluted tubules. Hemosiderosis.
Neck organs		See above under "External examination."
Peripheral nerves	For removal and specimen preparation, see Chapter 4.	Peripheral neuritis.

Poisoning, Bromide

Synonyms: Bromine poisoning; bromism.

NOTE: The lethal dose is about 0.2 g in children and 1 g in adults (ingested). After fatal methyl bromide poisoning, headspace gas chromatography revealed a subclavian blood concentration of 3.0 microgram/mL whereas inorganic bromide concentrations were 530 micrograms/mL in the blood *(1)*. Tissue concentrations were lower than those in the blood.

Organs and Tissues	*Procedures*	*Possible or Expected Findings*
External examination, skin, and eyes	Prepare photographs and histologic sections of skin lesions.	Chemical burns on face and conjunctivitis indicate direct exposure; skin pustules over body and nodose bromoderma of the legs indicate bromism.
Blood	Submit sample for toxicologic study.	Blood is best suited for bromide determination.
Urine	Submit sample for toxicologic study.	
Gastrointestinal tract	Submit gastric contents for toxicologic examination. Record appearance of gastro-intestinal mucosa.	After ingestion of bromide, necrosis with brown discoloration of mucosa of upper gastrointestinal tract may be present.
Trachea, bronchi, and lungs	If possible, remove lungs together with neck organs; open major airways posteriorly.	After inhalation of bromide, swelling and inflammation of mucous membranes in upper and lower respiratory tracts may be present. There may be pulmonary edema. Pneumonia occurs in bromism.
Other organs	Toxicologic samples should include liver and kidneys.	

Reference

1. Michalodimitrakis MN, Tsatsakis AM, Christakis-Hampsas MG, Trikilis N, Christodoulou P. Death following intentional methyl bromide poisoning: toxicological data and literature review. Vet Hum Toxicol 1997;39:30–34.

Poisoning, Cadmium

Organs to be analyzed for Cd should have no contact with water or be contaminated with blood; they should be sealed in polyethylene bags. Cd leaks into fixation fluid. Postmortem blood concentrations are very high and no indicator of the antemortem values *(1)*.

Organs and Tissues	*Procedures*	*Possible or Expected Findings*
External examination and oral cavity		Yellow gingival line in chronic poisoning.
Blood	Submit sample for toxicologic study.	
Urine	Submit sample for determination of cadmium concentration.	Elevated urinary cadmium concentrations *(2)*.
Lungs	Submit sample for toxicologic study and a portion of one lobe for microbiologic study. Perfuse one lung with formalin.	Pulmonary edema, alveolar wall damage, and interstitial pneumonia after acute inhalation. Severe pulmonary fibrosis may develop in chronic cases.
Gastrointestinal tract	Fix bowel as soon as possible.	Gastroenteritis after nonlethal food poisoning.
Kidneys	Collect renal tissue for light microscopic and electron microscopic study.	Degeneration of proximal tubules and proteinuria in acute poisoning; interstitial nephritis in chronic poisoning. Nephrolithiasis *(3)*.
Other organs	Sample for toxicologic study. Submit samples for histologic study also.	Degenerative changes of liver and myocardium.

References

1. Koizumi N, Hatayama F, Sumino K. Problems in the analysis of cadmium in autopsied tissues. Environm Res 1994;64:192–198.
2. Ando Y, Shibata E, Tsuchiyama F, Sakai S. Elevated urinary cadmium concentrations in a patient with acute cadmium pneumonitis. Scand J Work Environ Health 1996;22:150–153.
3. Savolainen H. Cadmium-associated renal disease. Ren Fail 1995;17: 483–487.

Poisoning, Carbon Monoxide

NOTE: If the victim had been in a fire, see also under "Burns." Carbon monoxide poisoning may rarely be responsible for automobile accidents. Relatively low carboxyhemoglobin concentrations may contribute to death if there is concomitant poisoning—for instance, with alcohol or drugs, particularly sedatives. Anemia, atherosclerotic heart disease, and chronic pulmonary disease also increase sensitivity to carbon monoxide.

If blood had been withdrawn at time of hospital admission—for instance, for crossmatching—submit this for carboxyhemoglobin determination. If no blood can be obtained, see under "Heart, kidneys, and other organs." For quick-orienting qualitative tests, for quantitative methods of carbon monoxide determi-nation, and for interpretation of toxicologic findings, see below. Request also determination of hemoglobin concentrations and of blood alcohol. Request drug screen. For shipping of blood and tissues for carbon monoxide determination, see Chapter 15. It should be noted that losses of up to 60% of the original saturation occurred when blood was kept in uncapped container at room temperature for 2 ½ wk or at 4°C for 3 wk.

Organs and Tissues	*Procedures*	*Possible or Expected Findings*
External examination	Record color of fingernails, particularly in heavily pigmented persons in whom lividity is difficult to discern.	Pink skin and fingernails; bullous edema of skin; decubital ulcers.
Blood	Record appearance of blood and submit sample of postmortem blood for toxicologic study. See also above under "Note."	Blood tends to be cherry red. For interpretation of toxicologic findings, see below.
Heart, kidneys, and other organs	If no blood can be obtained, prepare water extract of spleen, kidneys, or other organs. Request determination of carbon monoxide content and of carbon monoxide-binding capacity of this mixture. Submit tissue samples for histologic study.	Necrosis of papillary muscles in the heart or myocardial infarction may occur. Renal tubular degeneration may also be found. Acute kidney failure* has been observed after rhabdomyolysis complicated by compartment syndrome *(2)*.
Brain	For removal and specimen preparation, see Chapter 4.	Hemorrhagic necrosis of basal ganglia (lenticular nucleus in globus pallidus); diffuse petechial hemorrhages in white matter; cerebral edema. Acute hydrocephalus in infants *(3)*.

Methods of Carbon Monoxide Determination

Many methods of carbon monoxide determination have been described. Currently, carboxyhemoglobin is detected in most medical examiner toxicology laboratories by visible spectrophotometry or gas chromatography. In hospitals, carboxyhemoglobin is frequently detected and reported in the course of routine arterial blood gas analysis.

Pink discoloration of skin and organs usually indicates the presence of more than 30% carboxyhemoglobin (but rule out cyanide poisoning* and exposure to cold*).

In a healthy, middle-aged person, a carboxyhemoglobin concentration greater than 50–60% is usually fatal. If the victim was anemic or suffered from chronic lung disease, particularly emphysema* or atherosclerotic heart disease, the concentration may be lower. In association with alcohol, sedatives, and other drugs, carboxyhemoglobin levels may also be much lower and yet fatal.

A heavy cigarette smoker may have a carboxyhemoglobin concentration of 8–10%, and higher levels may occur in police officers and other persons exposed to automobile exhaust in dense traffic.

If the victim survived the carbon monoxide poisoning for several hours, postmortem blood samples usually will fail to show the presence of carboxyhemoglobin. In these instances, blood taken at the time of admission to the hospital may still be available and of particular value. If the victim had spent 1 h in fresh air before death, 40–50% of the carbon monoxide will have been removed, and 8–10% will have been removed during each subsequent hour. Even though clearance may be complete, death may still occur—primarily from brain damage and infectious complications in prolonged coma.

Physiologic Effects of Carbon Monoxide Poisoning†

% of carboxy-hemoglobin	*Clinical Signs/Symptoms*
10	No appreciable effect except shortness of breath on vigorous muscular exertion
20	In most cases, no appreciable effect except dyspnea, even on moderate exertion; slight headache in some cases

% of carboxy-hemoglobin	Clinical Signs/Symptoms
30	Decided headache; irritability; easy fatigability; disturbance of judgment
40–50	Headache; confusion; fainting and collapse on exertion
60–70	Unconsciousness, respiratory failure, and death if exposure is prolonged
80	Rapidly fatal
>80	Immediately fatal

†Modified from Henderson Y, Haggard HW. Noxious Gases. The Chemical Catalog Co., New York, 1927.

References

1. Ocak A, Valentour JC, Blanke RV. The effects of storage conditions on the stability of carbon monoxide in postmortem blood. J Anal Toxicol 1985;9:202–206.
2. Abdul-Ghaffar NU, Farghaly MM, Swamy AS. Acute renal failure, compartment syndrome, and systemic capillary leak syndrome complicating carbon monoxide poisoning. J Toxicol 1996;34:713–719.
3. So GM, Kosofsky BE, Southern JF. Acute hydrocephalus following carbon monoxide poisoning. Pediatr Neurol 1997;17:270–273.

Poisoning, Carbon Tetrachloride

Synonym: Tetrachloromethane poisoning.

NOTE: Toxicologic sampling of body fluids and organs should be done routinely in all cases. In many instances, however, death occurs 1 wk to 10 d after exposure, and by this time no carbon tetrachloride is demonstrable. Death may be sudden or delayed by only a few hours, particularly after inhalation of carbon tetrachloride. Sudden death probably is caused by cardiac dysrrhythmia.

Alcohol concentrations should be determined in all cases or, if death was delayed, evidence of drinking at the time of exposure should be sought. Alcohol considerably increases the hazards of carbon tetrachloride.

Organs and Tissues	*Procedures*	*Possible or Expected Findings*
External examination		Jaundice; pedal edema.
Heart	Submit samples for histologic study, and request frozen sections for Sudan stain.	Fatty changes of myocardium.
Liver	Record weight and photograph; submit samples for histologic study. Request frozen sections for Sudan stain.	Centrilobular or diffuse hepatic necrosis and fatty changes. Cirrhosis* after chronic exposure.
Kidneys	Photograph and submit samples for histologic study. Request frozen sections for Sudan stain.	Acute tubular necrosis (lower nephron nephrosis); fatty degeneration.
Adrenal glands	Sample for histologic study.	Necrosis in zona fasciculata and reticularis.
Brain	For removal and specimen preparation, see Chapter 4.	Perivenous necroses in cerebral white matter; cerebellar degeneration (Purkinje cells). Pontine necrosis.
Eyes	For removal and specimen preparation, see Chapter 5.	Optic neuritis in chronic cases.
Peripheral nerves	For sampling and specimen preparation, see Chapter 4.	Peripheral neuritis in chronic cases.

Poisoning, Chlorine or Hydrochloric Acid

Related Terms: Cl_2 poisoning; HCl poisoning.

NOTE: See also under "Bronchitis, acute chemical" and under "Poisoning, gas." Hydrochloric acid is sold by plumbing supply houses and pool supply companies as muriatic acid. It is a liquid. Chlorine is a water-soluble gas. As supplied for pool sanitation, liquid chlorine is usually acidic. For convenience, chlorine and hydrochloric acid are discussed here together.

Organs and Tissues	*Procedures*	*Possible or Expected Findings*
External examination and eyes	Prepare photographs of face.	Conjunctivitis and cyanosis in chlorine gas poisoning; burns of lips from hydrochloric acid.

Organs and Tissues	Procedures	Possible or Expected Findings
Lungs	Submit a portion of lung for toxicologic study (see under "Poisoning, gas"). Record lung weights. Formalin perfusion of lungs is not recommended; it may cause artifactual ballooning and internal ruptures of organ.	Severe pulmonary edema, bronchopneumonia, and swelling of mucous membranes in chlorine poisoning. Arterial thrombosis may occur. Pulmonary fibrosis may develop after prolonged survival.
Larynx and trachea	Leave esophagus and stomach attached to neck organs. Open larynx anteriorly and check whether a perforation has occurred.	Swelling and ulceration of mucous membranes in chlorine poisoning; acute laryngotracheitis. Tracheoesophageal perforation.
Esophagus and stomach	See also above under "Larynx and trachea." Photograph opened esophagus and stomach.	Corrosion of mucosa with thickening, hemorrhage, and blackish discoloration after ingestion of hydrochloric acid.
	Sample for histologic study, particularly if there is doubt whether a perforation was antemortem or postmortem.	Antemortem and postmortem perforation may occur.
Kidneys		Glomerular capillary thromboses.
Brain	For removal and specimen preparation, see Chapter 4.	Hemorrhages in white matter *(1)*.

Reference

1. Adelson L, Kaufman J. Fatal chlorine poisoning: report of two cases with clinicopathologic correlation. Am J Clin Pathol 1971;56:430–442.

Poisoning, Cyanide

Synonym: Hydrocyanic acid (hydrogen cyanide) poisoning.

NOTE: Hydrocyanic acid (hydrogen cyanide, HCN) is a water-soluble gas. Its salts, sodium cyanide and potassium cyanide are sold as "eggs" to the jewelry industry. Hydrocyanic acid is formed when cyanide salts are dissolved in acidic solutions. Containers from which the poison might have been ingested or inhaled should also be submitted for toxicologic examination. For cyanide screening tests in the autopsy room and for interpretation of findings, see below. Caution: Stomach may still contain cyanide gas, formed by acidic reaction of cyanide salt. It may be best to open the stomach under a hood *(1)*. The odor is quite characteristic for cyanide poisoning but most persons are unable to smell this odor. It is helpful to know in advance if any person in an office or laboratory can smell cyanide. Forensic pathologists who can smell the compound state that it has its own specific odor, which differs from the often quoted smell of bitter almonds. Autopsies also can be done in a negatively pressured isolation room *(1)*.

Organs and Tissues	Procedures	Possible or Expected Findings
External examination and oral cavity	Record color of skin and possible corrosion marks, as listed in right-hand column.	For odor, see above under "Note." Bright red skin color is not always present. Corrosion around mouth and in oral cavity may be found after ingestion of potassium or sodium cyanide.
Blood	Submit sample for toxicologic study. For autopsy screening tests, see below.	Blood is fluid and sometimes bright red.
Stomach	See above under "Note." Submit contents for toxicologic study. Sample for histologic study.	If potassium or sodium cyanide was ingested, brown-red mucosal corrosion may be present in stomach or in upper digestive tract.
Pharynx and esophagus	See above under "Stomach."	
Lungs	Record lung weights and submit one lung for toxicologic study. Submit samples from other lung for histologic study.	Pulmonary edema.
Liver	Submit portion for toxicologic study.	
Brain	For removal and specimen preparation, see Chapter 4.	For odor, see above under "Note." If death
	Submit portion for toxicologic study.	was not instantaneous, there may be hyaline thrombi in small blood vessels, minute hemorrhages, and necroses of lenticular nuclei.

Cyanide Screening Tests in the Autopsy Room

This test can be used for blood and gastric contents *(2)*. Dip squares of filter paper in a small amount of saturated picric acid. Let these squares dry until barely moist. Place a drop of the material to be tested—e.g., blood or gastric contents—on a piece of paper. Let material dry for a moment, and then place one drop of 10% sodium carbonate in the center of the material to be tested. If cyanide is present, a reddish purple color will chromatograph out from the material. The higher the concentration of cyanide the more blue the color will be. It is possible to recognize whole blood because the blood turns a rather dark brown and the reddish to purple color is clearly visible. High concentrations of sulfide interfere by giving a false-positive test.

Another screening test is done as follows *(3)*. Dip filter paper into normal blood. Then treat the paper with potassium chlorate, whereupon brown methemoglobin forms. Place this preparation into the fluid suspected of containing cyanide (e.g., blood, gastric contents, pulmonary edema fluid). If bright red cyanmethemoglobin forms, the reaction is positive.

Interpretation of Findings

If the concentration of cyanide in the stomach is high and the concentration in the lungs is low, cyanide was ingested. Alternatively, if the pulmonary cyanide concentration is high and the concentrtaion in the gastric contents is low, hydrogen cyanide most likely was inhaled. Occasionally, minimal cyanide levels will be present in decomposed bodies.

References

1. Nolte KB, Dasgupta A. Prevention of occupational cyanide exposure in autopsy prosectors. J Forens Sci 1996;41:146–147.
2. Camps FE. Gradwohl's Legal Medicine, 2nd ed. Williams & Wilkins Company, Baltimore, 1968, pp. 615–617.
3. Glaister J, Rentoul E. Medical Jurisprudence and Toxicology, 12th ed. E & S Livingstone, Edinburgh, 1966, p. 686.

Poisoning, Digitalis

Related Term: Digoxin toxicity.

NOTE: Certain drugs may interfere with correct digitalis determination.

Organs and Tissues	*Procedures*	*Possible or Expected Findings*
Blood	Submit sample of peripheral blood for digoxin radioimmunoassay.	Digoxin values in digitalis toxicity are greater than 2 ng/mL *(1)*.
Heart	Freeze fresh myocardium for digitalis extraction.	Increased digitalis concentrations *(2)*.
Vitreous	Submit sample for digoxin radioimmunoassay.	Digoxin concentration may be higher or lower than concentration in serum, depending on how long before death drug was taken *(1)*.

References

1. DiMaio VJM, Garriot JC, Putnam R. Digoxin concentrations in postmortem specimens after overdose and therapeutic use. J Forensic Sci 1975;20:340–347.
2. Jellifee RW, Stephenson RG. A fluorimetric determination of myocardial digoxin at autopsy, with identification of digitalis leaf, digitoxin and gitonin. Am J Clin Pathol 1969;51:347–357.

Poisoning, Drug(s) (See "Dependence, drug(s), all types or type unspecified" or under "Poisoning,..." followed by specific name of drug.)

Poisoning, Ethanol (Ethyl Alcohol) (See "Alcoholism and alcohol intoxication," "Cardiomyopathy, alcoholic," "Disease, alcoholic liver," "Syndrome, fetal alcoholic," and Syndrome, Wernicke-Korsakoff.")

Poisoning, Ethylene Glycol

Related Term: Antifreeze poisoning.

NOTE: Pulmonary and cerebral manifestations are the main findings in acute poisoning, and renal tubular necrosis is the primary finding in chronic poisoning. For general toxicologic sampling, see Chapter 13. Calcium oxalate crystals can be demonstrated in routine histologic sections but also in scanning electron micrographs of thick deparaffinized sections.

Organs and Tissues	*Procedures*	*Possible or Expected Findings*
Eyes	For removal and specimen preparation, see Chapter 5.	Papilledema; optic nerve atrophy.
Blood	In acute cases, submit sample for ethylene glycol determination; in chronic cases, request determination of calcium concentrations.	Ethylene glycol in serum *(1)*.
Urine	Prepare sediment.	Protein casts; calcium oxalate crystals *(2)*. Crystals are light yellow and birefringent, arranged as sheaves, rhomboids, or prisms.

Organs and Tissues	Procedures	Possible or Expected Findings
Heart	Sample for histologic study.	Myocardial degeneration; petechial hemorrhages.
Blood vessels	Submit samples of small vessels from multiple sites for histologic study. Request Verhoeff–van Gieson stain.	Oxalate crystals in media of small arteries, with associated ischemic lesions.
Lungs	Perfuse one lung with formalin.	Congestion; petechial hemorrhages; bronchopneumonia; edema.
Gastrointestinal tract	Submit at least contents for toxicologic study.	Petechial mucosal hemorrhages.
Liver	Record weight; submit samples for histologic study.	Hydropic hepatocellular degeneration; fatty changes and focal necroses.
Kidneys	See above under "Note."	Acute renal tubular necrosis;* intratubular crystals.
Brain	For removal and specimen preparation, see Chapter 4.	Petechial hemorrhages.

References

1. Eder AF, McGrath CM, Dowdy YG, Tomaszewski JE, Rosenberg FM, Wilson RB, et al. Ethylene glycol poisoning: toxicokinetic and analytical factors affecting laboratory diagnosis. Clin Chem 1998; 44:168–177.
2. Davis DP, Bramwell KJ, Hamilton RS, Williams SR. Ethylene glycol poisoning: case report of a record-high level and a review. J Emerg Med 1997;15:653–667.

Poisoning, Food

Related Terms: Bacillary dysentery* (*Shigella* food poisoning); botulism;* *Clostridium perfringens* food poisoning; favism; mushroom poisoning;* *Salmonella* food poisoning; staphylococcal food poisoning.

NOTE: If cause of food poisoning is unknown, submit suspected food for aerobic and anaerobic cultures, Gram stain of smears, and routine toxicologic study. This should include tests for heavy metals (antimony, cadmium, and lead) that may have leaked from old cooking utensils. Test for the presence of staphylococcal enterotoxin are done only in specialized laboratories. If botulism is suspected, follow procedures described under that heading. Mushroom poisoning also is listed as a separate entity. If *Salmonella* food poisoning is suspected, see under "Fever, typhoid." See also under "Enteritis" or "Enterocolitis" or under another specific heading such as "Dysentery, bacillary." Obtain sufficient material for microbiologic and histologic study to identify organisms such as *Chlamydia, Clostridium (type F strains), Salmonella, Shigella, verotoxic E. coli, Yersinia,* and others.

Organs and Tissues	Procedures	Possible or Expected Findings
External examination		Debilitated states; patients in extremes of life.
Gastrointestinal tract	Submit contents for aerobic and anaerobic cultures (see above under "Note"); prepare smears of contents for Gram stain. Submit samples for histologic study.	Enteritis or enterocolitis.

Poisoning, Gas

NOTE: Anesthesia-associated death,* carbon monoxide poisoning,* and sniffing and spray death* are presented under the appropriate headings. Procedures discussed here deal with other volatile substances, including chemical irritants such as ammonia (NH_3), chlorine or hydrochloric acid poisoning (see also under that heading); methylene chloride, phosgene ($COCl_2$), sulfurous acid (H_2SO_3), or sulfur dioxide (SO_2).

Gases from body cavities, heart chambers, or blood vessels can be removed as described under "Embolism, air." Gases can also be trapped with a rubber dam after cutting organs under water. Samples from various organs should be shipped in hermetically sealed nonplastic containers or in analyzing solutions.

Organs and Tissues	Procedures	Possible or Expected Findings
External examination, and oral cavity	Record extent of chemical burns.	Chemical burns in and around mouth or conjunctivas.
Blood	Submit sample for gas analysis. In many instances, inhaled gases can be demonstrated chromatographically in gas from head space above sealed blood specimen.	
Larynx and trachea		Chemical burns.

Organs and Tissues	*Procedures*	*Possible or Expected Findings*
Lungs	If gas was inhaled and is to be analyzed, submit intact lungs with bronchi ligated in airtight, nonplastic container to laboratory that can conduct gas analysis. If survival was short, formalin perfusion of lungs is not recommended; it may cause artifactual ballooning and internal ruptures of organ. Submit samples of tissue for routine histologic study.	Chemical pneumonia; pulmonary edema. After longer survival, obliterating fibrous bronchiolitis, chronic bronchitis, and saccular bronchiectasis* may occur.
Other organs	See above under "Note."	

Poisoning, Glycol (See "Poisoning, ethylene glycol.")

Poisoning, Halogen (See "Fluorosis," "Poisoning, bromide," "Poisoning, chlorine or hydrochloric acid," "Poisoning, gas," and "Poisoning, iodine.")

Poisoning, Heavy Metal (See "Poisoning, antimony," "Poisoning, arsenic," "Poisoning, cadmium," "Poisoning, lead," Poisoning, mercury," "Poisoning, thallium.")

Poisoning, Insecticide (See "Poisoning, organophosphate(s)*)

Poisoning, Iodine

Related Terms: Lugol's solution; tincture of iodine. For toxicologic sampling, see Chapter 13.

Organs and Tissues	*Procedures*	*Possible or Expected Findings*
External examination and eyes	Record color of skin and extent of corrosive lesions.	Perioral corrosive lesions; yellow discoloration of skin; conjunctivitis after exposure to vapors.
Urine, blood, and parenchymal organs	Submit samples for toxicologic study.	
Lungs and upper respiratory tract	Submit samples for histologic study.	Acute inflammation of respiratory tract after inhalation of vapors.
Stomach	Submit contents for toxicologic study; photograph mucosa; prepare histologic sections.	Corrosive gastritis; if starch was used as antidote, gastric lining will be bluish. Histologically, well-preserved mucosa is present because of in vivo fixation.
Intestinal tract	See above under "Stomach."	Mucosa may show same changes as stomach.
Kidneys		Swelling of tubular epithelium.

Poisoning, Isopropyl Alcohol

Synonyms: Propanol; rubbing alcohol.

Organs and Tissues	*Procedures*	*Possible or Expected Findings*
All organs	See under "Alcoholism and alcohol intoxication."	Nonspecific autopsy findings: visceral congestion; pulmonary and cerebral edema.

Poisoning, Lead

NOTE: Lead-free syringes and lead-free polyethylene containers should be used. Blood lead concentrations can be determined by inductively coupled plasma mass spectrometry *(1)*. For screening methods, see ref. *(2)*.

This is a **reportable** disease **in some states**.

Organs and Tissues	*Procedures*	*Possible or Expected Findings*
External examination, oral cavity, and hair		Bluish lead line at gingival margin in victims with poor oral hygiene.

Organs and Tissues	Procedures	Possible or Expected Findings
External examination, oral cavity, and hair *(continued)*	Prepare roentgenograms of long bones.	Densities at the ends of the shafts of long bones.
	For diagnosis of chronic plumbism, analysis of scalp hair may be useful. Analysis is done by neutron activation (see also under "Poisoning, arsenic").	Lead content of hair may be used to estimate time and duration of exposure. Evidence of old shotgun injury may explain chronic lead poisoning *(3)*.
Blood	Remove samples with lead-free syringe (see above under "Note") or 20-mL Vacutainer tubes (Becton, Dickinson and Company). Do not add anti-coagulant or preservative.	Normal concentration in children is less than 0.04 mg/100 g; values for "safe" industrial exposure in adults vary from 0.01–0.07 mg/100 g.
Urine	For collection procedures, see above under "Blood" and under "Note." Request also determination of coproporphyrin concentrations.	Values for "safe" industrial exposure in adults vary from 0.01–0.15 mg/L. Aminoaciduria and glycosuria after lead poisoning in children *(4)*.
Liver	Submit sample for histologic study; submit remaining tissue for toxicologic analysis.	Intranuclear inclusion bodies in acute poisoning.
Small and large bowel	Submit with contents for toxicologic study, particularly in acute poisoning.	
Kidneys	Submit sample from each kidney for histologic study; submit remaining tissue of both kidneys separately for toxicologic study.	Chronic nephritis; tubular degeneration with intranuclear inclusion bodies.
Bone	Submit at least 10 g of fresh bone for toxicologic study.	
Brain	For removal and specimen preparation, see Chapter 4.	Perivascular hemorrhages; cell necrosis; edema. Possibly increased risk of gliomas in chronic poisoning *(5)*.

References

1. Bergdahl IA, Schutz A, Gerhardsson L, Jensen A, Skerfving S. Lead concentrations in human plasma, urine and whole blood. Scand J Work Environ Health 1997;23:359–363.
2. Daher RT. Trace metals (lead and cadmium screening). Anal Chem 1995;67:405R–410R.
3. Wu PB, Kingery WS, Date ES. An EMG case report of lead neuropathy 19 years after a gunshot injury. Muscle Nerve 1995;18:326–329.
4. Loghman-Adham M. Aminoaciduria and glycosuria following severe childhood lead poisoning. Pediatr Nephrol 1998;12:218–221.
5. Anttila A, Heikkila P, Nykyri E, Kauppinen T, Pukkula E, Hernberg S, et al. Risk of nervous system cancer among workers exposed to lead. J Occup Environ Med 1996;38:131–136.

Poisoning, LSD (d-Lysergic Acid Diethylamide) (See "Abuse, hallucinogen(s).")

Poisoning, Lye

Related Terms: Ammonium hydroxide poisoning; calcium oxide or quicklime poisoning; poisoning by alkaline corrosives; potassium hydroxide poisoning; sodium hydroxide poisoning.

Organs and Tissues	Procedures	Possible or Expected Findings
External examination and oral cavity	Record extent of oral, perioral, and other facial corrosive injuries. Photograph lesions. Prepare histologic sections of tissue from inside of lips or mouth.	Lye burns on face and chest in acute cases; scars and manifestations of malnutrition* in chronic cases.
Blood	Submit sample for toxicologic study.	
Neck organs, esophagus, trachea, and lungs	After removal of heart, remove neck organs with hypopharynx, esophagus, larynx, and trachea. Leave stomach attached to esophagus. Open pharynx and esophagus along posterior midline. In acute cases, formalin perfusion of lungs is not recommended; it may cause artifactual ballooning and internal ruptures of organ.	Swelling, edema, and necrosis of mucous membranes in acute poisoning. Fibrosis and strictures in chronic cases. Bronchitis* and bronchopneumonia.

Organs and Tissues	*Procedures*	*Possible or Expected Findings*
Stomach	Remove gastric contents carefully from *in situ* incision. Caution—tissues are very friable. Leave stomach attached to esophagus (see above under "Neck organs,..."). Submit sample for pH determination. Submit sample for toxicologic study.	See below under "Intestinal tract."
Intestinal tract	Describe color of duodenal mucosa and odor of mucosa and contents.	Mucosal corrosion, with or without perforation.

Poisoning, Mercury

Related Term: Methylmercury poisoning (Minamata disease).

NOTE: For general toxicologic sampling, see Chapter 13. If kidney failure was present, see also under that heading. Analysis can be done by atomic absorption spectrophotometry *(1)*.

Organs and Tissues	*Procedures*	*Possible or Expected Findings*
External examination, skin, and oral cavity	Record extent of skin changes and prepare histologic sections.	Exfoliative dermatitis.
	Record appearance of oral cavity.	Blue line at gingival margin; hypertrophy of gum; acute and chronic gingivitis; exfoliation and loss of teeth *(2)*.
Blood	Submit sample for toxicologic study.	
Heart	Submit tissue for toxicologic study. Prepare histologic sections of myocardium.	Degeneration of myocardium.
Lungs	Submit samples for toxicologic and histologic study.	Increased concentrations of mercury *(1)*.
Esophagus	Submit sample for histologic study.	Induration of mucosa.
Liver and spleen	Submit samples for toxicologic and histologic study.	Congestion.
Stomach and colon	Submit samples for histologic study. Submit sample of colon for toxicologic study.	Erosive gastritis and colitis.
Kidneys	Submit samples for toxicologic and histologic study.	Increased concentrations of mercury *(1)*. Degeneration of proximal tubules; calcifications. Chronic kidney failure* may be the cause of death.
Neck organs	Submit specimen from pharynx for histologic study.	Induration of mucosa.
Brain and spinal cord	For removal and specimen preparation, see Chapter 4. Submit sample of brain for toxicologic study.	Increased concentrations of mercury *(1)*. Cortical hemorrhages.

References

1. Opitz H, Schweinsberg F, Grossmann T, Wendt-Gallitelli MF, Meyerman R. Demonstration of mercury in the human brain and other organs 17 years after metallic mercury exposure. Clin Neuropathol 1996;15:139–144.
2. Martin MD, Williams BJ, Charleston JD, Oda D. Spontaneous exfoliation of teeth following severe elemental mercury poisoning: case report and histological investigation for mechanism. Oral Surg Oral Med Oral Pathol 1997;84:495–501.

Poisoning, Metal (See "Poisoning, antimony," "Poisoning, arsenic," "Poisoning, cadmium," "Poisoning, lead," "Poisoning, mercury," and "Poisoning, thallium.")

Poisoning, Methanol (Methyl Alcohol)

Synonym: Wood alcohol.

NOTE: Autopsy findings are not diagnostic. Pulmonary and cerebral edema and edema of other viscera may be present. See also under "Alcoholism and alcohol intoxication."

Poisoning, Methylene Chloride (See "Poisoning, gas.")

Poisoning, Mushroom

NOTE: Fatalities usually are caused by members of the genus *Amanita*. The results of the autopsy may be less diagnostic than examination of the leftovers of the incriminated meal. If patient underwent liver *(1)* or kidney *(2)* transplantation, see also under these headings.

Organs and Tissues	*Procedures*	*Possible or Expected Findings*
Gastrointestinal tract	Submit gastric and intestinal contents for toxicologic study.	Usually, study of gastrointestinal contents gives no meaningful results because of the long interval between consumption of the poisoned meal and death.
Liver	Record size and weight. Submit samples for histologic and toxicologic study.	Massive or submassive hepatic necrosis, involving primarily zones 2 and 3 *(3)*.
Kidneys	Sample tissue for toxicologic study, and light microscopy.	Acute interstitial nephritis in *Cortinarius speciocissimus* poisoning. Acute tubular necrosis in *Amanita phalloides* poisoning *(3)* and in *Cortinarius speciocissimus* poisoning.
Other organs	For general toxicologic sampling, see Chapter 13. Histologic sections should include brain.	Hemorrhagic diathesis and cerebral edema in *Amanita phalloides* poisoning *(3)*.

References

1. Meunier B, Messner M, Bardaxoglou E, Spiliopoulos G, Terblanche J, Launois B. Liver transplantation for severe Lepiota helveola poisoning. Liver 1994;14:158–160.
2. Holmdahl J, Blohme I. Renal transplantation after Cortinarius speciocissimus poisoning. Nephrol Dialysis Transplant 1995;10:1920–1922.
3. Fineschi V, Di Paolo M, Centini F. Histological criteria for diagnosis of amanita phalloides poisoning. J Forens Sci 1996;41: 429–432.

Poisoning, Organophosphate(s)

Synonyms and Related Terms: Compounds include diazinon, dichlorvos, malathion, and parathion. For updates, consult poison hotlines.

NOTE: Organophosphate insecticides may produce rapid and severe toxic affects leading to coma and pulmonary edema and respiratory insufficiency. Interpretation of toxicologic findings, see below. For toxicologic sampling, Chapter 13.

Organs and Tissues	*Procedures*	*Possible or Expected Findings*
Blood and urine	Submit samples for toxicologic study and assay for cholinesterase activities.	Cholinesterase activity will be low.
Lungs	Record weights of lungs and contents of airways.	Pulmonary edema if poison was inhaled. Airways may contain aspirated material.
Gastrointestinal tract	Submit contents for toxicologic study.	
Liver and kidneys	Submit samples for toxicologic study.	
Skeletal muscles	Submit unfixed material for histochemical demonstration of reduced cholinesterase activity at motor end-plates.	Cholinesterase activity can be determined reliably even after decomposition and embalming.
Brain and spinal cord	For removal and specimen preparation, see Chapter 4.	Clinically, Guillain-Barré syndrome has been observed after poisoning with organophosphate.

Interpretation of Toxicologic Findings (1)

In acute poisoning, the cholinesterase levels may be 25% of the normal values (see below). The cholinesterase levels in the blood are not affected by the duration of the postmortem interval; measurement may be attempted even on decomposed or exhumed bodies.

Normal Cholinesterase Levels in Red Blood Cells (RBC) and in Whole Blood, Measured in Micromoles of Acetylcholine Hydrolyzed

Substrate	*Males*	*Females*	*Children*
RBC	0.74–2.38	0.90–2.33	0.72–2.25
Whole blood	0.78–3.88	1.33–3.32	1.52–2.88

Reference

1. Fatteh A. Organophosphates (parathion). In: Handbook of Forensic Pathology. J.B. Lippincott Company, Philadelphia, 1973, pp. 310–312.

Poisoning, Pesticide(s) (See "Poisoning, organophosphate(s).")

Poisoning, Phosphorus

NOTE: Fatal dose is about 2–3 g. Phosphorus is used in some rat poisons. Phosphorus can be detected in exhumed bodies.

Organs and Tissues	*Procedures*	*Possible or Expected Findings*
External examination, skin, and hair	Submit skin and hair for toxicologic study.	Jaundice (indicates subacute poisoning with severe hepatic changes).
Gastrointestinal tract	Tie stomach and various portions of intestinal tract and submit unopened for toxicologic study. If poisoning with yellow phosphorus is suspected, these viscera must be opened under nitrogen, just before analysis. Collect feces.	Gastric contents smell of garlic *(1)*.
Liver	Record weight. Photograph. Submit portion for toxicologic study. Request Sudan stain of frozen sections.	Severe fatty changes; periportal necroses.
Other organs	For general toxicologic sampling, see Chapter 13. Samples should include kidneys and pancreas. Submit samples for histologic study, and request Sudan-stained frozen sections.	Fatty changes in myocardium, skeletal muscles, and other organs.

Reference

1. Simon FA, Pickering LK. Acute yellow phosphorus poisoning: "smoking stool syndrome." JAMA 1976;235:1343–1344.

Poisoning, Strychnine

Organs and Tissues	*Procedures*	*Possible or Expected Findings*
External examination	Record extent and severity of rigor mortis and postmortem interval at time of recording.	Rigor mortis after fatal strychnine poisoning may occur very soon after death and may be very severe (opisthotonos); it may persist until decomposition sets in.
Organs and body fluids		Congestion of viscera; no characteristic morphologic autopsy findings. Acute pancreatitis has been observed *(1)*.
	For toxicologic sampling (gastric contents, urine, blood, brain, and other organs), see Chapter 13.	High strychnine concentrations (also demonstrable in exhumed bodies *[2]*).

References

1. Hernandez AF, Pomares J, Schiaffino S, Pla A, Villanueva E. Acute chemical pancreatitis associated with nonfatal strychnine poisoning. J Toxicol 1998;36:67–71.
2. Benomran FA, Henry JD. Homicide by strychnine poisoning. Med Sci Law 1996;36:271–273.

Poisoning, Thallium

NOTE: For toxicologic sampling, see below and Chapter 13. Thallium is used as a rodenticide and pesticide, and has some industrial applications.

Organs and Tissues	*Procedures*	*Possible or Expected Findings*
External examination and oral cavity	Record character and extent of skin and nail changes; record distribution of hair. Submit samples of skin for histologic study.	Dermatitis and trophic changes of fingernails; diffuse alopecia *(1)*. Stomatitis in acute poisoning.
	Examine hair under polarized light.	Dystrophic anagen hair with dark bands *(1)*.
Gastrointestinal tract	Submit samples of contents for toxicologic study. Prepare histologic sections of all segments.	Gastroenteritis in acute poisoning.
Liver	Record weight. Submit samples for toxicologic and histologic study.	Centrilobular hepatic necrosis; fatty changes.

Organs and Tissues	Procedures	Possible or Expected Findings
Kidneys	Submit samples for toxicologic and histologic study.	Fatty changes.
Brain and spinal cord; optic nerves	For removal and specimen preparation, see Chapter 4 and 5. Submit brain for toxicologic study. Submit sections of brain and optic nerves for histologic study.	Retrobulbar neuritis.
Skeletal muscles	Submit specimens for toxicologic study (take from lower extremity).	
Bones and bone marrow	For removal, prosthetic repair, and specimen preparation of bones, see Chapter 2. For preparation of sections and smears of bone marrow, see Chapter 2. Submit samples for toxicologic study.	Osteomalacia;* osteomyelofibrosis.

Reference

1. Tromme I, van Neste D, Dobbelaere F, Bouffioux B, Courin C, Dugernier T, et al. Skin signs in the diagnosis of thallium poisoning. Br J Dermatol 1998;138:321–325.

Poliomyelitis

Synonym: Acute anterior poliomyelitis.

NOTE: The disease has been nearly eliminated in the USA but not in many other countries.

(1) Collect all tissues that appear to be infected. (2) Request viral cultures. (3) Usually, special stains are not helpful. (4) Special **precautions** are indicated see Chapter 6. (5) Serologic studies may be helpful and are available from the Centers for Disease Control and Prevention, Atlanta, GA. (6) This is a **reportable** disease.

Organs and Tissues	Procedures	Possible or Expected Findings
External examination	If chronic paralysis had been present, record circumference of extremities on right and left sides.	Neurogenic atrophy of skeletal muscles in areas of paralysis.
Cerebrospinal fluid	In acute cases, submit for viral culture and cytologic study.	
Vitreous	If water or electrolyte disturbances are expected, submit for chemical study.	Electrolyte disorder.*
Heart	Record weight; submit samples for histologic study.	Hypertensive heart disease; myocarditis.*
Lungs	Submit one large sample for viral and bacterial cultures. Perfuse at least one lung with formalin.	Aspiration or bronchopneumonia (or both); edema; atelectasis; embolism;* alveolar wall necrosis (acute or organizing diffuse alveolar damage) after oxygen toxicity.
Esophagus		Acute ulcers.
Gastrointestinal tract	If there is blood in the lumen, record measured or estimated total volume.	Acute gastric dilatation; acute gastroduodenal ulcers; gastrointestinal erosions and hemorrhages. Dilatation of colon; perforation of cecum.
Kidneys and urinary bladder	Open renal pelves and ureters *in situ*; prepare photographs.	Urolithiasis and nephrolithiasis,* pyonephrosis and pyelonephritis.*
Veins	For removal of femoral veins, see Chapter 3.	Phlebothrombosis of legs, most commonly on left side.
Brain and spinal cord	For removal and specimen preparation, see Chapter 4. In acute cases, submit portions of brain and spinal cord for viral culture.	Necrosis of anterior horn cells of spinal cord, with neuronophagia and perivascular inflammatory reaction. Old lesions show neuronal loss and gliosis. Medulla ("bulbar polio") and other areas of brain stem, cerebellum, and cerebrum, particularly the motor cortex, may be affected in various degrees.

Organs and Tissues	*Procedures*	*Possible or Expected Findings*
Bones and joints	For removal, prosthetic repair, and specimen preparation, Chapter 2.	Arthritis* in acute cases; disuse osteoporosis* in chronic cases.
Skeletal muscles	For histologic sampling, see Chapter 4.	Neurogenic atrophy of affected muscles.
Eyes	For removal and specimen preparation, see Chapter 5.	Hypertensive retinopathy.

Polyarteritis Nodosa

Synonyms and Related Terms: Infantile polyarteritis nodosa; Kawasaki disease; mucocutaneous lymph node syndrome;* pan-arteritis nodosa; periarteritis nodosa. For other synonyms and related terms, see also under "Arteritis, all types or type unspecified."

Possible Associated Conditions: Acquired immunodeficiency syndrome* *(1)*; familial Mediterranean fever* *(2)*; polymyalgia rheumatica *(3)*; systemic lupus erythematosus* *(4)*; viral hepatitis B *(5)* or C *(6)*.* See also under "Arteritis, all types or type unspecified."

Organs and Tissues	*Procedures*	*Possible or Expected Findings*
External examination and skin	Record extent and character of skin lesions; submit samples of skin for histologic study.	Subcutaneous nodules (rare), sometimes with ulceration *(7)*.
Heart	For coronary arteriography, see Chapter 10. Record heart weight.	Coronary arteritis, with or without aneurysms and infarctions, primarily in childhood. Myocardial hypertrophy secondary to hypertension.*
Lungs	Perfuse with formalin and submit samples for histologic study.	Minimal or no involvement by polyarteritis nodosa; considerable involvement in other types of necrotizing vasculitis (see "Arteritis, all types or type unspecified").
Kidneys	Submit samples for light microscopic, electron microscopic, and fluorescent microscopic study.	Polyarteritis nodosa; glomerulitis; deposition of γ-globulin, fibrinogen, and albumin.
Other organs	Submit samples of liver, gallbladder, spleen, pancreas, esophagus, gastrointestinal tract (all segments, including appendix), mesentery; adrenals; urinary bladder, epididymis, and endocrine glands, particularly testes. Submit samples of all other tissues with infarctions and related gross lesions. Request Verhoeff–van Gieson stain. For special techniques, see above under "Kidneys."	Polyarteritis, with or without formation of aneurysms and infarctions, may occur in all organs. The liver may show bile duct injury and rarely, nodular regenerative hyperplasia *(8)*. Esophageal involvement *(9)*.
Aorta and other arteries	Submit samples for histologic study.	More frequently involved in giant cell elastic arteritis.*
Skeletal muscles	For removal and specimen preparation, see Chapter 4.	Polyarteritis of small muscular arteries, including vasa nervorum.
Joints	Submit samples of synovium for histologic study.	Arthritis* may rarely be present with swollen joints.
Brain and spinal cord	For removal and specimen preparation, see Chapter 4. For cerebral arteriography, see Chapter 4.	Infarctions;* subarachnoid hemorrhage; arteritis of cerebral arteries.
Eyes	For removal and specimen preparation, see Chapter 5.	Papillitis; retinal hemorrhages; hypertensive retinopathy.

References

1. Libman BS, Quismorio FP Jr, Stimmler MM. Polyarteritis nodosa-like vasculitis in human immunodeficiency virus infection. J Rheumatol 1995;22:351–355.
2. Kocak H, Cakar N, Hekimoglu B, Atakan C, Akkok N, Unal S. The coexistence of familial Mediterranian fever and polyarteritis nodosa: report of a case. Pediatr Nephrol 1996;10:631–633.
3. Uematsu-Yanagita M, Cho M, Hakamata Y, Tanaka M, Ishii K, Kume N, et al. Microscopic polyarteritis during polymyalgia rheumatica remission. Am J Kidney Dis 1996;28:289–291.
4. Vivancos J, Soler-Carrillo J, Ara-del Rey J, Font J. Development of polyarteritis nodosa in the course of inactive systemic lupus erythematosus. Lupus 1995; 4:494–495.

5. Guillevin L, Lhote F, Cohen P, Sauvaget F, Jarrousse B, Lortholary O, et al. Polyarteritis nodosa related to hepatitis B virus. A prospective study with long-term observation of 41 patients. Medicine 1995; 74:238–253.
6. Pateron D, Fain O, Sehonnou J, Trinchet JC, Beaugrand M. Severe necrotizing vasculitis in a patient with hepatitis C virus infection treated by interferon. Clin Exp Rheumatol 1996;14: 79–81.
7. Daoud MS, Hutton KP, Gibson LE. Cutaneous periarteritis nodosa: a clinicopathological study of 79 cases. Br J Dermatol 1997;136:706–713.
8. Goritsas CP, Repanti M, Papadaki E, Lazarou N, Andonopoulos AP. Intrahepatic bile duct injury and nodular regenerative hyperplasia of the liver in a patient with polyarteritis nodosa. J Hepatol 1997;26: 727–730.
9. Matsumoto M, et al. Esophageal involvement in microscopic polyangiitis: a case report and review of literature. Intern Med 2007;46:663–667.

Polychondritis, Relapsing

Possible Associated Conditions: Dermatomyositis; myelodysplastic syndrome *(1)*; rheumatoid arthritis;* Sjögren's syndrome* *(2)*.

Organs and Tissues	*Procedures*	*Possible or Expected Findings*
External examination and skin	Photograph and record appearance of head, chest, hands, and feet.	Chondritis involving nose (saddle nose) and ears (floppy ears); flail chest. Arthritic changes at any site.
	Submit sections of skin lesions for histologic study.	Erythemata nodosum; erythema multiforme; panniculitis *(3)*; vasculitis; venous thromboses.
	Prepare skeletal roentgenograms.	See below under "Bones and joints."
Blood	Submit sample for antibody study.	Antibodies to type II collagen.
Heart	Record weight; test competence of valves, and submit samples for histologic sudy.	Pericarditis.* Myocarditis.* Dilatation of aortic ring and destruction of cusps with aortic regurgitation.* Other valves may be affected *(4)* (mitral regurgitation)
	For dissection of the conduction system, see Chapter 3.	Conduction system abnormalities *(4)* with atrioventricular block.
Aorta	If an aortic aneurysm appears to be present, follow procedures described under that heading.	Aneurysm* of proximal thoracic or abdominal aorta.
Lungs, trachea, and neck organs	Larynx and trachea are best removed together with other neck organs, mediastinum, and lungs. Open airways in posterior midline, photograph areas of collapse or obstruction, and record mechanical state (pliability) of cartilage. Submit samples of all segments for histologic study.	Degeneration and inflammation of larynx and tracheobronchial tree with tracheal stenosis or collapse, which may be the cause of sudden death and suffocation. Aspiration bronchopneumonia.
Kidneys	Follow procedures described under "glomerulonephritis."	Segmental necrotizing glomerulonephritis* with crescent formation.
Lymph nodes	Submit samples for histologic study.	Castleman-like lymphadenopathy *(5)*.
Other organs		Vasculitis of small vessels; manifestations of Sjögren's syndrome.*
Eyes	For removal and specimen preparation, see Chapter 5.	Conjunctivitis; episcleritis; iritis; keratitis; cataracts; optic neuritis; retinal vasculitis.
Base of skull with middle and inner ear	For removal of middle and inner ear, see Chapter 4.	Swelling and occlusion of Eustachian tube; otitis media.* Cochleo-vestibular system may be affected by polychondritic changes.
Bones and joints	For removal, prosthetic repair, and specimen preparation, see Chapter 2.	Eburnation of bones; periostitis; osteoarthritis;* degeneration of cartilage of costochondral junctions and peripheral joints, with joint deformities.
	Prepare sections of bone marrow (Chapter 2).	Mylelodysplastic changes *(1)*.

References

1. Diebold L, Rauh G, Jager K, Lohrs U. Bone marrow pathology in relapsing polychondritis: high frequency of myelodysplastic syndrome. Br J Haematol 1995;89:820–830.
2. Harada M, Yoshida H, Mimura Y, Ohishi M, Miyazima I, Ichikawa F, et al. Relapsing polychondritis associated with subclinical Sjö-gren's syndrome and phlegmon of the neck. Intern Med 1995;34:768–771.

3. Disdier P, Andrac L, Swiader L, Veit V, Fuzibet JG, Weiller-Merli C, et al. Cutaneous panniculitis and relapsing polychonditis: two cases. Dermatology 1996:193:266–268.
4. Del Rosso A, Petix NR, Pratesi M, Bini A. Cardiovascular involvement in relapsing polychondritis. Semin Arthr Rheum 1997;26:840–844.
5. Manganelli P, Quaini F, Olivetti G, Savini M, Pileri S. Relapsing polychondritis with Castleman-like lymphadenopathy: a case report. Clin Rheumat 1997:16:480–484.

Polycythemia

Synonyms and Related Terms: Polycythemia vera; primary polycythemia; secondary polycythemia.

NOTE: If patient had recent radionuclide (^{32}P) treatment, special precautions are indicated (Chapter 11). Consult with radiation safety officer or other responsible person.

Possible Associated Conditions: For tumors producing erythropoietic substances and secondary polycythemia, see below under "Possible or Expected Findings." Certain drugs (androgens) or adrenal cortical hypersecretion also may cause polycythemia.

Organs and Tissues	*Procedures*	*Possible or Expected Findings*
Chest and abdomen	If large vessel thrombosis is suspected, remove chest and abdominal organs en masse. and open posterior aspect of inferior vena cava and aorta.	Thrombosis of inferior vena cava or hepatic veins (or both); aortic thrombosis or thrombosis at other sites.
Heart	For coronary arteriography, see Chapter 10. Other procedures depend on expected findings or grossly identified abnormalities as listed in right-hand column.	Coronary thrombosis; myocardial infarction. Chronic cardiac disease and right-to-left shunt may cause secondary polycythemia.
Lungs	Dissect one lung fresh and perfuse one lung with formalin.	Emboli;* chronic pulmonary disease with alveolar hypoventilation may cause secondary polycythemia.
Intestinal tract	Record volume of blood in lumen. Submit samples of all segments for histologic study.	Ulcer of the duodenum.* Gastrointestinal hemorrhage.* Venous infarction.
Esophagus and stomach	For demonstration of varices, see Chapter 2.	Esophageal varices;* gastric varices.
Liver; portal, mesenteric, and splenic veins	Dissect veins *in situ*.	Portal vein thrombosis (see also "Hypertension, portal").
	Record appearance of hepatic veins. Record weight of liver and submit samples for histologic study.	Budd-Chiari syndrome* (hepatic venous outflow obstruction); myeloid metaplasia or leukemic infiltrates (in primary polycythemia). Hepatocellular carcinoma may be a cause of secondary polycythemia.
Spleen	Record weight and submit samples for histologic study.	Congestive splenomegaly. Myeloid metaplasia or leukemic infiltrates (in primary polycythemia).
Lymph nodes	Record average size and submit samples for histologic study.	Infiltrative lymphadenopathy (see above under "Spleen").
Peripheral arteries and veins		Venous thrombosis;* thrombophlebitis. Leriche's syndrome.* Thromboses may occur in any vessel.
Kidneys	Procedures depend on expected findings or grossly identified abnormalities as listed in right-hand column.	Chronic renal disease (hydronephrosis, parenchymal disease, nephrotic syndrome), kidney transplantation;* renal cell carcinoma and Wilms tumor *(1)* may be causes of secondary polycythemia.
Brain and spinal cord	For cerebral arteriography, see Chapter 4.	Thrombotic or embolic vascular occlusions. Cerebral infarction.* Rarely, cerebellar hemangioblastoma may be a cause of secondary polycythemia.
Bone marrow	Prepare sections and smears, see Chapter 2.	Hyperplasia. Leukemic infiltrates in some patients with primary polycythemia. Rarely, multiple myeloma* may be a cause of secondary polycythemia. Myeloid fibrosis, myeloid metaplasia, and acute myeloid leukemia* are complications of polycythemia vera *(2)*.

Organs and Tissues	Procedures	Possible or Expected Findings
Other organs	Sample tumor tissue for histologic and electron microscopic study. (Snap-freeze material for determination of erythropoietic material).	Tumors of the prostate,* rectum, ovary,* uterus (leiomyoma) or breast,* as well as pheochromocytoma or malignant melanoma, rarely may be causes secondary polycythemia.

Reference

1. Lal A, Rice A, al Mahr M, Kern IB, Marshall GM. Wilms tumor associated with polycythemia: case report and review of the literature. J Pediatr Hematol/Oncol 1997;19:263–265.
2. Thiele JM, Kvasnicka HM. Diagnosis of polycythemia vera based on bone marrow pathology. Curr Hematol Rep 2005;4:218–223.

Polymyalgia Rheumatica

Possible Associated Condition: Giant cell arteritis* *(1)*.

Organs and Tissues	Procedures	Possible or Expected Findings
Blood	Submit sample for determination of rheumatoid factor, antinuclear factor, serum complement concentrations, immunoglobulins, and other serum proteins.	Immunologic tests are important for distinguishing polymyalgia rheumatica from systemic lupus erythematosus,* rheumatoid arthritis,* multiple myeloma,* and other diseases.
Other organs	Follow procedures described under "Arteritis, giant cell."	Giant cell arteritis* and polymyalgia rheumatica are commonly associated *(1)*. Other associations such as scleritis *(2)* or ankylosing spondylitis* *(3)* need further confirmation.
Skeletal muscles	For removal, prosthetic repair, and specimen preparation, see Chapter 2.	No diagnostic changes.
Joints		Focal synovitis, mostly in neck, shoulder, and hip area *(4)*.

References

1. Hunder GG. Giant cell arteritis and polymyalgia rheumatica. Med Clin North Am 1997;81:195–219.
2. Simmons IG, Kritzinger EE, Murray PI. Posterior scleritis and polymyalgia rheumatica. Eye 1997;11:727–728.
3. Elkayam O, Paran D, Yaron M, Caspi D. Polymyalgia rheumatica in patients with ankylosing spondylitis: a report of 5 cases. Clin Exp Rheumatol 1997;15:411–414.
4. Cantini F, et al. Inflammatory changes of hip synovial structures in polymyalgia rheumatica. Clin Exp Rheumatol 2005;23:462–468.

Polymyositis (See "Dermatomyositis.")

Polyneuritis (See "Syndrome, Guillain-Barré.")

Polyneuropathy (See "Beriberi.")

Polyposis, Familial, and Related Syndromes

Related Terms: Cowden's disease (multiple hamartoma syndrome); familial colonic polyposis; juvenile polyposis; Gardner's syndrome; non-polyposis syndrome (hereditary nonpolyposis colorectal cancer syndrome); Peutz-Jegher's syndrome; Turcot's syndrome.

NOTE: The conditions listed under "Related Terms" are hereditable (autosomal-dominant) polyp syndromes. The Cronkhite-Canada syndrome lacks a hereditary transmission.

Organs and Tissues	Procedures	Possible or Expected Findings
External examination and oral cavity	Record and photograph skin lesions, cutaneous tumors, and hair and nail abnormalities. Sampling for histologic study depends on expected findings or grossly identified abnormalities as listed in right-hand column. (See also below under "Soft tissues.")	Cachexia, edema, alopecia, hyperpigmentations and vitiligo, and onychodystrophy in Cronkhite-Canada syndrome; mucocutaneous pigmentations (buccal, perioral, priorbital, distal extremities) in Peutz-Jeghers syndrome;* papules in face and oral mucosa in Cowden's disease; tumors of skin and subcutis (see below under "Soft tissues...") in Gardner's syndrome.
	Prepare skeletal roentgenograms.	Osteomas or exostoses (mandible, calvara) in Gardner's syndrome.

Organs and Tissues	*Procedures*	*Possible or Expected Findings*
Soft tissues (skin, subcutis, mesentery, retroperitoneum)	Record size and distribution of tumors; submit samples for histologic study.	Epidermoid cysts, lipomas, desmoid tumors *(1)*, mesenteric fibromatosis, wound fibromatosis, other fibromas or leiomyomas, and fibrosarcomas in Gardner's syndrome.
Stomach	Prepare photographs of mucosa. Submit samples for histologic study.	Hamartomatous cystic-glandular polyps in Cronkhite-Canada syndrome and in Peutz-Jeghers syndrome.
Small bowel	For perfusion and specimen preparation, see Chapter 2. Photograph lesions. Submit samples for histologic study.	Hamartomatous cystic-glandular polyps in Cronkhite-Canada syndrome, in Peutz-Jeghers syndrome, and in juvenile polyposis. Adenomatous polyps in Gardner's syndrome.
Colon	Prepare photographs. Submit samples of several polyps for histologic study. Include regional lymph nodes for identification of metastases.	Adenomatous polyps in familial colonic polyposis, Gardner's syndrome, non-polyposis syndrome, and Turcot's syndrome. Colorectal carcinomas in familial polyposis, in Gardner's syndrome and in rare cases of juvenile polyposis *(2)*. Hamartomatous cystic-glandular polyps in Cronkhite-Canada syndrome, in Peutz-Jeghers syndrome, and in juvenile polyposis.
Liver and bile ducts	Open common bile duct *in situ*, prepare photographs and sample for histologic study.	Ampullary carcinoma *(3)* or adenoma of bile duct *(4)* in Gardner's syndrome.
Other organs	Procedures depend on expected findings or grossly identified abnormalities as listed in right-hand column.	Tumors of the breast, pancreas, ovary, and endometrium in Peutz-Jeghers syndrome; breast and thyroid tumors in Cowden's disease; endometrial adenocarcinoma in nonpolyposis syndrome. Adrenocortical adenomas or carcinomas or bilateral nodular hyperplasia also may occur, rarely with hypercortisolism.
Brain	For removal and specimen preparation, see Chapter 4.	Brain tumor* (e.g., glioblastoma multiforme) in Turcot syndrome.
Eyes	For removal and specimen preparation, see Chapter 5.	Orbital osteoma in Gardner's syndrome *(5)*.

References

1. Clark SK, Philips RK. Desmoid in familial adenomatous polyposis. Br J Surg 1996;83:1494–1504.
2. Coburn MC, Pricolo VE, DeLuca FG, Bland KI. Malignant potential in intestinal juvenile polyposis syndromes. Ann Surg Oncol 1995;2:386–391.
3. Tomia H, Fukunari H, Shibata M, Yoshinaga K, Iwama T, Mishima Y. Ampullary carcinoma in familial adenomatous polyposis. Surg Today 1996;26:522–526.
4. Futami H, Furuta T, Hanai H, Nakamura S, Baba S, Kaneko E. Adenoma of the common bile duct in Gardner's syndrome may cause relapsing acute pancreatitis. J Gastroenterol 1997;32:558–561.
5. McNab AA. Orbital osteoma in Gardner's syndrome. Austr NZ J Ophthalmol 1998;26:169–170.

Polyradiculoneuropathy (See "Encephalitis, all types or type unspecified," "Myelopathy/Myelitis," and "Syndrome, Guillain-Barré.")

Polyserositis, Familial Paroxysmal (See "Fever, familial Mediterranian.")

Porphyria, all Types or Type Unspecified (See "Porphyia,..." as listed in following entries, and "Protoporphria,...").

NOTE: A rare form of hepatic porphyria, delta-aminolevulinate dehydratase deficient porphyria, and the erythropoietic porphyria, X-linked sideroblastic anemia, have not been tabulated here.

Porphyria, Acute Intermittent

Related Terms: Hepatic porphyria; hydroxymethyl bilane synthase (HMB) deficiency; porphobilinogen deaminase deficiency *(1)*.

NOTE: Multiple drugs such as barbiturates or sulfonamides may precipitate attacks of the disease, which generally is not a fatal condition. Infections or surgery also may precipitate attacks.

Organs and Tissues	Procedures	Possible or Expected Findings
External examination	Record body weight and length. Record extent of pigmentation.	Pigmentation; emaciation.
Urine	Submit samples for determination of δ-aminolevulinic acid (ALA) and porphobilinogen (PBG).	Increased concentrations of ALA and PBG.
Heart and blood vessels	If hypertension is suspected, see under that heading.	Hypertensive cardiovascular disease.
Liver	Submit samples for histologic, electron microscopic, toxicologic, and porphyrin fluorescence study.	Porphyrin fluorescence usually not demonstrable. Hepatocellular carcinoma may be present.
Brain, spinal cord, and peripheral nerves		Peripheral motor neuropathy. Hypothalamic involvement may be a cause of hyponatremia.
Vitreous	If dehydration is suspected, submit sample for sodium, chloride, and urea nitrogen determination.	Manifestations of dehydration.*

Reference

1. Grandchamp B. Acute intermittent porphyria. Semin Liv Dis 1998;18:17–24.

Porphyria, Congenital Erythropoietic

Synonyms: Günther's disease; uroporphyrinogen III (URO) cosynthase deficiency.

NOTE: If bone marrow transplantation *(1)* was done, see also under that heading. Cord blood stem cell transplantation also has been done for this condition *(2)*.

Organs and Tissues	Procedures	Possible or Expected Findings
External examination and skin	Record extent and character of changes of hair, skin, and teeth. Prepare histologic sections of skin.	Hypertrichosis; erythrodontia; scarring and mutilation of hands and face.
Blood and bone marrow	For preparation of sections and smears, see Chapter 2. Submit fresh samples for porphyrin studies.	Hemolytic anemia. Erythrocytes contain large amounts of uroporphyrin I; normoblasts and reticulocytes exhibit intense red fluorescence. Erythrocyte inclusions *(4)*.
Urine	Submit sample for porphyrin study as listed in right-hand column.	Uroporphyrin I and coproporphyrin I in high concentrations.
Spleen	Record size and weight. Photograph spleen (with scale).	Splenomegaly (may have been treated by splenectomy).
Kidneys	Sample for histologic study; request Gomori's stain for iron.	Glomerulosclerosis and iron deposits *(3)*.

References

1. Thomas C, Ged C, Nordmann Y, de Verneuil H, Pellier I, Fischer A, Blanche S. Correction of congenital erythropoietic porphyria by bone marrow transplantation. J Pediatr 1996;129:453–456.
2. Zix-Kieffer I, Langer B, Eyer D, Acar G, Racadot E, Schlaeder G, et al. Successful cord blood stem cell transplantation for congenital erythropoietic porphyria (Gunther's disease). Bone Marrow Transpl 1996;18:217–220.
3. Lange B, Hofweber K, Waldherr R, Scharer K. Congenital erythropoietic porphyria associated with nephrotic syndrome. Acta Pediatr 1995;84: 1325–1328.
4. Merino A et al. Atypical red cell inclusions in congenital erythropoietic porphyria. Br J Haematol 2006;132:124.

Porphyria Cutanea Tarda

Synonyms and Related Terms: Hepatic porphyria; uroporphyrinogen decarboxylase deficiency.

Possible Associated Conditions: Adverse drug reaction; chronic alcoholism;* chronic hepatitis C *(1)*; human immunodeficiency virus infection (AIDS)* *(1)*.

Organs and Tissues	Procedures	Possible or Expected Findings
External examination and skin	Record extent and character of skin and hair changes. Prepare histologic sections of skin.	Vesicles and bullae in face and other sun-exposed areas. Thickening and scarring of skin, with or without calcifications; hyperpigmentation. Hypertrichosis.
Urine	Submit sample for porphyrin study as listed in right-hand column.	Increased concentrations of uroporphyrin and hepatocarboxylic porphyrin.
Liver	Submit fresh hepatic tissue for demonstration of porphyrin fluorescence in Wood's light. Record weight of liver and submit samples for histologic study. Request Gomori's iron stain. Prepare sample for electron microscopy. Needle-shaped inclusions are best seen by light microscopy in unstained paraffin sections or after staining with the ferric ferricyanide reduction test or Fontana-Masson silver stain.	Ultraviolet light reveals red hepatic porphyrin fluorescence. Fatty changes, fibrosis, cirrhosis,* and hepatocellular carcinoma. Hemosiderosis hemochromatosis *(3)*. Chronic hepatitis C may be a cause of porphyria cutanea tarda *(2)*. Needle shaped cytoplasmic inclusions (visible by light, fluorescence-, and electron microscopy).

References

1. O'Connor WJ, Badley AD, Dicken CH, Murphy GM. Porphyria cutanea tarda and human immunodeficiency virus: two cases associated with hepatitis C. Mayo Clin Proc 1998;73:895–897.
2. Lacour JP, Bodokh I, Castanet J, Bekri S, Ortonne JP. Porphyria cutanea tarda and antibodies to hepatitis C virus. Br J Dermatol 1993; 128:121–123.
3. Mogl MT et al. An unhappy triad: hemochromatosis, porphyria cutanea tarda and hepatocellular carcinoma-a case report. World J Gastroenterol 2007;13:1998–2001.

Porphyria, Variegate

Synonyms and Related Terms: Hepatic porphyria; protoporphyrinogen oxidase deficiency *(1)*.

NOTE: The manifestations of the disease closely resemble those in porphyria cutanea tarda and hereditary coproporphyria. Measurements of porphyrins and porphyrin precursors are the only clearly distinguishing features. For autopsy procedures, see under "Porphyria cutanea tarda."

Reference

1. Kirsch RE, Meissner PN, Hift RJ. Variegate porphyria. Semin Liv Dis 1998;18:33–41.

Potassium (See "Disorder, electrolyte(s)")

Preexcitation, Ventricular

Related Term: Aberrant atrioventricular conduction; Wolff-Parkinson-White syndrome.

Possible Associated Conditions: Ebstein's malformation of tricuspid valve.

Pregnancy

NOTE: In some instances, procedures described under "Death, abortion-associated," "Embolism, amniotic fluid," or "Toxemia of pregnancy" may be indicated.

Progeria

Synonym: Werner syndrome.

Organs and Tissues	Procedures	Possible or Expected Findings
External examination and skin	Record body weight and length; prepare histologic sections of skin. Prepare skeletal roentgenograms.	Growth retardation; short stature; alopecia; cutaneous atrophy; loss of subcutaneous fat. Premature fusion of epiphyses; large calvarium.
Cardiovascular system		Myocardial infarction; coronary and peripheral atherosclerosis.
Other organs	Record weights of endocrine organs and submit samples for histologic study. Other procedures depend on expected findings or grossly identified abnormalities as listed in right-hand column.	Manifestations of congestive heart failure;* normal endocrine system; osteoarthritis;* rare neoplasms, such as meningioma, soft tissue tumors, osteosarcoma, and myeloid tumors *(1)*.
Brain	For cerebral arteriography, and for removal and specimen preparation, see Chapter 4.	Cerebral atherosclerosis and hemorrhage.

Reference

1. Goto M, Miller RW, Ishikawa Y, Sugano H. Excess of rare cancers in Werner syndrome (adult progeria). Cancer Epid Biomarkers Prev 1996;5: 239–246.

Propanol (See "Poisoning, isopropyl alcohol.")

Proteinosis, Pulmonary alveolar (See "Lipoproteinosis, pulmonary alveolar.")

Protoporphyria, Erythropoietic

Synonym: Ferrochelatase deficiency *(1)*.

Organs and Tissues	*Procedures*	*Possible or Expected Findings*
External examination and skin	Record character and extent of skin lesions and prepare histologic sections of skin. Request PAS stain, with diastase digestion.	Chronic eczematous skin lesions or superficial scarring; nail changes. Perivascular PAS-positive hyaline *(2)*.
Blood	Submit sample for protoporphyrin study *(2)*.	High concentration of protoporphyrin IX in erythrocytes and plasma.
Feces and urine	Submit samples for protoporphyrin study.	High concentration of protoporphyrin IX in feces; normal concentration in urine.
Liver	Record weight. Submit samples for routine histologic study. Submit fresh material for biochemical study, and material for ultraviolet microscopy and transmission electron microscopy.	Intrahepatic cholestasis. Cirrhosis* and liver failure* is a rare complication *(3)*. Brown protoporphyrin deposits with red to yellow birefringence with a maltese cross configuration in hepatocytes, Kupffer cells, and bile canaliculi.
Gallbladder and bile	Submit stones for protoporphyrin analysis.	Cholelithiasis.* Increased protoporphyrin in bile.

References

1. Cox TM. Erythropoietic protoporphyria. J Inherit Metab Dis 1997;20:258–269.
2. Schleiffenbaum BE, Minder EI, Mohr P, Decurtins M, Schaffner A. Cytofluorometry as a diagnosis of protoporphyria. Gastroenterology 1992; 102:1044–1048.
3. Sarkany RPE, Alexander GJMA, Cox TM. Recessive inheritance of erythropoietic protoporphyria with liver failure. Lancet 1994;343: 1394–1396.

Pseudogout

Synonym: Calcium pyrophosphate dihydrate (CPPD) deposition disease.

Organs and Tissues	*Procedures*	*Possible or Expected Findings*
External examination	Prepare skeletal roentgenograms.	Punctate calcium deposits in knee joints and, less commonly, in joints of hips, ankles, shoulders, or wrists or in symphysis ossium pubis and intervertebral disks.
Joints	Puncture grossly affected joints and submit sample of synovial fluid for crystal analysis under compensated polarized light *(2)*. Consult roentgenograms (see above).	Arthritis* with synovitis. Crystals of calcium pyrophosphate dihydrate in periarticular tissue *(1)* and synovial fluid. Cartilage contains calcium salts of pyrophosphate, hydroxyapatite, and orthophosphate.
Other organs	Procedures depend on expected underlying disease, as listed in right-hand column.	Alkaptonuria;* gout;* hemochromatosis;* hyperparathyroidism.*

References

1. Luisiri P, Blair J, Ellman MH. Calcium pyrophosphate dihydrate deposition disease presenting as tumoral calcinosis (periarticular pseudogout). J Rheumatol 1996;23:1647–1650.
2. Joseph J, McGrath H. Gout or 'pseudogout': how to differentiate crystal-induced arthropathies. Geriatr 1995;50:33–39.

Pseudohyperparathyroidism

Synonyms: Ectopic hyperparathyroidism; hyperparathyroidism in malignancy.

NOTE: This condition is caused by pulmonary, renal, and other malignant tumors that secrete parathyroid hormone or a parathyroid hormone-like substance. If hormone assay is intended, snap-freeze tumor tissue. Other autopsy procedures are the same as in hyperparathyroidism. Parathyroid glands should be normal.

Pseudohypoparathyroidism

Related Term: Pseudopseudohypoparathyroidism.

Organs and Tissues	*Procedures*	*Possible or Expected Findings*
External examination and oral cavity	Record abnormalities of stature and appearance of teeth. Prepare roentgenograms of hands, feet, and skull.	Short stature, round face, brachydactyly with shortening of carpal and metatarsal bones and bowing of long bones, and heterotopic calcification (Albright's hereditary osteodystrophy). Coxa vara or coxa valga. Exostoses and thickening of calvaria may be found.
	Inspect mouth.	Dental aplasia and enamel defects.
Vitreous and urine	Submit samples for calcium and phosphate determination.	Decreased calcium and increased phosphate concentrations.
Neck organs	Dissect and record weights of parathyroid glands; submit samples for histologic study.	Parathyroid glands are normal or hyperplastic.
Other organs	Soft tissue roentgenograms may reveal calcium deposits. Sample for histologic study and request van Kossa stain.	Metastatic calcification or ossification in subcutaneous tissue, lungs, kidneys, basal ganglia of brain, and other organs.
Bones	For removal, prosthetic repair, and specimen preparation, see Chapter 2.	See above under "External examination and oral cavity."
Eyes	For removal and specimen preparation, see Chapter 5.	Cataracts.

Pseudomyxoma Peritonei

Related Terms: Disseminated peritoneal adenomucinosis *(1)*; peritoneal mucinous carcinomatosis *(1)*.

Organs and Tissues	*Procedures*	*Possible or Expected Findings*
Abdomen	Record volume of intraperitoneal fluid; prepare smears; submit samples of peritoneum for histologic study.	Colloid carcinoma of stomach or colon. Well-differentated adenocarcinoma of ovary or, rarely, of appendix; ruptured appendiceal mucinous adenoma is the most common cause of peritoneal adenomucinosis.

Reference

1. Ronnet BM, Shmookler BM, Sugarbaker PH, Kurman RJ. Pseudomyxoma peritonei: new concepts in diagnosis, origin, nomenclature, and relationship to mucinous borderline (low malignant potential) tumors of the ovary. Anat Pathol 1997;2:197–226.

Pseudotumor Cerebri

Synonym: Benign intracranial hypertension; meningeal hydrops.

NOTE: This condition, which generally affects young, obese females, is characterized by symptoms and signs of increased intracranial pressure without a demonstrable cause. Hence, intra-cranial mass lesions, infections, and related conditions should be excluded. Such conditions include adrenal insufficiency;* Guillain-Barré syndrome* (increased colloid-osmotic pressure); hyperadrenalism; hypervitaminosis A* (e.g., after treatment of acne); hypoparathyroidism;* hypothroidism;* infectious mono-nucleosis;* Lyme disease; pregnancy; Sydenham's chorea; throm-bus of the lateral or superior sagittal sinus (otitic hydrocephalus); and Wiskott-Aldrich syndrome.

Organs and Tissues	*Procedures*	*Possible or Expected Findings*
External examination	Record body weight and external features.	Obesity* (pickwickian syndrome).
Lungs	Perfuse one lung with formalin.	Emphysema.*
Genital organs	Procedures depend on expected findings or grossly identified abnormalities as listed in right-hand column.	Pregnancy* or postpartum changes.
Brain, spinal cord, base of skull	For removal and specimen preparation of brain and spinal cord, and dissection of base of skull, see Chapter 4.	Mastoiditis; lateral sinus thrombosis; marantic sinus thrombosis; head trauma.
Peripheral nerves	For removal and specimen preparation, see Chapter 4.	Polyneuritis.

Pseudoxanthoma elasticum

Synonym: Grönblad-Strandberg syndrome.

NOTE: This disease has not been studied thoroughly. Each autopsy should be regarded as a research procedure.

Organs and Tissues	*Procedures*	*Possible or Expected Findings*
External examination and skin	Record extent and character of skin lesions, photograph, and prepare histologic sections. Request von Kossa's and Verhoeff–van Gieson stains. For decalcification procedures, see Chapter 2.	Skin papules and plaques, particularly in neck, axillae, groins, and popliteal fossae. Telangiectases at edge of lesions. Hemorrhages (also in nose). Basophilic material and calcium deposits *(1)* in middle and lower dermis.
	Prepare soft tissue roentgenograms.	Calcifications in dermis; calcifications of blood vessels.
Abdomen		Diaphragmatic hernia.*
Heart	Record weight. Histologic samples should include pericardium, endocardium, and all valves. Photograph cardiac lesions. For special stains, see above under "External examination and skin."	Hypertensive cardiomegaly. Characteristic plaques in pericardium and endocardium, with or without mitral valve involvement. Coronary atherosclerosis may have been a cause of angina *(2)*. Coronary thrombosis and myocardial infarction may be present also.
Arteries	Submit samples of large and medium-sized arteries from various sites; request von Kossa's and Verhoeff–van Gieson stains.	Accelerated atherosclerosis; calcification of peripheral vessels.
Gastrointestinal tract	Record estimated or measured amount of blood in lumen.	Gastrointestinal hemorrhage;* peptic ulcer;* ulcerative colitis.*
Kidneys	Dissect renal arteries. For renal arteriography, see Chapter 2.	Hemangiomas; abnormalities of renal arteries.
Urinary bladder and uterus		Hemorrhages.
Other organs	Submit samples of all accessible organs and tissues, with or without gross lesions. Submit material for electron microscopy.	See above under "Note."
Brain		Subarachnoid and intracerebral hemorrhage; hypertensive cerebrovascular disease.
Eyes	For removal and specimen preparation, see Chapter 5.	Degeneration of Bruch's membrane with retinal hemorrhages; sclerosis of choroid vessels; angioid streaks; degenerative scleral changes, as in skin.
Joints	For removal, prosthetic repair, and specimen preparation, see Chapter 2.	Hemarthrosis.

References

1. Truter S, Rosenbaum-Fiedler J, Sapadin A, Lebwohl M. Calcification of elastic fibers in pseudoxanthoma elasticum. Mt Sinai J Med 1996;63:210–215.
2. Kevorkian JP, Masquet C, Kural-Menasche S, Le Dref O, Beaufils P. New report of severe coronary artery disease in an eighteen-year-old girl with pseudoxanthoma elasticum. Case report and review of the literature. Angiology 1997;48:735–741.

Psittacosis (See "Ornithosis.")

Psoriasis

Possible Associated Conditions: Acquired immunodeficiency syndrome* *(1)*; malabsorption syndrome.*

NOTE: The manifestations of psoriasis may be considerably aggravated if the patients have been infected with the human immunodeficiency virus.

Organs and Tissues	*Procedures*	*Possible or Expected Findings*
External examination	Record extent and character of skin lesions. Prepare histologic sections of skin.	Characteristic skin and nail changes.
	Prepare roentgenograms of joints.	Arthritis.*

Organs and Tissues	Procedures	Possible or Expected Findings
Heart	Procedures depend on expected findings or grossly identified abnormalities as listed in right-hand column.	Aortitis involving ascending aorta and aortic valve with regurgitation; mitral valve and adjacent myocardium and conduction system also may be involved.
Small bowel	Fix the bowel as soon as possible.	Sprue-like changes with loss of villi.
Liver	Record weight. Submit samples for histologic study.	Fibrosis or cirrhosis and other abnormalities, particularly in patients who had been taking methotrexate.
Bones and joints	For removal, prosthetic repair, and specimen preparation, see Chapter 2.	Psoriatic arthritis and spondylitis.

Reference

1. Weitzul S, Duvic M. HIV-related psoriasis and Reiter's syndrome. Semin Cut Med Surg 1997;16:213–218.

Purpura, Anaphylactoid (See "Purpura, Schönlein-Henoch.")

Purpura Fulminans

NOTE: This nonthrombocytopenic purpura occurs mainly in children, following an infectious disease, e.g., a staphylococcal infection. Skin hemorrhages, intravascular thromboses, and gangrene are major manifestations. For additional autopsy procedures, see under the name of the underlying infection.

Purpura, Schönlein-Henoch

Synonyms and Related Terms: Allergic purpura; anaphylactoid purpura; hypersensitivity vasculitis.

Organs and Tissues	Procedures	Possible or Expected Findings
External examination and skin	Record extent and character of skin lesions, and photograph lesions.	Macular, petechial, or vesicular purpura. Ulcers of skin and dermal nodules. Angioneurotic edema* of lips and neck.
	Prepare histologic sections of involved skin. Request Gomori's iron stain.	Angiitis (necrotizing vasculitis) involving capillaries, venules, and arterioles of dermis.
Gastrointestinal tract	Record estimated or measured volume of blood in lumen. Submit samples of all segments for histologic study.	Gastrointestinal hemorrhage.* Intussusception. Angiitis, as in skin.
Kidneys	Follow procedures described under "Glomerulonephritis."	Swollen cortex with subcapsular petechial hemorrhages. Acute focal glomerulonephritis with IgG, IgA, complement, and fibrinogen in mesangium. Angiitis, as in skin.
Neck organs	Open trachea and larynx in posterior midline.	Angioneurotic edema.*
Other organs		Findings may be similar to those described under "Polyarteritis nodosa" and "Failure, kidney."
Joints	Submit samples of synovium for histologic study.	Swelling of joints. Synovial angiitis (histologic manifestations as in skin).

Purpura, Thrombotic Thrombocytopenic

Synonyms and Related Term: Hemolytic uremic syndrome;* thrombotic microangiopathy.

Possible Associated Conditions: Acquired immunodeficiency syndrome* *(1)*; angiotropic large cell lymphoma *(2)*; glomerulonephritis;* polyarteritis nodosa;* rheumatoid arthritis;* Sjögren's syndrome;* systemic lupus erythematosus;* systemic sclerosis.*

Organs and Tissues	Procedures	Possible or Expected Findings
External examination and skin	Prepare histologic sections of skin with purpura; for special stains, see below.	Purpura; jaundice.

Organs and Tissues	Procedures	Possible or Expected Findings
Blood	Submit sample for microbiologic and serologic study.	
Other organs and tissues	Record extent of hemorrhages; submit samples from all viscera and tissues listed in right-hand column. Request phosphotungstic acid hematoxylin, PAS, and Verhoeff–van Gieson stain. Snap-freeze tissue samples for immunofluorescent study.	Fibrin and platelet thrombi, with or without microaneurysms and purpura in kidneys, adrenal glands, pancreas, heart, and brain; lesions may also be present in liver; spleen *(3)*, lymph nodes, muscle, bone marrow, and synovium. Fibrin thrombi can be demonstrated with labeled antihuman fibrin antibodies. Lesions in precapillary arterioles.

References

1. de Man AM, Smulders YM, Roozendaal KJ, Frissen PH. HIV-related thrombotic thrombocytopenic purpura: report of 2 cases and a review of the literature. Netherl J Med 1997;51:103–109.
2. Sill H, Hofler G, Kaufmann P, Horina J, Spuller E, Kleinert R, Beham-Schmid C. Angiotropic large cell lymphoma presenting as thrombotic micro-angiopathy (thrombotic thrombocytopenic purpura). Cancer 1995;75:1167–1170.
3. Saracco SM, Farhi DC. Splenic pathology in thrombotic thrombocytopenic purpura. Am J Surg Pathol 1990;14:223–229.

Pyelonephritis

Synonyms and Related Terms: Acute ascending pyelonephritis; calculous pyelonephritis; chronic interstitial nephritis; chronic pyelonephritis; emphysematous pyelonephritis; obstructive uropathy.

NOTE: If chronic renal insufficiency was diagnosed, see under "Failure, kidney."

Possible Associated Conditions: Diabetes mellitus* *(1)*. See also below under "Possible or Expected Findings."

Organs and Tissues	Procedures	Possible or Expected Findings
Abdominal cavity	Identify and record site of obstruction before removal of retroperitoneal and pelvic organs. For renal angiography and urography, see Chapter 2.	Aberrant vessels; adhesions (postradiation lesions). Perirenal abscess in acute pyelonephritis. Retroperitoneal fibrosis.* Tumor.
Urine	Submit sample for microbiologic study. Prepare smear of sediment.	Evidence of inflammation.
Urogenital system	Remove kidneys, ureters, and pelvic organs in one block. Record weight of both kidneys. Submit any grossly infected areas for microbiologic study.	Fistulas between kidney and other sites may be observed *(2,3)*.
	Record size of right and left renal pelves. Record character of contents. Cut kidneys in half and record number and size of abscesses and scars. Record appearance of papillae.	Hydronephrosis;* pyonephrosis; nephrolithiasis.* Necrotizing papillitis.
	Record width of ureters. Record size, contents, and degree of trabeculation of urinary bladder; record size and appearance of prostate.	Hydroureter; pyoureter. Urolithiasis; tumor of urinary bladder* or of adjacent organs; benign prostatic hyperplasia.
	If urethral valves are suspected to be present, see Chapter 2. Photograph all abnormalities.	Urethral valves. A dilated bladder in a woman without obvious obstruction may indicate presence of descensus of uterus (which is difficult to demonstrate at autopsy).
Other organs	Procedures depend on suspected underlying conditions.	Amyloidosis* *(4)*. Manifestations of diabetes mellitus* or sickle cell disease.*
Neck organs	Dissect parathyroid glands, record weights, and submit samples for histologic study.	Hyperplasia or adenoma(s) of parathyroid glands.
Brain and spinal cord		Abnormal findings may explain obstructive uropathy ("neurogenic bladder").
Bones	For sampling and specimen preparation, see Chapter 2.	Osteoclastic osteoporosis in primary or secondary hyperparathyroidism.*

References

1. Pontin AR, Barnes RD, Joffe J, Kahn D. Emphysematous pyelonephritis in diabetic patients. Br J Urol 1995;75:71–74.
2. O'Brien JD, Ettinger NA. Nephrobronchial fistula and lung abscess resulting from nephrolithiasis and pyelonephritis. Chest 1995;108:1166–1168.
3. Nayir A, Kadioglu A, Sirin A, Emre S, Oney V. A case of an enterorenal fistula and pyelonephritis with air in renal pelvis. Pediatr Radiol 1995;25: 229–230.
4. Mazuecos A, Araque A, Sanchez R, Martinez MA, Guesmes A, Rivero M, et al. Systemic amyloidosis secondary to pyonephrosis. Resolution after nephrectomy. Nephrol Dial Transplant 1996;11:875–878.

Pyothorax (See "Empyema, pleural.")

Q,R

Q Fever (See "Fever, Q")

Rabies

NOTE: (1) In most instances, an autopsy limited to the brain is sufficient to confirm the diagnosis. (2) Rabies virus is especially infectious and thus, universal **precautions** should be strictly followed (see Chapter 6). Avoid the use of scalpels whenever possible. The generation of aerosols should be assiduously avoided. (3) Consult the state health department prior to commencing the autopsy. (4) Request viral cultures. (5) Request immunofluorescent stain for rabies. (6) Serologic studies are available from the state health department laboratories. (7) This is a **reportable** disease.

Organs and Tissues	*Procedures*	*Possible or Expected Findings*
External examination	Photograph possible sites of animal bite.	
Chest and abdomen	See above under "Note." If a complete autopsy is done, sample heart, lungs, kidneys, pancreas, submaxillary salivary glands, and adrenal glands; freeze or refrigerate sampled tissues and submit for viral study (see below under "Brain and spinal cord").	Myocarditis with necrosis of muscle fibers and infiltrates of lymphocytes and histiocytes.
Blood	Obtain serum for serologic studies.	
Brain and spinal cord	Freeze or refrigerate cerebral tissue immediately after removal and submit frozen to special laboratory for fluorescent antibody staining. Take these sections from hippocampus or brain stem. Place the refrigerated tissues in 50% neutral glycerol saline solution for preservation. Fix remaining brain and spinal cord tissue in 15% formalin and submit for histologic study. As an alternative to freezing of tissue, immunoperoxidase methods for detection of rabies viral antigens can now be applied to formalin-fixed tissue *(1)*. Viral particles can be revealed by ultrastructural examination.	Rabies encephalitis. Generally, no external abnormalities. Perivascular cuffing and microglial hyperplasia as well as neuronophagia, predominantly in gray matters (pons and medulla). Negri bodies in neurons are pathognomonic; they are found primarily in hippocampal pyramidal neurons and cerebellar Purkinje cells. Absence of Negri bodies does not exclude diagnosis of rabies encephalitis. Inflammatory reaction may be completely lacking. In paralytic rabies, changes are most evident in spinal cord, with anterior horn neuronal degeneration.
Lacrimal glands	For technique of removal, see Chapter 5. Submit refrigerated sample for virologic study and fluorescent antibody testing.	
Ganglia	Submit samples of cranial, spinal, and sympathetic ganglia for histologic study.	Neural degeneration with neuronophagia and lymphocytic infiltrates.

Reference

1. Mrack RE, Young L. Rabies encephalitis in humans: pathology, pathogenesis, and pathophysiology. J Neuropathol Exp Neurol 1994;53:1–10.

From: *Handbook of Autopsy Practice,* 4th Ed. Edited by: B.L. Waters

Rachischisis (See "Meningocele.")

Radiation (See "Injury, radiation.")

Rape

Related Term: Sexual assault.

NOTE: In almost all instances, the procedures described under "Assault" and under "Homicide" must also be followed. See also refs. *(1)* and *(2)*. For the evaluation of bite marks, photographs with and without scales and black and white film should be used. A forensic dentist is required to compare the victim's bite marks to the teeth of suspects. Swabs of possible sperm or other fluids must be sent to the crime lab for proper evaluation.

Organs and Tissues	*Procedures*	*Possible or Expected Findings*
External examination	Comb pubic hair over a towel and then pull sample; also, pull samples of hair from head. Collect fingernail clippings and place in containers marked "right" and "left."	Blood, hair, and other material on the victim's body may be the assailant's and thus may become important legal evidence.
	Collect blood, hair, fibers, and residues of urine or saliva and/or semen that may have stained the victim's clothing or that may be found on the skin of the victim. For study of stains and scrapings, see below.	Saline swab may reveal saliva, particularly on breasts (areola, nipples). Photographs of the decedent's teets, with and without scales, may be useful if the victim may have bitten the assailant.
	Introduce sterile dry cotton swab into the posterior vault of the vagina or—preferably—into the cervical canal. Prepare smear on glass slide and send to crime laboratory for identification of sperm (see also above under "Note").	
	Keep a second swab dry for acid phosphatase determination and other tests (fluorescence *in situ* hybridization, DNA fingerprinting, Southern blot analysis, and polymerase chain reaction). These should be sent to the crime lab.	Material may be positive for acid phosphatase or p30 glycoprotein. Nonsperm male cells may be present, identified by Y-chromosome specific DNA probes.
	Repeat above tests with two other sets of swabs for study of lower rectum and anus (smears should be as thin as possible) and of oral cavity.	Spermatozoa and acid phosphatase-positive material may be found in rectum and oral cavity.
	A Woods lamp can be used to illuminate semen stains on the body or clothing.	Due to the flavin residues, seminal fluid appears green-yellow.
	Photograph face and oral cavity, if indicated. If a photocolposcope is available, vaginal vault and cervix can be photographed *in situ*.	Lips and buccal surfaces of cheeks may show evidence of trauma. Bite marks may be present (see above under "Note") and may help to identify the assailant.
Blood	Submit sample in EDTA tube for determination of blood groups. Retain specimens through end of office retention period. Further testing, e.g., for HIV or syphilis, may be requested during this period.	The victim's blood groups are important for comparison with specimens from the alleged assailant. Evidence of acquired immunodeficiency syndrome,* syphilis,* or intoxication at time of rape may have legal implications.
Other organs and tissues	Submit samples for toxicologic study.	
Genital organs	Photograph internal genitalia, anus, and vulva. Additional spermatic fluid may be retrieved from cervical canal during cervical dissection. Application of toluidine blue may enhance lacerations *(3)* (apply only after specimens for laboratory study have been obtained).	There may be perineal, perianal or vaginal lacerations, evidence of trauma to the cervix, or foreign bodies.
	Record appearance of all segments of genital tract. Prepare histologic sections of lacerations and wounds and of endometrium. If there is enough spermatic fluid, submit sample for microbiologic study.	Uterine contents and endometrium may reveal pregnancy.*

How Does One Examine Stains or Other Residues of Suspected Spermatic Fluid?

Using a sterile cotton swab moistened with sterile saline, lift suspected dried spermatic fluid from hair or skin of external genitalia, perineum, buttocks, or other sites. Stains on clothing will be extracted by forensic laboratory personnel. Let specimens air dry in absence of sunlight and then place in paper bags or envelopes and seal. Smears are made for the demonstration of spermatozoa, cytologic changes, bacteria, and other possible findings (Some crime labs prefer to make their own smears from the swabs). Other samples are used for the determination of acid phosphatase, as described below.

How Can One Estimate the Time Interval Between Intercourse and Removal for Freezing or Testing of the Specimen?

Usually, the survival time of morphologically recognizable spermatozoa in the vagina is less than 24 h, but on occasion this may be much longer. Thus, within the first 24 h after coitus, 64% of cervical smears have been found to be positive for spermatozoa. At day 10, spermatozoa have been found in 13% of the smears. Obviously, if the assailant had had a vasectomy, spermatozoa will not be found at any time.

Spermatozoa have been found in the vagina of some women several days or weeks after death. Dried stains (see above) may give positive results after longer intervals. Acid phosphatase activities greater than 5 Bodansky units (for method, see above) indicate that probably less than 12 h have elapsed since the time of intercourse *(1)*. In another study, vaginal swab specimens showed acid phosphatase activities of more than 2,000 King-Armstrong units/dL during the first 12 h after intercourse. Vaginal acid phosphatase activities returned to normal (<201 King-Armstrong units/dL) within approx 48 h. Regardless of the methods used, only very rough estimates can be made.

References

1. Spitz WU, Platt MS. Medicolegal Investigation of Death. Charles C. Thomas Publisher, Springfield, IL, 1993, pp. 716–722.
2. Collins KA. The laboratory's role in detecting sexual assault. Lab Med 1998;29:361–365.
3. Bays J, Lewman LV. Toluidine blue in the detection at autopsy of perineal and anal lacerations in victimes of sexual abuse. Arch Pathol Lab Med 1992;116:620–621.

Acknowledgement

Julia Martin, M.D., former Associate Medical Examiner, Hillsborough County Medical Examiner Department, has provided valuable advice on the procedures described in rape cases.

Reaction, Microgranulomatous Hypersensitivity, of Lungs (See "Pneumoconiosis" and "Pneumonia, interstitial.")

Reaction to Transfusion

NOTE: The autopsy should be done as soon as possible after death. Every attempt should be made to secure donor blood for typing and culture at 30°C and 37°C (see below).

Organs and Tissues	*Procedures*	*Possible or Expected Findings*
External examination	Record color of skin.	Jaundice.
	If air embolism is suspected, follow procedures described under that heading.	Air embolism.*
Blood	Submit samples for microbiologic and serologic study and for typing.	Gram-negative rods or other endotoxin-producing bacteria may have been perfused accidentally. More reliable is culture from residual donor blood (see above) at 30°C and 37°C. Some contaminants do not grow at the higher temperature.
Lungs	Record weights; submit samples for histologic study.	Shock lungs (see under "Syndrome, adult respiratory distress").
Kidneys	Photograph, record weights, and submit samples for histologic study.	Fibrin thrombi and platelet thrombi in small vessels; hemoglobinuric nephrosis.
Other organs	Procedures depend on expected findings or grossly identified abnormalities as listed in right-hand column.	Fibrin thrombi and platelet thrombi in small vessels (see under "Coagulation, disseminated intravascular").
Urine	Prepare sediment.	Hematuria.
Neck organs and trachea	Open larynx and trachea along posterior midline.	Angioneurotic edema; aspiration of vomitus.

Regurgitation, Aortic (See "Insufficiency, aortic [chronic or acute].")

Regurgitation, Mitral (See "Insufficiency, mitral [chronic or acute].")

Regurgitation, Pulmonary (See "Insufficiency, pulmonary valvular.")

Regurgitation, Tricuspid (See "Insufficiency, tricuspid [chronic or acute].")

Reticulosis, Midline Malignant (See "Granuloma, midline.")

Rhabdomyoma, Cardiac (See "Tumor of the heart.")

Rickets (See "Deficiency, vitamin D" and "Syndrome, Fanconi.")

Ring, Lower Esophageal

Synonym: Schatzki's ring.

Organs and Tissues	*Procedures*	*Possible or Expected Findings*
External examination	Prepare chest roentgenogram or follow other procedures for diagnosis of pneumothorax (see "Pneumothorax").	Pneumothorax.*
Esophagus	For postmortem demonstration of lower esophageal ring, see Chapter 2.	Bolus in esophagus; reflux esophagitis.

Rubella

Synonyms and Related Terms: Congenital rubella syndrome;* German measles; three-day measles.

NOTE: Congenital rubella syndrome is presented under "Syndrome, congenital rubella."

(1) The virus may be isolated from blood, urine, feces, tears, and CSF. (2) Collect any tissues that appear to be infected. (3) Usually, special stains are not helpful. (4) Serologic studies are available from local and state health department laboratories. (5) This is a **reportable** disease.

Organs and Tissues	*Procedures*	*Possible or Expected Findings*
External examination, skin, and eyes	Prepare histologic sections of skin lesions.	Dermatitis and exanthema; subconjunctival hemorrhages; lymphadenopathy.
Blood	Obtain serum for serologic study.	
Cerebrospinal fluid	Submit sample for cell count and determination of protein concentrations.	Increased cell count and elevated protein concentrations in presence of encephalitis.*
Gastrointestinal tract; kidneys		Hemorrhages.
Lymph nodes	Submit postauricular, suboccipital, and posterior cervical lymph nodes for histologic study.	Lymphadenitis.
Brain	For removal and specimen preparation, see Chapter 4. Submit sample for microbiologic study.	Acute rubella encephalitis with nonspecific perivascular infiltrates, cerebral edema, and neuronal degeneration. Rarely, severe hemorrhages.
Joints	For removal, prosthetic repair, and specimen preparation, see Chapter 2.	Arthritis (polyarthritis and tenosynovitis) of fingers, wrists, and knees.

Rubeola (See "Measles.")

S

St. Louis Encephalitis (See "Encephalitis, all types or type unspecified.")

Sarcoidosis

NOTE: The typical noncaseating granuloma of sarcoidosis is not pathognomonic. Fungal or mycobacterial infections, brucellosis,* hypersensitivity pneumonitis, pneumoconiosis* (in rare instances, sarcoid granulomas may contain calcium oxalate crystals), and Wegener's granulomatosis* must be ruled out. Metastatic calcifications may occur *(1)*.

Organs and Tissues	*Procedures*	*Possible or Expected Findings*
External examination and skin	Prepare histologic sections of skin lesions.	Erythema nodosum; lupus pernio; maculopapular eruptions; scars and keloids *(4)*.
	Prepare chest and skeletal roentgenograms.	Pulmonary and hilar infiltrates; cystic bone changes in phalanges of hands and feet.
Blood	Submit sample for determination of globulin concentrations.	Hyperglobulinemia; hypercalcemia.
Heart	Record weight. If there was a history of heart block, prepare histologic sections of conduction system.	Cor pulmonale; myocardial sarcoidosis, particularly of left ventricular wall (cardiomyopathy*). The conduction system may be involved also *(1)*.
Lungs	Submit any consolidated areas for microbiologic study. Perfuse at least one lung with formalin. If superinfection is expected, order Grocott's methenamine silver, acid fast, and Gram stain.	Noncaseating, noninfectious granulomas. Pulmonary fibrosis with honeycombing; aspergillomas or other mycetomas may be found. Pleural sarcoidosis. See also above under "Note."
Lymph nodes	Record size of hilar (mediastinal), abdominal, and peripheral lymph nodes (cervical, axillary, inguinal). Submit samples for histologic study.	Granulomatous lymphadenitis with epithelioid cells and giant cells (with or without asteroid and conchoid or Schaumann bodies).
Liver	Record weight; submit samples for histologic study.	Granulomatous hepatitis. Granulomatous cholangitis (chronic cholestasis of sarcoidosis) resembling primary biliary cirrhosis.
Spleen	Record weight; submit samples for histologic study. If there is splenomegaly or other evidence of portal hypertension,* follow procedures described under that heading.	Granulomatous splenitis. For histologic features, see under "Lymph nodes."
Kidneys	If there is evidence of kidney failure,* see under that heading.	Nephrolithiasis;* nephrocalcinosis.
Other tissues	Procedures depend on expected findings or grossly identified abnormalities as listed in right-hand column. If metastatic calcifications are found *(1)*, order von Kossa stain.	Manifestations of portal hypertension* or of kidney failure.* Granulomas and associated lesions may occur in many organs and tissues, such as nasal mucosa, tonsils, larynx with epiglottis, stomach, or rectum.

From: *Handbook of Autopsy Practice,* 4th Ed. Edited by: B.L. Waters

Organs and Tissues	*Procedures*	*Possible or Expected Findings*
Brain and spinal cord		Chronic meningitis; space-occupying lesions (submeningeal nodular granulomas).
Pituitary gland	If there is evidence of diabetes insipidus* or pituitary insufficiency,* see under those headings.	Granulomatosis.
Eyes, lacrimal glands, and other orbital tissues	For removal and specimen preparation, see Chapter 5.	Iridocyclitis; chorioretinitis; papilledema; posterior uveitis; keratoconjunctivitis sicca; conjunctival follicles; cataracts. Involvement of lacrimal glands and other orbital tissues *(2)*.
Parotid gland	If there is evidence of parotid involvement, other salivary glands should also be studied. Parotid gland can be biopsied from scalp incision. Submaxillary gland can be removed with floor of mouth.	Sarcoidosis of parotid gland is common.
Skeletal muscles and peripheral nerves	For sampling and specimen preparation, see Chapter 4.	Sarcoid neuropathy and sarcoid myopathy.
Bones and joints	For removal, prosthetic repair, and specimen preparation, see Chapter 2.	Cystic changes, primarily of small bones of hands and feet. Sarcoidosis of joints *(3)*.

References

1. Nelson JE, Kirschner PA, Teirstein AS. Sarcoidosis presenting as heart disease. Sarcoidosis Vasculitis Diffuse Lung Dis 1996;13:178–182.
2. Smith JA, Foster CS. Sarcoidosis and its ocular manifestations. Int Ophthalmol Clin 1996;36:109–125.
3. Pettersson T. Rheumatic features of sarcoidosis. Curr Opin Rheumatol 1998;10:73–78.
4. Fernandez-Faith E, Mc Donnell J. Cutaneous sarcoidosis: differential diagnosis. Clin Dermatol 2007;25:276–287.

Schistosomiasis

Synonyms and Related Terms: Bilharziasis; *Schistosoma haematobium* infection; *Schistosoma japonicum* infection; *Schis-tosoma mansoni* infection.

NOTE: Unless specifically stated, the changes listed below refer to chronic schistosomiasis mansoni and japonica.

(1) Collect all tissues that appear to be infected. (2) Request direct examination for *Schistosoma*. The following procedures have been described and recommended *(1)*. For demonstration of *Schistosoma* eggs, compress 4-mm tissue fragments—for instance, mucosa of the urinary bladder—between glass slides. If this gives negative results, digest a 5-g portion of tissue in potassium hydroxide.

For the recovery of adult worms of *Schistosoma mansoni* and *Schistosoma haematobium*, remove the viscera en bloc and rinse with water. Separate the intestines from the mesentery. Subsequently, perfuse the portal vein system, the liver, and one lung with saline *(2)*. Then pass the perfusion fluid through a monofilament nylon cloth with an aperture size of 180 μm. Submerge the cloth in water and examine with a dissecting microscope. Fix worms in formalin solution. Examine the intestinal mucosa directly.

From the urinary bladder, ureters, and surrounding connective tissue, worms can be recovered as follows. Inject water into the tissue until the tissue increases 2 or 3 times in thickness. Then compress the tissue gently with a glass plate. Cut slices 0.1–0.2 cm in thickness. Compress these slices between the glass plate and the stage of a dissecting microscope and examine for the presence of adult worms. Many worms also will be present in the fluid expressed from the tissue as it is cut. For the counting of eggs in tissues, urine, and feces, see ref. *(1)*. Immunodiagnostic methods (ELISA and immunoblot) also have been developed *(3)*. (3) Request Giemsa stain. (4) Usually, no special precautions are indicated. (5) Serologic studies are available from the Centers for Disease Control and Prevention, Atlanta, GA. (6) This is not a reportable disease.

Organs and Tissues	*Procedures*	*Possible or Expected Findings*
External examination and skin	Record extent and photograph skin lesions and prepare histologic sections.	Jaundice; edema and pyogenic infection of penis, scrotum, and perineum in *Schistosoma haematobium*. Clubbing of fingers and toes.
Blood	Collect serum for serologic studies.	
Heart	Record heart weight and thickness of ventricles.	Cor pulmonale.
Lungs	See above under "Note." Perfuse one lung with formalin. Request Verhoeff–van Gieson stain.	Embolized eggs with obstructive arteriolitis, angiomatoid lesions, granulomas, and arteriovenous fistulas. Arteriosclerosis; hyaline emboli in small pulmonary arteries.

Organs and Tissues	*Procedures*	*Possible or Expected Findings*
Peritoneal cavity	Submit samples with lesions for histologic study.	Subserosal granulomatous nodules; peritoneal and retroperitoneal fibrosis;* ascites.
Intestinal tract and mesentery	See above under "Note." Submit samples of all segments for histologic study.	Submucosal granulomas and submucosal fibrosis; mucosal ulcers; esophageal varices; inflammatory polyps.
Portal and splenic veins	See above under "Note." Dissect *in situ* or after en bloc removal of abdominal organs. If there is evidence of portal hypertension,* follow procedures described under that heading.	Thrombosis or cavernous transformation of portal vein system.
Liver	See above under "Note." Record weight, photograph, and submit samples for histologic study.	Hepatic fibrosis *(4)*. Hepatic thrombophlebitis.
Spleen	Record weight.	Congestive splenomegaly.
Kidneys, ureters, and pelvic organs	See above under "Note." Remove kidneys together with ureters and pelvic organs.	Hydronephrosis,* pyonephrosis, pyelonephritis,* granulomatous reaction to eggs and urinary bladder papillomas in *Schistosoma haematobium* infection. Ureteritis with strictures and scars; ureterolithiasis and urolithiasis; chronic constricting bilharzial cystitis and tumor of bladder in *Schistosoma haematobium* infection. The uterus and Fallopian tubes also may be involved *(5)*.
	For dissection of penis and urethra, see Chapter 2. Submit samples of prostate and seminal vesicles for histologic study.	Hyperplastic and fibrotic seminal vesiculitis and prostatitis; fibrotic granulomatous and suppurative infection of urethra and penis in *Schistosoma haematobium* infection.
	Submit samples of spermatic cord, epididymis, and testicles for histologic study.	Granulomatous infection by *Schistosoma haematobium.*
Other organs	Submit sections from all sites with grossly identifiable lesions.	*Schistosoma mansoni* infection may occur in every organ. Most frequent ectopic sites are spinal cord, brain, and genital tract.

References

1. Kamel IA, Cheever AW, Elwi AM, Mosimann JE, Danner R: *Schistosoma mansoni* and *S. haematobium* infections in Egypt. I. Evaluation of techniques for recovery of worms and eggs at necropsy. Am J Trop Med Hyg 1977;26:696–701.
2. Cheever AW. A quantitative post-mortem study of schistosomiasis mansoni in man. Am J Trop Med Hyg 1968;17:38–64.
3. Tsang VC, Wilkins PP. Immunodiagnosis of schistosomiasis. Screen with FAST-ELISA and confirm with immunoblot. Clin Lab Med 1991; 11(4):1029–1039.
4. Andrade ZA, Peixoto E, Guerret S, Grimaud JA. Hepatic connective tissue changes in hepatosplenic schistosomiasis. Hum Pathol 1992; 23(5):566–573.
5. Helling-Giese G, Kjetland EF, Gundersen SG, Poggensee G, Richter J, Krantz I, et al. Schistosomiasis in women: manifestations in the upper reproductive tract. Acta Trop 1996;62(4):225–238.

Scleroderma (See "Sclerosis, systemic.")

Sclerosis, Amyotrophic Lateral (See "Disease, motor neuron.")

Sclerosis, Diffuse (See "Sclerosis, Schilder's cerebral.")

Sclerosis, Multiple

Synonyms and Related Terms: Acute and subacute variants: Acute multiple sclerosis (Marburg type), acute necrotizing myelopathy; concentric sclerosis (Baló type); concentric lacunar leukoencephalopathy; encephalitis periaxialis diffusa (Schilder's type; see also next entry, "Sclerosis, Schilder's cerebral"*); neuromyelitis optica (Dèvic type).

Chronic Variants: Classic or Charcot type multiple sclerosis (relapsing and remitting, secondary progressive, arrested, benign, monosymptomatic and asymptomatic, primary progressive).

Possible Associated Conditions: Hypertrophic polyradicu -loneuropathy.

Organs and Tissues	Procedures	Possible or Expected Findings
Brain and spinal cord	For removal and specimen preparation, see Chapter 4. Record thickness of optic nerves. Request Luxol fast blue stain for myelin and Bielschowski's stain for axons.	Changes most commonly in cerebral white matter (periventricular), spinal cord white matter, and optic nerves. Appearance of plaques varies, depending on whether they are active, chronic active, or inactive. Myelin loss, accompanied by a variable histiocytic infiltrate and gliosis, are characteristic findings. Perivascular lymphocytic cuffs are present.
Other organs and tissues	Procedures depend on expected findings or grossly identified abnormalities as listed in right-hand column.	Aspiration bronchopneumonia; disuse atrophy of skeletal muscles.

Sclerosis, Schilder's Cerebral

Synonyms: Encephalitis periaxialis diffusa; multiple sclerosis, Schilder's type.

NOTE: The pathologic changes in adrenoleukodystrophy may resemble those in Schilder's disease (see also under "Leukodystrophy,...").

Organs and Tissues	Procedures	Possible or Expected Findings
Brain and spinal cord	For removal and specimen preparation, see Chapter 4. See also above under "Note."	Diffuse or large patches of demyelination in the cerebral white matter (>2 × 3 cm), with sudanophilic myelin breakdown products in macrophages.
	Submit wet tissue for determination of phospholipids and cholesterol esters.	Depletion of phospholipids and increase of cholesterol esters (nonspecific manifestations of myelin sheath breakdown).
Eye		Optic neuritis *(1)*.

Reference

1. Afifi AK, et al. Optic neuritis: a novel presentation of Schilder's disease. J Clin Neurol 2001;16:693–696.

Sclerosis, Systemic

Synonyms and Related Terms: Progressive systemic sclerosis; scleroderma.

Possible Associated Conditions: Sjögren's syndrome.*

Organs and Tissues	Procedures	Possible or Expected Findings
External examination	Record character and extent of skin lesions, photograph, and submit samples for histologic study, together with subcutaneous tissue.	Dermal sclerosis, primarily of face and fingers. Cutaneous calcium deposits with ulcerations. Ischemic ulcers of fingers.
	Prepare roentgenograms of jaws.	Thickening of periodontal membrane with replacement of the lamina dura.
Breast	If breast implants are present, record type and state whether they are intact.	Ruptured implants have been considered (probably erroneously) a possible cause of systemic sclerosis *(1)*.
Diaphragm		Diaphragmatic hernia.*
Blood	Freeze serum for possible serologic study.	
Heart	Measure volume of pericardial fluid. Record heart weight and measure thickness of ventricles.	Fibrinous pericarditis or hydropericardium. Cor pulmonale.
	For histologic study of the conduction system, see Chapter 3.	Interstitial fibrosis, which may involve the conduction system.
Lungs with hilar lymph nodes	Perfuse at least one lung with formalin. Submit samples of lungs and hilar lymph nodes for histologic study.	Diffuse alveolar damage *(2)*. Interstitial pulmonary fibrosis with honey-combing *(5)*. Vasculitis or intimal thickening of small pulmonary arteries and arterioles with pulmonary hypertension* (see "Heart").

Organs and Tissues	Procedures	Possible or Expected Findings
		Aspiration bronchopneumonia. Bronchiolo-alveolar carcinoma complicating advanced fibrosis.
Aorta and other elastic arteries		Rarely involved by vasculitis.
Esophagus	Leave esophagus attached to portion of stomach. Submit samples at various levels for histologic study.	Muscular fibrosis. Vasculitis. Dilatation and ulcers of lower esophagus; ulcers are secondary to systemic sclerosis or reflux.
Gastrointesinal tract	Open and fix bowel as soon as possible. Other procedures depend on expected findings or grossly identified abnormalities as listed in right-hand column.	Gastrointestinal fibrosis, most commonly of duodenum, jejunum, and colon; colonic muscular atrophy with large-mouth diverticula. Rarely, pneumatosis* of small intestine.
Kidneys	Follow procedures described under "Glomerulonephritis."	Intimal hyperplasia of interlobular arteries. Fibrinoid changes of afferent arterioles and glomeruli. Arteriolonecrosis. Cortical infarctions or ischemic scars. Hypertensive kidney failure* is a common cause of death.
Other organs	Procedures depend on expected findings or grossly identified abnormalities as listed in right-hand column.	Vasculitis in many organs and tissues—for instance, in pancreas, spleen, and central nervous system. Fibrosis of thyroid gland with hypothyroidism.*
Brain and spinal cord		Generally not affected. Rare cases of cerebrovascular calcification have been reported *(3)*.
Skeletal muscles		Polymyositis (overlap syndrome). Muscular fibrosis. Neurogenic changes also may occur *(4)*.
Bones and joints	For removal, prosthetic repair, and specimen preparation, see Chapter 2.	Osteoporosis.* Symmetric polyarthritis* with low-grade synovitis.

References

1. Anderson DR, Schwartz J, Cottrill CM, McClain AS, Ross JS, Magidson JG, et al. Silicone ganuloma in acral skin in a patient with silicone-gel implants and systemic sclerosis. Int J Dermatol 1996;35:36–38.
2. Muir TE, Tazelaar HD, Colby TV, Myers JL. Organizing diffuse alveolar damage associated with progressive systemic sclerosis. Mayo Clin Proc 1997;72:639–642.
3. Heron E, Fornes P, Rance A, Emmerich J, Bayle O, Fiessinger JN. Brain involvement in scleroderma: two autopsy cases. Stroke 1998;29:719–721.
4. Calore EE, Cavaliere MJ, Perez MN, Takayasu V, Wakamatsu A, Kiss MH. Skeletal muscle pathology in systemic sclerosis. J Rheumatol 1995;22:2246–2249.
5. du Bois RM. Mechanisms of scleroderma-induced lung disease. Proc Ann Thorac Soc 2007;4:434–438.

Sclerosis, Tuberous

Synonyms and Related Terms: Bourneville's disease; Bourneville-Pringle disease; neurocutaneous syndrome; phacomatosis.

NOTE: There are probably more abnormalities than the ones listed below and some may have not yet been described *(1)*.

Organs and Tissues	Procedures	Possible or Expected Findings
External examination and skin	Prepare photographs of face and pigment abnormalities at other sites. If accessible, prepare sections of skin tumors.	Angiofibromas with characteristic facial distribution (so-called facial adenoma sebaceum). Peri- and subungual "fibromas." Rough yellow skin in lumbosacral region (shagreen patch). Hypopigmented spots (white spots; hypomelanotic macules) over trunk and limbs.
	Prepare skeletal roentgenograms.	See below under "Bones."
Heart	Prepare photographs and sample tumors for electron microscopic study. See also under "Tumor of the heart."	Rhabdomyomas, often multiple.
Lungs	Unless a large sample or samples need to be submitted for microbiologic study, perfuse	Lymphangioleiomyomatosis characterized by multiple small cysts and honeycombing

Organs and Tissues	Procedures	Possible or Expected Findings
	both lungs with formalin.	with proliferation of connective tissue and smooth muscle.
Liver	Record weight; photograph cut sections and sample possible abnormalities for histologic study.	Focal fatty change. Angioleiomyomas.
Intestine	Fix intestinal wall samples on cork board and submit polyps for histologic study.	Microhamartomatous rectal polyps.
Kidneys	Record weights. Photograph outer surface and cut sections; submit tumor nodules for histologic study.	Angiomyolipomas; embryonal renal blastomas; microscopic cysts; cystic glomeruli; abnormal tubules.
Uterus	Sample for histologic study.	Abnormal proliferation of smooth muscle.
Neck organs	Open larynx in posterior midline.	Fibrous polyps of larynx.
Other organs and tissues	Procedures depend on expected findings or grossly identified abnormalities as listed in right-hand column.	Record size and character of all tumorous or other abnormal lesions. Angioleiomyomas in pancreas and adrenal glands.
Brain and spinal cord	For removal and specimen preparation, see Chapter 4.	Cortical tuber; subependymal nodules; white matter hamartomas; subependymal giant cell astrocytoma, callosal agenesis/dysplasia, hemimegalencephaly, schizencephaly, arachnoid cysts *(2)*.
Eyes	For removal and specimen preparation, see Chapter 5.	Retinal hamartoma; retinal giant cell astrocytoma; hypopigmented iris spot.
Bones		Rarefaction of phalanges; periosteal thickening of metacarpals and metatarsals; focal sclerosis of calvaria; melorheostosis-type changes.

Reference

1. Wiestler OD, Lopex PS, Crino PB. Tuberous sclerosis complex and subependymal giant cell astrocytoma. In: Pathology and Genetics of the Nervous System. Kleihues P, Cavence WK, eds. IARC, Lyon, 1997, pp. 182–184.
2. Tatli M, Guzel A. Bilateral temporal arachnoid cysts associated with tuberous sclerosis. J Child Neurol 2007;22:775–779.

Scopolamine (See "Poisoning, alkaloid.")

Scuba (See "Accident, diving [skin or scuba].")

Scurvy (See "Deficiency, vitamin C.")

Shigellosis (See "Dysentery, bacillary.")

Shingles (See "Infection, Herpes zoster.")

Shock

Related Terms: Anaphylactic shock; bacteremic shock; cardiogenic shock; electric shock; hypovolemic shock; septic shock; and many others.

NOTE: See also under name of suspected underlying condition, such as "Burns," "Death, anaphylactic," "Injury, electrical," and "Stroke, heat."

Organs and Tissues	Procedures	Possible or Expected Findings
Blood	Submit sample for bacterial culture.	Bacteremia or septicemia may be either the cause or the effect of shock.
Heart	Dissection procedures depend on type of heart disease. Sample myocardium for histologic study.	Heart disease causing cardiogenic shock. Other types of shock may cause subendocardial and subepicardial interstitial hemorrhages, minute necroses, and patchy contraction band changes.
Lungs	Record weights. Perfuse at least one lung with formalin.	Shock lungs (wet lungs). See also under "Syndrome, respiratory distress, of adult." Pulmonary embolism* may be the cause of shock.

Organs and Tissues	Procedures	Possible or Expected Findings
Gastrointestinal tract	Record intestinal abnormalities and estimated amount of intraluminal blood.	Mucosal hemorrhages and necroses; erosions and ulcers.
Liver	Record weight and sample for histologic study.	Centrilobular (zone 3) necroses, with or without fatty changes.
Kidneys	Record weights. Submit samples of cortex and papillae for histologic study.	Acute tubular necrosis.
Adrenal glands	Record weights; record appearance of cortex.	Cortical lipid depletion and atrophy.
Brain		Hypoxic encephalopathy with neuronal damage.

Sickness, Decompression: Caisson disease. (see Accident diving)

Sickness, Serum

Related Term: Immune complex disease.

NOTE: This is a nonfatal, self-limited disease, characterized by swelling of the face, rash, lymphadenopathy, and arthritis, mainly of large joints.* Globulin antibodies may be demonstrable. There may be proteinuria. Fatalities are caused by acute ana-phylactic reactions, which may occur in the course of serum therapy. See under "Death, anaphylactic."

Sickness, Sleeping (See "Trypanosomiasis, African.")

Silicosis (See "Pneumoconiosis.")

Snakebite

Organs and Tissues	Procedures	Possible or Expected Findings
External examination and skin (wound)	Photograph and submit material from wound for histologic and possible toxicologic study. Use Gram stains if superinfection (e.g., with clostridia) appears to be present.	Necrosis, edema, and hemorrhage around bite wound; bleeding from body orifices. Mild jaundice. Superinfection of wounds with or without gangrene.
Kidneys	Record weights, photograph, and sample for histologic study.	Renal cortical and tubular necrosis. Myoglobin or hemoglobin in tubules.
Other organs	Procedures depend on expected findings or grossly identified abnormalities as listed in right-hand column.	Features of disseminated intravascular coagulation.* Hemorrhages.

Sodium (See "Disorder, electrolyte(s)")

Spherocytosis (See "Anemia, hemolytic.")

Sphingolipidosis (See "Gangliosidosis.")

Spina Bifida (See "Meningocele.")

Splenomegaly, Chronic Congestive (See "Hypertension, portal.")

Spondylitis, Ankylosing

Synonyms and Related Terms: Bechterew's disease; Marie-Strümpell spondylitis; rheumatoid spondylitis; spondylarthropathy *(1)*.

Possible Associated Conditions: Amyloidosis;* isolated heart block.

Organs and Tissues	*Procedures*	*Possible or Expected Findings*
External examination, skin, and subcutaneous tissue	Prepare skeletal roentgenograms.	Deformities of rheumatoid arthritis.* Kyphosis. See below under "Bones and joints."
Blood	There are no diagnostic laboratory tests but it still is advisable to save a blood sample.	The HLA-B27 gene is present in most cases. Rheumatoid factor and antinuclear antibodies are absent.
Heart and aorta	Record heart weight. Test competence of valves (Chapter 3). Open heart in line of blood flow. Photograph and measure valvular lesions. Prepare sections of valves, myocardium, conduction system (if there was a history of heart block), and ascending aorta.	Thickening of supravalvular aortic wall. Thickening of aortic cusps. Subaortic bump. Thickening of anterior mitral leaflet. Aortic and mitral insufficiency,* with signs of regurgitation. Aortitis.
Lungs	Perfuse at least one lung with formalin. Submit any consolidated area for microbiologic study.	Interstitial fibrosis and cysts in upper lobes. Pleuritis, pleural effusions,* fibrobullous lesions, and cavitating lesions with fungal (Aspergillus) or bacterial infections.
Intestine	Fix intestines as soon as possible. abnormalities as listed in right-hand column.	Chronic ulcerative colitis. Crohn's disease.* Granulomatous inflammation *(2, 4)*.
Kidneys and prostate	Sample for histologic study and request amyloid stains or renal parenchyma.	Amyloid nephropathy. Prostatitis.
Bones and joints	Prepare roentgenograms of spine, sacroiliac joints, symphysis ossium pubis, and manubriosternal, sternoclavicular, and humeroscapular joints.	Fusion of sacroiliac and intervertebral joints and disks ("bamboo spine"). These changes often are associated with severe spinal osteoporosis.* The involvement of the sacroiliac joint is pathognomonic *(3)*.
	If spine cannot be removed in its entirety, it can be split in midline and one half can be removed, with costovertebral and costotransversal joints. Hip joints should be exposed.	Cervical spinal fracture may be a cause of quadriplegia.
	Histologic sections should include synovia and periarticular tissue.	Secondary and peripheral osteoarthritis* may be present.
Bone marrow	For preparation of sections and smears, see Chapter 2.	Leukemia* developed in some patients who had had radiation treatment (1950 or earlier).
Eyes	For removal and specimen preparation, see Chapter 5.	Acute anterior uveitis.

References

1. Schumacher HR, Bardin T. The spondyloarthropathies: classification and diagnosis. Do we need new terminologies? Bailliers Clin Rheumatol 1998;12:551–565.
2. Porzio V, Biasi G, Corrado A, De Santi M, Vindigni C, Viti S, et al. Intestinal histological and ultrastructural inflammatory changes in spondyloarthropathy and rheumatoid arthritis. Scand J Rheumatol 1997;26:92–98.
3. Braun J, Sieper J. The sacroiliac joint in the spondyloarthropathies. Curr Opin Rheumatol 1996;8:275–287.
4. Adebavo D et al. Granulomatous ileitis in a patient with ankylosing spondylitis. Nat Clin Pract Gastroenterol Hepatol 2007;4:347–351.

Sporotrichosis

Synonym: *Sporothrix (Sporotrichum) schenckii* infection.

NOTE: (1) Collect all tissues that appear to be infected.

(2) Request fungal culture. (3) Request Grocott's methenamine silver stain. (4) No special precautions are indicated. (5) Serologic studies are available on a research basis from the Centers for Disease Control and Prevention, Atlanta, GA. (6) This is not a reportable disease.

Possible Associated Conditions: Sarcoidosis;* tuberculosis.*

Organs and Tissues	*Procedures*	*Possible or Expected Findings*
External examination and skin	Prepare sections of cutaneous and subcutaneous lesions. Prepare skeletal roentgenograms.	Acute or chronic skin infection, with or without granulomas and suppuration. Osteomyelitis* (metacarpals, phalanges, and tibiae) and arthritis.*
Lymph nodes	Dissect lymph nodes that drain cutaneous and subcutaneous infections. Submit samples for microbiologic and histologic study. See also above under "Note."	Lymphadenitis.
Chest cavity	Record volume of pleural effusions.	Pleural effusions* may be associated with pulmonary sporotrichosis.
Lungs	Submit consolidated areas for culture. Perfuse both lungs with formalin.	Few sporadic cases with cavities and fungus ball. Pulmonary fibrosis.
Other organs	See above under "Note." Other procedures depend on expected findings or grossly identified abnormalities as listed in right-hand column.	Gastrointestinal tract, central nervous system, eyes, and skeletal system—among others—may be involved by hematogenous dissemination.

Sprue, Celiac

Synonyms and Related Terms: Adult celiac disease; collagenous sprue; gluten-sensitive enteropathy; idiopathic steatorrhea; nontropical sprue; protein-losing enteropathy; sprue syndrome.

Possible Associated Conditions: Chronic ulcerative colitis;* dermatitis herpetiformis; diabetes mellitus;* IgA deficiency; insufficiency, adrenal;* lipodystrophy *(1)*; lymphoma* *(2)*; primary biliary cirrhosis;* primary sclerosing cholangitis* (See also below under "Possible or Expected Findings.")

Organs and Tissues	*Procedures*	*Possible or Expected Findings*
External examination and skin	Submit samples of grossly normal and of abnormal skin for histologic study.	Baldness; perianal and perioral erosions; cutaneous vasculitis; dermatitis herpetiformis; eczema; psoriasis;* other skin diseases. Facial, upper extremity and truncal lipodystrophy *(1)*.
	Prepare skeletal roentgenograms.	Osteomalacia with compression fractures; kyphoskoliosis.
Heart		Ischemic heart disease.*
Lungs	Perfuse at least one lung with formalin. Request Gomori's iron stain.	Idiopathic pulmonary hemosiderosis; interstitial pneumonia.*
Esophagus and stomach	See "Tumor of the esophagus" and "Tumor of the stomach."	Carcinoma may be found in both organs.
Intestinal tract	Open and fix bowel as soon as possible. Record sites in small intestine from where histologic material was sampled (in centimeters	Volvulus; mucosal diaphragms; villous atrophy. Sprue-like changes in patients with carcinoma or lymphoma, with or without

Organs and Tissues	Procedures	Possible or Expected Findings
Intestinal tract (continued)	from duodenojejunal junction or from ileocecal valve).	intestinal ulceration and perforation.
	Submit samples of colonic mucosa for histologic study. Request PAS and azure-eosin stains.	Ulcerative colitis. Lymphocytic or microscopic colitis.
Other organs	Procedures depend on expected findings or grossly identified abnormalities as listed in right-hand column.	Manifestations of malabsorption syndrome* with osteomalacia.*

References

1. O'Mahony D, O'Mahony S, Whelton MJ, McKiernan J. Partial lipodystrophy in coeliac disease. Gut 1990;31:717–718.
2. Mathus-Vliegen EM. Coeliac disease and lymphoma: current status. Netherlands J Med 1996;49:212–220.

Sprue, Tropical

NOTE: This term is not well-defined and has been applied to a variety of diseases.

Organs and Tissues	Procedures	Possible or Expected Findings
Intestinal tract	For preparation for study under dissecting microscope, see Chapter 2. Submit samples for histologic study.	Partial mucosal atrophy of whole length of the small bowel. Many geographic variations; probably infectious etiology in many instances.
Stomach		Atrophic gastritis.
Bone marrow	For preparation of sections and smears, see Chapter 2.	Macrocytic megaloblastic anemia.*

Stabbing (See "Injury, stabbing.")

Stannosis (See "Pneumoconiosis.")

Starvation

NOTE: In developed countries, psychiatric conditions such as anorexia nervosa* or organic diseases such as malignancies are the most common causes of starvation. See also under "Malnutrition."

Organs and Tissues	Procedures	Possible or Expected Findings
External examination and skin	Record body weight and length and location of edema. Prepare sections of skin lesions.	Hunger edema; skin changes secondary to vitamin deficiencies.
Blood	Submit sample for biochemical studies.	Hypoproteinemia.
Liver and spleen	Record weights.	Atrophy; hemosiderosis of spleen.
Other organs and tissues	Record weight of all organs (for expected weights, see Part III). Submit samples of all major organs, including endocrine glands, lymphatic and fat tissue, bone, and bone marrow for histologic study.	Degree of atrophy varies from organ to organ; atrophy of fat tissue, lymphoid tissue, and gonads usually is most pronounced. Severe infections, such as tuberculosis,* may be present without having been apparent clinically.

Steatohepatitis, Nonalcoholic (NASH)

NOTE: The morphologic findings in the liver are indistinguishable from those in alcoholic liver disease* *(1)*. Follow autopsy procedures described under "Disease, alcoholic liver." If the patient had received a liver transplant, procedures described under "Transplantation, liver" should be followed also.

Possible Associated Conditions: Celiac sprue (rare); diabetes mellitus* (type 2); hyperlipidemia; malnutrition* from bulemia (rare); morbid obesity with liver failure particularly after episodes of rapid weight loss (e.g., after recent gastroplasty); lipodystrophy; mild obesity;* short bowel syndrome (rare); total parenteral nutrition.*

Organs and Tissues	Procedures	Possible or Expected Findings
External examination and skin	Record body weight and length.	Obesity,* which may be mild or severe *(3)*.
Liver	Record weight and sample for histologic study.	Chronic steatohepatitis with or without cirrhosis. Submassive hepatic necrosis.
Other organs	Procedures depend on expected findings or grossly identified abnormalities as listed in right-hand column.	Manifestations of portal hypertension.* See also above under "Possible Associated Conditions."
Brain and spinal cord	For removal and specimen preparation, see Chapter 4.	Wernicke's encephalopathy *(2)*.

References

1. Ludwig J, McGill DB, Lindor KD. Review: nonalcoholic steatohepatitis. J Gastroenterol Hepatol 1997;12:398–403.
2. Yamamoto T. Alcoholic and non-alcoholic Wernicke's encephalopathy. Be alert to the preventable and treatable disease. Intern Med 1996;35:754–755.
3. Palasciano G, et al. Non-alcoholic fatty liver disease in the metabolic syndrome. Curr Pharm Des 2007;13:2193–2198.

Steatorrhea, Idiopathic (See "Sprue, celiac.")

Stenosis, Acquired Valvular Aortic

Related Terms: Acquired calcification of congenitally bicuspid aortic valve; degenerative (or senile) calcific aortic stenosis; rheumatic aortic stenosis.

NOTE: See also "Stenosis, congenital valvular aortic."

Organs and Tissues	Procedures	Possible or Expected Findings
Heart	Follow procedures described under "Stenosis, congenital valvular aortic."	Bicuspid aortic valve;* calcific nodular aortic stenosis. Chronic rheumatic mitral and tricuspid valvulitis.

Stenosis, Acquired Valvular Pulmonary

NOTE: Record weight of heart, thickness of ventricles, and valve circumferences.

Possible Associated Conditions: Carcinoid heart disease (both the pulmonary valve and the tricuspid valve may be involved).

Stenosis, Congenital Supravalvular Aortic

Synonyms: Supravalvular aortic stenosis, diffuse type; supravalvular aortic stenosis, discrete; Williams-Beuren syndrome.

NOTE: Sudden death may occur, as may acute aortic dissection. For acquired forms, see "Arteritis, Takayasu's."

Possible Associated Conditions: Adhesions of aortic valve cusps; obstruction of coronary ostia and brachiocephalic branches of the aortic arch; supravalvular pulmonary stenosis; Williams-Beuren syndrome.

Organs and Tissues	Procedures	Possible or Expected Findings
External examination	Prepare photograph of face.	Unusual elfin-like facial features.
Blood	Submit sample for microbiologic study. Postmortem calcium values are unreliable.	Hypercalcemia; septicemia.
Heart	If infective aortitis is suspected, expose stenosed area through sterilized aortic wall (similar to procedure suggested for valvular aortic endocarditis, Chapter 7). Culture vegetations, prepare smears and sections, and request Gram stain.	Infective aortitis.
	Remove heart together with aortic arch and adjacent great neck vessels. Measure diameters of stenosed and nonstenosed portions of aorta (calipers work best); record extent and nature of stenosis. For coronary arteriography, see Chapter 10. Prepare histologic sections of multiple segments of coronary arteries. Request Verhoeff–van Gieson stain.	Diffuse or discrete type of aortic stenosis. Increased heart weight. Substantial thickening and stenosis of involved arteries. Microscopic arterial dysplasia with merged intima and media, and with haphazard interlacing of elastic layers.
Other organs		Manifestations of congestive heart failure.*

Stenosis, Congenital Supravalvular Pulmonary

Synonyms: Williams-Beuren syndrome.

NOTE: Follow procedures described under "Stenosis, congenital valvular pulmonary." For acquired forms, see "Arteritis, Takayasu's."

Possible Associated Conditions: Supravalvular aortic stenosis.*

Stenosis, Congenital Valvular Aortic

Synonyms: Acommissural (dome-shaped) aortic valve; unicommissural aortic valve; unicuspid aortic valve (either acommissural or unicommissural).

NOTE: Congenital aortic stenosis may cause sudden death in infancy and childhood. Most valves are unicommissural, hypo-plastic, and dysplastic (thickened and malformed). Occasionally, bicuspid aortic valves are stenotic at birth.

Possible Associated Conditions: Coarctation of aorta;* endocardial fibroelastosis* of left ventricle; hypoplasia of left ventricle;* interrupted aortic arch;* tubular hypoplasia of aortic arch.*

Organs and Tissues	*Procedures*	*Possible or Expected Findings*
Heart	If infective endocarditis is suspected, follow procedures described in Chapter 7.	Infective endocarditis.*
	Remove heart with ascending aorta; record weight of heart and open in ventricular cross-sections. Test competence of valves (Chapter 3). Leave aortic valve intact. Record size of valve orifice and thickness of heart chambers.	Hypertrophy of left and right ventricles; dilatation of left atrium.
	Histologic samples should include endocardium and area(s) of fusion of aortic cusp(s). Request Verhoeff–van Gieson stain.	Endocardial fibroelastosis* of left ventricle. Infarction of mitral papillary muscles. Subendocardial fibrosis, biventricular.
Lungs	Perfuse one lung with formalin. Request Verhoeff–van Gieson stain.	Chronic pulmonary venous changes.

Stenosis, Congenital Valvular Pulmonary

Related Terms: Isolated (pure, simple, or dome-shaped) pulmonary stenosis.

NOTE: The pulmonary valve is usually acommissural in isolated congenital pulmonary stenosis. With other coexistant congenital heart disease (such as tetralogy), the pulmonary valve is usually bicuspid and hypoplastic, but may be unicommissural or dys-plastic and tricuspid.

Organs and Tissues	*Procedures*	*Possible or Expected Findings*
Heart and great vessels; peripheral pulmonary arteries	Culture any grossly infected valve. For general dissection techniques, see Chapter 3.	Infective endocarditis* of pulmonary valve and tricuspid valve; infective endarteritis at bifurcation of pulmonary trunk.
	Record weight of heart, thickness of ventricles, and annular circumferences.	Thickened and incompetent tricuspid valve; right ventricular hypertrophy; poststenotic dilatation of pulmonary trunk; peripheral pulmonary artery stenosis.
Brain	For removal and specimen preparation, see Chapter 4.	Cerebral abscess* (would indicate presence of right-to-left shunt).

Stenosis, Mitral

Synonyms and Related Terms: Acquired mitral stenosis; congenital mitral stenosis; rheumatic mitral stenosis.

Possible Associated Conditions: Acquired mitral stenosis generally is the result of rheumatic carditis (often decades earlier). Congenital mitral stenosis may be associated with bicuspid aortic valve;* coarctation of the aorta;* parachute mitral valve; Shone's syndrome; subaortic stenosis;* supravalvular stenosing ring of the left atrium; and ventricular septal defect.*

Organs and Tissues	Procedures	Possible or Expected Findings
External examination	Record color of skin. Prepare chest roentgenogram.	Cyanosis. Cardiomegaly; calcification in and around mitral valve.
Blood	If infective endocarditis* is suspected, submit sample for microbiologic study.	Septicemia.
Heart and great vessels	For general dissection techniques in congenital mitral stenosis, see Chapter 3. If infective endocarditis is suspected, submit any possible vegetations for culture, after photographing the lesion. Record weight and measurements of heart; record size of left atrium; record appearance and size of mitral orifice.	See above under "Possible Associated Conditions." Infective endocarditis.* Cardiomegaly; dilatation of left atrium; thrombi in atrial appendages. Rheumatic valvulitis.
Lungs	Perfuse lungs with formalin; prepare sections of bronchi, pulmonary arteries, and pulmonary veins. Request Verhoeff–van Gieson stain.	Pulmonary congestion, emboli, and infarctions; bronchopneumonia; manifestations of pulmonary venous hypertension.* Elevated left bronchus.
Other organs	Procedures depend on expected findings or grossly identified abnormalities as listed in right-hand column.	Manifestations of congestive heart failure;* systemic emboli; cholelithiasis* and chronic cholecystitis.*

Stenosis, Renal Artery

Organs and Tissues	Procedures	Possible or Expected Findings
Retroperitoneal organs	For renal arteriography, see Chapter 2. Open aorta lengthwise *in situ*; record width of renal artery orifices. Probe renal arteries, record width of lumen, and open lengthwise. Photograph; submit samples for histologic study; request Verhoeff–van Gieson stain.	Dissection, embolus, or thrombus of renal artery. Fibromuscular renal artery dysplasia. Atherosclerotic plaques. Some lesions may have been induced by previous percutaneous transluminal angioplasty. Fibromuscular dysplasia with renal artery stenosis must be shown in longitudinal histologic sections of the artery.
Kidneys	Prepare histologic sections of both kidneys (it is important to identify the side, right or left, from which the sample was taken.	Ischemic damage with scarring in affected kidney. Hypertensive vascular changes in unprotected kidney. Abnormalities of juxtaglomerular apparatus.
Other organs		Manifestations of hypertension.*

Stenosis, Subvalvular Aortic

Synonyms and Related Terms: Discrete congenital subvalvular aortic stenosis; idiopathic hypertrophic subaortic stenosis (see "Cardiomyopathy, hypertrophic"); subaortic stenosis; subaortic stenosis of membranous type; subaortic stenosis of muscular type; tunnel subaortic stenosis.

Possible Associated Conditions: Accessory tissue (windsock deformity) of the mitral valve; age-related angled (sigmoid) ventricular septum; complete atrioventricular septal defect;* congenital rhabdomyoma; infundibular stenosis of right ventricle; mitral insufficiency;* supravalvular stenosis of left atrium, parachute mitral valve, and coarctation of aorta;* ventricular septal defect* (malalignment type); Shone's syndrome.

Organs and Tissues	Procedures	Possible or Expected Findings
Heart	Before opening outflow tract, measure diameter of stenosis. Dissect by short axis or long-axis method (see Chapter 3). Compare septal thickness with thickness of lateral ventricular wall. Histologic samples should include ventricular septum. For fixation for electron microscopy, see Chapter 15.	Membranous or muscular subaortic (subvalvular) stenosis. Increased heart weight. Ventricular septum may be thicker than lateral wall of left ventricle (normal ratio <1.3).

Stenosis, Subvalvular Pulmonary

Synonyms: Right ventricular infundibular stenosis; stenosis of ostium infundibuli; double-chambered right ventricle; dynamic right ventricular outflow tract obstruction.

NOTE: Infective endocarditis* may occur on the wall of the right infundibular chamber above the localized area of infundibular stenosis.

Possible Associated Conditions: Congenital valvular pulmonary stenosis;* double outlet right ventricle;* tetralogy of Fallot;* ventricular septal defect.*

Stillbirth

It is preferable to have autopsies of fetuses and stillborns performed by pathologists experienced in perinatal pathology. If such personnel are not immediately available, the attending pathologist may nevertheless collect important information. If attempts to induce abortion appear to have caused the death of the mother, see "Death, abortion-associated."

The placenta should be immediately procured from the delivery room should it not arrive in the laboratory with the fetus. This will avoid the possibility of the placenta being discarded by the delivery room staff. No fetal autopsy is complete without a careful examination of the placenta (see Part I, Chapter 2). Pathologic changes of placenta that are causative of stillbirth are summarized in Ref. 1.

Fascia lata or other aseptically obtained tissue should be collected for tissue culture for karyotype analysis. If the fetus is at all autolyzed, then the fascia lata cells may not grow in tissue culture. Therefore, if the fetus shows any evidence of autolysis, tissue should be taken aseptically, from placenta immediately beneath the chorionic plate. A portion of placenta and liver should also be snap-frozen for possible molecular analysis.

The initial stage of the autopsy should include photography and radiography, taking anterior-posterior and lateral views. The photographs will record the degree of maceration, which can be roughly correlated with the duration of fetal demise before delivery *[1]* External measurements should include body weight, circumference of head, chest and abdomen, crown-rump length, crown-heel length, and foot length. These measurements are compared with Tables of standards for normal fetuses (see Part III of this book). Assessment of growth retardation may be based on these data. A careful external examination should search for abnormalities such as jaundice, bulging fontanel, cranial bone softening, hyper- or hypotelorism, choanal atresia, external ear anomalies, cleft lip, cleft palate, macroglossia, micrognathia, colobomata, cystic hygroma, shortened neck, contractures, omphalocele, gastroschisis, abnormal external genitalia, anal atresia, absent vagina, sacral pits, open neural tube defects, hemihypertrophy, syndactyly, clinodactyly, transverse palmar creases, or incomplete descent of testes.

The organ bloc may be removed in the manner similar to the adult, using the technique of Letulle (see Chapter 2). If the thyroid gland is noted to be in its usual location and if it appears normal, then the tongue may be left in the body. In macerated fetuses, it is suggested that the organ bloc be fixed overnight in formalin solution prior to dissection. To aid adequate fixation, the following simple steps may be done: 1) wash the organ bloc thoroughly prior to fixation; 2) place multiple transverse cuts through the liver and lungs; 3) dissect the posterior leaves of the diaphragm away from the adrenal glands and kidneys; 4) bivalve the adrenal glands and kidneys in the coronal plane; 5) instill formalin in the lumen of the intestine, using a syringe; and 6) gently instill formalin into both ventricles of the heart, being careful to avoid the ventricular septum.

The procedure for dissection of the organs is similar to that of the adult except: 1) The venous and arterial connections of the heart, including the patency of the ductus arteriosus must be determined before the heart is removed; 2) The esophagus must be opened posteriorly prior to its complete removal so that esophageal atresia or tracheo-esophageal fistula may be recognized and photographed prior to further dissection; 3) The location of the appendix and of the testes should be recorded. Until the intestine has been examined for stenosis or atresia, the mesentery should be left attached.

The degree of autolysis as seen grossly and with histologic examination of both the fetus and the placenta can be used to estimate the duration of time between fetal death and delivery *(2,3,4)*. Trichrome stain is useful for better visualizing histologic features in severely autolyzed tissue.

To remove the brain, Benecke's technique of one of its modifications may be used.

Stillbirth vs Livebirth. A decision has to be made whether the infant was born alive or was stillborn. The hydrostatic lung test, described in the previous edition, appears unreliable. The presence of gas in the lungs does not rule out stillbirth. After death, air can be introduced into the lungs, or putrefaction gases might be present. However, air artificially introduced after death will not distend the alveoli and can be squeezed out, whereas this does not seem to be the case after active ventilation. The distribution of fat in the fetal zone of the adrenal cortex may indicate whether intrauterine death was acute, more prolonged, or chronic *(3)*. This is particularly helpful if the stillborn baby is macerated. If the mother died also, see under "Death, abortion-associated"

References

1. Khong YT. The placenta in stillbirth. Curr Diagn Pathol 2006;12:161–172.
2. Genest DR, Williams MA, Greene MF. Estimating the time of death in stillborn fetuses: I. Histologic examination of fetal organs: an autopsy study of 150 stillborns. Obstet Gynecol 1992;80:575–584.
3. Genest DR. Estimating the time of death in stillborn fetuses: II. Histologic evaluation of the placenta; a study of 71 stillborns. Obstet Gynecol 1992;80:585–92.
4. Genest DR, Singer DB. Estimating the time of death in stillborn fetuses: III. External fetal examination; a study of 86 stillborns. Obstet Gynecol 1992;80:593–600.
5. Becker MJ, Becker AE. Fat distribution in the adrenal cortex as an indication of the mode of intrauterine death. Hum Pathol 1976;7:495– 504.

Stimulant(s) (See "Dependence, drug(s), all types or type undetermined.")

Sting, Insect (See "Death, anaphylactic.")

Strangulation

NOTE: In many instances, procedures described under "Hom-icide" must also be followed. If a rope or some other material had been used (see also under "Hanging"), leave ligature in place until autopsy can be done. See also under "Hypoxia." Toxicologic sampling, particularly for alcohol, should be done in all instances (Chapter 13).

Organs and Tissues	*Procedures*	*Possible or Expected Findings*
External examination and skin	If identity of victim is unknown, follow procedures described in Chapter 13.	
	If a ligature and knot are present, record and photograph their position. Do not disturb knot but cut ligature at some distance and bind ends together.	Strangulation ligatures tend to run horizontally.
	Photograph skin and neck and prepare histologic sections of strap muscles and fascia for demonstration of vital reaction. Collect fingernail scrapings.	Abrasions; fingernail marks; laceration. Defense marks.
Neck organs	Photograph sequentially during layer-wise dissection. Handle neck organs carefully.	
	Prepare roentgenogram of hyoid bone and submit tissues with evidence of trauma for histologic study.	Contusions in soft tissues. Fracture of hyoid bone; laryngeal injury.

Stroke, Cerebrovascular (See "Infarction, cerebral.")

Stroke, Heat (See "Heatstroke.")

Strychnine (See "Poisoning, strychnine.")

Sulfur (Dioxide or Sulfurous Acid) (See "Bronchitis, acute chemical" and "Poisoning, gas.")

Surgery (See following entries and under "Transplantation,..." See also under "Postoperative Autopsies.")

Surgery, Aortocoronary Bypass

Organs and Tissues	*Procedures*	*Possible or Expected Findings*
Heart and ascending aorta	Record *in situ* appearance of heart and ascending aorta. Remove heart with ascending aorta and graft(s) attached.	Cardiomegaly. Injury to ascending aorta.
	Record weight of heart.	
	Prepare angiograms—first of saphenous vein or internal mammary artery graft(s) and then of coronary arteries. If native coronary arteries are calcified, remove them, submit them for decalcification and then thoroughly examine with multiple transverse cuts along their length.	Focal or diffuse graft obstruction. Aneurysm(s) of venous graft(s). Twisting or kinking of graft(s).
	Record patency of distal and proximal anastomoses of graft(s). Remove venous graft(s) for histologic study, including the distal anastomoses.	
	Request Verhoeff-van Gieson stain. Prepare 1-cm-thick transverse (coronal) slices of myocardium.	Obstructive coronary atherosclerosis. Thrombosis, intimal proliferation, calcification, and atherosclerosis of venous graft(s). Scars, recent myocardial infarctions, myocardial aneurysm, mural thromboses.

Surgery, Cardiac Valvular Replacement

Organs and Tissues	*Procedures*	*Possible or Expected Findings*
External examination	Prepare chest roentgenogram.	Abnormal position of prosthesis or catheter.
Blood	Submit sample for microbiologic study.	Septicemia.
Heart	If infective endocarditis is suspected, follow procedures described in Chapter 7.	Prosthetic infective endocarditis.* *Staphylococcus aureus* and Gram-negative bacilli are the most common microorganisms in early-onset endocarditis, and viridans streptococci and Gram-negative bacilli are the most common in late-onset cases. Poppet variance or dislodgement; paravalvular leak; thrombosed valve; calcification of bioprosthetic valve.
	Record weight of heart.	Cardiac hypertrophy.* Mural thrombi.
	For coronary arteriography, see Chapter 10.	Myocardial infarction.
	Open heart in cross sections. Leave valve prosthesis in place. For identification of valve type, see Chapter 3. Test function and record appearance of valves that had not been replaced.	Mechanical valve damage. Dislodged valve. Rheumatic and other diseases of valves that had not been replaced.
Lungs	Perfuse lungs with formalin. Request Verhoeff-van Gieson stain.	Emboli; diffuse alveolar damage. Chronic pulmonary venous hypertensive changes. Pneumonia.
Other organs	Procedures depend on expected findings or grossly identified abnormalities as listed in right-hand column.	Systemic emboli. Escaped poppet, usually at bifurcation of aorta. Hemorrhages secondary to coagulopathy or excessive anticoagulation.

Surgery, Heart Transplantation (See "Transplantation, heart.")

Surgery, Kidney Transplantation (See "Transplantation, kidney.")

Surgery, Liver Transplantation (See "Transplantation, liver.")

Surgery, Lung Transplantation (See "Transplantation, lung.")

Syndrome (See also under "Disease, . . ." and "Sickness,...")

Syndrome, Acquired Immunodeficiency (AIDS)

Synonyms: Human immunodeficiency virus (HIV) infection; HIV infection.

NOTE: For a general review of findings, see ref. *(1)*. Collect all tissues that appear to be infected. Tissue yields better culture results than body fluids. (2) Universal **precautions** should be strictly followed. The generation of aerosols should be minimized. To sterilize tissue surfaces in preparation for culture, swab the surface with povidone iodine. Avoid searing the tissue surface since this will produce an aerosol. Keep no more than one scalpel in the dissecting area at any one time. Have an assistant available with clean, gloved hands to receive specimens in containers, so as to minimize the degree of contamination on the outside of the containers. For cleaning procedures and related information, see Chapter 6. (3) HIV-1 in tissue may be demonstrated using polymerase chain reaction (PCR), immunohistochemistry, *in situ* hybridization, or immunofluorescence. (4) For immunocytochemical and molecular studies, fix tissue in ethanol or Carnoy's solution. The virus can be identified using PCR in most tissues, whether fresh, frozen, or fixed in ethanol. (5) Serologic tests as well as direct fluorescent antibody tests are avail-able for many of the expected infections. (6) This is not a reportable disease.

In Adults:

Organs and Tissues	*Procedures*	*Possible or Expected Findings*
External examination and skin	Record body weight and evidence of lipodystrophy following AIDS medications.	Cachexia. Severe loss of subcutaneous fat in face and extremities, associated with large fat deposits on upper back and upper abdomen ("protease paunch").
	Record and photograph any skin lesions. Examine oral cavity.	Cutaneous Kaposi's sarcoma *(1)*.
Blood and vitreous	If the diagnosis is in doubt, samples can be submitted for enzyme immunoassay.	Test may be positive for many weeks after death *(2)*.

Organs and Tissues	Procedures	Possible or Expected Findings
Cardiovascular system	Procedures depend on expected findings or grossly identified abnormalities as listed in right-hand column.	Increased lipochrome deposition; toxoplasmosis of myocardium; *Cytomegalovirus* and atypical mycobacterial infections *(2)*.
Respiratory tract	Culture any consolidated areas. If none can be identified, take a random section for viral culture.	Many routine and opportunistic infections; diffuse alveolar damage; diffuse interstitial fibrosis; malignant lymphoma;* foreign body granulomas (in parenteral drug users).
Gastrointestinal tract	Open and examine as soon as removed to minimize autolysis. Promptly fix any lesion. Submit sections for electron microscopy.	Villous atrophy and crypt hyperplasia of small bowel; cryptosporidiosis; microsporidiosis; *Mycobacterium avium-intracellulare* and other opportunistic infections; lymphoma.*
Liver	Record weight; sample for microbiologic and histologic study. If indicated, request acid fast stains, Grocott's methenamine silver stain, immunostains for hepatitis antigen, and Gomori's iron stain.	Hepatitis *(3)* due to hepatitis A,B,C,delta, *Mycobacterium avium-intracellulare, Cytomegalovirus, Cryptococcus;* Kaposi's sarcoma; lymphoma; erythrophagocytosis; increased hemosiderin.
Pancreas	Sample for histologic study.	*Cytomegalovirus* pancreatitis.
Adrenal glands	Record weights. Sample for histologic study.	Medullary necrosis with *Cytomegalovirus*; lipid depletion.
Lymph nodes and bone marrow	Sample enlarged lymph nodes for histologic study.	Lymphadenopathy; follicular hyperplasia; absent germinal centers; sinus histiocytosis; hemophagocytosis. Bone marrow with plasmacytosis; variable cellularity; lymphoma;* lymphoproliferative disorder.
Spleen	Record weight and sample for histologic study.	Opportunistic infections; lymphoma;* depletion of white pulp with fibrosis; increased plasma cells; hemophagocytosis; increased hemosiderin in macrophages.
Kidneys		BK virus-associated renal disease *(7)*.
Brain	For removal and specimen preparation, see Chapter 4. The saw should be used within a plastic bag or it should be fitted with a vacuum to collect aerosolized bone particles. Other procedures, including requests for special stains, depend on expected findings or grossly identified abnormalities as listed in right-hand column.	Viral (HIV encephalitis *(4)*; progressive herpes simplex, or varicella/zoster infection, multifocal leukoencephalopathy;* CMV), bacterial (*Mycobacterium avium intra-cellulare* infection; Whipple's disease; Nocardia), and fungal (*Aspergillus fumigatus; Candida albicans*; Coccidioidomycosis; Cryptococcosis; mucormycosis; histoplasmosis). Syphilis and infection with *Toxoplasma gondii* also may be found. Lymphoma;* Kaposi's sarcoma; vacuolar myelopathy; lymphocytic meningitis; cerebral hemorrhage or infarction.
Spinal cord	For removal, see Chapter 4. The saw should be fitted with a vacuum or used under a plastic cover sheet to collect aerosolized bone particles.	Demyelination of posterior columns and pyramidal tracts (vacuolar myelopathy) *(5)*; lymphoma; opportunistic infections.

[a]Vitreous tested up to 34 h postmortem and blood tested up to 58 d postmortem were consistently positive for HIV. No false-negatives *(6)*.

References

1. Fisher BK, Warner LC. Cutaneous manifestations of the acquired immunodeficiency syndrome. Intl J Dermatol 1987;26(10):615–630.
2. Lewis W. AIDS: cardiac findings from 115 autopsies. Prog Cardiovasc Dis 1989;32(3):207–215.
3. Schaffner F. The liver in HIV infection. Prog Liver Dis 1990;9:505–522.
4. Kanzer MD. Neuropathology of AIDS. Crit Rev Neurobiol 1990:5(4):313–362.
5. Hénin D, Smith TW, De Girolami U, Sughayer M, Hauw J-J. Neuropathology of the spinal cord in the acquired immunodeficiency syndrome. Hum Pathol 1992;23:1106–1114.
6. Klatt EC, Shibata D, Strigle SM. Postmortem enzyme immunoassay for human immunodeficiency virus. Arch Pathol Lab Med 1989;113:485–487.
7. Crum-Cianflone N, et al. BK virus-associated renal failure among HIV patients. AIDS 2007;21:1501–1502.

In Children ***(1,2)*****:**

Organs and Tissues	*Procedures*	*Possible or Expected Findings*
External examination and skin	Obtain body weight and external measurements. Photograph all abnormalities. Perform whole body radiographs.	Developmental delay; cachexia.
Oral cavity	Obtain exudate of ulcers for smears and culture. Scrape ulcers for Tzanck prep and viral culture.	Candidal, cytomegalovirus and herpetic ulcers; EBV-induced oral hairy leukoplakia; oral warts due to papillomavirus; bacteria-induced necrotizing ulcerative gingivitis.
Salivary glands	Submit portion of parotid gland for histologic study. The parotid gland may be obtained via the scalp incision (see Chapter 4).	Lymphocytic infiltration; infectious sialoadenitis.
Thymus	Weigh and submit for histologic study.	Precocious involution *(3)*; dysinvolution (decrease or absence of Hassall's corpuscles); thymitis with giant cells.
Cardiovascular system	Procedures depend on expected findings or grossly identified abnormalities as listed in right-hand column.	Dilated cardiomyopathy;* myocarditis;* pericardial effusion; myocardial interstitial fibrosis; opportunistic infections; fibrocalcific vasculopathy; aneurysms.
	Prepare sections for electron microscopy.	Myelin-like figures within myocytes.
Respiratory tract	Culture any consolidated areas for viruses, fungi, and bacteria. Submit sections for histologic study. Photograph any lesion suspicious for neoplasm.	Bacterial, fungal, viral, and mycobacterial pneumonias; diffuse alveolar damage; lymphoid hyperplasia; malignant lymphoma;* lymphoproliferative disorder; Kaposi's sarcoma.
Gastrointestinal tract	Open and examine intestines as soon as they are removed, so as to limit autolysis. Promptly photograph and immerse lesions in fixative. Sample lesions for histologic study.	Infections due to parasites, viruses, fungi, bacteria, and mycobacteria; ulcers; necrotizing inflammation; lymphoproliferative disorder; lymphoma (including MALT [mucosea associated lymphoid tissue] lymphoma); Kaposi's sarcoma; calcific arteriopathy.
Liver	Photograph any grossly evident lesions. Submit lesions and grossly normal liver for histologic study.	Chronic hepatitis;* opportunistic infections; cholestasis; steatosis; Kupffer cell hyperplasia; lymphoproliferative disorder; Kaposi's sarcoma.
Pancreas	Submit for histologic study.	Drug-related acute pancreatitis; chronic pancreatitis; opportunistic infections.
Lymph nodes, bone marrow		Persistent generalized lymphadenopathy (hyperplasia, involution, or lymphoid depletion); lymphoproliferative disorder; Kaposi's sarcoma; opportunistic infections; hypercellular bone marrow with increased megakaryocytes, plasmacytosis, hematophagocytosis; increased iron stores; lymphoma;* leukemia.*
Spleen	Record weight and sample for histologic study.	Concentric vascular sclerosis; depletion of red/white pulp.
Urinary system	Submit kidney for histologic study. Follow procedures described under "Glomerulonephritis." Submit sections for electron microscopy.	Focal segmental glomerulosclerosis; tubulo-Interstitial nephritis; mesangial hypercellularrity; cytomegalovirus, candidal infection.
Brain and spinal cord	For removal and specimen preparation, see Chapter 4. For prevention of aerosolization of bone particles, see previous page under "Brain" and "Spinal Cord."	Micrencephaly *(4)*; enlarged ventricles; delayed myelination; interstitial mineralization of putamen, globus pallidus, frontal lobe white matter; mononuclear glial and microglial nodules with giant cells; leptomeningitis; lymphoma;* opportunistic infections. Spinal cord with pallor of corticospinal tracts; vacuolar myelopathy.

Organs and Tissues	Procedures	Possible or Expected Findings
Placenta	Record weight and photograph all gross lesions.	Retroplacental hematoma; infarcts; acute chorioamnionitis; funisitis; abnormal villous maturation; villitis due to *Cytomegalovirus, Toxoplasma*.

References

1. Systemic Pathology of HIV Infection and AIDS in Children. Moran C, Mullick FG, eds. Armed Forces Institute of Pathology. American Registry of Pathology, Washington, DC, 1997. (To order copies, call: 202-782-2100 or write to American Registry of Pathology Sales Office, AFIP, Room 1077, Washington, DC 20306-6000.)
2. Joshi W. Pathology of acquired immunodeficiency syndrome (AIDS) in children. Keio J Med 1996;45:306–312.
3. Grody WW, Fligiel S, Naeim F. Thymus involution in the acquired immunodeficiency syndrome. Am J Clin Pathol 1985;84:85–95.
4. Kozlowski PB, Brudkowska J, Kraszpulski M, Sersen EA, Wrzolek MA, Anzil AP, et al. Micrencephaly in children congenitally infected with human immunodeficiency virus—a gross-anatomical morphometric study. Acta Neuropathol 1997;93:136–145.

Syndrome, Adams-Stokes (See "Arrhythmia, cardiac.")

Syndrome, Adult Respiratory Distress [ARDS]

Related Term: Diffuse alveolar damage; shock lung.

NOTE: For related changes in infancy, see "Syndrome, respiratory distress, of infant."

Possible Associated Conditions: Amniotic fluid embolism;* aspiration (e.g., in near-drowning accidents*); burns;* inhalation of toxic gases; major trauma (with or without fat embolism*); malignancies; pancreatitis;* radiation injury;* severe infections, and many other potentially fatal conditions may cause ARDS, particularly if they are associated with shock.*

Organs and Tissues	Procedures	Possible or Expected Findings
External examination	Prepare chest roentgenogram.	Pneumothorax* (including tension pneumothorax); pneumomediastinum.
Blood	Submit sample for microbiologic study, particularly if septicemia is suspected.	Septicemia.
	Toxicologic studies (drug screen) are indicated in some instances.	Illicit drug use; paraquat or salicylate poisoning.
Heart	If the patient had cardiopulmonary surgery, see also under name of underlying condition.	Surgical procedures that required cardiopulmonary bypass may cause ARDS.
Trachea and lungs	Determine position of endotracheal tube.	Endotracheal tube may become dislodged.
	Record lung weights. Submit samples for microbiologic study, particularly if septicemia is suspected. Perfuse one lung with formalin. For the demonstration of edema, some samples should be fixed in Bouin's solution.	Diffuse alveolar damage, with or without evidence of underlying condition such as trauma, fat embolism,* viral infection, damage from toxic inhalants (e.g., smoke, oxygen or nitrogen oxides), or aspiration (gastric acid or swimming pool water in near-drowning accidents).
Other organs	Procedures depend on expected associated conditions.	Manifestations of conditions listed above under "Possible Associated Conditions"

Syndrome, Afferent Loop

Possible Associated Conditions: Malabsorption syndrome* in patients with stasis and bacterial overgrowth in afferent loop.

Organs and Tissues	Procedures	Possible or Expected Findings
Stomach, duodenum, and jejunum	Dissect stomach and intestines *in situ*.	Previous Billroth II operation. Distension, lengthening, and kinking of afferent duodenal loop.

Syndrome, Albright's (See "Dysplasia, fibrous, of bone.")

Syndrome, Alport

Synonyms and Related Terms: Classic (X-linked) Alport syndrome; hereditary congenital hemorrhagic nephritis; hereditary nephritis with nerve deafness; nonclassic (autosomal) Alport syndrome without deafness or eye changes.

Organs and Tissues	Procedures	Possible or Expected Findings
All organs	Follow procedures described under "Glomerulonephritis" and "Failure, kidney."	Chronic glomerulonephritis* with foam cells.
Eyes	For removal and specimen preparation, see Chapter 5.	Conical deformation of the anterior surface of the lens (lenticonus) in classic Alport syndrome.

Syndrome, Aortic Arch (See "Arteritis, Takayasu's.")

Syndrome, Asplenia (See "Syndrome, polysplenia and asplenia.")

Syndrome, Ataxia-Telangiectasia

Synonym: Louis-Bar syndrome.

NOTE: See also under "Syndrome, immunodeficiency." Chronic pulmonary disease and malignancy (see below) are the most common causes of death.

Possible Associated Conditions: Malignant lymphomas* and, rarely, carcinomas.

Organs and Tissues	Procedures	Possible or Expected Findings
External examination and skin; oral cavity	Record body weight and height. Prepare photographs and histologic sections of skin lesions.	Growth retardation. Telangiectases of conjunctivas, face, ears, neck, and antecubital and popliteal fossae. Telangiectases of palate. Café au lait spots.
Thymus	Record weight and submit samples for histologic study.	Atrophy of thymus (embryonic appearance of thymus).
Blood	Submit sample for immunoglobulin determination.	IgA deficiency.
Lungs	Perfuse one lung with formalin. Submit one lobe for microbiologic study. Submit samples of all lobes for histologic study.	Bronchopulmonary infection, often with bronchiectasis. Characteristic cells in ataxia-telangiectasia (generalized nucleomegaly).
Small bowel	Record size of Peyer's plaques and prepare histologic sections.	Atrophy of Peyer's plaques.
Liver and kidneys	Record weights and sample for histologic study.	Characteristic cells in ataxia-telangiectasia (generalized nucleomegaly).
Lymph nodes	Submit samples for histologic study.	Atrophy.
Ovaries	Record presence or absence.	May be absent (agenesis).
Neck organs	Submit samples of tonsils and lymph nodes for histologic study. Record sizes.	Atrophy of tonsils and cervical lymph nodes.
Brain and spinal cord	For removal and specimen preparation, see Chapter 4.	Atrophy of cerebellar cortex with loss of Purkinje and granular cells; irregular dendritic expansions and eosinophilic cytoplasmic inclusions in some of the remaining Purkinje cells. Degeneration of posterior columns (fasciculus gracilis more than fasciculus cuneatus) of spinal cord.
Peripheral nerves	For removal and specimen preparation, see Chapter 4.	Abnormal and large cells with bizarre nuclei.

Syndrome, Banti's (See "Hypertension, portal.")

Syndrome, Barrett's (See "Esophagus, Barrett's.")

Syndrome, Bartter's (See "Aldosteronism.")

Syndrome, Bassen-Kornzweig (See "Abetalipoproteinemia.")

Syndrome, Beckwith-Wiedemann

NOTE: This cellular overgrowth syndrome may be sporadic or autosomal dominant. In some patients, a duplication of chro-mosome 11p15.5 is present.

Organs and Tissues	Procedures	Possible or Expected Findings
External examination and skin	Record body weight, as well as head, abdomen, and chest circumference, crown-heel length, crown-rump length. Record and photograph all anomalies.	Hemihypertrophy; macroglossia; infraorbital hypoplasia; grooved ear lobules; capillary nevus flammeus; large fontanels; prominent occiput; malocclusion of teeth; cliteromegaly; hypospadias.
Abdominal organs	Carefully examine organs and photograph anomalies. Submit tissue for histologic study. Submit fascia, tissue, such as liver or lung, or blood for karotype analysis.	Portal-biliary dysgenesis; hepatoblastoma; islet cell hyperplasia; cytomegaly of adrenal cortical cells; dysplastic renal medulla; Wilms tumor. Large ovaries, uterus, kidneys, and bladder; bicornuate uterus, vascular malformations *(1)*.
Brain	For removal and specimen preparation, see Chapter 4.	Brain stem gliomas. Choroid plexus adrenal heterotopias *(1)*.
Placenta and umbilical cord	Record weight. Submit sections away from periphery for histologic study.	Large placenta; edematous umbilical cord.

Reference

1. Drut R, et al. Vascular malformation and choroid plexus adrenal heterotopia: new findings in Beckwith-Wiedemann Syndrome? Fetal Pediatr Pathol 2006;25:191–197.

Syndrome, Behçet's

Organs and Tissues	Procedures	Possible or Expected Findings
External examination and skin	Record extent and character of skin and mucosal lesions. Prepare photographs; prepare sections of skin.	Ulcers *(1)* of oral mucosa; ulcers of perianal region and genitalia; erythema nodosum *(2)*; skin ulcers; subungual infarctions.
	Prepare roentgenograms of joints.	Monarthritis or polyarthritis (without deformations).
Central and peripheral and veins	For removal of femoral vessels, see Chapter 3.	Aortitis and other forms of arteritis;* arterial thromboses and peripheral arterial aneurysms; thrombophlebitis or thrombosis,* primarily of thigh and calf veins *(2)*.
Lungs		Pulmonary embolism.*
Esophagus	Remove together with stomach.	Ulcers.
Colon, rectum, and pelvic organs	Open rectum in posterior midline.	Colitis; rectovaginal fistula.
Pancreas	Sample for histologic study.	Pancreatitis.*
Neck organs	Prepare sections of cricoarytenoid joint (Chapter 2), particularly if peripheral joints cannot be studied.	Ulcer of pharynx; scarring and stenosis of hypopharynx. Laryngeal arthritis.
Brain		Encephalitis;* pseudotumor cerebri.*
Base of skull	Expose venous sinuses (see Chapter 4).	Thrombophlebitis of dural venous sinuses.
Eyes	For removal and specimen preparation, see Chapter 5.	Corneal ulceration; uveitis with hypopyon; iridocyclitis; thrombosis of central retinal vein. Eye changes may have caused blindness.
Peripheral nerves	For sampling and specimen preparation, see Chapter 4.	Peripheral neuropathy.
Skeletal muscles	For sampling and specimen preparation, see Chapter 2.	Vasculitis; inflammatory lesions; fibrosis.
Joints	For removal and specimen preparation, see Chapter 2. For proper sampling, consult roentgenograms and clinical records.	Monarthritis—for instance, of a sacroiliac joint—or polyarthritis.

Reference

1. Criteria for diagnosis of Behçet's Disease. International Study Group for Behçet's Disease. Lancet 1990;335:1078–1080.
2. Yazici H, et al. Behçet's syndrome: disease manifestations, management and advances in treatment. Nat Clin Pract Rheumatol 2007;3:148–155.

Syndrome, Bloom's

Possible Associated Condition: Acute leukemia* and other malignancies.

Organs and Tissues	*Procedures*	*Possible or Expected Findings*
External examination, oral cavity, and skin	Record facial features and status of teeth; appearance of hands; body weight and length. Record and photograph skin abnormalities and prepare sections.	Small, narrow face with prominent nose and ears; telangiectases on face, hands, forearms. Defective dentition; polysyndactyly of hands. Stunted growth or dwarfism;* ichthyosis, café au lait spots.
Blood or fascia lata	Submit blood for immunoglobulin study. For sampling for chromosome analysis, see Chapter 9. Snap-freeze tissue for identification of BLM gene *(1)*.	Reduced immunoglobulin concentrations in blood. Chromatid breaks and gaps.
Other organs		Multiple malignancies.
Eye		Macular drusen; diabetic retinopathy; leukemic retinopathy *(2)*.

References

1. Straughen JE, Johnson J, McLaren D, Proytcheva M, Ellis N, German J, Groden J. A rapid method for detecting the predominant Ashkenazi Jewish mutation in the Bloom's syndrome gene. Hum Mutation 1998;11:175–178.
2. Bhisitkul RB, Rizen M. Bloom syndrome: multiple retinopathies in a chromosome breakage disorder. Br J Opthalmol 2004;88:354–357.

Syndrome, Bonnevie-Ullrich (See "Syndrome, Turner's.")

Syndrome, Budd-Chiari

Synonyms and Related Terms: Acute veno-occlusive disease of the liver; hepatic vein thrombosis; hepatic venous outflow obstruction.

Possible Associated Conditions: Antithrombin III deficiency; oral contraceptive use; paroxysmal nocturnal hemoglobinuria;* polycythemia rubra vera;* pregnancy;* protein C deficiency.

Organs and Tissues	*Procedures*	*Possible or Expected Findings*
External examination		Dilatation of abdominal veins. Edema of extremities.
Chest organs	In most cases, it seems best to remove chest organs together with abdominal organs (see below under "Portal and inferior vena cava system; heart").	Constrictive pericarditis or right atrial myxoma may be causes of hepatic venous outflow obstruction.
Abdominal and chest cavities	Measure volume of effusions and submit for culture.	Ascites.
	For lymphangiography and dissection of the thoracic duct, see Chapter 2.	Dilatation of retroperitoneal, hepatic capsular, and anterior mediastinal lymphatics and of the thoracic duct. Dilatation (in suprahepatic obstruction) or intrahepatic obstruction of hepatic veins.
Portal and inferior vena cava system; heart	After removal of intestines, dissect mesenteric, splenic, and portal veins *in situ*. Remove chest and abdominal organs en masse. Open inferior vena cava and its branches along posterior midline from iliac veins to right atrium.	Thromboses. Tumor of right atrium. Compression of intrathoracic inferior vena cava by constrictive (calcific) pericarditis.
Hepatic veins	Identify right, middle, and left hepatic veins. Record type and location of obstruction.	Thrombosis, tumor, or webs on or near hepatic ostia. Webs usually obstruct left and middle hepatic veins and the inferior vena cava just cephalad to the patent right hepatic vein.
	Record appearance of venous ostia of caudate lobe.	Veins of caudate lobe are not involved by disease process.

Organs and Tissues	Procedures	Possible or Expected Findings
Liver	Record weight and size. Photograph venous ostia and cut section of liver. Submit samples for histologic study. Request Verhoeff–van Gieson and Gomori's iron stains. If condition was treated by liver transplantation,* search for thromboses in allograft.	Hepatic and vein thromboses *(1)*. Congestive fibrosis with uninvolved or hypertrophic caudate lobe. Hemosiderosis. Tumor(s) of the liver;* amebic abscesses, and other lesions may have caused hepatic venous outflow obstruction.
Spleen	Record weight and size.	Congestive splenomegaly. Hemosiderosis.
Esophagus and stomach	Remove together. For demonstration of esophageal varices, see Chapter 2.	Esophageal varices.*
Bone marrow	For preparation of sections and smears, see Chapter 2.	Hyperplasia. See also under "Polycythemia."
Extremities	For phlebography and for removal of femoral and popliteal vessels, see Chapter 10 and Chapter 4, respectively.	Phlebothrombosis or arterial thromboses. Thrombophlebitis migrans. Buerger's disease.*

Reference

1. Bayraktar UD, et al. Hepatic venous outflow obstruction: three similar syndromes. World J Gastroenterol 2007;13:1912–1927.

Syndrome, Caplan's

Synonyms and Related Terms: Complicated pneumoconiosis;* conglomerate silicosis; progressive massive fibrosis of coal workers.

Organs and Tissues	Procedures	Possible or Expected Findings
External examination	Prepare roentgenograms of the chest and peripheral joints.	Pulmonary nodules, often perihilar. Joint changes of rheumatoid arthritis.*
Lungs	Submit a portion of lung for microbiologic study. Perfuse one lung with formalin. Photograph slices. Request Verhoeff–van Gieson stain.	Rheumatoid-type pulmonary nodules (0.5–2.0 cm) often with necrotic center. Multiple small silicotic nodules.
Joints	For removal, prosthetic repair, and specimen preparation, see Chapter 2.	Rheumatoid arthritis.*
Other organs		Systemic manifestations of rheumatoid arthritis.*

Syndrome, Carcinoid

Synonyms and Related Terms: Argentaffinoma syndrome; carcinoid tumor; Cassidy-Scholte syndrome; malignant carcinoid syndrome.

NOTE: Autopsy should be performed as soon as possible, and tumor material should be removed first. Argentaffin cell reaction disappears within 3–6 h after death. If patient had undergone liver transplantation, see also under that heading.

Possible Associated Conditions: Cushing's syndrome;* multiple endocrine neoplasia.*

Organs and Tissues	Procedures	Possible or Expected Findings
External examination	Record extend of skin changes and prepare histologic sections of skin.	Hyperpigmentation and keratosis of skin (pellagra dermatosis).
Heart and inferior vena cava system	Remove chest and abdominal organs en masse.	
	Open inferior vena cava posteriorly and expose hepatic vein orifices, right atrium of the heart, and tricuspid valve. Photograph intimal lesions and submit samples for histologic study. Request Verhoeff–van Gieson stain. Test competence of tricuspid and pulmonary valves (Chapter 3). Open heart in direction of blood flow.	Intimal fibrosis may involve hepatic veins, upper inferior vena cava, right atrium, coronary sinus, superior vena cava, tricuspid valve, right ventricle, pulmonary valve, and, rarely, the left heart chambers. Appreciable involvement of the left heart chambers indicates active pulmonary tumor or right-to-left shunt. Tricuspid stenosis* and insufficiency,* pulmonary stenosis,* and mild mitral and aortic fibrosis may occur.

Organs and Tissues	Procedures	Possible or Expected Findings
Lungs	If primary tumor is suspected in lungs, dissect and snap-freeze fresh tumor tissue for chemical analysis. For staining, see below under "Gastrointestinal tract."	Small cell (oat cell) carcinoma. Bronchial carcinoid.
	Perfuse tumor-free lung with formalin. Request Verhoeff–van Gieson stain.	Intimal fibrosis and fibroelastosis of small pulmonary arteries.
Peritoneum	Submit samples for histologic study.	Fibrosis (rare).
Urine	Submit sample for chemical analysis.	Increased concentration of 5-hydroxyindoleacetic acid (5-HIAA). Results are not always reliable.
Gastrointestinal tract		Endocrine-active carcinoid tumor may occur in all segments except in rectum. Most frequent in ileum; occurs also in Meckel's diverticulum.
	Freeze fresh tumor for chemical analysis. For formalin-fixed tissue, request Bodian stain for argyrophil cell reaction and Fontana-Masson stain for argentaffin cell reaction. Prepare tumor samples for electron microscopy.	High concentratios of 5-hydroxyindoles. Argyrophil cell reaction may persist for 24 h after death; argentaffin cell reaction disappears within 3–6 h. Autofluorescence in ultraviolet light.
		Peptic ulcer of stomach.* If malabsorption syndrome* was present, see under that heading.
Liver	Record weight. Photograph cut section and submit samples for histologic study.	Massive metastatic involvement in most instances.
Bile ducts and gallbladder	Dissect extrahepatic bile ducts *in situ*.	May contain active tumor tissue.
Pancreas	If tumor is present, submit samples as described above under "Gastrointestinal tract."	Carcinoid tumor. Islet cell tumor.
Lymph nodes	Submit samples for histologic and chemical study.	Massive para-aortic metastases may produce carcinoid syndrome in absence of hepatic metastases.
Ovaries	If ovaries appear abnormal, record sizes and weights and sample for histologic study.	Primary carcinoid tumors may occur in teratomas. Ovaries also may be site of metastases.
Testes		Rarely, primary carcinoid tumors may occur in teratomas.
Bones and joints	For removal, prosthetic repair, and specimen preparation, see Chapter 2.	Osteogenic metastases (rare). Rheumatoid arthritis.*

Syndrome, Chédiak-Higashi

Synonyms and Related Terms: Chédiak-Higashi anomaly; Béguez-César disease; hereditary neutrophil granule dysfunction syndrome.

Possible Associated Condition: Lymphoma.*

Organs and Tissues	Procedures	Possible or Expected Findings
External examination and skin	Record extent of hypopigmented areas and of hemorrhagic and infected skin. Photograph and take sections of abnormal and of pigmented skin. Request Fontana-Masson silver stain.	Decreased pigmentation of skin and hair (albinism). Pyoderma gangrenosum. Staphylococcal skin infection. Skin hemorrhages. Enlarged melanin granules in melanocytes of pigmented areas.
Blood	Submit sample for microbiologic study and for study of immunoglobulins. Prepare smears. If fresh specimens are available, submit sample for electron microscopic study (Chapter 15).	Bacteremia; septicemia. Hypogammaglobulinemia. Large azurophilic peroxidase-positive granules (giant lysosomes) in neutrophils. Granules in lymphocytes are peroxidase-negative and periodic acid–Schiff-positive.

Organs and Tissues	Procedures	Possible or Expected Findings
Lungs	Submit any consolidated areas for bacterial culture.	Bacterial pneumonia.
Liver and spleen	Record sizes and weights. Submit samples for histologic study.	Hepatosplenomegaly. Lymphohistiocytic infiltrates.
Lymph nodes	Request Wright stain for touch preparations. Use B Plus® fixative for paraffin sections.	Lymphohistiocytic infiltrates.
Kidneys	Snap-freeze tissue for histochemical study.	Glycolipid inclusions in tubular epithelial cells.
Other organs	Procedures depend on expected findings or grossly identified abnormalities as listed in right-hand column.	Infections, particularly of upper respiratory tract, and hemorrhages caused by thrombocytopenia and coagulation factor deficiencies.
Bone marrow	For preparation of sections and smears, see p. 96. Snap-freeze material for histochemical study. Prepare sample for electron microscopy.	Large azurophilic granules in promyelocytes. Granules positive for acid phosphatase and myeloperoxidase. Lymphocytic infiltrates in accelerated phase of disease. Megaloblastic changes.
Brain and spinal cord	For removal and specimen preparation, see Chapter 4. Snap-freeze material for histochemical study. Prepare sample for electron microscopy.	Lymphohistiocytic infiltrates. Glycolipid inclusions in neurons and histiocytes. Giant lysosomes.
Peripheral nerves	For sampling and specimen preparation, see Chapter 4. Prepare sample for electron microscopic study.	Lymphohistiocytic infiltrates. Degeneration of nerve tissue. Giant lysosomes.
Eyes	For removal and specimen preparation, see Chapter 5.	Decreased pigmentation (oculocutaneous albinism) of uvea and particularly of retina.

Syndrome, Churg-Strauss (See "Granulomatosis, allergic, and angiitis (Churg-Strauss syndrome).")

Syndrome, Congenital Rubella

Synonym and Related Term: Congenital rubella; rubella.*

NOTE: See also "Rubella." (1) Collect all tissues that appear to be infected. (2) Request viral cultures. (3) Usually, special stains are not helpful. (4) No special precautions are indicated. (5) Serologic studies are available from local or state health department laboratories. (6) This is a **reportable** disease.

Organs and Tissues	Procedures	Possible or Expected Findings
External examination and umbilical cord; oral cavity	Record body weight and length. Record and photograph abnormalities as listed in right-hand column.	Intrauterine growth retardation; failure to thrive; purpura; jaundice; hypoplastic mandible; microcephaly; enamel hypoplasia; caries; delayed eruption of deciduous teeth; skin dimples; abnormal dermatoglyphics; skin pigmentation.
	Record appearance of external genitalia.	Hypospadias; cryptorchidism.
Cardiovascular system	Procedures depend on expected findings or grossly identified abnormalities as listed in right-hand column.	Congenital heart disease; myocarditis;* pulmonary artery branch stenosis; systemic arterial hypoplasia and stenosis due to intimal proliferation.
Lungs	Perfuse at least one lung with formalin.	Interstitial pneumonia.*
Liver	Record weight. Submit samples for histologic study. For cholangiography, see Chapter 2.	Giant cell hepatitis; cholestasis; fibrosis; cirrhosis;* necrosis; extramedullary hematopoiesis; bile duct proliferation mimicking biliary atresia.
Spleen	Record weight and sample for histologic study.	Splenomegaly with extramedullary hematopoiesis.
Blood	Submit sample for determination of IgM and IgG antibodies.	

Organs and Tissues	Procedures	Possible or Expected Findings
Lymph nodes	Submit samples for histologic study.	Lymphadenopathy with enlarged germinal centers or lymphoid depletion.
Kidneys	Submit samples for histologic study.	Extramedullary hematopoiesis; glomerulonephritis.
Pancreas	Submit samples for histologic study.	Lymphocytic infiltration of islets.
Brain and spinal cord	For removal and specimen preparation, see Chapter 4.	Microcephaly; meningoencephalitis;* ischemic necrosis; later in life, progressive panencephalitis; perivascular mononuclear infiltrates; glial nodules in white matter.
Ears	For removal and specimen preparation, see Chapter 4.	Otitis media;* inflammation and scarring of cochlea.
Eyes	For removal and specimen preparation, see Chapter 5.	Microphthalmia; iridocyclitis; cataracts; chorioretinitis.
Skeletal muscles	For specimen preparation, see Chapter 2.	Myositis.
Bones	For removal and specimen preparation, see Chapter 2.	Metaphyseal osteoporosis;* retardation of ossification.
Placenta	Record weight and sample for histologic study.	Villus vessel necrosis; villus edema; necrosis of syncytiotrophoblast with fibrin accretion; plasma cell deciduitis. With infection late in gestation, villus sclerosis and small placenta.

Syndrome, Conn's (See "Aldosteronism.")

Syndrome, Cronkhite-Canada (See "Polyposis, familial, and related syndromes.")

Syndrome, Cushing's

Related Terms: Cushing's disease (associated with ACTH-producing pituitary tumor); hypercorticism.

NOTE: Glucocorticoid therapy is the most common cause of Cushing's syndrome and thus, the autopsy also may show the features of the condition that had been treated—for example, an allograft with signs of rejection.

Organs and Tissues	Procedures	Possible or Expected Findings
External examination and skin	Record body weight and length, abdominal circumference, skeletal muscle development, and hair distribution. Prepare sections of skin and smears of infectious skin lesions. Request Gram and Grocott's methenamine silver stains.	"Moon face"; obesity of trunk; edema and striae of abdomen, hips, and shoulders. Muscle wasting. Virilism in women (acne and hirsutism) and children. Ecchymoses. Skin infections.
	Prepare skeletal roentgenograms.	Osteoporosis.*
Blood	Submit sample for biochemical study.	Increased concentrations of cortisol or adrenocorticotropic hormone (ACTH)-like substances. (There is diurnal variability.)
Heart	Record weight.	Hypertrophy secondary to hypertension.*
Lungs	Snap-freeze tumor tissue for determination of ACTH-like substances.	Bronchogenic carcinoma (oat cell type) or malignant bronchial carcinoid, producing ACTH-like substances.
Pancreas	See above under "Lungs."	Malignant islet cell tumor, producing ACTH-like substances.
Adrenal glands	Record weight, size, and thickness of cortex of both adrenal glands. Snap-freeze tumor tissue for biochemical study. See also under "Tumor of the adrenal glands." Submit samples of both glands for histologic study.	Adrenal nodular hyperplasia; adrenal cortical adenoma or carcinoma. Pheochromocytoma, producing ACTH-like substances. Adrenocortical hypertrophy secondary to ACTH stimulation. Atrophy of adrenal cortex after steroid therapy or secondary to effects of adrenocortical tumor.

Organs and Tissues	Procedures	Possible or Expected Findings
Kidneys		Nephrolithiasis.*
Ovaries	Record sizes and weights. If tumor is present, snap-freeze sample for determination of ACTH-like substances. Submit samples for histologic study.	Ovarian tumor, producing ACTH-like substances.
Thyroid gland	See above under "Ovaries."	Carcinoma of thyroid gland, producing ACTH-like substances.
Other organs	See above under "Lungs," "Pancreas," "Ovaries," and "Thyroid gland."	ACTH-like substances may be produced by tumors at various sites.
Pituitary gland	For removal and specimen preparation, see Chapter 4. Submit samples for histologic study. Snap-freeze tumor tissue for biochemical study. See also under "Tumor of the pituitary gland."	A normal pituitary gland is compatible with increased secretion of ACTH and with Cushing's disease. Pituitary micro- or macroadenoma (Cushing's disease), basophilic or chromophobic type. Crooke's hyaline degeneration in adenohypophysis indicates that excessive amounts of glucocorticoids had been present.
Bones	For removal and specimen preparation, see Chapter 2.	Osteoporosis.*
Skeletal muscles	For sampling and specimen preparation.	Steroid myopathy and atrophy.
Vitreous	Submit sample for glucose, sodium, and chloride determination.	Hyperglycemia or electrolyte abnormalities may be present.

Syndrome, DiGeorge's

Synonyms and Related Terms: Harrington syndrome; 3rd and 4th pharyngeal pouch syndrome; thymic agenesis, 22q11.2 deletion syndrome.

NOTE: See also "Syndrome, primary immunodeficiency."

Organs and Tissues	Procedures	Possible or Expected Findings
External examination	Record body weight and length. Record and photograph abnormalities as listed in right-hand column.	Growth retardation. Hypertelorism; anti-mongoloid slant of eyes; short philtrum; small and low set ears; notched pinnae; micrognathia. Eczema *(1)*.
Heart	See under specific lesion as listed in right-hand column.	Conotruncal and aortic arch anomalies.
Lungs	If any consolidated areas are identified, submit for culture.	Pneumonia; pulmonary abscess.
Other organs and tissues	Record and photograph abnormalities and submit possible infectious lesions for culture.	Infections at various sites.
Neck organs	Carefully search for thymus, parathyroid glands, and isthmus of thyroid.	Absence of thymus and parathyroid glands (3rd and 4th pharyngeal pouch derivatives) *(2)*. Absence of thyroid gland (rare) or of isthmus of thyroid.
Brain	For removal see Chapter 4.	Basal ganglia calcification *(3)*.

References

1. Archer E, Chuang TY, Hong R. Severe eczema in a patient with DiGeorge's syndrome. Cutis 1990;45:455–459.
2. Robinson HB Jr. DiGeorge's syndrome or the III - IV pharyngeal pouch syndrome: pathology and a theory of pathogenesis. Perspect Pediatr Pathol 1975;3:773–206.
3. Sieberer M, et al. Basal ganglia calcification and psychosis in 22q11.2 deletion syndrome. Eur Psychiatry 2005;20:567–569.

Syndrome, Down's

Synonyms and Related Terms: Mongolism; trisomy 21; trisomy G syndrome.

Possible Associated Conditions: Acute lymphocytic, myelocytic or megakaryocytic leukemia;* atresia of esophagus;* atre-sia or stenosis of duodenum;* congenital heart disease (especially ventricular septal defects and atrioventricular canal defects*).

Organs and Tissues	*Procedures*	*Possible or Expected Findings*
External examination and oral cavity	Record and photograph abnormalities as listed in right-hand column.	Epicanthal folds; cleft lip/palate; high arched palate; furrowed tongue; rhagades. Depressed nasal bridge; dysplastic ears; small, broad or flat nose; slanted palpebral fissures; flat occiput; brachycephaly; palmar "simian crease"; short fifth middle finger; short limbs; abnormal dermatoglyphics;
	Prepare radiographs of pelvis.	Horizontal acetabular roof.
Blood; fascia lata	Submit samples for chromosome study.	Complete trisomy 21 or trisomy 12q due to a translocation.
Heart	Procedures depend on grossly identified abnormalities as listed in right-hand column.	Ventricular septal defect;* complete atrioventricular septal defect* *(1)*.
Gastrointestinal tract	Open stomach and duodenum *in situ*; if indicated, probe anus.	Duodenal stenosis and atresia; imperforate anus.
Brain and spinal cord	For removal and specimen preparation, see Chapter 4.	Microcephaly; poorly developed secondary gyri; open operculum; hypoplastic superior temporal gyrus *(2)*; short corpus callosum; hypoplastic brain stem, medulla and cerebellum; polymicrogyria; neurofibrillary tangles; meningomyelocoele.
Bone marrow	For preparation of sections and smears, see Chapter 2.	Acute lymphocytic leukemia; acute myelocytic leukemia; acute megakaryocytic leukemia.

References

1. Spicer RL. Cardiovascular disease in Down syndrome. Pediatr Clin North Am 1984;31(6):1331–1344.
2. Jay V. Brain and eye pathology in an infant with Down syndrome and tuberous sclerosis. Pediatr Neurol 1996;15:57–59.

Syndrome, Dystonia

Synonyms or Related Terms: Dopa-responsive dystonia (Segawa's syndrome); inherited or sporadic primary (or idiopathic) dystonia; primary torsion dystonia (dystonia musculorum deformans); secondary (or symptomatic) dystonia.

NOTE: Primary dystonia includes primary torsion dystonia (autosomal-dominant), an X-linked form, and Dopa responsive dystonia. The condition may be focal, multifocal, segmental, generalized, or appear as hemidystonia.

Organs and Tissues	*Procedures*	*Possible or Expected Findings*
Brain, spinal cord, and spinal ganglia	For removal and specimen preparation, see Chapter 4. Autopsy in cases of primary torsion dystonia should be considered a research procedure; extensive collection of tissue is indicated, including frozen samples.	No diagnostic pathologic changes in primary torsion dystonia. In hemidystonia, changes in the basal ganglia may be found, such as infarcts, tumors, or effects of trauma or toxic damage. These last findings may have medicolegal implications.

Syndrome, Eaton-Lambert (See "Myasthenia gravis.")

Syndrome, Ehlers-Danlos

NOTE: Nine subtypes have been distinguished, based primarily on the extent of the disease. However much overlap exists.

Organs and Tissues	*Procedures*	*Possible or Expected Findings*
External examination, skin, and oral cavity	Record body weight, length, stature; record and photograph all abnormal features, as listed in right-hand column. Procure subcutaneous tissue to establish cell line for genetic testing.	Widely spaced eyes; epicanthal folds; broad nasal bridge; lop ears. Flatfeet or clubfeet; genu recurvatum; arachnodactyly; pigeon breast; kyphoscoliosis. Umbilical and inguinal hernias. Subcutaneous emphysema (see below under "Chest cavity"). Poorly formed teeth. High arched palate.

Organs and Tissues	Procedures	Possible or Expected Findings
External examination, skin, and oral cavity *(continued)*	Prepare sections of skin and request Verhoeff–van Gieson stain. Submit samples of skin for electron microscopic study.	Hyperelasticity of skin, bruises or scars, hemorrhages, and hyperpigmentation. Lipomatous pseudotumors that may be calcified or ossified. Normal or abnormal amounts and fragmentation of elastic tissue. Abnormalities of collagen.
	Prepare skeletal roentgenograms.	Dislocation of hip, shoulder, patella, radius, or clavicle. Loose-end clavicles; spondylolisthesis; osteolytic changes in distal phalanges. Degenerative arthritis.
Chest cavity	Record appearance of pleural surfaces *in situ*.	Rupture of lung with mediastinal and subcutaneous emphysema (see above).
Heart and great vessels	Procedures depend on grossly identified abnormalities as listed in right-hand column.	Congenital malformations of the heart. Mitral valve prolapse; Aortic insufficiency.* Aortic dissection, aneurysm, ectasia, occlusion *(1)*.
Lungs	Perfuse at least one lung with formalin.	Various congenital anomalies.
Other organs and tissues	Procedures depend on expected findings or grossly identified abnormalities as listed in right-hand column.	Congenital anomalies of gastrointestinal and genitourinary tracts.
	Record size and location of hematomas. Prepare tissue samples with small vessels for electron microscopic study (see Chapter 15).	Bleeding from various organ sites.
Joints	For removal, prosthetic repair, and specimen preparation, see Chapter 2.	Arthritis;* hemarthrosis. Effusions. Hyperextensibility of joints.

Reference

1. Zilocchi M, et al. Vascular Ehlers-Danlos syndrome: imaging findings. Am J Roentgenol 2007;189:712–719.

Syndrome, Ellis-Van Creveld

Synonyms and Related Terms: Chondrodysplasia;* chondroectodermal dysplasia; short-rib polydactyly chondrodysplasia.

NOTE: This syndrome belongs to a large family (with more than 30 subtypes) of chondrodysplasias. The suggested autopsy procedures are essentially the same in all chondrodysplasias. See also under "Chondrodysplasia."

Organs and Tissues	Procedures	Possible or Expected Findings
External examination	Record and photograph abnormal features as listed in right-hand column.	Short-limb dwarfism* with narrowing of the rib cage; polydactyly; dysplasia of fingernails; thin and sparse hair; premature eruption of teeth; defective dentition; eye abnormalities; upper lip bound down by multiple frenula.
	Record appearance of external genitalia.	Cryptorchidism; epispadias; hypospadias.
	Prepare skeletal roentgenograms.	Chondrodysplasia with acromelic micromelia (shortening of the distal segment of the limb); fusion of capitate and hamate bones of wrist; defects of lateral aspect of proximal tibia.
Heart		Congenital heart disease (atrial septal defect*).
Bones	Procure long bones and vertebral bodies	See lesions listed above under "External examination." Delayed ossification with or without disorganization.

Syndrome, Empty Sella

Synonyms and Related Terms: Primary empty sella syndrome; secondary empty sella syndrome (e.g., after surgical removal or spontaneous infarction of pituitary adenoma).

Organs and Tissues	Procedures	Possible or Expected Findings
External examination	Record body weight and length.	Empty sella syndrome relatively common in obese females.
	Prepare roentgenogram of skull.	Enlargement of pituitary fossa visible on lateral roentgenograms of the skull.
Base of skull and pituitary gland	For exposure and specimen preparation, see Chapter 4. Photograph sella.	Flattening and postero-inferior displacement of the gland. Necrosis of pituitary gland (Sheehan's syndrome*) or of pituitary adenoma.
Other organs		Manifestations of pituitary insufficiency* (mostly in association with secondary empty sella syndrome).

Syndrome, Eosinophilic (Unspecified) (See "Cardiomyopathy, restrictive [eosinophilic type]," "Gastroenteritis, eosinophilic," and "Syndrome, eosinophilic pulmonary.")

Syndrome, Eosinophilic Pulmonary

Synonyms and Related Terms: Acute eosinophilic pneumonia with respiratory failure *(1)*; allergic bronchopulmonary aspergillosis; Carrington's chronic eosinophilic pneumonia; Churg-Strauss syndrome; eosinophilic pneumonia; hypereosinophilic syndrome; idiopathic acute eosinophilic pneumonia; Löffler's syndrome; pulmonary infiltration with eosinophilia (PIE syndrome); tropical pulmonary eosinophilia.

NOTE: For review of eosinophilic lung diseases, see Ref *(4)*.

Organs and Tissues	Procedures	Possible or Expected Findings
External examination	Prepare chest roentgenogram.	Pulmonary infiltrates.
Lungs	Submit a section for culture. Freeze portion of same lung for special studies. Prepare smears. Perfuse one lung with formalin. Request Giemsa or azure-eosin stain for demonstration of eosinophilic leukocytes.	Ascariasis and hookworm (pulmonary larval migration) infestation *(2)*; other parasitic diseases or fungal infections. Bronchiolitis obliterans; eosinophilic microabscesses *(3)*.
Other organs	Procedures depend on expected findings or grossly identified abnormalities as listed in right-hand column.	Systemic manifestations of eosinophilia; parasitic or other infectious or allergic disease.

References

1. Tazelaar H, Linz LJ, Colby TV, Myers JL, Limper AH. Acute eosinophilic pneumonia: Histopathologic features in nine cases. Am Rev Resp Crit Care Med 1997;155:296–302.
2. Sarinas PS, Chitkara RK. Ascariasis and hookworm. Semin Resp Inf 1997;12:130–137.
3. Jederlinic PJ, Sicilian L, Gaensler EA. Chronic eosinophilic pneumonia. A report of 19 cases and a review of the literature. Medicine 1988;67:154–162.
4. Jeong YJ et al. Eosinophilic lung diseases: a clinical, radiologic, and pathologic overview. Radiographics 2007;27:617–637.

Syndrome, Extrapyramidal (See "Chorea, acute," "Chorea, hereditary," and "Disease, Parkinson's.")

Syndrome, Fanconi

Related Terms: Aminoaciduria;* cystinosis;* familial hypophosphatemic vitamin D-resistant rickets; galactosemia;* proximal tubular transport defect; tyrosinemia.* Excludes Fanconi's anemia (sometimes also called Fanconi's syndrome) due to a defect in DNA repair.

Organs and Tissues	Procedures	Possible or Expected Findings
External examination	Record body weight and external measurements; record and photograph abnormalities as listed in right-hand column.	Red/blond hair, fair skin (diminished pigmentation); dehydration;* stigmata of hypothyroidism;* delay of sexual maturation.
	Prepare skeletal roentgenograms. Radiographs of long bones.	Rickets; osteomalacia.*
Fascia lata	Submit for tissue culture for possible enzyme analysis.	

Organs and Tissues	Procedures	Possible or Expected Findings
Blood	Obtain sample for possible assay of heavy metals. Obtain sample for protein electrophoresis and parathyroid hormone assay.	Lead,* mercury,* cadmium,* uranium poisoning; myeloma;* parathyroid hyperplasia (primary or secondary).
Kidney	Photograph lesions. Submit for histologic study. nephrolithiasis.*	Cysts; nephrocalcinosis; pyelonephritis;*
Urine	Obtain sample for biochemical analysis.	Glucosuria; phosphaturia; aminoaciduria.

Syndrome, Felty's

Related Terms: Pseudo-Felty syndrome *(1)*; rheumatoid arthritis.*

Organs and Tissues	Procedures	Possible or Expected Findings
External examination, skin, and oral cavity	Record body weight and length.	Cachexia.
	Record extent and character of skin infections and ulcers, appearance of eyes and oral cavity, and character of pigmentation. Sample skin lesions for histologic study.	Infections involving skin, oral cavity, and eyes (corneas). Chronic leg ulcers. Brown pigmentation over exposed areas of extremities.
Subcutaneous tissues and lymph nodes	Submit samples of axillary, cervical, and other enlarged lymph nodes and all subcutaneous nodules for histologic study.	Lymphadenopathy. Rheumatoid nodules.
Blood	Submit sample for serologic study.	Positive rheumatoid factor.
Lungs	Submit a section for bacterial and fungal cultures. Perfuse one lung with formalin.	Various types of pneumonia. Bronchiectasis.*
Liver	Record weight and sample for histologic study.	Nodular regenerative hyperplasia *(2)*; sinusoidal lymphocytosis *(3)*.
Spleen	Record size and weight. If splenectomy had been done, record presence or absence of accessory spleens.	Splenomegaly *(4)*. After splenectomy, presence of accessory spleen may account for treatment failure.
Other organs		Manifestations of portal hypertension.*
Mediastinal and retroperitoneal lymph nodes	Submit samples for histologic study.	Lymphadenopathy of mediastinal and para-aortic lymph nodes.
Bone marrow, bones, and joints	For preparation of bone marrow sections and smears, see Chapter 2.	Anemia;* neutropenia; thrombocytopenia.
	For removal, prosthetic repair, and specimen preparation of bones and joints, see Chapter 2.	Rheumatoid arthritis.*

References

1. Rosenstein ED, Kramer N. Felty's and pseudo-Felty's syndrome. Semin Arthritis Rheum 1991;21:129–142.
2. Perez-Ruiz F, Orte Martinez FJ, Zea Mendoza AC, Ruiz del Arbol L, Moreno Caparros A. Nodular regenerative hyperplasia of the liver in rheu-matic diseases: report of seven cases and review of the literature. Semin Arthritis Rheum 1991;21:47–54.
3. Cohen ML, Manier JW, Bredfeldt JE. Sinusoidal lymphocytosis of the liver in Felty's syndrome with a review of the liver involvement in Felty's syndrome. J Clin Gastroenterol 1989;11:92–94.
4. Fishman D, Isenberg DA. Splenic involvement in rheumatic diseases. Semin Arthritis Rheum 1997;27:141–155.

Syndrome, Fetal Alcoholic

Organs and Tissues	Procedures	Possible or Expected Findings
External examination and oral cavity	Record body weight and length, and head circumference. Record and photograph all abnormalities as listed in right-hand column.	Growth retardation; microcephaly; depressed nasal bridge; thin upper lip; smooth philtrum; epicanthal folds; small palpebral fissures; strabismus; midfacial hypoplasia; cleft palate; pectus excavatum; small nails; abnormal palmar creases; hirsutism; contractures; spina bifida; pigmented nevi.

Organs and Tissues	*Procedures*	*Possible or Expected Findings*
Diaphragm	Record location, character, and size of defects.	Anomalies of diaphragm.
Liver	Record weight and sample for histologic study.	Steatosis; fibrosis.
Heart		Ventricular and atrial septal defects.*
Brain		Hydrocephalus; micrencephaly; small frontal lobes; irregular convolutions or microgyria; small third ventricle; arhinencephaly; abnormal lamination of cortical cells; malorientaton of neurons; cerebellar heterotopias *(1)*.
Eyes	For removal and specimen preparation, see Chapter 5.	Hypoplasia of optic nerve head; increased tortuosity of retinal vessels.

Reference

1. Johnson VP, Swayze VW II, Sato Y, Andreasen NC. Fetal alcohol syndrome: craniofacial and central nervous system manifestations. Am J Med Genet 1996;61(4):329–339.

Syndrome, Fibrosing

Synonyms and Related Terms: Dupuytren's contracture; mediastinal fibrosis; multifocal fibrosclerosis; periureteral fibrosis; Peyronie's disease; pseudotumor of the orbit; retroperitoneal fibrosis,* Riedel's thyroiditis; sclerosing cholangitis;* sclerosing mediastinitis.*

NOTE: In rare instances, the conditions listed under "Synonyms and Related Terms" appear to occur together or overlap. Autopsy procedures in the most important conditions are listed under the specific title (see names with *). In all cases, other possible sites of fibrosis should be carefully studied.

Organs and Tissues	*Procedures*	*Possible or Expected Findings*
Mediastinum	If there is evidence of fibrosis, submit tissues for culture of *Histoplasma capsulatum*. Prepare horizontal sections through fixed tissues.	Superior vena cava obstruction. Sclerosing mediastinitis.* Histoplasmosis.*
Biliary system		Sclerosing cholangitis.*
Retroperitoneum		Retroperitoneal fibrosis.* Periureteral fibrosis.
Other organs and tissues	Procedures depend on expected findings or grossly identified abnormalities as listed in right-hand column. Use cultures and special stains to rule out underlying infection or tumor.	Dupuytren's contracture; pseudotumor of the orbit; Riedel's thyroiditis; Peyronie's disease; and possibly other fibrosing conditions.

Syndrome, Foix-Alajouanine (See "Malformation, arteriovenous, cerebral or spinal [or both].")

Syndrome, Gardner's (See "Polyposis, familial, and related syndromes.")

Syndrome, Gasser's (See "Syndrome, hemolytic uremic.")

Syndrome, Goodpasture's

Related Term: Goodpasture's disease.

NOTE: For a pertinent review, see ref. *(1)*.

Organs and Tissues	*Procedures*	*Possible or Expected Findings*
Lungs	Record weights. Photograph surface of lungs. Submit a portion for general bacterial and viral cultures.	Influenza virus infection.

Organs and Tissues	Procedures	Possible or Expected Findings
Lungs *(continued)*	Photograph cut surface of fresh lung. Snap-freeze tissue block for immunofluorescent study. Perfuse one lung with formalin. Request Gomori's iron and Verhoeff–van Gieson stains. Prepare samples for electron microscopic study (Chapter 15).	Pulmonary hemorrhages. Interstitial pulmonary fibrosis.
Kidneys	Follow procedures described under "Glomerulonephritis."	Anti-basement membrane antibody mediated nephritis (Goodpasture's disease). Glomeruli may appear normal or show focal proliferative or necrotizing changes. Linear immunofluorescence of glomerular basement membrane, indicating presence of IgG (or rarely IgA) *(2)*.
Urine	Submit sample for protein determination and study of sediment.	Proteinuria; hematuria; casts.
Other organs	Histologic samples should include heart, liver, spleen, lymph nodes, intestine, testes, and tissue from nasopharynx.	Histologic study of multiple organs may be needed to rule out other systemic diseases such as Wegener's granulomatosis.*

Reference

1. Bolton WK. Goodpasture's syndrome. Kidney Intl 1996;50:1753–1766.
2. Fischer EG, Lager DJ. Anti-glomerular basement membrane glomerulonephritis: a morphologic study of 80 cases. Am J Clin Path 2006;125:445–450.

Syndrome, Grönblad-Strandberg (See "Pseudoxanthoma elasticum.")

Syndrome, Guillain-Barré

Synonyms: Acute inflammatory polyradiculoneuropathy; Guillain-Barré-Strohl syndrome; idiopathic polyneuritis; Landry's ascending paralysis.

Organs and Tissues	Procedures	Possible or Expected Findings
Cerebrospinal fluid	For removal, see Chapter 7.	Increased proteins; normocellular.
Brain, spinal cord, dorsal and ventral roots of spinal cord, and spinal ganglia	For removal and specimen preparation, see Chapter 4. Request Luxol fast blue stain for demonstration of myelin and Bielschowky's stain for axons. Embed samples in plastic for thick, toluidin-stained sections and for electron microscopic study.	Segmental demyelination and mononuclear infiltrates in cranial and spinal nerve roots. If axons are involved, there is chromatolysis of lower motor neurons (spinal cord and brain stem).
Peripheral nerves	For sampling and specimen preparation, see Chapter 4 and above under "Brain, spinal cord,..."	Segmental demyelination and mononuclear infiltrates.
Eyes	For removal and specimen preparation, see Chapter 5.	Papilledema.
Urinary bladder and kidneys	Procedures depend on grossly identified abnormalities as listed in right-hand column.	Urinary retention with urocystitis and pyelonephritis.*

Syndrome, Hamman-Rich (See "Pneumonia, interstitial.")

Syndrome, Hand-Schüller-Christian (See "Histiocytosis, Langerhans cell.")

Syndrome, Hemolytic Uremic

Related Term: Thrombotic thrombocytopenic purpura *(1)*.

NOTE: If the patient underwent organ transplantation, see under "Transplantation,..."; use of cyclosporine may be a cause of hemolytic uremic syndrome *(2)*. Antineoplastics may have a similar effect.

Organs and Tissues	Procedures	Possible or Expected Findings
Kidney	Record weights, photograph, and sample for histologic study.	Renal cortical necrosis;* thromboses of glomerular arterioles and capillaries.
Gastrointestinal tract	If indicated, submit intestinal contents for microbiologic study.	Enterohemorrhagic *E. coli* 0157:H7 infection *(3)*.
Pancreas	Submit for histologic study.	Pancreatitis may be a complication or, rarely, a cause of the disease.
Other organs and tissues	Procedures depend on expected findings or grossly identified abnormalities as listed in right-hand column.	Childhood infection. Disseminated intravascular coagulation.* Toxemia of pregnancy.* Premature separation of placenta. Manifes-festations of HIV infection *(4)*. Malignancies such as carcinoma of prostate *(5)*.

References

1. Neild GH. Hemolytic uremic syndrome/thrombotic thrombocytopenic purpura: pathophysiology and treatment. Kidney Intl 1998;64:S45–S49.
2. Katznelson S, Wilkinson A, Rosenthal TR, Cohen A, Nast C, Danovitch GM. Cyclosporin-induced hemolytic uremic syndrome: factors that obscure its diagnosis. Transpl Proc 1994;26:2608–2609.
3. Koutkia P, Mylonakis E, Flanigan T. Enterohemorrhagic Escherichia coli 0157:H7: an emerging pathogen. Am Family Physician 1997;56: 853–856.
4. Badesha PS, Saklayen MG. Hemolytic uremic syndrome as a presenting form of HIV infection. Nephron 1996;72:472–475.
5. Muller NJ, Pestalozzi BC. Hemolytic uremic syndrome in prostatic carcinoma. Oncol 1998;55:174–176.

Syndrome, Hepatorenal

NOTE: Decompensated cirrhosis* of the liver with ascites is almost always present. Most possible causes of hepatorenal failure, such as intrarenal shunting or reduced plasma volume, have no anatomic substrate. A possible and demonstrable mech-anical cause is enlargement of the caudate lobe, which may compress the hepatic fossa of the inferior vena cava. For roentgenologic demonstration of this system, see Chapter 2 (renal venography). See also under "Obstruction, inferior vena cava." The kidneys are often autolytic—particularly if jaundice is severe—but usually fail to show other morphologic abnormalities.

Syndrome, Heterotaxy (See "Syndrome, polysplenia and asplenia.")

Syndrome, Hunter-Hurler (See "Mucopolysaccharidosis.")

Syndrome, Hypereosinophilic (See "Cardiomyopathy, restrictive [with eosinophilia]," "Gastroenteritis, eosinophilic," and "Syndrome, eosinophilic pulmonary.")

Syndrome, Hypoplastic Left Heart (See "Atresia, aortic valvular.")

Syndrome, Immunodeficiency (See "Syndrome, acquired immunodeficiency (AIDS)" and "Syndrome, primary immunodeficiency.")

Syndrome, Intravascular Coagulation and Fibrinolysis (See "Coagulation, disseminated intravascular.")

Syndrome, Kimmelstiel-Wilson (See "Diabetes mellitus.")

Syndrome, Klinefelter's

Synonym: Seminiferous tubule dysgenesis.

Possible Associated Conditions: Carcinoma; chronic pulmonary disease; congenital malformations; diabetes mellitus* *(1)*; Down's syndrome;* leukemia;* malignant lymphoma;* Osler's disease;* progressive systemic sclerosis;* Sjögren's syndrome;* systemic lupus erythematosus.*

Organs and Tissues	Procedures	Possible or Expected Findings
External examination and breast tissue	Record body weight and length and length of lower extremities.	Tall person with long lower extremities; eunuchoidism; varicose veins.
	Record appearance of external genitalia.	Hypoplastic external genitalia; cryptorchidism; hypospadias.
	Prepare histologic sections of breast tissue.	Gynecomastia.
	Prepare skeletal roentgenograms.	Deformities—for instance, radioulnar synostosis.
Blood or fascia lata	Submit tissue or blood for chromosome analysis. Refrigerate blood sample for possible hormone assay.	47, XXY and less common variants, including sex chromosome mosaicism.
Urine	Refrigerate specimen for possible hormone assay.	
Endocrine organs	Record weights and dimensions of both testes.	Germ cell deficiency or hyalinization of seminiferous tubules. Usually, longitudinal axis of testes is smaller than 2 cm.
	Record weights of all endocrine glands. Prepare histologic sections of adrenal glands and of pituitary gland.	

Organs and Tissues	Procedures	Possible or Expected Findings
Other organs and tissues	Procedures depend on expected findings or grossly identified abnormalities as listed in right-hand column.	Suprasellar tumors of maldevelopmental origin *(2)*. Extragonodal germ cell tumors *(3, 4)*.

References

1. Robinson S, Kessling A. Diabetes secondary to genetic disorders. Baillieres Clin Endocrin Metabol 1992;6:867–898.
2. Hamed LM, Maria BL, Quisling R, Fanous MM, Mickle P. Suprasellar tumors of maldevelopmental origin in Klinefelter's syndrome. A report of two cases. J Clin Neuro-Ophthalmol 1992;12:192–197.
3. Tay HP, Bidair M, Shabaik A, Gilbaugh JH 3rd, Schmidt JD. Primary yolk sac tumor of the prostate in a patient with Klinefelter's syndrome. J Urol 1995;153:1066–1069.
4. Aguirre D, et al. Extragonodal germ cell tumors are often associated with Klinefelter syndrome. Hum Pathol 2006;37:477–480.

Syndrome, Klippel-Feil

Synonym: Congenital fusion of cervical vertebrae.

Organs and Tissues	Procedures	Possible or Expected Findings
External examination		Short neck. Disorders with dysraphia (see below).
	Prepare roentgenograms of chest, neck, and head.	Fusion of cervical vertebrae. Congenital elevation of the scapula (Sprengel's deformity).
Skull, spine, brain, and spinal cord		Arnold-Chiari malformation;* basilar impression;* meningomyelocele; platybasia;* spinal cord compression; syringomyelia.*

Syndrome, Korsakoff (See "Syndrome, Wernicke-Korsakoff.")

Syndrome, Lambert-Eaton (See "Myasthenia gravis.")

Syndrome, Laurence-Moon-Biedl

Related Term: Bardet-Biedl syndrome *(1)*.

Organs and Tissues	Procedures	Possible or Expected Findings
External examination	Record body weight and length; record and photograph abnormalities as listed in right-hand column.	Obesity;* polydactyly; developmental delay in infants. Dysmorphic extremities. Hypogonadism in males *(1)*.
Liver	Record weight and sample for histologic study.	Congenital hepatic fibrosis* *(2)*.
Kidneys	If renal transplantation *(3)* had been carried out, see also under that heading. Follow procedures described under "glomerulonephritis."	Renal cysts, tubulointerstitial nephritis and focal sclerosing glomerulonephritis. Calyceal clubbing and blunting *(4)*.
Gonads	Submit samples for histologic study.	Hypogonadism.
Eyes	For removal and specimen preparation, see Chapter 5.	Retinal dystrophy *(1)* and other retinal changes.

References

1. Green JS, Parfrey PS, Harnett JD, Farid NR, Cramer BC, Johnson G, et al. The cardinal manifestations of Bardet-Biedl syndrome, a form of Laurence-Moon-Biedl syndrome. N Engl J Med 1989;321:1002–1009.
2. Nakamura F, Sasaki H, Kajihara H, Yamanoue M. Laurence-Moon-Biedl syndrome accompanied by congenital hepatic fibrosis. J Gastroenterol Hepatol 1990;5:206–210.
3. Collins CM, Mendoza SA, Griswold WR, Tanney D, Liebermann E, Reznik VM. Pediatric renal transplantation in Laurence-Moon-Biedl syn-drome. Pediatr Nephrol 1994;8:221–222.
4. Ucar B, et al. Renal involvement in the Laurence-Moon-Bardet-Biedl syndrome: report of five cases. Pediatr Nephrol 1997;11:31–35.

Syndrome, Leriche's

NOTE: The morphologic substrate is isolated aortoiliac atherosclerosis. Remove aorta together with common and external iliac arteries. For arteriography of lower extremities, see Chapter 10.

Syndrome, Letterer-Siwe (See "Histiocytosis, Langerhans cell.")

Syndrome, Löffler's (See "Cardiomyopathy, restrictive [eosinophilic type] and "Syndrome, eosinophilic pulmonary.")

Syndrome, Louis-Bar (See "Syndrome, primary immunodeficiency.")

Syndrome, Malabsorption

NOTE: If malabsorption is suspected to have been caused by a systemic disease, see also under that entry. Such systemic dis-eases include abetalipoproteinemia,* amyloidosis,* Degos' disease, diabetes mellitus,* hyperthyroidism,* hypoparathyroidism,* hypothyroidism,* mastocytosis,* polyarteritis nodosa,* and systemic lupus erythematosus.*

Organs and Tissues	*Procedures*	*Possible or Expected Findings*
External examination and oral cavity	Record character and extent of skin and oral changes. Prepare histologic sections of affected skin. Prepare skeletal roentgenograms.	Brownish discoloration of skin; dermatitis; cheilosis; glossitis. Clubbing of fingers and toes. Osteomalacia;* rickets.
Intestinal tract	If an infectious or parasitic intestinal disorder is suspected, submit portions for microbiologic study.	Bacterial, fungal, viral, or parasitic infection.
	For mesenteric angiography, see Chapter 2.	Mesenteric atherosclerosis,* vasculitis, thromboembolism, or other occlusive changes.
	Open and fix intestine as soon as possible. If there were surgical resections, anastomoses, or blind loops, record length of remaining intestine, size and location of anastomoses, and length of blind loops. Submit samples of all segments for dissecting microscopic and histologic study. Identify exact location of samples in relation to ligament of Treitz or other anatomic landmarks.	Previous intestinal resection ("short bowel syndrome"), anastomoses, and blind loops. Diverticula;* strictures; fistulas; carcinoid tumors. Granulomatous or nongranulomatous enteritis; eosinophilic enteritis; radiation enteritis; sprue;* Whipple's disease.* Intestinal lymphangiectasia. Lymphoma,* carcinoma, and many other diseases and conditions (see also above under "Note").
Mesentery	See also above under "Intestinal tract." Prepare histologic sections of arteries, veins, and lymph nodes.	Lymphoma.* Granulomatous lymphadenitis. Vascular disease or other condition, as listed above under "Intestinal tract" and under "Note."
Liver and extrahepatic bile ducts	For postmortem cholangiography, see Chapter 2. Dissect extrahepatic bile ducts *in situ*.	Biliary obstruction.
Pancreas	For roentgenologic study of duct system, see Chapter 2. Prepare thin slices in order to detect minute lesions. If appropriate, see also under "Tumor of the pancreas."	Pancreatitis.* Non-beta islet cell tumor.
Other organs and tissues	Procedures depend on expected findings or grossly identified abnormalities as listed above under "Note."	Manifestations of systemic diseases that may have caused malabsorption. See above under "Note."
Bones, bone marrow, and joints	For removal, prosthetic repair, and specimen preparation of bones and joints, see Chapter 2. For preparation of sections and smears of bone marrow, see Chapter 2.	Bone changes related to vitamin D deficiency.* Megaloblastic bone marrow.
Vitreous	Submit sample for sodium, calcium, chloride, magnesium phosphate, and urea nitrogen determination.	Manifestations of dehydration.* Electrolyte changes associated with vitamin D deficiency.*

Syndrome, Marfan's

Synonyms and Related Terms: Arachnodactyly; dolichostenomelia.

Organs and Tissues	Procedures	Possible or Expected Findings
External examination	Record body weight and length, arm span, pubis-to-sole distance, and pubis-to-vertex distance.	Typical skeletal proportions. Arachnodactyly; pectus excavatum; pigeon breast; dolichocephaly; kyphoscoliosis; genu recurvatum; dislocation of joints; striae of skin.
Diaphragm		Diaphragmatic hernia.*
Heart and aorta	If infective endocarditis is suspected, follow procedures described in Chapter 7. Leave aorta attached to heart. Test competence of mitral and aortic valves (Chapter 3). Record circumference of aorta and pulmonary artery just above valves and further distally.	Infective endocarditis.* Atrial septal defect.* Myxomatous transformation of mitral ring. Mitral valve prolapse. Aortic and pulmonary dilatation and valvular insufficiency.* Aortic dissection* with dissection of adjacent vessels. Ascending aortic aneurysm (rarely with aortopulmonary fistula *[1]*). Myocardial infarction *(2)*.
	Request PAS, toluidine blue, and Verhoeff–van Gieson stains of sections of vascular walls.	Cystic change of media.
Lungs	Perfuse one or both lungs with formalin.	Multiple cysts (see "Cyst(s), pulmonary").
Colon	Record extent of diverticulosis.	Diverticulosis.
Neck organs	Inspect carotid arteries.	Aneurysms *(3)*.
Eyes	For removal and specimen preparation, see Chapter 5.	Subluxation of lens.

References

1. Massetti M, Babatasi G, Rossi A, Kapadia N, Neri E, Bhoyroo S, et al. Aortopulmonary fistula: an uncommon complication in dystrophic aortic aneurysm. Ann Thor Surg 1995;59:1563–1564.
2. Santucci JJ, Katz S, Pogo GJ, Boxer R. Peripartum acute myocardial infarction in Marfan's syndrome. Am Heart J 1994;127:1404–1407.
3. Ohyama T, Ohara S, Momma F. Aneurysm of the cervical internal carotid artery associated with Marfan's syndrome—case report. Neurologia Medico-Chirrugica 1992;32:965–968.

Syndrome, Mucocutaneous Lymph Node

Synonyms and Related Terms: Infantile polyarteritis nodosa;* Kawasaki disease.

NOTE: This syndrome is rarely fatal. The morphologic changes found at autopsy are identical to those seen in infantile polyarteritis nodosa.* The disease might be caused by an infectious agent *(1)*. The disease is reportable in some states.

Organs and Tissues	Procedures	Possible or Expected Findings
External examination and skin	Record and photograph abnormalities listed in right-hand column.	Congestion of conjunctivas. Fissuring of lips; protuberance of lingual papillae; edema of hands and feet; desquamation at junction of nails and skin of the fingers and toes; furrowing of the nails. Mild jaundice may be present.
Heart	For coronary arteriography, see Chapter 10. Submit samples of all coronary arteries for histologic study, and request Verhoeff–van Gieson' stain.	Coronary thromboarteritis with coronary occlusion, indistinguishable from infantile polyarteritis nodosa.* Coronary artery aneurysms. Myocarditis and valvulitis in early phases of the disease *(1)*.
Other organs	Follow procedures described under "Polyarteritis nodosa."	Early in the disease, lymphocytic or mixed interstitial infiltrates in hilar area of liver, spleen, pancreas, and kidneys.
Neck organs	Remove together with tongue. Submit samples of tongue and of cervical lymph nodes for histologic study.	Protuberance of lingual papillae. Cervical lymphadenopathy.
Urine	Submit sample for study of sediment.	Proteinuria; increased number of leukocytes.

Organs and Tissues	Procedures	Possible or Expected Findings
Joints	For removal, prosthetic repair, and specimen preparation, see Chapter 2.	Arthritis.*
Brain	For removal and specimen preparation, see Chapter 4.	Aseptic meningitis.*

Reference

1. Landing BH, Larson EJ. Pathological features of Kawasaki disease (mucocutaneous lymph node syndrome). Am J Cardiovasc Pathol 1987;1: 218–229.

Syndrome, Myasthenia (See "Myasthenia gravis.")

Syndrome, Myelodysplastic

Synonyms and Related Terms: Chronic myelomonocytic leukemia;* refractory anemia; refractory anemia with excess of blasts; refractory anemia with excess of blasts in transformation; refractory anemia with ringed sideroblasts; refractory dysmyelopoietic anemias.

NOTE: The myelodysplastic syndromes are represented by a heterogeneous group of normocytic anemias, often with neutropenia, thrombocytopenia, and monocytosis. For expected bone marrow changes, see above under "Synonyms and Related Terms." Autopsy procedures are similar to those recommended for most cases of leukemia, with particular attention paid to intercurrent infections and thrombocytopenic hemorrhages. In all instances, material should be collected using aseptic technique for tissue culture for chromosome analysis. Common findings in these conditions are deletion of the long arm of chromosome 5, deletion of chromosome 5 or 7, or trisomy 8.

Syndrome, Nephrotic

NOTE: See under name of suspected underlying condition, such as amyloidosis,* anaphylactoid purpura,* diabetes mellitus,* glomerulonephritis,* Goodpasture's syndrome,* heavy metal poisoning, hemolytic uremic syndrome,* infective endo-carditis,* polyarteritis nodosa,* syphilis,* or systemic lupus erythematosus.* If accelerated hypertension or constrictive pericarditis is the suspected underlying condition, see under "Hypertension (arterial), all types or type unspecified" or "Pericarditis," respectively.

In all instances, the renal veins and the inferior vena cava should be opened *in situ*. "En masse" removal of organs is recommended for this purpose. If thrombosis is found, record exact location and size of clot and submit sample of clot with wall of veins for histologic study. See also under "Thrombosis, venous." Coronary atherosclerosis and its complications seem to be increased in patients with the nephrotic syndrome.

Syndrome, Neurocutaneous (See "Disease, Sturge-Weber-Dimitri," "Disease, von Hippel-Lindau," "Neurofibromatosis," and "Sclerosis, tuberous.")

Syndrome, Neutrophil Dysfunction (See "Disease, chronic granulomatous," and "Syndrome, Chédiak-Higashi.")

Syndrome, Noonan's

Possible Associated Conditions: Acute leukemia *(1)*.

NOTE: Snap freeze tissue for identification of PTPN11 gene mutation *(5)*.

Organs and Tissues	Procedures	Possible or Expected Findings
External examination	Record body weight and length. Record and prepare photographs of all abnormalities listed in right-hand column.	Small stature; neck webbing or nuchal edema; antimongoloid slant of palpebral fissures; micrognathia; hypertelorism; cubitus valgus; short curved fifth finger; broad, short fingernails; undescended testes. Hydrops fetalis* due to lymphatic dysplasia *(2)*.
	Prepare skeletal roentgenograms.	Pectus excavatum and other skeletal malformations;
Blood or fascia lata	These specimens should be collected using aseptic technique for tissue culture for chromosome analysis (see Chapter 9).	Normal karyotype in most instances.
Heart	Dissection techniques depend on expected abnormalities as shown in right-hand column.	Congenital valvular pulmonary stenosis.* Congestive obstructive or nonobstructive hypertrophic cardiomyopathy.* Left ventricular hypoplasia;* aneurysms of the sinuses of valsalva *(3)*.
	For coronary arteriography, see Chapter 10.	Congenital coronary anomalies.
Lungs	Perfuse lungs with formalin.	Pulmonary lymphangiectasis.

Organs and Tissues	Procedures	Possible or Expected Findings
Kidneys	See "Cyst(s), renal."	Cystic renal disease.
Brain		Cerebral arteriovenous malformation *(4)*.

References

1. Johannes JM, Garcia CR, De Vaan GA, Weening RS. Noonan's syndrome in association with acute leukemia. Pediatr Hematol Oncol 1995;12:571–575.
2. Bloomfield FH, Hadden W, Gunn TR. Lymphatic dysplasia in a neonate with Noonan's syndrome. Pediatr Radiol 1997;27:321–323.
3. Noonan J, O'Connor W. Noonan syndrome: a clinical description emphasizing the cardiac findings. Acta Pediatr Japn 1996;38:76–83.
4. Schon F, Bowler J, Baraitser M. Cerebral arteriovenous malformation in Noonan's syndrome. Postgrad Med J 1992;68:37–40.
5. Bertola DR et al. Clinical variability in a Noonan syndrome family with a new PTPN11 gene mutation. Am J Med Gen A 2004;130:378–383.

Syndrome, Obesity-Hypoventilation (See "Obesity.")

Syndrome, Parkinson's (See "Disease, Parkinson's.")

Syndrome, Peutz-Jeghers

NOTE: For the gene location, see ref. *(1)*.

Organs and Tissues	Procedures	Possible or Expected Findings
External examination, skin, and oral cavity	Record extent of pigmentations; photograph and prepare histologic sections of skin.	Mucocutaneous pigmentations around lips and of buccal mucosa, forearms, hands, feet, and umbilical area.
Gastrointestinal tract and regional lymph nodes		Intussusception and hemorrhage.
	Record location and size of polypoid lesions. Leave polyps attached to wall of intestine until after fixation is completed. Histologic section should include polyps and wall of intestine. Request van Gieson's and mucicarmine stains.	Hamartomatous polyps in jejunum and ileum and less commonly in stomach, duodenum, appendix, and colon. Adenocarcinomas may arise from the polyps.
	Submit samples of regional lymph nodes for histologic study.	Metastases in rare cases in which carcinoma had developed.
Other organs	Procedures depend on expected findings or grossly identified abnormalities as listed in right-hand column.	Rarely, hamartomatous polyps in pharynx, urinary bladder, and other sites. Gonadal tumors have been observed *(2,3)*.

References

1. Tomlinson IP, Houlston RS. Peutz-Jeghers syndrome. J Med Genet 1997;34:1007–1011.
2. Dreyer L, Jacyk WK, du Plessis DJ. Bilateral large-cell calcifying Sertoli cell tumor of the testes in Peutz-Jeghers syndrome: a case report. Pediatr Dermatol 1994;11:335–337.
3. Dozois RR, Kempers RD, Dahlin DC, Batholomew LG. Ovarian tumors associated with the Peutz-Jeghers syndrome. Ann Surg 1970;172:233–238.

Syndrome, Pickwickian (Obesity-Hypoventilation syndrome) (See "Obesity.")

Syndrome, Pierre Robin

Related Terms: Catel-Manzke syndrome (Pierre Robin complex with accessory metacarpal of index finger); Pierre-Robin sequence; Trisomy 18.

NOTE: The Pierre-Robin phenotype (i.e., micrognathia with resulting retroglossia and cleft palate) may be present in numerous other malformation complexes. Other abnormalities comprising these malformation complexes are listed below.

Organs and Tissues	Procedures	Possible or Expected Findings
External examination; oral and nasal cavities; soft tissues	Record and prepare photographs of all abnormalities as listed in right-hand column.	Micrognathia; cleft palate; bulging of upper rib cage; bifid uvula; choanal atresia; hypertelorism; hypertrophy of soft tissues of the neck; caudal regression syndrome *(4)*.
	Prepare skeletal roentgenograms, including hands.	Rib defects; syndactyly; hypoplastic digits; extra metacarpal of index finger; hypoplastic femora.

Organs and Tissues	*Procedures*	*Possible or Expected Findings*
Chest		Pneumothorax.*
Blood or fascia lata	These specimens should be collected using aseptic technique for tissue culture for chromosome analysis (see Chapter 9). This is particularly important if condition must be distinguished from trisomy 18 or cri-du-chat syndrome.	Usually normal karyotype but chromosomal deletions may occur *(1)*.
Heart	For dissection techniques, see Chapter 3.	Congenital heart disease *(2)*. Cor pulmonale.
Liver	Record weight and sample for histologic study.	Congenital hepatic fibrosis.
Neck organs and tongue	Record size of tongue; record presence or absence of signs of asphyxiation from malformed organs and tissues.	Tongue size normal or decreased. Rarely, aglossia. Glossoptosis may lead to acute airways obstruction *(3)*.
Brain	For removal and specimen preparation, see Chapter 4.	Hypoxic encephalopathy. Chiari I malformation *(4)*.
Eyes	For removal and specimen preparation, see Chapter 5.	Glaucomatous cupping of optic disk; myopic disk changes; cataract; retinal detachment; microphthalmia.

References

1. Menk FH, Madan K, Baart JA, Beukenhorst HL. Robin sequence and a deficiency of the left forearm in a girl with a deletion of chromosome 4g33-gter. Am J Med Genet 1992;44:696–694.
2. Pearl W. Congenital heart disease in the Pierre Robin syndrome. Pediatr Cardiol 1982;2:307–309.
3. Cozzi F, Pierro A. Glossoptosis-apnea syndrome. Pediatr 1985;75:836–843.
4. Tubbs RS, Oakes WJ. Chiari I malformation, caudal regression syndrome, and Pierre Robin syndrome: previously unreported combination. Childs Nerv Syst 2006;22:1507–1508.

Syndrome, Plummer-Vinson

Synonym: Sideropenic dysphagia.

Organs and Tissues	*Procedures*	*Possible or Expected Findings*
External examination		Koilonychia.
Esophagus and stomach	Request PAS-alcian blue stain of histologic samples.	Squamous cell carcinoma of esophagus *(1)*. Chronic gastritis.
Neck organs	Remove together with base of tongue and oropharynx. Open esophagus in posterior midline, photograph, and take sections of grossly identifiable lesions and random sections at various levels.	Web formation; postcricoid carcinoma.
Other organs	For preparation of sections and smears of bone marrow, see Chapter 2.	Manifestations of hypochromic anemia.* Blood smears reveal microsytosis.

Reference

1. Ribeiro U Jr, Posner MC, Safatle-Ribeiro AV, Reynolds JC. Risk factors for squamous cell carcinoma of the esophagus. Br J Surg 1996;83:1174–1185.

Syndrome, Polysplenia and Asplenia

Synonyms: Heterotaxy syndrome; Ivemark's syndrome; visceral isomerism.

Possible Associated Conditions: With *asplenia*: Right isomerism (bilateral mirror-image right-sided symmetry) of heart, lungs, and abdominal viscera; common atrium; total anomalous pulmonary venous connection; absent coronary sinus; complete atrioventricular septal defect;* subpulmonary stenosis;* pulmonary valve atresia;* midline symmetric liver; malrotation of bowel; absent spleen.

With *polysplenia*: Left isomerism (bilateral mirror-image left-sided symmetry) of heart and lungs, with variable sidedness of abdominal viscera; anomalous pulmonary venous connection; ventricular inversion; subpulmonary stenosis;* transposition of the great arteries;* bilateral superior caval veins; azygos continuation of inferior vena cava; multiple spleens of variable size, all on same side as stomach and pancreas.

Organs and Tissues	Procedures	Possible or Expected Findings
Blood	Prepare smears.	Howell-Jolly bodies occur in asplenia syndrome and, rarely, in polysplenia.
Chest and abdominal cavity, cardiovascular system, and lungs	Procedures depend on expected findings or grossly identified abnormalities as listed in right-hand column and under "Possible Associated Conditions."	Two pulmonary lobes occur bilaterally in polysplenia, and three lobes in asplenia syndrome. If inferior vena cava is interrupted, hepatic veins unite to form a vessel or vessels that empty into either atrium. See also under "Possible Associated Conditions."
Spleen	Dissect splenic artery and vein *in situ*. For celiac arteriography, see Chapter 2.	In polysplenia, there are two or more splenic masses but no normal-sized spleen.
Liver, gallbladder, bile ducts	For postmortem cholangiography, see Chapter 2.	Rarely, absence of gallbladder; biliary atresia* in polysplenia. Large midline liver in asplenia.

Syndrome, Primary Immunodeficiency

Synonyms and Related Terms *(1)*: *T-cell defects*—Alymphocytosis (a severe combined immunodeficiency); ataxia telangiectasia; Bloom's syndrome;* deficit of T and NK cells (a severe combined immunodeficiency); DiGeorge's syndrome;* HLA-class I or II deficiency; hyper-IgM syndrome; Wiskott-Aldrich syndrome; xeroderma pigmentosum; reticular dysgenesis (a severe combined immunodeficiency); and several others. *B-cell defects*—Bruton's agammaglobulinemia; common variable immunodeficiency; hyper IgE syndrome; IgA deficiency or IgG subclass deficiency, lymphoproliferative syndrome (X-linked or autoimmunity); and several others. *Phagocytic defects*—Chédiak-Higashi syndrome;* chronic granulomatous disease;* leukocyte adhesion deficiency; and several others. *Complement deficiencies* also belong here.

NOTE:

For the usual complications, such as skin diseases, hematologic diseases, and various types of infections, see above under "Synonyms and Related Terms" and below under "Possible or Expected Findings." For the *acquired* immunodeficiency syndrome, see under "Syndrome, acquired immunodeficiency."

Possible Associated Conditions (syndromes associated with immunodeficiency): Chromosome abnormalities (Bloom's syndrome,* Down's syndrome,* or Fanconi syndrome*); hereditary metabolic defects (acrodermatitis enteropathica [zinc deficiency], biotin dependent carboxylase deficiency, transcobalamin II deficiency, and type I orotic aciduria); hypercatabolism of Ig (familial hypercatabolism of Ig, intestinal lymphangiectasia, and myotonic dystrophy); multiple organ system abnormalities (agenesis of the corpus callosum, cartilage hair hypoplasia, partial albinism, or short-limbed dwarfism); and other defi-ciences (chronic mucocutaneous candidiasis, hyper IgE syndrome, immunodeficiency following hereditarily determined susceptibility to Epstein-Barr virus, and thymoma).

Conditions that are more common in immunodeficient patients: Infectious mononucleosis (with or without B cell lymphoma in X-linked lymphoproliferative syndrome); rheumatoid arthritis;* systemic lupus erythematosus.*

Organs and Tissues	Procedures	Possible or Expected Findings
External examination, skin, and oral cavity	Record body weight and length; record and photograph abnormalities as listed in right-hand column. Prepare histologic sections of skin and oral mucosa, particularly of infected or eczematous areas.	Malformed ears, micrognathia, hypertelorism and short philtrum in Di George's syndrome.* Dermatomyositis* in immunoglobulin deficiency. Immunodeficiency may be associated with short-limbed dwarfism with absence of scalp hair, eyelashes, and eyebrows, ichthyosiform skin lesions, and erythroderma. Eczema in Wiskott-Aldrich syndrome; oculocutaneous telangiectasia (Louis-Bar syndrome); mucocutaneous infections, such as candidiasis* (chronic mucocutaneous candidiasis).
Thymus	Record weight of intact organ. Record presence or absence of ectopic thymic tissue in neck organs. Submit samples for histologic study, and snap-freeze fresh material for immunofluorescent study.	Thymus may be normal, hypoplastic (e.g., in ataxia telangiectasia), aplastic (for instance, in DiGeorge's syndrome*) or ectopic (see "Neck organs"). Spindle cell thymoma in hypogammaglobulinemia patients.

Organs and Tissues	*Procedures*	*Possible or Expected Findings*
Blood	Submit sample for microbiologic study.	Bacterial or fungal septicemia; viremia.
	Submit samples for determination of immunoglobulins in serum and for B and T lymphocyte counts.	Hypogammaglobulinemia; dysgammaglobulinemia; hyperimmunoglobulinemia.
	Blood or fascia lata should be collected using aseptic technique for tissue culture for chromosome analysis (see Chapter 9).	See above under "Possible Associated Conditions..."
Heart and great vessels		Malformations of aortic arch and/or conotruncus in DiGeorge's syndrome.
Lungs	Submit any consolidated area for culture. Stain touch preparations for *Pneumocystis carinii.** Perfuse one lung with formalin. Request Gram and Grocott's methenamine silver stain.	Bacterial, fungal, or viral pneumonia. *Pneumocystis carinii* infection.* Herpesvirus infection. Bronchiectasis,* e.g., in transient hypogammaglobulinemia of infancy or common variable immunodeficiency.
Gastrointestinal tract	For study under the dissecting microscope, see Chapter 2. Submit contents for microbiologic study. Submit samples of ileum, jejunum, appendix, and colon for histologic study.	Atrophy of intestinal villi and peripheral lymphoid tissue, most pronounced in Peyer's patches and appendix. Atrophic gastritis with megaloblastic anemia* or gastrointestinal infection, including giardiasis, may be present, e.g., in common variable immundeficiency.
Lymph nodes and spleen	Place specimens in B-Plus Fixative™. If lymphoma is suspected, follow procedures described under that heading.	T cells, primarily in paracortical zone of lymph nodes and in periarteriolar sheaths of the spleen. There may be generalized lymphadenopathy with or without lymphoma.*
Neck organs	Remove together with base of tongue, tonsils, soft palate, and pharyngeal wall. Prepare histologic sections of lingual tonsils, palatine tonsils, and pharyngeal lymphatic tissue (see also above under "Thymus" and "Lymph nodes and spleen").	Upper respiratory infections. Ectopic thymus may occur near the base of the tongue, or in or around thyroid and parathyroid glands.
	Dissect and record weights of thyroid gland and parathyroid glands. Submit samples for histologic study.	Agenesis of parathyroid glands and—rarely—of thyroid gland in DiGeorge's syndrome.
Other organs	Procedures depend on expected findings or grossly identified abnormalities as listed in right-hand column.	Manifestations of malabsorption syndrome.* Infections. Ovarian agenesis in ataxia telangiectasia.
Middle ears and sinuses	For exposure and specimen preparation,	Otitis media* and sinusitis.
Eyes	For removal and specimen preparation, see Chapter 5.	Oculocutaneous telangiectasias in ataxia telangiectasia.
Bone marrow	For preparation of sections and smears, see Chapter 2. If bone marrow had been transplanted (e.g., in severe combined immunodeficiency), see also under "Transplantation, bone marrow."	Hypoplasia (may be associated with agranulocytosis*). Leukemia* or related neoplastic disease. Megaloblastic anemia* in idiopathic late-onset immunoglobulin deficiency.
Joints	If infectious arthritis is suspected, submit exudate for microbiologic study.	*Mycoplasma* infection in agammaglobulinemia.

Reference

1. Ten RM. Primary immunodeficiencies. Mayo Clin Proc 1998;73:865–872.

Syndrome, Reifenstein's

Related Term: Hereditary familial hypogonadism; male pseudohermaphroditism.

Organs and Tissues	*Procedures*	*Possible or Expected Findings*
External examination	Record and prepare photographs of all abnormalities as listed in right-hand column.	Microphallus; hypospadias; absent vas deferens; incomplete fusion of labioscrotal folds; gynecomastia.
Blood and fascia lata	These specimens should be collected using aseptic technique for tissue culture for chromosome analysis (see Chapter 9).	Normal karyotype.
Gonads	Record weights and prepare histologic sections.	Testicular atrophy; crytorchidism; germ cell neoplasia.

Syndrome, Reiter's

Synonym: Urethritis-arthritis-conjunctivitis syndrome.

NOTE: AIDS-related psoriasiform dermatitis may show clinical features of Reiter's syndrome *(1)*.

Possible Associated Condition: Ankylosing spondylitis.*; syndrome, acquired immune deficiency*.

Organs and Tissues	*Procedures*	*Possible or Expected Findings*
External examination, skin, and oral cavity	Record character and extent of lesions of skin, external genitalia, and oral mucosa. Prepare photographs of lesions. Prepare histologic sections of skin and mucosal lesions.	Keratoderma (keratosis blennorrhagica) with vasculitis *(2)* of sole of feet, of palms, and of circumcised glans penis.
	Prepare roentgenograms of joints.	Arthritis* of knees, ankles, and metatarsal and midtarsal joints, with or without ankylosis. Osteoporosis.*
Blood	Submit sample for bacteriologic, viral, and serologic study.	Usually, sterile culture.
Heart	Record weight and submit samples for histologic study. If heart block was present, submit samples of conduction system for histologic study (Chapter 4).	Pericarditis;* myocarditis.* Aortic valve lesions.
Lungs	Submit consolidated areas for microbiologic study. Perfuse at least one lung with formalin.	Pleuritis and pneumonia.* Pulmonary fibrosis involving upper lobes.
Urinary bladder and urethra	For removal of urethra, see Chapter 2.	Erosions, papules, and plaques in urethral or bladder mucosa.
Other organs	Procedures depend on expected findings or grossly identified abnormalities as listed in right-hand column.	Enteritis. Thrombophlebitis.
Eyes	For removal and specimen preparation, see Chapter 5.	Conjunctivitis; multifocal choroiditis; acute anterior uveitis; iritis; keratitis.
Joints	Consult roentgenograms (see above under "External examination, skin, and oral cavity").	Arthritis* (see above under "External examination, skin, and oral cavity") resembling rheumatoid arthritis.* Nonspecific synovitis.

References

1. Romani J, Puig L, Baselga E, De Moragas JM. Reiter's syndrome-like pattern in AIDS-associated psoriasiform dermatitis. Intl J Dermatol 1996; 35:484–488.
2. Magro CM, Crowson AN, Peeling R. Vasculitis as the basis of cutaneous lesions in Reiter's disease. Hum Path 1995;26: 633–638.

Syndrome, Respiratory Distress, of Adult (ARDS) (See "Syndrome, adult respiratory distress (ARDS).")

Syndrome, Respiratory Distress, of Infant

Related Terms: Hyaline membrane disease; bronchopulmonary dysplasia.

Organs and Tissues	*Procedures*	*Possible or Expected Findings*
External examination	Prepare chest and abdominal roentgenograms.	Pneumothorax;* pneumomediastinum;* pneumoperitoneum.
Blood	Submit sample for microbiologic study if sepsis is suspected.	Septicemia.
Heart	Record weight of heart and thickness of ventricles.	Right ventricular hypertrophy and/or dilatation.
Trachea, major bronchi, and lungs	Submit a section for culture. Perfuse lungs with formalin. Submit multiple sections for histologic study.	Intubation trauma and mural edema and hemorrhage in trachea; hyaline membrane disease; pulmonary interstitial emphysema; bronchopulmonary dysplasia *(1)*, arrested acinar development *(2)*.
Neck organs	Prepare cross-sections that include larynx, thyroid, esophagus, and adjacent structures.	Intubation trauma.
Brain	For removal and specimen preparation, see Chapter 4.	Hemorrhages or other evidence of birth trauma; germinal matrix hemorrhages in premature infants; infarctions of subcortical white matter in term infants.
Eyes	For removal and specimen preparation, see Chapter 5.	Retinopathy of prematurity (a vasoproliferative disorder).

Reference

1. Coalson JJ. Pathology of bronchopulmonary dysplasia. Semin Perinatol 2006;30:179–180.
2. Husain AN, et al. Pathology of arrested acinar development in postsurfactant bronchopulmonary dysplasia, Hum Pathol 1998;29:710–717.

Syndrome, Reye's

NOTE: Hypoglycemia* may have been present, but that condition is difficult or impossible to confirm after death. An immediate autopsy is indicated (see below under "Liver" and "Pancreas").

Organs and Tissues	*Procedures*	*Possible or Expected Findings*
Vitreous	Submit sample for sodium, chloride, and urea nitrogen determination.	Manifestations of dehydration.*
Blood	Submit sample for microbiologic (viral) and serologic study, for ammonia and bilirubin determination, and for determination of salicylate levels if there is a history of treatment with this drug.	Influenza;* varicella.* Manifestations of liver failure. Evidence of salicylate administration.
Urine	Obtain sample for biochemical and toxicologic analysis.	Assay for organic acids should rule out acyl-coenzyme A dehydrogenase deficiency, and toxicity, e.g., of acetaminophen and valproic acid *(1)*.
Heart	Record weight. Request frozen sections for Sudan stain.	Cardiomegaly; fatty changes of myocardium and patchy myocytolysis.
Lungs	Submit fresh tissue for bacterial and viral culture.	Viral pneumonia rarely present.
	Request paraffin sections and frozen sections for fat stain (see above under "Heart").	Acute interstitial pneumonia;* bronchitis;* hemorrhages. Lipid-laden histiocytes in alveoli.

Organs and Tissues	Procedures	Possible or Expected Findings
Liver	Record weight and photograph; submit sample for microbiologic (viral) study. Request frozen sections for fat stain (see above under "Heart").	Hepatomegaly; microvesicular fatty changes (they are not specific); zonal degeneration and necrosis *(2,3)*.
	If tissue can be obtained immediately after death, prepare sample for electron microscopic study.	Increase of peroxisomes; proliferation of smooth endoplasmic reticulum; swelling of mitochondria.
Pancreas	If tissue can be obtained immediately after death, prepare sample electron microscopic study.	Intranuclear inclusions *(4)*.
Kidneys	See above under "Liver."	Tubular fatty changes.
Brain and spinal cord	For removal and specimen preparation, see Chapter 4. See also under "Encephalopathy, hepatic."	Hepatic encephalopathy.* Cerebral edema *(5)*.

References

1. Greene CL, Blitzer MG, Shapira E. Inborn errors of metabolism and Reye's syndrome: differential diagnosis. J Pediatr 11988;113:156–159.
2. Fraser JL, Antonioli DA, Chopra S, Wang HH. Prevalence and non-specificity of microvesicular fatty changes. Mod Pathol 1995; 8:65–70.
3. Kimura S, Kobayashi T, Tanaka Y, Sasaki Y. Liver histopathology in clinical Reye syndrome. Brain Dev 1991;13:95–100.
4. Collins DN. Ultrastructural study of intranuclear inclusions in the exo-crine pancreas in Reye's syndrome. Lab Invest 1974;30:333–340.
5. Blisard KS, Davis LE. Neuropathologic findings in Reye syndrome. J Child Neurol 1991;6:41–44.

Syndrome, Sanfilippo's (See "Mucopolysaccharidosis.")

Syndrome, Scheie's (See "Mucopolysaccharidosis.")

Syndrome, Segawa's (See "Syndrome, dystonia.")

Syndrome, Severe Acute Respiratory (SARS)

Note: This highly contagious illness, caused by a coronavirus (SARS-CoV), has a mortality rate of up to 10%. Any autopsies planned for suspected SARS cases must be conducted in a specially designed biosafety level 3 (BSL-3) autopsy laboratory (for details, see http://www.who.int/csr/resources/publications/biosafety/Biosafety7.pdf) and *Ref (1)*. Other tests, such as RT-PCR, *in situ* hybridization, immunohistochemistry, electron microscopy and viral culture are also available. An excellent review article on this topic is listed as *Ref (2)*. This is a reportable disease.

Organs and tissues	Procedures	Possible or Expected Findings
Respiratory tract	Weigh and perfuse lungs.	Diffuse alveolar damage, mixed cellular infiltration, giant cells, atypical reactive pneumocytes, vascular injury.
Heart		Atrophy and edema.
Spleen, lymph nodes		Lymphocyte depletion, splenic white pulp atrophy.
Intestines	Remove and fix digestive tract as soon as possible.	Depletion of mucosal lymphoid tissue.
Liver		Necrosis, evidence of apoptosis.
Kidneys		Acute tubular necrosis.
Bone marrow	Procure from multiple sites and fix in B-Plus®,	Reactive hemophagocytosis.
Adrenal glands		Necrosis and mononuclear cell infiltration.
Thyroid gland		Destruction of epithelial cells and disruption of architecture.
Skeletal muscle		Myofiber necrosis, atrophy, regenerative changes.
Testes		Germ cell destruction and apoptosis.

References

1. Li, L et al. Biosafety level 3 laboratory for autopsies of patients with severe acute respiratory syndrome: principles, practices, and prospects. Clin Infect Dis 2005;41:815–2.
2. Gu J, Korteweg C. Pathology and pathogenesis of severe acute respiratory syndrome. Am J Pathol 2007;170:1136–47.

Syndrome, Sézary's (See "Lymphoma.")

Syndrome, Sheehan's

Synonyms: Postpartum pituitary necrosis; Sheehan's disease.

NOTE: Follow procedures described under "Insufficiency, pituitary." In early stages, the pituitary gland shows subtotal or total infarction; in late stages, fibrosis with residual small nests of normal chromophils is present. For *in situ* cerebral arteriography, see Chapter 4.

Syndrome, Shy-Drager (See "Atrophy, multiple system.")

Syndrome, Sick Sinus

Organs and Tissues	*Procedures*	*Possible or Expected Findings*
Heart	For histologic study of conduction system, see Chapter 3.	Excessive fibrosis of sinus node or adjacent myocardium.

Syndrome, Sipple's (See "Neoplasia, multiple endocrine.")

Syndrome, Sjögren's

Related Terms: Mikulicz's disease; sicca complex.

Possible Associated Conditions: Chronic hepatitis;* discoid lupus erythematosus; generalized or pulmonary amyloidosis* *(1)*; Hashimoto's thyroiditis; polyarteritis nodosa (necrotizing arteritis);* polymyositis; primary biliary cirrhosis; rheumatoid arthritis;* systemic lupus erythematosus* *(4)*; systemic sclerosis.*

Organs and Tissues	*Procedures*	*Possible or Expected Findings*
External examination and skin	Prepare histologic sections of skin.	Sweat gland atrophy. Cutaneous focal amyloidosis *(6)*.
Blood	Submit sample for determination of IgA, IgM, and IgG concentrations and of rheumatoid factor.	
Heart	Record volume and appearance of pericardial fluid.	Fibrinous or serofibrinous pericarditis.*
Trachea, bronchi, and lungs	Submit consolidated areas for microbiologic study. Perfuse one lung with formalin. If much inspissated mucus appears to be present, perfuse also through pulmonary artery. Submit samples for histologic study. Request Verhoeff–van Gieson and amyloid stains.	Mucosal glandular atrophy. Inspissated mucous secretions. Pulmonary arterial hypertension;* lymphoma* or pseudo-lymphoma *(1)*; Bronchopneumonia. Bronchiolitis obliterans organizing pneumonia *(2)*; interstitial pulmonary fibrosis;* amyloidosis.*
Esophagus	Submit samples for histologic study (pin on cork board, fix in formalin, and cut on edge).	Submucosal glandular atrophy. Atrophy of mucosa with infiltrates of lymphocytes and plasma cells.
Stomach and duodenum	Submit samples for histologic study (pin on cork board, fix in formalin, and cut on edge).	Chronic atrophic gastritis *(3)*; lymphocytosis of pyloric and Brunner's glands.
Liver and spleen	Record weights and sample for histologic study.	Hepatosplenomegaly. Primary biliary cirrhosis *(3)*.
Kidneys	Follow procedures described under "Glomerulonephritis."	Focal or membranous glomerulonephritis;* interstitial nephritis;* nephrocalcinosis; tubular atrophy.
Neck organs and tongue; salivary glands	Thyroid, submaxillary salivary gland, base of tongue, pharynx, and soft palate should be sampled for histologic study.	Atrophic sialadenitis (see below under "Eyes and lacrimal glands"); loss of taste buds of tongue; thyroiditis.*
Eyes and lacrimal glands	For removal and specimen preparation of eyes, see Chapter 5. Submit samples of lacrimal glands for histologic study.	Keratoconjunctivitis. Lymphocytic, hyalinizing, atrophic dacryoadenitis with benign lymphoepithelial lesions (Mikulicz's disease).
Skeletal muscles	For sampling and specimen preparation, see Chapter 2.	Myopathy. Polymyositis *(2)*.

Organs and Tissues	Procedures	Possible or Expected Findings
Other organs and tissues	Procedures depend on expected findings or grossly identified abnormalities as listed in right-hand column.	Lymphomas *(4)* and pseudolymphomas. See also under "Possible Associated Conditions."
Brain and spinal cord	For removal and specimen preparation, see Chapter 4.	Transverse myelopathy *(5)*.

References

1. Quismorio FP Jr. Pulmonary involvement in primary Sjögren's syndrome. Curr Opin Pulm Med 1996;2:424–428.
2. Imasaki T, Yoshii A, Tanaka S, Ogura T, Ishikawa A, Takahashi T. Polymyositis and Sjögren's syndrome associated with bronchiolitis obliterans organizing pneumonia. Intern Med 1996;35:231–235.
3. Sheikh SH, Shaw-Stiffel TA. The gastrointestinal manifestations of Sjögren's syndrome. Am J Gastroenterol 1995;90:9–14.
4. Anaya JM, McGuff HS, Banks PM, Talal N. Clinicopathological factors relating malignant lymphoma with Sjögren's syndrome. Semin Arthritis Rheumat 1996;25:337–346.
5. Lyu RK, Chen ST, Tank LM, Chen TC. Acute transverse myelopathy and cutaneous vasculopathy in primary Sjögren's syndrome. Euro Neurol 1995;35:359–362.
6. Konishi A, et al. Primary localized cutaneous amyloidosis with unusual clinical features in a patient with Sjögren's syndrome. J Dermatol 2007;34:394–396.

Syndrome, Steele-Richardson **(See "Disease, Parkinson's.")**

Syndrome, Stevens-Johnson **(See "Erythema multiforme.")**

Syndrome, Stiff-Man

Related Terms: Armadillo disease; continuous muscle fiber activity; neuromyotonia; paraneoplastic opsoclonus *(1)*; quantal squander.

Organs and Tissues	Procedures	Possible or Expected Findings
Brain, spinal cord, and peripheral nerves	For removal and specimen preparation, see Chapter 4.	No diagnostic findings.
Skeletal muscles	For sampling and specimen preparation, see Chapter 2.	Variable but not diagnostic findings.

Reference

1. Dropcho EJ. Autoimmune central nervous system paraneoplastic disorders: mechanisms, diagnosis, and therapeutic options. Ann Neurol 1995; 37:S102–S113.

Syndrome, Sudden Infant Death (SIDS) **(See "Death, Sudden unexpected, of Infant.")**

Syndrome, Superior Vena Cava

Related Term: Superior vena cava obstruction.

Organs and Tissues	Procedures	Possible or Expected Findings
Chest cavity	Dissect superior vena cava and its tributaries *in situ*, with head and neck of deceased well-extended (place wooden block or some other support under scapulas). Continue dissection of veins into neck and axillas. Record and photograph site of thrombosis or of compression by surrounding pathologic conditions. Submit samples for histologic study.	Benign or malignant tumors; fibrosing mediastinitis;* postradiation fibrosis; infectious disease (tuberculosis,* histoplasmosis*); thoracic aortic aneurysm;* chronic constrictive pericarditis;* chest trauma; arteriovenous fistula between ascending aorta and superior vena cava; congenital anomaly of superior vena cava.

Syndrome, Toxic Shock

Synonyms and Related Terms: Staphylococcal scarlet fever.

NOTE: (1) Collect all tissues that appear to be infected. (2) Request aerobic and anaerobic cultures. (3) Request Gram stain. (4) Usually, no special precautions are indicated. (5) Serologic studies are available from the Centers for Disease Control and Prevention, Atlanta, GA. (6) This is a **reportable** disease.

Organs and Tissues	*Procedures*	*Possible or Expected Findings*
External examination, skin, oral cavity, and vagina	Record extent and character of skin and oral lesions; prepare photographs.	Erythematous, deep red "sun burn" rash; oral mucosal hyperemia; desquamation; conjunctival hyperemia.
	Culture vaginal discharge, if present. Culture cervix. Culture tampon, if present.	Infected tampon and vaginal discharge.
Other organs	Procedures depend on expected findings or grossly identified abnormalities as listed in right-hand column.	Periportal inflammation of liver; acute tubular necrosis of kidneys; hyaline membranes in lungs; evidence of coagulopathy.
Pelvic organs	Remove pelvic organs; open vagina and cervix with uterus in posterior midline; photograph and sample for histologic study.	Vaginal hyperemia; desquamation/ulceration of vaginal or cervical mucosa.

Syndrome, Turcot (See "Polyposis, familial, and related syndromes.")

Syndrome, Turner

Synonyms and Related Terms: Gonadal dysgenesis; primary ovarian failure.

Organs and Tissues	*Procedures*	*Possible or Expected Findings*
External examination	Record body weight and length, stature, and distribution of head, axillary, and pubic hair. Record and prepare photographs of features of face and neck. Prepare skeletal roentgenograms.	Premature aging; increased number of pigmented nevi; infantile sex organs; webbed neck; broad chest with wide spacing of nipples. Short fourth metacarpal; abnormal epiphyseal fusions; osteochondrosis-like changes of spine. Osteoporosis.*
Breasts	Submit samples of breast tissues for histologic study.	Infantile breast tissue.
Blood and fascia lata	These specimens should be collected using aseptic technique for tissue culture for chromosome analysis (see Chapter 9).	45, X(XO).
Heart and aorta	Procedures depend on expected findings or grossly identified abnormalities as listed in right-hand column.	Bicuspid aortic valve;* coarctation of aorta.* Rarely other anomalies *(1)*.
Ovaries	Submit for histologic study.	Decreased/absent follicles.
Intestinal tract	Submit samples of all portions for histologic study.	Intestinal telangiectases.
Liver and extrahepatic bile ducts	If biliary atresia is suspected, follow procedures described under that heading.	Biliary atresia.*
Kidneys and ureters	Dissect kidneys and ureters *in situ* and record findings.	Horseshoe kidney; double ureters.
Pelvic organs	Submit samples of gonads or—if gonads cannot be identified—equivalent ridges on mesosalpinx for histologic study. Also submit samples of endometrium, cervix, and vagina.	Streak gonads without germ cells or follicles.
Thyroid gland	Record weight and submit sample for histologic study.	Hashimoto's thyroiditis.*
Other organs	Procedures depend on expected findings or grossly identified abnormalities as listed in right-hand column.	Manifestations of diabetes mellitus,* hypertension,* or thyrotoxicosis. Neuroblastoma and related tumors *(2)*.
Eyes	For removal and specimen preparation, see Chapter 5.	Keratoconus; retinal detachments *(3)*.

References

1. Oohara K, Yamazaki T, Sakaguchi K, Nakayama M, Kobayashi A. Acute aortic dissection, aortic insufficiency, and a single coronary artery in a patient with Turner's syndrome. J Cardiovasc Surg 1995;36:273–275.
2. Blatt J, Olshan AF, Lee PA, Ross JL. Neuroblastoma and related tumors in Turner's syndrome. J Pediatr 1997;131:666–670.
3. Mason JO III, Tasman W. Turner's syndrome associated with bilateral retinal detachments. Am J Ophthalmol 1996;122:742–743.

Syndrome, Waterhouse-Friderichsen (See "Disease, meningococcal.")

Syndrome, Weil's (See "Leptospirosis.")

Syndrome, Wernicke-Korsakoff

Related Terms: Alcoholic Wernicke's encephalopathy; Korsakoff's psychosis; nonalcoholic Wernicke's encephalopathy *(1,2)*; Wernicke's disease.

Organs and Tissues	*Procedures*	*Possible or Expected Findings*
Brain and spinal cord	For removal and specimen preparation, see Chapter 4. For selection of histologic samples, see right-hand column. Request LFB stain to highlight areas of acute necrosis.	Hypervascularity, neuronal degeneration, neuronal necrosis of mammillary bodies, periventricular regions of 3rd and 4th ventricles, anterior cerebellum and aqueduct. Hemorrhage and necrosis are typical of acute stage; shrinkage and brown discoloration of mammillary bodies suggest chronic disease.
Other organs	Procedures depend on expected findings or grossly identified abnormalities as listed in right-hand column.	Other manifestations of chronic alcoholism (see under "Alcoholism and alcohol intoxication") or of nonalcoholic steatohepatitis *(1,2)*.
Peripheral nerves	For sampling and specimen preparation, see Chapter 4.	Peripheral neuropathy. See also under "Beriberi."

References

1. Christodoulakis M, Maris T, Plaitakis A, Melissas J. Wernicke's encephalopathy after vertical banded gastroplasty for morbid obesity. Eur J Surg 1997;163:473–474.
2. Yamamoto T. Alcoholic and non-alcoholic Wernicke's encephalopathy. Be alert to the preventable and treatable disease. Internal Med 1996;35:754–755.

Syndrome, Wilson-Mikity (See "Syndrome, respiratory distress, of infant.")

Syndrome, Wiskott-Aldrich (See "Syndrome, primary immunodeficiency.")

Syndrome, Wolff-Parkinson-White (See "Malformation, Ebstein's" and "Preexcitation, ventricular.")

Syndrome, Zellweger

Synonyms and Related Terms: Adrenoleucodystrophy; cerebro-hepato-renal syndrome; infantile Refsum's disease.*

NOTE: This congenital familial cholestatic syndrome results from impaired assembly of peroxisomes and has its main manifestations in the brain, liver, and kidneys *(1)*. Craniofacial dysmorphia and hepatomegaly with siderosis are typical findings.

Reference

1. Lindhard A, Graem N, Skovby F, Jeppesen D. Postmortem findings and prenatal diagnosis of Zellweger syndrome. Case report. APMIS 1993;101:226–228.

Syndrome, Zieve (See "Alcoholism and alcohol intoxication" and "Disease, alcoholic liver.")

Syndrome, Zollinger-Ellison

Related Term: Endocrine hyperfunction and ulcer disease.

Possible Associated Condition: Multiple endocrine neoplasia.*

Organs and Tissues	*Procedures*	*Possible or Expected Findings*
Vitreous	Submit sample for sodium, chloride, urea nitrogen, and potassium determination.	Manifestations of dehydration* and hypokalemia. Postmortem values of potassium are not reliable.
Esophagus and gastrointestinal tract	Record character and location of ulcers. Histologic sections should include ulcers and all portions of stomach. Before samples are sectioned, pin stomach and other involved hollow viscera on corkboard for fixation.	Peptic ulcers in esophagus, stomach, duodenum, jejunum, and ileum. Usually, ulcers are at or near duodenal bulb. Parietal cells in corpus and fundus of stomach may be increased.
	Request PAS-alcian blue stain for sections of gastric mucosa. If there is a tumor in the gastric or duodenal wall, follow procedures described below under "Pancreas."	Gastrinoma in cardia/fundus of stomach *(1)* or wall of duodenum *(2)*. Fundic argyrophil carcinoid tumors (in patients with type 1 multiple endocrine neoplasia) *(3)*.
Pancreas	If tumor is not immediately identifiable, prepare 2-mm sagittal slices of whole organ. Examine slices under dissecting microscope.	Gastrinoma or increased number of islets of Langerhans with high proportion of non-beta cells.
	Request aldehyde-thionin stain. which stains islet B cells and frequently insulinoma cells. Request Grimelius silver stain. Silver techniques for islet D or A (A_1 or A_2) cells are also indicated.	Insulinomas may give positive aldehyde-thionin stain. Gastrinomas give positive Grimelius silver stain.
	Snap-freeze fresh tumor tissue for immunohistologic study. Submit tissue samples for electron microscopy.	Peroxidase-labeled gastrin antibodies seem to react with cells in all gastrinomas.
Other organs	Submit extrapancreatic primary or metastatic tumor tissue for biochemical and other studies, as described above. Other procedures depend on expected findings or grossly identified abnormalities as listed in right-hand column.	Aberrant gastrinoma may occur at hilus of spleen. Metastases are found in regional lymph nodes and liver. There may be manifestations of multiple endocrine neoplasia.*

References

1. Gibril F, Curtis LT, Termanini B, Fritsch MK, Lubensky IA, Doppman JL, et al. Primary cardiac gastrinoma causing Zollinger-Ellison syndrome. Gastroenterology 1997;112:567–574.
2. Kisker O, Bastian D, Bartsch D, Nies C, Rothmund M. Localization, malignant potential, and surgical management of gastrinoma. World J Surg 1998;22:651–657.
3. Cadiot G, Vissuzaine C, Potet F, Mignon M. Fundic argyrophil carcinoid tumor in a patient with sporadic-type Zollinger-Ellison syndrome. Dig Dis Sci 1995;40:1275–1278.

Syphilis, Acquired

Synonym: *Treponema pallidum* infection.

NOTE: Congenital syphilis is presented below under a separate heading.

(1) Collect all tissues that appear to be infected. (2) Culture methods are not available, but animal inoculation can be performed. Consultation with a microbiology laboratory is recommended. (3) Special stains for *Treponema pallidum* rarely are positive except with material from fresh lesions of primary or secondary syphilis. Levaditi's stain or Warthin-Starry stain is recommended for paraffin sections, and labeled fluorescent antibody techniques are recommended for frozen sections. India ink preparations or the Fontana-Masson silver stain has been used for the study of fresh lesions, and electron microscopy has also been employed. (4) In adult autopsies, no special precautions are indicated (see below under "Liver"). (5) Serologic studies are available from local and state health department laboratories. (6) This is a **reportable** disease.

Organs and Tissues	*Procedures*	*Possible or Expected Findings*
External examination	Record and prepare photographs of all abnormalities listed in right-hand column. Prepare smears and sections of acute lesions; prepare sections of older skin lesions or anogenital mucosal lesions.	Hunterian chancre in primary syphilis; condylomata lata. Noduloulcerative gummas and scarring in later stages.

Organs and Tissues	Procedures	Possible or Expected Findings
	Prepare skeletal roentgenograms.	Syphilitic periostitis; gummas; arthritis (Charcot joints of knees, hips, ankles, and lumbar and thoracic spine).
Cerebrospinal fluid	Obtain sample for laboratiory study.	Lymphocytosis and increased protein concentrations.
Lymph nodes		Syphilitic lymphadenitis.
Heart and aorta	For coronary arteriography (see Chapter 10), inject contrast medium into the clamped, ascending aorta to show takeoff of coronary arteries. Record competence of aortic valve (Chapter 3). Leave aorta attached to heart. Request Verhoeff–van Gieson stain for histologic sections of aorta.	Intimal proliferation with narrowing of coronary orifices; myocarditis. Syphilitic aortic valvulitis and aortic insufficiency.* Syphilitic aortitis with arteritis of vasa vasorum. Saccular thoracic aortic aneurysm.*
Other organs and tissues	Procedures depend on expected findings or grossly identified abnormalities. Submit samples for histologic study of small arteries.	
Brain and spinal cord	For removal and specimen preparation, see Chapter 4.	Meningitis with mononuclear cells mainly in adventitial/perivascular distribution. Infarcts; focal cortical atrophy; gliosis of floor of 4th ventricle. Tabes dorsalis.*
Bones and joints	For removal, prosthetic repair, and specimen preparation, see Chapter 2.	See above under "External examination and skin."

Syphilis, Congenital

Related Term: Congenital neurosyphilis.*

NOTE: Prior to 20 wk gestation, the destructive effects of syphilis may not be seen. Gummata are rare in neonates. Tabes dorsalis is also uncommon. Serologic diagnosis is difficult in the neonate because of transplacental transfer of maternal IgG antibodies. Acquired syphilis (syphilis in adulthood) is presented above under a separate heading.

(1) Collect all tissues that appear to be infected. (2) Culture methods are not available, but animal inoculation can be performed. Consultation with a microbiology laboratory is recommended. (3) Special stains for *Treponema pallidum* rarely are positive except with material from fresh lesions of primary or secondary syphilis and of syphilitic hepatitis of the newborn. Levaditi's stain or Warthin-Starry stain is recommended for paraffin sections, and labeled fluorescent antibody tech-niques are recommended for frozen sections. India ink preparations or the Fontana-Masson silver stain has been used for the study of fresh lesions, and electron microscopy has also been employed. (4) In neonates, special **precautions** are indicated (see below under "Liver") (5) Serologic studies are available from local and state health department laboratories. (6) This is a **reportable** disease.

Organs and Tissues	Procedures	Possible or Expected Findings
Placenta	Record weight and submit samples for histologic study.	Villous edema; plasma cell villitis and chorioamnionitis.
External examination, skin, oral and nasal cavity	Record and prepare photographs of all abnormalities listed in right-hand column. Prepare histologic sections of skin lesions.	Growth retardation; jaundice; maculopapular rash; bullae; condylomata lata; hydrocephalus;* dental deformities (Hutchinson's teeth); saddle nose; frontal bossing of skull; saber shins; snuffles; nasal septal perforation; rhagades; ulnar deviation of fingers; hydrops fetalis *(1)*.
	Prepare skeletal roentgenograms.	Irregular radiolucencies in the metaphyses and diaphyses *(2)*.
Cerebrospinal fluid	Submit samples for serologic biochemical, cytologic, and microbiologic study.	A detectable fluorescent antitreponemal antibody (absorbed) titer.[a]
Blood	Submit sample for serologic study.	A detectable fluorescent antitreponemal antibody (absorbed) titer.[a]
Liver	Record weight and sample for histologic	Syphilitic hepatitis. Histologic sections show

Organs and Tissues	*Procedures*	*Possible or Expected Findings*
	study. For special stains and infectious precautions, see above under "Note."	abundance of *Treponema* organisms.
Other organs	Procedures depend on expected findings or grossly identified abnormalities as listed in right-hand column. Submit samples for histologic study.	Fibrosing pneumonia; thymic abscesses; splenomegaly; thickening of bowel wall by inflammation and fibrosis *(2)*; splenomegaly; interstitial fibrosis and inflammation of pancreas *(2)*.
Brain and spinal cord	For removal and specimen preparation, see Chapter 4. For histologic sections, request Warthin-Starry stain for spirochetes.	Chronic meningitis, encephalitis, and myelitis. For details, see under "Neurosyphilis, congenital."
Eyes	For removal and specimen preparations, see Chapter 5.	Interstitial keratitis; choroiditis; uveitis; optic atrophy.
Bones and joints	For removal, prosthetic repair and specimen preparation, see Chapter 2.	Mononuclear periostitis; osteochondritis; "Clutton's joints" (fused joints).

[a]Immunofluorescent antigen testing is more sensitive than silver staining for the detection of Treponema pallidum *(3)*.

References

1. Levine Z, Sherer DM, Jacobs A, Rotenberg O. Nonimmune hydrops fetalis due to congenital syphilis associated with negative intrapartum mater-nal serology screening. Am J Perinatol 1998;15:233–236.
2. Oppenheimer EH, Dahms BB. Congenital syphilis in the fetus and neonate. Perspectives Pediatr Pathol 1981;6:115–138.
3. Rawstron SA, Vetrano J, Tannis G, Bromberg K. Congenital syphilis: detection of Treponema pallidum in stillborns. Clin Infect Dis 1997;24:24–27.

Syringomyelia

Synonyms and Related Term: Hydromyelia; idiopathic syringomyelia; secondary syringomyelia; syringobulbia.

Possible Associated Conditions: With idiopathic syringomyelia—Arnold Chiari malformation, type I;* basilar impression;* Klippel-Feil syndrome;* spina bifida. With secondary syringomyelia—Intramedullary gliomas (ependymoma, pilocytic astrocytoma) and vascular tumors; spinal arachnoiditis and pachymeningitis; traumatic myelopathy.

Organs and Tissues	*Procedures*	*Possible or Expected Findings*
External examination	Record and prepare photographs of all abnormalities as listed in right-hand column.	Hypertrophy of body parts. Muscle atrophy of upper extremities and hands. Cyanosis, hyperkeratosis, and other trophic changes of hands.
	Prepare roentgenograms of spine and joints.	Kyphoscoliosis. Clubfoot deformities. Cervical rib. Traumatic osteoarthropathy (Charcot joints).
Brain and spinal cord	For removal and specimen preparation, see Chapter 4. For histologic sampling, see right-hand column.	Hydrocephalus.* Cervical spinal cord is swollen and tense, with cavitation (syrinx) containing clear fluid. Wall of cavity consists of degenerated glial and neural elements, with marked gliosis. Spinal cord parenchyma is markedly compressed. See also above under "Possible Associated Conditions."

T

Tabes Dorsalis

Related Terms: General paralysis; locomotor ataxia; parenchymatous neurosyphilis; taboparesis.

Possible Associated Conditions: Acquired immunodeficiency syndrome.*

Organs and Tissues	*Procedures*	*Possible or Expected Findings*
External examination		Ulcers of feet.
	Prepare roentgenograms of major joints.	Degenerative arthritis (Charcot joints).
Cerebrospinal fluid	Submit sample for serologic study, cell count, and determination of protein concentrations.	Late in the disease, serologic tests for syphilis* may be negative. Pleocytosis and increased protein concentrations may indicate presence of meningitis.*
Brain, spinal cord, spinal ganglia, and nerves of lumbar plexus	For removal and specimen preparation of brain, spinal cord, and spinal ganglia, see Chapter 4. Request Luxol fast blue stain for myelin and Bielschowsky's stain for axons.	Syphilitic meningoencephalitis (general paresis) may also be present. Degeneration of dorsal root ganglia and posterior nerve roots (mainly lumbosacral) with Wallerian degeneration of posterior columns. Posterior roots are grey and shrunken and the spinal cord is atrophic with excavated posterior surface.
Eyes and optic nerves	For removal and specimen preparation, see Chapter 5.	Optic nerve atrophy.

Talcosis (See "Pneumoconiosis.")

Telangiectasia, Hereditary Hemorrhagic (See "Disease, Osler-Rendu-Weber.")

Tetanus

Synonym: *Clostridium tetani* infection; lockjaw.

NOTE: (1) Collect all tissues that appear infected. (2) Request aerobic and anaerobic cultures. However, the presence of tetanus bacilli established in culture is not diagnostic, since spores of *C. tetani* frequently contaminate wounds. (3) Request Gram stain. (4) Usually, no special precautions are indicated. (5) Serologic studies are available from the Centers of Disease Control and Prevention, Atlanta, GA. (6) This is a **reportable** disease.

Organs and Tissues	*Procedures*	*Possible or Expected Findings*
External examination	Record body weight and length and appearance of wound(s); photograph and excise wound(s) for histologic study.	Evidence of weight loss; subcutaneous abscesses.
	Record evidence of parenteral drug abuse, especially subcutaneous injection (i.e., "skin popping").	Tetanus may occur in drug addicts.
	Prepare chest roentgenogram.	Tension pneumothorax* after mechanical ventilation.

From: *Handbook of Autopsy Practice,* 4th Ed. Edited by: B.L. Waters

Organs and Tissues	*Procedures*	*Possible or Expected Findings*
Cerebrospinal fluid	Submit sample for microbiologic study.	Bacterial meningitis must be ruled out.
Lungs	Submit any consolidated area for microbiologic study.	Aspiration and bronchopneumonia; embolism;* atelectasis.

Tetany

NOTE: See under name of suspected underlying conditions, such as hyperparathyroidism,* malabsorption syndrome,* or vitamin D deficiency.* Respiratory or metabolic alkalosis* cannot be confirmed after death; determination of blood pH is not helpful because acidity increases rapidly after death. The concentration of serum phosphates also increases after death.

Tetralogy of Fallot

Synonym: Large ventricular septal defect with pulmonary stenosis* or atresia.*

NOTE: The basic anomaly consists of subpulmonary stenosis, ventricular septal defect, overriding aorta, and secondary right ventricular hypertrophy. For general dissection techniques, see Chapter 3. Surgical interventions include modified Blalock-Taus-sig subclavian-to-pulmonary arterial shunt; complete repair with patch closure of ventricular septal defect, and reconstruction of right ventricular outflow tract (with a patch or with an extracardial conduit).

Possible Associated Conditions: Origin of left pulmonary artery from aorta; minor abnormalities of the tricuspid valve; absent ductal artery (25%); atrial septal defect* (in 20%; pentalogy of Fallot); bicuspid pulmonary valve;* dextroposition of aorta; double aortic arch; hypoplastic pulmonary arteries; patent ductal artery;* patent oval foramen; complete atrioven-tricular septal defect* (usually with Down's syndrome*); persis-tent left superior vena cava; pulmonary valve atresia (see "Atresia, pulmonary valve, with ventricular septal defect"); right aortic arch (25%); second ventricular septal defect; origin of left anterior descending (LAD) or right coronary artery (RCA) from contralateral aortic sinus or coronary artery (5%); syndrome with absent pulmonary valve and massively dilated pulmonary arteries (rare).

Organs and Tissues	*Procedures*	*Possible or Expected Findings*
Chest cavity	Record course of superior vena cava and of its tributaries.	Persistent left superior vena cava.
	Record course of thoracic aorta and of its main branches.	Right aortic arch with or without right-sided ductal artery; double aortic arch; absent ductal artery.
	Record origin of pulmonary arteries.	Origin of the left pulmonary artery from descending aorta. For possible additional findings, see above under "Note" and under "Possible Associated Conditions."
Heart	If infective endocarditis is suspected, follow procedures described under that heading (Chapter 7). For coronary arteriography, see Chapter 10.	Infective endocarditis* (usually of pulmonary or aortic valve). See also above under "Possible Associated Conditions." Marked right ventricular hypertrophy. Right ventricular dilatation and fibrosis with late postoperative right-sided heart failure or sudden death due to arrhythmia.
Lungs	Perfuse both lungs with formalin. Request Verhoeff–van Gieson stain.	Old *in situ* thrombosis of small pulmonary artery branches.
Other organs	Procedures depend on expected findings or grossly identified abnormalities as listed in right-hand column.	Paradoxic embolism; cerebral abscess.*

Thalassemia

Synonyms and Related Terms: Congenital hemolytic anemia; alpha-thalassemia; beta-thalassemia major (Cooley's anemia); beta thalassemia minor (beta-thalassemia trait).

NOTE: The changes described below are observed primarily in beta-thalassemia major.

Organs and Tissues	Procedures	Possible or Expected Findings
External examination	Record body weight and length; record and prepare photographs of other abnormalities as listed in right-hand column.	Evidence of wasting with peculiar brownish skin pigmentation. Hydrops fetalis *(1)* and limb deformities *(2)* in rare forms of alpha-thalassemia.
	Prepare roentgenogram of skull and, if indicated, of deformed extremities.	Malocclusion of jaws due to enlargement of malar bones; bone deformities of calvaria. Deformed extremities.
All organs	Procedures depend on expected findings or grossly identified abnormalities as listed in right-hand column. See also under "Anemia, hemolytic."	Cardiomegaly and myocardial hemosiderosis with manifestations of congestive heart failure.* Pancreatic hemosiderosis (with or without diabetes mellitus); hepatosplenomegaly. Uneven iron deposition in liver *(3)*.

References

1. Chui DH, Waye JS. Hydrops fetalis caused by alpha-thalassemia: an emerging health care problem. Blood 1998;91:2213–2222.
2. Chitayat D, Silver MM, O'Brien K, Wyatt P, Waye JS, Chiu DH, et al. Limb defects in homozygous alpha-thalassemia: report of three cases. Am J Med Genet 1997;68:162–167.
3. Ambu R, et al. Uneven hepatic iron and phosphorus distribution in beta-thalasemia. J Hepatol 1995;23:544–549.

Thallium (See "Poisoning, thallium.")

Thirst (See "Dehydration.")

Thromboangiitis Obliterans (See "Disease, Buerger's.")

Thrombocytopenia (See "Purpura, thrombotic thrombocytopenic" and "Syndrome, hemolytic uremic.")

Thrombophlebitis, Ileofemoral (See "Thrombosis, venous.")

Thrombophlebitis Migrans (See "Phlebitis.")

Thrombosis, Cavernous Sinus (See "Thrombosis, cerebral venous sinus.")

Thrombosis, Cerebral Venous Sinus

Related Term: Cavernous sinus thrombosis.

NOTE: Idiopathic recurrent venous thrombosis also may affect the cerebral venous sinuses.

Organs and Tissues	Procedures	Possible or Expected Findings
External examination	Record body weight and length and skin turgor. Prepare photograph of face.	In infants, manifestations of marasmus and dehydration.* Head injury;* infection of skin in upper half of face. Presence of edema of forehead and eyelids, proptosis, and chemosis indicate cavernous sinus thrombosis.
Vitreous and eyes	If dehydration is suspected, submit samples of vitreous for electrolyte studies.	In infants, manifestations of dehydration.*
	For removal and specimen preparation of eyes, see Chapter 5.	Thrombosis of angular and superior ophthalmic veins may be associated with cavernous sinus thrombosis.
Cerebrospinal fluid	Submit sample for microbiologic study (see Chapter 7).	See below under "Brain and meninges."
Brain and meninges	For removal and specimen preparation, see Chapter 4.	Cerebral abscess* or tumor; meningitis.* Venous infarction of brain may be caused by superior sagittal sinus thrombosis *(1)*. Epidural and subdural empyema* may be present.
Calvaria and base of skull with venous sinuses	For exposure of venous sinuses, see Chapter 4. Submit contents of affected sinuses for microbiologic study. Prepare smears of contents and submit samples of sinus walls for histologic study.	Superior sagittal sinus thrombosis may be associated with terminal diseases with marasmus, with osteomyelitis,* or a tumor of the skull. (See also below under "Systemic veins.") Thrombosis and thrombophlebitis may occur in all venous sinuses.
Pituitary gland	For dissection and specimen preparation, see Chapter 4.	Infarction or abscess of pituitary gland may be caused by cavernous sinus thrombosis.

Organs and Tissues	Procedures	Possible or Expected Findings
Paranasal sinuses, middle ears, and mastoid cells	For exposure of middle ears and paranasal sinuses, see Chapter 4. If there is evidence of infection, prepare smears of contents and submit for microbiologic study.	Acute and chronic otitis media* and interna; mastoiditis; paranasal sinusitis.
Systemic veins	Procedures depend on expected findings or grossly identified abnormalities as listed in right-hand column.	Thrombosis—for instance, of pelvic veins in presence of pelvic infection. Pelvic infections and pregnancy may be associated with superior sagittal sinus thrombosis.

Reference

1. Shintaku M, Yasui N. Chronic superior sagittal sinus thrombosis with phlebosclerotic changes of the subarachnoid and intercerebral veins. Neuropath 2006;26:323–328.

Thrombosis, Lateral Sinus

NOTE: Possible causes include cholesteatoma, infections in the neck or pharynx, mastoiditis, and otitis media.* For general autopsy procedures, see "Thrombosis, cerebral venous sinus."

Thrombosis, Portal Vein (See "Hypertension, portal.")

Thrombosis, Renal Vein

NOTE: In infants, inquire about birth injury, maternal diabetes mellitus,* toxemia,* or anoxia.

Organs and Tissues	Procedures	Possible or Expected Findings
Vitreous	Submit samples of vitreous of infants for determination of sodium, chloride, and urea nitrogen concentrations.	In infants, manifestations of dehydration.*
Lungs		Pulmonary embolism.*
Retroperitoneal space and femoral veins	Procedures depend on expected findings or grossly identified abnormalities as listed in right-hand column. For renal venography, see Chapter 2. Open veins *in situ*. Dissect testicular or ovarian veins—particularly on left—and adrenal veins. For removal of femoral vessels, see Chapter 3.	Tumor of the kidney* (renal cell carcinoma); aortic aneurysm; lymphadenopathy; other mass lesions. Inferior vena cava thrombosis involving orifice or whole length of renal veins. Tumor thrombus (e.g., from renal cell carcinoma). Femoral vein thrombosis. Rare venous malformations also may cause renal vein thrombosis *(1)*.
Kidneys	Unless the cause of the renal vein thrombosis and the nature of the complicating or underlying renal disease are known, follow procedures described under "Glomerulonephritis."	Hemorrhagic infartion. Parenchymal renal disease with nephrotic syndrome,* including amyloidosis* and vasculitis* (these last conditions may be associated with renal vein thrombosis).
Other organs	Procedures depend on expected findings or grossly identified abnormalities as listed in right-hand column.	Acute gastroenteritis in infancy. Hyperparathyroidism,* pregnancy,* trauma, and other conditions.

Reference

1. Lash C, Radhakrishnan J, McFadden JC. Renal vein thrombosis secondary to absent inferior vena cava. Urol 1998;51:829–830.

Thrombosis, Venous

NOTE: For peripheral venous thrombosis, the autopsy procedures are essentially similar to those described under "Phlebitis." See also under "Hypertension, portal," "Syndrome, Budd-Chiari," "Thrombosis, cerebral venous sinus," "Thrombosis, lateral sinus," and "Thrombosis, renal vein."

Thymoma (See "Tumor of the thymus.")

Thyroiditis

Synonyms and Related Terms: Chronic fibrosing thyroiditis (Riedel's struma); chronic thyroiditis with transient thyrotoxicosis; Hashimoto's thyroiditis; pyogenic thyroiditis; subacute (granulomatous, giant cell, de Quervain's) thyroiditis.

Possible Associated Conditions: With Hashimoto's thyroiditis—autoimmune (chronic) hepatitis,* megaloblastic anemia,* rheumatoid arthritis,* Sjögren's syndrome,* and systemic lupus erythematosus.* With Riedel's struma—retroperitoneal fibrosis,* sclerosing cholangitis,* sclerosing mediastinitis,* and other conditions with idiopathic fibrosis. With subacute thyroiditis—viral infection.

Organs and Tissues	*Procedures*	*Possible or Expected Findings*
Blood	Submit sample for serologic study.	Viral antibodies in subacute (de Quervain) thyroiditis; tissue antibodies in Hashimoto's thyroiditis.
Thymus	Record weight and submit sample for histologic study.	Enlarged thymus with multiple germinal centers with Hashimoto's thyroiditis.
Neck organs	Remove together with tongue. If there is evidence of pyogenic infection, submit material for culture. Record weight of thyroid and of parathyroid glands and submit samples for histologic study, together with cervical lymph nodes. Record presence or absence of compression of trachea by struma.	Acute suppurative thyroiditis. Acute nonsuppurative thyroiditis after irradiation. Struma and lymphadenopathy in Hashimoto's thyroiditis. Fibrosis with tracheal compression associated with Riedel's struma.
Other organs	Submit samples of all endocrine glands for histologic study.	If hypothyroidism* is suspected, see also under that entry. Encephalopathy *(1)*.

Reference

1. Mocellin R, et al. Hashimoto's encephalopathy: epidemiology, pathogenesis and management. CNS Drugs 2007;21:799–811.

Thyrotoxicosis (See "Hyperthyroidism.")

Torticollis, Spasmodic

Related Terms: Dystonia musculorum deformans; torsion dystonia.

Organs and Tissues	*Procedures*	*Possible or Expected Findings*
Brain		No diagnostic pathologic lesions.

Torulosis (See "Cryptococcosis.")

Toxemia of Pregnancy

Related Terms: Eclampsia or preeclampsia; postpartum hemolytic uremic syndrome; postpartum renal failure.

NOTE: See also "Failure, kidney."

Organs and Tissues	*Procedures*	*Possible or Expected Findings*
External examination	Record body weight, extent and location of edema, and level of fundus of uterus.	Edema involving periorbital region, hands, and ankles; hemorrhagic foci in conjunctivas and fingernails.
	Prepare chest roentgenogram.	Infiltrates.
Blood	Submit sample for microbiologic study. Refrigerate sample for possible serologic, toxicologic, or biochemical study.	Evidence of infection, poisoning, electrolyte abnormalities, and other conditions.
Heart	Record weight; submit samples for histologic study.	Cardiac hypertrophy; hemorrhagic necroses caused by small-vessel thromboses.
Lungs	Submit a portion for microbiologic study. perfuse both lungs with formalin.	Hemorrhagic necroses.
Liver	Record weight; submit samples for histologic study. For the demonstration of fibrin depositis, request phosphotungstic acid hematoxylin (PTAH) stain.	Periportal fibrin deposition with hemorrhages; centrilobular and midzonal necroses or cell dropout. Infarction *(1)* and one-time or recurrent hemorrhages *(2)*.
Adrenal glands	Submit samples for histologic study (see also "Liver").	Hemorrhagic necroses.

Organs and Tissues	Procedures	Possible or Expected Findings
Kidneys	Follow procedures described under "Glomerulonephritis."	Thromboses of small vessels. Glomerulonephritis.* Hemorrhagic necroses.
Urine	Submit sample for determination of protein concentration; record appearance of sediment.	Proteinuria; abnormal sediment.
Placenta		Abruptio placentae, small placenta with accelerated maturation of villi; infarcts; fibrinoid necrosis of decidual arterioles.
Brain and spinal cord; pituitary gland	For removal and specimen preparation, see Chapter 4.	Thrombotic occlusion of small vessels with hemorrhagic necroses; anterior lobe of pituitary gland may contain necroses (see also "Syndrome, Sheehan's").

References

1. Krueger KJ, Hoffman BJ, Lee WM. Hepatic infarction associated with ecclampsia. Am J Gastroenterol 1990;85:588–592.
2. Greenstein D, Henerson JM, Boyer TD. Liver hemorrhage: recurrent episodes during pregnancy complicated by eclampsia. Gastroenterol 1994; 106:1668–1671.

Toxoplasmosis

Synonyms: Adult toxoplasmosis; congenital toxoplasmosis; disseminated toxoplasmosis; latent toxoplasmosis; *Toxoplasma gondii* infection.

NOTE: (1) Collect all tissues that appear to be infected. (2) Culturing requires animal inoculation in specialized laboratories. Consult microbiology laboratory before performing autopsy. (3) Request Giemsa stain and *Toxoplasma* immunoperoxidase or immunofluorescent stain. (4) No special precautions are indicated. (5) Serologic studies are available from local and state health department laboratories. (6) This is not a reportable disease.

Possible Associated Conditions: Acquired immunodeficiency syndrome (AIDS)* *(1,2)*.

Organs and Tissues	Procedures	Possible or Expected Findings
External examination	Record head circumference of infant. Prepare radiograph of cranium of infants.	Jaundice and hydrocephalus* in congenital toxoplasmosis.
Blood	Submit sample for serologic study.	See above under "Note."
Heart	Record weight; submit samples for histologic study and request PAS stain. Snap-freeze myocardium for immunofluorescent study.	Myocarditis* in adult form of toxoplasmosis. Trophozoites of *Toxoplasma* stain well with PAS. Coinfection with parvovirus *(4)*.
Lungs	Prepare smears and request Giemsa and immunofluorescent stains. Perfuse at least one lung with formalin.	Interstitial pneumonitis* in adult toxoplasmosis *(1)*.
Liver	Record weight. Submit sample for histologic study.	*Toxoplasma* hepatitis, with hepatocellular giant cell transformation in congenital toxoplasmosis.
	In diagnostically difficult cases, submit material for electron microscopic study (see Chapter 15).	Electron micrographs allow distinction between *Toxoplasma* and *Sarcocystis*, oval yeasts, and other organisms.
Spleen	Record weight.	Splenomegaly in congenital toxoplasmosis.
Lymph nodes	Submit samples for histologic study.	Marked follicular hyperplasia with histiocytes inside and around follicles *(3)*.
Skeletal muscles	For sampling and specimen preparation, see Chapter 2.	Myositis occurs in adult toxoplasmosis.
Placenta	Record weight and sample for histologic study.	Diffuse lymphoplasmacytic villitis with sclerosis of villi. Cysts may be found.
Other organs and tissues	Procedures depend on expected findings or grossly identified abnormalities as mentioned in right-hand column.	Infections may occur in many organs and tissues.

Organs and Tissues	Procedures	Possible or Expected Findings
Brain and spinal cord	For removal and specimen preparation, see Chapter 4.	Cerebral calcifications; periventricular necrosis. Hydrocephalus* in congenital toxoplasmosis; meningoencephalitis in adult form.
Eyes	For removal and specimen preparation, see Chapter 5.	Chorioretinitis; uveitis.

References

1. Nash G, Kerschmann RL, Herndier B, Dubey JP. The pathological manifestations of pulmonary toxoplasmosis in the acquired immunodeficiency syndrome. Hum Pathol 1994;25:652–658.
2. Bertoli F, Espino M, Arosemena JR 5th, Fishback JL, Frenkel JK. A spectrum in the pathology of toxoplasmosis in patients with acquired immu-nodeficiency syndrome. Arch Pathol Lab Med 1995;119:214–224.
3. Rose I. Morphology and diagnostics of human toxoplasmosis. General Diagn Pathol 1997;142:257–270.
4. Chimenti C, et al. Fatal myocardial coinfection by Toxoplasma gondii and Parvovirus B19 in an HIV patient. AIDS 2007;21:1386–1388.

Transfusion (See "Reaction to transfusion.")

Transplantation, Bone Marrow

NOTE: If the patient had symptoms of acute or chronic graft-versus-host disease (GVHD), see "Disease, graft-versus-host." If the patient developed recurrent leukemia, see under "Leukemia,..." Cytogenetic and other techniques can be used in such cases to determine whether the leukemic cells are of donor or host origin. If the patient developed post-transplant lymphoproliferative disease (PTLD), see under "Lymphoma."

Organs and Tissues	Procedures	Possible or Expected Findings
External examination and skin	Record skin abnormalities and sample for histologic study.	Manifestations of graft-versus-host disease (e.g., scleroderma-like changes).*
Blood	Submit sample for microbiologic study.	Septicemia.
Lungs	Submit samples for microbiologic (bacterial, fungal, and viral) and histologic studies. Request Grocott's methenamine silver stain to detect *Pneumocystis carinii* organisms. If complicating toxoplasmosis is suspected, see under that heading.	Interstitial pneumonia* and cytomegalovirus infection* or human herpesvirus 6 infection *(1)*. Bacterial, fungal, or protozoal infections. Pulmonary veno-occlusive disease (see "Hypertension, pulmonary") *(2)*.
Liver	Record weight; sample for histologic study.	Hepatic veno-occlusive disease. Viral hepatitis (hepatitis C; herpesvirus hepatitis). Cholangitis or ductopenia and other manifestations of GVHD.
Kidneys	If indicated, see also "Failure, kidney."	Kidney failure* associated with tumor lysis syndrome, hepatorenal syndrome,* cyclosporine nephrotoxicity, or bone marrow-transplant associated nephropathy *(3)*.
Other organs and tissues	If there is evidence of infection, submit material for microbiologic studies. If there is evidence of recurrent leukemia or lymphoma, sample as described under those headings.	Bacterial or fungal infections in GVHD.* Other manifestations of GVHD.* Recurrent leukemia,* lymphoma* (including post-transplant, Epstein-Barr virus associated lymphoproliferative disorder). Recurrent solid tumor, e.g., carcinoma of breast, lung (small cell carcinoma), ovary, or testis.
	If the patient had symptoms of thrombotic thrombocytopenic purpura (TTP) or hemolytic uremic syndrome (HUS), see these headings.	Manifestations of TTP, HUS *(4)*, or thrombotic microangiopathy *(5)*.
Lymph nodes	Record average size. Fix specimens in B-Plus®. Make touch preparations. Request Giemsa or Wright stain.	Lymphomatous or leukemic infiltrates.
Bone marrow	For preparation of sections and smears (imprints), see Chapter 2.	Myeloid cells may be absent in marrow graft rejection or nonimmunologic marrow graft failure.

Organs and Tissues	*Procedures*	*Possible or Expected Findings*
Brain and spinal cord; peripheral nerves	For removal and specimen preparation, see Chapter 4.	Hematomas; hemorrhagic necroses; infarcts; bacterial or fungal infections; leukoencephal-opathy; vascular siderocalcinosis; neuro-axonal spheroids *(6)*. Peripheral neuropathy.

References

1. Kadakia MP. Human herpesvirus 6 infection and associated pathogenesis following bone marrow transplantation. Leukemia Lymphoma 1998;31:251–266.
2. Williams LM, Fussell S, Veith RW, Nelson S, Mason CM. Pulmonary veno-occlusive disease in an adult following bone marrow transplantation. Case report and review of the literature. Chest 1996;109:1388–1391.
3. Pulla B, Barri YM, Anaissie E. Acute renal failure following bone mar-row transplantation. Renal Failure 1998;20:421–435.
4. Schriber JR, Herzig GP. Transplantation-associated thrombotic thrombocytopenic purpura and hemolytic uremic syndrome. Semin Hematol 1997;34:126–133.
5. Moake JL, Byrness JJ. Thrombotic microangiopathies associated with drugs and bone marrow transplantation. Hematol Oncol Clin North Am 1996:485–497.
6. Mohrmann RL, Mah V, Vinters HV. Neuropathologic findings after bone marrow transplantation: an autopsy study. Hum Pathol 1990;21: 630–639.

Transplantation, Heart

Organs and Tissues	*Procedures*	*Possible or Expected Findings*
External examination	Record abnormalities, e.g., after high-dose steroid therapy.	Cushingoid features (see "Syndrome, Cushing's") after steroid therapy.
Chest cavity	Record status of all vascular anstomoses. If there are hemorrhages, record volume and site.	Suture dehiscence. Hemothorax or hemomediastinum in recent cases.
Heart	Record weight, ventricular thickness, and valve circumferences. Take multiple sections from all areas of myocardium. Cut coronary arteries in cross sections; request Verhoeff–van Gieson stain.	Left ventricular hypertrophy, from cyclosporine-related hypertension. Acute transplant rejection (for grading, see ref. *1*). Chronic transplant vasculopathy with coronary artery stenosis *(2)*. Old or recent myocardial infarction. Recurrence of native cardiac disease (e.g., amyloidosis* or giant cell myocarditis). Infection.
Other organs	Procedures depend on expected findings or grossly identified abnormalities as listed in right-hand column.	Post-transplant lymphoproliferative disorder *(1)*. Opportunistic infection *(1)*. Pneumonia; septicemia. Fulminant toxoplasma infection *(3)*.

References

1. Billingham ME, Cary NRB, Hammond ME, Kemnitz J, Marboe C, McCallister HA, et al. A working formulation for the standardization of nomenclature in the diagnosis of heart and lung rejection: Heart and Lung Rejection Study Group. J Heart Transplant 1990;9:587–593.
2. Graham A. Autopsy findings in cardiac transplant patients: a 10-year experience. Am J Clin Pathol 1992;97:369–375.
3. Cunningham KS, Veinot JP. Fulminant toxoplasmosis following heart transplantation. Pathol 2007;39:188–189.

Transplantation, Kidney

Organs and Tissues	*Procedures*	*Possible or Expected Findings*
External examination	Record abnormalities, e.g., after high-dose steroid therapy.	Cushingoid features (see "Syndrome, Cushing's") after steroid therapy.
Blood	Submit sample for bacterial, fungal, and viral cultures. Submit samples for tests for hepatitis B and C antigens.	Septicemia (see below under "Other organs").
Other organs	If systemic infection is suspected, sample material for microbiologic study. Other procedures depend on expected findings or	Bacterial, fungal, or viral infections may be observed. There may be evidence of post-transplant lymphoproliferative disorder.

Organs and Tissues	Procedures	Possible or Expected Findings
	grossly identified abnormalities as listed in right-hand column.	
Kidneys	Dissect renal allograft *in situ* and record whether vascular and ureteral anastomoses were competent. For renal arteriography, see Chapter 2. For the processing of samples from the allograft and the native kidneys (if they had been left *in situ*), follow procedures described under "Glomerulonephritis."	Leaking anastomoses; infection; acute or chronic graft rejection. Recurrent primary disease.
Lymph nodes, bone marrow and bone	Fix samples in B-Plus® solution. For preparation of sections and smears of bone marrow, see Chapter 2.	Post-transplant lymphoproliferative disorder. Decrease in bone mineral density *(1)*.

Reference

1. Weisinger JR, et al. Bone disease after renal transplantation. Clin J Am Soc Nephrol 2006;1:1300–1313.

Transplantation, Liver

Organs and Tissues	Procedures	Possible or Expected Findings
External examination	Record abnormalities, e.g., after high-dose steroid therapy.	Cushingoid features (see "Syndrome, Cushing's") after steroid therapy.
Chest organs	Open right atrium *in situ* and probe sub-diaphragmatic inferior vena cava anastomosis; leave thoracic inferior vena cava with sleeve of right atrium attached to liver.	Dehiscence or stricture of subdiaphragmatic vena cava anastomosis. Leave esophagus attached to stomach, particularly if varices might be present.
Liver, hepatic artery, portal vein, hepatic veins, and bile ducts	Remove abdominal organs en block (intestines can be removed earlier to debulk organ block) and partially open inferior vena cava to inspect anastomoses with the graft. Dissect hepatic artery anastomosis, portal vein anastomosis, and bile duct anastomosis.	Dehiscence or stricture of anastomoses.
	If there is evidence of hepatic infection, sample material for microbiologic and histologic study. Perfuse entire liver with formalin or slice fresh organ horizontally with long-bladed knive. Obtain multiple samples for histologic study.	Nonsupporative cholangitis *(2)*; hematogenous infections; ischemic lesions, including infected infarcts; recurrent primary disease such as primary biliary cirrhosis, viral hepatitis, or tumors. Acute-cellular or chronic-ductopenic rejection (for grading of rejection, see ref. *1*).
Other organs and blood	If systemic infection is suspected, sample material for microbiologic study. Other procedures depend on expected findings or grossly identified abnormalities as listed in right-hand column.	Bacterial, fungal, or viral infections may be observed. Septicemia. Post-transplant lymphoproliferative disorder.

Reference

1. Anonymous. Banff schema for grading liver allograft rejection: an international consensus document. Hepatology 1997;25:658–663.
2. Lin CC, et al. Subacute nonsuppurative cholangitis (cholangitis lenta) in pediatric liver transplant patients. J Pediatr Gastroenterol 2007;45:228–233.

Transplantation, Lung

Organs and Tissues	Procedures	Possible or Expected Findings
External examination	Record abnormalities, e.g., after high-dose steroid therapy.	Cushingoid features (see "Syndrome, Cushing's") after steroid therapy.
Chest cavity	Record status of all vascular anstomoses. If there are hemorrhages, record volume and site.	Suture dehiscence. Hemothorax or hemomediastinum in recent cases.
Lungs	Record lung weights separately. If lung infection is suspected, submit material for microbiologic	Opportunistic infection (in patients with a single lung transplant, infections may involve

Organs and Tissues	Procedures	Possible or Expected Findings
	study. Perfuse both lungs through the bronchial tree. Cut lungs in frontal sections. Submit sections of proximal airways and of distal parenchyma for histologic study. Request Verhoeff–van Gieson and Gomori's methenamine silver stains.	the nontransplant lung, as well). Chronic bronchitis* and bronchiectasis.* Acute rejection (rare); chronic airway rejection (obliterative bronchiolitis); chronic vascular rejection. (For grading of rejection, see *ref. 1.) Post-transplant lymphoproliferative* disorder. Recurrence of primary disease (e.g., sarcoidosis,* lymphangioleiomyomatosis).
Kidneys	Submit samples for histologic study.	Manifestations of cyclosporine toxicity.
Other organs	If infection is expected, submit material for microbiologic study. Other procedures depend on expected findings or grossly identified abnormalities as listed in right-hand column.	Infection *(2)* or septicemia. Post-transplant lymphoproliferative disorder.

References

1. Billingham ME, Cary NRB, Hammond ME, Kemnitz J, Marboe C, McCallister HA, et al. A working formulation for the standardization of nomenclature in the diagnosis of heart and lung rejection: Heart and Lung Rejection Study Group. J Heart Transplant 1990;9:587–593.
2. Tazelaar HD, Yousem SA. The pathology of combined heart-lung transplantation: an autopsy study. Hum Pathol 1988;19:1403–1416.

Transposition, Complete, of the Great Arteries

NOTE: The basic anomaly is the origin of the aorta from the right ventricle, and of the pulmonary artery from the left ventricle, with a shunt, and usually with a right anterior aorta. There are four major types: (1) with an intact ventricular septum (65%), (2) with a ventricular septal defect* (20%), (3) with a ventricular septal defect and subvalvular pulmonary stenosis* (10%), and (4) with an intact ventricular septum and subvalvular pulmonary stenosis* (5%). For general dissection techniques, see Chapter 3. Interventions include atrial septostomy or septectomy; Mustard or Senning atrial switch procedure; Rastelli-type repair with a valved extracardiac conduit; and Jatene arterial switch procedure with LeCompte maneuver.

Possible Associated Conditions: Abnormal origin of coronary arteries (10%); atrial septal defect* (5%); coarctation of the aorta;* interrution of the aortic arch;* juxtaposition of atrial appendages (4%); overriding aorta (5%); overriding pulmonary artery (10%); patent ductal artery;* patent oval foramen; subvalvular pulmonary stenosis* (15%); tubular hypoplasia of the aortic arch;* ventricular septal defect* (30%), often mal-alignment type (50%).

Transposition, Physiologically Corrected, of the Great Arteries

Synonyms: Atrioventricular and ventriculoarterial discordance; L-transposition.

NOTE: The basic anomaly is a mirror-image ventricular inversion, with a left anterior aorta, and with blood flow from right atrium to left ventricle to pulmonary artery, and from left atrium to right ventricle to aorta. For general dissection techniques, see Chapter 3. Interventions include patch closure of the ventricular septal defect; relief of pulmonary stenosis; relief of tricuspid insufficiency; and insertion of pacemakers.

Possible Associated Conditions: Anterior and posterior AV nodes (100%), prone to develop complete heart block; dysplasia or Epstein's malformation* of left-sided tricuspid valve (40%); mirror-image epicardial coronary artery distribution (100%); right-sided mitral valve anomalies; subvalvular pulmonary stenosis* (40%); ventricular septal defect* (65%).

Trichinosis

Synonyms: *Trichinella spiralis* infection; trichinelliasis; trichiniasis.

NOTE: (1) Collect all tissues that appear infected. (2) Request direct examination for *Trichinella.* (3) Request Giemsa stain. (4) No special precautions are indicated. (5) Serologic studies are available from local and state health department laboratories. (6) This is a **reportable** disease.

Organs and Tissues	Procedures	Possible or Expected Findings
External examination and skin	Record abnormalities and photopgraph edema and hemorrhages.	Palpebral and facial edema; splinter hemorrhages under the nails.
Blood	Obtain sample for quantification of IgE and eosinophils.	Increased IgE concentration and eosinophilia.
Heart	Record weight and submit samples of myocardium for histologic study.	Interstitial myocarditis early in the disease; focal necroses; no cysts can be seen.

Organs and Tissues	Procedures	Possible or Expected Findings
Duodenum, jejunum, and ileum	For preparation for study under the dissecting microscope, see Chapter 2. Submit samples for histologic study.	Mild partial villous atrophy; acute and chronic infiltrate with eosinophils in mucosa and submucosa; mucosal edema; punctate hemorrhages; prominent Peyer's plaques.
Lungs, kidney, liver, pancreas, and soft tissues	Submit samples for histologic study. In older infections, decalcification of cysts and larvae may be required.	Resorption granulomas around migrating larvae.
	Prepare roentgenograms of organs and soft tissues.	Calcified cysts.
Kidneys	Follow procedures described under "Glomerulonephritis."	Immune-mediated glomerulonephritis.*
Lymph nodes	Submit samples for histologic study.	Resorption granulomas around migrating larvae.
Brain and spinal cord	For removal and specimen preparation, see Chapter 4. For decalcification, see Chapter 2.	Mononuclear meningitis; tiny foci of gliosis around capillaries; encephalitis.
Skeletal muscles	Submit samples for histologic study, especially from diaphragm, gastrocnemius, intercostal, deltoid, gluteus, and pectoral muscles.	Encysted larvae; cysts in varying stages of lymphocytic and eosinophilic inflammation and degeneration.
	Prepare roentgenograms.	Calcified cysts.
Bone marrow	For preparation of sections and smears, see Chapter 2.	Hyperplasia and eosinophilia.

Trisomy 21 (See "Syndrome, Down's.")

Truncus Arteriosus (See "Artery, persistent truncal.")

Trypanosomiasis, African

Synonyms: African sleeping sickness; *Trypanosoma brucei gambiense* infection (West African trypanosomiasis); *Trypanosoma brucei rhodesiense* infection (East African trypanosomiasis).

NOTE: (1) Collect all tissues that appear infected. (2) Request direct examination for trypanosomes. (3) Request Giemsa stain. (4) No special precautions are indicated. (5) Serologic studies are available from the Centers for Disease Control and Prevention, Atlanta, GA. (6) This is not a reportable disease.

Organs and Tissues	Procedures	Possible or Expected Findings
External examination	Record abnormalities and photograph skin changes.	Cachexia. Facial edema; rash, especially on rump.
Cerebrospinal fluid	Submit sample for biochemical analysis and prepare sediment.	Increased IgM protein concentrations; trypanosomes may be present, especially in late Gambian disease; plasma cells with Russell bodies (Mott cells).
Chest and abdomen	Record volume of effusions and prepare smears of sediment.	Ascites; pleural* and pericardial effusions with trypanosomes.
Blood	Prepare thick, unfixed film and request Giemsa stain.	Trypanosomes may be present, particularly in Rhodesian disease.
Heart	Record weight and submit samples for histologic study.	Acute and chronic pancarditis, or both, with cardiac hypertrophy* and dilatation.
Lymph nodes	Submit touch preparations and material in B-Plus® fixative (see Chapter 15) for histologic study.	Reactive hyperplasia in early stages; perivascular mononuclear infiltration; fibrosis in later stages.
Brain and spinal cord	For removal and specimen preparation, see Chapter 4. Histologic sections should include cortex, basal ganglia, cerebellum, brain stem, and spinal cord.	Cerebral edema; diffuse perivascular lymphoplasmacytic meningoencephalitis in cortex; characteristic are Mott cells (see above) in brain and spinal cord; inflamed choroid plexus; hydrocephalus.*

Trypanosomiasis, American (See "Disease, Chagas.")

Tuberculosis

Synonyms and Related Terms: *Mycobacterium tuberculosis, M. bovis, M. africanum* infection; scrofula; lupus vulgaris.

NOTE: (1) Collect all tissues that appear infected. (2) Request mycobacterial cultures. (3) Request Ziehl-Neelsen, Kinyoun's, or other acid-fast stains. Polymerase chain reaction for mycobacterial DNA may be helpful in the differential diagnosis of granulomas *(1)*. (4) Universal **precautions** should be strictly followed and aerolization should be avoided. (5) Reliable serologic studies are not available. A definite diagnosis requires isolation of the organism. (6) This is a **reportable** disease.

Organs and Tissues	*Procedures*	*Possible or Expected Findings*
External examination and skin	Record abnormalities and prepare photographs. Submit sections of skin lesions for histologic study; if there are fistulas, obtain curettings for smears for acid fast stains (see "Note" above) and for culture. Fill fistulas with contrast medium and prepare roentgenograms.	Tuberculosis of skin (lupus vulgaris).
	Prepare chest and skeletal roentgenograms.	Pulmonary infiltrates and cavities; effusions; manifestations of tuberculous osteomyelitis and arthritis.
Chest and abdomen	Record volume of effusions or exudates; submit sections of serosal surfaces for histologic study.	Tuberculous pleuritis, pericarditis,* and peritonitis.
Lungs with hilar lymph nodes	If diagnosis was confirmed clinically, perfuse both lungs with formalin; if not, submit consolidated or cavitated areas for culture and histologic study with acid-fast stains.	Cavitary, fibrocalcific, miliary, bronchial, and other types of pulmonary tuberculosis; granulomas in hilar lymph nodes.
Other organs	Procedures depend on expected findings or grossly identified abnormalities as listed in right-hand column. See also above under "Lungs with hilar lymph nodes."	Most organs and tissues may be involved, including liver, pancreas, spleen, kidneys, adrenal glands and other endocrine glands, gonads, and lymph nodes.
Brain and spinal cord	For removal and specimen preparation, see Chapter 4. If material is to be submitted for culture, follow procedures described under "Meningitis", in this section.	Tuberculous meningitis; tuberculoma.
Eyes	For removal and specimen preparation, see Chapter 5.	Iridocyclitis or panophthalmitis.
Bones and joints	Submit sample of synovial fluid for culture. For removal, prosthetic repair, and specimen preparation, see Chapter 2.	Tuberculous arthritis and synovitis (hips, spine, knee); tuberculous osteomyelitis (anterior aspect of vertebrae; metaphysis of long bones).

Reference

1. Trauner M, Grasmug E, Stauber RE, Hammer HF, Hoefler G, Reisinger EC. Recurrent Salmonella enteritidis and hepatic tuberculosis. Gut 1995;37:136–139.

Tularemia

Synonyms and Related Terms: *Francisella tularensis* infection; *Pasteurella tularensis* infection; typhoidal tularemia; ulceroglandular tularemia; rabbit fever.

NOTE: (1) Collect all tissues that appear infected. (2) Request aerobic bacterial cultures. (3) Request Gram stain. (4) Special **precautions** are indicated. (5) Serologic studies are available from local and state health department laboratories. (6) This is not a reportable disease.

Organs and Tissues	Procedures	Possible or Expected Findings
External examination, skin, and eyes	Record abnormalities and photograph skin changes; submit for histologic study.	Skin ulcers of hands, feet or perineal area; necrotizing lesions of eye and purulent conjunctivitis.
Chest and abdomen	Submit samples of serosal surfaces for histologic study.	Peritonitis;* perisplenitis; pleural effusions.*
Heart	If infective endocarditis is suspected, follow procedures described in Chapter 7.	Infective endocarditis;* pericarditis.*
Lungs	Record lung weights. Submit consolidated areas for bacterial culture.	Necrotizing bronchopneumonia.
Liver and spleen	Record weights. Submit samples for histologic study.	Hepatosplenomegaly; characteristic granulomas.
Lymph nodes	Submit enlarged lymph nodes (particularly those with draining skin lesions) for histologic and microbiologic study. Prepare smears for Gram stain.	Lymphadenopathy; granulomatous lymphadenitis.
Brain and spinal cord		Meningitis.* Cerebral abscesses *(1)*.
Nasopharynx	Remove neck organs together with portions of pharynx. Nasal cavities will be accessible after removal of brain (Chapter 4).	Necrotizing nasopharyngeal lesions.
Bones		Osteomyelitis.*

Reference

1. Gangat N. Cerebral abscesses complicating tularemia meningitis. Scand J Infect Dis 2007;39:258–261.

Tumor, Carcinoid (See "Syndrome, carcinoid.")

Tumor, Endocrine (See "Neoplasia, multiple endocrine," "Syndrome, carcinoid," and "Tumor, of the [name of affected gland].")

Tumor, Malignant, Any Type

NOTE: If the tumor had been treated by surgery, irradiation, chemotherapy, or other means (the most common situation at autopsy), record possible adverse treatment effects and presence or absence of recurrent or metastatic malignancy. If the patient had participated in a treatment trial, contact investigator or consult study protocol to provide optimal autopsy documentation.

For classification and terminology of tumors and their histologic features, the tumor fascicles of the Armed Forces Institute of Pathology are recommended references. Of course, many other excellent textbooks of tumor pathology are available.

For some tumors, possible associated or underlying conditions are listed. However, many additional associations do or might exist and therefore, careful documentation of all autopsy findings is recommended, even if abnormalities do not appear clearly tumor-related.

Tumor of the Adrenal Gland(s)

NOTE: See also "Tumor, malignant, any type."

Possible Associated Conditions: With adrenocortical adenoma—Conn's syndrome (primary hyperaldosteronism); Cush-ing's syndrome* with virilization. With adrenocortical carci-noma—Cushing's syndrome;* hypoglycemia;* virilization. With pheochromocytoma—cerebellar hemangioblastoma; ery-throcytosis; hypercalcemia; hypertension,* multiple endocrine neoplasia* (with medullary carcinoma of the thyroid in types 2a and 2b and with hyperparathyroidism in type 2a); neurofibromatosis* (von Recklinghausen's disease); von Hippel-Lindau disease.*

Organs and Tissues	Procedures	Possible or Expected Findings
External examination	Record body weight and abnormal features. Photograph skin changes.	Cachexia. Virilization or cushingoid features (see above under "Possible Associated Conditions.")
Heart and arteries	Record heart weight and thickness of ventricles. Procure multiple sections of myocardium.	Focal myocarditis.* Hypertensive cardiovascular disease (See "Hypertension [arterial], all types or type unspecified"). Myocardial infarction without severe coronary artery disease (with pheochromocytoma).

Organs and Tissues	*Procedures*	*Possible or Expected Findings*
Gallbladder	Record contents of gallbladder.	Cholelithiasis* with pheochromocytoma.
Urine	Refrigerate sample for biochemical study—for instance, of catecholamines in cases with pheochromocytoma, or 17-ketosteroids and 17-hydroxy-corticosteroids with adrenocortical carcinoma.	Abnormal metabolites.
Retroperitoneal space	Photograph and record size of tumor(s). Snap-freeze portion of fresh tumor tissue for biochemical study. Submit samples of both tumor and adjacent tissues for histologic study. For fixation in Orth's solution and gross staining procedures for pheochromocytoma, see Chapter 15.	Pheochromocytoma may be bilateral and multiple. The tumor may also occur in other sites of the retroperitoneal space (organ of Zuckerkandl) and pelvis.
Other organs and tissues	Chemodectomas and carotid body tumors rarely may produce large amounts of catecholamines. Tumors of this type must be searched for if adrenal glands appear normal.	Pheochromocytoma may occur in paravertebral areas of thorax and neck and, rarely, in the urinary bladder. Widespread metastases may occur with pheochromocytoma and with adrenocortical carcinoma.
Bone marrow	For preparation of sections and smears, see Chapter 2.	Hyperplasia in association with pheochromocytoma. Extramedullary hematopoiesis may also be present. Hyperplasia would indicate the presence of an erythropoiesis-stimulating factor in tumor and plasma.

Tumor of the Bile Ducts (Extrahepatic or Hilar or of Papilla of Vater)

Possible Associated Conditions: Clonorchiasis;* fibropolycystic disease of the liver and biliary tract;* inflammatory bowel disease;* primary sclerosing cholangitis.*

Organs and Tissues	*Procedures*	*Possible or Expected Findings*
External examination	Record body weight.	Cachexia; jaundice.
Duodenum	Open and fix as soon as possible.	Tumor of papilla of Vater.
Bile ducts	Expose extrahepatic bile ducts *in situ*. Record width of lumen at area of obstruction and proximal and distal to it. Record and collect contents of bile duct (sludge, concrements, parasites).	Usually, bile ducts proximal to the obstruction are dilated. Choledochal cyst* *(1)*. Primary sclerosing cholangitis.* Infestation with *Clonorchis sinensis* or *Opisthorchis viverrini* (rarely observed in North America) *(2)*.
Lymph nodes	Dissect all hepatoduodenal lymph nodes and submit samples for histologic study, even if no metastatic tumor is grossly evident.	Lymph nodes seldom compress bile ducts to such an extent that they cause bile duct obstruction.
Portal vein	Dissect vein *in situ*.	Thrombosis* (blood clot or tumor or both); pylephlebitis.
Gallbladder	Record volume and character of contents. Search for primary tumor (with or without cholelithiasis) or tumor infiltration of gallbladder.	Dilatation of gallbladder (Courvoisier's sign); cholecystitis;* cholelithiasis.* White bile.
Liver	Record weight. Submit samples for histologic and microbiologic study.	Ascending cholangitis. Cholangitic and pylephlebitic abscesses; cholestasis. Primary sclerosing cholangitis* (PSC) with or without biliary cirrhosis. Secondary (obstructive) biliary cirrhosis without PSC. Intrahepatic metastases.

Organs and Tissues	Procedures	Possible or Expected Findings
Colon	Procedures depend on expected findings or grossly identified abnormalities as listed in right-hand column.	Chronic ulcerative colitis may be associated with carcinoma of bile ducts, typically arising in PSC.*
Other organs	Procedures depend on expected findings or grossly identified abnormalities as listed in right-hand column.	Metastases common in regional lymph nodes and lungs.

References

1. Fieber SS, Nance FC. Choledochal cyst and neoplasm: a comprehensive review of 106 cases and presentation of two original cases. Am Surgeon 1997;63:982–987.
2. Elkins DB, Mairiang E, Sithithaworn P, Mairiang P, Chaiyakum J, Chamadol N, et al. Cross sectional patterns of hepatobiliary abnormalities and possible precursor conditions of cholangiocarcinoma associated with Opisthorchis viverrini infections in humans. Am J Trop Med Hyg 1996;55: 295–301.

Tumor of Bone or Cartilage

Possible Associated Conditions: Bone infarction; chronic osteomyelitis;* fibrous dysplasia of bone; Paget's disease of bone.*

Organs and Tissues	Procedures	Possible or Expected Findings
External examination	Record body weight.	Cachexia.
Vitreous	Submit for determination of electrolyte concentrations. Postmortem calcium value in blood is unreliable.	Evidence of hypercalcemia (particularly in presence of osteolytic metastases).
Bones and joints	Prepare roentgenograms or review clinical films. For removal, prosthetic repair, and specimen preparation and decalcification procedures, see Chapter 2. If *osteoblastic* metastases appear to be present, search for primary tumor in prostate and breast, carcinoid tumors and Hodgkin's lymphoma.	Metastases to bone (e.g., from carcinoma of prostate, breast, bronchi, thyroid gland, kidney, or urinary bladder) usually involve red bone marrow. Therefore, distal extremities are rarely involved by metastatic tumors in adults.
Other organs	Procedures depend on expected findings or grossly identified abnormalities as listed in right-hand column.	Metastases, commonly in lungs.

Tumor of the Brain

For pituitary tumors or tumors of the spinal cord, see under these headings.

Possible Associated Conditions: Neurofibromatosis;* tuberous sclerosis;* von Hippel-Lindau Disease.*

Organs and Tissues	Procedures	Possible or Expected Findings
External examination	Record body weight.	Cachexia.
Brain and spinal cord	For removal and specimen preparation, and for cerebral arteriography, see Chapter 4.	
	If tumor showed endocrine activity, submit fresh sample (snap-freeze) for biochemical study.	Cerebellar hemangioblastoma with erythropoiesis-stimulating factor. Other endocrine-active tumors. See also "Tumor of the pituitary gland."

Tumor of the Breast

Possible Associated Conditions: Acanthosis nigricans; cerebellar cortical degeneration;* dermatomyositis;* subacute spinocerebellar degeneration.* See also below under "Possible or Expected Findings."

Organs and Tissues	*Procedures*	*Possible or Expected Findings*
External examination and skin	Record body weight. Record skin abnormalities, prepare photographs of these lesions, and sample for histologic study.	Cachexia. Acanthosis nigricans; herpes zoster infection;* dermatomyositis.* Carcinoma metastases to skin.
Breasts and axillary lymph nodes	Record size and location of tumor. Submit tumor tissue for histologic study. Grossly uninvolved breast tissue as well as sentinel and other axillary lymph nodes of both sides should be cut into thin slices to detect tumor.	Metastases or secondary primary tumor may occur in opposite breast.
	If a mastectomy or other breast surgery had been done, explore site for local recurrence.	Local recurrence of breast tumor.
Other organs	Histologic samples should include right and left supraclavicular and retrosternal lymph nodes, lungs, liver, bone marrow, and endocrine (pituitary) glands.	Regional and systemic metastases frequent at sites listed in middle column. Eosinophilic infiltrates may be present in many tissues.
Brain and spinal cord	For removal and specimen preparation, see Chapter 2.	Cerebellar cortical degeneration.* Subacute spinocerebellar degeneration.*
Skeletal muscles	For sampling and specimen preparation, see Chapter 2.	Myopathy;* dermatomyositis.*

Tumor of the Colon

Possible Associated Conditions: With adenocarcinoma of the colon—Barrett's esophagus *(1)*; chronic ulcerative colitis; Crohn's disease;* familial colonic polyposis;* Gardner's syndrome; juvenile polyposis; non-polyposis syndrome; Peutz-Jeghers syndrome;* Turcot's syndrome.

Organs and Tissues	*Procedures*	*Possible or Expected Findings*
External examination	Record body weight.	Cachexia.
Blood and vitreous	Submit blood sample for microbiologic study. Submit vitreous for determination of calcium and glucose concentration. Postmortem calcium values in blood are unreliable.	Increased incidence of colonic cancer in the presence of *S. bovis* bacteremia. Hypercalcemia. Hypoglycemia* may be present but usually cannot be diagnosed at autopsy.
	Circulating carcinoembryonic antigen can be determined in blood sample.	Carcinoembryonic antigen not specific for carcinoma of the colon.
Heart	If endocarditis is suspected, see under that heading.	Increased incidence of colonic cancer in the presence of *S.bovis* endocarditis.
Colon	Record exact location, size, and shape of tumor and width of lumen in area of tumor and proximal and distal to it.	See above under "Possible Associated Conditions." Muscular hypertrophy of colon proximal to tumor. Mixed adeno endocrine carcinoma *(3)*.
	Record presence of ureterosigmoidostomy (for congenital extrophy of bladder).	Increased incidence of colon cancer after ureterosigmoidostomy.
Other organs	Procedures depend on expected findings or grossly identified abnormalities as listed in right-hand column. For decalcification methods, see Chapter 2.	Metastatic calcification in patients with hypercalcemia. Eosinophilia. Myopathy.* Metastases in liver and regional lymph nodes. See also above under "Possible Associated Conditions." Malakoplakia (rare) *(2)*.

References

1. HowdenCW,HornungCA.Asystematicreviewoftheassociationbetween Barrett's esophagus and colon neoplasm. Am J Gastroenterol 1995;90: 1814–1819.
2. Bates AW, Dev S, Baithun SI. Malakoplakia and colorectal adenocarcinoma. Postgrad Med J 1997;73:171–173.
3. Pecorella I, et al. An unusual case of colonic mixed adenoendocrine carcinoma: collision vs composite tumor. A case report and review of the literature. Ann Diagn Pathol 2007;11:285–290.

Tumor of the Esophagus

Possible Associated Conditions: Barrett's esophagus;* Plummer-Vinson syndrome;* tylosis of palms and soles. See also below under "Possible or Expected Findings."

Organs and Tissues	*Procedures*	*Possible or Expected Findings*
External examination and skin	Record body weight.	Cachexia.
	Record skin changes, prepare photographs, and sample for histologic study.	Congenital hyperkeratosis and pitting of the palms and soles (tylosis of palms and soles).
Chest	Record volume and character of fluid in pleural cavities.	Pleural empyema.*
		Tracheoesophageal fistula. Mediastinitis, with or without mediastinal emphysema. Metastases.
	Submit lymph nodes for histologic study.	
Esophagus with neck organs and stomach	Remove neck organs with tongue together with esophagus. Open pharynx and esophagus in posterior midline. If fistulas and abscesses are suspected, dissect esophagus but leave attached to mediastinum, stomach and diaphragm.	Esophageal web and glossitis in Plummer-Vinson syndrome.*
	Record width of lumen of esophagus at various levels. Photograph and record size and location of tumor; sample tumor and uninvolved esophagus for histologic study. Request PAS stain of uninvolved esophagus (sample from all levels).	Esophagus dilated proximal to obstruction, with or without retained food or medications. Stricture or total luminal occlusion by tumor. Reflux esophagitis (distal) and Barrett's esophagus* with low-grade and high-grade dysplasia (distal or at all levels).
Other organs	Procedures depend on expected findings or grossly identified abnormalities as listed in right-hand column.	Metastases in regional lymph nodes and lungs.

Tumor of the Gallbladder

NOTE: Follow procedures described under "Tumor of the bile ducts (extrahepatic or hilar or of papilla of Vater").

Tumor of the Heart

Possible Associated Conditions: Carney's syndrome with cardiac myxomas; LAMB syndrome (lentigines, atrial myxoma, blue nevi); NAME syndrome (pigmented nevi, atrial myxoma, myxoid neurofibroma, and ephelids); also with myxoma of the heart: Adrenal cortical nodules with or without Cushing's syndrome;* pituitary adenomas; and testicular tumors. With cardiac rhabdomyoma(s): Adenoma sebaceum; benign kidney tumors;* tuberous sclerosis.*

Organs and Tissues	*Procedures*	*Possible or Expected Findings*
External examination	Record and prepare photographs of skin lesions.	Freckles (ephelides); pigmented spots (lentigines) or pigmented nevi; clubbing of fingers (with cardiac myxoma).
Heart	If rhabdomyoma is suspected, submit tumor samples in absolute alcohol or other water-free fixative for demonstration of glycogen. Record size and location of	Glycogen in rhabdomyoma is extractable with dilute trichloracetic acid. Tumor types include fibroma, lipoma, myxoma; primary or metastatic sarcoma; lymphoma;*

Organs and Tissues	Procedures	Possible or Expected Findings
	tumor(s). If tumor is within a heart chamber (usually a myxoma), record extent of mobility and capability of tumor to obstruct a valvular orifice. Submit samples of tumor(s) for histologic study and, particularly if the tumor is of unknown type, for immunohistochemical study and electron microscopy (Chapter 15).	metastatic carcinoma or melanoma. Secondary cardiac effects by tumors include carcinoid heart disease, amyloid heart disease in multiple myeloma, and lymphocytic myocarditis in pheochromocytoma. Treatment effects such as adriamycin cardiotoxicity may be noted also.
Other organs and peripheral arteries	Procedures depend on expected findings or grossly identified abnormalities as listed in right-hand column.	Tumor (myxoma) emboli in pulmonary or peripheral vessels *(1)*. Multiple aneurysms* of cerebral and other arteries may rarely be associated with atrial myxomas.

Reference

1. Lee VH et al. Central nervous system manifestations of cardiac myxoma Arch Neurol 2007;64:1115–1120.

Tumor of the Hematopoietic or Lymphatic Tissue (See "Leukemia" or "Lymphoma.")

Tumor of the Intestines (See "Tumor of the colon" and "Tumor of the small intestine.")

Tumor of the Kidney(s)

Possible Associated Conditions: With adult renal cell carcinoma—amyloidosis,* hepatomegaly (Stauffer's syndrome), von Hippel Lindau disease;* also leukemoid reaction and plasmacytosis; with either adult renal cell carcinoma or nephroblastoma—manifestations of hypertension* or polycythemia;* with Wilms tumor—polycythemia* *(1)*; with renal medullary carcinoma—sickle cell disease* *(2)*. See also below under "Possible or Expected Findings."

Organs and Tissues	Procedures	Possible or Expected Findings
External examination and skin	Record body weight.	Cachexia.
	Record skin changes, prepare photographs, and sample for histologic study.	Eczematoid dermatitis with adult renal cell carcinoma. Cushing's syndrome,* galactorrhea or feminization or masculinization in some cases of renal cell carcinoma.
Blood	Submit sample for biochemical study.	Evidence of hyperalcemia.
Lungs	Inspect lumen of pulmonary arteries prior to dissection (fresh emboli may fall out).	Pulmonary tumor embolism after invasion of renal vein and inferior vena cava.
Retroperitoneal space and kidneys	Renal veins and inferior vena cava should be opened *in situ* or after removal of organ block. Photograph tumor; record size of tumor and extent of tumor invasion. Snap-freeze portion of tumor tissue for possible biochemical	Acquired renal cystic disease (mainly in dialysis patients) with renal cell carcinoma *(3)*. Tumor thrombus in renal vein and inferior vena cava.
	or molecular study. For arteriography of kidneys, see Chapter 2.	Erythropoietin, gonadotropins, parathyroid hormone, prolactin, renin, and prostaglandins in some renal cell carcinomas.
Other organs	Procedures depend on expected findings or grossly identified abnormalities as listed above and in right-hand column.	See above under "Possible Associated Conditions." Metastases are common in lungs and regional lymph nodes.

References

1. Lal A, Rice A, al Mahr M, Kern IB, Marshall GM. Wilms tumor associated with polycythemia: case report and review of the literature. J Pediatr Hematol/Oncol 1997;19:263–265.
2. Wesche WA, Wilimas J, Khare V, Parham DM. Renal medullary carcinoma: a potential sickle cell nephropathy of children and adolescents. Pediatr Pathol Lab Med 1998;18:97–113.
3. Levine E. Acquired cystic kidney disease. Radiol Clin North Am 1996;34:947–964.

Tumor of the Liver

Possible Associated Conditions: With hepatocellular carcinoma (HCC)—Alagille's syndrome (arteriohepatic dysplasia), $alpha_1$-antitrypsin deficiency,* alpha-fetoproteinemia, ataxia telangiectasia, Byler's disease, carcinoid syndrome,* cirrhosis* of any type (mostly nonbiliary), congenital hepatic fibrosis,* Cushing's syndrome,* erythrocytosis, genetic hemochromatosis,* glycogen storage disease (type I),* hepatitis B or C virus infection, hereditary tyrosinemia (type I),* hypercalcemia, hypercholesterolemia, hypoglycemia,* neurofibromatosis,* Osler-Rendu-Weber disease* (hereditary hemorrhagic telangiectasia), polycythemia,* porphyria (acute intermittent and porphyria cutanea tarda),* pseudohyperparathyroidism,* and thorium (thorotrast) deposition.

With bile duct carcinoma (cholangiocarcinoma)—*Clonorchis sinensis* or *Opisthorchis viverrini* infection, fibropolycystic liver and biliary tract disease,* hepatolithiasis, hypercalcemia, pri-mary sclerosing cholangitis,* and thorium (thorotrast) deposition.

With hepatoblastoma—Alpha-fetoproteinemia, cardiac and renal malformations, cleft palate, diaphragmatic hernia,* Down's syndrome,* familial colonic polyposis,* hemihypertrophy, nephroblastoma.

With angiosarcoma—Thorium (thorotrast) deposition.

See also below under "Possible or Expected Findings."

Organs and Tissues	*Procedures*	*Possible or Expected Findings*
External examination and skin	Record body weight. Record abnormal features as listed in right-hand column; prepare photographs.	Cachexia. Precocious puberty. Feminization and gynecomastia in rare cases of HCC. Spider angiomas; clubbing of fingers.
Blood	Refrigerate sample for possible biochemical study.	See above under "Possible Associated Conditions."
Abdominal cavity	Record volume and character of contents; determine hematocrit of hemorrhagic fluid.	Hemoperitoneum or ascites (which may be hemorrhagic).
Liver	For hepatic angiography, see Chapter 2. Record weight and size of liver and size and location of tumor(s). Describe and photograph cut surfaces. Sample tumor and nonneoplastic liver for histologic study. If thorium deposition is suspected, prepare roentgenograms of liver slices and submit samples for energy-dispersive x-ray microanalysis of paraffin sections.	Tumor thrombi or thromboses in hepatic and portal veins. Hemorrhages after rupture of tumor (HCC and angiosarcoma). Evidence of chronic viral hepatitis B or C;* cirrhosis* of any type (mostly nonbiliary). Thorotrast storage may cause cirrhosis, HCC, bile duct carcinoma, or angiosarcoma.
Other organs	Procedures depend on expected findings or grossly identified abnormalities as listed above and in right-hand column.	See above under "Possible Associated Conditions." Metastases most common in lungs and regional lymph nodes.

Tumor of the Lung or Bronchus

Possible Associated Conditions: Abnormal concentrations of hormons or other metabolites in blood and tumor tissue (adrenocorticotropic, antidiuretic, growth hormone, parathyroid-like substances, or 5-hydroxyindolacetic acid); acanthosis nigricans; acromegaloid features; carcinoid syndrome;* Cushing's syndrome;* dermal hyperpigmentation; feminization; hyperglycemia; hypercalcemia; hypoglycemia;* hypokalemia; hyponatremia; precocious puberty. For syndromes affecting the brain, peripheral nerves or muscles, see below under "Possible or Expected Findings." (Most paracarcinomatous syndromes are associated with small cell or other types of bronchogenic carcinoma.)

Organs and Tissues	*Procedures*	*Possible or Expected Findings*
External examination and skin	Record body weight. Record abnormal features as listed in right-hand column; prepare photographs. Prepare histologic sections of normal and grossly abnormal skin. Prepare skeletal roentgenograms.	Cachexia. Skin metastases. Clubbing of fingers; spider angiomas. For other rare tumor-related changes, see above under "Possible Associated Conditions." Hypertrophic osteoarthropathy;* pachydermoperiostosis. Bone marrow metastases.

Organs and Tissues	*Procedures*	*Possible or Expected Findings*
Blood and vitreous	Submit samples of vitreous for study of electrolyte and sugar concentrations. Submit sample of serum for possible hormon assay.	See above under "Possible Associated Conditions." Note that hypoglycemia* generally cannot be confirmed at autopsy.
Heart	Inspect valves and prepare photographs and sections of vegetations.	Nonbacterial thrombotic endocarditis.*
Lungs	For pulmonary arteriography and bronchography, see Chapter 2. Record size and location of tumor(s). If there was evidence of endocrine activity (see above), snap-freeze portion of fresh tumor for hormone assay. Perfuse lungs with formalin. Sample neoplastic and non-neoplastic tissue for histologic study.	Carcinoma may be associated with asbestosis or other types of pneumoconiosis,* chronic bronchitis,* emphysema,* interstitial pneumonia,* and many other broncho-pulmonary diseases.
Other organs and tissues	Procedures depend on expected findings or grossly identified abnormalities as listed above and in right-hand column.	See above under "Possible Associated Conditions." Metastases (regional lymph nodes, liver, bones, brain, and many other sites) and metastatic calcification.
Peripheral veins	For removal and specimen preparation, see Chapter 4.	Migratory thrombophlebitis.*
Brain and spinal cord	For removal and specimen preparation, see Chapter 4.	Encephalomyelitis;* cerebellar corticoid degeneration;* subacute spinocerebellar degeneration.*
Pituitary gland	For removal and specimen preparation, see Chapter 4.	Crooke cell hyperplasia.
Skeletal muscles and peripheral nerves	For removal and specimen preparation, see Chapter 4.	Myasthenic syndrome (Eaton-Lambert syndrome); myopathy;* dermatomyositis.* Peripheral neuropathy.
Bones	For removal and specimen preparation, see Chapter 2.	See above under "External examination and skin." Bones (with red marrow) are common sites of metastases.

Tumor of the Ovary (or Ovaries)

Possible Associated Conditions: Cushing's syndrome,* dermal hyperpigmentation; dermatomyositis.* See also below under "Possible or Expected Findings."

Organs and Tissues	*Procedures*	*Possible or Expected Findings*
External examination and skin	Record body weight. Record and prepare photographs of abnormal features as listed in right-hand column. Prepare histologic sections of normal and grossly abnormal skin.	Cachexia. Dermal hyperpigmentation; dermato-myositis.* Cushingoid features. Gangrene of fingers *(1)*.
Vitreous	Submit samples for electrolyte analysis. Post-mortem calcium values in blood are unreliable.	Hypercalcemia.
Abdominal cavity and pelvic organs	Record appearance of peritoneum and volume and character of intraabdominal fluid. If possible, remove pelvic organs with tumor(s) en block. Record size, weight, and appearance of ovarian tumor.	Peritoneal carcinomatosis; ascites. Tumors may be bilateral or may be so large (e.g., cystadenocarcinoma) that they are difficult to remove with pelvic organs.
Other organs and tissues, including skeletal muscles		See above under "Possible Associated Conditions."

Organs and Tissues	Procedures	Possible or Expected Findings
Peripheral veins		Venous thromboses.*
Brain and spinal cord	For removal and specimen preparation, see Chapter 4.	Cerebellar cortical degeneration.*

Reference

1. Chow SF, McKenna CH. Ovarian cancer and gangrene of the digits: case report and review of the literature. Mayo Clin Proc 1996;71:253–258.

Tumor of the Pancreas

Possible Associated Conditions: With carcinoma of the exocrine pancreas—Cushing's syndrome;* diabetes mellitus* (rare); hypercalcemia; hyperglycemia; dermal hyperpigmentation; pemphigus* *(1)*; Peutz-Jeghers syndrome* *(2)*; venous thromboses or thrombophlebitis.

With islet cell tumor—Abnormal concentrations of hormons in blood and tumor tissue (see below under "pancreas"); carcinoid syndrome;* Cushing's syndrome;* diabetes mellitus;* hypoglycemia;* hypokalemia; Zollinger-Ellison syndrome.*

Organs and Tissues	Procedures	Possible or Expected Findings
External examination and skin	Record body weight.	Cachexia; jaundice.
	Record abnormal features as listed in right-hand column; prepare photographs. Prepare histologic sections of normal and grossly abnormal skin.	Cushingoid features. Dermal hyper-pigmentation. For other rare tumor-related changes, see above under "Possible Associated Conditions."
Blood and vitreous	Submit samples of vitreous for determination of electrolyte and glucose concentrations. Blood values are often unreliable. Snap-freeze serum for possible hormone assay.	See above under "Possible Associated Conditions." Note that hypoglycemia generally cannot be confirmed at autopsy.
Heart	Inspect valves and prepare photographs and sections of vegetations.	Nonbacterial thrombotic endocarditis.*
Esophagus and gastrointestinal tract	Record or estimate volume of blood in lumen.	Esophageal varices.* Gastrointestinal hemorrhage.
Pancreas	For pancreatography, see Chapter 2. Dissect common bile duct *in situ*. Record size and location of tumor in relationship to head, body, and tail of pancreas.	Biliary obstruction caused by tumor in head of pancreas.
	Portions of primary or metastatic endocrine tumors should be snap-frozen for biochemical and histochemical study and for hormone assay. For preparation of tissue for electron microscopy, see Chapter 15.	Islet cell tumor with adrenocorticotropic hormone, gastrin, glucagon, insulin, or other peptide hormones.
Other organs	Procedures depend on expected findings or grossly identified abnormalities as listed above and in right-hand column.	See above under "Possible Associated Conditions." Regional lymph nodes and liver are common sites of metastases.
Veins	For phlebography and removal of femoral veins, see Chapters 3 and 10.	Venous thrombosis or migratory thrombophlebitis associated with carcinoma of exocrine pancreas.

References

1. Matz H, Milner Y, Frusic-Zlotkin M, Brenner S. Paraneoplastic pemphigus associated with pancreatic carcinoma. Acta-Dermato-Venereol 1997;77:289–291.

2. Pauwels M, Delcenserie R, Yzet T, Duchmann JC, Capron JP. Pancreatic cystadenocarcinoma in Peutz-Jeghers syndrome. J Clin Gastroenterol 1997;25:485–486.

Tumor of the Peripheral Nerves

Possible Associated Conditions: Abnormal concentrations of metabolites in urine and tumor tissue (with ganglioneuroma or neuroblastoma); neurofibromatosis;* pheochromocytoma.

Organs and Tissues	*Procedures*	*Possible or Expected Findings*
External examination and skin	Record abnormal pigmentations and presence of skin tumors.	Manifestations of neurofibromatosis.*
Urine	If ganglioneuroma or neuroblastoma is suspected, submit sample for determination of catecholamin concentration.	Abnormal concentrations of catecholamine in association with ganglioneuroma or neuroblastoma.
Peripheral nerves and tumor tissue	Record size and location. If biochemical study is intended, snap-freeze tumor tissue. For removal and specimen preparation of peripheral nerves, see Chapter 4.	Catecholamine may be found in ganglioneuroma or neuroblastoma.
Other organs and tissues	Procedures depend on expected findings or grossly identified abnormalities as listed above.	See above under "Possible Associated Conditions."

Tumor of the Pituitary Gland

NOTE: See also "Tumor, malignant, any type."

Possible Associated Conditions: Acromegaly;* Cushing's syndrome.* See also below under "Possible or Expected Findings."

Organs and Tissues	*Procedures*	*Possible or Expected Findings*
External examination	Record abnormal features as listed in right-hand column.	Features of acromegaly* or of Cushing's syndrome.*
Pituitary gland	Record size, weight, and boundaries of tumor; photograph tumor *in situ* and after removal. If hormone assay is intended, snap-freeze portion of tumor. Prolactin and growth hormone cells can be localized by the immunoperoxidase method. If an adenoma of unknown type is suspected, submit sample for electron microscopic study (Chapter 15).	Carcinoma metastases in the pituitary gland most commonly originate from breast carcinoma. Usually, metastases are found in the posterior lobe, whereas adenomas are anterior lobe tumors. Schwannoma *(1)*.
Other organs and tissues	Procedures depend on expected findings or grossly identified abnormalities as listed in right-hand column.	Manifestations of pituitary insufficiency* or of excessive hormone production (acromegaly,* Cushing's syndrome*).

Reference

1. Rodriguez FJ, et al. Massive sellar and parasellar schwannoma. Arch Neurol 2007;64:1198–1199.

Tumor of the Pleura

Organs and Tissues	*Procedures*	*Possible or Expected Findings*
External examination	Record abnormal features as listed in right-hand column. Prepare roentgenograms of chest and extremities.	Hypertrophic osteoarthropathy* (with pleural mesothelioma).
Chest cavity	Record character and volume of pleural effusions. Record size and location of tumor(s). Submit sample of tumor tissue and of non-neoplastic lung tissue for analysis of asbestos bodies.	Pleural effusions.* Asbestosis may be complicated by pleural mesothelioma.

Organs and Tissues	Procedures	Possible or Expected Findings
Other organs and tissue	Document absence of tumor that might have metastasized to pleurae.	Pleural metastases from distant primary tumors may mimic mesothelioma.

Tumor of the Prostate

Possible Associated Conditions: Cushing's syndrome;* disseminated intravascular coagulation;* hemolytic uremic syndrome* *(1)*; osteomalacia* *(2)*.

Organs and Tissues	Procedures	Possible or Expected Findings
External examination	Record body weight. Record abnormal features as listed in right-hand column. Prepare roentgenograms of chest, thoracic and lumbar spine, and extremities.	Cachexia. Dermal hyperpigmentation; Cushingoid features. Osteomalacia *(2)*. Osteoblastic bone metastases.
Pelvic organs with prostate; testes	 Record presence or absence of testes.	Infiltrating carcinoma of prostate may cause obstructive uropathy and other complications. Testes may have been surgically removed to achieve androgen deprivation.
Other organs	Procedures depend on expected findings or grossly identified abnormalities as listed in right-hand column.	Urinary obstruction and hydronephrosis.* Osteoblastic metastases, particularly in vertebral bodies. See also above under "Possible Associated Conditions."

References

1. Muller NJ, Pestalozzi BC. Hemolytic uremic syndrome in prostatic carcinoma. Oncol 1998;55:174–176.
2. Reese DM, Rosen PJ. Oncogenic osteomalacia associated with prostatic cancer. J Urol 1997;158:887.

Tumor of the Small Intestine

Possible Associated Conditions: Acquired immunodeficiency syndrome* (AIDS) in patients with small bowel lymphoma;* Carcinoid syndrome;* familial polyposis and related syndromes* (Cronkhite-Canada syndrome; Gardner's syndrome); Peutz-Jeghers syndrome.*

Organs and Tissues	Procedures	Possible or Expected Findings
External examination	Record body weight. Record abnormal features as listed above.	Cachexia. Mucocutaneous pigmentations associated with Peutz-Jeghers syndrome.*
Small and large bowel	For mesenteric angiography, see Chapter 2. If there is a history of carcinoid syndrome,* see under that entry. A frozen section diagnosis of the tumor may help to determine how to process the tumor tissue and what stains to order. Submit sample of non-neoplastic small bowel for histologic study.	 Carcinoid tumor. Lymphoma (see also above under "Possible Associated Conditions"). Familial polyposis or related syndrome.* Celiac sprue.* Crohn's disease.*
Other organs and tissues	Procedures depend on expected findings or grossly identified abnormalities as listed above.	See above under "Possible Associated Conditions." Regional lymph nodes and liver are common sites of metastases.

Tumor of the Soft Tissues

The possible sites and characteristics of soft tissue tumors vary so much that no universally applicable autopsy techniques can be presented. In all instances, the size, weight, and location of the tumor(s) must be recorded and tissue must be sampled for histologic study. If the tumor had not been classified prior to death, samples should be snap-frozen for immunohistochemical study. Other samples should be prepared for electron microscopic study. Evidence of paraneoplastic syndromes (see below) may require additional procedures.

Possible Associated Conditions: Only a few paraneoplastic syndromes or systemic complications can be presented here. For the type of soft tissue tumor that was associated with each condition, see title of reference. Kasabach-Merritt syndrome *(1)* (thrombocytopenia, microangiopathic hemolytic anemia, and acute or chronic coagulopathy associated with a rapidly enlarging hemangioma); liver function abnormalities *(2)*; neurofibromatosis *(3)*; osteomalacia *(4)*.

References

1. Esterly NB. Kasabach Merritt syndrome in infants. J Am Acad Dermatol 1983;8:504–513.
2. Sharara AI, Panella TJ, Fitz JG. Paraneoplastic hepatopathy associated with soft tissue sarcoma. Gastroenterol 1992;103:330–332.
3. Hartley AL, Birch JM, Marsden HB, Harris M, Blair V. Neurofibromatosis in children with soft tissue sarcoma. Pediatr Hematol Oncol 1988;5:7–16.
4. Zura RD, Minasi JS, Kahler DM. Tumor-induced osteomalacia and symptomatic looser zones secondary to mesenchymal chondrosarcoma. J Surg Oncol 1999;71:58–62.

Tumor of the Spinal Cord

Possible Associated Conditions: With angioma—cerebellar hemangioblastoma; segmental cutaneous vascular nevi; with hemangioblastoma—von Hippel-Lindau disease;* with arteriovenous malformation—vertebral hemangioma(s).

Organs and Tissues	*Procedures*	*Possible or Expected Findings*
External examination and skin	Record abnormal features; photograph and submit nevi for histologic study.	Segmental cutaneous vascular nevi (associated with spinal cord angiomas).
Brain and spinal cord	For removal and specimen preparation, see Chapter 4. See also below under "Vertebral column." Describe gross appearance, location, and size of spinal cord tumor and status of adjacent spinal cord.	Subarachnoid hemorrhage.* Spinal cord compression; ischemic spinal cord changes. See also above under "Possible Associated Conditions."
Vertebral column	Record and photograph changes listed in right-hand column.	Bone erosion and calcification of spinal canal. Vertebral hemangiomas may be associated with arteriovenous malformation of spinal cord.
Other organs and tissues	Procedures depend on expected findings or grossly identified abnormalities as listed in right-hand column.	Manifestations of von Hippel-Lindau disease.*

Tumor of the Stomach

Possible Associated Conditions: Hypoglycemia;* megaloblastic anemia;* skin changes (as listed under "Possible or Expected Findings); venous thromboses.

Organs and Tissues	*Procedures*	*Possible or Expected Findings*
External examination and skin	Record body weight. Record abnormal features; photograph and submit samples of normal and abnormal skin for histologic study.	Cachexia; lower leg lymphoedema *(3)*. Acanthosis nigricans; hyperkeratosis palmaris and plantaris *(1)*. Pyoderma gangrenosum. Dermatomyositis;* herpes zoster.* Periumbilical metastases.

Organs and Tissues	Procedures	Possible or Expected Findings
Blood and vitreous	In most instances, determination of vitreous sugar concentration and of blood group is not indicated.	Hypoglycemia may have been present but this condition generally cannot be confirmed at autopsy. Blood group A is more common in patients with carcinoma of stomach than in controls.
Heart	Inspect valves and prepare photographs and sections of vegetations.	Nonbacterial thrombotic endocarditis.*
Esophagus, stomach, and duodenum	Leave esophagus and part of duodenum attached to stomach.	Acanthosis of the esophagus *(1)*.
	Submit samples of tumor and of grossly uninvolved stomach for histologic study. Request PAS stain and Warthin-Starry stain for identification of *H. pylori.*	Chronic gastritis with or without intestinal metaplasia. Infection with *H. pylori* (with carcinoma or lymphoma *[2]*).
	Portions of endocrine gastric tumor should be snap-frozen for immunohistochemical study and possible hormone assay.	Gastric carcinoid tumors; neuroendocrine carcinoma (rare).
Other organs and tissues		Eosinophilia. Manifestations of paraneoplastic syndromes as listed above under "Possible Associated Conditions."
	Record location of tumor metastases.	Metastases common in liver, retroperitoneal and supraclavicular lymph nodes (Virchow's node), ovaries (Krukenberg tumor), and peritoneal cul de sac (Blumer's shelf").

References

1. Murata I, Ogami Y, Nagai Y, Furuma K, Yoshikawa I, Otsuli M. Carcinoma of the stomach with hyperkeratosis palmaris and plantaris and acanthosis of the esophagus. Am J Gastroenterol 1998;93:449–451.
2. Wotherspoon AC. Gastric lymphoma of mucosa-associated lymphoid tissue and Helicobacter pylori. Ann Rev Med 1998;49:289–299.
3. Lanznaster G, et al. Gastric signet-ring cell carcinoma: unilateral lower extremity lymphoedema as the presenting feature. Scientific World J 2007;7:1189–1192.

Tumor of the Testis

Possible Associated Conditions: Demyelinating neuropathy *(1)*; dermatomyositis* *(2)*; Down's syndrome;* eosinophilia; herpes zoster;* megaloblastic anemia.*

Organs and Tissues	Procedures	Possible or Expected Findings
External examination	Record body weight.	Cachexia.
	Record genital abnormalities as listed in right-hand column.	Cryptorchism; hypospadia.
	Submit breast tissue for histologic study.	Gynecomastia.
Blood and urine	Freeze samples for hormone assay.	Increased concentrations of alpha-fetoprotein and human chorionic gonadotropin.
Kidneys	If indicated, follow procedures described under "glomerulonephritis."	Glomerulonephritis;* developmental anomalies *(3)*.
Testes	Record location, size, and weight of both testes and of testicular tumor. Submit samples of tumor and of ininvolved testis and epididymis for histologic study. Snap-freeze tumor tissue for hormone assay.	Cryptorchid testis with tumor or contralateral to testicular tumor. Testicular microlithiasis. Secondary testicular tumors (metastases to the testes) are rare, except in association with leukemia* in children.

Other organs	Procedures depend on expected findings or grossly identified abnormalities as listed in right-hand column. For dissection of the thoracic duct (for search of tumor cell clusters), see Chapter 3.	Pulmonari embolism.* Paraneoplastic diseases as listed above under "Possible Associated Conditions." Metastases are found primarily in retroperitoneal lymph nodes, left supraclavicular lymph nodes, and lungs.

References

1. Greenspan BN, Felice KJ. Chronic inflammatory demyelinating polyneuropathy (CIDP) associated with seminoma. Eur Neurol 1998;39:57–58.
2. Hayami S, Kubota Y, Sasagawa I, Suzuki H, Nakada N, Motoyama T. Dermatomyositis associated with intratubular germ cell tumor and metastatic germ cell cancer. J Urol 1998;159:2096–2097.
3. Klein EA, Chen RN, Levin HS, Rackley RR, Williams BR. Testicular cancer in association with developmental renal anomalies and hypospadias. Urol 1996;47:82–87.

Tumor of the Thymus

Possible Associated Conditions: Anemia (autoimmune hemolytic or aplastic);* Cushing's syndrome;* dermal hyperpigmentation; hypogammaglobulinemia (and other immunoglobulin abnormalities); myasthenia gravis;* pancytopenia;* pemphigus foliaceus; polymyositis;* Sjögren's syndrome;* thrombotic thrombocytopenic purpura* *(1)*. See also below under "Other organs."

Organs and Tissues	*Procedures*	*Possible or Expected Findings*
External examination	Record body weight. Record and prepare photographs of skin abnormalities; sample for histologic study.	Cachexia. Dermal hyperpigmentation. Pemphigus foliaceus (rare).
Blood	Submit samples for protein analysis.	Hypogammaglobulinemia and other immunoglobulin abnormalities.
Chest	Photograph and dissect tumor *in situ*. Record size, weight, gross appearance, and relationship to thoracic veins, pericardium, lungs, and other tissues. Sample for histologic and electron microscopic study.	Usually, thymoma presents as an infiltrating, anterior mediastinal mass that rarely metastasizes. Carcinoid tumor, malignant lymphoma* (Hodgkin's disease), and metastases from carcinoma of the breast* and other tumors also may occur in this location.
Heart	Record weight. Submit samples for histologic study.	Idiopathic granulomatous myocarditis.*
Kidneys	Follow procedures described under "Glomerulonephritis."	Minimal-change or membranous nephropathy; extracapillary glomerulonephritis* *(2)*.
Other organs	Submit samples of lymph nodes, spleen, Peyer's plaques, and bone marrow for histologic study. Other procedures depend on expected findings or grossly identified abnormalities as listed in right-hand column.	Viral (e.g., herpes simplex*) and fungal infections (e.g., candidiasis*) due to thymoma-related immunodeficiency *(3)*. Manifestations of paraneoplastic diseases and conditions as listed above under "Possible Associated Conditions."

References

1. Hatama S, Kumagai H, Iwato K, Fujiwara M, Fujishima M. Thrombotic thrombocytopenic purpura accompanied by transient pure red cell aplasia and thymoma. Clin Nephrol 1998;49:193–197.
2. Valli G, Fogazzi GB, Cappelari A, Rivolta E. Glomerulonephritis associated with myasthenia gravis. Am J Kidney Dis 1998;31:350–355.
3. Sicherer SH, Cabana MD, Perlman EJ, Lederman HM, Matsakis RR, Winkelstein JA. Thymoma and cellular immune deficiency in an adolescent. Pediatr Allergy Immunol 1998;9:49–52.

Tumor of the Thyroid Gland

NOTE: See also "Tumor, malignant, any type."

Possible Associated Conditions: With papillary carcinoma—Familial adenomatous polyposis* *(1)*; with medullary thyroid carcinoma—Multiple endocrine neoplasia (MEN, type 2A or 2B).*

Organs and Tissues	Procedures	Possible or Expected Findings
External examination	Record abnormal features.	Acromegaly* *(2)*.
Neck organs with thyroid gland	Leave thyroid gland and tumor attached to trachea until degree of tracheal compression can be recorded. Identify exact location of cervical lymph nodes that are submitted for histologic study.	Upper airway obstruction *(3)*. Benign nodular goiter or adenoma(s); carcinoma or lymphoma. Hashimoto's thyroiditis with lymphoma. Metastasis from prostate cancer *(4)*.
	If medullary carcinoma is suspected, snap-freeze portion of fresh tumor for hormone assay.	Thyrocalcitonin in medullary carcinoma of thyroid.
Other organs	Samples of thymic tissue, lymph nodes, and endocrine glands should be submitted for histologic study. Other procedures depend on expected findings or grossly identified abnormalities as listed in right-hand column.	Manifestations of hyperthyroidism,* which may be associated with metastasizing follicular carcinoma. Manifestations of MEN (see above under "Possible Associated Conditions").

References

1. Cetta F, Toti P, Petracci M, Montalto G, Disanto A, Lore F, Fusco A. Thyroid carcinoma associated with familial adenomatous polyposis. Histo-pathology 1997;31:231–236.
2. Balkany C, Cushing GW. An association between acromegaly and thyroid carcinoma. Thyroid 1995;5:47–50.
3. Carter N, Milroy CM. Thyroid carcinoma causing fatal laryngeal obstruction. J Laryngol Otol 1996;110:1176–1178.
4. Selimoglu H, et al. Prostate cancer metastasis to thyroid gland. Tumori 2007;93:292–295.

Tumor of the Urinary Bladder

Organs and Tissues	Procedures	Possible or Expected Findings
External examination	Record body weight.	Cachexia.
Kidneys and ureters	Leave these organs attached to urinary bladder, particularly if hydronephrosis and hydroureter are noted. En block removal of abdominal organs generally is the best approach.	Hydronephrosis* (obstructive uropathy) and hydroureter, usually caused by distal ureteral obstruction. Recurrent nephrolithiasis* or pyelitis may have been present and is a risk factor for urinary bladder carcinoma.
Pelvic organs with urinary bladder	Sample bladder tumor and uninvolved urinary bladder for histologic study.	Chronic urocystitis; infestation with *Schistosoma haematobium (1)* (uncommon in North America).
Other organs		Manifestations of uremia (see "Failure, kidney").

Reference

1. Bedwani R, Renganathan E, El Kwhsky F, Braga C, Abu Seif HH, Abul Azm T, et al. Schistosomiasis and the risk of bladder cancer in Alexandria, Egypt. Br J Canc 1998;77:1186–1189.

Tumor of the Uterus (with Cervix)

Possible Associated Conditions: Acquired immunodeficiency syndrome* (AIDS) *(1)*. With carcinoma of the uterus—Cerebellar cortical degeneration;* with carcinoma of the cervix—Myopathy.*

Organs and Tissues	Procedures	Possible or Expected Findings
External examination	Record body weight.	Cachexia.
Vitreous	Submit samples for determination of calcium concentrations. Postmortem calcium values in blood are unreliable.	Evidence of hypercalcemia.

Organs and Tissues	*Procedures*	*Possible or Expected Findings*
Kidneys and ureters	Leave these organs attached to urinary bladder, particularly if there is evidence of hydronephrosis and hydroureter. En block removal of abdominal organs generally is the best approach.	Hydronephrosis* (obstructive uropathy) and hydroureter, usually caused by distal ureteral obstruction.
Pelvic organs	Record size and location of tumor; sample tumor and non-neoplastic uterus and cervix for histologic study. If indicated, submit samples for electron microscopic study.	Fistulas to urinary bladder or rectum or both. Human papilloma virus infection *(2)* or herpesvirus infection *(3)* with invasive cervical carcinoma.
	If hormone assay is intended, snap-freeze portion of tumor.	Erythropoietin may be found in some tumors.
Veins	For removal of femoral veins, see Chapter 3.	Thrombosis.*
Skeletal muscles		Myopathy* may be associated with carcinoma of the cervix.
Brain and spinal cord	For removal and specimen preparation, see Chapter 4.	Cerebellar cortical degeneration* may be associated with carcinoma of the uterus.
Other organs	Procedures depend on expected findings or grossly identified abnormalities as listed in right-hand column.	Manifestations of uremia (see "Failure, kidney"). Manifestations of acquired immunodeficiency syndrome* (AIDS).

References

1. Chin KM, Sidhu JS, Janssen RS, Weber JT. Invasive cervical cancer in human immunodeficiency virus-infected and uninfected hospital patients. Obstetr Gynecol 1998;92:83–87.
2. Ursic-Vrscaj M, Kovacic J, Poljak M, Marin J. Association of risk factors for cervical cancer and human papilloma viruses in invasive cervical cancer. Eur J Gynaecol Oncol 1996;17:368–371.
3. Koffa M, Koumantakis E, Ergazaki M, Tsatsanis C, Spandidos DA. Association of herpesvirus infection with the development of genital cancer. Intl J Canc 1995;63:58–62.

Tumor, Wilms (See "Tumor of the kidney(s).")

Tyrosinemia

Synonyms and Related Terms: Fumarylacetoacetate hydrolase deficiency; aminoaciduria.*

Organs and Tissues	*Procedures*	*Possible or Expected Findings*
External examination and skin	Record body weight. Note odor.	Growth delay. The body may have a "fishy" odor.
	Sample skin for histologic study.	Hyperkeratosis of skin *(1)*. Vesicles on fingers *(3)*.
	Prepare skeletal roentgenograms (especially of epiphyses).	Hypophosphatemic rickets.
Fascia lata	Specimens should be collected using aseptic technique for tissue culture for biochemical studies (see Chapter 9).	Enzyme deficiency (see above under "Synonyms and Related Terms").
Blood	Submit samples for culture and biochemical analysis.	Sepsis. Increased concentrations of methionine, tyrosine, alpha-fetoprotein, and delta-aminolevulinic acid.
Urine	Submit sample for biochemical analysis.	Evidence of aminoaciduria (see above under "Blood"); tyrosine metabolites.
Liver	Record weight, photograph cut surfaces, and sample for histologic study (include nodules that might be neoplastic).	Enlarged liver with lobular disarray, fibrosis or cirrhosis;* steatosis; cholestasis; hepatocellular carcinoma *(2)*.
Kidneys	Weigh both kidneys and submit for histologic study.	Tubular ectasia; tubular calcification.
Other organs	Procedures depend on expected findings or grossly identified abnormalities as listed in right-hand column.	Evidence of bleeding. Islet cell hyperplasia and mineralization of pancreas; hepatic encephalopathy.*

Organs and Tissues	Procedures	Possible or Expected Findings
Bones	Prepare sections of epiphyses for histologic study.	See above under "External examination."

References

1. Benoldi D, Orsoni JB, Allegra F. Tyrosinemia type II: a challenge for ophthalmologists and dermatologists. Ped Dermatol 1997;14:110–112.
2. Dehner LP, Snover DC, Sharp HL, Ascher N, Nakhleh R, Day DL. Hereditary tyrosinemia type I (chronic form): Pathologic findings in the liver. Hum Pathol 1989;20:149–158.
3. Viglizzo GM, et al. Richner-Hanhart syndrome (tyrosinemia II): early diagnosis of an incomplete presentation with unusual findings. Pediatr Dermatol 2006;23:259–261.

U

Ulcer, Peptic, of Stomach or Duodenum

Possible Associated Conditions: Multiple endocrine neoplasia;* rheumatoid arthritis;* Zollinger-Ellison syndrome.* acute pancreatitis *(1)*.

Organs and Tissues	*Procedures*	*Possible or Expected Findings*
External examination	Prepare roentgenograms of chest and abdomen.	Free air in abdomen suggests perforation of ulcer.
Peritoneal cavity	If peritonitis is present, submit exudate for bacteriologic study. Record volume of exudate and location of perforation.	Peritonitis.* Perforation of ulcer.
Heart	See "Disease, ischemic heart."	Coronary atherosclerosis and manifestations of coronary insufficiency are commonly associated with peptic ulcer disease.
	Other procedures depend on grossly identified abnormalities as listed in right-hand column.	In rare instances, pericardial fistula may be present from ulcer in hiatus hernia.
Lungs	Procedures depend on expected findings or grossly identified abnormalities as listed in right-hand column. Perfuse at least one lung with formalin.	Peptic ulcers may be associated with emphysema,* tuberculosis,* and other chronic pulmonary diseases.
Stomach and duodenum	For celiac arteriography, see Chapter 2. Open stomach and duodenum *in situ* and record site of perforation or penetration. Record measured or estimated volume of blood in gastrointestinal tract. Rinse ulcer with saline to locate eroded vessel(s).	Perforating or penetrating peptic ulcer. Infiltrating and ulcerating carcinoma or lymphoma of stomach.* Gastrointestinal hemorrhage.*
	Pin stomach and duodenum on corckboard (serosa toward board) and fix specimen in formalin before sectioning. Prepare histologic sections of ulcer(s) and of remainder of stomach. Request Warthin-Starry stain for *H. pylori.*	Chronic gastritis (with *H. pylori* infection) and duodenitis.
Other organs	Procedures depend on expected findings or grossly identified abnormalities as listed in right-hand column.	Manifestations of multiple endocrine neoplasia;* Zollinger-Ellison syndrome,* and rheumatoid arthritis.*

Reference

1. Chen TA et al. Acute pancreatitis-associated acute gastrointestinal mucosal lesions: incidence, characteristics, and clinical significance. J Clin Gastroenterol 2007;41:630–634.

Uncinariasis (See "Ancylostomiasis.")

Uremia (See "Failure, kidney.")

From: *Handbook of Autopsy Practice,* 4th Ed. Edited by: B.L. Waters

Uropathy, Obstructive (See "Hydronephrosis.")

Urticaria Pigmentosa of Childhood (See "Mastocytosis, systemic.")

V–Z

Valve, Congenitally Bicuspid Aortic

Possible Associated Conditions: Acute aortic dissection;* aneurysma(s) of cerebral arteries; aortic insufficiency;* calcific aortic stenosis,* coarctation of the aorta;* infective endocarditis;* Shone's syndrome; Turner's syndrome.*

Organs and Tissues	*Procedures*	*Possible or Expected Findings*
Heart	If infective endocarditis is suspected, see Chapter 7. Open heart in cross-sections (see Chapter 3). Photograph aortic valve and test valvular competence (Chapter 3). Prepare histologic section of aortic valve, if infected; request Gram and Grocott's methenamine silver stains.	Infective endocarditis* of bicuspid aortic valve. Aortic valvular insufficiency*. Ascending aorta dilation *(1)*.

Reference

1. Keane MG, et al. Bicuspid aortic valves are associated with aortic dilatation out of proportion to coexistent valvular lesions. Circulation 2000;102(19 Suppl 3):III35–39.

Valve, Congenitally Bicuspid Pulmonary

Possible Associated Conditions: Double outlet left ventricle; tetralogy of Fallot;* complete or congenitally corrected transposition of the great arteries;* tricuspid atresia;* congenitally bicuspid aortic valve.*

Valve, Congenitally Quadricuspid Aortic

NOTE: The condition may be complicated by infective endocarditis.* Follow procedures described under that heading.

Varicella

Synonyms and Related Terms: Chickenpox; congenital varicella syndrome; varicella gangrenosa; varicella-zoster virus infection.

NOTE:

Reye's syndrome* is a possible postviral complication of varicella that must be distinguished from varicella encephalitis. Varicella may also cause exacerbation of tuberculosis.*

(1) Collect all tissues that appear infected. (2) Request viral cultures. (3) Usually, special stains are not helpful. (4) Special **precautions** are indicated (Chapter 6). (5) Serologic studies are avail-able from state health department laboratories. (6) This is not a reportable disease.

Possible Associated Conditions: Human immunodeficiency virus (HIV) infection *(1)*; leukemia;* lymphoma;* other immunodeficient conditions. See also above under "Note."

Organs and Tissues	*Procedures*	*Possible or Expected Findings*
External examination, skin, and oral cavity	Record extent and character of skin and oral mucosal lesions; photograph lesions and submit samples for histologic study (preferably lesions without evidence of superinfection).	Vesicular crusting rash; vesicles with type A intranuclear inclusions in surrounding epithelial cells, endothelial cells and fibroblasts; evidence of disseminated intravascular coagulation;* purpura fulminans.* (See also below under "Eyes, orbitae, and surrounding skin.")
Cerebrospinal fluid	Submit sample for viral culture and for cell count.	Evidence of meningitis.
Chest cavity	Record volume of fluid.	Pleural effusions.*
Blood	Submit sample for microbiologic study.	Septicemia (e.g., group A beta-hemolytic streptococcus; *Staphylococcus aureus*).
Heart	Submit samples for histologic study.	Pancarditis (usually mild).

From: *Handbook of Autopsy Practice,* 4th Ed. Edited by: B.L. Waters

Organs and Tissues	*Procedures*	*Possible or Expected Findings*
Lungs	Record weights. Submit consolidated areas for bacterial and viral cultures. Perfuse lungs with formalin.	Varicella pneumonia, with or without bacterial superinfection; intranuclear inclusions in epithelial, mesothelial, and endothelial cells; pulmonary edema; hemorrhages and abscesses; fibrosis and calcification in late stages. Mediastinitis *(6)*.
Liver	Record weight and submit samples for histologic study.	Varicella hepatitis.
Spleen	Inspect carefully *in situ* to detect evidence of rupture. Record weight and consistency; sample for histologic study.	Splenitis, with or without rupture of spleen.
Stomach	Examine as soon as possible to minimize autolysis. Submit sections for histologic study.	Ulcerative gastritis.
Kidneys	Follow procedures described under "Glomerulonephritis."	Glomerulonephritis.*
Testes	Record weights; submit samples for histologic study.	Orchitis.
Neck organs	Open in posterior midline. (See also under "Laryngitis.")	Bacterial epiglottitis *(2)*.
Brain and spinal cord	For removal and specimen preparation, see Chapter 4.	Encephalitis with cerebral edema; petechial hemorrhages; perivenous demyelination; acute cerebellitis; aseptic meningitis;* transverse myelitis.*
Eyes, orbitae, and surrounding skin	For removal and specimen preparation, see Chapter 5.	Keratitis; vesicular conjunctivitis; optic neuritis *(3)*. Periorbital varicella gangrenosa *(4)*.
Peripheral nerves	For removal and specimen preparation, see Chapter 4.	Acute motor axonal neuropathy *(5)*.
Skeletal muscles, joints and soft tissues	Procedures depend on expected findings or grossly identified abnormalities as listed in right-hand column. For specimen preparation of muscles, and joints see Chapter 2.	Rhabdomyolysis; necrotizing fasciitis (varicella gangrenosa). Arthritis

References

1. Gershon AA, Mervish N, LaRussa P, Steinberg S, Lo SH, Hodes D, et al. Varicella-zoster virus infection in children with underlying immunodeficiency virus infection. J Infect Dis 1997;176:1496–1500.
2. Belfer RA. Group A beta-hemolytic streptococcal epiglottitis as a complication of varicella infection. Pediatr Emerg Care 1996;12:202–204.
3. Lee CC, Venketasubramanian N, Lam MS. Optic neuritis: a rare complication of primary varicella infection. Clin Infect Dis 1997;24:515–516.
4. Tornervy NR, Fomsgaard A, Nielsen NV. HSV-1-induced acute retinal necrosis syndrome presenting with severe inflammatory orbitopathy, proptosis, and optic nerve involvement. Opthal 2000;107:397–400.
5. Picard F, Gericke CA, Frey M, Collard M. Varicella with acute motor axonal neuropathy. Euro Neurol 1997;38:68–71.
6. Macarrón CP, et al. Descending necrotizing mediastinitis in a child with chicken pox. J Thorac Cardiovasc Surg 2007;133:271–272.

Varices, Esophageal

NOTE: See also under "Hypertension, portal."

Organs and Tissues	*Procedures*	*Possible or Expected Findings*
Chest	Dissect major veins *in situ.*	Superior vena cava obstruction; other venous abnormalities such as unilateral pulmonary vein atresia.
Esophagus and stomach	Remove esophagus and stomach together as one specimen. Record volume and character of blood in stomach. For demonstration of esophageal varices, see Chapter 2.	Gastric varices; blood in stomach. Esophageal varices with or without evidence of rupture.

Organs and Tissues	*Procedures*	*Possible or Expected Findings*
Esophagus and stomach *(continued)*	Record effects of sclerotherapy or evidence of surgical esophageal transection.	Evidence of sclerotherapy or esophageal transection surgery may be found.
Intestinal tract	Record measured or estimated amount of blood in lumen.	Blood in intestinal tract.
Portal vein system	Dissect all accessible veins *in situ.* Submit samples of veins for histologic study. Request Verhoeff–van Gieson stain. If surgical shunts had been created, record type, location, and patency of anastomoses.	Portal vein thrombosis; other conditions causing portal vein obstruction. Sclerosis associated with idiopathic portal hypertension. Shunt surgery (portacaval and proximal or distal splenorenal shunts.)
Liver	Record weight and submit samples for histologic study. If a transjugular intrahepatic portasystemic shunt had been placed, document location and patency. For portal venography, see Chapter 2.	Cirrhosis;* chronic alcoholic hepatitis; congenital hepatic fibrosis* and other fibropolycystic liver diseases;* nodular regenerative hyperplasia, veno-occlusive disease, and other liver diseases.
Spleen	Record weight.	Congestive splenomegaly.

Vasculitis (See "Aortitis," "Arteritis, ...," "Phlebitis," and "Purpura,...")

Ventricle, Double Inlet Left *(1)*

Synonyms: Single functional ventricle; univentricular heart; univentricular atrioventricular connection; Holmes heart.

NOTE: The basic anomaly is the connection of both atrioventricular valves to the left ventricle, often with transposed great arteries and a restrictive ventricular septal defect. There are four major types, based on the ventriculoarterial connection: (1) with congenitally corrected transposition (60%); (2) with complete transposition (30%); (3) with normally related great arteries (Holmes heart; 5%); and (4) double outlet, persistent truncal artery, or pulmonary atresia (5%). For general dissection techniques, see Chapter 3.

Possible Associated Conditions: Bicuspid pulmonary valve; bilateral mirror-image mitral valves (without tricuspid morphology); subvalvular aortic stenosis,* often with hypoplasia, coarctation, or interruption of the aortic arch; subvalvular pulmonary stenosis;* dual AV nodes and progressive heart block in patients with congenitally corrected transposition.

Reference

1. Cook AC, Anderson RH. The anatomy of hearts with double inlet ventricle. Cardiol Young 2006;16Suppl 1:22–26.

Ventricle, Double Outlet Right

Synonym: Origin of both great arteries from right ventricle; Taussig-Bing anomaly.

NOTE: The basic anomaly is the origin of the aorta and pulmonary artery primarily from the right ventricle, usually with a ventricular septal defect, and often with subpulmonary stenosis. For general dissection techniques, see Chapter 3.

Possible Associated Conditions: Complete atrioventricular septal defect (often with asplenia syndrome); muscular discontinuity between aortic and mitral valves; right ventricular infundibular stenosis; ventricular septal defect* that may be subaortic, subpulmonary, doubly committed, or remote.

Reference

1. Sakurai N, et al. Double outlet right ventricle with intact ventricular septum. Pediatr Int 2007;49:248–250.

Virus, Respiratory Syncytial (See "Pneumonia, all types or type unspecified.")

Virus, Salivary Gland (See "Infection, cytomegalovirus.")

Vitamin A (See "Deficiency, vitamin A" and "Hypervitaminosis A.")

Vitamin B1 (Thiamine) (See "Syndrome, Wernicke-Korsakoff.")

Vitamin B6 (See "Beriberi.")

Vitamin B12 (See "Anemia, megaloblastic.")

Vitamin C (See "Deficiency, vitamin C.")

Vitamin D (See "Deficiency, vitamin D" and "Hypervitaminosis D.")

Waldenström's macroglobulinemia (See "Macroglobulinemia, Waldenström's.)

Waterhouse-Friderichsen syndrome (See "Disease, meningococcal.")

Weber-Christian disease (See "Disease, Weber-Christian.")

Wegener's granulomatosis (See "Granulomatosis, Wegener's.")

Werdnig-Hoffman disease (See "Disease, motor neuron.")

Whipple's disease (See "Disease, Whipple's.")

Whooping cough (See "Pertussis.")
Wilson's disease (See "Disease, Wilson's.")

Wiscott-Aldrich syndrome (See "Syndrome, primary immunodeficiency.")
Wolman's Disease

Xanthoma Tuberosum (See "Hyperlipoproteinemia.")

Organs and tissues	*Procedures*	*Possible or Expected Findings*
External examination		Hepatomegaly and splenomegaly, jaundice.
Skin fibroblasts	Establish cell culture for enzyme assay.	Deficiency of acid lipase (1).
Gastrointestinal tract	Remove and fix portions of bowel as soon as possible.	Foam cells in the lamina propria.
Liver	Examine histologically with H&E and oil red O stains.	Hepatomegaly, severe steatosis with cholesterol clefts in hepatocytes and Kupffer cells. Fibrosis.
Spleen		Splenomegaly with lipid-laden foam cells.
Adrenal glands		Symmetric enlargement with dystrophic calcifications, giving the adrenals a gritty texture. Vacuolated cells of the inner zona fasciculata and entire zona reticularis with cholesterol clefts.
Other organs		Foam cells may be found in the lungs, bone marrow, lymph nodes, vessel walls, as well as Schwann and ganglion cells.

Reference

1. Guy, GJ, Butterworth J. Acid esterase activity in cultured skin fibroblasts and amniotic fluid cells using 4-methylumbelliferyl palmitate. Clin Chim Acta 1978;84:361–71.

Yaws

Organs and tissues	*Procedures*	*Possible or Expected Findings*
External examination	Gross inspection and darkfield microscopy of lesion scrapings	Papular, ulcerated, hyperkeratotic lesions, which may be secondarily infected by bacteria. Dark field microscopy will identify the organism.
Bone and Joints		Gummatous lesions.

Yellow fever (See "Fever, yellow.")
Yersinia enterocolitica infection

Organs and tissues	*Procedures*	*Possible or Expected Findings*
Intestines	Remove and fix bowel as soon as possible.	Mucosal ulcers, resembling those of typhoid fever, primarily of distal ileum and colon. Villous shortening, crypt hyperplasia with mucosal microabscesses. Microabscesses in regional mesenteric lymph nodes, rimmed by macrophages.

Zellweger's syndrome (See "Syndrome, Zellweger.")
Zollinger-Ellison syndrome (See "Syndrome, Zollinger-Ellison.")
Zygomycosis (See "Mucormycosis" and procedures under "Diabetes mellitus.")
Xanthoma Tuberosum (See "Hyperlipoproteinemia.")

NORMAL WEIGHTS AND MEASUREMENTS

III

Conversion Table

Hagen Blaszyk, William D. Edwards, Jurgen Ludwig, and Brenda L. Waters

Conversion Factors

To convert from	*To*	*Multiply by*
Metric to English		
Centimeters (cm)	Inches (US) (in)	0.394
Centimeters (cm)	Feet (US) (ft)	0.033
Square meters (m^2)	Square feet (US) (ft)	10.753
Grams (g)	Ounces (avoirdupois) (oz)	0.035
Grams (g)	Pounds (avoirdupois) (lb)	0.002
Kilograms (kg)	Ounces (avoirdupois) (oz)	35.274
Kilograms (kg)	Pounds (avoirdupois) (lb)	2.202
Milliliters (mL)*	Ounces (US fluid) (fl oz)	0.034
Liters (L)	Quarts (US liquid) (qt)	1.057
Liters (L)	Gallons (US) (gal)	0.264
English to Metric		
Inches (US) (in)	Centimeters (cm)	2.54
Feet (US) (ft)	Centimeters (cm)	30.480
Square feet (US) (ft)	Square meters (m^2)	0.093
Ounces (avoirdupois) (oz)	Grams (g)	28.350
Pounds (avoirdupois) (lb)	Grams (g)	453.592
Ounces (avoirdupois) (oz)	Kilograms (kg)	0.028
Pounds (avoirdupois) (lb)	Kilograms (kg)	0.454
Ounces (US fluid) (fl oz)	Milliliters (mL)*	29.57
Quarts (US liquid) (qt)	Liters (L)	0.946
Gallons (US) (gal)	Liters (L)	3.785
Pressure Conversion		
cm H_2O	mm Hg	0.760
mm Hg	cm H_2O	1.316
	Temperature Conversion	
°C	°F	°F = (1.8 × °C) + 32
°F	°C	$°C = \frac{(°F - 32)}{1.8}$

Concentration Conversion for Ethyl Alcohol:

1,000 ug/mL = 100 mg/dL = 21.74 mmol/Liter = 1.0 promille = 0.1%

*For most purposes, cubic centimeter (cc) is equal to milliliter (mL).

From: *Handbook of Autopsy Practice,* 4th Ed. Edited by: B.L. Waters

BODY MASS INDEX

Body Mass Index (BMI) is the ratio of a person's weight in kilograms over the square of his/her height in centimeters. The formula to use when measuring in the English system is provided below. BMI does not measure body fat directly, but research has shown that it correlates well with direct measures of body fat, such as underwater weighing and dual energy x-ray absorptiometry. When documented in autopsy reports, the numerical value should be followed by the unit, kg/m^2

$$\text{BMI} = \frac{\text{pounds}}{\text{inches}^2} \times 703.1$$

BMI	*Weight Status*
Below 18.5	Underweight
18.5–24.9	Normal
25.0–29.9	Overweight
Above 30	Obese

Acknowledgment is given to the Centers for Disease Control and Prevention.

In children, recommendations for weight control should be focused primarily on those with a BMI above the 95th percentile, and those with a BMI above the 85th percentile who show even minimal signs of physical impairment.

Weights and Measurements in Fetuses, Infants, Children, and Adolescents

Birth to 36 months: Girls
Length-for-age and Weight-for-age percentiles

NAME ____________________

RECORD # ____________

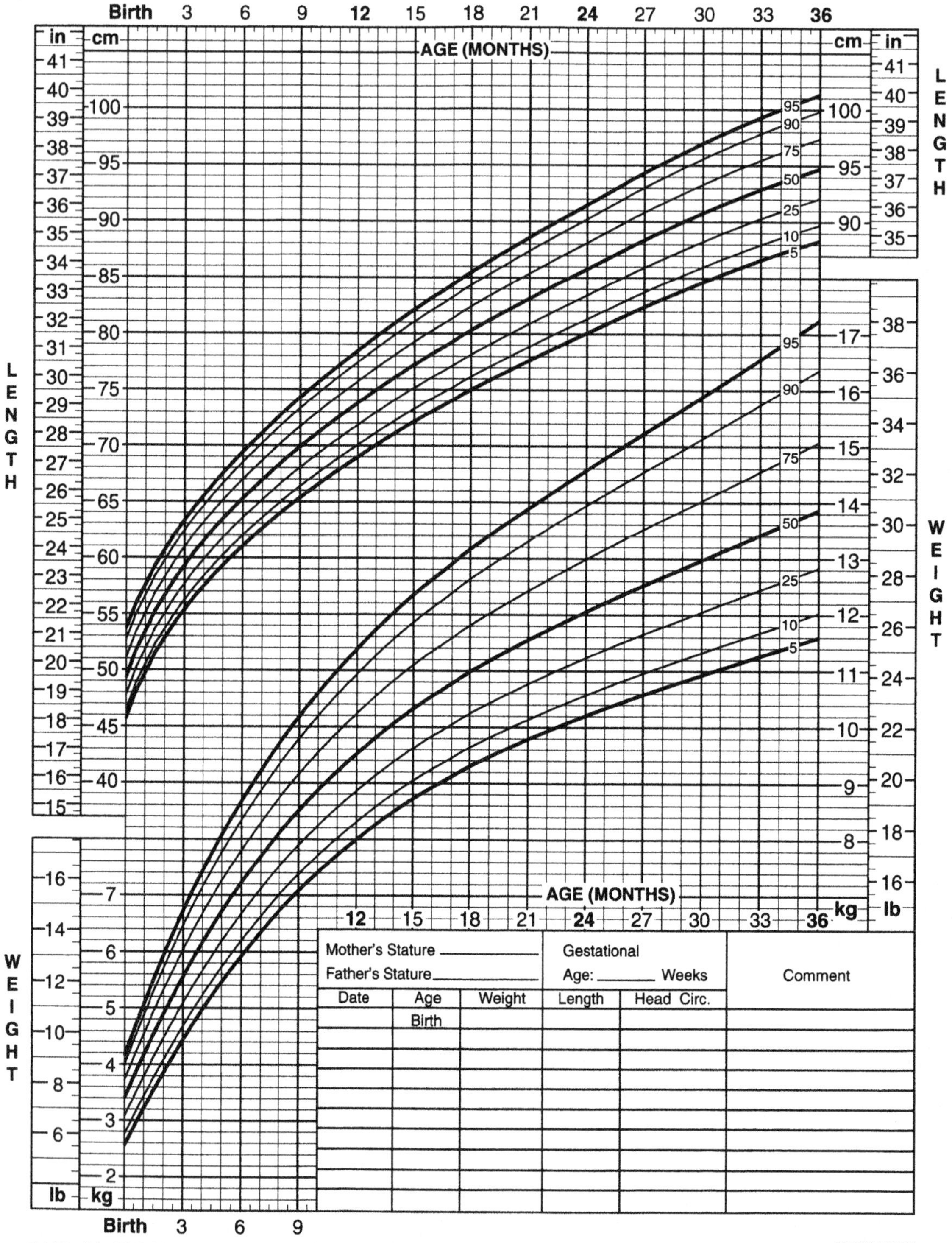

Birth 3 6 9 12 15 18 21 24 27 30 33 36

AGE (MONTHS)

LENGTH (in / cm) — WEIGHT (kg / lb)

Percentiles: 95, 90, 75, 50, 25, 10, 5

Mother's Stature ____________

Father's Stature ____________

Gestational Age: ________ Weeks

Date	Age	Weight	Length	Head Circ.	Comment
	Birth				

Published May 30, 2000 (modified 4/20/01).
SOURCE: Developed by the National Center for Health Statistics in collaboration with the National Center for Chronic Disease Prevention and Health Promotion (2000).
http://www.cdc.gov/growthcharts

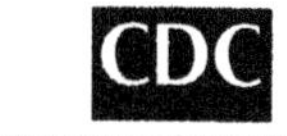

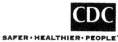

SAFER • HEALTHIER • PEOPLE™

2 to 20 years: Girls
Stature-for-age and Weight-for-age percentiles

NAME ____________________

RECORD # ____________

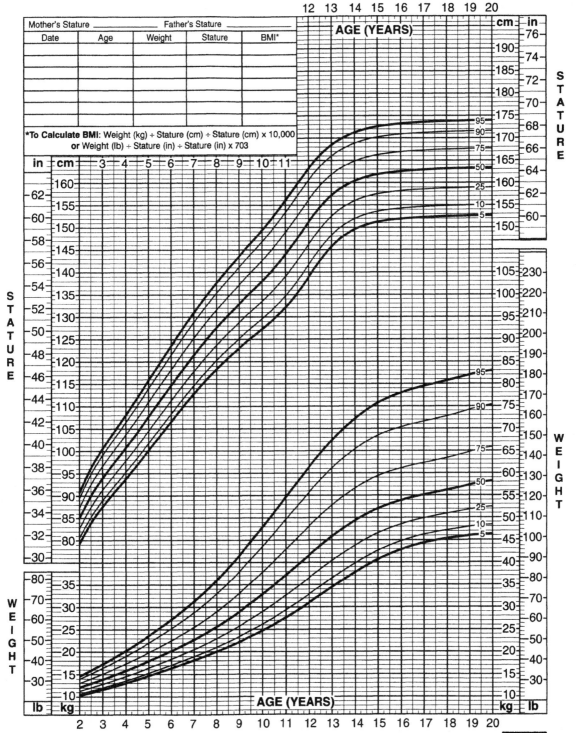

Mother's Stature ____________ Father's Stature ____________

Date	Age	Weight	Stature	BMI*

***To Calculate BMI:** Weight (kg) ÷ Stature (cm) ÷ Stature (cm) x 10,000
or Weight (lb) ÷ Stature (in) ÷ Stature (in) x 703

AGE (YEARS)

STATURE

WEIGHT

Published May 30, 2000 (modified 11/21/00).
SOURCE: Developed by the National Center for Health Statistics in collaboration with the National Center for Chronic Disease Prevention and Health Promotion (2000).
http://www.cdc.gov/growthcharts

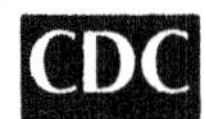

SAFER · HEALTHIER · PEOPLE™

Birth to 36 months: Boys
Length-for-age and Weight-for-age percentiles

NAME ______________________

RECORD # ____________

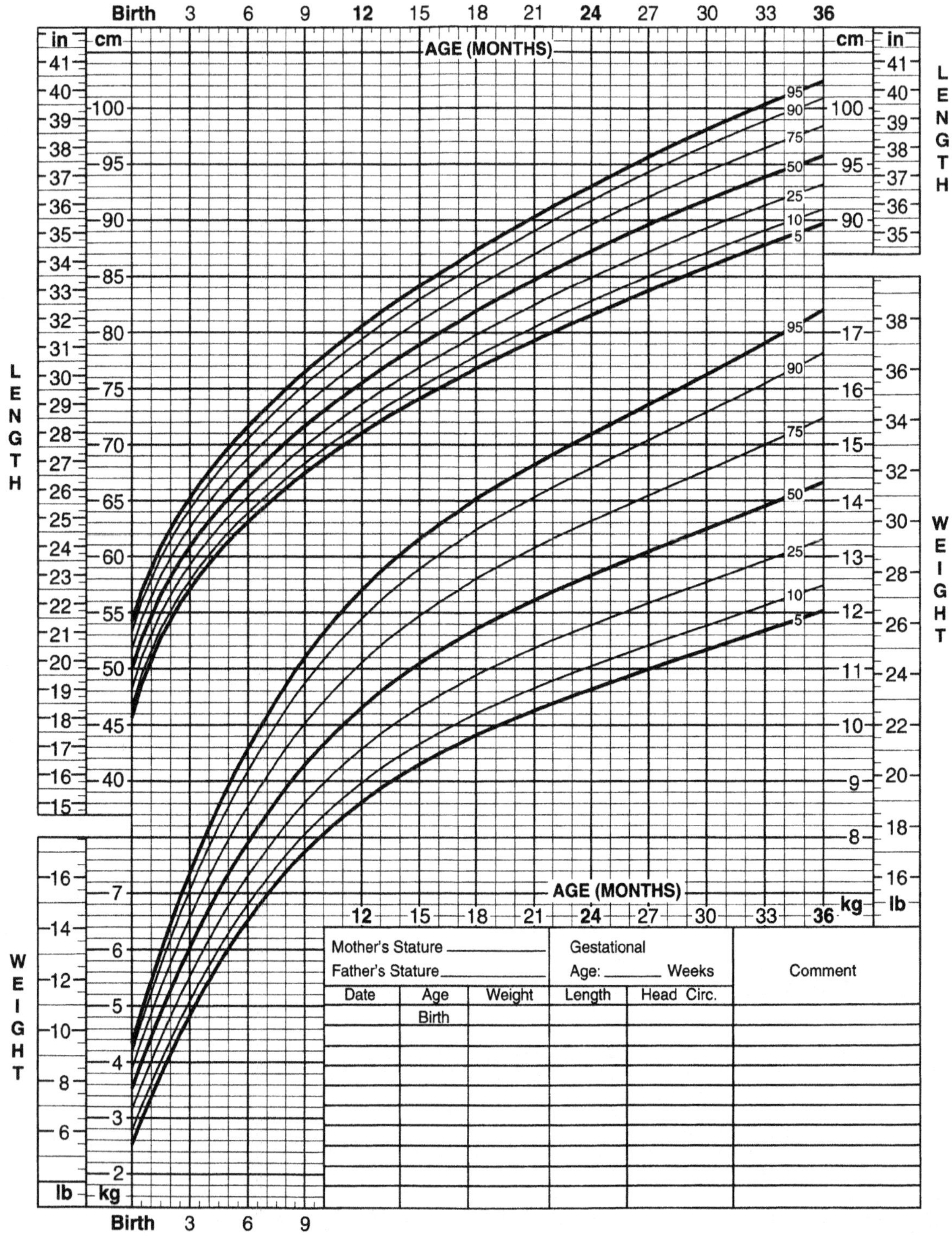

Mother's Stature ______ Father's Stature ______			Gestational Age: ____ Weeks		Comment
Date	Age	Weight	Length	Head Circ.	
	Birth				

Published May 30, 2000 (modified 4/20/01).
SOURCE: Developed by the National Center for Health Statistics in collaboration with the National Center for Chronic Disease Prevention and Health Promotion (2000).
http://www.cdc.gov/growthcharts

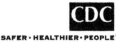

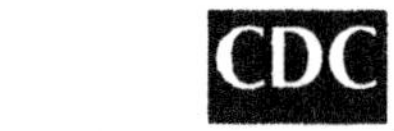

2 to 20 years: Boys
Stature-for-age and Weight-for-age percentiles

NAME ____________________

RECORD # ____________

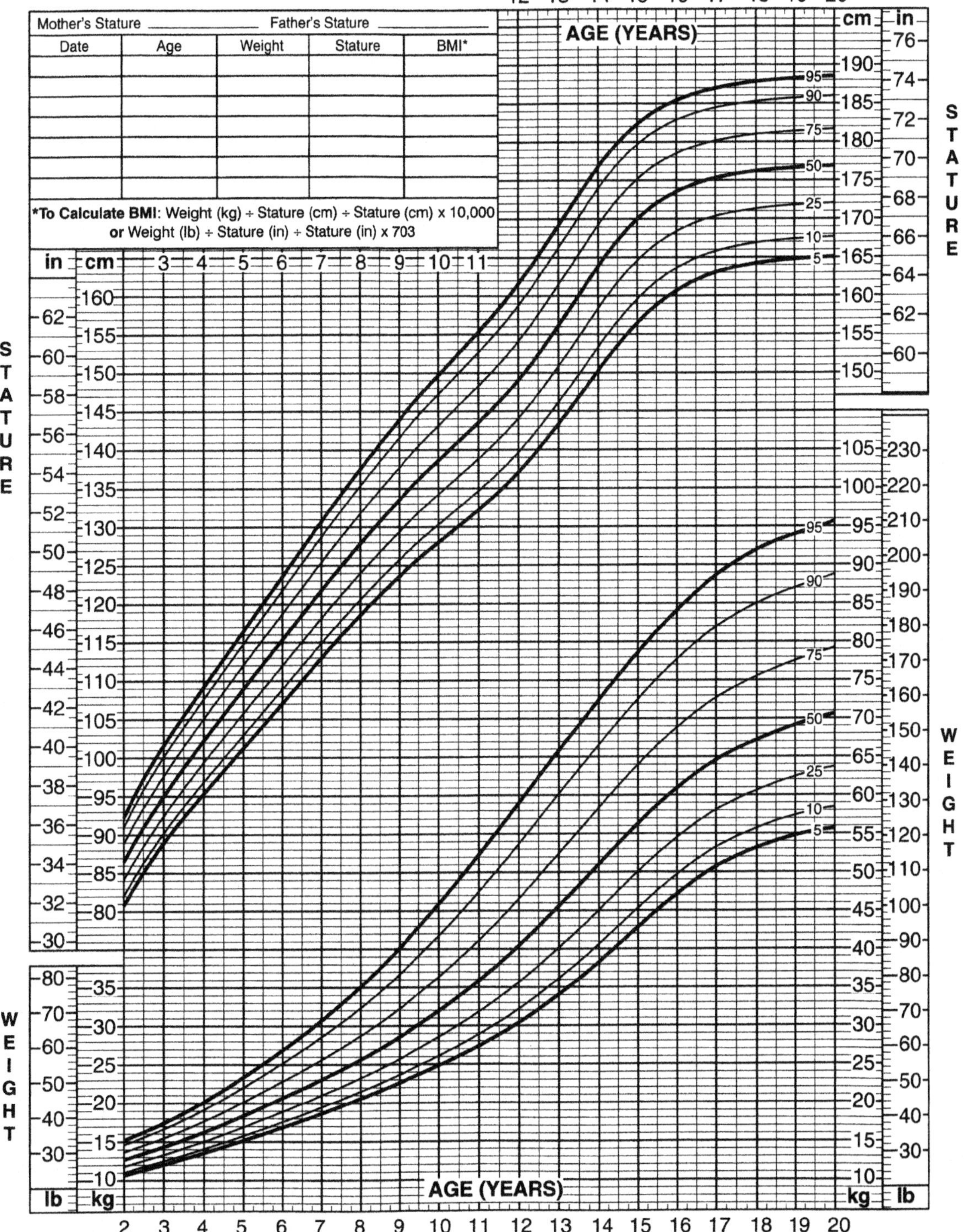

Published May 30, 2000 (modified 11/21/00).

SOURCE: Developed by the National Center for Health Statistics in collaboration with the National Center for Chronic Disease Prevention and Health Promotion (2000).

http://www.cdc.gov/growthcharts

CDC

SAFER · HEALTHIER · PEOPLE™

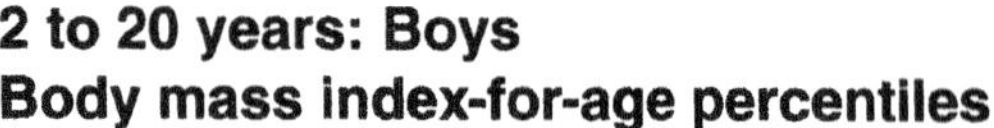

2 to 20 years: Boys
Body mass index-for-age percentiles

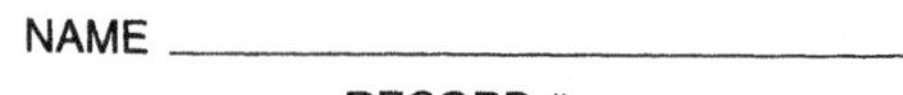

NAME ______________________

RECORD # ____________

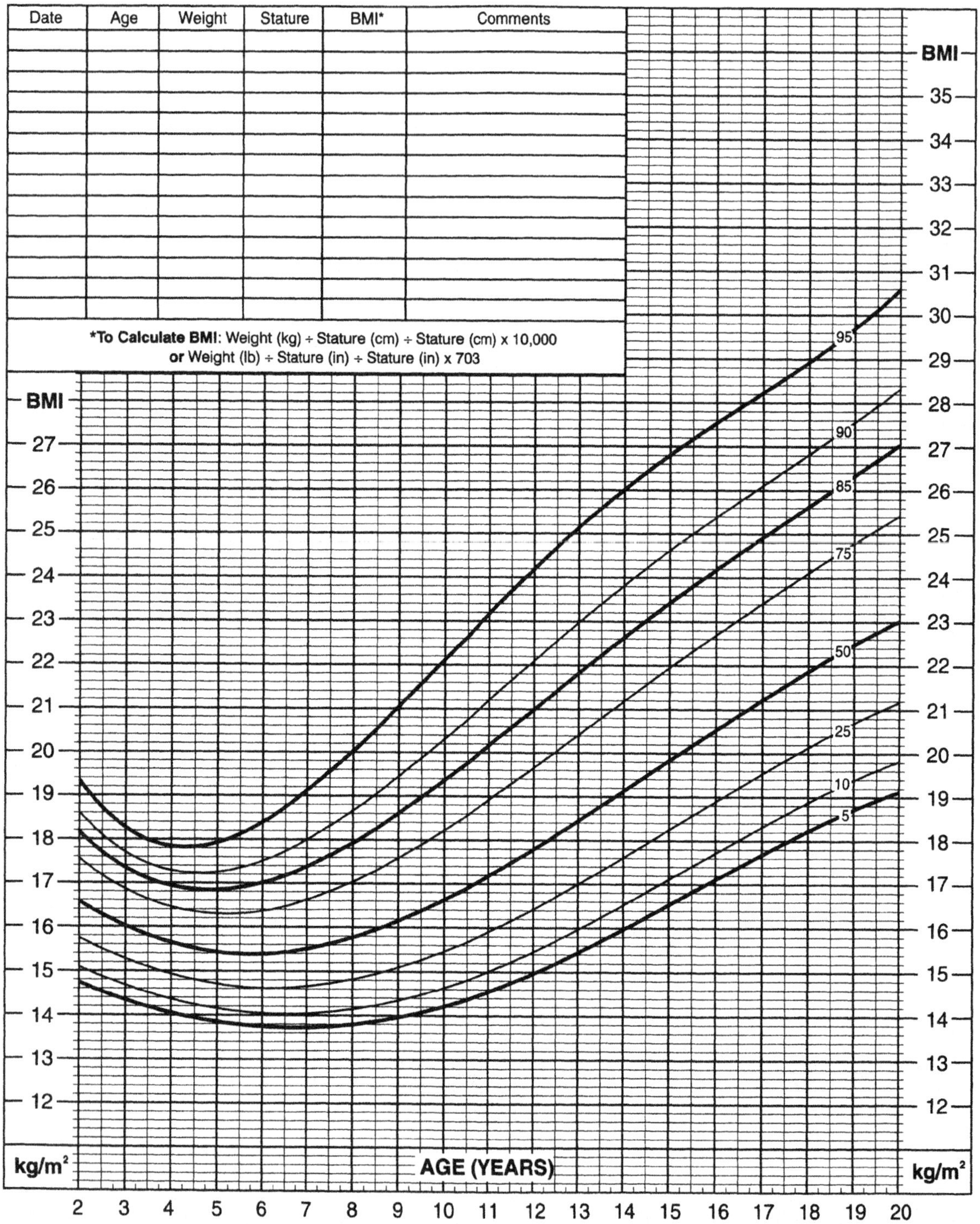

Date	Age	Weight	Stature	BMI*	Comments

***To Calculate BMI**: Weight (kg) ÷ Stature (cm) ÷ Stature (cm) x 10,000
or Weight (lb) ÷ Stature (in) ÷ Stature (in) x 703

BMI

35 34 33 32 31 30 29 28 27 26 25 24 23 22 21 20 19 18 17 16 15 14 13 12

95 90 85 75 50 25 10 5

kg/m²

AGE (YEARS)

2 3 4 5 6 7 8 9 10 11 12 13 14 15 16 17 18 19 20

Published May 30, 2000 (modified 10/16/00).
SOURCE: Developed by the National Center for Health Statistics in collaboration with the National Center for Chronic Disease Prevention and Health Promotion (2000).
http://www.cdc.gov/growthcharts

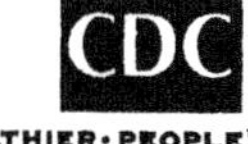

SAFER • HEALTHIER • PEOPLE™

Heart Weight as a Function of Body Weight: Infants and Adolescents*

Body Height		*Heart Weight*			
		Females		*Males*	
		Mean	*Range*	*Mean*	*Range*
(cm)	*(in)*	*(g)*		*(g)*	
40	16	12	8–19	14	8–26
45	18	15	10–24	18	10–32
50	20	19	12–29	22	12–39
55	22	24	14–35	26	14–46
60	24	27	17–42	35	20–63
70	28	36	23–56	40	23–72
75	30	41	26–64	46	26–81
80	31	46	30–72	51	29–92
85	33	52	33–81	58	32–103
90	35	58	37–90	64	36–114
95	37	64	41–100	71	40–126
100	39	71	45–111	78	44–138
105	41	78	50–122	85	48–151
110	43	85	55–133	93	52–165
115	45	93	59–145	100	56–179
120	47	101	64–157	109	61–194
125	49	109	70–170	117	66–209
130	51	117	75–183	126	71–224
135	53	126	81–197	135	76–240
140	55	135	87–211	144	81–257
145	57	145	93–226	154	86–274
150	59	154	99–241	164	92–292
155	61	165	105–257	174	98–310
160	63	175	112–273	184	103–329
165	65	185	119–290	195	109–348
170	67	196	126–307	206	116–367
175	69	208	133–324	217	122–388
180	71	219	140–342	229	128–408
185	73	231	148–361	241	135–429
190	75	243	156–380	253	142–451
195	77	256	164–399	265	149–473
200	79	268	172–419	278	156–495

*Data adapted with permission from Scholz DG, Kitzman DW, Hagen PT, Ilstrup DM, Edwards WD. Age-related changes in normal human hearts during the first 10 decades of life. Part I (Growth): A quantitative anatomic study of 200 specimens from subjects from birth to 19 years old. Mayo Clin Proc 1988;63:126–136.

Heart Weight as a Function of Body Height: Infants and Adolescents*

Body Weight		*Heart Weight*			
		Females		*Males*	
		Mean	*Range*	*Mean*	*Range*
(kg)	*(lb)*	*(g)*		*(g)*	
3	7	19	13–29	16	11–24
4	9	24	16–37	21	14–31
5	11	29	19–44	26	18–38
6	13	33	22–51	30	21–45
7	15	38	25–58	35	24–51
8	18	42	28–64	39	27–58
9	20	46	30–71	44	30–64
10	22	50	33–77	48	33–71
12	26	58	38–89	57	39–83
14	31	66	43–101	65	45–96
16	35	74	48–113	74	50–108
18	40	81	53–124	82	56–120
20	44	88	58–135	90	61–132
22	49	95	62–146	98	67–143
24	53	102	67–156	106	72–155
26	57	109	71–166	114	78–167
28	62	116	76–177	122	83–178
30	66	122	80–187	130	89–190
32	71	129	84–197	137	94–201
34	75	135	88–207	145	99–212
36	79	148	97–226	160	110–235
40	88	154	101–236	168	115–246
42	93	160	105–245	175	120–257
44	97	166	109–254	183	125–268
46	101	172	113–264	190	130–279
48	106	179	117–273	198	135–289
50	110	184	121–282	205	140–300
55	121	199	130–304	224	153–327
60	132	214	140–326	242	165–354
65	143	228	149–348	260	178–380
70	154	242	158–370	278	190–406
75	165	256	167–391	295	202–432
80	176	269	176–412	313	214–458
85	187	283	185–432	331	226–484
90	198	296	194–453	348	238–509
95	209	309	202–473	365	250–535
100	220	322	211–493	383	262–560

*Data adapted with permission from Scholz DG, Kitzman DW, Hagen PT, Ilstrup DM, Edwards WD. Age-related changes in normal human hearts during the first 10 decades of life. Part I (Growth): A quantitative anatomic study of 200 specimens from subjects from birth to 19 years old. Mayo Clin Proc 1988;63:126–136.

Heart Valve Circumferences (cm) as a Function of Age: Infants and Adolescents*

Age (yr)	*Aortic valve*				*Mitral valve*				*Pulmonary valve*				*Tricuspid valve*			
	Female		*Male*		*Female*		*Male*		*Female*		*Male*		*Female*		*Male*	
	Mean	*Range*	*Mean*	*Range*	*Mean*	*Range*	*Mean*	*Range*	*Mean*	*Range*	*Mean*	*Range*	*Mean*	*Range*	*Mean*	*Range*
0	2.2	1.33–3.00	2.2	1.35–3.02	2.8	1.31–4.31	2.6	0.83–4.44	2.2	1.13–3.23	2.1	0.83–3.32	3.0	1.11–4.88	2.5	0.66–4.38
1	3.0	2.11–3.79	3.0	2.20–3.87	4.1	2.57–5.57	4.1	2.24–5.86	3.0	1.97–4.07	3.0	1.78–4.27	4.7	2.80–6.56	4.5	2.67–6.39
2	3.4	2.53–4.21	3.5	2.65–4.32	4.7	3.25–6.24	4.8	3.00–6.62	3.5	2.42–4.52	3.5	2.29–4.78	5.6	3.70–7.46	5.6	3.75–7.47
3	3.7	2.82–4.50	3.8	2.96–4.63	5.2	3.71–6.70	5.3	3.52–7.13	3.8	2.72–4.82	3.9	2.64–5.13	6.2	4.31–8.08	6.3	4.48–8.20
4	3.9	3.04–4.72	4.0	3.20–4.87	5.6	4.06–7.06	5.7	3.91–7.53	4.0	2.96–5.06	4.2	2.91–5.40	6.7	4.78–8.55	6.9	5.04–8.77
5	4.1	3.22–4.89	4.2	3.39–5.06	5.8	4.34–7.34	6.0	4.23–7.85	4.2	3.14–5.24	4.4	3.12–5.61	7.1	5.17–8.93	7.4	5.50–9.22
6	4.2	3.37–5.04	4.4	3.55–5.22	6.1	4.58–7.58	6.3	4.50–8.12	4.4	3.30–5.40	4.6	3.30–5.79	7.4	5.48–9.25	7.7	5.88–9.60
7	4.3	3.49–5.17	4.5	3.69–5.36	6.3	4.79–7.78	6.5	4.73–8.35	4.5	3.49–5.54	4.7	3.46–5.95	7.6	5.76–9.53	8.1	6.21–9.93
8	4.5	3.61–5.28	4.7	3.81–5.48	6.5	4.97–7.96	6.7	4.93–8.55	4.6	3.56–5.66	4.8	3.59–6.08	7.8	6.00–9.77	8.4	6.50–10.2
9	4.6	3.71–5.38	4.8	3.92–5.59	6.6	5.13–8.13	6.9	5.12–8.73	4.7	3.67–5.77	5.0	3.71–6.21	8.1	6.22–9.98	8.6	6.75–10.5
10	4.6	3.88–5.47	4.9	4.02–5.69	6.8	5.27–8.27	7.1	5.28–8.89	4.8	3.76–5.86	5.1	3.82–6.32	8.3	6.41–10.2	8.9	6.99–10.7
11	4.7	3.92–5.56	4.9	4.11–5.78	6.9	5.40–8.40	7.2	5.43–9.04	4.9	3.85–5.95	5.2	3.92–6.42	8.5	6.59–10.3	9.1	7.20–10.9
12	4.8	3.96–5.63	5.0	4.19–5.86	7.0	5.53–8.52	7.4	5.56–9.18	5.0	3.93–6.03	5.3	4.02–6.51	8.6	6.75–10.5	9.3	7.39–11.1
13	4.9	4.03–5.70	5.1	4.27–5.93	7.1	5.64–8.64	7.5	5.69–9.31	5.1	4.01–6.11	5.4	4.10–6.59	8.8	6.90–10.7	9.4	7.57–11.3
14	4.9	4.09–5.77	5.2	4.34–6.00	7.2	5.74–8.74	7.6	5.81–9.42	5.1	4.07–6.17	5.4	4.18–6.67	8.9	7.04–10.8	9.6	7.74–11.5
15	5.0	4.15–5.83	5.2	4.40–6.07	7.3	5.84–8.84	7.7	5.92–9.53	5.2	4.14–6.24	5.5	4.25–6.74	9.1	7.17–10.9	9.8	7.89–11.6
16	5.1	4.21–5.89	5.3	4.46–6.13	7.4	5.93–8.93	7.8	6.02–9.64	5.3	4.20–6.30	5.6	4.32–6.81	9.2	7.29–11.1	9.9	8.04–11.8
17	5.1	4.26–5.94	5.4	4.52–6.19	7.5	6.02–9.02	7.9	6.12–9.73	5.3	4.26–6.36	5.6	4.39–6.88	9.3	7.41–11.2	10.0	8.18–11.9
18	5.2	4.32–5.99	5.4	4.58–6.25	7.6	6.10–9.10	8.0	6.21–9.83	5.4	4.31–6.41	5.7	4.45–6.94	9.4	7.52–11.3	10.2	8.31–12.0
19	5.2	4.36–6.04	5.5	4.63–6.30	7.7	6.18–9.17	8.1	6.30–9.91	5.4	4.36–6.46	5.8	4.51–7.00	9.5	7.62–11.4	10.3	8.43–12.1

*Data adapted with permission from Scholz DG, Kitzman DW, Hagen PT, Ilstrup DM, Edwards WD. Age-related changes in normal human hearts during the first 10 decades of life. Part I (Growth): A quantitative anatomic study of 200 specimens from subjects from birth to 19 years old. Mayo Clin Proc 1988;63:126–136.

Brain Weight as a Function of Age in Children and Adolescents*

Age	Females		Males	
	Body Height (cm)	Brain Weight (g)	Body Height (cm)	Brain Weight (g)
0 mo	49	372	51	448
1 mo	54	516	54	523
2 mo	57	560	58	609
4 mo	60	645	62	718
7 mo	66	755	68	871
9 mo	71	935	72	999
13 mo	75	961	79	1,141
16 mo	78	1,117	83	1,176
19 mo	82	1,121	83	1,109
22 mo	87	1,063	83	1,088
2 yr	87	1,176	90	1,249
3 yr	98	1,213	99	1,317
4 yr	99	1,243	107	1,419
5 yr	109	1,284	114	1,480
6 yr	118	1,286	117	1,437
7 yr	123	1,328	128	1,424
8 yr	130	1,400	133	1,457
9 yr	132	1,360	138	1,489
10 yr	135	1,550	135	1,501
11 yr	145	1,380	148	1,397
12 yr	157	1,356	154	1,483
13 yr	163	1,453	159	1,564
14 yr	164	1,322	166	1,484
15 yr	166	1,378	168	1,483
16 yr	164	1,383	175	1,547
17 yr	166	1,380	174	1,528
18 yr	166	1,359	176	1,491

*Data adapted with permission from Voigt J, Pakkenberg H. Brain weight of Danish children. Acta Anat 1983;116:290–301.

Fetal Organ weights, Guihard Costa
Mean, standard deviation, and 5th and 95th percentiles of organ weight in relation to gestational age

Age interval (GW)	*Mean*	*SD*	*5th percentile*	*95th percentile*
Body weight				
11–12	9.1	7.9	−3.8	22.0
13–14	55.8	14.4	32.2	79.4
15–16	108.6	24.7	68.0	149.3
17–18	176.1	39.0	112.0	240.3
19–20	267.7	57.1	173.7	361.7
21–22	392.7	79.2	262.5	522.9
23–24	559.6	105.1	386.7	732.5
25–26	773.9	134.9	552.0	995.8
27–28	1038.2	168.6	760.9	1315.5
29–30	1350.4	206.1	1011.3	1689.5
31–32	1702.5	247.6	1295.2	2109.7
33–34	2080.2	292.9	1598.3	2562.0
35–36	2460.8	342.1	1898.0	3023.7
37–38	2813.1	395.3	2162.9	3463.3
39–40	3095.1	452.2	2351.2	3839.1
41–42	3254.9	513.1	2410.9	4099.0
Brain				
13–14	9.09	2.49	5.00	13.18
15–16	18.98	4.60	11.42	26.54
17–18	31.37	7.11	19.67	43.06
19–20	47.93	10.03	31.43	64.43
21–22	69.90	13.35	47.93	91.87
23–24	97.98	17.08	69.88	126.08
25–26	132.43	21.21	97.53	167.33
27–28	172.98	25.75	130.62	215.34
29–30	218.89	30.69	168.41	269.38
31–32	268.95	36.04	209.67	328.23
33–34	321.43	41.79	252.69	390.17
35–36	374.13	47.94	295.27	453.00
37–38	424.37	54.50	334.72	514.02
39–40	468.96	61.46	367.85	570.07
41–42	504.23	68.83	391.01	617.46
Heart				
13–14	0.24	0.13	0.02	0.46
15–16	0.82	0.23	0.45	1.20
17–18	1.44	0.37	0.83	2.05
19–20	2.21	0.56	1.29	3.12
21–22	3.23	0.79	1.93	4.52
23–24	4.55	1.07	2.79	6.30
25–26	6.21	1.39	3.92	8.49
27–28	8.20	1.76	5.31	11.09
29–30	10.48	2.17	6.90	14.05
31–32	12.98	2.63	8.65	17.31
33–34	15.60	3.14	10.44	20.76
35–36	18.21	3.69	12.15	24.27
37–38	20.63	4.28	13.59	27.67
39–40	22.68	4.92	14.58	30.77
41–42	24.49	5.58	15.31	33.67

(continued)

(continued)

Age interval (GW)	*Mean*	*SD*	*5th percentile*	*95th percentile*
Liver				
13–14	3.09	0.27	2.64	3.54
15–16	5.81	1.71	3.00	8.62
17–18	9.39	3.33	3.91	14.87
19–20	14.33	5.15	5.87	22.80
21–22	21.00	7.15	9.23	32.77
23–24	29.63	9.35	14.24	45.02
25–26	40.27	11.75	20.95	59.60
27–28	52.89	14.33	29.32	76.46
29–30	67.29	17.10	39.15	95.42
31–32	83.10	20.07	50.09	116.12
33–34	99.87	23.23	61.67	138.08
35–36	116.97	26.58	73.25	160.69
37–38	133.64	30.12	84.10	183.18
39–40	148.97	33.85	93.29	204.66
41–42	161.94	37.78	99.80	224.08
Pancreas				
13–14	0.09	0.01	0.08	0.11
15–16	0.28	0.08	0.15	0.41
17–18	0.42	0.16	0.16	0.68
19–20	0.57	0.24	0.17	0.98
21–22	0.78	0.34	0.22	1.35
23–24	1.08	0.45	0.33	1.82
25–26	1.47	0.57	0.54	2.41
27–28	1.98	0.70	0.83	3.13
29–30	2.58	0.84	1.21	3.96
31–32	3.26	0.98	1.64	4.87
33–34	3.97	1.14	2.09	5.84
35–36	4.66	1.31	2.50	6.81
37–38	5.26	1.49	2.82	7.71
39–40	5.71	1.67	2.96	8.46
41–42	5.90	1.87	2.82	8.97
Spleen				
13–14	0.06	0.04	–0.01	0.14
15–16	0.12	0.08	–0.00	0.25
17–18	0.23	0.13	0.02	0.44
19–20	0.38	0.20	0.06	0.71
21–22	0.62	0.29	0.14	1.11
23–24	0.96	0.42	0.27	1.66
25–26	1.44	0.59	0.48	2.41
27–28	2.09	0.80	0.78	3.41
29–30	2.95	1.06	1.21	4.70
31–32	4.08	1.39	1.80	6.36
33–34	5.53	1.78	2.59	8.46
35–36	7.35	2.25	3.64	11.06
37–38	9.63	2.82	4.99	14.26
39–40	12.43	3.48	6.71	18.16
41–42	15.85	4.25	8.86	22.85

(continued)

(continued)

Age interval (GW)	*Mean*	*SD*	*5th percentile*	*95th percentile*
Thymus				
13–14	0.09	0.07	–	0.20
15–16	0.17	0.12	–	0.37
17–18	0.31	0.19	–	0.63
19–20	0.53	0.30	0.04	1.03
21–22	0.87	0.45	0.13	1.60
23–24	1.35	0.64	0.29	2.40
25–26	2.01	0.89	0.55	3.48
27–28	2.92	1.21	0.93	4.92
29–30	4.14	1.61	1.49	6.79
31–32	5.72	2.10	2.26	9.18
33–34	7.75	2.70	3.31	12.20
35–36	10.33	3.42	4.71	15.95
37–38	13.54	4.27	6.52	20.56
39–40	17.50	5.27	8.84	26.17
41–42	22.34	6.44	11.75	32.93
Thyroid				
15–16	0.13	0.08	–0.00	0.27
17–18	0.19	0.10	0.02	0.36
19–20	0.25	0.13	0.04	0.46
21–22	0.33	0.16	0.08	0.59
23–24	0.42	0.18	0.12	0.73
25–26	0.53	0.22	0.18	0.89
27–28	0.66	0.25	0.24	1.07
29–30	0.80	0.29	0.32	1.27
31–32	0.95	0.33	0.42	1.49
33–34	1.13	0.37	0.53	1.73
35–36	1.33	0.41	0.65	2.00
37–38	1.54	0.46	0.79	2.30
39–40	1.78	0.51	0.95	2.61
41–42	2.04	0.56	1.13	2.96

Age interval (GW)	*Left*				*Right*			
	Mean	*SD*	*5th percentile*	*95th percentile*	*Mean*	*SD*	*5th percentile*	*95th percentile*
Adrenals								
13–14	0.13	0.03	0.08	0.17	0.16	0.08	0.03	0.29
15–16	0.28	0.10	0.12	0.45	0.28	0.09	0.13	0.43
17–18	0.47	0.18	0.18	0.76	0.44	0.13	0.22	0.66
19–20	0.69	0.26	0.27	1.11	0.63	0.20	0.30	0.96
21–22	0.93	0.34	0.38	1.48	0.86	0.29	0.38	1.33
23–24	1.21	0.42	0.51	1.90	1.12	0.39	0.47	1.76
25–26	1.51	0.51	0.67	2.34	1.41	0.50	0.58	2.24
27–28	1.84	0.60	0.86	2.82	1.73	0.62	0.71	2.76

(continued)

(continued)

Age interval (GW)	Left				Right			
	Mean	SD	5th percentile	95th percentile	Mean	SD	5th percentile	95th percentile
29–30	2.21	0.69	1.07	3.34	2.09	0.74	0.88	3.31
31–32	2.60	0.78	1.31	3.89	2.48	0.85	1.09	3.88
33–34	3.02	0.88	1.57	4.47	2.91	0.95	1.34	4.47
37–38	3.95	1.08	2.17	5.74	3.84	1.10	2.04	5.65
39–40	4.47	1.19	2.51	6.42	4.36	1.14	2.49	6.23
41–42	5.01	1.30	2.87	7.14	4.91	1.15	3.02	6.79
Kidneys								
13–14	0.19	0.12	−0.01	0.39	0.22	0.10	0.05	0.38
15–16	0.37	0.18	0.08	0.66	0.34	0.17	0.05	0.62
17–18	0.71	0.26	0.28	1.13	0.67	0.27	0.22	1.11
19–20	1.21	0.37	0.60	1.83	1.20	0.39	0.55	1.85
21–22	1.91	0.51	1.07	2.75	1.93	0.54	1.03	2.82
23–24	2.81	0.68	1.69	3.92	2.83	0.72	1.65	4.01
25–26	3.89	0.87	2.45	5.32	3.89	0.92	2.38	5.40
27–28	5.14	1.09	3.34	6.94	5.08	1.15	3.20	6.97
29–30	6.52	1.34	4.31	8.73	6.38	1.40	4.07	8.68
31–32	7.99	1.62	5.32	10.65	7.74	1.68	4.98	10.51
33–34	9.48	1.93	6.32	12.65	9.14	1.99	5.87	12.40
35–36	10.94	2.26	7.22	14.65	10.52	2.32	6.71	14.33
37–38	12.27	2.62	7.96	16.58	11.85	2.67	7.45	16.25
39–40	13.38	3.01	8.43	18.33	13.07	3.06	8.04	18.10
41–42	14.16	3.42	8.53	19.79	14.12	3.47	8.42	19.82
Lungs								
13–14	0.70	0.25	0.29	1.12	0.56	0.25	0.15	0.97
15–16	1.52	0.55	0.62	2.42	1.47	0.53	0.59	2.35
17–18	2.42	0.88	0.97	3.87	2.67	0.93	1.13	4.20
19–20	3.53	1.26	1.46	5.59	4.15	1.42	1.81	6.49
21–22	4.92	1.67	2.18	7.67	5.92	2.00	2.64	9.20
23–24	6.67	2.12	3.19	10.15	7.98	2.63	3.65	12.31
25–26	8.77	2.60	4.48	13.05	10.32	3.32	4.87	15.78
27–28	11.20	3.13	6.05	16.35	12.95	4.03	6.32	19.59
29–30	13.92	3.70	7.84	20.00	15.87	4.77	8.03	23.71
31–32	16.82	4.30	9.75	23.90	19.08	5.50	10.02	28.13
33–34	19.79	4.94	11.66	27.91	22.57	6.23	12.33	32.81
35–36	22.64	5.62	13.39	31.88	26.34	6.92	14.97	37.72
37–38	25.18	6.34	14.75	35.61	30.41	7.56	17.97	42.85
39–40	27.18	7.10	15.51	38.85	34.76	8.15	21.36	48.16
41–42	28.36	7.89	15.38	41.33	39.24	8.66	25.00	53.47

Used with permission from Guihard Costa, A-M Ménez F, Delezoide AL, Organ weights in human fetuses after formalin fixation: standards by gestational age and body weight. Ped and Dev Pathology 2002;5:559–578.

PART III: Fetal Organ weights, Guihard Costa
Mean, standard deviation, and 5th and 95th percentiles of organ weight in relation to body weight

Body weight (g)	Mean	SD	5th percentile	95th percentile
Brain				
1–200	25.2	7.9	12.3	38.1
201–400	55.0	11.2	36.5	73.5
401–600	85.6	14.6	61.5	109.7
601–800	117.0	18.0	87.3	146.6
801–1000	149.0	21.4	113.8	184.2
1001–1200	181.4	24.8	140.7	222.2

(continued)

(continued)

Body weight (g)	*Mean*	*SD*	*5th percentile*	*95th percentile*
1201–1400	214.1	28.2	167.8	260.5
1401–1600	246.9	31.6	195.0	298.8
1601–1800	279.4	34.9	221.9	336.8
1801–2000	311.2	38.3	248.2	374.2
2001–2200	342.1	41.7	273.5	410.7
2201–2400	371.5	45.1	297.3	445.7
2401–2600	399.1	48.5	319.3	478.8
2601–2800	424.3	51.9	338.9	509.6
2801–3000	446.5	55.2	355.6	537.4
3001–3200	465.2	58.6	368.8	561.6
3201–3400	479.7	62.0	377.7	581.7
3401–3600	489.4	65.4	381.8	597.0
3601–3800	496.9	68.8	383.7	610.0
3801–4000	504.4	72.2	385.7	623.1
4001–4200	511.9	75.6	387.6	636.1
Heart				
1–200	9.4	5.1	1.0	17.8
201–400	25.3	7.1	13.6	37.1
401–600	41.0	9.2	26.0	56.1
601–800	56.5	11.1	38.2	74.8
801–1000	71.8	13.0	50.4	93.3
1001–1200	86.9	14.9	62.3	111.4
1201–1400	101.8	16.8	74.2	129.3
1401–1600	116.4	18.6	85.9	146.9
1601–1800	130.8	20.3	97.4	164.2
1801–2000	145.1	22.0	108.8	181.3
2001–2200	159.1	23.7	120.1	198.0
2201–2400	172.8	25.3	131.2	214.5
2401–2600	186.4	26.9	142.2	230.6
2601–2800	199.8	28.4	153.0	246.5
2801–3000	212.9	29.9	163.7	262.1
3001–3200	225.9	31.4	174.3	277.4
3201–3400	238.6	32.8	184.7	292.5
3401–3600	251.1	34.1	195.0	307.2
3601–3800	263.4	35.4	205.1	321.7
3801–4000	275.5	36.7	215.1	335.8
4001–4200	287.3	37.9	224.9	349.7
Liver				
1–200	8.2	4.0	1.7	14.8
201–400	17.7	5.5	8.6	26.8
401–600	27.2	7.1	15.6	38.8
601–800	36.6	8.6	22.5	50.8
801–1000	46.1	10.1	29.5	62.7
1001–1200	55.6	11.6	36.5	74.7
1201–1400	65.1	13.2	43.4	86.7
1401–1600	74.5	14.7	50.4	98.7
1601–1800	84.0	16.2	57.3	110.7
1801–2000	93.5	17.7	64.3	122.6
2001–2200	102.9	19.3	71.3	134.6
2201–2400	112.4	20.8	78.2	146.6
2401–2600	121.9	22.3	85.2	158.6
2601–2800	131.3	23.8	92.1	170.6
2801–3000	140.8	25.4	99.1	182.5
3001–3200	150.3	26.9	106.1	194.5

(continued)

(continued)

Body weight (g)	*Mean*	*SD*	*5th percentile*	*95th percentile*
3201–3400	159.8	28.4	113.0	206.5
3401–3600	169.2	29.9	120.0	218.5
3601–3800	178.7	31.5	126.9	230.5
3801–4000	188.2	33.0	133.9	242.4
4001–4200	197.6	34.5	140.9	254.4
Pancreas				
1–200	0.32	0.11	0.14	0.50
201–400	0.67	0.21	0.34	1.01
401–600	1.03	0.30	0.53	1.53
601–800	1.38	0.40	0.72	2.04
801–1000	1.73	0.50	0.92	2.55
1001–1200	2.09	0.59	1.11	3.06
1201–1400	2.44	0.69	1.31	3.58
1401–1600	2.79	0.79	1.50	4.09
1601–1800	3.15	0.88	1.69	4.60
1801–2000	3.50	0.98	1.89	5.11
2001–2200	3.85	1.08	2.08	5.63
2201–2400	4.21	1.17	2.28	6.14
2401–2600	4.56	1.27	2.47	6.65
2601–2800	4.91	1.37	2.66	7.16
2801–3000	5.27	1.46	2.86	7.68
3001–3200	5.62	1.56	3.05	8.19
3201–3400	5.97	1.66	3.25	8.70
3401–3600	6.33	1.75	3.44	9.22
3601–3800	6.68	1.85	3.64	9.73
3801–4000	7.04	1.95	3.83	10.24
4001–4200	7.39	2.05	4.02	10.75
Spleen				
1–200	0.10	0.07	–0.02	0.22
201–400	0.46	0.24	0.07	0.86
401–600	0.93	0.42	0.25	1.61
601–800	1.47	0.60	0.49	2.45
801–1000	2.07	0.78	0.79	3.36
1001–1200	2.73	0.97	1.13	4.32
1201–1400	3.43	1.16	1.52	5.34
1401–1600	4.17	1.35	1.94	6.40
1601–1800	4.95	1.55	2.40	7.50
1801–2000	5.76	1.75	2.89	8.63
2001–2200	6.60	1.94	3.41	9.80
2201–2400	7.48	2.14	3.95	11.00
2401–2600	8.38	2.35	4.52	12.24
2601–2800	9.31	2.55	5.12	13.50
2801–3000	10.26	2.75	5.74	14.79
3001–3200	11.24	2.96	6.38	16.11
3201–3400	12.25	3.16	7.05	17.45
3401–3600	13.27	3.37	7.73	18.81
3601–3800	14.32	3.58	8.44	20.20
3801–4000	15.38	3.78	9.15	21.60
4001–4200	16.43	3.99	9.86	23.00
Thymus				
1–200	0.18	0.12	–0.01	0.38
201–400	0.73	0.36	0.14	1.32
401–600	1.39	0.60	0.40	2.37
601–800	2.12	0.84	0.74	3.51

(continued)

(continued)

Body weight (g)	Mean	SD	5th percentile	95th percentile
801–1000	2.91	1.09	1.13	4.70
1001–1200	3.75	1.33	1.57	5.94
1201–1400	4.64	1.57	2.05	7.23
1401–1600	5.55	1.82	2.56	8.55
1601–1800	6.51	2.06	3.11	9.90
1801–2000	7.49	2.31	3.69	11.29
2001–2200	8.49	2.56	4.29	12.70
2201–2400	9.53	2.80	4.92	14.14
2401–2600	10.59	3.05	5.57	15.60
2601–2800	11.67	3.29	6.25	17.08
2801–3000	12.77	3.54	6.94	18.59
3001–3200	13.89	3.79	7.66	20.12
3201–3400	15.03	4.04	8.39	21.67
3401–3600	16.19	4.28	9.14	23.23
3601–3800	17.36	4.53	9.91	24.82
3801–4000	18.55	4.78	10.69	26.41
4001–4200	19.73	5.02	11.46	28.00
Thyroid				
1–200	0.16	0.11	–0.03	0.35
201–400	0.27	0.14	0.05	0.50
401–600	0.38	0.16	0.12	0.64
601–800	0.49	0.18	0.20	0.79
801–1000	0.60	0.20	0.26	0.93
1001–1200	0.70	0.23	0.33	1.07
1201–1400	0.80	0.25	0.39	1.21
1401–1600	0.90	0.27	0.45	1.34
1601–1800	0.99	0.29	0.51	1.47
1801–2000	1.08	0.31	0.56	1.60
2001–2200	1.17	0.34	0.62	1.73
2201–2400	1.26	0.36	0.67	1.85
2401–2600	1.34	0.38	0.71	1.97
2601–2800	1.42	0.40	0.75	2.08
2801–3000	1.50	0.43	0.79	2.20
3001–3200	1.57	0.45	0.83	2.31
3201–3400	1.64	0.47	0.87	2.42
3401–3600	1.71	0.49	0.90	2.52
3601–3800	1.78	0.52	0.93	2.63
3801–4000	1.84	0.54	0.96	2.73
4001–4200	1.91	0.56	0.98	2.83

Body weight (g)	Right				Left			
	Mean	SD	5th percentile	95th percentile	Mean	SD	5th percentile	95th percentile
Adrenals								
1–200	0.41	0.26	–0.02	0.83	0.43	0.26	0.00	0.86
201–400	0.68	0.32	0.15	1.20	0.71	0.32	0.19	1.23
401–600	0.94	0.38	0.32	1.57	0.99	0.37	0.38	1.60
601–800	1.21	0.44	0.49	1.93	1.27	0.42	0.58	1.97
801–1000	1.48	0.50	0.67	2.30	1.55	0.48	0.77	2.34
1001–1200	1.75	0.56	0.84	2.67	1.83	0.53	0.96	2.71
1201–1400	2.02	0.62	1.01	3.04	2.11	0.59	1.15	3.08
1401–1600	2.29	0.68	1.18	3.40	2.40	0.64	1.34	3.45
1601–1800	2.56	0.73	1.35	3.77	2.68	0.69	1.53	3.82
1801–2000	2.83	0.79	1.52	4.14	2.96	0.75	1.73	4.19

(continued)

(continued)

Body weight (g)	Right				Left			
	Mean	SD	5th percentile	95th percentile	Mean	SD	5th percentile	95th percentile
2001–2200	3.10	0.85	1.70	4.50	3.24	0.80	1.92	4.56
2201–2400	3.37	0.91	1.87	4.87	3.52	0.86	2.11	4.93
2401–2600	3.64	0.97	2.04	5.24	3.80	0.91	2.30	5.30
2601–2800	3.91	1.03	2.21	5.60	4.08	0.96	2.49	5.67
2801–3000	4.18	1.09	2.38	5.97	4.36	1.02	2.68	6.04
3001–3200	4.44	1.15	2.55	6.34	4.64	1.07	2.88	6.40
3401–3600	4.98	1.27	2.90	7.07	5.20	1.18	3.26	7.14
3601–3800	5.25	1.33	3.07	7.44	5.48	1.24	3.45	7.51
3801–4000	5.52	1.39	3.24	7.80	5.76	1.29	3.64	7.88
4001–4200	5.79	1.45	3.41	8.17	6.04	1.34	3.83	8.25
Kidneys								
1–200	0.66	0.28	0.20	1.12	0.56	0.31	0.05	1.08
201–400	1.58	0.43	0.87	2.28	1.55	0.46	0.80	2.30
401–600	2.48	0.58	1.53	3.43	2.52	0.60	1.53	3.51
601–800	3.37	0.73	2.18	4.57	3.47	0.74	2.25	4.69
801–1000	4.26	0.87	2.82	5.70	4.41	0.89	2.95	5.86
1001–1200	5.14	1.02	3.46	6.82	5.32	1.03	3.63	7.02
1201–1400	6.00	1.17	4.08	7.93	6.22	1.17	4.30	8.15
1401–1600	6.86	1.32	4.69	9.03	7.11	1.31	4.94	9.27
1601–1800	7.71	1.47	5.30	10.13	7.97	1.46	5.58	10.37
1801–2000	8.55	1.62	5.89	11.21	8.82	1.60	6.19	11.45
2001–2200	9.38	1.76	6.48	12.29	9.65	1.74	6.78	12.52
2201–2400	10.20	1.91	7.06	13.35	10.47	1.89	7.36	13.57
2401–2600	11.02	2.06	7.62	14.41	11.26	2.03	7.92	14.60
2601–2800	11.82	2.21	8.18	15.46	12.04	2.17	8.47	15.62
2801–3000	12.61	2.36	8.73	16.49	12.80	2.32	8.99	16.61
3001–3200	13.40	2.51	9.27	17.52	13.55	2.46	9.50	17.59
3201–3400	14.18	2.66	9.81	18.54	14.27	2.60	9.99	18.55
3401–3600	14.94	2.80	10.33	19.56	14.98	2.75	10.47	19.50
3601–3800	15.70	2.95	10.84	20.56	15.68	2.89	10.92	20.43
3801–4000	16.45	3.10	11.35	21.56	16.36	3.03	11.37	21.35
4001–4200	17.21	3.25	11.86	22.56	17.05	3.17	11.82	22.27
Lungs								
1–200	2.76	1.49	0.32	5.21	1.45	0.78	0.16	2.73
201–400	4.87	1.88	1.78	7.96	3.87	1.15	1.98	5.75
401–600	6.98	2.27	3.24	10.72	6.18	1.51	3.70	8.67
601–800	9.08	2.67	4.70	13.47	8.39	1.88	5.30	11.47
801–1000	11.19	3.06	6.15	16.23	10.49	2.24	6.80	14.17
1001–1200	13.30	3.46	7.61	18.98	12.47	2.61	8.19	16.76
1201–1400	15.40	3.85	9.07	21.73	14.35	2.97	9.47	19.24
1401–1600	17.51	4.24	10.53	24.49	16.12	3.33	10.64	21.61
1601–1800	19.62	4.64	11.99	27.24	17.78	3.70	11.70	23.87
1801–2000	21.72	5.03	13.45	30.00	19.34	4.06	12.65	26.02
2001–2200	23.83	5.42	14.90	32.75	20.78	4.43	13.49	28.06
2201–2400	25.93	5.82	16.36	35.51	22.11	4.79	14.23	30.00
2401–2600	28.04	6.21	17.82	38.26	23.34	5.16	14.85	32.82
2601–2800	30.15	6.61	19.28	41.01	24.45	5.52	15.37	33.54
2801–3000	32.25	7.00	20.74	43.77	25.46	5.89	15.78	35.15
3001–3200	34.36	7.39	22.20	46.52	26.36	6.25	16.08	36.64
3201–3400	36.47	7.79	23.66	49.28	27.15	6.62	16.27	38.03
3401–3600	38.57	8.18	25.11	52.03	27.83	6.98	16.35	39.32
3601–3800	40.68	8.58	26.57	54.79	28.47	7.35	16.38	40.55
3801–4000	42.79	8.97	28.03	57.54	29.10	7.71	16.42	41.79
4001–4200	44.89	9.36	29.49	60.29	29.74	8.08	16.45	43.02

PART III: Fetal Organ weights, Guihard Costa
Mean, standard deviation, and 5th and 95th percentiles of body dimensions (mm) in relation to gestational age

Age interval (GW)	*Mean*	*SD*	*5th percentile*	*95th percentile*
Crown–heel length				
11–12	91.7	14.6	67.6	115.8
13–14	131.8	15.4	106.4	157.2
15–16	170.4	16.2	143.7	197.1
17–18	207.4	17.0	179.4	235.4
19–20	242.9	17.8	213.6	272.2
21–22	276.8	18.6	246.2	307.4
23–24	309.2	19.4	277.3	341.1
25–26	340.0	20.2	306.8	373.2
27–28	369.3	21.0	334.8	403.8
29–30	397.0	21.8	361.2	432.8
31–32	423.2	22.6	386.1	460.3
33–34	447.8	23.4	409.4	486.3
35–36	470.9	24.2	431.2	510.7
37–38	492.5	24.9	451.4	533.5
39–40	512.5	25.7	470.1	554.8
41–42	530.9	26.5	487.3	574.6
Crown-rump length				
11–12	62.1	11.2	43.6	80.5
13–14	89.6	11.7	70.4	108.9
15–16	116.2	12.2	96.1	136.2
17–18	141.7	12.7	120.9	162.5
19–20	166.2	13.1	144.6	187.9
21–22	189.8	13.6	167.4	212.2
23–24	212.3	14.1	189.1	235.5
25–26	233.8	14.6	209.9	257.8
27–28	254.4	15.1	229.6	279.1
29–30	273.9	15.5	248.3	299.5
31–32	292.4	16.0	266.1	318.8
33–34	309.9	16.5	282.8	337.1
35–36	326.5	17.0	298.5	354.4
37–38	342.0	17.5	313.3	370.7
39–40	356.5	17.9	327.0	386.0
41–42	370.0	18.4	339.7	400.3
Foot length				
11–12	8.9	2.8	4.3	13.0
13–14	14.0	2.9	9.0	19.0
15–16	19.0	3.0	14.0	24.0
17–18	25.0	3.2	19.0	30.0
19–20	30.0	3.3	25.0	36.0
21–22	36.0	3.5	30.0	42.0
23–24	42.0	3.6	36.0	48.0
25–26	48.0	3.8	41.0	54.0
27–28	53.0	3.9	47.0	59.0
29–30	58.0	4.1	51.0	65.0
31–32	63.0	4.2	56.0	70.0
33–34	67.0	4.4	60.0	74.0
35–36	71.0	4.6	63.0	78.0
37–38	74.0	4.7	66.0	82.0
39–40	76.0	4.9	68.0	84.0
41–42	77.0	5.1	69.0	86.0

(continued)

(continued)

Age interval (GW)	*Mean*	*SD*	*5th percentile*	*95th percentile*
Head circumference				
11–12	60.3	11.5	41.4	79.2
13–14	89.2	11.8	69.7	108.7
15–16	116.7	12.2	96.6	136.8
17–18	142.8	12.6	122.1	163.5
19–20	167.5	12.9	146.2	188.8
21–22	190.9	13.3	169.0	212.8
23–24	212.8	13.7	190.3	235.3
25–26	233.4	14.0	210.3	256.5
27–28	252.7	14.4	229.0	276.4
29–30	270.5	14.8	246.2	294.8
31–32	287.0	15.1	262.1	311.9
33–34	302.1	15.5	276.5	327.6
35–36	315.8	15.9	289.7	341.9
37–38	328.1	16.2	301.4	354.8
39–40	339.1	16.6	311.7	366.4
41–42	348.6	17.0	320.7	376.6

Used with permission from Guihard Costa, A-M, Ménez F, Delezoide A-L, Organ weights in human fetuses after formalinfixation: standards by gestational age and body weight. Ped and Dev Pathology 2002;5:559–578.

WEIGHTS AND MEASUREMENTS IN ADULTS

Comparative data of organ weight (g) of males and females

	Males (n=355)		*Females (n=329)*	
	Mean±S.D.	*Range*	*Mean±S.D.*	*Range*
Heart	365 ± 71	90-630	312 ± 78	174-590
Right lung	663 ± 239	200-1593	546 ± 207	173-1700
Left lung	583 ± 216	206-1718	467 ± 174	178-1350
Liver	1677 ± 396	670-2900	1475 ± 362	508-3081
Spleen	156 ± 87	30-580	140 ± 78	33-481
Pancreas	144 ± 39	65-243	122 ± 35	60-250
Right kidney	162 ± 39	53-320	135 ± 39	45-360
Left kidney	160 ± 41	50-410	136 ± 37	40-300
Thyroid	25 ± 11	12-87	20 ± 9	5-88

Mean and standard deviation of organ weight (g) according to height (cm)

	Males			**Females**		
	144=H=165	165=H=175	176=H=190	126=H=155	156=H=165	166=H=180
Heart	344 ± 75	360 ± 75	381 ± 56	320 ± 88	308 ± 79	311 ± 67
Right lung	616 ± 210	625 ± 207	741 ± 274	494 ± 202	545 ± 183	597 ± 243
Left lung	523 ± 190	551 ± 178	658 ± 257	450 ± 146	472 ± 181	491 ± 204
Liver	1455 ± 370	1637 ± 369	1831 ± 384	1275 ± 321	1496 ± 331	1624 ± 380
Spleen	120 ± 51	150 ± 88	180 ± 90	122 ± 67	39 ± 79	160 ± 82
Pancreas	138 ± 35	143 ± 39	147 ± 39	111 ± 25	122 ± 35	138 ± 41
Right kidney	150 ± 49	157 ± 36	170 ± 37	117 ± 32	137 ± 40	148 ± 36
Left kidney	155 ± 53	164 ± 38	175 ± 38	120 ± 41	136 ± 35	148 ± 33
Thyroid	25 ± 7	25 ± 13	25 ± 9	20 ± 11	18 ± 6	20 ± 11

Mean and standard deviation of organ weight (g) according to BMI (kg/m2)

	Males			**Females**		
	14=BMI=21	22=BMI=24	25=BMI=34	13=BMI=20	21=BMI=24	25=BMI=40
Heart	342 ± 58	370 ± 75	400 ± 69	287 ± 74	308 ± 68	362 ± 77
Right lung	670 ± 249	651 ± 241	663 ± 217	536 ± 178	547 ± 203	561 ± 256
Left lung	593 ± 224	579 ± 201	569 ± 221	450 ± 146	472 ± 181	491 ± 204
Liver	1581 ± 372	1730 ± 405	1769 ± 390	1346 ± 328	1521 ± 331	1609 ± 419
Spleen	143 ± 83	157 ± 83	175 ± 93	126 ± 70	150 ± 93	152 ± 67
Pancreas	131 ± 38	143 ± 34	162 ± 38	114 ± 33	129 ± 38	125 ± 32
Right kidney	156 ± 40	163 ± 37	169 ± 37	126 ± 35	139 ± 40	144 ± 40
Left kidney	158 ± 43	170 ± 41	174 ± 35	126 ± 32	139 ± 38	146 ± 38
Thyroid	24 ± 11	25 ± 7	28 ± 13	19 ± 7	19 ± 8	20 ± 11

Reprinted from: Organ weight in 684 adult autopsies: new tables for Caucasoid population. Forensic Science International, de la Grandmaison Geoffroy Lorin, Clairand Isabelle and Durigon Michel.

Heart Weight as a Function of Body Weight: Adults*

Body Weight		*Heart Weight*			
		Females		*Males*	
		Mean	*Range*	*Mean*	*Range*
(kg)	*(lbs)*	*(g)*		*(g)*	
30	66	196	133–287	213	162–282
32	71	201	137–295	220	167–291
34	75	206	141–302	227	172–300
36	79	211	144–310	234	177–309
38	84	216	148–317	240	182–317
40	88	221	151–324	247	187–325
42	93	226	154–331	253	191–334
44	97	230	157–337	259	196–341
46	101	234	160–344	265	200–349
48	106	239	163–350	270	205–357
50	110	243	166–356	276	209–364
52	115	247	169–362	281	213–371
54	119	251	171–368	287	217–379
56	123	255	174–374	292	221–386
58	128	259	177–379	297	225–392
60	132	262	179–385	302	229–399
62	137	266	182–390	307	233–406
64	141	270	184–395	312	237–412
66	146	273	187–401	317	240–419
68	150	277	189–406	322	244–425
70	154	280	191–411	327	248–431
72	159	284	194–416	331	251–437
74	163	287	196–420	336	255–444
76	168	290	198–425	341	258–450
78	172	293	200–430	345	261–455
80	176	297	202–435	349	265–461
82	181	300	205–439	354	268–467
84	185	303	207–444	358	271–473
86	190	306	209–448	362	275–478
88	194	309	211–453	367	278–484
90	198	312	213–457	371	281–489
92	203	315	215–461	375	284–495
94	207	318	217–465	379	287–500
96	212	320	219–470	383	290–506
98	216	323	221–474	387	293–511
100	220	326	222–478	391	296–516
102	225	329	224–482	395	299–521
104	229	331	226–486	399	302–526
106	234	334	228–490	403	305–531
108	238	337	230–494	406	308–536
110	243	339	232–497	410	311–541
112	247	342	233–501	414	314–546
114	251	345	235–505	418	316–551
116	256	347	237–509	421	319–556
118	260	350	239–513	425	322–561
120	265	352	240–516	429	325–566
125	275	359	244–525	437	331–577
130	287	364	249–534	446	338–589
135	297	370	252–542	455	345–600
140	309	376	257–551	463	351–611
145	320	382	260–560	472	357–622
150	331	387	264–567	479	363–633

*Data adapted with permission from Kitzman DW, Scholz DG, Hagen PT, Ilstrup DM, Edwards WD. Age-related changes in normal human hearts during the first 10 decades of life. Part II: (Maturity): A quantitative anatomic study of 765 specimens from subjects 20 to 99 years old. Mayo Clin Proc 1988;63:137–146. The title of the publication indicates that the hearts were normal, but subjects with hypertension were not excluded. The table should probably not be used as a reference norm against which to exclude the diagnosis of hypertensive heart disease.

Heart Measurements in Adults*

	Age 20–60 yr		*Age > 60 yr*	
	Men	*Women*	*Men*	*Women*
1. Valve Circumference (cm)	*mean (range)*	*mean (range)*	*mean (range)*	*mean (range)*
Aortic Valve	6.7 (6.0–7.4)	6.3 (5.7–6.9)	8.3 (8.1–8.5)	7.6 (7.3–7.9)
Pulmonary Valve	6.6 (6.1–7.1)	6.2 (5.7–6.7)	7.3 (7.2–7.5)	7.1 (6.8–7.4)
Mitral Valve	9.6 (9.4–9.9)	8.6 (8.2–9.1)	9.5 (9.2–9.8)	8.6 (8.2–9.0)
Tricuspid Valve	11.4 (11.2-11.7)	10.6 (10.2-10.9)	11.6 (11.4-11.8)	10.5 (10.0-11.1)
2. Wall Thickness (cm)	*mean*	*range*	*mean*	*range*
Left Ventricle	1.25	1.00–1.50	1.15	1.05–1.25
Right Ventricle	0.40	0.25–0.50	0.38	0.35–0.40
Ventricular Septum	1.35	1.20–1.60	1.35	1.20–1.60
Atrial Muscle	0.20	0.10–0.30	0.20	0.10–0.30

*Modified with permission from Sunderman FW, Boerner F. Normal Values in Clinical Medicine. W.B. Saunders Company, Philadelphia, 1949; and from Kitzman DW, Scholz DG, Hagen PT, Ilstrup DM, Edwards WD. Age-related changes in normal human hearts. Part II: (Maturity): A quantitative anatomic study of 765 specimens from subjects 20 to 99 years old. Mayo Clin Proc 1988;63:137–146.

Factors for Calculation of Cardiac Muscle Mass from Specific Gravity*

Spec Grav	*x*	*Spec Grav*	*x*	*Spec Grav*	*x*	*Spec Grav*	*x*	*Spec Grav*	*x*
1.055	1.000	1.032	0.798	1.009	0.569	0.986	0.395	0.963	0.193
1.054	0.991	1.031	0.789	1.008	0.588	0.985	0.386	0.962	0.184
1.053	0.982	1.030	0.781	1.007	0.579	0.984	0.377	0.961	0.175
1.052	0.974	1.029	0.772	1.006	0.570	0.983	0.368	0.960	0.167
1.051	0.965	1.028	0.763	1.005	0.561	0.982	0.360	0.959	0.158
1.050	0.956	1.027	0.754	1.004	0.553	0.981	0.351	0.958	0.149
1.049	0.947	1.026	0.746	1.003	0.544	0.980	0.342	0.957	0.140
1.048	0.939	1.025	0.737	1.002	0.535	0.979	0.333	0.956	0.132
1.047	0.930	1.024	0.728	1.001	0.526	0.978	0.325	0.955	0.123
1.046	0.921	1.023	0.719	1.000	0.518	0.977	0.316	0.954	0.114
1.045	0.912	1.022	0.711	0.999	0.509	0.976	0.307	0.953	0.105
1.044	0.904	1.021	0.702	0.998	0.500	0.975	0.298	0.952	0.096
1.043	0.895	1.020	0.693	0.997	0.491	0.974	0.289	0.951	0.088
1.042	0.886	1.019	0.684	0.996	0.482	0.973	0.281	0.950	0.079
1.041	0.877	1.018	0.675	0.995	0.474	0.972	0.272	0.949	0.070
1.040	0.868	1.017	0.667	0.994	0.465	0.971	0.263	0.948	0.061
1.039	0.860	1.016	0.658	0.993	0.456	0.970	0.254	0.947	0.053
1.038	0.851	1.015	0.649	0.992	0.447	0.969	0.246	0.946	0.044
1.037	0.842	1.014	0.640	0.991	0.439	0.968	0.237	0.945	0.035
1.036	0.833	1.013	0.632	0.990	0.430	0.967	0.228	0.944	0.026
1.035	0.825	1.012	0.623	0.989	0.421	0.966	0.219	0.943	0.018
1.034	0.816	1.011	0.614	0.988	0.412	0.965	0.211	0.942	0.009
1.033	0.807	1.010	0.605	0.987	0.404	0.964	0.202	0.941	0.000

*The Heart is weighed in isotonic saline for this determination. From the table above, one uses the specific gravity to find the factor that, when multiplied by heart weight, gives the cardiac muscle mass. *Example:* A heart weighing 700 g has a specific gravity of 1.032. The table shows a factor (X) of 0.798, or 79.8%. The muscle mass of this heart is 79.8% of 700 g, or 558.6 g.

Data adapted with permission from: Masshoff W, Scheidt D, Reimers HF. Quantitative Bestimmung des Fett- und Myokardgewebes im Leichenherzen. Virchows Arch [Pathol Anat] 1967;342:184–189.

Extent of Left Ventricular Hypertrophy and Dilatation in Adult Hearts*

Extent of left ventricular hypertrophy	*Percent increase in total heart weight*[a]
None	0–25
Mild	26–50
Moderate	51–100
Severe	>100

[a]Based on the expected normal mean value for the subject's gender and body size. For example, if the expected mean heart weight is 300 g, then hearts weighing 375–450 g have mild left ventricular hypertrophy (LVH), those weighing 451–600 g show moderate LVH, and hearts weighing >600 g have severe LVH. (Note: There may be some overlap between the upper range of normal heart weight and the lower range of mild hypertrophy.)

Extent of left ventricular dilatation	*Left ventricular short-axis diameter (cm)*[b]
None	0–2.5
Mild	2.6–4.0
Moderate	4.1–5.5
Severe	>5.5

[b]For an adult of average size, with rigor mortis. (Note: Once rigor mortis has abated, artifactual dilatation of all four cardiac chambers commonly occurs and may be substantial, such that this table no longer applies.)

*Data adapted with permission from Edwards WD. Applied anatomy of the heart. In: Mayo Clinic Practice of Cardiology, 3rd ed. Giuliani ER, et al., eds. Mosby, St. Louis, 1996, pp. 422-489.

Spleen Weight as a Function of Age in Adults*

Spleen weight (g) in men				*Spleen weight (g) in women*			
Age (yr)	*Race*	*Mean*	*Range*	*Age (yr)*	*Race*	*Mean*	*Range*
15–24	White	190	105–280	15–59	White	120	60–185
25–39	White	155	75–250	60+	White	110	55–195
40–54	White	145	75–230	All	White	115	55–190
55+	White	145	70–225				
15–39	White	170	85–275				
40+	White	145	70–225				
All	White	145	75–245				
15–24	Black	120	60–190	15–36	Black	100	35–190
25–39	Black	115	50–225	37+	Black	95	45–150
40–54	Black	110	50–210	All	Black	95	35–190
55+	Black	90	40–135				
15–39	Black	115	55–220				
40+	Black	105	45–190				
All	Black	105	40–200				

*Data adapted with permission from Myers J, Segal RJ. Weight of the spleen. Range of normal in a nonhospital population. Arch Pathol 1974;98:33–38.

Brain Weight as a Function of Age in Adults*

	Brain Weight (g)			
	Men		*Women*	
Age (yr)	*Mean*	*Range*	*Mean*	*Range*
17–19	1,340	1,170–1,527	1,242	1,120–1,420
20–29	1,396	1,158–1,620	1,234	1,057–1,565
30–39	1,365	1,075–1,685	1,233	1,038–1,440
40–49	1,366	1,069–1,605	1,240	995–1,543
50–59	1,375	1,113–1,665	1,200	820–1,447
60–69	1,323	1,018–1,610	1,178	920–1,372
70–85	1,279	1,039–1,485	1,121	832–1,370

*Data adapted with permission from Sunderman FW, Boerner F. Normal Values in Clinical Medicine. W.B. Saunders, Philadelphia, 1949.

Miscellaneous Weights and Measurements of Adults*

	Weight (g)		*Weight*	*Size or Length*
	mean	*range*	*(% of Body Weight)*	*(cm)*
Adrenal glands, combined	11.5	8.3–16.7	–	–
Bones	–	–	11.6	–
Brain	–	–	1.4	–
Carotid bodies, combined	0.02	0.004–0.034	–	–
Colon	–	–	–	150–170
Duodenum	–	–	–	30
Esophagus	–	–	–	25
Heart	–	–	0.40–0.45	–
Kidneys, combined	–	–	0.3	11.5 × 5.5 × 3.5
Male	313	230–440	–	–
Female	288	240–350	–	–
Liver				
Male	–	–	1.9–3.0	–
Female	–	–	2.2–2.9	–
Lung				
Combined	–	–	1	–
Right	450	360–570	–	–
Left	375	325–480	–	–
Ovary	7	–	–	3.4 × 1.5 × 0.8
Pancreas	110	60–135	0.1	23 × 4.5 × 3.8
Parathyroid glands, combined	0.15	0.12–0.18	–	–
Pineal gland	0.14	0.10–0.18	–	0.7 × 0.45 × 0.4
Pituitary gland	–	–	–	2.1 × 1.4 × 0.5
Ages 10–20 yr	0.56	–	–	–
Ages 20–70 yr	0.61	–	–	–
Pregnancy	0.95	–	–	–
Placenta	500	–	–	18 × 2.8
Prostate	–	–	–	3.6 × 2.8 × 1.9
Ages 21–25 yr	18	–	–	–
Ages 51–60 yr	20	–	–	–
Ages 71–80 yr	40	–	–	–
Seminal vesicle	–	–	–	4.3 × 1.7 × 0.9
Skeletal muscle	–	–	28.7	–
Small intestine	–	–	–	550–650
Spinal cord	27	–	–	45
Spleen	–	–	0.16	–
Testis	25	20–27	–	4.5 × 3.0 × 2.4
Thymus				
Ages <25 yr	25	–	–	–
Ages 26–35 yr	20	–	–	–
Ages >65 yr	6	–	–	–
Thyroid gland	40	30–70	–	6.5 × 3.5 × 2.0
Uterus				
Multiparus	110	102–117	–	9.0 × 5.7 × 3.4
Nulliparus	35	33–41	–	7.9 × 3.9 × 2.3

*Modified with permission from Furbank RA. Conversion data, normal values, normograms and other standards. In: Modern Trends in Forensic Medicine. Simpson K, ed. Appleton-Century-Crofts, New York, 1967, pp. 344–364; and Sunderman FW, Boerner F. Normal Values in Clinical Medicine. W.B. Saunders, Philadelphia, 1949.

Mean weights and percentiles for singleton placentas

Gestational age (wk)	*90th percentile*	*75th percentile*	*Mean singleton placental wt.*	*25th percentile*	*10th percentile*	*No. of cases*
21	172	158	143	128	114	3
22	191	175	157	138	122	6
23	211	193	172	151	133	7
24	233	212	189	166	145	9
25	256	233	208	182	159	19
26	280	255	227	200	175	14
27	305	278	248	219	192	9
28	331	302	270	238	210	16
29	357	327	293	259	229	11
30	384	352	316	281	249	12
31	411	377	340	303	269	14
32	438	403	364	325	290	24
33	464	428	387	347	311	30
34	491	453	411	369	331	32
35	516	477	434	391	352	44
36	542	501	457	412	372	36
37	566	524	478	432	391	32
38	589	547	499	452	409	62
39	611	567	519	470	426	103
40	632	587	537	487	442	193
41	651	605	553	502	456	87

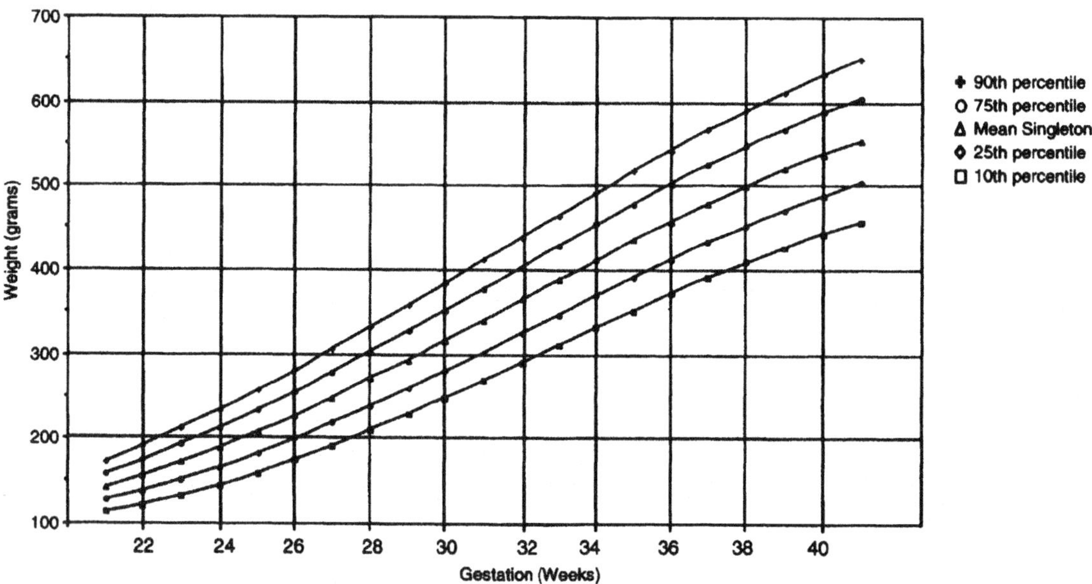

Singleton placental weights and ranges.

Used with permission from Pinar H, Sung CJ, Oyer CE and Singer DB. Pediatric Pathology and Laboratory Medicine 1996;16:910–907.

Mean weights and percentiles for singleton placentas

Gestational age (wk)	*90th percentile*	*75th percentile*	*Mean singleton placental wt.*	*25th percentile*	*10th percentile*	*No. of cases*
21	172	158	143	128	114	3
22	191	175	157	138	122	6
23	211	193	172	151	133	7
24	233	212	189	166	145	9
25	256	233	208	182	159	19
26	280	255	227	200	175	14
27	305	278	248	219	192	9
28	331	302	270	238	210	16
29	357	327	293	259	229	11
30	384	352	316	281	249	12
31	411	377	340	303	269	14
32	438	403	364	325	290	24
33	464	428	387	347	311	30
34	491	453	411	369	331	32
35	516	477	434	391	352	44
36	542	501	457	412	372	36
37	566	524	478	432	391	32
38	589	547	499	452	409	62
39	611	567	519	470	426	103
40	632	587	537	487	442	193
41	651	605	553	502	456	87

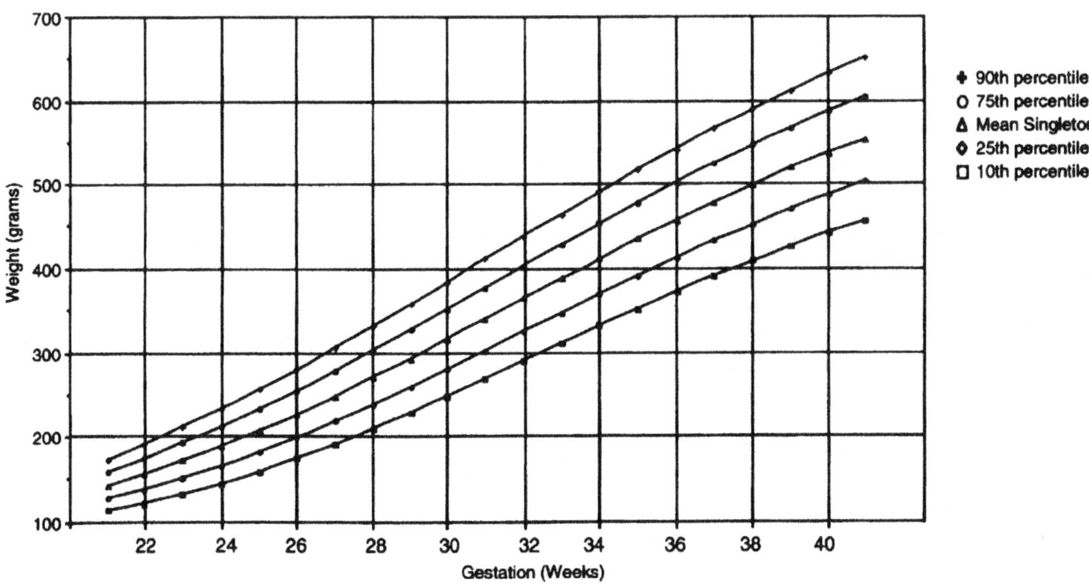

Figure 1. Singleton placental weights and ranges.

Mean weights and percentiles for twin placentas

Gestational age (wk)	*90th percentile*	*75th percentile*	*Mean twin placental wt.*	*25th percentile*	*10th percentile*	*No. of cases*
19	263	239	212	185	161	2
20	270	245	218	190	166	3
21	286	260	231	202	176	2
22	310	282	251	219	191	5
23	343	311	276	241	210	2
24	382	346	307	267	232	3
25	426	386	341	297	257	5
26	475	430	380	330	284	4
27	528	478	421	365	314	8
28	584	527	464	401	345	7
29	641	579	509	439	377	12
30	700	631	554	478	409	17
31	758	683	600	516	441	13
32	815	734	644	554	472	29
33	870	783	687	590	503	27
34	923	830	727	624	531	53
35	971	873	764	656	558	52
36	1014	912	798	684	582	66
37	1051	945	827	708	602	58
38	1082	972	850	728	619	54
39	1105	993	868	743	631	38
40	1118	1005	879	753	639	47
41	1123	1009	882	756	642	12

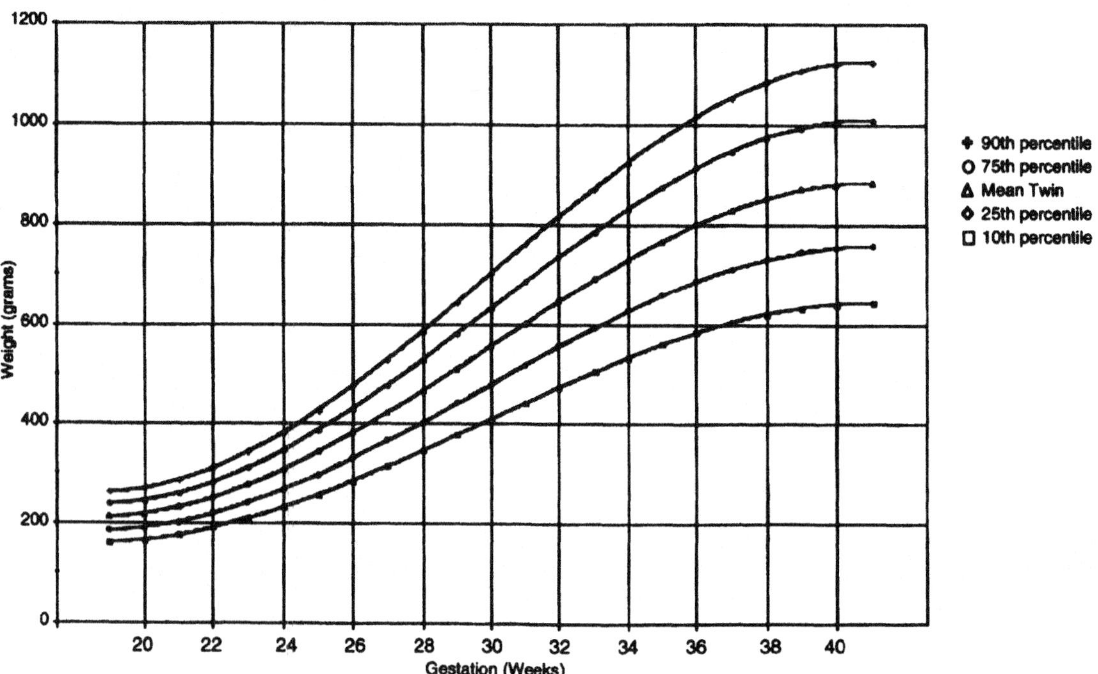

Figure 2. Mean twin placental weights and ranges.

Comparison of twin placental weights

Group	*P value*
All twins vs. Di-Di twins	.774
All twins vs. Di-Mo twins	.867
Di-Di twins vs. Di-Mo twins	.9293

Comparison of placental weights with the data in the literature

Ratio	*Range*	*Mean*
Twin placental wts/singleton placental wts	1.59–1.77	1.69
Twin placental wts/Naeye'ssingleton placental wts [4]	1.89–1.99	1.94
Singleton placental wts/Naeye's singleton placental wts	1.08–1.20	1.12
Singleton placental wts/Boyd and Hamilton's singleton placental wts [8]	1.02–1.17	1.12
Singleton placental wts/Molteni's AGA (appropriate for gestational age) placental wts [9]	1.18–1.64	1.26

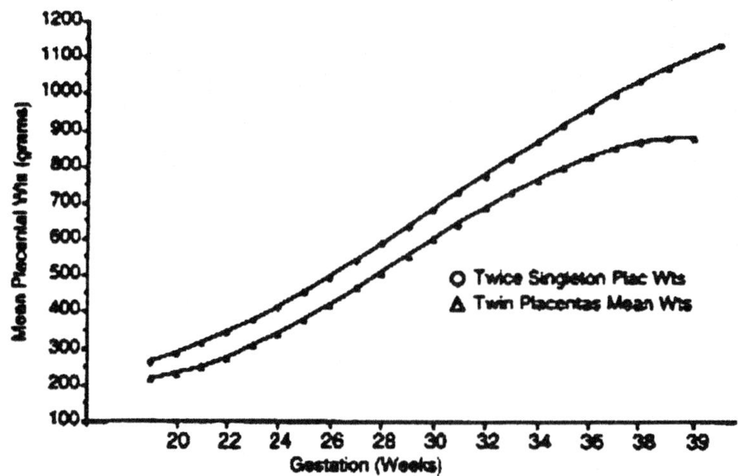

Figure 3. Comparison of twin placental weights with singleton placental weights.

Weight Changes of Organs after Formalin Fixation*

Organ	*Weight after fixation*	*% Weight change*	
		Mean	*Range*
Heart			
Adults	Decreased	4.0	0.4–9.0
Children	Decreased	5.8	0.9–19.2
Lung	Increased or decreased	6.6	0.4–17.1
Liver			
Adults	Decreased	4.0	0.5–7.6
Children	Decreased	4.0	0.7–6.6
Spleen			
Adults	Increased or decreased	2.1	0.1–6.2
Children	Decreased	3.1	0.2–6.6
Kidney			
Adults	Increased or decreased	1.9	0.1–6.4
Children	Decreased	3.3	0.2–6.0
Thyroid gland	Increased	14.8	6.2–34.0
Testis	Increased or decreased	3.2	0.0–8.8
Placenta	Increased	9.9	0.7–23.0
Skeletal muscle	Decreased	7.0	0.8–13.3
Adipose tissue	Increased	2.2	0.1–4.8
Brain			
Adults	Increased	8.8	3.3–19.2
Children	Increased	14.1	8.0–22.3
Dura mater cerebri	Decreased	3.9	0.2–10.0

*Weight changes were determined after 10 d of fixation in 10% buffered formalin. Adapted with permission from Schremmer C-N. Gewichtsänderungen verschiedener Gewebe nach Formalinfixierung. Frankf Z Pathol 1967;77:299–304.

Index

E

CPSIA information can be obtained
at www.ICGtesting.com
Printed in the USA
BVOW09*0220281216
472012BV00006B/27/P

9 781588 298416